Contents

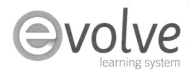
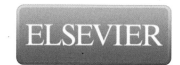
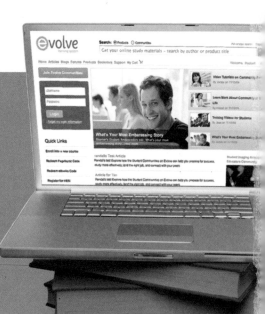

Physical Examination & Health Assessment

Second Canadian Edition

JARVIS

Physical Examination & Health Assessment

Second Canadian Edition

Carolyn Jarvis, PhD, APN, CNP

Professor of Nursing
School of Nursing
Illinois Wesleyan University
Bloomington, Illinois

Family Nurse Practitioner
Bloomington, Illinois

Original Illustrations by
Pat Thomas, CMI, FAMI

Oak Park, Illinois

Assessment Photographs by
Kevin Strandberg

Professor of Art
Illinois Wesleyan University
Bloomington, Illinois

Canadian Editors

Annette J. Browne, PhD, RN

Professor
School of Nursing
University of British Columbia
Vancouver, British Columbia

June MacDonald-Jenkins, RN, BScN, MSc

Professor, School of Health and Community Studies
Durham College
Assistant Adjunct Professor
Faculty of Health Science
University of Ontario Institute of Technology
Oshawa, Ontario

Marian Luctkar-Flude, RN, MScN, PhD(c)

Lecturer
School of Nursing
Queen's University
Kingston, Ontario

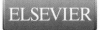
ELSEVIER

Notice

Knowledge and best practice in this field are constantly changing. As new research and expertise broaden our knowledge, changes in practice, treatment, and drug therapy may become necessary or appropriate. Readers are advised to check the most current information provided (i) on procedures featured or (ii) by the manufacturer of each product to be administered and to verify the recommended dose or formula, the method and duration of administration, and contraindications. It is the responsibility of practitioners, relying on their own experience and knowledge of the client, to make diagnoses, to determine dosages and the best treatment for each individual patient, and to take all appropriate safety precautions. To the fullest extent of the law, neither the Publisher nor the Authors assumes any liability for any injury and/or damage to persons or property arising out of or related to any use of the material contained in this book.

The Publisher

Library and Archives Canada Cataloguing in Publication
Jarvis, Carolyn
    Physical examination & health assessment / Carolyn Jarvis; Canadian editors, Annette J. Browne, June MacDonald-Jenkins, Marian Luctkar-Flude; original illustrations by Pat Thomas; assessment photographs by Kevin Strandberg.—2nd Canadian ed.
Includes bibliographical references.
ISBN 978-1-926648-72-9
    1. Physical diagnosis.   2. Nursing assessment.   I. Browne, Annette J   II. MacDonald-Jenkins, June, 1965-   III. Luctkar-Flude, Marian, 1961-   IV. Title.   V. Title: Physical examination and health assessment.
RC76.J37 2013   616.07′5   C2013-901415-2

ISBN: 978-1-926648-72-9
Ebook ISBN: 978-1-926648-79-8

Vice President, Publishing: Ann Millar
Managing Developmental Editor: Martina van de Velde
Publishing Services Manager: Deborah L. Vogel
Project Manager: John W. Gabbert
Copy Editor: Anne Ostroff
Design Direction: Teresa McBryan
Typesetting and Assembly: Toppan Best-set Premedia Limited
Printing and Binding: Transcontinental

Elsevier Canada
905 King Street West, 4th Floor
Toronto, ON, Canada M6K 3G9
Phone: 1-866-896-3331
Fax: 1-866-359-9534

Printed in Canada

4   5   6   19   18   17   16

To my mother, Frances,
With gratitude
—Carolyn Jarvis

This book is dedicated to Rachel (Ray) Browne, whom I dearly love.
—Annette J. Browne

I would like to dedicate my work in this edition in memory of my sister Sandra,
my very best friend and cheerleader.
—June MacDonald-Jenkins

My work on this book is dedicated to the memory of my mother, Annemarie,
who first encouraged me to pursue a career in nursing, and to my nursing students,
past and future, who keep me going.
—Marian Luctkar-Flude

About the Author

Carolyn Jarvis received her BSN cum laude from the University of Iowa, her MSN from Loyola University (Chicago), and her PhD from the University of Illinois at Chicago, with a research interest in the physiological effect of alcohol on the cardiovascular system. She has taught physical assessment and critical care nursing at Rush University (Chicago), the University of Missouri (Columbia), and the University of Illinois (Urbana), and she has taught physical assessment, pharmacology, and pathophysiology at Illinois Wesleyan University (Bloomington).

Dr. Jarvis is a recipient of the University of Missouri's Superior Teaching Award; has taught physical assessment to thousands of baccalaureate students, graduate students, and nursing professionals; has held 150 continuing education seminars; and is the author of numerous articles and textbook contributions.

Dr. Jarvis has maintained a clinical practice in advanced practice roles—first as a cardiovascular clinical specialist in various critical care settings and as a certified family nurse practitioner in primary care. She is currently a professor at Illinois Wesleyan University; a nurse practitioner in Bloomington, Illinois; and licensed as an advanced practice nurse in the state of Illinois. During the past 6 years, her enthusiasm has focused on speaking Spanish to provide health care in rural Guatemala and in a local Bloomington clinic.

ABOUT THE CANADIAN EDITORS

Annette J. Browne's career began as an outpost nurse, living and working in northern First Nations and Inuit communities in Canada. She holds a master's degree as a family nurse practitioner from the University of Rhode Island and a PhD in nursing from the University of British Columbia (UBC). Dr. Browne is a professor at the UBC School of Nursing and has taught advanced health assessment to nurse practitioners and post-RNs for many years. Dr. Browne is an active researcher who focuses on health and health care inequities, with a particular focus on fostering health equity with Indigenous peoples. She conducts research on access to health care, women's health, cultural safety, and primary health care interventions to improve health outcomes. Her work is aimed at promoting health equity through improvements in nursing practice, health care delivery, and health policy.

June MacDonald-Jenkins is a recognized expert in hybrid course delivery e-learning, having worked in this field for many years. As a nursing professor in the Durham College/University of Ontario Institute of Technology (UOIT) BScN program, Ms. MacDonald-Jenkins brings strong education experience to the team. She has taught health assessment to thousands of students, from those enrolled in diploma to advanced practice programs. She is also an accomplished practitioner and researcher on the subject of technology and hybrid course delivery use in nursing education. She has recently been seconded as Dean of Police Education and Innovation for a two-year period to enhance policing education through customization of the learning environment. Ms. MacDonald-Jenkins's research interests are primarily in the areas of assessing core competencies across curriculum, simulation, and e-learning course delivery. She is the recipient of the 2007 Elsevier Canada Resource Award, which recognizes exemplary use of technology resources in the academic environment. Ms. MacDonald-Jenkins has presented across the country to numerous nursing faculties and internationally on the concept of creating engaging hybrid learning environments. She is a faculty member with SIM_One–Ontario Simulation Network focusing on the enhancement of e-Learning strategies.

Marian Luctkar-Flude received her BScN and MScN from the University of Ottawa, her critical care nursing diploma from St. Lawrence College (Kingston), and is currently working on her PhD in Rehabilitation Sciences at Queen's University. She has more than 20 years' medical–surgical nursing experience in various clinical settings and, in particular, in general surgery and urology nursing. She has taught clinically in the St. Lawrence College and Queen's University (Kingston) nursing programs and is now a faculty member of the Queen's University School of Nursing where she has provided a leadership role in the integration of patient simulation throughout the undergraduate program, including the *Nursing Health Assessment* course. She currently teaches the *Nursing Research*, and the *Common Health Challenges and Implications for Care* courses and is actively involved in interprofessional education and curriculum development.

Her research interests include older persons with cancer, cancer fatigue and physical activity, breast cancer survivorship care, knowledge translation interventions for primary care providers, and the use of patient simulation in undergraduate nursing, with a focus on interprofessional education. She has presented at local, national, and international nursing conferences and has acted as a peer reviewer for several nursing and medical journals.

Contributors

Ian M. Camera, MSN, ND, RN

Ian Camera is an associate professor in the Division of Nursing Education at Holyoke Community College in Massachusetts, where he teaches the fundamentals and advanced medical–surgical courses. His work experience includes long-term care, summer camp nursing, and inpatient medical–surgical nursing. His doctoral research has focused on the impact of for-profit penetration into the home health care market in Ohio, using a human ecology framework.

Chapter 29: Bedside Assessment of the Hospitalized Adult

Martha Driessnack, PhD, PNP-BC, RN

Martha Driessnack is a Pediatric Nurse Practitioner with more than 25 years of experience in teaching, practice, and research. She received her PhD from Oregon Health & Science University, completed a post-doctoral research fellowship in Clinical Genetics from the University of Iowa, and is an Assistant Professor in the College of Nursing at the University of Iowa.

Promoting Health feature boxes from the U.S. 6th edition

Dana S. Edge, PhD, RN

Dana Edge received her BSN from the University of Iowa, her MSN from the University of North Carolina at Chapel Hill, and her doctorate in epidemiology from the University of Toronto. She has taught health assessment to undergraduate students at Memorial University of Newfoundland and at the University of Northern British Columbia, and to both undergraduate and graduate students at the University of Calgary. Dr. Edge practised nursing in Minnesota, Colorado, Alaska, and North Carolina before moving to Newfoundland and Labrador in 1986. In Canada she has practised in nursing stations in Labrador and in a rural hospital in northern British Columbia. She is currently an associate professor at Queen's University in Kingston, Ontario.

Chapter 2: Health Promotion in the Context of Health Assessment

Carla Graf, MS, RN, CNS-BC

Carla Graf is a board-certified geriatric clinical nurse specialist at the University of California, San Francisco (UCSF), and is an assistant clinical professor at the UCSF School of Nursing. She is currently a doctoral student at UCSF, with a research focus on functional decline in hospitalized older adults.

Chapter 31: Functional Assessment of the Older Adult

Dianne Groll, PhD, RN, BA, BScH, MScH

Dianne Groll is an assistant professor with the Faculty of Health Sciences at Queen's University in Kingston. Her research interests include factors affecting physical function and patient quality of life and the impact of comorbid illness on patient outcomes. Her doctoral research focused on the influence of comorbidity on physical function and how best to quantify the impact of chronic illness. She is involved with studies of older patients in orthopedics, oncology, cardiology, and psychiatry. She received her undergraduate and master's degrees from Queen's University and her PhD from the University of Toronto.

Chapter 31: Functional Assessment of the Older Adult

Lynn Haslam, RN(EC), MN

Lynn Haslam is a Nurse Practitioner currently working on the Trauma unit at St. Michael's Hospital in Toronto. Lynn has over 8 years of experience working as an NP for the Acute Pain Service at Sunnybrook Hospital in Toronto. She has presented nationally and internationally on pain and focuses her research on both pain in the critically ill who are unable to self-report, and also trauma patients. She was one of the first graduates of the Canadian NP in Anesthesia Certificate Program through the Lawrence S. Bloomberg Faculty of Nursing, University of Toronto, where she is also an Adjunct Lecturer.

Chapter 11: Pain Assessment

Joyce K. Keithley, DNSc, RN, FAAN

Joyce Keithley is a professor in the Department of Adult Health Nursing, Rush University College of Nursing and Rush University Medical Center in Chicago. Having worked in both clinical and instructional settings, she is an experienced and well-known practitioner, teacher, researcher, and author in the area of clinical nutrition.

Chapter 12: Nutritional Assessment and Nursing Practice

Melissa A. Lee, MS, RN, CNS-BC

Melissa Lee is a clinical nurse specialist at the University of California San Francisco Medical Center. She has experience in medical–surgical and telemetry nursing and education. She is certified in geriatrics by the American Nurses Credentialing Center.

Chapter 31: Functional Assessment of the Older Adult

Freda O'Bannon Lemmi, RN, MS, ANP-C, FNP

Images of normal and abnormal conditions are original photographs from patients in her clinical practice, students, relatives, and friends. She has been teaching physical assessment and curriculum of nurse practitioner programs as Professor of Nursing at California State University and at UCLA. She taught physical assessment classes in England to help prepare faculty to teach advanced nursing practice roles at the Royal Brompton Hospital in London in 1995 and at Oxford University in 1996. Carlos A.E. Lemmi, PhD, has taught microscopic anatomy to medical, dental, and graduate students at the UCLA school of medicine for over 15 years. His medical background and knowledge of computer graphics helped prepare the images for this book.

Laraine Michalson, MSN, RN

Laraine Michalson has worked for 15 years as a Public Health Nurse at the Sheway Program in Vancouver, British Columbia. Sheway is a community-based program that provides health and social services to pregnant and parenting women who have addiction issues. Laraine is an Adjunct Professor at the University of British Columbia School of Nursing.

Chapter 7: Substance Use in the Context of Health Assessment

Andrea Miller, MHSc, RD

Andrea Miller is a registered dietitian with over 20 years of experience. Over her career, Andrea has coordinated a dietetic internship program, managed the nutrition care program in a number of long-term care homes across Ontario, and written for a family practice medical journal. Andrea currently owns and operates a private nutrition counselling practice, where she counsels individuals for a variety of nutrition related concerns including eating disorders, diabetes, weight management, and food allergies and intolerances. Andrea is in the Board of Directors of Dietitians of Canada and is a sessional instructor at the University of Ontario Institute of Technology.

Chapter 12: Nutritional Assessment and Nursing Practice

Shawna S. Mudd, MSN, CRNP

Shawna Mudd is a pediatric nurse practitioner in the Pediatric Emergency Department at the Johns Hopkins Hospital. She is also a member of the hospital's child protection team, which provides inpatient and outpatient consultation for cases of suspected child abuse and neglect. She is also faculty at the Johns Hopkins University School of Nursing.

Chapter 7: Domestic Violence Assessment (U.S. Sixth Edition)

Daniel Sheridan, PhD, RN, FAAN

Daniel Sheridan is an associate professor in the Johns Hopkins University School of Nursing, where he coordinates a forensic clinical nurse specialist graduate degree programs at the Masters, DNP, and PhD levels. Dr. Sheridan has 25 years of experience working with survivors of family abuse and sexual assault, and he lectures and consults nationally and internationally on these topics.

Chapter 7: Domestic Violence Assessment (U.S. Sixth Edition)

Deborah E. Swenson, MSN, ARNP, C-WHCNP

Deborah Swenson is a certified women's health care nurse practitioner with Swedish Medical Center's Perinatal Medicine Clinic and OBSTETRIX Medical Group of Washington, Inc., PS, in Seattle, Washington. She holds certification from the NCC as a women's health care nurse practitioner. She is the author of *Telephone Triage for the Obstetric Patient: A Nursing Guide.*

Chapter 30: Pregnancy

Denise Tarlier, PhD, MSN, NP(F), NCMP

Denise Tarlier is a family nurse practitioner in British Columbia and has also held national U.S. NP certification since 1998. She is a certified menopause practitioner with the North American Menopause Society. Her clinical practice over many years has been primarily in remote and northern Aboriginal communities across Canada. Denise is currently practicing as a family nurse practitioner in Kamloops, British Columbia. She is also a member of the Nurse Practitioner Leadership Team in the Family Nurse Practitioner program at the University of Northern British Columbia in Prince George. Her scholarship and teaching are guided by a strong clinical practice orientation to primary health care, rural and remote health care services, Aboriginal health issues, and primary care and nurse practitioner nursing roles.

Chapter 18: Breasts and Regional Lymphatics

Christina Vaillancourt, MHSc, RD, CDE

Christina Vaillancourt completed her Masters of Health Sciences at University of Ontario's Institute of Technology. She is a Registered Dietitian and a Certified Diabetes Educator currently working in management role in the areas of nephrology and diabetes. She has taught nutrition courses for Durham College, Georgian College, and the University of Ontario Institute of Technology.

Chapter 12: Nutritional Assessment and Nursing Practice

Colleen Varcoe, PhD, RN

Colleen Varcoe teaches at undergraduate and graduate levels with a focus on culture, ethics, inequity, and policy at the University of British Columbia. Her research focuses on women's health, with an emphasis on violence and inequity; and on the culture of health care, with an emphasis on ethical practice. Her program of research is aimed at promoting ethical practice and policy in the context of violence and inequity. She recently co-led a longitudinal study of the health and economic effects of violence against women after women have left abusive partners. She is currently leading a study of a health care intervention for Aboriginal women who have experienced violence and co-leading an intervention study to promote equity in primary health care. She has more than 90 peer-reviewed publications and is writing a textbook on nursing as relational inquiry, with co-author Gweneth Hartrick Doane.

Chapter 3: Cultural and Social Considerations in Health Assessment; Chapter 7: Substance Use in the Context of Health Assessment; and Chapter 8: Interpersonal Violence Assessment

Ellen Vogel, PhD, RD, FDC

Ellen Vogel is dean and associate professor in the Faculty of Health Sciences at the University of Ontario Institute of Technology, located in Oshawa, Ontario. Dr. Vogel completed a PhD in nutrition and metabolism at the University of Alberta (2001). In 2003 she was awarded a postdoctoral fellowship from the Office of the Chief Scientist at Health Canada. Dr. Vogel is a fellow with Dietitians of Canada, a past chair of the Dietitians of Canada's Board of Directors, and the recipient of numerous awards for leadership and innovation in dietetics practice. Dr. Vogel has a broad base of practice, applied research, and networking experience. She is well known for her work in the field of community health and her involvement with the Canada Prenatal Nutrition Program. Dr. Vogel has led, or co-led, a variety of national research studies tackling topics such as the effectiveness of community-based programs and building capacity for food security through policy change. She was recently involved with a three-year Canadian study examining social issues in nutritional genomics, such as the design of appropriate regulatory systems, ethical considerations, and consumers' understandings.

Chapter 12: Nutritional Assessment and Nursing Practice

Nancy Watts, RN, MN

Nancy Watts has worked in various nursing settings with a primary focus in obstetrical nursing. Her education includes a master's degree in Nursing and certification in Perinatal Nursing. Nancy has pursued learning in family-centred care, adult learning, and complex care planning. She is currently the President of the Canadian Association of Perinatal and Women's Health Nurses (CAPWHN). She has been the author of various publications including chapters on Pregnancy and High Risk Labour/Birth in recent textbooks.

Chapter 30: Pregnancy

Kathryn Weaver, PhD, RN

Dr. Kathryn Weaver received her undergraduate education at Dalhousie University, Halifax, Nova Scotia; her master's degree at the University of New Brunswick, Fredericton, New Brunswick; her PhD (Nursing) at the University of Alberta, Edmonton, Alberta; and postdoctoral fellowships through the International Institute for Qualitative Methodology and Alberta Foundation for Medical Research, Faculty of Nursing, University of Alberta. She is a Harrison-McCain Young Scholar, Associate Professor with the Faculty of Nursing, University of New Brunswick, Associate Editor of the International Journal of Interdisciplinary Health Sciences, and Nurse Psychotherapist with an independent practice counseling women and adolescents suffering from eating disorders. Her teaching and research interests include qualitative and mixed methods research, psychiatric-mental health nursing, community development, ethical sensitivity in professional practice, and eating disorders. She is principal investigator of the video documentary *Through True Eyes: Recovery from Eating Disorders* produced by Atlantic Mediaworks, Fredericton, New Brunswick (2009).

Chapter 6: Mental Health Assessment

Barbara Wilson-Keates, RN, PhD

Barbara Wilson-Keates has experience in adult medicine and cardiac and critical care nursing in acute care hospitals across Canada and the United States. Over the past 25 years, she has worked in a variety of nursing positions, including clinical nurse, research assistant, and nursing instructor for clinical and classroom courses for undergraduate and graduate nursing students. Dr. Wilson-Keates has assisted in the development and implementation of nursing and interprofessional simulation teaching modules for numerous Ontario colleges and universities. Her PhD dissertation examined the predictors of a nurse's trust in one's manager. She is currently a clinical policy consultant with Alberta Health Services.

Chapter 17: Nose, Mouth, and Throat

Reviewers of the Second Canadian Edition

Monique Mallet Boucher, RN, MN, MEd, PhD(c)
Senior Teaching Associate
University of New Brunswick
Moncton, New Brunswick

Catherine Bowman, BScN, MN, RN, ENC(C)
Faculty of Health and Community Studies
Grant MacEwan University
Edmonton, Alberta

Karen Furlong, MN, RN, CNN(C)
Full-Time Doctoral Student, Faculty of Education
University of New Brunswick—Fredericton
Senior Teaching Associate, Department of Nursing &
   Health Research
University of New Brunswick—Saint John

Dawn Inman-Flynn, RN, BScN, MN
Clinical Nursing Instructor
University of Prince Edward Island
Charlottetown, Prince Edward Island

Neemera Jamani, RN, BScN
Assistant Lecturer
School of Nursing
York University
Toronto, Ontario

Paul Jeffrey, RN(EC), BScN, MN, NP
Adult Program Coordinator and Professor of
   Health Sciences
Nursing Program
Sheridan College
Brampton, Ontario

Tania Killian, RN, BScN, BEd, MEd, CCN
Lecturer, Seneca/York Collaborative Degree Program
Faculty of Health Sciences
Seneca College
King City, Ontario

Debora Kirschbaum-Nitkin, BScN, MEd, PhD
Lecturer
Lawrence S. Bloomberg Faculty of Nursing
University of Toronto
Toronto, Ontario

Jennifer Lapum, PhD, MN, BScN
Associate Professor
Daphne Cockwell School of Nursing
Ryerson University
Toronto, Ontario

Maureen MacInnis-Wheatley, RN, MN
Learning Resource Coordinator & Instructor;
   Sessional Lecturer
School of Nursing
University of Prince Edward Island
Charlottetown, Prince Edward Island

Faith Richardson, DNP, MSN-FNP
Assistant Professor
School of Nursing
Trinity Western University
Langley, British Columbia

Lori Schindel-Martin, RN, PhD
Associate Professor, Daphne Cockwell School of Nursing
Associate Director—Scholarship, Research & Creative
   Activities, Faculty of Community Services
Ryerson University
Toronto, Ontario

Karen Silvester, RN, BSN, MN(c)
Nursing Faculty
Baccalaureate Nursing Program
North Island College
Courtenay, British Columbia

Lisa Sworts, RN, BSN
Lab Resource Nurse
Vancouver Island University
Nanaimo, British Columbia

Margaret Verkuyl, NP-PHC, MN, AGD:ANP
Nursing Professor
Centennial College
Toronto, Ontario

It is important that students develop, practise, and then learn to trust their health history and physical examination skills. In this book we give you the tools to do that. Learn to listen to the patient—most often he or she will tell you what is wrong (and right) and what you can do to meet his or her health care needs. Then learn to inspect, examine, and listen to the person's body. The data are all there and are accessible to you by using just a few extra tools. High-technological machinery is a smart and sophisticated adjunct, but it cannot replace your own bedside assessment of your patient.

Whether you are a beginning examiner or an advanced-practice student, this book holds the content you need to develop and refine your clinical skills. The **Second Canadian Edition** of *Physical Examination & Health Assessment* is a comprehensive textbook of health history-taking methods, physical examination skills, health promotion techniques, and clinical assessment tools.

Thank you for your enthusiastic anticipation of this second Canadian edition. We are excited to be able to bring you an established, successful text with a focus on Canadian issues and content to further meet the needs of both novice and advanced practitioners in Canada.

DUAL FOCUS AS TEXT AND REFERENCE

Physical Examination & Health Assessment is both a **text for beginning students** of physical examination and also a **text and reference for advanced practitioners such as nurse practitioners and clinical nurse specialists.** The chapter progression and format permit this scope without sacrificing one use for the other.

Chapters 1 through 8 focus on **health assessment of individuals and families,** including developmental tasks and health promotion for all age groups; the importance of **relational practice** in health assessment; **cultural and social considerations in assessment;** interviewing and complete health history gathering; and the social context of **mental health assessment, substance use assessment,** and **interpersonal violence assessment.**

Chapters 9 through 12 begin the approach to the **clinical care setting,** describing physical data-gathering techniques, how to set up the examination site, body measurement and vital signs, pain assessment, and nutritional assessment.

Chapters 13 through 27 focus on the **physical examination and related health history** in a body-systems approach. This is the most efficient method of performing the examination and is the most systematic and logical method for student

learning and retrieval of data. **Each chapter has five major sections:** Structure and Function, Subjective Data (history), Objective Data (examination skills and findings), Documentation and Critical Thinking, and Abnormal Findings. The novice practitioner can review anatomy and physiology and learn the skills, expected findings, and common variations for generally healthy people and selected abnormal findings in the Objective Data sections. New to this edition is **a sixth section,** Special Considerations for Advanced Practice, in selected relevant chapters. The sections on Special Considerations for Advanced Practice were created to address assessment approaches that are particularly relevant for **advanced practice nurses.** These sections also help to delineate the boundaries between basic assessments and more advanced assessments that may be conducted by advanced practice nurses.

Chapters 28 through 31 **integrate the complete health assessment.** Chapters 28 and 29 present the choreography of the head-to-toe examination for a complete screening examination in various age groups and for the focused examination of a hospitalized adult. Special populations are addressed in Chapters 30 and 31—the health assessment of the pregnant woman and the functional assessment of the older adult.

Students continue to use this text in subsequent courses throughout their education, and experienced clinicians will use this text as part of their advanced nursing practice. Given that each course demands more advanced skills and techniques, students can review the detailed presentation and the additional techniques in the Objective Data sections as well as variations for different age levels. Students can also study the extensive pathology illustrations and detailed text in the Abnormal Findings sections.

This text is valuable to both advanced practice students and experienced clinicians because of its comprehensive approach. *Physical Examination & Health Assessment* can help clinicians learn the skills for advanced practice, refresh their memory, review a specific examination technique when confronted with an unfamiliar clinical situation, and compare and label a diagnostic finding.

NEW TO THE SECOND CANADIAN EDITION

All chapters are **revised and updated** to include Canadian concepts, terminology, statistics, standards and guidelines, and assessment tools commonly used in Canadian health care settings. Four newly written chapters and several new features that span various chapters are presented in this Second

Canadian Edition. Three new and 15 revised **Promoting Health** boxes are presented, at least one in each of the physical examination chapters. These boxes describe an important health promotion topic related to the system discussed in each chapter—a topic you can use to enhance patient education initiatives.

New **Special Considerations for Advanced Practice** sections provided in selected chapters identify assessment approaches that are particularly relevant for advanced practice nurses. New **Critical Findings** textboxes are placed strategically throughout the chapters to alert practitioners to assessment findings that require immediate attention, action, and decision-making. The **Cultural and Social Considerations** sections have been newly written in each chapter to reflect content relevant to Canada. The cultural and social factors that influence health, illness, and access to health care are discussed, and implications requiring consideration in the context of health assessment are identified. Highlights of Canadian content in each chapter are outlined below.

Chapter 1, **Critical Thinking and Evidence-Informed Assessment,** includes new perspectives on critical thinking and diagnostic reasoning as integral to health assessment. The relevance of conducting assessments based on evidence-informed decisions is emphasized. Relational approaches to nursing practice are discussed to foster nurses' capacities to convey respect, and as a means to avoid objectifying people in the process of health assessment.

Chapter 2, **Health Promotion in the Context of Health Assessment,** is newly written and integrates the latest Canadian guidelines for health promotion, illness prevention, screening, immunizations, developmental assessment, and health education and patient counseling across the lifespan. Emphasis is placed on health promotion opportunities and actions that can be taken in the process of conducting health assessments.

Chapter 3, **Cultural and Social Considerations in Health Assessment,** is newly written to reflect the ethnocultural and social diversity within the Canadian population. Examples of current trends in health, social, and gender inequities are reviewed and discussed in terms of the implications for health assessment. Guidelines are provided for assessing culturally based understandings and the social and economic contexts shaping people's lives.

Chapter 6, **Mental Health Assessment,** is newly written to provide content reflecting Canadian perspectives on the personal and social factors that shape people's mental health. The chapter provides strategies for conducting mental health assessments, including mental status examinations and risk assessments for suicide. The developmental adaptations that are required to conduct respectful assessments across the lifespan are also discussed.

Chapter 7, **Substance Use in the Context of Health Assessment,** is a cutting-edge, new chapter—one of the first of its kind in a nursing health assessment textbook. It provides clinicians with the knowledge and skills to integrate assessments regarding substance use across a range of practice settings and with patients of all ages. Factors influencing the use of substances and the health effects of substance use are

discussed. Emphasis is placed on nonjudgemental, respectful approaches and techniques for assessing substance use.

Chapter 8, **Interpersonal Violence Assessment,** has also been heavily revised to include guidelines for assessing intimate partner violence, sexual assault, child abuse, and elder abuse as important problems for health care professionals to recognize and respond to. The chapter discusses the long-term effects of violence on health and the implications in the context of health assessment. Mandatory reporting requirements are also discussed, and strategies for assessing violence in a nonjudgemental and accepting manner are emphasized.

Chapter 9, **Assessment Techniques and the Clinical Setting,** focuses on assessment techniques and includes the Canadian Hypertensive Education Program guidelines for diagnosis. The chapter will help both novice and advanced practitioners make clinical decisions based on accurate assessment techniques.

Chapter 11, **Pain Assessment,** has been updated to include assessment tools for both conscious and unconscious patients. These additions reflect a growing trend toward caring for palliative patients in the community setting and the increased complexity of caring for the patient found outside the intensive care environment.

Chapter 12, **Nutritional Assessment and Nursing Practice,** has been updated to reflect developmental considerations with regard to nutrition, address determinants of health, and reinforce the latest information concerning dietary reference intakes and nutrition labeling in Canada.

Chapter 30, **Pregnancy,** incorporates Canadian screening and diagnostic tests for the pregnant woman and guidelines for health promotion.

Chapter 31, **Functional Assessment of the Older Adult,** includes Canadian statistics on aging; guidelines for screening for elder abuse and prevention of falls; and content related to caregiver, environmental, and spiritual assessments. Tools for assessment of activities of daily living, instrumental activities of daily living, and advanced activities of daily living are discussed.

APPROACHES USED IN THIS EDITION

The Second Canadian Edition of *Physical Examination & Health Assessment* builds on the strengths of the U.S. Sixth Edition and is designed to engage students and enhance learning:

1. **Method of examination** (Objective Data section) is clear, orderly, and easy to follow. Hundreds of original examination illustrations are placed directly with the text to demonstrate the physical examination in a step-by-step format.

2. **Two-column format** begins in the Subjective Data section, where the running column highlights the rationales for asking various history questions. In the Objective Data section, the running column highlights selected abnormal findings to show a clear relationship between normal and abnormal findings.

3. **Abnormal Findings tables** organize and expand on material in the examination section. These have been

revised and updated with many new clinical photos. The atlas format of these extensive collections of pathology and original illustrations helps students recognize, sort, and describe abnormal findings. When applicable, the text under a table entry is presented in a Subjective Data–Objective Data format.

4. **Developmental approach** in each chapter presents prototypical content on the adult, then age-specific content for the infant, child, adolescent, pregnant woman, and older adult so that students can learn common variations for all age groups.

5. **Cultural and social considerations** are discussed throughout as factors that shape health, illness, and access to health care. In addition to Chapter 3, where these issues are discussed in depth, cultural and social considerations are included throughout the chapters to orient readers to relevant issues in the Canadian context.

   Readers will note that literature citations based on U.S. or British research continue to use the terms "Black" (to refer to people of African American descent) and "White" (for people of European descent). In Canada, there has been a shift away from identifying people on the basis of "race," and these issues are discussed in more depth in Chapter 3. When U.S. or British literature is cited, however, the terms "Black" and "White" are retained in keeping with the original reference sources.

6. **Stunning full-colour art** shows detailed human anatomy, physiology, examination techniques, and abnormal findings.

7. **Health history** (Subjective Data) appears in two places: Chapter 4, The Interview, has the most complete discussion available on the process of communication and on interviewing skills, techniques, and potential traps to avoid. This chapter includes guidelines for communicating with people whose primary language differs from yours and for working with interpreters to conduct sensitive and accurate health assessments. In Chapter 5, The Complete Health History, and in pertinent history questions that are repeated and expanded in each chapter, history questions are included that highlight health promotion opportunities and activities. This approach to emphasizing history questions helps students to understand the relationship between subjective and objective data. Because the history and examination data are considered together, as they would be in the clinical setting, each chapter can stand on its own if a person has a specific problem related to that body system.

8. **Summary checklists** toward the end of each chapter provide a quick review of examination steps to help you develop a mental checklist.

9. **Sample recordings** of normal findings show the written language you should use to ensure that charting is complete yet succinct.

10. **Focused assessment and clinical case studies** of frequently encountered situations demonstrate the application of assessment techniques to patients of different ages in differing clinical situations. These case histories, in subjective-objective-assessment-plan (SOAP) format, ending in diagnosis, are presented in the language actually used during recording.

11. **Integration of the complete health assessment** for the adult, infant, and child is presented as an illustrated essay in Chapter 28. This approach integrates all the steps into a choreographed whole. Included is a complete write-up of a health history and physical examination.

12. **User-friendly design** makes the book easy to use. Frequent subheadings and instructional headings help readers to easily retrieve content.

13. Bedside Assessment of the Hospitalized Adult, in Chapter 29, provides a unique photo sequence that **illustrates a head-to-toe assessment** suitable for each daily shift of care. It would be neither possible nor pertinent to perform a complete head-to-toe examination on every patient during every 24-hour stay in the hospital; therefore, this sequence shows a consistent specialized examination for each 8-hour shift that focuses on certain parameters pertinent to areas of medical, surgical, and cardiac step-down care.

The Canadian content that appears in the book—particularly the content about dealing with hospitalized patients, older adults, and pain assessment; relating to substance use and interpersonal violence; and cultural and social considerations—form part of the standard repertoire of knowledge from which Canadian examiners can draw.

CONCEPTUAL APPROACH

The Second Canadian Edition of *Physical Examination & Health Assessment* reflects a commitment to the following approaches:

- **Relational practice** in clinical practice recognizes that health, illness, and the meanings they hold for people are shaped by one's gender, age, ability, and social, cultural, familial, historical, and geographical contexts. These contexts influence how nurses and other health care professionals view, relate, and work with patients and families. By practising relationally, health care professionals will be optimally prepared to conduct accurate health assessments and to respond meaningfully to the patient's health, illness, and health promotion needs.

- **Health promotion** is discussed in depth in Chapter 2, with an emphasis on how to integrate health promotion into the process of health assessment. Health promotion textboxes are also provided in most chapters outlining the latest health promoting practices.

- Engaging with the patient as an **active participant in health care** involves encouraging discussion of what the person is currently doing to promote his or her health and supporting people to participate in health promoting practices given the social contexts of their lives.

- **Cultural and social considerations** take into account our global society and the wide range of ethnocultural and social diversity within Canada.

- Assessing individuals **across the lifespan** reflects the understanding that a person's state of health must be considered in light of his or her developmental stage.

Developmental anatomy; modifications of examination techniques; and expected findings for infants and children, adolescents, pregnant women, and older adults are provided. **Developmental Considerations** are provided in each relevant chapter, along with strategies for adapting health assessment approaches and techniques across the lifespan.

ANCILLARIES

- The *Pocket Companion for Physical Examination & Health Assessment* continues to be a handy and current clinical reference that provides pertinent material in full colour, with over 150 illustrations from the textbook.
- The *Student Laboratory Manual* with physical examination forms is a workbook that includes a student study guide, glossary of key terms, clinical objectives, regional write-up forms, and review questions for each chapter. The pages are perforated so that students can use the regional write-up forms in the skills laboratory or in the clinical setting and turn them in to the instructor.
- The new revised *Health Assessment Online* resource is an innovative and dynamic teaching and learning tool with more than **8000 electronic assets,** including video clips, anatomic overlays, animations, audio clips, interactive exercises, laboratory/diagnostic tests, review questions, and new **electronic charting activities.** Comprehensive **Self-Paced Learning Modules** offer increased flexibility to faculty who wish to provide students with tutorial learning modules and in-depth capstone cases for each body system chapter in the text. The **Capstone Case Studies** now include **Quality and Safety Challenge** activities. Additional **Advance Practice Case Studies** put the student in the exam room and test history taking and documentation skills. The comprehensive **video clip library** shows exam procedures across the life span and is expanded to now include clips on the pregnant woman. Animations, sounds, images, interactive activities, and video clips are embedded in the learning modules and cases to provide a dynamic, multimodal learning environment for today's learners.
- *Physical Examination & Health Assessment Video Series* is an 18-video package developed in conjunction with this text. There are 12 body system videos and 6 head-to-toe videos, with the latter containing complete examinations of the neonate, child, adult, older adult, and pregnant woman, and the bedside examination of the hospitalized adult. This series is available in DVD or streaming online formats. There are over 5 hours of video footage with highlighted Cross-Cultural Care Considerations, Developmental Considerations, and Health Promotion Tips, as well as Instructor Booklets with video overviews, outlines, learning objectives, discussion topics, and questions with answers.
- The companion *EVOLVE Web site* (http://evolve.elsevier.com/Canada/Jarvis/examination/) contains learning objectives: more than 150 multiple-choice review questions; new

system-by-system examination summaries and bedside examination summaries that are downloadable into audio CD or MP3 player files; a comprehensive physical examination form for the adult; and numerous reference appendices from previous editions that have been updated and moved online, including immunization schedules, standard precautions, growth charts, and blood pressure levels. **Case studies**—including a variety of developmental and cultural variables—help students apply health assessment skills and knowledge. These include 25 in-depth case studies with critical thinking questions and answer guidelines, as well as printable health promotion handouts. Also included is a complete Head-to-Toe Video examination of the adult that can be viewed in its entirety or by systems, as well as a new printable section on Quick Assessments for Common Conditions.
- *Simulation Learning System.* The new *Simulation Learning System* (SLS) is an online toolkit that incorporates medium- to high-fidelity simulation with scenarios that enhance the clinical decision-making skills of students. The SLS offers a comprehensive package of resources, including leveled patient scenarios, detailed instructions for preparation and implementation of the simulation experience, debriefing questions that encourage critical thinking, and learning resources to reinforce student comprehension.
- For instructors, the Evolve website presents an Instructor's Manual and PowerPoint slides, a comprehensive Image Collection, and a Test Bank. The **Instructor's Manual** provides annotated learning objectives; key terms; and teaching strategies for the classroom in a revised section with strategies for both clinical and simulation lab use, critical thinking exercises, websites, and performance checklists. The **PowerPoint slides** include 2000 slides with integrated images. A separate 1200-illustration **Image Collection** is featured. Finally, the **ExamView Test Bank** has more than 850 multiple choice questions with coded answers and rationales. Instructors also have access to the accompanying online course, Health Assessment Online.

IN CONCLUSION

Throughout all stages of manuscript preparation and production, every effort has been made to develop a book that is readable, informative, instructive, and vital. Your comments and suggestions have been important to this task and continue to be welcome for this new Canadian edition.

Carolyn Jarvis
Annette J. Browne
June MacDonald-Jenkins
Marian Luctkar-Flude
c/o Elsevier Canada
905 King Street West, 4th Floor
Toronto, ON M6K 3G9

Acknowledgements for the U.S. Sixth Edition

It is my pleasure to recognize the many wonderful friends and colleagues who helped make the revision of this textbook possible. For their help and support I send my gratitude:

To my artistic colleagues, who made this book the vibrant visual display it is. Pat Thomas, medical illustrator, is a gifted artist with an eye for detail and clarity. Kevin Strandberg is a clever and careful photographer who has endless patience for capturing the images of children and adults in just the right moment of the examination. It is wonderful to collaborate with these two professionals. Our team has worked together for six editions, providing an artistic unity and clarity to this latest textbook. We are joined in this edition by Ronnie Lemmi, who contributed many photos of abnormal conditions, gathered through her clinical practice.

To my research assistants, whose tireless help enabled me to survive and proceed through manuscript preparation and revision. Erin Kugler and Abby Koestra searched for and retrieved countless articles. Abby read and reread endless copies of galley and page proofs, making astute suggestions and finding errors.

To the faculty and students who took the time to write letters of encouragement and suggestions—your comments are gratefully received and are very helpful. To the reviewers who spent considerable time reading the chapter manuscript and filling out response questionnaires—your suggestions and ideas are very important for this sixth edition.

Thank you to the remarkable professional team at Elsevier. I am grateful to Sally Schrefer, Managing Director, Nursing and Health Professions, for her guidance and support for the book and its ancillaries. Sally knows the text well and has been personally involved in its advancement and promotion. Robin Carter, Executive Editor, has been a beacon of support for me and for the book. Robin always has sound suggestions for new ideas for the book and is everlastingly prompt and positive.

Many people worked very hard to guide this book through production. I am grateful to Debbie Vogel, Publishing Services Manager, for supervising the schedule for book production and making all the contacts to keep everyone on schedule. My thanks go especially to Jodi Willard, Senior Project Manager, who has been so organized and positive in our day-to-day production schedule. Her messages are always welcome. I know readers will share my pleasure in the striking colors and design of the sixth edition. I am grateful to Teresa McBryan, Design Manager, for coordinating the beautiful interior design. The design draws the reader into the book and guides one through all the subsections. The dramatic illustration on the cover is the work of Max Fischer. The individual page layout is the wonderful work of Leslie Foster, Illustrator/Designer. Leslie crafts every page, always planning how the page can be made even better. Finally, I am so fortunate to have the support of Laurie Gower, Managing Editor. Laurie is so prompt and efficient and cheerful in directing the countless details of moving along the manuscript. It is always my pleasure to work with Deanna Dedeke, Developmental Editor. Deanna has worked tirelessly to guide the instructor ancillaries, the Pocket Companion, and the Student Laboratory Manual. I am very grateful to Laurie and Deanna.

Most important are the members of my wonderful family for their help, love, and complete support. Their constant belief in me and their encouragement have kept me going throughout this process.

Carolyn Jarvis

ACKNOWLEDGEMENTS FOR THE SECOND CANADIAN EDITION

Carolyn Jarvis's text has been a constant companion throughout my clinical and teaching career. The opportunity to adapt this classic textbook to reflect Canadian perspectives, content, and guidelines is a major honour. I have thoroughly enjoyed thinking critically about the range of content to include, especially given the diverse range of students, clinicians, and faculty who may use this text. I want to thank Dr. Sally Thorne, a professor at the University of British Columbia School of Nursing, for encouraging me to take on this project, and Ann Millar at Elsevier for her expert guidance throughout this process. I am also grateful to June MacDonald-Jenkins and Marian Luctkar-Flude for adapting this text in significant ways to reflect the unique context of nursing practice in Canada. I am fortunate to be able to draw on the expertise of Dr. Colleen Varcoe, Dr. Dana Edge, Dr. Denise Tarlier, and Dr. Kate Weaver as chapter authors and contributors, and I thank them for providing highly pertinent and cutting-edge content. To John, whose loving support makes this work possible.

Annette J. Browne

What a pleasure to have been given the opportunity to potentially influence the learning of students across the country. My thanks to every student who risked taking a stance of inquiry, looked for more, and sought the answers; you are the reason that editing this text was such a pleasure. I, too, would like to thank the editorial team at Elsevier Canada; they have been gracious and supportive while ensuring that we met timelines for publication of the Second Canadian Edition. I would like to thank my colleagues Dr. Ellen Vogel, Christina Vaillancourt, and Andrea Miller for contributing to Chapter 12, Nutritional Assessment and Nursing Practice, and to Lynn Haslam for her work on Chapter 11, Pain. I extend my thanks to these four professionals for hours of collaboration and consultation to ensure the inclusion of a truly national perspective. Many thanks, as well, to my co-editors Annette and Marian; your knowledge and insight have truly shaped the perspective of this text. I would like to thank my family for their endless support and indulgence of my "adventures:" my husband, Dean, and my three daughters, Sarah, Emily, and Mackenzie.

June MacDonald-Jenkins

I am truly grateful for having had the opportunity to participate in the development of the Second Canadian Edition of Jarvis's *Physical Examination & Health Assessment*. The support of the Elsevier Canada staff throughout this challenging process has been invaluable. In particular, I would like to thank the publisher, Ann Millar, the managing developmental editor, Martina van de Velde, and the project manager, John Gabbert, for their guidance. I would also like to thank my colleagues Barbara Wilson-Keates and Dianne Groll for their contributions to the Nose, Mouth, and Throat, and Functional Assessment of the Older Adult chapters; and Nancy Watts for contributing to the Pregnancy chapter, as these are not my areas of expertise. I would like to thank my Canadian coeditors, Annette J. Browne and June MacDonald-Jenkins, for their long-distance collaboration, for sharing their knowledge, contacts, and resources, and for providing helpful feedback on my revisions. It has been a pleasure and a great learning experience to work with each of you. And, finally, I would like to acknowledge the support of those dearest to me: Richard, Curtis and Sarena, Cameron and Katurah, Corey, and Brianna.

Marian Luctkar-Flude

JARVIS

Physical Examination & Health Assessment

Second Canadian Edition

Critical Thinking and Evidence-Informed Assessment

Written by Carolyn Jarvis, PhD, APN, CNP
Adapted by Annette J. Browne, PhD, RN

⊝volve WEBSITE

http://evolve.elsevier.com/Canada/Jarvis/examination/
- Appendices
- Examination Review Questions
- Key Points

OUTLINE

The ability to conduct a high-quality health assessment and physical examination is foundational to nursing practice. Similarly, in order to provide relevant, timely, and appropriate nursing and health care, nurses must be able to accurately describe assessment findings to patients, families, and other members of the interprofessional team. Assessments must be conducted in ways that convey respect for the whole person, to avoid objectifying people. Learning to conduct systematic assessments is integral to developing confidence in clinical abilities and capacity to respond effectively to patients' needs.

You work in a primary health care clinic in a Canadian city. Ellen K. is a 23-year-old woman whom you have seen several times over the past 2 months (Figure 1-1). She has been admitted for observation at the Emergency Department because of sudden onset of shortness of breath.

The health care provider in the Emergency Department documented a health history and performed a complete physical examination. Examples of the preliminary list of significant findings recorded in her health record are as follows:
- *Appearance: Sitting quietly alone in the examination room. Facial expression appears sad. Eyes fill with tears when she discusses her boyfriend.*
- *Elevated BP [blood pressure]; 142/100 at end of examination today*
- *Diminished breath sounds, with moderate expiratory wheeze and scattered rhonchi at both bases*

- *Grade II/VI systolic heart murmur, left lower sternal border*
- *Resolving hematoma, 2 to 3 cm, R [right] infraorbital ridge*
- *Missing R lower first molar, gums receding on lower incisors, multiple dark spots on front upper teeth*
- *Well-healed scar, 28 cm long × 2 cm wide, R lower leg, with R leg 3 cm shorter than L [left], sequelae of auto accident at age 12*
- *Altered nutrition: omits breakfast; daily intake has no fruits, no vegetables; meals at fast food restaurants most days*
- *Oral contraceptives for birth control × 3 years, last pelvic examination 1 year ago*
- *Smokes a half PPD [pack of cigarettes per day] × 2 years, prior use one PPD × 4 years.*
- *Alcohol use started age 16. For past 2 years, has equivalent of 3–4 drinks per day × 4–5 days a week. Last intake of alcohol was yesterday.*
- *Currently is unemployed × 6 months. Receives employment insurance (≈$680/month). Previous work as cashier in large department store.*
- *History of emotional and physical abuse related to current relationship with boyfriend. Today has orbital hematoma as a result of being struck by boyfriend with the back of his hand. States, "We had a big fight—I probably deserved it"*
- *Relationships: Over past 12 months, has not been in communication with her parents, who live in another city. Has*

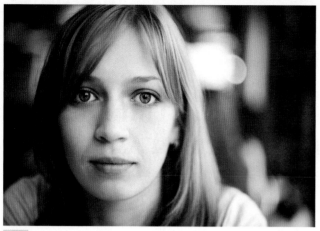

1-1

one close woman friend who lives nearby. Significant relationship is with boyfriend of 2 years, with whom she resides in a rented small basement suite.

The examiner analyzed and interpreted all the data; clustered the information, sorting out which data to refer and which to treat; and identified the diagnoses. Of interest is how many significant findings are derived from data the examiner collected. Not just physical data but also cognitive, psychosocial, and behavioural data are significant for an analysis of Ellen's health state. Also, the findings are interesting when considered from a life cycle perspective; that is, Ellen is a young adult who normally should be concerned with the developmental tasks of emancipation from parents, building an economically stable life, and developing caring relationships.

*A body of clinical **evidence** has validated the importance of using the assessment techniques in Ellen's case. For example, measuring blood pressure is a way to screen for hypertension, and early intervention can ward off heart attack and stroke. Listening to breath sounds is a way to screen (in Ellen's case) for asthma, which is compounded by her smoking. Listening to heart sounds reveals Ellen's heart murmur, which could be "innocent" or a sign of a structural abnormality in a heart valve; further examination will yield further data. The physical examination is not just a rote formality. Its parts are determined by the best clinical evidence available and documented in the professional literature.*

ASSESSMENT: POINT OF ENTRY IN AN ONGOING PROCESS

Assessment is the collection of data about an individual's health state. Throughout this text, you will study the techniques of collecting and analyzing **subjective data** (i.e., what the person *says* about himself or herself during history taking) and **objective data** (i.e., what you as the health care provider *observe* by inspecting, percussing, palpating, and auscultating during the physical examination). Together with the patient's record and laboratory studies, these elements form the **database.** For example, in the case of Ellen, above, an example of subjective data is "History of emotional and physical abuse in current relationship with boyfriend." An example

of objective data is "Resolving hematoma, 2 to 3 cm, R infraorbital ridge."

From the database, you make a clinical judgement or diagnosis about the individual's health state or response to actual health problems or risk factors and life processes, as well as diagnoses about overall levels of wellness. Thus, the purpose of assessment is to make a judgement or diagnosis on the basis of data from various sources.

An organized assessment is the starting point of diagnostic reasoning. Because all health care diagnoses, decisions, and treatments are based on the data you gather during assessment, it is paramount that your assessment be factual and complete.

Diagnostic Reasoning

The step from data collection to diagnosis can be a difficult one. Most beginning examiners perform well in gathering the data, with adequate practice, but then treat all the data as being equally important. This makes decision making slow and laboured.

Diagnostic reasoning, the process of analyzing health data and drawing conclusions to identify diagnoses, is based on the scientific method. It has four major components: (a) attending to initially available cues; (b) formulating diagnostic hypotheses; (c) gathering data relative to the tentative hypotheses; and (d) evaluating each hypothesis with the new data collected, thus arriving at a final diagnosis. A *cue* is a piece of information, a sign or symptom, or a piece of laboratory data. A *hypothesis* is a tentative explanation for a cue or a set of cues that can be used as a basis for further investigation.

For example, Ellen K., the patient described at the beginning of this chapter, presents with a number of initial cues, one of which is the resolving hematoma under her eye. (a) You can recognize this cue even before history documentation begins. Is it significant? (b) If Ellen were to say she ran into a door, mumbles as she speaks, and avoids eye contact, you formulate a hypothesis of trauma. (c) During the history documentation and physical examination, you gather data to support or reject the tentative hypothesis. (d) You synthesize the new data collected, which support the hypothesis of trauma but eliminate the accidental cause. The final diagnoses are "resolving right orbital contusion" and "risk for trauma."

Diagnostic hypotheses are activated very early in the reasoning process. Consider a hunch that Ellen has suffered physical trauma. A hunch helps diagnosticians adapt to large amounts of information because it clusters cues into meaningful groups and directs subsequent data collection. Later, you can accept your hunch or rule it out.

Once you complete data collection, develop a preliminary list of significant signs and symptoms and all patient health needs. This is less formal in structure than your final list of diagnoses will be and is in no particular order. (Such a list for Ellen is found on p. 1–2.) In some institutions, it is easier to generate such a list if you use a conceptual model. Examples of conceptual models are described later in this chapter.

Cluster or group together the assessment data that appear to be causal or associated. For example, for a person in acute pain, associated data may include rapid heart rate and anxiety.

Organizing the data into meaningful clusters is slow at first; experienced examiners cluster data more rapidly because they recall proven results of earlier patient situations (Benner, 2001). Use of a conceptual model helps to organize data.

Validate the data you collect to make sure they are accurate. As you validate your information, look for gaps in data collection. Be sure to find the missing information because identifying missing information is an essential critical thinking skill. How you validate your data depends on experience. If you are unsure of the blood pressure, validate it by repeating the measurement yourself. Eliminate any extraneous variables that could influence blood pressure results, such as recent activity or anxiety over admission. If you have less experience analyzing breath sounds or heart murmurs, ask an expert to listen. Even for nurses with years of clinical experience, some signs always require validation (e.g., a breast lump).

Critical Thinking and the Diagnostic Process

The standards of practice in nursing, traditionally termed the **nursing process,** include six phases: assessment, diagnosis, outcome identification, planning, implementation, and evaluation (American Nurses Association, 2004; Canadian Nurses Association, 2010). In the 1970s and 1980s, the nursing process was considered a clear, stepwise, linear approach that started with assessment and ended with evaluation. Now it is considered a more dynamic, interactive process; in today's complex clinical setting, practitioners move back and forth within the steps (Figure 1-2).

Although the nursing process is a problem-solving approach to clinical judgements, the way in which a nurse applies the process depends on level and time of experience. *Novice* nurses have no experience with a specified patient population and use rules to guide performance (Benner, 2001). It takes time, perhaps 2 to 3 years in similar clinical situations, to achieve *competency,* whereby nurses see actions in the context of arching goals or daily plans for patients. *Proficient* nurses, who have had more time and experience, understand a patient's situation as a whole rather than as a list of tasks. These nurses envision long-term goals for the patient and how today's nursing actions apply to achieving those goals in, for example, 6 weeks. Finally, *expert* nurses appear to vault over the steps and arrive at a clinical judgement in one leap. Expert nurses have an intuitive grasp of a clinical situation and pinpoint the accurate solution (Benner, 2001).

This is true particularly with expert nurses in critical care situations in which patient status changes rapidly and accurate decisions are paramount. The stakes are high, and nursing autonomy is strong. In these cases, expert nurses focus on patients' responses and prevent complications by vigilant monitoring (Dains, Ciofu Baumann, & Scheibel, 2012). Expert nurses have well-developed physical assessment skills and trust these physical assessment skills, even if their conclusions conflict with technologically driven data. For example, consider the expert nurse's actions in assessing a woman with a drug overdose who had an endotracheal tube and was receiving mechanical ventilation:

> *The expert nurse examined the woman's posterior chest during medical rounds. She said to the medical team, "Mrs. Potter has bronchial breath sounds and dullness to percussion here and here (pointing to an area the size of a nickel and to another area the size of a quarter over the right lower lobe). Do you think she aspirated?" The physicians said, "No, her chest x-ray is normal." Three physicians took turns auscultating and percussing Mrs. Potter's chest. None of them could hear the changes, even when the expert [nurse] drew circles around the areas. The medical conclusion was that Mrs. Potter had not aspirated. Undaunted, the expert nurse initiated a regimen of pulmonary interventions. On rounds the next day, the medical team ordered antibiotics and frequent pulmonary treatments based on the early morning chest x-ray findings of right lower lobe consolidation.*
>
> *(Hanneman, 1996, p. 332)*

Functioning at the level of expert in clinical judgement includes using intuition: that is, knowledge received as a whole. Intuition is characterized by immediate recognition of patterns; expert practitioners learn to attend to a pattern of assessment data and act without consciously labelling it. Whereas the beginning nurse operates more from a set of defined, structured rules, the expert practitioner uses intuitive links, has the ability to perceive salient issues in a patient situation, and knows instant therapeutic responses (Benner, 2001). The expert nurse has a storehouse of experience about which interventions have been successful in the past.

For example, compare the actions of the nonexpert nurse and the expert nurse in the following situation of a young man with *Pneumocystis jiroveci (P. carinii)* pneumonia:

> *He was banging the side rails, making gurgling sounds, and pointing to his endotracheal tube. He was diaphoretic, gasping, and frantic. The nurse put her hand on his arm and tried to ascertain whether he had a sore throat from the tube. While she was away from the bedside retrieving an analgesic, the expert nurse strolled by, hesitated, listened, went to the man's bedside, re-inflated the endotracheal cuff, and accepted the patient's look of gratitude because he was able to breathe again. The nonexpert nurse was distressed that she had misread the situation. The expert reviewed the signs of a leaky cuff with the nonexpert and pointed out that banging the side rails and panic help differentiate acute respiratory distress from pain.*
>
> *(Hanneman, 1996, p. 333)*

The method of moving from novice to becoming an expert practitioner is through the use of critical thinking. All nurses start as novices, when clear-cut rules are needed to guide actions. Critical thinking is the means by which nurses learn to assess and modify, if indicated, before acting.

Critical thinking is required for sound diagnostic reasoning and clinical judgement. During your career, you will need to sort through vast amounts of data and information in

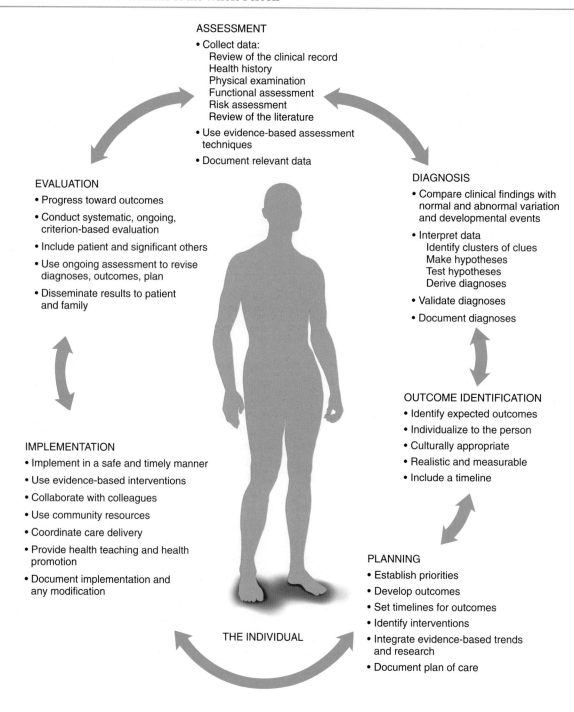

ASSESSMENT
- Collect data:
  Review of the clinical record
  Health history
  Physical examination
  Functional assessment
  Risk assessment
  Review of the literature
- Use evidence-based assessment techniques
- Document relevant data

EVALUATION
- Progress toward outcomes
- Conduct systematic, ongoing, criterion-based evaluation
- Include patient and significant others
- Use ongoing assessment to revise diagnoses, outcomes, plan
- Disseminate results to patient and family

DIAGNOSIS
- Compare clinical findings with normal and abnormal variation and developmental events
- Interpret data
  Identify clusters of clues
  Make hypotheses
  Test hypotheses
  Derive diagnoses
- Validate diagnoses
- Document diagnoses

OUTCOME IDENTIFICATION
- Identify expected outcomes
- Individualize to the person
- Culturally appropriate
- Realistic and measurable
- Include a timeline

IMPLEMENTATION
- Implement in a safe and timely manner
- Use evidence-based interventions
- Collaborate with colleagues
- Use community resources
- Coordinate care delivery
- Provide health teaching and health promotion
- Document implementation and any modification

THE INDIVIDUAL

PLANNING
- Establish priorities
- Develop outcomes
- Set timelines for outcomes
- Identify interventions
- Integrate evidence-based trends and research
- Document plan of care

1-2

order to make the sound judgements to manage patient care. This data will be dynamic, unpredictable, and ever changing. No single protocol that you can memorize will apply to every situation.

The following critical thinking skills are organized in a logical progression of the ways the skills might be used in the nursing process (Alfaro-LeFevre, 2009). Although each skill here is described separately, they are not used that way in the clinical area. Rather than a step-by-step linear process, critical thinking is a multidimensional thinking process. With experience, you will be able to apply these skills in a rapid, dynamic, and interactive way. You will also be able to conduct health assessments and physical examinations in ways that

convey genuine positive regard and acceptance toward the person, in ways that show you are not viewing people with regard merely to their bodily parts. For now, follow Ellen's case study through the steps.

1. *Identifying assumptions;* that is, recognize that you could take information for granted or see it as fact when actually there is no evidence for it. Ask yourself what you may be taking for granted here. For example, in Ellen's situation, you might have assumptions of a "typical profile" of a person who uses alcohol or who experiences physical violence on the basis of your past experience or exposure to media coverage. However, the facts of Ellen's situation are unique.

2. *Identifying an organized and comprehensive approach* to assessment. This approach depends on the patient's priority needs and your personal or institutional preference. Ellen has many physical and psychosocial issues, but at her time of admission, she is not acutely physically ill. Thus you may use any organized format for assessment that is feasible for you: a head-to-toe approach, a body systems approach (e.g., cardiovascular, gastrointestinal), a regional area approach (e.g., pelvic examination), or the use of a preprinted assessment form developed by the hospital or clinic.

3. *Validation* or checking the accuracy and reliability of data. For example, in addiction treatment, a clinician corroborates data with a family member or friend in order to verify the accuracy of Ellen's history. In Ellen's particular case, her significant others are absent or non-supportive, and the corroborative interview may need to be with a social worker.

4. *Distinguishing normal from abnormal* when signs and symptoms are identified. This is the first step in problem identification, and your ease will grow with study, practice, and experience. Increased blood pressure, wheezing, and heart murmur are among the many abnormal findings in Ellen's case.

5. *Making inferences* or hypotheses. This involves interpreting the data and deriving a correct conclusion about the health status. This is a challenge for the beginning examiner because both a baseline amount of knowledge and experience are needed. Is Ellen's blood pressure increased as a result of the stress of admission or as a result of a chronic condition? Is the heart murmur "innocent" or a sign of heart valve disease?

6. *Clustering related cues,* which helps you see relationships among the data. For example, heavy alcohol use, social and interpersonal consequences of alcohol use, academic consequences, and occupational consequences are a clustering of cues that suggest a maladaptive pattern of alcohol use.

7. *Distinguishing relevant from irrelevant.* A complete history and physical examination yield a vast amount of data. Look at the clusters of data, and consider which data are important for a health problem or a health promotion need. This skill is also a challenge for beginning examiners and one area in which the expertise of a clinical mentor can be invaluable.

8. *Recognizing inconsistencies.* Ellen's explanation that she ran into a door (subjective data) is at odds with the location of the infraorbital hematoma (objective data). With this kind of conflicting information, you can investigate and further clarify the situation.

9. *Identifying patterns.* Awareness of patterns helps you fill in the whole picture and discover missing pieces of information. To decide whether the systolic murmur is a problem for Ellen, you need to know the usual function of the heart, characteristics of innocent murmurs, and risk factors for abnormal or pathological murmurs.

10. *Identifying missing information,* gaps in data, or a need for more data to make a diagnosis. Ellen needs more interviewing regarding any increasing tolerance to alcohol, any withdrawal signs or symptoms, and laboratory data regarding liver enzyme levels and blood cell count, in order to specify a diagnosis.

11. *Promoting health* by identifying priorities with the patient, assessing risk factors, and considering a patient's social contexts. This applies to generally healthy people and concerns disease prevention and health promotion. To accomplish this skill, you need to identify and work with each patient to manage known risk factors for the individual's age group and social context. Managing risk factors drives the health promotion goals and priorities. For example, safety planning is an important intervention for Ellen, inasmuch as she identified interpersonal violence as an immediate concern. Following Ellen's lead, you would convey acceptance of her and a willingness to listen, and you would tell Ellen that the abuse she experiences is not her fault (see Chapter 8). You would ask Ellen whether she is interested in developing a safety plan to ensure that she has a safe place to go to if her boyfriend becomes abusive, or whether she is interested in discussing other issues that she identifies as priorities. You might ask her whether she would like to talk to a social worker who could help her address her social, economic, or housing needs. Depending on her priorities, you might also refer Ellen to a dental clinic that provides low-cost or no-cost dental care.

12. *Diagnosing actual and potential (risk) problems* from the assessment data. All diagnoses (both medical and nursing) derived from Ellen K.'s health history and physical examination findings are listed in Chapter 28.

   Nursing diagnoses can be conceptualized as clinical judgements about a person's response to an actual or potential health state and identification of their health concerns, risks, and goals in response to the nurse's analysis of assessment data. The 2012–2014 North American Nursing Diagnosis Association (NANDA) list is provided in Appendix H on the Evolve Web site. The NANDA listing has become popular as a device to organize nursing care because it allows for efficient categorization of patients' problems or diagnoses into computer databases that can then help prepare standardized nursing care plans (Thorne, 2006). Despite its popularity with health care administrators in some jurisdictions, the NANDA list is not used uniformly and can create challenges for nurses who prefer to develop more individualized ways of identifying and responding to unique patient problems. Note that the list includes (a) *actual diagnoses,* which are existing problems that are amenable to independent nursing interventions; (b) *risk diagnoses,* which are potential problems that an individual does not currently have but is particularly vulnerable to developing; and (c) *wellness diagnoses,* which focus on strengths and reflect an individual's transition to a higher level of wellness. Throughout this book, appropriate diagnoses from this list are presented and developed as they pertain to related content in each chapter. In Chapter 28, as noted previously, the findings for Ellen K. are analyzed and rewritten as diagnoses.

Medical and nursing diagnoses should not be considered isolated from each other; interprofessional perspectives and assessment data are needed to fully understand a person's health status. **Nurse practitioners,** for example, have expanded scopes of practice. Nurse practitioners are registered nurses who typically have master's degrees and have advanced education in health assessment and the diagnosis and management of illnesses and injuries, including the ability to prescribe medications. Nurse practitioners provide a direct point of entry to the health care system for case management, diagnosis, treatment, prevention and promotion, and, in some cases, palliative care (Canadian Nurses Association, 2009). It makes sense that the medical diagnosis of asthma be reflected in the nursing diagnoses, in view of the nurse's knowledge of the signs of asthma. In this book, common nursing diagnoses are presented along with medical diagnoses to illustrate common abnormalities. It is important to observe how these two types of diagnoses are interrelated.

With regard to Ellen's case, for example, the medical diagnosis is used to evaluate the cause of disease. The nursing diagnosis is used to evaluate the response of the whole person to actual or potential health problems. Note that the admitting nurse and later the physician auscultate Ellen's lung sounds and determine that they are diminished and that wheezing is present. This is both a medical problem and a nursing clinical problem. The physician or nurse practitioner listens to diagnose the cause of the abnormal sounds (in this case, asthma) and to order specific drug treatment. The nurse listens to detect abnormal sounds early, to monitor Ellen's response to treatment, and to initiate supportive measures and health education.

13. *Setting priorities* when a patient has more than one health or illness issue occurring concurrently (which is often the case). In the acute care hospital setting, the initial problems are usually related to the reason for admission. However, the acuity of illness, as well as the person's social and family context, often determines the order of priorities of the person's problems (Table 1-1).

For example, **first-level priority problems** are those that are emergencies, life-threatening, and immediate, such as establishing an airway or supporting breathing.

Second-level priority problems are those that are next in urgency: those necessitating your prompt intervention to forestall further deterioration, such as mental status change, acute pain, acute urinary elimination problems, untreated medical problems, abnormal laboratory values, risks of infection, or risk to safety or security. Ellen has abnormal physical signs that fit in the category of untreated medical problems. For example, Ellen's adventitious breath sounds are a cue to further assess respiratory status to determine the final diagnosis. Ellen's mildly elevated blood pressure also needs monitoring.

TABLE 1-1	**Identifying Immediate Priorities**

PRINCIPLES OF SETTING PRIORITIES

1. **Make a complete list of current medications, medical problems, allergies, and reasons for seeking care.** Refer to them frequently because they may affect how you set priorities.
2. **Determine the *relationships* among the problems:** If problem Y causes problem Z, problem Y takes priority over problem Z. **Example:** If pain is causing immobility, *pain management* is a high priority.

Setting priorities is a dynamic, changing process; at times, the order of priority changes, depending on the seriousness and relationship of the problems. **Example:** If abnormal laboratory values are at life-threatening levels, they become a higher priority; if the patient is having trouble breathing because of acute rib pain, managing the pain may be a higher priority than dealing with a rapid pulse (first-level priority, listed in the following section of this table).

STEPS TO SETTING PRIORITIES

1. Assign high priority to *first-level* priority problems (immediate priorities): Remember the "ABCs plus V":
   - **A**irway problems
   - **B**reathing problems
   - **C**ardiac/circulation problems
   - **V**ital sign concerns (e.g., high fever)

Exception: With cardiopulmonary resuscitation (CPR) for cardiac arrest, begin chest compressions immediately. Go online to *http://www.heartandstroke.com/site/c.iklQLcMWJtE/b.6301495/k.940B/CPRguidelines.htm* for the most current CPR guidelines.

2. Next, attend to *second-level* priority problems:
   - Mental status change (e.g., confusion, decreased alertness)
   - Untreated medical problems that necessitate immediate attention (e.g., for a diabetic patient who has not had insulin)
   - Acute pain
   - Acute urinary elimination problems
   - Abnormal laboratory values
   - Risks of infection, to safety, or to security (for the patient or for others)

3. Address *third-level* priority problems (later priorities):
   - Health problems that do not fit into the previous categories (e.g., problems with lack of knowledge, activity, rest, family coping)

Adapted from Alfaro-LeFevre, R. (2009). *Critical thinking and clinical judgment: A practical approach* (4th ed.). Philadelphia: W. B. Saunders.

Third-level priority problems are those that are important to the patient's health but can be addressed after more urgent health problems are addressed. In Ellen's case, the data indicating diagnoses of knowledge deficit, social isolation, risk for other-directed violence, and risk for situational low self-esteem fit in this category. Interventions to treat these problems are lengthier, and the response to treatment is expected to take more time.

Collaborative problems are those in which the approach to treatment involves multiple disciplines. Collaborative problems are certain physiological complications in which nurses have the primary responsibility to diagnose the onset and monitor the changes in status (Carpenito-Moyet, 2004). For example, the data regarding alcohol abuse represent a collaborative problem. With this problem, the sudden withdrawal of alcohol has profound implications on the central nervous and cardiovascular systems. Ellen's response to the rebound effects of these systems is managed.

14. *Identifying patient-centred expected outcomes.* What specific, measurable results that will show an improvement in the person's problem after treatment will you expect? The outcome statement should include a specific time frame. For example, before discharge from the emergency department, Ellen will identify a safety plan for dealing with interpersonal violence that fits with her life context.

15. *Determining specific interventions* that will achieve positive outcomes. These interventions aim to prevent, manage, or resolve health problems. They constitute the health care plan. For specific interventions, state who should perform the intervention, when and how often, and the method used.

16. *Evaluating and revising your thinking.* Observe the actual outcomes, and evaluate them in relation to the expected outcomes (do the stated outcomes match the individual's actual progress?). Then, analyze whether your interventions were successful or not. Continually think about what you could be doing differently or better.

17. *Determining a comprehensive plan* or evaluating and updating the plan. Record the revised plan of care and keep it up to date. The use of electronic health records is widespread in Canada; nurses play an important role in influencing the flow, use, and management of information. Communicate the plan to the multidisciplinary team. Be aware that the plan of care is a legal document, and accurate recording is important for accountability purposes, billing purposes, evaluation, and research.

EVIDENCE-INFORMED ASSESSMENT

Does honey help burn wounds heal more quickly? Is St. John's wort effective in relieving the symptoms of major depression? Does male circumcision reduce the risk of transmitting human immunodeficiency virus (HIV) in heterosexual men? Can magnesium sulphate reduce risk for cerebral palsy in premature infants? Can infusing hearts with stem cells help heal tissue damage after a heart attack?

Health care in Canada is increasingly shaped by corporatization, cost constraints, and cutbacks of community-based health and social services (Varcoe & Rodney, 2009). Lack of timely access to primary care services is linked to the increasingly acute conditions among hospitalized patients, many of whom are discharged earlier than traditionally and without adequate supports in their home or communities. Despite these realities, studies show that nurses and nursing continue to find ways of ensuring that patients are provided with high-quality clinical care (see, for example, Laschinger, Wong, Grau, Read, & Stam, 2011; Tourangeau et al., 2011; Tourangeau, Cranley, Laschinger, & Pachis, 2010).

All patients deserve to be treated with the most current best-practice techniques. It is this conviction that led to the development of **evidence-based practice** (EBP).* In 1972, a British epidemiologist and early proponent of EBP, Archie Cochrane, identified a pressing need for systematic reviews of randomized clinical trials. In a landmark case, Dr. Cochrane noted that multiple clinical trials published between 1972 and 1981 showed that the use of corticosteroids to treat women in premature labour reduced the incidence of infant mortality. A short course of corticosteroid stimulates fetal lung development, thus preventing respiratory distress syndrome, a serious and common complication of premature birth. However, these findings had not been implemented into daily practice, and thousands of premature infants of low birth weight were needlessly dying. After a systematic review of the evidence in 1989, obstetricians were finally aware that the corticosteroid treatment was effective. Corticosteroid treatment has since been shown to reduce the risk of infant mortality by 30% to 50% (Crowther, McKinlay, Middleton, & Harding, 2011).

The term **evidence-informed practice** (EIP) is increasingly used in the literature to encompass a more inclusive view of what "counts" as evidence than is conventionally implied when using the term evidence-based practice (Rycroft-Malone, 2008). While the literature on evidence-based practice recognizes the appropriateness of the randomized controlled trial for evidence of effectiveness of nursing and medical interventions, other forms of evidence also inform clinical decision making and the delivery of nursing care—hence the relevance of the term evidence-informed practice (Rycroft-Malone, 2008). EIP is more than the use of best-practice techniques to treat patients; it is "a systematic approach to practice that emphasizes the use of best evidence in combination with the clinician's experience, as well as the patient preferences and values, to make decisions about care and treatment" (Leufer, 2009; Figure 1-3). This definition is comprehensive and inclusive of the various factors and contexts that shape the delivery of nursing care. Note how clinical decision making depends on all four factors: the best and most appropriate evidence from a critical review of research literature; the patient's own context and preferences; the clinician's experience and expertise; and finally, physical examination and assessment. Assessment skills must be practised with hands-on experience and refined to a high level.

Although assessment skills are foundational to EIP, it is important to question tradition when no compelling research evidence exists to support it. Some time-honoured assessment techniques have been omitted from the examination repertoire because clinical evidence has shown them to be less than useful. For example, the traditional practice of auscultating bowel sounds was found not to be the best indicator of returning gastrointestinal motility in patients having abdominal surgery (Madsen, Sebolt, Cullen, Folkedahl, Mueller, Richardson, & Titler, 2005). Madsen and colleagues first reviewed earlier studies suggesting that early postoperative bowel sounds probably do not represent the return of normal gastrointestinal motility and that listening to the abdomen is therefore not useful in this situation. Research

---

*In this chapter, evidence-informed practice is used interchangeably with evidence-based practice.

In acute hospital care, the complete database also is compiled after the patient's admission to the hospital. In the hospital, data related specifically to disease may be collected by the admitting physician. You collect additional information about the patient's perception of illness, functional ability or patterns of living, activities of daily living, health maintenance behaviours, response to health problems, coping patterns, interaction patterns, and health goals. This information completes the database from which the nursing diagnoses can be made.

Episodic or Problem-Centred Database

The episodic database is for a limited or short-term problem. It is a "mini-database," smaller in scope and more focused than the complete database. It concerns mainly one problem, one cue complex, or one body system. It is used in all settings: hospital, primary care, or long-term care. For example, 2 days after surgery, a hospitalized person suddenly has a congested cough, shortness of breath, and fatigue. The history and examination focus primarily on the respiratory and cardiovascular systems. In another example, a person presents with a rash in an outpatient clinic. The history and examination follow the direction of this presenting concern, such as whether the rash had an acute or chronic onset, was associated with a fever, and was localized or generalized. Documentation of the history and examination must include a clear description of the rash.

Follow-Up Database

The status of any identified problems should be evaluated at regular and appropriate intervals. What change has occurred? Is the problem getting better or worse? What coping strategies are used? The follow-up database is used in all settings to monitor short-term or chronic health problems.

Emergency Database

The emergency database calls for a rapid collection of the data, often compiled while life-saving measures are occurring. Diagnosis must be swift and sure. For example, in a hospital emergency department, a person is brought in with suspected substance overdose. The first history questions are "What did you take?", "How much did you take?", and "When did you take it?" The person is questioned simultaneously while his or her airway, breathing, circulation, level of consciousness, and disability are being assessed. Clearly, the emergency database requires more rapid collection of data than does the episodic database.

FREQUENCY OF ASSESSMENT

The frequency of assessment varies with the person's age, gender, social context, and illness and wellness needs. Most ill people seek care because of pain or some abnormal signs and symptoms they have noticed. This prompts an assessment: gathering a complete, an episodic, or an emergency database.

For the well person, however, opinions are changing about assessment intervals. The term *annual checkup* is vague. What does it constitute? Is it necessary or cost effective? Does it

sometimes give an implicit promise of health and thus provide false security? What about the classic situation in which a person suffers a heart attack 2 weeks after a routine checkup that includes normal findings on an electrocardiogram? The timing of some formerly accepted recommendations have now changed; for example, the Papanicolaou (Pap) test for cervical cancer in women is no longer required annually depending on past test results and the woman's health history (Canadian Task Force on Preventive Health Care, 2013b). Screening guidelines for the use of mammography, breast self-exam, and clinical breast exam to screen for breast cancer have also recently changed, and recommendations vary significantly in different provinces (Canadian Task Force on Preventive Health Care, 2013c). The same annual routine physical examination cannot be recommended for all persons because health priorities vary among individuals, different age groups, and risk categories.

In Canada, there are various guidelines for disease prevention and health promotion. New national and provincial guidelines are developed regularly for particular populations; an example is the 2007 human papillomavirus (HPV) vaccine guidelines for adolescents (HPV Consensus Guidelines Committee, 2007). Many of these guidelines are outlined in Chapter 2.

National standards for **immunizations** are contained in the *Canadian Immunization Guide* (Public Health Agency of Canada, 2012). Each province and territory adapts these standards slightly according to its population's needs. In addition, there are ongoing updates posted by the National Advisory Committee on Immunizations (2012). It is important to check the provincial or territorial guidelines where you practise. **Periodic health examinations** are designed to prevent morbidity and mortality by identifying modifiable risk factors and early signs of treatable conditions (Milone & Lopes Milone, 2006). In 1980, the Canadian Task Force on the Periodic Health Examination produced its first evidence-informed clinical practice guidelines. The task force was renamed the *Canadian Task Force on Preventive Health Care* in 1984, and many of the guidelines were updated in 2006 and again in 2013 (Canadian Task Force on Preventive Health Care, 2013a).

Since 2006, the Public Health Agency of Canada (2011) has taken the lead in developing and distributing health promotion, disease prevention, and other guidelines for children, adults, pregnant women, and older adults. The Canadian Medical Association's (2012) *Clinical Practice Guidelines* are also updated regularly and include prevention, promotion, and treatment guidelines for use by nurses, nurse practitioners, and physicians.

For infants and children, clinical practice guidelines developed at the provincial and territorial level are accessible; these guidelines include the following:
- Developmental screening tools
- Schedules for periodic well-child assessments
- Health promotion, injury prevention, and disease prevention strategies for various age groups
- Depression screening tools for adolescents
- Strategies to promote healthy parenting
- Strategies to support psychosocial and emotional development in children

For example, the *Rourke Baby Record* (Rourke, Leduc, & Rourke, 2011) is an evidence-informed health maintenance and prevention guide that can be used by community health nurses, nurse practitioners, and physicians caring for children during the first 5 years of life. The Canadian Paediatric Society (2012) and the World Health Organization (2012) also have evidence-informed developmental and preventive screening guidelines.

The United States has taken a lead in developing evidence-informed guidelines for age-specific periodic health visits and preventive services in the *Guide to Clinical Preventive Services, Second Edition* (U.S. Preventive Services Task Force, 2006). Aspects of these guidelines can be adapted for use with Canadian populations; for example,

- Screening for major risk factors
- Age-specific and gender-specific items for physical examination and laboratory procedures
- Health promotion guidelines (however, nurses should follow the Canadian rather than the U.S. immunization schedule)
- Health education and counselling topics

Tables 1-2, 1-3, 1-4, and 1-5 contain examples of clinical preventive health care recommendations per age group, beginning with birth to 9 years of age. These recommendations are periodically updated, and they vary from one province or territory to another, as noted previously; however, these tables provide a good overview of preventive guidelines over the life span. Addressing health promotion in the context of health assessment is discussed in depth in Chapter 2.

ASSESSMENT THROUGHOUT THE LIFE CYCLE

It makes good sense to consider health assessment from a life cycle approach. First, you must be familiar with the usual and expected developmental tasks for each age group. This alerts you to which physical, psychosocial, cognitive, and behavioural tasks are currently important for each person. For example, an adult in Ellen K.'s age group has developmental tasks that include growing independent from the parents' home and care, establishing a career, forming an intimate bond with another person, making friends, and establishing a social group.

Next, once assessment skills are learned, they are more meaningful when considered from a developmental perspective. Your knowledge of communication skills and health history content is enhanced as you consider how they apply to individuals throughout the life cycle. The physical examination also is more relevant when you consider age-specific data about anatomy, the method of examination, normal findings, and abnormal findings. For example, an average normal blood pressure for a woman Ellen K.'s age is 116/70 mm Hg (see Figure 10-18 on p. 174).

For each age group, the approach to health assessment arises from an orientation toward wellness, quality of life, and health maintenance. The nurse learns to capitalize on the patient's strengths. What is the patient already doing that promotes health? What other areas are amenable to health teaching so that the patient can further build his or her potential for health?

CULTURAL AND SOCIAL CONSIDERATIONS

Cultural and social considerations are critical in health and physical assessments. An introduction to key concepts is provided in Chapter 3. These concepts are threaded throughout the text as they relate to specific chapters. Of importance is that a relational stance in your clinical practice will help you to attend to the varying contexts that shape people's health and well-being.

Canada's population, estimated at 35,002,447 in 2012, is very diverse (Statistics Canada, 2012). The Canadian population grew more rapidly between 2001 and 2006 than it did in the previous 5-year interval, and this acceleration was attributable primarily to an increase in international migration (Statistics Canada, 2007a, 2007b). During 2001 to 2006, it was estimated that just over 1 million people immigrated to Canada. Canada's Aboriginal population is also relatively large, accounting for almost 4% of the total population (Statistics Canada, 2008). Aboriginal people in Canada include the First Nations, Métis, and Inuit groups, which are recognized as three separate groups with unique histories, cultural backgrounds, and languages spoken.

A disturbing trend is the increasing divisions between people who are wealthy and those who are poor (Beiser & Stewart, 2005). At least 15% of Canadians live in impoverished circumstances, and these rates are dramatically higher for lone-mother families (51%; Raphael, 2007). Of concern is the fact that as poverty rates increase, health status declines (Raphael, 2010). Nurses and other health care providers therefore require the skills and knowledge to effectively—and respectfully—explore these interrelated biological, social, cultural, and economic factors.

TABLE 1-2	Clinical Preventive Health Care Recommendations: Birth to Age 9 Years

LEADING CAUSES OF DEATH (2004)[1]

Conditions originating in perinatal period
Congenital anomalies
Sudden infant death syndrome (SIDS)
Unintentional injuries
Cancer

Source of immunization schedule: Public Health Agency of Canada (2012).
[1]Data from Public Health Agency of Canada (2008). *Leading causes of death and hospitalization in Canada.* Retrieved from *http://www.phac-aspc.gc.ca/publicat/lcd-pcd97/.*

Continued

TABLE 1-2	Clinical Preventive Health Care Recommendations: Birth to Age 9 Years—cont'd

INTERVENTIONS FOR THE PEDIATRIC POPULATION[2]

Screening

Hip examination, serial (first year)
Eye examination (infants)
Hearing examination, serial (first year)
Vision screen (age 3 or 4 yr)
Serial height, weight, head circumference measurements (infants)
Phenylalanine level (birth)
Thyroid stimulating hormone (TSH) (at birth)

Counselling

Injury Prevention:

Child safety car seats (<5 yr)
Seatbelts (<5 yr)
Smoke detector, flame-retardant sleepwear
Set hot water heater temperature below 48.9 C (120 F)
Window and stair guards, pool fence
Poison control phone number (see Web site of the Canadian Association of Poison Control Centres: *http://www.capcc.ca/index.html*)

Diet and Exercise:

Breast milk, iron-enriched formula, and foods (infants and toddlers)
Regular exercise: 60 min of moderate physical activity (bike riding, skating) and 30 min of vigorous activity (running, basketball, soccer) per day[3]

Anticipatory Guidance:

Inquiries about developmental milestones
Night-time crying
Skin cancer:
- Sun exposure and protective clothing
Substance abuse:
- Effects of passive smoking
- Antismoking message
Dental health:
- Community fluoridation
- Regular visits to dental care provider
- Flossing, brushing with fluoride toothpaste daily

Immunizations (examples)[4]

Diphtheria–tetanus–acellular pertussis–inactivated poliovirus (DTaP-IPV)[5]
Haemophilus influenzae type b (Hib) conjugate[6]
Measles-mumps-rubella (MMR)[7]
Varicella (Var)[8]
Hepatitis B (HB)[9]
Pneumococcal conjugate (Pneu-C-7)[10]
Meningococcal C conjugate (Men-C)[11]
Influenza (Inf)[12]

Chemoprophylaxis

Ocular prophylaxis (birth)

[2]Review latest recommendations by the Canadian Task Force on Preventive Health Care (2013). *Guidelines.* Retrieved from *http://canadiantaskforce.ca/*.
[3]Data from Public Health Agency of Canada. (2011). *Canada's physical activity guides for children and youth.* Retrieved from *http://www.phac-aspc.gc.ca/pau-uap/paguide/child_youth/index.html.* Source of immunization schedule: Public Health Agency of Canada (2006, pp. 93-95).
[4]Based on the Canada National Advisory Committee on Immunization. (2006) *Canadian Immunization Guide 2006, Seventh Edition* (please note that the 2006 *Canadian Immunization Guide* is currently under review and being converted into an online version with chapters updated as needed (referred to as the Evergreen version). As chapter updates become available, they will be posted online at the following website: *http://www.phac-aspc.gc.ca/publicat/cig-gci/errarta-eng.php.* Be sure to consult more specific provincial and territorial guidelines in your local area.
[5]At ages 2, 4, 6, and 18 mo and 4–6 yr.
[6]At ages 2, 4, 6, and 18 mo.
[7]At ages 12 and 18 mo or 4–6 yr.
[8]At age 12 mo.
[9]Three doses in infancy or two or three doses in preteen or teen years.
[10]At ages 2, 4, 6, and 12–15 mo.
[11]Infancy: 2, 6, or 12 mo. At least one dose in primary infant series should be given after age 5 months. If the provincial policy is to give the vaccine at 12 months or older, then only one dose is required.
[12]One dose at age 6–23 months.

INTERVENTIONS FOR POPULATIONS AT HIGH RISK[2]

Population	Potential Interventions
First-time mothers of low socioeconomic status (SES); lone parents or teenage mothers at risk for child maltreatment	Home visitation by nurses during perinatal period through infancy
Children at high risk for dental caries	Fissure sealants
Infants at high risk for iron deficiency anemia	Routine hemoglobin testing
Children at high risk for exposure to lead	Blood lead screening
Recent immigrants from endemic areas; Canadian-born Aboriginal children; parental history of intravenous (IV) drug use, HIV-positive status, or alcohol abuse	Tuberculin (TB) skin test

---

TABLE 1-3   Clinical Preventive Health Care Recommendations: Ages 10 to 19 Years

LEADING CAUSES OF DEATH (2004)[1]

Unintentional injuries
Suicide
Cancer
Homicide
Nervous system diseases

INTERVENTIONS FOR THE PREADOLESCENT AND ADOLESCENT POPULATION[2]

Screening

Height, weight measurements
Blood pressure
Papanicolaou (Pap) test[3] (girls)
Assessment for problem drinking

Counselling

Injury Prevention:

Seatbelts
Avoidance of the combination of alcohol and drug use with activities such as driving, swimming, and boating
Smoke detector

Diet and Exercise:

Limiting fat and cholesterol; maintaining caloric balance; emphasizing grains, fruits, vegetables
Adequate calcium intake
Regular exercise: 60 min of moderate physical activity (bike riding, skating) and 30 min of vigorous activity (running, basketball, soccer) per day[4]
Skin cancer:
  • Limiting sun exposure and wearing protective clothing
Substance abuse:
  • Antismoking message
  • Avoidance of underage drinking and illicit drugs
Sexual behaviour:
  • STI prevention: avoiding high-risk behaviour; abstinence; using condoms and barrier with spermicide
  • Prevention of unintended pregnancy: using contraception
Dental health:
  • Regular visits to dental care provider
  • Flossing, brushing with fluoride toothpaste daily

Immunizations (examples)

Diphtheria–tetanus–acellular pertussis (Tdap)[5]

INTERVENTIONS FOR POPULATIONS AT HIGH RISK[2]

Population	Potential Interventions
Recent immigrants from endemic areas; Canadian-born Aboriginal children; parental history of IV drug use, HIV-positive status, or alcohol abuse	Tuberculin (TB) skin test

[1]Data from Public Health Agency of Canada. (2008). *Leading causes of death and hospitalization in Canada.* Retrieved from *http://www.phac-aspc.gc.ca/publicat/lcd-pcd97/.*

[2]Data from Canadian Task Force on Preventive Health Care. (2013). *Guidelines.* Retrieved from *http://canadiantaskforce.ca/.*

[3]Recommendations are presented for screening asymptomatic women who are or have been sexually active. They do not apply to women with symptoms of cervical cancer, previous abnormal screening results (until they have been cleared to resume normal screening), those who do not have a cervix (due to hysterectomy), or who are immunosuppressed (Canadian Task Force on Preventive Health Care, 2013b). For women aged <20 we recommend not routinely screening for cervical cancer. (Strong recommendation; high-quality evidence)

[4]Data from Public Health Agency of Canada (2011). Source of immunization schedule: Public Health Agency of Canada (2006, pp. 93-95).

[5]14–16 yr; "adult-like" preparation. Based on the Canada National Advisory Committee on Immunization. (2006) *Canadian Immunization Guide 2006, Seventh Edition* (Please note that the 2006 *Canadian Immunization Guide* is currently under review and being converted into an online version with chapters updated as needed. As chapter updates become available, they will be posted online at the following website: *http://www.phac-aspc.gc.ca/publicat/cig-gci/errarta-eng.php.* Be sure to consult more specific provincial and territorial guidelines in your local area.

TABLE 1-4   Clinical Preventive Health Care Recommendations: Ages 20 to 64 Years

LEADING CAUSES OF DEATH (2004)[1]

Ages 20–44
Unintentional injuries
Cancer
Suicide

Ages 45–64
Cancer
Circulatory system diseases
Endocrine, nutritional, and metabolic diseases

INTERVENTIONS FOR THE ADULT POPULATION[2]

Screening

Height, weight measurements
Blood pressure
Papanicolaou (Pap) test (women)[3]
Fecal occult blood test[4] (≥50 yr)
Mammography ± clinical breast examination[5]
Screening for depression[6]
Clinical and risk factor screening for osteoporosis (≥50 yr)[7]
Assessment for problem drinking

Counselling

Injury Prevention:

Seatbelts
Avoidance of the combination of alcohol and drug use with activities such as driving, swimming, and boating
Smoke detector

Diet and Exercise:

Limiting fat and cholesterol; maintaining caloric balance; emphasizing grains, fruits, vegetables
Adequate calcium intake
Regular physical activity

Sexual Behaviour:

STI prevention: avoidance of high-risk behaviour; use of condoms and barrier with spermicide
Prevention of unintended pregnancy: contraception

Skin Cancer:

Limiting sun exposure and wearing protective clothing

Substance Abuse:

Smoking cessation

Dental Health:

Regular visits to dental care provider
Flossing, brushing with fluoride toothpaste daily

[1]Data from Public Health Agency of Canada. (2008). *Leading causes of death and hospitalization in Canada.* Retrieved from *http://www.phac-aspc.gc.ca/publicat/lcd-pcd97/.*

[2]Data from Canadian Task Force on Preventive Health Care. (2013). *Guidelines.* Retrieved from *http://canadiantaskforce.ca/.*

[3]Recommendations are presented for screening asymptomatic women who are or have been sexually active. They do not apply to women with symptoms of cervical cancer, previous abnormal screening results (until they have been cleared to resume normal screening), those who do not have a cervix (due to hysterectomy), or who are immunosuppressed (Canadian Task Force on Preventive Health Care, 2013b).
- For women aged 20 to 24 we recommend not routinely screening for cervical cancer. (Weak recommendation; moderate-quality evidence)
- For women aged 25 to 29 we recommend routine screening for cervical cancer every 3 years. (Weak recommendation; moderate-quality evidence)
- For women aged 30 to 69 we recommend routine screening for cervical cancer every 3 years. (Strong recommendation; high-quality evidence)

[4]At least once every 2 years.

[5]Recommendations vary in different provinces: be sure to check your local guidelines. The following recommendations are presented for the use of mammography and clinical breast exam to screen for breast cancer (Canadian Task Force on Preventive Health Care, 2013c). These recommendations apply only to women at average risk of breast cancer aged 40 to 74 years. They do not apply to women at higher risk due to personal history of breast cancer, history of breast cancer in first degree relative, known BRCA1/BRCA2 mutation, or prior chest wall radiation. No recommendations are made for women aged 75 and older, given the lack of data.
- For women aged 40–49 we recommend not routinely screening with mammography. (Weak recommendation; moderate-quality evidence)
- For women aged 50–69 years we recommend routinely screening with mammography every 2 to 3 years. (Weak recommendation; moderate quality evidence)

They recommend not routinely performing clinical breast exam alone or in conjunction with mammography to screen for breast cancer. (Weak recommendation; low-quality evidence)

[6]The Canadian Task Force on Preventive Health Care concludes that there is fair evidence to recommend screening adults for depression in primary care settings since screening improves health outcomes when linked to effective follow-up and treatment (Canadian Task Force on Preventive Health Care, 2013e).

[7]The four key predictors of fracture related to osteoporosis are low bone mineral density (BMD), prior fragility fracture, age, and family history. BMD testing is appropriate for targeted case finding among people younger than 65 and for all women aged 65 and older.

TABLE 1-4	Clinical Preventive Health Care Recommendations: Ages 20 to 64 Years—cont'd

Immunizations (examples)

Diphtheria-tetanus (Td)[8]

Chemoprophylaxis

Multivitamin with folic acid (women planning or capable of pregnancy)
Calcium and vitamin D supplements (≥50 yr)

INTERVENTIONS FOR HIGH-RISK POPULATIONS[2]

Population	Potential Interventions
• Recent immigrants from endemic areas; Canadian-born Aboriginal children; parental history of IV drug use, HIV-positive status, or alcohol abuse	Tuberculin (TB) skin test
• Individuals at high risk for type 2 diabetes (e.g., hypertension, hyperlipidemia)	Fasting plasma glucose test

[8]Td booster every 10 years. Based on the Canada National Advisory Committee on Immunization. (2006) *Canadian Immunization Guide 2006, Seventh Edition* (Please note that the 2006 *Canadian Immunization Guide* is currently under review and being converted into an online version with chapters updated as needed. As chapter updates become available, they will be posted online at the following website: *http://www.phac-aspc.gc.ca/publicat/cig-gci/errarta-eng.php*. Be sure to consult more specific provincial and territorial guidelines in your local area.

TABLE 1-5	Clinical Preventive Health Care Recommendations: Ages 65 Years and Older

LEADING CAUSES OF DEATH (2004)[1]

Circulatory system diseases
Cancer
Respiratory system diseases
Nervous system diseases
Endocrine, nutritional, and metabolic diseases

INTERVENTIONS FOR THE LATE ADULT POPULATION[2]

Screening

Height, weight measurements
Blood pressure
Papanicolaou (Pap) test (women)[3]
Fecal occult blood test[4]
Mammography ± clinical breast examination[5]
Screening for depression[6]
Visual screening (Snellen sight card)
Hearing screening
Fall prevention (postfall multidisciplinary team assessment)
Bone mineral density (BMD)[7]
Assessment for problem drinking

[1]Data from Public Health Agency of Canada. (2008). *Leading causes of death and hospitalization in Canada.* Retrieved from *http://www.phac-aspc.gc.ca/publicat/lcd-pcd97/.*

[2]Data from Canadian Task Force on Preventive Health Care. (2013). *Guidelines.* Retrieved from *http://canadiantaskforce.ca/.*

[3]Recommendations are presented for screening asymptomatic women who are or have been sexually active. They do not apply to women with symptoms of cervical cancer, previous abnormal screening results (until they have been cleared to resume normal screening), those who do not have a cervix (due to hysterectomy), or who are immunosuppressed (Canadian Task Force on Preventive Health Care, 2013b). For women aged ≥70 who have been adequately screened (i.e., 3 successive negative Pap tests in the last 10 years), we recommend that routine screening may cease. For women aged 70 or over who have not been adequately screened, we recommend continued screening until 3 negative test results have been obtained. (Weak recommendation; low-quality evidence)

[4]At least once every 2 years.

[5]Recommendations vary in different provinces: be sure to check your local guidelines. The following recommendations are presented for the use of mammography and clinical breast exam by the Canadian Task Force on Preventive Health Care (2013c). These recommendations apply only to women at average risk of breast cancer aged 40 to 74 years. They do not apply to women at higher risk due to personal history of breast cancer, history of breast cancer in first-degree relative, known BRCA1/BRCA2 mutation, or prior chest wall radiation. No recommendations are made for women aged 75 and older, given the lack of data.

• For women aged 50–69 years, we recommend routinely screening with mammography every 2 to 3 years. (Weak recommendation; moderate-quality evidence)

• For women aged 70–74, we recommend routinely screening with mammography every 2 to 3 years. (Weak recommendation; low-quality evidence) They recommend not routinely performing clinical breast exam alone or in conjunction with mammography to screen for breast cancer. (Weak recommendation; low-quality evidence)

[6]The Canadian Task Force on Preventive Health Care concludes that there is fair evidence to recommend screening adults for depression in primary care settings since screening improves health outcomes when linked to effective follow-up and treatment (Canadian Task Force on Preventive Health Care (2013e).

[7]The four key predictors of fracture related to osteoporosis are low BMD, prior fragility fracture, age, and family history. BMD testing is appropriate for targeted case-finding among people younger than 65 and for all women aged 65 and older.

Continued

TABLE 1-5	Clinical Preventive Health Care Recommendations: Ages 65 Years and Older—cont'd

Counselling

Injury Prevention:

Seatbelts
Avoidance of the combination of alcohol and drug use with activities such as driving, swimming, and boating
Smoke detector

Diet and Exercise:

Limiting fat and cholesterol; maintaining caloric balance; emphasizing grains, fruits, vegetables
Adequate calcium intake
Regular physical activity

Sexual Behaviour:

STI prevention: avoidance of high-risk behaviour; use of condoms

Skin Cancer:

Limiting sun exposure and wearing protective clothing

Substance Abuse:

Smoking cessation

Dental Health:

Regular visits to dental care provider
Flossing, brushing with fluoride toothpaste daily

Immunizations (examples)

Diphtheria-tetanus (Td)[8]
Influenza[9]
Pneumococcal vaccine[10]

Chemoprophylaxis

Calcium and vitamin D supplements[11]

INTERVENTIONS FOR HIGH-RISK POPULATIONS[2]

Population	Potential Interventions
Informants or caregivers describe cognitive decline of individual or corroborate self-reported memory complaint	Cognitive assessment and careful follow-up required
Vascular risk factors for dementia (elevated systolic blood pressure, hyperlipidemia)[12]	Management of hypertension; physical exercise
Individuals at high risk for type 2 diabetes (e.g., hypertension, hyperlipidemia)	Fasting plasma glucose test
Recent immigrants from endemic areas; Canadian-born Aboriginal children; parental history of IV drug use, HIV-positive status, or alcohol abuse	Tuberculin (TB) skin test

[8]Td booster every 10 years. Based on the Canada National Advisory Committee on Immunization. (2006) *Canadian Immunization Guide 2006, Seventh Edition* (Please note that the 2006 *Canadian Immunization Guide* is currently under review and being converted into an online version with chapters updated as needed. As chapter updates become available, they will be posted online at the following website: *http://www.phac-aspc.gc.ca/publicat/cig-gci/errarta-eng.php*. Be sure to consult more specific provincial and territorial guidelines in your local area.
[9]Annually.
[10]Given once after age 65.
[11]For women without documented osteoporosis, there is fair evidence that calcium and vitamin D supplementation alone prevents osteoporotic fractures (grade B recommendation). Canadian Task Force on Preventive Health Care. (2013d).

REFERENCES

Alfaro-LeFevre, R. (2009). *Critical thinking and clinical judgment: A practical approach* (4th ed.). Philadelphia: W. B. Saunders.

American Nurses Association. (2004). *Nursing scope and standards of performance and standards of clinical practice*. Washington, DC: American Nurses Publishing.

Baumbusch, J., Reimer Kirkham, S., Khan, K. B., McDonald, H., Semeniuk, P., & Anderson, J. (2008). Pursuing common agendas: A collaborative model for knowledge translation in clinical settings. *Research in Nursing & Health, 31*, 130–140.

Beiser, M., & Stewart, M. (2005). Reducing health disparities: A priority for Canada. *Canadian Journal of Public Health, 96*(2), 4–5.

Benner, P. (2001). *From novice to expert: Excellence and power in clinical nursing practice*. Upper Saddle River, NJ: Prentice Hall.

Canadian Medical Association. (2012). *Clinical practice guidelines*. Retrieved from *http://www.cma.ca/cpgs*.

Canadian Nurses Association. (2005). *Social determinants of health and nursing: A summary of the issues*. Ottawa, ON: Author.

Canadian Nurses Association. (2009). *Position statement: The nurse practitioner*. Ottawa: Author. Retrieved from *http://www. cna-aiic.ca/CNA/documents/pdf/publications/PS_Nurse_ Practitioner_e.pdf*.

Canadian Nurses Association. (2010). *Canadian Registered Nurse examination: Competencies*. Retrieved from *http://www. cna-aiic.ca/CNA/nursing/rnexam/competencies/default_e.aspx*.

Canadian Paediatric Society. (2012). *News and publications*. Retrieved from *http://www.cps.ca/english/index.htm*.

Canadian Task Force on Preventive Health Care. (2013a). *All guidelines*. Retrieved from *http://canadiantaskforce.ca/guidelines/ all-guidelines/*.

Canadian Task Force on Preventive Health Care. (2013b). Screening for cervical cancer. *Canadian Medical Association Journal*, *185*(1), 35–45.

Canadian Task Force on Preventive Health Care. (2013c). *Screening for breast cancer*. Retrieved from *http:// canadiantaskforce.ca/guidelines/2011-breast-cancer/*.

Canadian Task Force on Preventive Health Care. (2013d). *Prevention of osteoporosis and osteoporotic fractures in postmenopausal women*. Retrieved from *http:// canadiantaskforce.ca/guidelines/all-guidelines/2002-prevention- of-osteoporosis-and-osteoporotic-fractures-in-postmenopausal- women/*.

Canadian Task Force on Preventive Health Care. (2013e). *Screening for depression in primary care*. Retrieved from *http:// canadiantaskforce.ca/guidelines/all-guidelines/2005-screening- for-depression-in-primary-care/*.

Carpenito-Moyet, L. (2004). *Nursing diagnosis: Application to clinical practice* (10th ed.). Philadelphia: Lippincott Williams & Wilkins.

Crowther, C., McKinlay, C., Middleton, P., & Harding, J. (2011). Repeat doses of prenatal corticosteroids for women at risk of preterm birth for improving neonatal health outcomes. *Cochrane Database of Systematic Reviews*, (6), doi: 10.1002/14651858.CD003935.pub3

Dains, J. E., Ciofu Baumann, L., & Scheibel, P. (2012). *Advanced health assessment and clinical diagnosis in primary care* (4th ed.). St. Louis: Elsevier Mosby.

DiCenso, A., Guyatt, G., & Ciliska, D. (2005). *Evidence-based nursing: A guide to clinical practice*. St. Louis: Mosby.

Doane, G. H., & Varcoe, C. (2005). *Family nursing as relational inquiry: Developing health-promoting practice*. Philadelphia: Lippincott Williams & Wilkins.

Estabrooks, C. A., Squires, J. E., Strandberg, E., Nilsson-Kajermo, K., Scott, S. D., …, Wallin, L. (2011). Towards better measures of research utilization: A collaborative study in Canada and Sweden. *Journal of Advanced Nursing*, *67*(8), 1705–1718. doi:10.1111/j.1365–2648.2011.05610.x

Hanneman, S. K. (1996). Advancing nursing practice with a unit-based clinical expert. *Image*, *28*, 331–337.

HPV Consensus Guidelines Committee. (2007). Canadian consensus guidelines on human papillomavirus. *Journal of Obstetrics and Gynaecology Canada*, *29*(8, Suppl. 3).

Laschinger, H. K. S., Wong, C., Grau, A., Read, E., & Stam, L. (2011). The influence of leadership practices and empowerment on Canadian nurse managers. *Journal of Nursing Management*, *20*(7), 877–888.

Leufer, T. C. (2009). Evidence-based practice: Improving patient outcomes. *Nursing Standard*, *23*(32), 35–39.

Madsen, D., Sebolt, T., Cullen, L., Folkedahl, B., Mueller, T., Richardson, C., & Titler, M. (2005). Listening to bowel sounds: An evidence-based practice project: Nurses find that a traditional practice isn't the best indicator of returning gastrointestinal motility in patients who've undergone abdominal surgery. *American Journal of Nursing*, *105*(12), 40–50.

Milone, D., & Lopes Milone, S. (2006). Evidence-based periodic health examination of adults: Memory aid for primary care physicians. *Canadian Family Physician*, *52*(1), 40–47.

National Advisory Committee on Immunization (NACI) (2013). *About NACI*. Retrieved from *http://www.phac-aspc.gc.ca/ naci-ccni/*.

Public Health Agency of Canada. (2006). *Canadian immunization guide* (7th ed.). Public Health Agency of Canada: Ottawa.

Public Health Agency of Canada. (2011). *Health promotion*. Retrieved from *http://www.phac-aspc.gc.ca/hp-ps/index-eng.php*.

Public Health Agency of Canada. (2012). *Canadian immunization guide* (Evergreen edition). Retrieved from *http://www. phac-aspc.gc.ca/publicat/cig-gci/index-eng.php*.

Raphael, D. (2007). *Poverty and policy in Canada: Implications for health and quality of life*. Toronto: Canadian Scholars' Press.

Raphael, D. (Ed.) (2009). *Social determinants of health: Canadian perspectives* (2nd ed.). Toronto: Canadian Scholars' Press.

Raphael, D. (Ed.) (2010). *Health promotion and quality of life in Canada: Essential readings*. Toronto: Canadian Scholars' Press.

Rourke, L., Leduc, D., & Rourke, J. (2011). *Rourke baby record: Evidence-based infant/child health maintenance record*. Retrieved from *http://www.rourkebabyrecord.ca/pdf/ RBR2011Nat_Eng.pdf*.

Rycroft-Malone, J. (2008). Evidence-informed practice: From individual to context. *Journal of Nursing Management*, *16*(4, Special Issue), 404–408.

Statistics Canada. (2007a). *Immigration in Canada: A portrait of the foreign-born population, 2006 census*. Ottawa: Author. Retrieved from *http://www.statcan.ca/bsolc/english/ bsolc?catno=97-557-XIE2006001#formatdisp*.

Statistics Canada. (2007b). *Portrait of the Canadian population in 2006. Population and dwelling counts*. Ottawa: Author. Retrieved from *http://www12.statcan.ca/english/census06/analysis/ popdwell/index.cfm*.

Statistics Canada. (2008). *Aboriginal peoples in Canada in 2006: Inuit, Métis and First Nations, 2006 census*. Ottawa: Author. Retrieved from *http://www12.statcan.ca/english/census06/ analysis/aboriginal/pdf/97-558-XIE2006001.pdf*.

Statistics Canada. (2012). *Quarterly Population Estimates, Canada, Provinces and Territories, 1971 to 2012*. Ottawa: Statistics Canada. Retrieved from *http://www.stats.gov.nl.ca/statistics/ population/pdf/quarterly_pop_prov.pdf*.

Thorne, S. (2006). Theoretical foundations of nursing. In P. Potter, A. G. Perry, J. Ross-Kerr, & M. Wood (Eds.), *Canadian fundamentals of nursing* (3rd ed., pp. 67–79). Toronto: Elsevier Canada.

Tourangeau, A. E. (2011). Mortality rate as a nursing sensitive outcome. In D. Doran (Ed.), *Nursing sensitive outcomes: State of the science* (2nd ed.), (pp. 409–437). Sudbury, MA: Jones & Bartlett.

Tourangeau, A. E., Cranley, L., Laschinger, H. S., & Pachis, J. (2010). Relationships among leadership practices, work environments, staff communication and outcomes in long-term care. *Journal of Nursing Management*, *18*, 1060–1072.

U.S. Preventive Services Task Force. (2006). *Guide to clinical preventive services*. Baltimore: Williams & Wilkins.

Varcoe, C., & Rodney, P. (2009). Constrained agency: The social structure of nurses' work. In S. Bolaria & H. D. Dickinson (Eds.), *Health, illness, and health care in Canada* (4th ed., pp. 122–151). Toronto: Nelson Education Ltd.

World Health Organization. (1986). *Ottawa charter for health promotion*. Retrieved from *http://www.who.int/healthpromotion/ conferences/previous/ottawa/en/*.

World Health Organization. (2012). *The WHO child growth standards*. Retrieved from *http://www.who.int/childgrowth/en/*.

2

Health Promotion in the Context of Health Assessment

Written by Dana S. Edge, PhD, RN

⊖volve WEBSITE

http://evolve.elsevier.com/Canada/Jarvis/examination/
- Appendices
- Examination Review Questions
- Key Points

OUTLINE

Changes in the conceptualization about the meaning of health began with the World Health Organization's (1946) declaration that health is "not merely the absence of disease." Since that time, the definition of health has transformed from being a two-dimensional concept to one that accounts for the importance of the environment, both physical and social, in defining health. It is not enough simply to have access to good health care services. In this chapter, you are introduced to the role that Canada has played in health promotion, the foundational concepts of disease prevention and health promotion, and how nurses assess health-promoting behaviours in clinical settings.

HEALTH PROMOTION: DEVELOPMENT AND CONCEPT

Prevalent patterns of disease and mortality in North America changed from infectious diseases in the early 1900s to chronic conditions by the late 1950s. Sanitation improvements and the discovery of penicillin played a role in this shift. Many individuals were spared contracting potentially fatal cases of polio, diphtheria, and pertussis with the development of vaccines in the 1940s and early 1950s. Sanitation and immunization are examples of **primary prevention,** whereby people and populations are prevented from becoming ill, sick, or injured in the first place (Figure 2-1).

Primary prevention was first discussed by American academics Hugh R. Leavell and Edwin G. Clark in the 1940s; they further described **secondary prevention** as early detection of

disease, before symptoms emerge, and **tertiary prevention** as the prevention of complications when a condition or disease is present or has progressed (Cohen, Chávez, & Chehimi, 2010). Screening tests, such as mammography, lipid profiles, and the Papanicolaou (Pap) test, are examples of secondary prevention. As you teach a patient with newly diagnosed diabetes how to care for his or her feet, you are engaging in tertiary prevention activities designed to help the patient avoid complications of diabetes, such as a diabetic ulcer or infection. Box 2-1 illustrates the levels of prevention for tobacco-related illnesses.

Nurses' ability to understand the natural history of a particular disease, to know the patterns of disease occurrence, and to detect a condition early all factor into how they intervene to prevent disease. Prevention strategies are not static; as the understanding about a condition evolves, so do the prevention and treatment approaches. For example, before

---

BOX 2-1 PREVENTION OF THE DAMAGING EFFECTS OF TOBACCO

Primary: Teaching a group of third-grade students about the harmful effects of tobacco use.
Secondary: Providing tobacco cessation strategies to a current smoker who has expressed an interest in attempting to quit or cut down.
Tertiary: Limiting second-hand smoke exposure to a patient with chronic obstructive lung disease.

1982, peptic ulcer disease was attributed to oversecretion of gastric acid, and stress was considered to be a major contributor to the excess acid. Treatment with antacids and, in severe cases, surgery was the norm. The discovery that a bacterium, *Helicobacter pylori*, was responsible for the development of peptic ulcers totally shifted the management and prevention of the condition, including nurses' approach to health teaching (Lynch, n.d.).

Despite medical breakthroughs and advances in technology, curative approaches to health have limits (Illich, 1976;

Raphael, 2009). The 1974 *Lalonde Report* highlighted the limitations of the health care system to Canadians and to the international community. The traditional approach to health shifted from biomedical responses to the influences of lifestyle, human biology, and the environment with this development (Lalonde, 1974; MacDonald, 2002). The report laid the foundation for future health promotion initiatives in Canada. The *Declaration of Alma Ata* reinforced health promotion principles in 1978, which heralded a shift in power from health care providers to consumers of health care and their communities (Catford, 2004). **Health promotion** as defined by the *Ottawa Charter for Health Promotion* (World Health Organization, 1986, p. 1) is "the process of enabling people to increase control over, and to improve their health" (Figure 2-2).

How broad is this view of environmental and biological influences? The **social determinants of health** as outlined by the Public Health Agency of Canada (PHAC) include the following elements: the socioeconomic environment; the physical environment; healthy childhood development; personal health practices; individual capacity and coping skills; biology and genetics; health services; gender; and culture (PHAC, 2012). The socioeconomic environment, in particular, has a profound influence on individuals' health. Income, social status, social support networks, education, employment, and social environments are components of the socioeconomic environment. Five principles underpin health

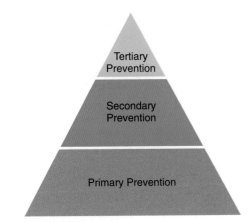

2-1 Levels of health promotion.

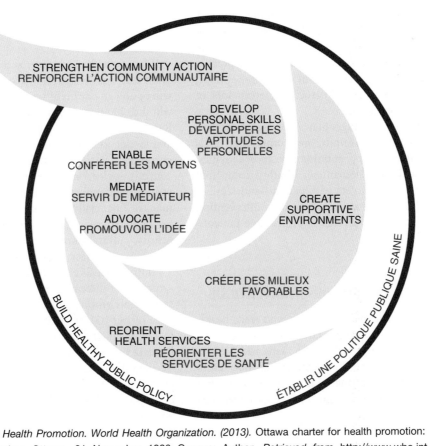

2-2 The *Ottawa Charter for Health Promotion. World Health Organization. (2013).* Ottawa charter for health promotion: First International Conference on Health Promotion, Ottawa, 21 November 1986 Geneva: Author. *Retrieved from* http://www.who.int/healthpromotion/conferences/previous/ottawa/en/.

promotion activities. According to Catford (2004), these activities

- Involve the population as a whole in the context of their everyday lives
- Are directed toward action on the social determinants of health
- Combine diverse but complementary methods
- Aim at effective and concrete public participation
- Are nurtured and enabled by health professionals, particularly in primary health care

Certain populations in Canada are at increased risk for disease and disability as a result of the growing social inequities. As discussed in Chapter 3, First Nations and Inuit peoples also have shorter life expectancy, higher infant mortality rates, and higher rates of morbidity from infectious diseases, such as tuberculosis, than do the rest of Canadians (Health Council of Canada, 2005). Temporary worker immigration has increased in Canada since 2007, and concerns have been raised about the working conditions of these immigrants (Canadian Food and Commercial Workers Union, 2011). Questionable working conditions, inadequate housing, and vulnerability affect their ability to work and, ultimately, their health (Preibisch & Hennebry, 2011). These health indicators can be linked directly to social and economic conditions such as overcrowding, low income, and lack of access to nutritious foods, particularly for those living on reserve or in remote locations. Health promotion forces nurses to focus upstream* to the root causes of health conditions; health care providers alone cannot tackle many of the barriers to adequate health in populations. Instead, public policy must promote sustainable employment, sound education, food security, environmental protection, political stability, and affordable health care; enacting such policies necessitates that multiple players, including the public, understand the importance of the social determinants of health and act to improve them.

However, health care providers play a pivotal role in promoting health at individual, family, and community levels through counselling, screening, and immunization activities. Inquiry into the social determinants of health is completed during health history encounters with patients and families (Table 2-1). Health education is one specific intervention strategy that is employed by all nurses to promote patients' health.

SPECIFIC HEALTH PROMOTION INTERVENTIONS

Consider Randy, a 45-year-old single man who seeks health care for recurrent early morning insomnia. During your interview with him, Randy reports that he falls asleep easily at night but awakens around 3:00 A.M. and spends hours unable to fall back asleep, sitting in front of the television in his armchair. As the interview proceeds, Randy indicates

---

*Taking action to avoid a problem before it occurs is referred to as "moving upstream" and is the hallmark of primary prevention (Cohen, Chávez, & Chehimi, 2010, p. 5).

TABLE 2-1	Social Determinants of Health and the Health History
Social Determinants of Health	**Corresponding Components of the Health History***
Socioeconomic environment • Income • Social status • Social support network • Education • Employment • Social environments	Biographical data; functional assessment (interpersonal relationships; social and economic contexts; spiritual resources)
Physical environment	Functional assessment (environmental hazards; occupational health)
Healthy childhood development	Developmental history
Personal health practices	Health promotion and harm reduction approaches
Individual capacity and coping skills	Functional assessment (self-concept; coping and stress management)
Biology and genetics	Family history
Health services	Most recent examination (medical, dental, immunizations)
Gender	Biographical data
Culture and social considerations	Biographical data; perception of health

*Chapter 5 in this book.

that he was a chief engineer at a major automobile assembly plant but was "let go" 4 weeks ago; he is not sure how he will be able to pay his bills or his mortgage. His aging parents, who live in another province, are not aware of his situation. Randy reveals that he has lost 5 kg during the past month and is not interested much in eating. At this point in the encounter, you have information about his presenting concern, socioeconomic status, and his coping skills. At this visit, more detail about his social supports and how he can manage financially is required. Future visits could explore his physical environment, personal health practices, family history, cultural and social contexts, and use of preventive health care services.

Your diagnosis and intervention about Randy's presenting symptom of insomnia are affected by the knowledge that the suicide rate among Canadians is highest between ages 45 and 54 (17.9 per 100,000; PHAC, 2008). Randy is experiencing the loss of a valued occupational role and social isolation, which increase the risk for self-harm. Your interventions today focus on identifying any deviations from health in your physical examination that could explain the insomnia, screening for depression and suicidal ideation (see Chapter 6), and working with Randy on a plan to support him during this period of upheaval in his life. The approach used with Randy is illustrative of a counselling intervention to achieve healthy behaviours and promote overall health. Depending on Randy's responses, screening for suicidal ideation may be required (see Chapter 6). From the previous description, several domains of the social determinants of health have been assessed in this one encounter between you and Randy.

COUNSELLING ACTIVITIES IN HEALTH PROMOTION

Injury prevention, diet, exercise, sexual health, substance use, dental health, anticipatory guidance, and primary prevention of specific cancers are all important topics to be discussed with patients during health encounters. The counselling intervention will be informed by the developmental level and the cultural, social, and economic context of the individual (and the family); the readiness of the person to engage in discussions related to health information; availability of local resources; and the prevalent health conditions for which the individual may be at risk. For example, men younger than 20 are at risk for injuries during recreational and organized sports activities (PHAC, 2010); during a health care visit by a young man, you are provided with the opportunity to learn the man's interests, his health-protective behaviours (e.g., protective gear), and his beliefs about vulnerability, and you can tailor your health messages accordingly.

SCREENING

Early detection of a condition or disease is possible when a sensitive and effective tool for detection is available; when the natural history of the condition has a long latency period before symptoms appear; and when an acceptable treatment method is available (Fletcher & Fletcher, 2005). Some malignancies are amenable to early detection, including cervical, breast, colon, skin, and prostate tumours. Nurses can also screen to identify individuals at risk for falls, depression, visual acuity loss, problematic alcohol or substance use, and hearing loss. Screening is based on the prevalence of the disease in the population; therefore, routine screening is reasonable when the prevalence is relatively high in a specific age group, gender, or ethnic population. The natural history of disease, the pattern of the disease in the population, and other epidemiological indicators, in addition to the individual's risk profile, provide the evidence to support the decision of whether to screen.

IMMUNIZATIONS

Active immunization through the use of either vaccines or toxoid preparations elicits immunological self-response within the host body that provides protection at a later exposure date. The measles-mumps-rubella (MMR) immunization is an example of a vaccine, whereas protection against diphtheria and tetanus is provided through the administration of a toxoid (McDonnell & Askari, 1997; Moss & Griffin, 2012; PHAC, 2012). In some instances, antibodies are administered in the form of immune globulin to people who have already been exposed to a disease; this action

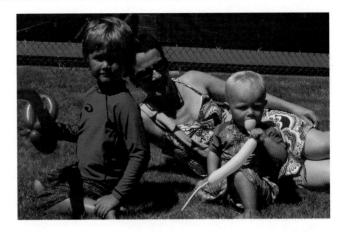

is known as *passive immunization,* and the effects are shortlived. As mentioned previously, immunization is a primary prevention activity. Opportunities to check immunization status with patients occur with nearly every health encounter, and yet it is an opportunity frequently missed in many health care settings (Turner, Grant, Goodyear-Smith, & Pertousis-Harris, 2009).

TOOLS TO ASSESS DEVELOPMENTAL TASKS

Before its revision in 1989, public health nurses in Canada used the Denver Developmental Screening Test (DDST), a professionally administered test, extensively. By the early 1990s, however, the Canadian Task Force on Preventive Health Care (2013) had reported insufficient evidence for the routine developmental screening of children. Because of the lack of evidence of effectiveness, as well as funding cuts in public health, the routine use of the DDST ceased. In its place, several provincial programs now use the Nipissing District Developmental Screen (NDDS), a parent-report screening tool (Figure 2-3).

The NDDS originated in 1993 from the work of a multidisciplinary committee of health professionals within the Nipissing District of Ontario; by 1997, the screen was being used across Canada, and since that time, the tool has been revised and analyzed for cultural sensitivity, grade 5 literacy level, and reliability. Currently, Ontario, New Brunswick, and the Northwest Territories have endorsed the NDDS as the screening tool of choice in provincial programs (see the Web Sites of Interest at the end of this chapter), and the forms are free of charge to Ontario residents. Translated versions in French, Spanish, and Vietnamese are available, and the tool can be accessed electronically, with interactive screens. The NDDS elicits a "yes" or "no" response from parents for a set of developmental milestones appropriate to the age of the child; a "no" response highlights a potential developmental delay. Other available parent-report developmental screening tools that were developed in North America include the Ages and Stages Questionnaires (ASQ), the Child Development Inventory (CDI), and the Parents' Evaluation of Developmental Status (PEDS). Weighing the evolving discoveries in neuroscience and the effects of environment on early childhood development, the Canadian Paediatric Society endorsed the systematic use of a developmental screening tool (e.g., NDDS, ASQ, PEDS) at each 18-month well-baby visit (Williams, Clinton, & Canadian Paediatric Society, Early Years Task Force, 2011). An overview of developmental tasks for each age group can be found on the Evolve Web site.

USE OF A HEALTH PROMOTION MODEL IN NURSING ASSESSMENT

In the early 1980s, Nola Pender first described the Health Promotion Model, which used a competence, or strength-based, approach to describe motivation for behaviour change, rather than threats (Pender, Murdaugh, & Parsons, 2006). The

---

Nipissing District Developmental Screen™

Child's Name _____

Birth Date _____   Today's Date _____

The Nipissing, Nipissing District Developmental Screen, and NDDS are trademarks of NDDS Intellectual Property Association, used under license. All rights reserved.

The Nipissing District Developmental Screen™ is a checklist designed to help monitor your child's development.

✔ Yes   ✔ No   *By **Two Years** of age, does your child...*

1. Usually have healthy ears and seem to hear well?
2. Point to at least two familiar objects when asked (e.g. car, bowl)?
3. Ask for help using words or actions?
4. Learn and use one or more new words a week (may only be understood by family)?
5. Join two words together like "want cookie", "more milk", "my hat"?
6. Eat most foods without coughing and choking?
7. Eat with a utensil with little spilling?*
8. Take off own shoes, socks or hat?*
9. Try to run?
10. Play in a squat position? (Picture A)
11. Walk backwards or sideways pulling a toy?
12. Make scribbles and dots on paper or in sand?
13. Put objects into a small container? (Picture B)
14. Like to watch and play near other children?
15. Say "no", and like to do some things without help?*
16. Recognize the use of familiar objects (e.g. drink from cup, hug doll)?
17. Use skills already learned and develop new ones (i.e. no loss of skills)?
18. Copy your actions (i.e. you clap your hands and he/she claps hands)?

* item may not be common to all cultures

2 YEARS Always talk to your health care or child care professional if you have any questions about your child's development or well being. See reverse side for instructions, limitation of liability, and product license.

2-3 Nipissing District Developmental Screen.

ACTIVITIES FOR YOUR CHILD...

♡ Emotional 🖐 Fine Muscle ⚡ Large Muscle 🔤 Learning/Thinking
🧦 Self-Help 👥 Social 👄 Speech/Language

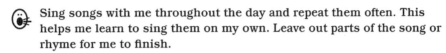
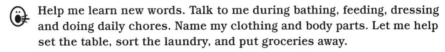

Nipissing District
Developmental Screen™

The following activities will help you play your part in your child's development.

👄 Sing songs with me throughout the day and repeat them often. This helps me learn to sing them on my own. Leave out parts of the song or rhyme for me to finish.

👄 Help me learn new words. Talk to me during bathing, feeding, dressing and doing daily chores. Name my clothing and body parts. Let me help set the table, sort the laundry, and put groceries away.

👥 Let's play a game. Use two shoeboxes and two toys. We each get a box and a toy. Let's take turns putting our toy in the box, over, under, behind, and on. Talk to me about what we are doing.

⚡ Provide me with toys that allow me to push or pedal with my feet. This will help me learn to climb on and off and to pedal. Make sure I have lots of room. Praise my efforts.

⚡ Let's practice climbing and jumping. I love to get in and out of a box or jump from a bottom step. We can have fun together.

⚡ Let's sing Old MacDonald and move our bodies like the animals: hop like a frog or bunny, squat or waddle like a duck or jump up and down like a kangaroo; etc.

🔤 I like to play sorting games with you. We can sort objects by shape, touch, colour, and size. Use spoons, blocks, toys, and clothing.

🖐 Let me open and close plastic containers by twisting and turning the lids. Help me find the right lid to put on each container.

🖐 I love to pour water from containers during my bath.

🖐 I enjoy stringing beads or buttons on a shoelace, string or pipe cleaner. Talk to me about the colour and count the beads as I lace them. Remember, I may still put things in my mouth – so watch me.

🧦 I want to become independent. Encourage me to get dressed and undressed, do household tasks, turn lights on and off, and open and close doors.

♡ I am learning about my feelings. Give me words for my feelings and show that you understand.

👥 I love sharing storybooks with you. Cuddle me while we read together.

I am learning to make decisions. Offer me simple choices throughout the day. For example, "Do you want juice or milk?"

2 YEARS

Always talk to your health care or child care professional if you have any questions about your child's development or well being. See reverse side for instructions, limitation of liability, and product license.

2-3 cont'd.

---

model, which was designed to be holistic, incorporated elements from social cognitive theory and expectancy-value theory. The 1996 revised version of the Health Promotion Model identifies interrelated elements of individual characteristics and expectations that influence behaviour-specific cognitions and affect, which then drive the individual's commitment to a plan of action and the desired behavioural outcomes (Figure 2-4). Although this model is widely used, it has limitations: Its individualistic orientation draws attention away from the social, economic, and political factors that influence people's abilities to engage in health promotion activities. However, Pender's model is useful for identifying a range of health promotion interventions that can be considered during health assessments.

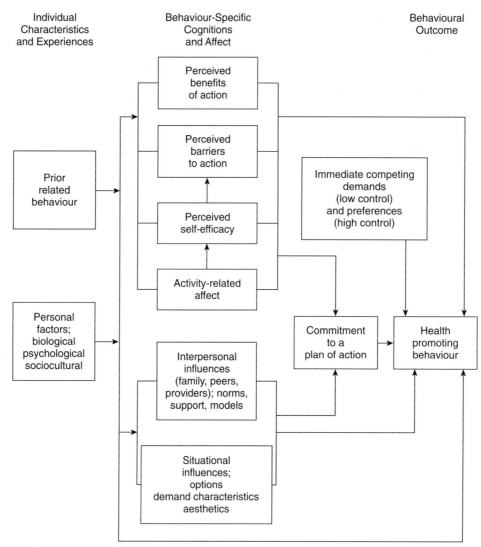

2-4   Pender's Health Promotion Model.

Pender and colleagues (2006) described six interventions for assisting patients with behaviour change, a process that involves time and frequently multiple attempts. These interventions are (a) raising consciousness by providing health information; (b) helping patients re-evaluate their actions; (c) giving positive feedback about efforts to promote self-efficacy; (d) enhancing the benefits of change by supporting patients' efforts; (e) shifting the environment when possible to support change efforts; and (f) assisting patients to think through ways of addressing the barriers to change. Pender's Health Promotion Model can serve as a guide in assessment during a patient encounter and can assist in planning health promotion interventions. Solid assessments lead to effective health promotion strategies when (a) they are systematic and thorough; (b) they involve the use of a strength-based approach; (c) developmental levels are considered; d) the patient's and family's cultural and social context are taken into account; and (e) the patient is involved in decision making and care is patient-centred.

HEALTH PROMOTION: CASE EXAMPLE

Mary is a 72-year-old Cree woman who is living with five members of her extended family in a three-bedroom bungalow on reserve. For the past 10 years, Mary has been living with type 2 diabetes and has been seen by health care professionals on a regular basis. Over the past 6 months, her glucose levels have not been at target, despite the adjustment of her oral hypoglycemic agent. She has come today to clinic because she just does not feel "right." You check her glucose level and find that it is moderately elevated. What information do you need to gather to properly care for Mary? What else might be happening in her environment that might be contributing to her diabetes being out of control? How will you determine the focus of your health education message?

You need to begin by reviewing with Mary what her typical day has been like over the past 6 months, particularly with regard to her diet, medication, and exercise patterns. Mary's understanding of the disease process, her social support, factors potentially impeding her ability to walk in the community (as her form of exercise), plus your understanding of local food availability, all contribute to a better understanding of the situational influences affecting Mary. You can pose to Mary several questions: "You told me that you don't feel 'right.' Can you describe what you mean by 'not right'?" "You've been told you have diabetes, Mary. Tell me what diabetes means to you." "How do the diabetes pills make you feel? Any problems with taking them?" "Mary, tell me about what you ate yesterday. Today?" "How often are you able to eat traditional food?" "Mary, who prepares the meals in your home?" "What do you think may be wrong, Mary?" Inquiry into Mary's daily activities and any recent departures from her routines, along with her beliefs about what might be causing her to feel "not right," can provide immeasurable insights into her beliefs and behaviours. These assessment data are critical for beginning a plan with Mary to develop health promotion strategies that are acceptable to her.

SUMMARY

Individuals and their families reside in communities that are part of a much larger sociopolitical environment. As you focus on caring for an individual, you must remain mindful of the larger context and engage in upstream thinking to more fully understand the person's particular situation. Health care providers frequently undervalue the influence of a well-placed question or comment to a patient. Even short health assessment encounters offer the opportunity to inquire about health-promoting behaviours within the context of the visit (e.g., asking about bicycle helmet use during an assessment of a minor sports-related injury). The key is to attend to what is being said and not said, to appreciate the environmental context, and to demonstrate genuine respect. The effect of the social determinants of health on an individual's health status cannot be underestimated, and the opportunities to promote health are endless.

REFERENCES

Canadian Food and Commercial Workers Union. (2011). *Report on the status of migrant workers in Canada, 2011.* Retrieved from *http://www.ufcw.ca/templates/ufcwcanada/images/Report-on-The-Status-of-Migrant-Workers-in-Canada-2011.pdf.*

Catford, J. (2004). Health promotion's record card: How principled are we 20 years on? *Health Promotion International, 19*(1), 1–4.

Cohen, L., Chávez, V., & Chehimi, S. (Eds). (2010). *Prevention is primary: Strategies for community well-being* (2nd ed.). San Francisco: Jossey-Bass.

Fletcher, R. H., & Fletcher, S. W. (2005). *Clinical epidemiology: The essentials* (4th ed.). Philadelphia: Lippincott Williams & Wilkins.

Health Council of Canada. (2005, January). *The health status of Canada's First Nations, Métis and Inuit peoples. A background paper to accompany Health Care Renewal in Canada: Accelerating Change.* Toronto: Author.

Illich, I. (1976). *Limits to medicine. Medical nemesis: The expropriation of health.* New York: Penguin Books.

Lalonde, M. (1974, April). *A new perspective on the health of Canadians.* Ottawa: Minister of Supply and Services Canada.

Lynch, N. A. (n.d.). *Helicobacter pylori and ulcers: A paradigm revised. Breakthroughs in Bioscience.* Bethesda, MD: Federation of American Societies for Experimental Biology. Retrieved from *http://www.faseb.org/portals/0/pdfs/opa/pylori.pdf.*

MacDonald, M. (2002). Health promotion: Historical, philosophical and theoretical perspectives. In L. E. Young & V. Hayes (Eds.), *Transforming health promotion practice: Concepts, issues and applications* (pp. 22–45). Philadelphia: F. A. Davis.

McDonnell, W. M., & Askari, F. K. (1997). Immunization. *JAMA, 278*(22), 2000–2007.

Moss, W. J., & Griffin, D. E. (2012). Measles. *The Lancet, 379,* 153–164. doi:10.1016/S0140-6736(10)62352-5

Pender, N., Murdaugh, C. L., & Parsons, M. A. (2006). *Health promotion in nursing practice* (5th ed.). Upper Saddle River, NJ: Pearson, Prentice Hall.

Preibisch, K., & Hennebry, J. (2011). Temporary migration, chronic effects: The health of international migrant workers in Canada. *Canadian Medical Association Journal, 183*(9), 1033–1038.

Public Health Agency of Canada. (2012). *Canadian immunization guide* (Evergreen edition). Retrieved from *http://www.phac-aspc.gc.ca/publicat/cig-gci/index-eng.php.*

Public Health Agency of Canada. (2008). *Leading causes of death and hospitalization in Canada, 2005, males and females combined: Counts [Table 1].* Retrieved from *http://phac-aspc.gc.ca/publicat/lcd-pcd97/table1-eng.php.*

Public Health Agency of Canada. (2010). *Data sampler: Injuries associated with sport & recreation.* Ottawa: Author. Retrieved from *http://www.phac-aspc.gc.ca/injury-bles/chirpp/injrep-rapbles/pdf/sports_rec_e.pdf.*

Public Health Agency of Canada. (2012). *Key element 2: Address the determinants of health and their interactions.* Retrieved from *http://cbpp-pcpe.phac-aspc.gc.ca/population_health/key_element_2-eng.html.*

Raphael, D. (2009). Poverty, human development, and health in Canada: Research, practice, and advocacy dilemmas. *Canadian Journal of Nursing Research, 41*(2), 7–18.

Turner, N., Grant, C., Goodyear-Smith, F., & Pertousis-Harris, H. (2009). Seize the moment: Missed opportunities to immunize at the family practice level. *Family Practice, 26*(4), 275–278.

Williams, R., Clinton, J., & Canadian Paediatric Society, Early Years Task Force. (2011). Getting it right at 18 months: In support of an enhanced well-baby visit. *Paediatrics & Child Health, 16*(10), 647–650. Retrieved from *http://www.cps.ca/english/statements/ECD/ECD11-01.htm.*

World Health Organization. (1986). *Ottawa charter for health promotion: First International Conference on Health Promotion, Ottawa, 21 November 1986* Geneva: Author. Retrieved from *http://www.who.int/healthpromotion/conferences/previous/ottawa/en/.*

World Health Organization. (1946). *Preamble to the Constitution of the World Health Organization as adopted by the International Health Conference, New York, 19-22 June, 1946; signed on 22 July 1946 by the representatives of 61 States (Official Records of the World Health Organization, no. 2, p. 100) and entered into force on 7 April 1948.* Retrieved from *http://www.who.int/kobe_centre/about/faq/en/.*

Web Sites of Interest

Canadian Best Practices Portal, Public Health Agency of Canada: *http://cbpp-pcpe.phac-aspc.gc.ca/.*

Canadian Consortium for Health Promotion Research: *http://www.utoronto.ca/chp/CCHPR/introe.htm.*

Canadian Stroke Network, Heart & Stroke Foundation: Canadian Best Practices for Stroke Care: *http://www.strokebestpractices.ca/index.php/managing-stroke-care-transitions-new-for-2010/patient-and-family-education/*.

Canadian Task Force on Preventive Health Care. (2013a). *History*. Retrieved from *http://canadiantaskforce.ca/about-us/history/*.

Canadian Women's Health Network. About us: *http://www.cwhn.ca/*.

College of Family Physicians of Canada—Resources for Patients: *http://www.cfpc.ca/ForPatients/*.

Government of Nunavut: *http://www.gov.nu.ca/en/Home.aspx*.

Health Closer to Home: *http://www.gov.nu.ca/files/Health%20Closer%20to%20Home.pdf*.

Health Canada: *First Nations and Inuit Health: http://www.hc-sc.gc.ca/fniah-spnia/index-eng.php*.

Mayo Clinical: *Mayo Clinic Health Assessment: Overview: http://www.mayoclinichealthsolutions.com/products/Health-Assessment.cfm*.

Nipissing District Developmental Screen (NDDS): *http://www.ndds.ca/usa/*.

Nutrition North Canada: *http://www.nutritionnorthcanada.ca/index-eng.asp*.

Physical Activity Line: *Health Promotion Activties http://www.physicalactivityline.com/index.php?option=com_content&view=article&id=62:health-promotion-strategies-&catid=51:getting-started-and-staying-motivated&Itemid=66*.

Registered Nurses Association of Ontario (RNAO). (2008). *Best practices toolkit. Implementing and sustaining change in long-term care: http://ltctoolkit.rnao.ca/*.

RNAO. (2004). *Clinical Practice Guidelines: Reducing foot complications with people with diabetes: http://www.rnao.org/Page.asp?PageID=924&ContentID=815*.

RNAO. (2008). *Clinical Practice Guidelines. Oral health: Nursing assessment and interventions: http://www.rnao.org/Page.asp?PageID=122&ContentID=1567*.

RNAO. (2010). *Clinical Practice Guidelines. Enhancing healthy adolescent development: http://www.rnao.org/Page.asp?PageID=924&ContentID=800*.

Tools for Community Action, U.S. Centers for Disease Control and Prevention (CDC) Healthy Communities Program: *http://www.cdc.gov/healthycommunitiesprogram/tools/#ag*.

Cultural and Social Considerations in Health Assessment

Written by Annette J. Browne, PhD, RN, and Colleen Varcoe, PhD, RN

Evolve WEBSITE

http://evolve.elsevier.com/Canada/Jarvis/examination/
• Examination Review Questions
• Key Points

• Quick Assessment for Common Conditions:
  • Sickle Cell Anemia

OUTLINE

Who is the person you are meeting for the first time? Where does he or she come from? What is the person's heritage? What is the person's cultural, social, and family background—his or her ethnicity and religion? Does the person understand, speak, and read English or French? What language does the person understand, speak, and read? What are the person's health* and illness beliefs and practices? Operating from a relational† standpoint, you would also want to ask yourself, "Who am I? Where do I come from? What is my social, cultural, or family background? What is my heritage, ethnicity, and religion? What is my primary language? Do I understand, speak, and read a language other than English? What are my health and illness beliefs and practices?"

A relational approach to health assessment prompts you to ask, "How do my social, cultural, and professional backgrounds shape my ability to relate to, and my assumptions about, the various people I encounter in my practice?"

Approaching cultural and social considerations in health assessment from a relational stance helps you understand and attend to the contexts that shape patterns of health and illness. These contexts include people's past experiences, culture, heritage, socioeconomic status, and history and their understanding of health, illness, and pathways to healing. By recognizing and attending to these contexts, you will be optimally prepared to conduct accurate health assessments and respond meaningfully to people's health, illness, and health promotion needs.

Over the course of your professional education, you will study the developmental tasks and the principles of health promotion across the life span and learn to conduct numerous assessments, such as documentation of a complete health history, a mental health assessment, an assessment of risks for violence, a nutritional assessment, a pain assessment, and a physical examination of a patient. As a health care provider, you will continually experience similarities and differences between you and the people and families with whom you come in contact. These differences are based on a wide range of factors: life experiences, opportunities and circumstances, and the linguistic, social, and cultural traditions of all persons, including you. A relational approach is aimed at making similarities and differences more transparent to us so that we can be as responsive as possible to people's varying needs.

The purposes of this chapter are as follows:
1. To describe concepts that are central to understanding cultural and social considerations in health assessment
2. To distinguish between cultural sensitivity and cultural safety

---

*The World Health Organization (2012) defines health as "a state of complete physical, mental and social well-being and not merely the absence of disease or infirmity."

†As introduced in Chapter 1, a "relational" approach refers to more than interpersonal relationships among people (Doane & Varcoe, 2005). According to a relational approach, health, illness, and the meanings they hold for people are shaped by gender, age, ability, and social, cultural, family, historical, and geographical contexts. Similarly, these contexts influence how nurses and other health care providers view, relate, and work with patients and families. Nurses and other health care providers therefore must remain critically attuned to the significance of these contexts during the process of health assessment.

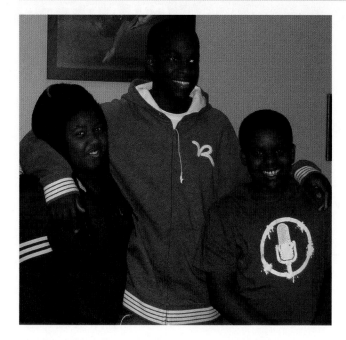

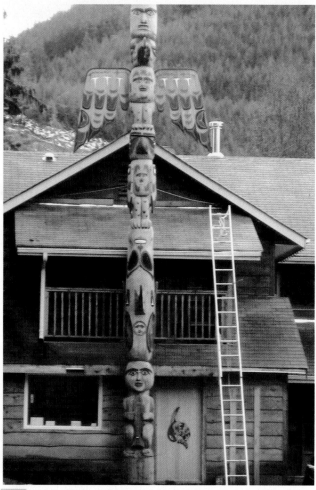

3. To review demographic trends within the Canadian population
4. To provide examples of ethnocultural diversity within the Canadian population
5. To review trends in health, social, and gender inequities in Canada
6. To identify guidelines for assessing culturally based understandings and the social and economic contexts that shape people's lives

As you encounter the various questions we pose in this chapter, take a few minutes to reflect on the thoughts and feelings that may arise.

CULTURAL AND SOCIAL CONSIDERATIONS: CENTRAL CONCEPTS

Culture and Culturalism

No single definition of **culture** exists, and all too often, definitions tend to be so general that they lack any real meaning or erase the complexity and shifting nature of culture. Culture is not something that is external to people; it is a universal phenomenon that shapes the health and well-being of every person. An individual person's cultural orientation, however, develops in distinctive and specific ways depending on where he or she lives (Figure 3-1), family background, socioeconomic circumstances, languages spoken, spiritual orientation, ancestry, and history as an individual and as a member of specific groups. Within any given group, people have varying health practices, differing levels of knowledge about health-related issues, and diverse family norms.

In disciplines such as anthropology, culture is understood as an inherently complex dimension of people's lives. In health care, however, culture tends to be viewed in very narrow and prescriptive terms, as the values, beliefs, and customs and practices characteristic of particular

3-1 What aspects of culture do you see in this picture? Do you tend to think of the Aboriginal carvings as "cultural" and overlook the ways in which the house's architecture, the logging slash behind the house, and the various items (ladder, chimney) also reflect culture?

ethnocultural group members (Figure 3-2). These assumed "cultural traits" are typically those identified as different from "ours," the unspoken comparison being made with the assumed dominant norm. In this narrow view, people tend to equate culture with ideas about ethnicity or "race," overlooking most sociocultural aspects relevant to health.

Because health care in Canada and the United States has drawn so heavily on narrowly defined ideas about culture, there has been a proliferation of textbooks in nursing and medicine that provide health care providers with systematized descriptions or lists of cultural characteristics for various groups. Although these culturally based characteristics are applicable to some people, they most certainly do not apply to all members of a group. For example, Chinese or Iranian communities in Canada are extremely diverse. There is no "recipe" or predefined approach for a Canadian-born person to follow in interacting with people who have recently immigrated from China or Iran. Furthermore, there are often significant differences between generations, including differences after migration. Regardless of country of birth, language, or religion, people have diverse points of view,

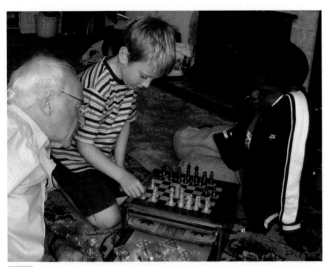

3-2 What definition of "culture" comes to your mind when looking at this picture?

educational levels, economic levels, and religions (Behjati-Sabet & Chambers, 2005; Yue, 2005). The dangers of applying lists of cultural traits to patients whom you encounter lies in drawing on stereotypes and making assumptions about particular people, which, in turn, lead to unsafe health assessment practices. Health care providers must therefore find ways of learning about all their patients, and their contexts, to understand how best to address their health needs (Gustafson, 2008).

This process of conceptualizing culture in fairly narrow terms, or assuming that people act in particular ways because of their culture, is known as **culturalism.** From a culturalist perspective, culture, in the narrow sense, is often given as the primary explanation for why certain people or populations experience various health, social, or economic problems. For example, research has shown that health care providers frequently attribute people's social problems to their cultural characteristics (Anderson et al., 2003; Browne, 2005, 2007; Varcoe, 2008). This would lead them to wrongly assume that violence toward women may be acceptable in particular cultural groups or that some people are more prone to using drugs or alcohol because of "their culture." Similarly, you cannot make accurate assumptions about people's health beliefs on the basis of their ethnicity; for example, it would be wrong to assume that people from China necessarily embrace the hot–cold theory of health and illness (an explanatory model in which the treatment of illness requires cold, heat, dryness, or wetness to restore balance). Such assumptions are culturalist because they are based on (a) popularized (and often stereotypical) ideas about culture as something fixed and inherent to particular groups defined by language, country of origin, or physical characteristics and (b) the notion that culture is the primary explanation for people's health-related practices or decisions. Of most importance is that such assumptions do not lead to useful information.

To counter this tendency toward culturalism in health care, it can be useful to define culture from a **critical cultural perspective** (Browne & Varcoe, 2006; Browne, McDonald, &

Elliott, 2009). According to a critical cultural perspective, culture is a relational aspect of individuals that shifts and changes over time, depending on an individual's history, social context, past experiences, gender, professional identity, and so on. As Anderson and Reimer-Kirkham (1999, p. 63) explain,

> [Culture] is located in a constantly shifting network of meanings enmeshed within historical, social, economic and political relationships and processes. It is not therefore reduced to an easily identifiable set of characteristics, nor is it a politically neutral concept.

Viewing culture in this way does not imply that health care providers should not pay attention to patient's values, beliefs, and practices. From a critical perspective of culture, these are viewed as highly significant: not as determining factors in people's lives but as intersecting with broader social determinants of health. For example, rather than viewing people's diet (or other health-related practices) as determined by their "culture," a critical cultural perspective is that what people eat is equally influenced by their income, access to food resources, ability to afford fresh fruits and vegetables, geographical location, and educational levels. In many rural or remote communities, high-carbohydrate fast foods or drinks are often less expensive than milk, fresh fruits, and fresh vegetables. This explains why people in these communities can have difficulties purchasing fresh foods that would be beneficial to, for example, those with diabetes or heart disease. It also explains, in part, why rates of type 2 diabetes are high in some Aboriginal communities, where access to traditional foods (e.g., berries, fish, game) has been denied by policies (e.g., the reserve system and land appropriation) and environmental damage (e.g., collapse of fisheries). Similarly, people who immigrate to Canada may have difficulty accessing the ingredients with which they are familiar and therefore turn to less healthy, prepackaged foods. Thus when a nurse documents a health history, understanding whether a person or family can afford healthy food choices is as important as understanding their culturally based preferences for particular foods.

Just as each individual has a particular cultural orientation, health care has a particular culture. For example, Western-educated health care providers tend to attribute illness to individual behaviours or factors, such as bacteria and viruses, poor lifestyle practices, or failure to exercise (Waxler-Morrison & Anderson, 2005). They also tend to view the individual as responsible for getting well and to value "adherence" to medical recommendations, such as technical diagnostic procedures, medications, and surgeries. However, the extent to which patients and their family members ascribe to the values of the **dominant health care culture** varies greatly. For some patients, the Western-style approach to history-taking (asking questions in quick succession) is not part of their pattern of communication. For some, taking a prescribed medication requires consultations with other members of the family. If you are alert to and respectful of the wide variety of health care practices and understandings about health, you will more easily find a mutually acceptable way to address people's concerns. This requires you to remain critically reflective about how you may be conveying the dominant culture of health care in ways that can make patients feel uncomfortable or hesitant to share their perspectives.

Culture, Ethnicity, and "Race"

Culture is often wrongly equated with ethnicity, and because ethnicity is often based on ideas about "race," culture is also often confused with "race." **Ethnicity** is a complex concept that often implies geographical and national affiliation. An **ethnic group** is a group or "community maintained by a shared heritage, culture, language or religion" (Henry, Tator, Mattis, & Rees, 2005, p. 350).

However, ethnicity is an ambiguous concept because it can encompass multiple different aspects such as "race," origin or ancestry, identity, language, and religion. Statistics Canada (2006) noted that ethnicity is dynamic and in a constant state of flux, changing as a result of new immigration flows and the development of new identities. In the context of health assessment, it is important to remember that people's ethnic identities depend on how they perceive themselves. In some contexts, people may choose to report that they are, for example, Iranian, Greek, Sri Lankan, Latino, Canadian, or Jewish. In other situations, they may feel that if they reveal their ethnicity to the health care providers or the admissions clerk, they may be treated differently on the basis of assumptions about them.

In health care and other sectors of Canadian society, the concept of ethnicity is often used as a substitute for the idea of "race." **"Race"** is defined as follows (Henry et al., 2005, p. 351):

> *A socially constructed category used to classify humankind according to common ancestry and reliant on differentiation by such physical characteristics as colour of skin, hair texture, stature and facial characteristics. The concept of race has no basis in biological reality and, as such, has no meaning independent of its social definitions.*

Although the United Nations Educational, Scientific and Cultural Organization (UNESCO) released its first statement on "race" in 1952, dismissing it as a biological category (UNESCO, 1952) and continuing to do so as recently as 1997, and despite the ongoing scientific evidence that dispels the existence of "races," the tendency in nursing, medicine, and health care is to continue to confuse "race" with genetic characteristics.

All people, regardless of the colour of their skin or other physical appearances, are a mixture of populations (Henry et al., 2005). As stated in the 1952 UNESCO declaration, "biological differences between human beings within a single [so called] 'race' may be as great as, or greater than, the same biological differences between races" (p. 15). Although skin colour, eye shape, and hair texture are genetically determined and reflect heredity and ancestry, those features do not signify any meaningful biological groupings. Rather, "race," like ethnicity, is a way of categorizing people socially.

In the United States, the terms *race* and *ethnicity* are often used interchangeably to categorize people as, for example,

"Black," "White," "Hispanic," or "Asian." These categories signal social classifications rather than genetically linked groups of people. Although "race" is not a biological entity, the social dynamics that occur in societies because of racialization (for example, discrimination against people with dark skin or against those who are thought to be descended from people with dark skin) have a profound effect on patterns of health and illness. The health effects of these social dynamics can be profound. For example, research has demonstrated that the increased incidence of high blood pressure experienced among African Americans in the United States, when socioeconomic and other factors are controlled, is attributable to experiences of discrimination (Krieger, 2011). In Canada, people from Nova Scotia who are descended from African ancestors have been shown to have a higher incidence of circulatory disease, diabetes, and mental health problems, that cannot be explained by socioeconomic characteristics or distance to a hospital (Kisely, Terashima, & Langille, 2008), which suggests that psychosocial stress and discrimination may explain the differences. The prevalence of certain diseases, such as hypertension, diabetes, and circulatory disease, can be higher in particular population groups and can vary according to genetic, biological, and family history; however, those factors intersect in significant ways with social factors, such as socioeconomic characteristics, gender roles, and exposure to stressful experiences, including discrimination.

Racialization continues to affect people in many ways: in health care and in the wider social world. **Racialization** is "a process by which ethno-racial groups are categorized, stigmatized, inferiorized, and marginalized as the 'others'" (Henry et al., 2005, p. 352). Racialization may be conscious and deliberate (an act of racism in which discrimination is overt) or unconscious and unintended. It exerts its power through everyday actions and attitudes and from institutionalized policies and practices that marginalize individuals and groups on the basis of presumed biological, physical, or genetic differences. For example, in our research, we have observed situations in which health care providers have erroneously assumed that alcoholism is "genetic" among Aboriginal people, which leads them to presume that an Aboriginal patient exhibiting bizarre behaviour is drunk when, in fact, the patient is experiencing cerebral bleeding, severe dehydration, a seizure disorder, or ataxia as a side effect of prescription medication.

Racialization is closely linked to culturalism and **discrimination,** the denial of equitable treatment and opportunities to individuals or groups with regard to education, accommodation, health care, employment, services, goods, and facilities (Henry et al., 2005, p. 349). Of significance in the General Social Survey of 2009 was that 50.2% of women and 49.3% of men aged 15 years and older and who were part of a "visible minority" reported that they had experienced discrimination or unfair treatment at work or when applying for a job or promotion in the previous 5 years (Chui & Maheux, 2011). The *Employment Equity Act* defines **visible minorities** as "persons, other than Aboriginal peoples, who are non-Caucasian in race or non-white in colour." Such persons belong to a visible minority group, and the *Employment*

Equity Act defines the various visible minority groups (Statistics Canada, 2011a). According to Statistics Canada, "the visible minority population consists mainly of the following groups: Chinese, South Asian, Black, Arab, West Asian, Filipino, Southeast Asian, Latin American, Japanese, and Korean" Using the term *visible minority* is a classification of people by skin colour or other physical characteristics and, as such, is a racializing process. As a health care provider, you need to think critically about these processes and examine the categories and assumptions that you may be using (sometimes unconsciously) in relation to particular patients and families (Browne, Varcoe, Wong, Smye, & Khan, in press; Varcoe, Browne, Wong, & Smye, 2009). In health assessments, it is usually not necessary to ask people to identify their ethnicity. Rather, focusing on an individual's particular understandings, explanations, values, and practices related to health and illness will help you obtain information relevant to health and avoid making assumptions—in other words, provide culturally safe care.

CULTURAL SENSITIVITY, CULTURAL COMPETENCE, AND CULTURAL SAFETY

Health care providers are increasingly called on to provide culturally sensitive health care services. **Cultural sensitivity** reflects the idea that health care providers should be aware of and accommodate people's values, beliefs, customs, and practices. Being culturally sensitive can be useful if it is done in a way that does not demean people or their differences from the dominant norm. However, a critical cultural perspective emphasizes that health care providers must go beyond being passively sensitive to examine how values, beliefs, customs, and practices intersect with broader social determinants and the power relations that shape health and health care (Figure 3-3). The Canadian Nurses Association (CNA) (CNA, 2010) "believes that cultural competence is an entry-to-practice level competence for registered nurses" (p. 1) and defines **cultural competence** as "the application of knowledge, skills, attitudes or personal attributes required by nurses to maximize respectful relationships with diverse populations of clients and co-workers" (p. 1). The CNA also recognizes "that cultural issues are intertwined with socioeconomic and

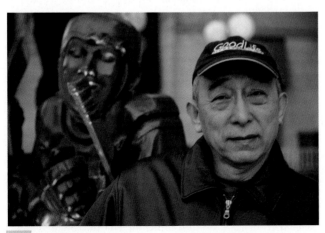

3-3 How can you counter your own assumptions?

political issues," and the organization "is committed to social justice as central to the social mandate of nursing" (p. 1). Similarly, Srivastava (2007) used the idea of cultural competence to draw attention to power relations and to consider culture in ways that directly address issues of racism and inequity. Regardless of the terminology used or the school of thought, you cannot develop knowledge about cultural and social considerations through quick one-lesson programs or brief "cross-cultural training" alone. Rather, you must develop knowledge in several areas, such as the following:

1. Your own personal ethnocultural and social background
2. The culture of nursing and related professions
3. The culture of the health care system
4. The significance of social, economic, and cultural contexts
5. Your ability to critically examine your assumptions about each of these areas.

The idea of *cultural safety* is a form of cultural competence that assists you in obtaining knowledge in these areas.

Cultural Safety

The concept of cultural safety emerged in the nursing literature in the 1990s in New Zealand as a concept that was developed by Maori nurse leaders and educators who were concerned by the persistent health and health care inequities affecting Maori people (the indigenous people of New Zealand) (Papps & Ramsden, 1996; Ramsden, 1993, 2002; Wepa, 2005). The CNA (2010) recognizes **cultural safety** "as both a process and an outcome whose goal is to promote greater equity" (p. 1) by focusing on the root causes of "power imbalances and inequitable social relationships in health care" (p. 168). Cultural safety is increasingly being incorporated in nursing, medicine, and other health care disciplines to provide care that takes into account the social, economic, political, and historical contexts of people's lives and how those contexts affect their health and health care experiences (Anderson et al., 2003; Association of Faculties of Medicine of Canada, 2007; Browne, Varcoe, et al., 2009; CNA, 2010; Smye, Rameka, & Willis, 2006). In the practice of cultural safety, health care providers acknowledge that culturally based meanings and practices must be respected; however, health care providers are also directed to change the culture of health care, especially the practices and policies that perpetuate culturalism, racialization, and inequities.

Some of the main principles of cultural safety are as follows:

- The cultural, social, economic, and historical positioning of people intersect to shape their health status and access to health care.
- Individual and institutional discrimination, culturalism, and racialization create risks for patients, particularly when people from a particular group perceive they are "demeaned, diminished or disempowered by the actions and delivery systems" of providers within the health care system (Ramsden & Spoonley, 1994, p. 164).
- How members of a group are treated and perceived within the health care system is more important than the

As you approach a new patient who is different from you in terms of appearance, age, skin colour, clothing, socio-economic status, accent, or primary language spoken, take the time to ask yourself the following questions:
- What biases, assumptions, or stereotypes are influencing my verbal and nonverbal behaviours and decisions?
- What am I paying attention to, and how is that causing me to overlook certain things?
- How does the work environment (e.g., norms, colleagues, workload) contribute to, or challenge, the formation of these stereotypes and assumptions?

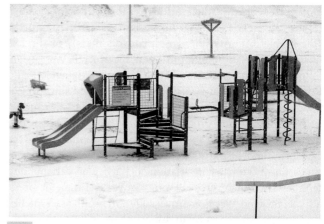

3-4 How does our geography shape health?

cataloguing of culturally specific beliefs or practices (Polaschek, 1998).
- Nurses and other health care providers must reflect on their own personal and cultural histories, and the values, beliefs, and assumptions that they bring to health care encounters and must avoid uncritically imposing their understandings, assumptions, or beliefs on others (Anderson et al., 2003).

Because relational approaches are concerned with relationships among providers and patients within particular historical, economic, social, and cultural contexts, relational approaches are integral to cultural safety (Box 3-1).

DEMOGRAPHIC PROFILE OF CANADA

As of January 1, 2012, Canada's population was estimated at 35,002,447 (Statistics Canada, 2012d). Canada's population is diverse in terms of where people live, languages spoken, age distributions, and ethnocultural identities. Although the majority of the population is Canadian born, the Canadian population is increasing primarily as a result of international migration. Of significance is the fact that 70% of people who immigrated to Canada in 2013 reported a mother tongue* other than English or French (Statistics Canada, 2012).

Canada's two official languages, English and French, are entrenched in the country's history, which confers rights and institutional support for Anglophones and Francophones. In 2006, 58% of the population in Canada reported English and 22% reported French as their mother tongues (Statistics Canada, 2007a). Many distinct Aboriginal language families and dialects also exist. Strategies for communicating effectively with people whose primary language is different from yours are discussed in depth in Chapter 4.

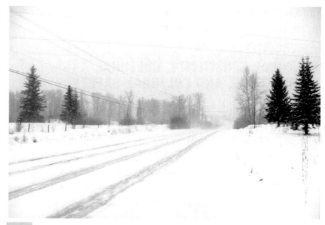

3-5 How does our geography shape health care access?

Canadians live primarily in urban areas. In 2011, 81.1% of the population lived in urban areas and 18.9% in rural areas (Statistics Canada, 2012a); 69.1% of Canadians were living in one of Canada's 33 large census metropolitan areas (CMAs)[†] (Statistics Canada, 2012b; Figures 3-4 and 3-5). In 2006, Canada had six CMAs whose populations exceeded 1 million: Toronto, Montreal, Vancouver, Ottawa-Gatineau, and, for the first time, Calgary and Edmonton; together, these cities contained 45% of Canada's total population (Statistics Canada, 2007b).

Canada's population as a whole is aging (Statistics Canada, 2012c). In 2011, people aged 65 and older constituted 14.8% of the total population, up from 13.7% 5 years earlier; this was a record high. In contrast, in 2006, the proportion of the population younger than 15 fell to 17.7%, its lowest level ever (Statistics Canada, 2007b). In 2011, for the first time in Canadian history, the number of people aged 55 to 64 exceeded that of people aged 15 to 24 (Statistics Canada, 2012c). Because life expectancy is longer for women (82.5 years for

---

Mother tongue is defined by Statistics Canada as the first language learned at home in childhood and still understood by the individual at the time the data were collected (Statistics Canada, 2011b). If the person no longer understands the first language learned, the mother tongue is the second language learned. For a person who learned two languages at the same time in early childhood, the mother tongue is the language this person spoke most often at home before starting school.

[†]A CMA is an area consisting of one or more neighbouring municipalities situated around a major urban core. A CMA must have a total population of at least 100,000, of which 50,000 or more live in the urban core.

BOX 3-2 STANDARDS FOR CULTURALLY, LINGUISTICALLY, AND SOCIALLY APPROPRIATE SERVICES IN HEALTH CARE

1. Promote and support the attitudes, openness, knowledge, behaviours, and skills necessary for staff to work respectfully and effectively with patients and each other in a culturally, linguistically, and socially diverse work environment.
2. Have a comprehensive management strategy to address culturally, linguistically, and socially appropriate services, including strategic goals, plans, policies, procedures, and designated staff responsible for implementation.
3. Use formal mechanisms for community and consumer involvement in the design and execution of service delivery, including planning, policymaking, operations, evaluation, training, and, as appropriate, treatment planning.
4. Develop and implement a strategy to recruit, retain, and promote diverse administrative, clinical, and support staff who are trained and qualified to address the needs of the various communities being served.
5. Require and arrange for continuing education and training for administrative, clinical, and support staff in how to foster respectful and responsive services for culturally, linguistically, and socially diverse people.
6. Provide all patients who have limited English or French proficiency with access to interpretation services.
7. Provide oral and written notices, including translated signage at key points of contact, to patients in their primary languages, and inform them of their right to receive interpreter services free of charge.
8. Translate signage and commonly used written patient educational material and other material for members of the predominant language groups in the local service areas, and make these translated materials available.
9. Ensure that interpreters and bilingual staff can demonstrate bilingual proficiency and receive training that includes the skills and ethics of interpreting and knowledge of the terms and concepts relevant to clinical or nonclinical encounters. Family and friends are not considered adequate substitutes because they usually lack these abilities.
10. Ensure that the patient's primary language spoken is included in the health care organization's information system and in any patient records used by staff or health care providers.
11. Use a variety of methods to collect and make use of accurate demographic, epidemiological, and clinical outcome data for groups and populations in the service area, and become informed about the cultural, linguistic, and social needs, resources, and assets of the surrounding community.
12. Undertake continuing organizational self-assessments, internal audits, and performance improvement programs, and integrate measures of access, quality, and outcomes of services particularly for culturally, linguistically, and socially diverse people.
13. Develop structures and procedures to address ethical and legal conflicts in health care delivery and complaints or grievances by patients and staff about unfair, insensitive, or discriminatory treatment, inequities in accessing services, or denial of services.
14. Prepare an annual progress report documenting the organization's progress with implementing services that are culturally, linguistically, and socially responsive, including information on programs, staffing, and resources.

Source: Adapted from Office of Minority Health. (2001). *National standards for culturally and linguistically appropriate services in health care. Final report.* Washington, DC: Office of Minority Health, U.S. Department of Health and Human Services.

women, in comparison with 77.7 years for men), nearly two thirds of people aged 80 and older are women (Statistics Canada, 2007b).

The increasing ethnocultural, linguistic, and social diversity within society necessitates health care policies and practices that support providers in working across differences. Box 3-2 lists guidelines adapted from standards developed in the United States to support services for culturally and linguistically diverse populations (Office of Minority Health, 2001). Many hospitals and health care agencies in Canada have similar policies.

ETHNOCULTURAL DIVERSITY WITHIN THE CANADIAN POPULATION

As suggested by the demographic profile in the preceding section, Canada is one of the most diverse countries in the world along many dimensions. Ethnocultural diversity is part of Canada's national identity. As the demographics indicate,

the majority of Canadians associate themselves with the dominant linguistic groups (English and French) and with the dominant European ancestry. These patterns create both the potential for "Othering"* (Peternelj-Taylor, 2005) in health care, as well as the potential for modelling culturally safe, actively respectful ways of working across differences in health care. Differences are most evident when members of dominant groups provide care to people who are from racialized groups or visible minorities, such as Aboriginal people or some people who have immigrated to Canada, particularly if those persons cannot communicate in the official languages. Therefore, to provide culturally safe care, health care providers require particular knowledge pertaining to Aboriginal people and immigrants.

---

*Othering refers to the projection of assumed cultural characteristics, differences, or identities onto members of particular groups. These projections are not based on actual differences; rather, they are based on stereotypes.

Aboriginal Populations in Canada

The term *Aboriginal people* is used to refer generally to the indigenous inhabitants of Canada, including First Nations, Métis, and Inuit people (Royal Commission on Aboriginal Peoples, 1996, p. xii). These three groups reflect "political and cultural entities that stem historically from the original peoples of North America, rather than collections of individuals united by so-called 'racial' characteristics" (p. xii). Of the 3.8% of the population in Canada who self-identified as Aboriginal, 60% identified as First Nations, 33% identified as Métis, and 4% identified as Inuit (Statistics Canada, 2008b). Although the terms *Indian* and *Native* are used in federal legislation (e.g., the *Indian Act*) and by the federal government (e.g., Indian and Northern Affairs Canada [INAC], which has recently been renamed Aboriginal Affairs and Northern Development Canada [AANDC]), the term *First Nations* is often viewed as more respectful than the colonial term *Indian*. *Inuit* replaces the colonial term *Eskimo*, and *Métis* refers to people of mixed European and Aboriginal ancestry. It is important to recognize that there is a great deal of diversity within First Nations, Métis, and Inuit people, reflected, in part, by the more than 50 Aboriginal languages currently spoken that belong to 11 Aboriginal language families (Norris, 2008).

Increasing numbers of Aboriginal people are moving from rural and northern communities into urban areas, often to seek employment that is not available in other regions. In 2006, the proportion of First Nations people living off reserve (60%) exceeded those living on reserve (40%; Statistics Canada, 2008b). Winnipeg was home to the largest urban Aboriginal population, and Saskatoon, Regina, Edmonton, Vancouver, Toronto, and Calgary also had high proportions of Aboriginal residents. Among the Inuit population, however, 78% continued to reside in the northern regions of Canada, with 49% living in Nunavut, 19% in Nunavik in northern Quebec, 6% in the Inuvialuit region of the Northwest Territories, and 4% in Nunatsiavut in northern Labrador (Statistics Canada, 2008b). Very few sources of data, however, pertain strictly to urban/off-reserve First Nations health and well-being, which makes assessing health trends as a population level challenging (Browne, McDonald, & Elliott, 2009).

Policies Affecting Aboriginal Peoples in Canada

In Canada, the complex history of colonialism and current policies and practices have resulted in profound social disruption within many Aboriginal communities. This has contributed to the lack of employment opportunities, limited access to educational programs, inadequate and often crowded housing, and high levels of poverty (Waldram, Herring, & Young, 2006). The regulation of First Nations people's lives through the policies of the *Indian Act* and the ongoing restrictions placed on self-government, land claims, and economic development in Aboriginal communities continue to shape life opportunities, economic conditions, and the overall health and social status of individuals and families (Figure 3-6).

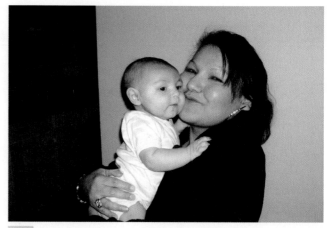

3-6 What do you imagine about this woman? She is the grandmother of a great-great-grandchild of a renowned traditional medicine woman, Mrs. Sophie Thomas, from Saik'uz First Nation, British Columbia.

The **Indian Act,** originally developed in 1876, was founded on the paternalistic motivation to assimilate and govern "Indians" (now often referred to as First Nations people). The original *Indian Act* has been amended several times, but it remains an actively applied set of legislation and contains all the federal policies and regulations pertaining to "registered status Indians" (a term used in the *Indian Act*). The *Indian Act* classifies First Nations people into registered status Indians or nonstatus Indians to distinguish people who receive legal recognition as First Nations citizens in Canada from those who do not (AANDC, 2012). The process of obtaining registered status (hereafter referred to as *status*) is complex and requires a series of paperwork submissions to AANDC, the federal department responsible for meeting the government's constitutional, treaty, political, and legal responsibilities to First Nations people.

Some First Nations people do not have status (e.g., approximately 20% of the total First Nations population), but they identify themselves as First Nations and are often members of a First Nation community (Statistics Canada, 2008b). They are not, however, recognized by the federal government under the *Indian Act,* either because they are unable to prove their status or because they have lost their status rights. For example, many First Nations women in Canada lost their status when they married nonstatus men. Although the *Act* was changed in 1985 to repeal these discriminatory policies, it is still possible for the grandchildren of status First Nations women to lose their status designation. The issue of who has status and who does not is relevant to health care providers because people who are nonstatus are not entitled to the limited benefits available to people with status.

Currently, First Nations people with status and Inuit people receive limited health care benefits (called *noninsured health benefits* [NIHBs]) not covered by provincial health insurance plans (Health Canada, 2012). NIHBs are administered by Health Canada and include selected prescription drugs, limited medical supplies and equipment, short-term crisis counselling, limited coverage for glasses and vision care, medical transportation, and dental care (although many dentists do not provide services to people who have status because the dentist must wait to be reimbursed by the federal government, as opposed to receiving payment directly from the patient). Unfortunately, many members of the public, including health care providers, are unaware that the services provided through NIHBs are very limited and that these benefits do not apply to nonstatus or Métis people.

Another prevalent misconception is that Aboriginal people in Canada do not pay taxes. This can be a source of resentment for some Canadians. In general, Aboriginal people are required to pay taxes on the same basis as other people in Canada, except where limited exemptions are defined by the *Indian Act* for people with status (AANDC, 2012). Status First Nations people are not required to pay provincial or federal taxes for goods, services, income, and property on reserve. However, this exemption does not apply to 60% of First Nations people in Canada who live off reserve. Nonstatus and Inuit people are subject to taxation, like all other Canadians.

Inequities in Health Status

In the past, discriminatory practices and policies were aimed at assimilating Aboriginal people into the dominant Canadian society. First Nations lands were appropriated and **reserves** were created, often in regions where economic development was limited. Cultural and spiritual practices were outlawed, including the work of traditional healers. Although it is not commonly known among the Canadian public, status First Nations people were not permitted to vote in federal elections until 1960, despite the fact that historically they were among the most intensively governed members of Canadian society (Furniss, 1999). Indoctrination into the dominant culture was attempted through church- or state-run **residential schools**. Residential schools included industrial schools, boarding schools, student residences, and hostels and were located in every province and territory except New Brunswick and Prince Edward Island. The last residential school, located in Saskatchewan, closed in 1996. Many individuals and their family members have since come forward with painful stories of physical and sexual abuse at residential schools. In response, in 2006, the federal government announced the approval of the Indian Residential Schools Settlement Agreement and the new Truth and Reconciliation Commission (Indian Residential Schools Resolution Canada, 2008).

The inequities of the past continue to influence people's health status in the present. Despite improvements over the past three decades, the health of many Aboriginal people continues to lag behind that of the overall Canadian population on virtually every measure (Adelson, 2005; Reading, 2009; Richmond & Ross, 2009). In the year 2000, life expectancy at birth for the status First Nations population was estimated at 68.9 years for men and 76.6 years for women, 7.4 and 5.2 years less, respectively, than that of the total Canadian population. The poverty rate among First Nations children is at least double the national average (Campaign 2000 Report Card, 2012). Infant mortality rates, one of the most

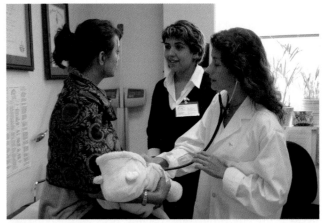

3-7 What do you miss when you make assumptions based on appearances about the social influences on health?

powerful indicators of the social determinants of health, are almost twice as high among status First Nations infants as for other Canadians.

These health and social status indicators cannot be understood outside of their social, historical, and economic contexts or viewed as "cultural" problems. Rather, they are manifestations of the complex interplay of historical, social, political, and economic determinants influencing health status and access to equitable health care. For example, health care providers often fail to see how social conditions, systemic racism, and discrimination have shaped substance use and suicide among Aboriginal people (Kirmayer et al., 2007). Other research shows that prenatal care for Aboriginal women in some settings is hampered by judgemental discriminatory attitudes and, for many, by poverty and limited resources in rural settings (Brown, Varcoe, Calam, 2011). Nevertheless, health care providers may judge these women for not accessing care (Browne, 2005, 2007; Browne et al., 2011). This is an area in which relational approaches in clinical practice can make a difference: It is important for you to remain critically reflective about the assumptions that you may have and also to remain focused on the historical and social contexts and current living conditions that continue to shape people's health, access to health care, and overall well-being (Figure 3-7).

People Who Immigrate to Canada

Canada's population is becoming increasingly diverse; immigration contributes to two thirds of the nation's population growth (Statistics Canada, 2008a). Canada continues to be the country of choice for many people, and in 2006, one per five people living in Canada was born outside of Canada. This means you have the opportunity to work with increasingly diverse groups of patients, particularly if you work in urban areas.

Since the 1970s, patterns of immigration have shifted significantly. In the past, European nations such as the United Kingdom, Italy, Germany, and The Netherlands, as well as the United States, were the primary sources of immigrants to

Canada (Statistics Canada, 2008a). In 2006, people emigrating from Asia and the Middle East made up the largest proportion (58.3%) of newcomers to Canada (Statistics Canada, 2008a). People born in Europe constituted the second largest group (16.1%) of recent immigrants. The next largest groups were from India (≈11.6%), Central and South America and the Caribbean (10.8%), Africa (10.6%), and the Philippines (7%).

It is important to be aware of the terms used to refer to the diverse groups of people who move to Canada. The term *immigrant* refers to "a person who is or has ever been a landed immigrant. A landed immigrant or permanent resident is a person who has been granted the right to live in Canada permanently by immigration authorities. Immigrants are either Canadian citizens by naturalization (the citizenship process) or permanent residents (landed immigrants) under Canadian legislation. Some immigrants have resided in Canada for a number of years, while others have arrived recently. Most immigrants are born outside Canada, but a small number are born in Canada" (Statistics Canada, 2012). The term *visible minority* is sometimes confused with the term *immigrant*. Many people in Canada who fulfill the definition of visible minority are not immigrants but are from families who have resided in Canada for many generations. Nurses and other clinicians cannot assume that a person's appearance or accent has anything to do with a person's country of birth or citizenship. Rather, they need to remain amenable to learning about people's unique and multifaceted contexts, including their ethnocultural backgrounds, family origins, and social circumstances. Health care providers should also realize that some people view the term *visible minority* as demeaning because it does not account for people's various histories. Recognizing this as an issue, organizations such as the Ontario Human Rights Commission use the term *racialized groups* to acknowledge the dynamic and complex processes by which racial categories are socially produced and used in ways that entrench social inequities (Access Alliance, 2007).

In the Longitudinal Survey of Immigrants to Canada, Schellenberg and Maheux (2007) asked people why they chose to immigrate to Canada. Of the respondents, more than half (55%) said they wanted to reside here because of the "quality of life" in Canada, and 39% planned to stay because of the positive future for their family here (Schellenberg & Maheux, 2007). People's decisions to migrate can be voluntary, involuntary, or a blend of both (Vissandjée, Thurston, Apale, & Nahar, 2007). The "push–pull" factors in immigration are often the need to explore new economic opportunities, family reunification, or forced relocation as a result of persecution or ecological disasters. Refugees often come from countries where conflict and war are ongoing, and they seek safer conditions in Canada. The decision and ability to migrate is never easy: Immigration involves complex applications, classification, and landing procedures. Immigration applications can take many years to process. With changing eligibility requirements, those who immigrate generally must come with significant economic resources. On the other hand, people who are refugees may come with few or no resources. After immigration, the processes of integration and adaptation into a new society are often lengthy and may take an entire lifetime or many generations. The development of a healthy and vibrant society requires the ongoing commitment of both recent immigrants and Canadians already residing in Canada (Vissandjée et al., 2007).

Most recent immigrants to Canada (97.2%) live in either a CMA or a census agglomeration (i.e., an urban community; Statistics Canada, 2008a). Among these population groups, two thirds reside in Canada's three largest CMAs: Toronto, Montreal, and Vancouver. People who were born in countries other than Canada accounted for 45.7% of Toronto's population, 39.6% of Vancouver's, and 20.6% of Montreal's (Statistics Canada, 2008a). In these three cities, immigration continues to be the major contributor to population growth. The most common reasons for settling in Toronto, Vancouver, or Montreal were to join social support networks of family and friends or because of the employment prospects. Most recently, an increasing number of new immigrants are settling in CMAs other than the three largest, including Calgary, Ottawa-Gatineau, Edmonton, Winnipeg, Hamilton, and London.

The Process of Immigration and Effects on Health

As a clinician, you need to recognize how the processes of migration and resettlement to another country can affect people's health and social status. Although many people are healthy when they first arrive in Canada, research shows that the health of immigrants, particularly non-Europeans, deteriorates over time in comparison with that of Canadian-born residents and immigrants from Europe (Pederson & Raphael, 2006). This pattern of declining health status has a number of causes. Some health problems are linked to the stress of immigration itself, which involves finding suitable employment and establishing a new social support network (Ng, Wilkins, Gendron, & Berthelot, 2005). The likelihood of a deterioration in health is also related to socioeconomic status, specifically low education and low household income. Vissandjée and colleagues (2007) showed that immigrant women, in particular, are often vulnerable to the stress that comes from trying to meet the basic needs of their families in a new country, learning a new language, and the social isolation that results from leaving family and friends behind.

People who immigrate to Canada often experience difficulties getting the help they need from health care providers, hospitals, and other health care agencies (Waxler-Morrison & Anderson, 2005). Immigrants can feel frustrated because few health care providers can communicate in the family's language and few interpreter services are available. Immigrants may also lack a basic understanding of how the Canadian health care system works. Some people experience discrimination or prejudice in hospitals and clinics, which can lead to situations of mistrust. Clinicians, in turn, may believe that families are not following their instructions or are not abiding by hospital policies in terms of the numbers of visitors. Despite these frustrations, most people who immigrate to Canada are very appreciative of the health care

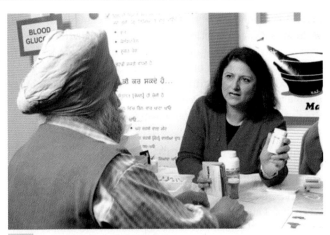

3-8 What situations most challenge you when trying to shift from the stance of expert to that of inquirer?

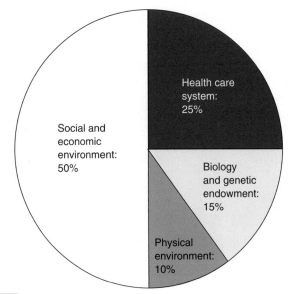

3-9 Estimated effect of determinants of health on the health status of the population.

they receive, particularly if services were scarce or limited in their countries of origin (Figure 3-8).

People also face challenges accessing health and social services because they have limited proficiency in English or French, despite their ability to speak other languages (often several). Waiting periods to qualify for provincial health care coverage can extend to several years, compromising access to health care services for children and families (Caulford & Vali, 2006). Studies of immigrants' economic integration in Canada have shown that those with non-European origins are more likely than those with European origins to have low-paying jobs that require little education. It has been shown that despite higher levels of education, immigrants have greater difficulties finding meaningful employment and are often forced to take low-paying jobs. These factors—in combination with experiences of racism, discrimination, and lower levels of social support—contribute to declining health status. Together, these social and economic trends have a profound effect on health status and can limit access to the resources and services necessary to maintain health in Canada.

It is important to remember that people who come from the same country may nevertheless be very diverse culturally, socially, and linguistically. People have varying levels of education and proficiency in Canada's two official languages, varied socioeconomic backgrounds, and varied understandings of Western health care services. Applying relational approaches in clinical practice will help you assess the unique contexts, histories, and experiences that shape an individual's or a family's overall health and well-being.

HEALTH, SOCIAL, AND GENDER INEQUITIES

To understand how inequities affect health, it is useful to distinguish between concepts such as health inequality and inequity. **Health inequality** is a generic term used to designate differences, variations, and disparities in the health status of individuals and groups (Varcoe, Pauly, Laliberté, & MacPherson, 2011). An example of health inequality is the higher incidence of deaths in the prime of life among women in Canada than among men, largely because of breast and

other cancers (Varcoe, Hankivsky, & Morrrow, 2007). **Health inequity** refers to the inequalities in health that are unnecessary and avoidable and differences that are considered unfair and unjust (Baum, Bégin, Houweling, & Taylor, 2009; Marmot, 2007). In Canada and elsewhere, many of the health care services are inequitable because they reflect an unfair distribution of the underlying social determinants of health: for example, access to educational opportunities and meaningful employment, adequate income for people with physical or intellectual disabilities, access to needed health care, the ability to afford nutritious foods, and respectful treatment free of discrimination.

As indicated in Figure 3-9, the economic, social, and political conditions in which people live are the major determinants of whether they are healthy or not. Rates of ill health are especially high among particular populations because of social, economic, and historical conditions. For example, people living in poverty, lone mothers in low-income brackets, older women, people who experience discrimination or racism, significant numbers of the Aboriginal population, women experiencing abuse, people with severe or persistent mental illnesses or addictions, refugees, and some immigrant groups are more likely than others to become ill and are less likely to receive appropriate health care services (Henry et al., 2005; Krieger, 2005; Raphael, 2009, 2011). Assessing risk factors and promoting health therefore require consideration of the intersecting social and economic factors that go far beyond the immediately identifiable behavioural or biological risk factors (e.g., smoking, a diet high in processed foods, high blood pressure, high cholesterol levels).

Evidence continues to show that at both the population and individual levels, poverty is the primary cause of poor health among Canadians (Raphael, 2011; Figure 3-10). For example, Canadians who live in the poorest 20% of urban neighbourhoods have significantly shorter life expectancies than do other Canadians. Of major concern is the ongoing

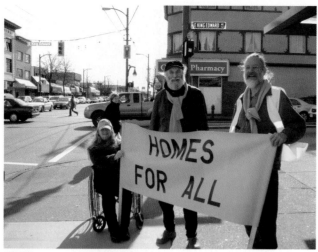

3-10 How do gender, disability, and poverty intersect to affect health?

evidence indicating that inequities in health and social status are continuing to grow, despite Canada's official commitment to equity and access.

In wealthy industrialized nations such as Canada, **relative poverty** is defined as the situation in which individuals are unable to carry out or participate in the activities expected in a wealthy developed nation such as Canada. These deficits manifest themselves in a variety of ways, including access to the food, clothing, and other amenities typical of most Canadians; involvement in occupational and leisure activities; and participation in decision making and in civil, social, and cultural life (Raphael, 2011, p. 58). In 2008, 13.6% of Canadian adults, 14.2% of children, and 13.1% of older Canadians were living in poverty (Raphael, 2011, p. 63). Poverty rates also differ by family type and gender, as shown in Figure 3-11.

Women's poverty in Canada is of particular concern. For example, for **lone-mother families,** the poverty rate in 2004 was 51%, which is exceptionally high in comparison with those of other wealthy industrialized nations. Living in poverty is an especially significant threat to the health of children inasmuch as it has both immediate and long-lasting effects. For women, the main causes of poverty are labour market inequities, family circumstances such as marriage

breakdown or lone parenting, cutting of welfare payments for women with small children, and wage disparities between women and men (Reid, 2007). These are important factors to consider in the context of health assessment. Recognizing how health and social inequities intersect to differentially affect people will help you to recognize and be more responsive to the range of factors that influence health and well-being.

HEALTH CARE PRACTICES

Health care practices vary among individuals and groups and cannot be determined on the basis of assumptions regarding ethnicity. The extent to which any individual subscribes to the tenets of Western medicine depends on the totality of his or her own life experiences, including experience with and exposure to Western medicine. Today, Canadians of all backgrounds draw upon a range of traditions as part of their health care. Some wholeheartedly ascribe to the full range of allopathic medicine (referring to the dominant Western practice of medicine), including some aspects (e.g., cosmetic surgery) that many others would not embrace. Most people also draw on other approaches, such as the use of chiropractic medicine, massage therapy, vitamins, or herbs such as Echinacea (Figure 3-12).

Perspectives on what are acceptable health care practices change over time and are culturally and socially bound. Whereas in the past, few people were familiar with the practice of acupuncture, many today seek the services of qualified acupuncturists or traditional Chinese medicine practitioners. Your responsibility is to inform patients about the potential effects of particular practices (e.g., the potential for some nutritional supplements to potentiate certain anticoagulants) but not to judge the acceptability of those practices.

More and more Canadians are turning to **complementary and alternative health care** and **natural health products** to treat illness and promote health (Health Canada, 2005). As defined by Health Canada (2005), *complementary and alternative health care* is an umbrella term that encompasses numerous individual therapies and health care approaches, including traditional Chinese medicine, reflexology, homeopathy, therapeutic massage, chiropractic services, relaxation therapy, and Aboriginal traditional medicines and healing

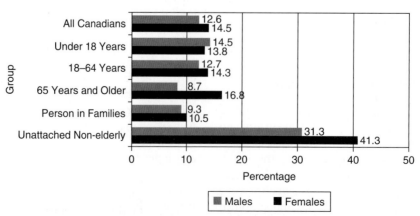

3-11 Percentage of Canadians living in poverty, by age, gender, and family situation, 2008.

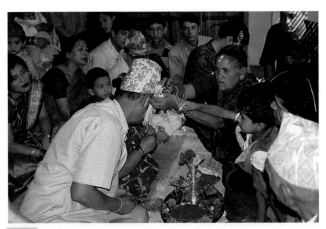

3-12 How does a "critical cultural" lens shape your view differently than a "culturalist" lens?

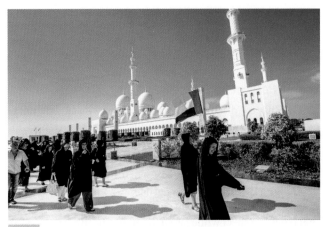

3-13 How does your understanding of religion and spirituality shape your health assessments?

practices. The term *natural health products* describes a variety of products, such as herbal medicines, homeopathic remedies, nutritional supplements, vitamins, and minerals.

When conducting a health assessment, remember that people may draw on a combination of approaches. However, the ability to access and engage in complementary and alternative approaches varies greatly, depending on people's economic and social resources and their geographical locale. For example, acupuncture, chiropractic medicine, massage, and natural health products can be prohibitively expensive. In general, most of these approaches are not covered by provincial or territorial health care plans.

Spirituality and Health

The significance of **spirituality** in people's health and healing has long been recognized. Although spirituality commonly tends to be perceived as an offshoot of religion, it is important to distinguish between religion and spirituality (Fowler, 2011). Spirituality has always been more central to the human experience than religion. Religions are often established by formal institutional structures, rituals, and beliefs, whereas spirituality may refer more generally to the search for meaning. Both religion and spirituality can play a significant role in the ways people deal with health and illness (Reimer-Kirkham, 2011; Figure 3-13). As a health care provider, you do not need to know the specifics of various religious and spiritual traditions. However, it is important to convey openness, interest, and acceptance. First, you must check your own assumptions and biases. If you call places of worship "churches" in your work with patients, you are conveying a Christian bias that may discourage communication by patients who call their places of worship by other names (e.g., "temples," "mosques," or "synagogues"). Second, you need to avoid making assumptions about particular people. A person may be part of an ethnocultural group but not part of an associated religion. During the health assessment, conveying openness and inviting patients to identify what is important to them is most effective in eliciting data. For example, you might ask, "Do you have any religious beliefs or practices that you would like me to know about in relation to your health?"

GUIDELINES FOR CLINICAL PRACTICE

Assess Culturally Based Understandings and Practices

A health assessment can be performed over time. Regardless of whether you are completing a health assessment rapidly in the context of a single encounter or as part of a long-term professional relationship, building trust, engaging through listening, conveying respect for differences, and paying attention to the context of people's lives are key to culturally safe health assessments.

Work to Build Trust

Although certain data must be collected in the initial interview to address the patient's presenting health issues, patients should not be expected to share sensitive information until trust has been established (Anderson et al., 2005). Patients may be reluctant to reveal their understandings or beliefs for fear of being dismissed as providing information that is less than legitimate. Clinicians can find out more by asking questions phrased in a nonjudgemental way, such as "Have you found anything else that has helped you?" rather than "Are you taking medications besides those prescribed by the doctor?" (Anderson et al., 2005, p. 339).

Engage Through Listening

Engaging in conversations with patients or their family members during the process of establishing trust helps you obtain a deeper understanding of their explanatory models: that is, how they understand their world and health, illness, and approaches to healing. Kleinman (1980) and colleagues (Kleinman & Benson, 2006) and Anderson and associates (2005, p. 343) provided some questions that can assist clinicians in assessing patients' culturally based understandings. These are not always asked as direct questions but can be used as cues for listening and, in some cases, as follow-up questions:

- What do you call this health problem? What term or name do you give it?
- What do you think may have brought on this health problem?

- What concerns you most about this illness?
- What do you usually do to stay healthy (e.g., activities, foods, medications)? Have you been able to continue with those?

Convey Respect for Differences

As this chapter discusses, you will engage with a wide range of people from diverse backgrounds. Conveying respect for differences helps build trust and welcomes patients to share their understandings. Research continues to show that patients are very quick to sense when health care providers are judging them negatively, particularly through verbal and nonverbal communications conveyed to patients. Questions that convey respect while people's varying health practices are explored can focus on what the patients themselves have done to address their health or illness concerns. For example:

- Have you found any treatments or medications that have worked for you in the past?
- How did they help you?
- Are you using them now? If so, are they helping?
- (For people who have recently immigrated to Canada) Did you use any special treatments or medicines in your home country that seemed to work for you?

Questions that convey an interest in hearing about traditional or complementary healing practices include the following:

- Have you used any traditional medicines or healing methods that you found helpful?
- Are you able to access those medicines or healing methods?

Pay Attention to the Social and Economic Contexts of Patients' and Families' Lives

For all patients and families, it is important to consider how people are managing with jobs, housing, child care, financial resources, care of older parents or relatives, transportation, and access to health care services (Anderson et al., 2005). These considerations are relevant whether you are working in a community health care setting or in an acute care or long-term care facility. Conveying interest in the circumstances of people's lives with a simple question such as "How have things been going for you?" is not "small talk" but rather an opportunity for you to assess a person's overall health in a nonjudgemental way (Figure 3-14).

Assessing a patient's social and economic context requires tact and effective listening and interviewing skills (as discussed in Chapter 4). Depending on the context, it may or may not be appropriate to explore this during your first meeting with a patient or family. Asking direct questions about a person's finances may be seen as intrusive, and many people are embarrassed by such questions. However, inquiring about the person's ability to deal with the health, illness, or health promotion issues may be a good way to start the discussion. Anderson and associates (2005) have suggested the following questions as helpful for assessing people's social and economic contexts:

- What is particularly challenging or difficult, or what is needed to manage your health or illness?

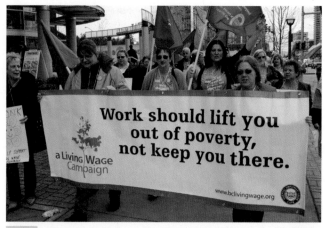

3-14 How can health care providers participate in social change?

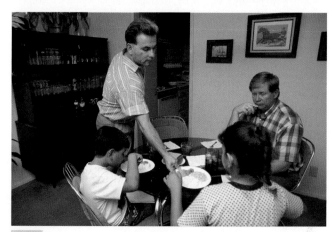

3-15 How do dominant ideas about families shape your assessments?

- Are you working currently? Can you tell me a bit about the job you have?
- What do you need help with at home in order to manage (with your health or illness issues)?
- Whom do you rely on to help you at home? Do you live alone?
- Do you have family or friends nearby who can help you if needed?
- What kinds of things do you need help with?
- Are you able to afford the things you need to stay healthy, such as medications, glasses, dental work, and assistive devices such as a cane or wheelchair?
- Are you able to travel as necessary to access services or support?

Many families in Canada are required to take on the extra work of caring for family members in their homes because of shortened hospital stays for acutely ill patients; the lack of affordable, high-quality long-term care facilities; and, in some cases, families' personal commitments to care for older parents in the home (Baumbusch & Shaw, 2011; Cohen, Tate, & Baumbusch, 2009). The financial circumstances of the family influence whether and how they are able to take on these caregiving responsibilities. Research has shown that health care providers in hospitals are often not familiar with patients' home environments (Figure 3-15) and may assume that a family has the resources to care for a sick or older person at home (Anderson et al., 2005). However, nurses must remember that for many people, staying at home to care for a relative probably means loss of wages, which many families cannot afford. Social circumstances therefore have a profound effect on how people can manage illness and the changes that are associated with aging. These are important aspects to consider in the process of health assessment.

SUMMARY: CONNECTING ACROSS DIFFERENCES

The notion of "connecting across differences" comes from Doane and Varcoe (2005), who emphasized that "relational practice requires that you connect across differences by joining people as they are and where they are" (p. 295). This can be easier said than done, and the integration of knowledge and reflection will take time. In preparing to work across differences, the first step is to anticipate your own biases and assumptions by reflecting on your own social, cultural, economic, and family backgrounds relative to health, illness, and health promotion (Figure 3-16). In the process, you need to critically examine and, in some cases, challenge your own biases, perceptions, and prejudices about particular groups, practices, and health behaviours. Second, learn to critically reflect on the culture of the health care system, how it works, its taken-for-granted practices and policies, and their consequences for patients. Third, become knowledgeable about the social and economic conditions and policies in Canada that influence people's ability to maintain their health or to access the resources necessary to stay healthy. Such knowledge includes information about immigration trends, racism, discrimination, socioeconomic trends, gender inequities, welfare reforms, child care availability, and issues affecting older people in relation to your practice area. Finally, as discussed in Chapter 4, you need the skills to communicate effectively with people from a variety of backgrounds, including those whose primary language is different from yours.

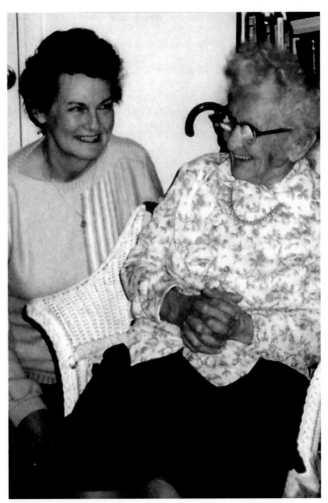

3-16 What stereotypes about women, aging, and caregiving does this photo of a 101-year-old woman and her daughter challenge?

REFERENCES

Aboriginal Affairs and Northern Development Canada. (2012a). *Frequently asked questions about Aboriginal peoples.* Retrieved from *http://www.aadnc-aandc.gc.ca/eng /1100100013800/1100100013801.*

Aboriginal Affairs and Northern Development Canada. (2012b). *Indian Residential Schools Resolution Canada. Frequently asked questions.* Retrieved from *http://www.aadnc-aandc.gc.ca/eng /1100100015798/1100100015799.*

Access Alliance. (2007). *Racialization and health inequalities: Focus on children. City of Toronto and neighbourhood highlights.* Toronto: Access Alliance Multicultural Community Health Centre.

Adelson, N. (2005). The embodiment of inequity: Health disparities in Aboriginal Canada. *Canadian Journal of Public Health, 96*(Suppl 2), S45–S61. Retrieved from *http:// pubs.cpha.ca/PDF/P24/22247.pdf.*

Anderson, J., Perry, J., Blue, C., Browne, A., Henderson, A., Khan, K., … Smye, V. (2003). "Rewriting" cultural safety within the postcolonial and postnational feminist project. *Advances in Nursing Science 26*(3), 196–214.

Anderson, J. M., & Reimer-Kirkham, S. (1999). Discourses on health: A critical perspective. In H. Coward & P. Ratanakul (Eds.), *A cross-cultural dialogue on health care ethics* (pp. 47–67). Waterloo, ON: Wilfrid Laurier University Press.

Anderson, J. M., Reimer-Kirkham, S., Waxler-Morrison, N., Herbert, C., Murphy, M., & Richardson, E. (2005). Conclusion. In N. Waxler-Morrison, J. M. Anderson, E. Richardson, & N. Chambers (Eds.), *Cross-cultural caring: A handbook for health providers* (2nd ed., pp. 323–352). Vancouver: UBC Press.

Association of Faculties of Medicine of Canada. (2007). Cultural awareness, sensitivity, and safety. In *AFMC primer on population health: A virtual textbook on public health concepts for clinicians.* Ottawa: Author. Retrieved from *http://phprimer.afmc.ca/Part1-TheoryThinkingAboutHealth/Chapter3CulturalCompetenceAndCommunication/Culturalawarenesssensitivityandsafety.*

Baum, F. E., Bégin, M., Houweling, T. A. J., & Taylor, S. (2009). Changes not for the fainthearted: Reorienting health care systems toward health equity through action on the social determinants of health. *American Journal of Public Health, 99*(11), 1967-1974. doi:10.2105/AJPH.2008.154856

Baumbusch, J., & Shaw, M. (2011). Geriatric emergency nurses: Addressing the needs of an aging population. *Journal of Emergency Nursing, 37*(4), 321–327. doi:10.1016/j.jen.2010.04.013

Behjati-Sabet, A., & Chambers, N. (2005). People of Iranian descent. In N. Waxler-Morrison, J. M. Anderson, E. Richardson, & N. Chambers (Eds.), *Cross-cultural caring: A handbook for health providers* (2nd ed., pp. 127–162). Vancouver: UBC Press.

Brown, H., Varcoe, C., & Calam, B. (2011). The birthing experiences of rural Aboriginal women in context: Implications for nursing. *Canadian Journal of Nursing Research, 43*(4), 100–117.

Browne, A. J. (2005). Discourses influencing nurses' perceptions of First Nations patients. *Canadian Journal of Nursing Research, 37*(4), 62–87. Retrieved from *http://cjnr.mcgill.ca/TOC/37-4.htm.*

Browne, A. J. (2007). Clinical encounters between nurses and First Nations women in a Western Canadian hospital. *Social Science and Medicine, 64*(10), 2165–2176. doi:10.1016/j.socscimed.2007.02.006

Browne, A. J., McDonald, H., & Elliott, D. (2009). *Urban First Nations health research discussion paper. A report for the First Nations Centre of the National Aboriginal Health Organization (NAHO).* Ottawa: National Aboriginal Health Organization. Retrieved from *http://www.naho.ca/documents/fnc/english/UrbanFirstNationsHealthResearchDiscussionPaper.pdf.*

Browne, A. J., Smye, V., Rodney, P., Tang, S., Mussell, B., & O'Neil, J. (2011). Access to primary care from the perspective of Aboriginal patients at an urban emergency department. *Qualitative Health Research, 21*(3), 333–348. doi:10.1177/1049732310385824

Browne, A. J., & Varcoe, C. (2006). Critical cultural perspectives and health care involving Aboriginal peoples. *Contemporary Nurse, 22*(2), 155–167.

Browne, A. J., Varcoe, C., Smye, V., Reimer-Kirkham, S., Lynam, J. M., & Wong, S. (2009). Cultural safety and the challenges of translating critically-oriented knowledge in practice. *Nursing Philosophy: An International Journal for Health Care Providers, 10*, 167–179. doi:10.1111/j.1466-769X.2009.00406.x

Browne, A. J., Varcoe, C., Wong, S., & Smye, V. L. (in press). Can ethnicity data collected at an organizational level be useful in addressing health and healthcare inequities? *Ethnicity & Health.*

Campaign 2000. (2012). *2012 report card on child and family poverty in Canada.* Family Service Toronto: Toronto. Retrieved from *http://www.campaign2000.ca/reportCards/national/C2000ReportCardNov2012.pdf.*

Canadian Nurses Association (CNA). (2010). *Position statement: Promoting cultural competence in nursing.* Ottawa: Author. Retrieved from *http://www2.cna-aiic.ca/CNA/documents/pdf/publications/PS114_Cultural_Competence_2010_e.pdf.*

Caulford, P., & Vali, Y. (2006). Providing health care to medically uninsured immigrants and refugees. *Canadian Medical Association Journal, 174*(9), 1253–1254. doi:10.1503/cmaj.051206

Chui, T. (2011). *Women in Canada: A gender-based statistical report. Immigrant women.* Statistics Canada: Ottawa. Retrieved from *http://www.statcan.gc.ca/pub/89-503-x/2010001/article/11528-eng.htm#a26.*

Chui, T., & Maheux, H. (2011). *Visible Minority Women.* Ottawa: Statistics Canada.

Cohen, M., Tate, J., & Baumbusch, J. (2009). *An uncertain future for seniors: BC's restructuring of home and community care, 2001–2008.* Vancouver: Canadian Centre for Policy Alternatives.

Doane, G. H., & Varcoe, C. (2005). *Family nursing as relational inquiry: Developing health-promoting practice.* Philadelphia: Lippincott Williams & Wilkins.

Fowler, M. D. (2011). Religion and nursing. In M. Fowler, S. Reimer-Kirkham, R. Sawatzky, & E. Johnson Taylor (Eds.), *Religion, religious ethics, and nursing* (pp. 1–26). New York: Springer.

Furniss, E. (1999). *The burden of history: Colonialism and the frontier myth in a rural Canadian community.* Vancouver: UBC Press.

Gustafson, D. L. (2008). Are sensitivity and tolerance enough? Comparing two theoretical approaches to caring for newcomer women with mental health problems. In S. Guruge & E. Collins (Eds.), *Working with immigrant women: Issues and strategies for mental health providers* (pp. 39–63). Toronto: Canadian Centre for Addiction & Mental Health.

Health Canada. (2005). *Complementary and alternative health care: The other mainstream?* Retrieved from *http://www.hc-sc.gc.ca/sr-sr/pubs/hpr-rpms/bull/2003-7-complement/index-eng.php.*

Health Canada. (2012). NIHB (*Non-insured health benefits) reimbursement question and answer.* Retrieved from *http://www.hc-sc.gc.ca/fniah-spnia/nihb-ssna/benefit-prestation/form_questions-eng.php.*

Henry, F., Tator, C., Mattis, W., & Rees, T. (2005). *The colour of democracy: Racism in Canadian society* (3rd ed.). Toronto: Nelson.

Indian Residential Schools Resolution Canada. (2008). *Frequently asked questions* Retrieved from *http://www.irsrrqpi.gc.ca/english/truth_reconciliation_commission.html.*

Kirmayer, L., Brass, G., Holton, T., Paul, K., Simpson, C., & Tait, C. (2007). *Suicide among Aboriginal people in Canada.* Ottawa: Aboriginal Healing Foundation.

Kisely, S., Terashima, M., & Langille, D. (2008). A population-based analysis of the health experience of African Nova Scotians. *CMAJ: Canadian Medical Association Journal, 179*, 653–658. doi:10.1503/cmaj.071279

Kleinman, A. (1980). *Patients and healers in the context of culture.* Berkeley: University of California Press.

Kleinman, A., & Benson, P. (2006). Anthropology in the clinic: The problem of cultural competency and how to fix it. *PLoS Medicine—A Peer-Reviewed Open-Access Journal, 3*(1), 1673–1676. doi:10.1371/journal.pmed.0030294

Krieger, N. (2005). Defining and investigating social disparities in cancer: Critical issues. *Cancer Causes and Control, 16*(1), 5–14.

Krieger, N. (2011). *Epidemiology and the people's health: Theory and context.* Oxford, UK: Oxford University Press.

Marmot, M. (2007). Achieving health equity: From root causes to fair outcomes. *The Lancet, 370*(9593), 1153–1163. doi:10.1016/S0140-6736(07)61385-3

Ng, E., Wilkins, R., Gendron, F., & Berthelot, J. M. (2005). *Dynamics of immigrants' health in Canada: Evidence from the National Population Health Survey.* Ottawa: Statistics Canada.

Norris, M. J. (2008). Aboriginal languages in Canada: Emerging trends and perspectives on second language acquisition. *Canadian Social Trends,* Cat. no. 11–008, pp. 19–27. Ottawa: Statistics Canada. Retrieved from *http://www.statcan.gc.ca/pub/11-008-x/2007001/pdf/9628-eng.pdf.*

Office of Minority Health. (2001). *National standards for culturally and linguistically appropriate services in health care: Final report.* Washington, DC: Office of Minority Health, U.S. Department of Health and Human Services.

Papps, E., & Ramsden, I. (1996). Cultural safety in nursing: The New Zealand experience. *International Journal for Quality in Health Care, 8*(5), 491–497.

Pederson, A., & Raphael, D. (2006). Gender, race and health inequities. In D. Raphael, T. Bryant, & M. Rioux (Eds.), *Staying alive: Critical perspectives on health, illness and health care* (pp. 159–191). Toronto: Canadian Scholars' Press.

Peternelj-Taylor, C. (2005). An exploration of othering in forensic psychiatric and correctional nursing. *Canadian Journal of Nursing Research, 36*(4), 130–147.

Polaschek, N. R. (1998). Cultural safety: A new concept in nursing people of different ethnicities. *Journal of Advanced Nursing, 27*(3), 452–457.

Ramsden, I. (1993). Kawa Whakaruruhau: Cultural safety in nursing education in Aotearoa (New Zealand). *Nursing Praxis in New Zealand, 8*(3), 4–10.

Ramsden, I. (2002). *Cultural safety and nursing education in Aotearoa and Te Waipounamu*. Wellington, New Zealand: University of Wellington.

Ramsden, I., & Spoonley, P. (1994). The cultural safety debate in nursing education in Aotearoa. *New Zealand Annual Review of Education, 3*, 161–174.

Raphael, D. (Ed.). (2009). *Social determinants of health: Canadian perspectives* (2nd ed.). Toronto: Canadian Scholars' Press.

Raphael, D. (2011). *Poverty in Canada: Implications for health and quality of life* (2nd ed.). Toronto: Canadian Scholars' Press.

Reading, J. (2009). *The crisis of chronic disease among Aboriginal peoples: A challenge for public health, population health and social policy*. Victoria, BC: Centre for Aboriginal Health Research and the University of Victoria.

Reid, C. (2007). Women's heath and the politics of policy and exclusion. In M. Morrow, O. Hankivsky, & C. Varcoe (Eds.), *Women's health in Canada: Critical theory, policy and practice* (pp. 199–220). Toronto: University of Toronto Press.

Reimer-Kirkham, S. (2011). A critical reading across religion and spirituality: Contributions of postcolonial theory to nursing ethics. In M. Fowler, S. Reimer-Kirkham, R. Sawatzky, & E. Johnson Taylor (Eds.), *Religion, religious ethics, and nursing* (pp. 93–112). New York: Springer.

Richmond, C., & Ross, N. (2009). The determinants of First Nation and Inuit health: A critical population health approach. *Health & Place, 15*, 403–411. doi:10.1016/j.healthplace.2008.07.004

Royal Commission on Aboriginal Peoples. (1996). *Report of the Royal Commission on Aboriginal peoples: Vol. 3. Gathering strength*. Ottawa: Author.

Schellenberg, G., & Maheux, H. (2007). Immigrants' perspectives on their first four years in Canada: Highlights from three waves of the Longitudinal Survey of Immigrants to Canada. *Canadian Social Trends,* Cat. no. 11-008 (Special Edition). Ottawa: Statistics Canada/Minister of Industry. Retrieved from *http://www.statcan.gc.ca/pub/11-008-x/2007000/pdf/9627-eng.pdf*.

Smye, V., Rameka, M., & Willis, E. (2006). Indigenous health care. Advances in nursing practice: An introduction. *Contemporary Nurse, 22*(2), 142–154.

Srivastava, R. H. (2007). *The healthcare provider's guide to clinical cultural competence*. Toronto: Elsevier Canada.

Statistics Canada. (2006). *Concept: Ethnicity*. Ottawa: Author. Retrieved from *http://www.statcan.ca/english/concepts/definitions/ethnicity.htm*.

Statistics Canada. (2007a). *Profile of language, immigration, citizenship, mobility and migration, 2006 census*. Ottawa: Author. Retrieved from *http://www.statcan.gc.ca/bsolc/olc-cel/olc-cel?lang=eng&catno=94-577-X*.

Statistics Canada. (2007b). *Portrait of the Canadian population in 2006: Population and dwelling counts*. Ottawa: Author. Retrieved from *http://www12.statcan.ca/english/census06/analysis/popdwell/index.cfm*.

Statistics Canada. (2008a). *Census snapshot—Immigration in Canada: A portrait of the foreign-born population, 2006 census*. Ottawa: Author. Retrieved from *http://www.statcan.gc.ca/pub/11-008-x/2008001/article/10556-eng.htm#2*.

Statistics Canada. (2008b). *Aboriginal peoples in Canada in 2006: Inuit, Métis and First Nations, 2006 census*. Ottawa: Author. Retrieved from *http://www12.statcan.ca/english/census06/analysis/aboriginal/pdf/97-558-XIE2006001.pdf*.

Statistics Canada. (2011a). Visible minority of person. Retrieved from *http://www.statcan.gc.ca/concepts/definitions/minority-minorite1-eng.htm*.

Statistics Canada. (2011b). *Mother tongue of person*. Ottawa: Author. Retrieved from *http://www.statcan.gc.ca/concepts/definitions/language-langue01-eng.htm*.

Statistics Canada. (2012). *Census of population: Linguistic characteristics of Canadians*. Statistics Canada: Ottawa. Retrieved from *http://www.statcan.gc.ca/daily-quotidien/121024/dq121024a-eng.htm*

Statistics Canada. (2012a). *Canada's rural population since 1851: Population and dwelling counts, 2011 census* (Cat. no. 98-310-X2011003). Ottawa: Author. Retrieved from *http://www12.statcan.gc.ca/census-recensement/2011/as-sa/98-310-x/98-310-x2011003_2-eng.pdf*.

Statistics Canada. (2012b). *The Canadian population in 2011: Age and sex* (Cat. no. 98-311-X2011001). Ottawa: Statistics Canada. Retrieved from *http://www12.statcan.gc.ca/census-recensement/2011/as-sa/98-311-x/98-311-x2011001-eng.pdf*.

Statistics Canada. (2012c). *The Canadian population in 2011: Population counts and growth* (Cat. no. 98-310-X2011001). Ottawa: Author. Retrieved from *http://www12.statcan.gc.ca/census-recensement/2011/as-sa/98-310-x/98-310-x2011001-eng.pdf*.

Statistics Canada. (2012d). *Quarterly population estimates, Canada, provinces and territories, 1971 to 2012*. Ottawa: Statistics Canada. Retrieved from *http://www.stats.gov.nl.ca/statistics/population/pdf/quarterly_pop_prov.pdf*.

United Nations Educational, Scientific and Cultural Organization. (1952). *The race concept: Results of an inquiry*. Retrieved from *http://unesdoc.unesco.org/images/0007/000733/073351eo.pdf*.

Varcoe, C. (2008). Inequality, violence and women's health. In B. S. Bolaria & H. Dickinson (Eds.), *Health, illness and health care in Canada* (4th ed., pp. 211–230). Toronto: Nelson.

Varcoe, C., Browne, A. J., Wong, S., & Smye, V. L. (2009). Harms and benefits: Collecting ethnicity data in a clinical context. *Social Science & Medicine, 68*(9), 1659–1666. doi:10.1016/j.socscimed.2009.02.034

Varcoe, C., Hankivsky, O., & Morrow, M. (2007). Beyond gender matters: An introduction. In M. Morrow, O. Hankivsky, & C. Varcoe (Eds.), *Women's health in Canada: Critical theory, policy and practice* (pp. 3–30). Toronto: University of Toronto Press.

Varcoe, C., Pauly, B., Laliberté, S., & MacPherson, G. (2011). Intersectionality, justice, and influencing policy. In O. Hankivsky (Ed.), *Health inequities in Canada: Intersectional frameworks and practices* (pp. 331–348). Vancouver: UBC Press.

Vissandjée, B., Thurston, W., Apale, A., & Nahar, K. (2007). Women's health at the intersection of gender and the experience of international migration. In M. Morrow, O. Hankivsky, & C. Varcoe (Eds.), *Women's health in Canada: Critical theory, policy and practice* (pp. 221–243). Toronto: University of Toronto Press.

Waldram, J. B., Herring, A., & Young, T. K. (2006). *Aboriginal health in Canada: Historical, cultural and epidemiological perspectives* (2nd ed.). Toronto: University of Toronto Press.

Waxler-Morrison, N., & Anderson, J. (2005). Introduction: The need for culturally sensitive health care. In N. Waxler-Morrison, J. M. Anderson, E. Richardson, & N. Chambers (Eds.), *Crosscultural caring: A handbook for health professional* (2nd ed., pp. 1–10). Vancouver: UBC Press.

Wepa, D. (Ed.). (2005). *Cultural safety in Aotearoa New Zealand*. Auckland, New Zealand: Pearson New Zealand Limited.

World Health Organization. (2012). *Frequently asked questions.* Retrieved from *http://www.who.int/suggestions/faq/en/index.html.*

Yue, K. K. (2005). People of Chinese descent. In N. Waxler-Morrison, J. M. Anderson, E. Richardson, & N. Chambers (Eds.), *Crosscultural caring: A handbook for health providers* (2nd ed., pp. 127–162). Vancouver: UBC Press.

Web Sites of Interest

Aboriginal Nurses Association of Canada: *http://www.anac.on.ca/*

Access Alliance: Multicultural Health and Community Services: *http://www.accessalliance.ca/*

Assembly of First Nations: *http://www.afn.ca/index.php/en*

British Columbia Centre of Excellence for Women's Health: *http://www.bccewh.bc.ca/*

Canadian Institute for Health Information: *http://secure.cihi.ca/cihiweb/dispPage.jsp?cw_page=home_e*

Canadian Nurses Association: *http://www.cna-nurses.ca/cna/*

Canadian Women's Health Network: *http://www.cwhn.ca/*

Citizenship and Immigration Canada: *http://www.cic.gc.ca/english/index.asp*

Congress of Aboriginal Peoples: *http://www.abo-peoples.org/*

Inuit Tapiriit Kanatami: *http://www.itk.ca/*

Métis National Council: *http://www.metisnation.ca/*

National Aboriginal Health Organization: *http://www.naho.ca*

Native Women's Association of Canada: *http://www.nwac.ca/*

Public Health Agency of Canada: *http://www.phac-aspc.gc.ca/index-eng.php*

Statistics Canada: *http://cansim2.statcan.ca*

Status of Women Canada: *http://www.swc-cfc.gc.ca/*

World Health Organization: *http://www.who.int/about/en/*

The Interview

Written by Carolyn Jarvis, PhD, APN, CNP
Adapted by Annette J. Browne, PhD, RN

⊖volve WEBSITE

OUTLINE

The Process of Communication
Techniques of Communication
Interviewing in Challenging Situations

Communicating Across Cultures
Overcoming Communication Barriers

The interview is a meeting between you and your patient. The goal of this meeting is to record a complete health history. The health history helps you begin to identify the patient's health strengths and problems and contextual influences, and it functions as a bridge to the next step in data collection: the physical examination.

The interview is the first, and really the most important, part of data collection. It entails the collection of **subjective data:** what the patient says about himself or herself. The interview is the optimal way to learn about the patient's perceptions of, understandings of, and reactions to their health state. Once people enter the acute care system, power relations may change, and opportunities for relational practice may shift. The initial interview, however, is the ideal opportunity to build trust, establish rapport, and engage in relational practice. Your skill in interviewing, your nonverbal behaviours, and the attitude you convey will affect the kinds of information you elicit. If the interview is well-planned and implemented, you will be able to glean most of the necessary information needed to plan the next steps in the assessment process. The interview therefore forms the basis of a successful working relationship. To accomplish a successful interview, you must perform the following tasks:

1. Gather complete and accurate data about the patient's health state, including the description and chronology of any symptoms of illness.
2. Establish rapport and trust, and convey respect, so that the patient feels accepted (versus judged by you) and thus free to share all relevant data.
3. Teach the patient about his or her health state so that the patient can participate in identifying problems.

4. Build rapport for a continuing therapeutic relationship; this rapport facilitates future opportunities for assessment, diagnoses, planning, and treatment.
5. Look for opportunities to engage in teaching for health promotion and disease prevention

Consider the interview as being similar to forming a contract between you and your patient. A contract consists of spoken or unspoken rules for behaviour. In this case, the contract concerns what the patient needs and expects from the health care system and what you, the health care provider, have to offer. Your mutual goal is optimal health and health care for the patient. The contract's terms include the following:

- Time and place of the interview and subsequent physical examination. In some cases, the interview may occur in outreach settings, in people's homes, or on the streets (for example, when assessments are conducted by street nurses).
- Introduction of yourself and a brief explanation of your role.
- The purpose of the interview.
- How long it will take.
- An indication of what will occur during the interview.
- Presence of any other people (e.g., patient's family, other health care providers, students).
- Confidentiality and to what extent it may be limited.
- Any other information specific to the organizational setting in which you are working, including potential costs that the patient must pay (for example, services, dental work, or prescription or over-the-counter pharmaceuticals that are not covered by medicare or insurance premiums).

Although the patient may know some of this information already through telephone contact with receptionists (or office assistant) or the admitting office, these points of clarification need to be stated clearly at the outset as a way of fostering openness and trust as you facilitate the interview.

THE PROCESS OF COMMUNICATION

The vehicle that carries you and your patient through the interview is communication. Communication is exchanging information so that each person clearly understands the other. If you do not understand each other, if you have not conveyed *meaning*, no communication has occurred.

It is challenging to teach the skill of interviewing because initially most students think little needs to be learned. They assume that if they can talk and hear, they can communicate. However, much more than talking and hearing is necessary. Communication is all behaviour, conscious and unconscious, verbal and nonverbal, including, for example, tone of voice, facial expressions, gestures, and body posture. *All* behaviour has meaning.

The contexts in which nurses practise can also profoundly shape how they engage in the interview process. To more consciously choose how you will practise requires that you develop the skill of reflectivity. Critical reflection is one of the central skills of relational practice, as discussed in Chapter 1. It involves "a combination of self-observation, critical scrutiny, and conscious participation … and paying attention to whom, how, and what you are doing in the moment" as you work with patients and families (Doane & Varcoe, 2005, p. 150). By paying attention to how you are acting and what you are feeling in any particular situation, you can begin to see how your behaviours and responses affect other people. By observing yourself and paying attention to your thoughts, emotions, tone of voice, facial expressions, posture, and bodily responses during the health assessment process, you will more consciously and intentionally choose how to act and respond.

Sending

You are probably most aware of *verbal* communication: the words you speak, vocalizations, the tone of voice. *Nonverbal* communication also occurs; this is your body language: posture, gestures, facial expression, eye contact, foot tapping, touch, what you do with your hands, even where you place your chair. Because nonverbal communication is under less conscious control than verbal communication, nonverbal communication is probably more reflective of your true feelings. A high degree of critical reflection is necessary to remain attuned to your nonverbal communication during the interview and physical examination.

Receiving

Being aware of the messages you send is only part of the process. Your words and gestures must be interpreted in a *specific context* in order to have meaning. You have a specific context in mind when you send your words. The receiver has his or her own interpretation of them. The receiver attaches meaning determined by his or her past experiences, social and family contexts, culture, and self-concept, as well as current physical and emotional states. Sometimes these contexts do not coincide. Remember how frustrating it may have been to try to communicate something to a friend, only to have your message totally misunderstood? Your message can be misinterpreted by the listener. Mutual understanding by the sender and receiver is necessary for communication to be successful.

Even greater risk for misunderstanding exists in the health care setting than in a social setting. In this setting, most patients have a health problem, and this factor emotionally charges your professional relationship. It *intensifies* the communication because the patient feels dependent on you to get better.

Communication and critical self-reflection are *foundational skills* that can be learned and continually improved over the course of your career. As a foundational skill, communication is as essential in high-quality health care as the tools of inspection, palpation, and diagnosis.

Attending to Power Differentials

Nurses and other health care providers are usually in a position of power in relation to patients and families (Doane & Varcoe, 2005). They usually have more knowledge about the health care system and have influence over the access that patients have to health care. Health care providers also have advantages such as education, language skills, and employment, which can position them as relatively powerful in relation to patients. At the same time, nurses and health care providers are also diverse in terms of their experiences, social contexts, knowledge, and so on. On an ongoing basis, it is important to be aware of how your power and privilege in relation to patients, families, and colleagues are reflected in the way you communicate, both verbally and nonverbally. You must continually assess how you may be using your power in relation to patients as you facilitate their access to the health care system.

Communication Skills

Cultivating the skills of relational practice during the interview involves particular communication skills. These skills include unconditional positive regard, empathy, and active listening.

Unconditional Positive Regard

One essential feature of effective communication is the ability to meet patients, individuals, and families with "unconditional positive regard" (Doane & Varcoe, 2005, p. 280). Although it may be challenging, you need to develop the skills and capacity to convey unconditional positive regard to engage therapeutically with people. This means a generally optimistic view of people: an assumption of their strengths and an acceptance of their limitations. An atmosphere of warmth and caring is necessary. The patient must feel that he or she is accepted unconditionally, even if you think he or she may be engaging in behaviours or making choices that seem to be unhealthy (Browne, Doane, Reimer, MacLeod, & McLellan, 2010). Conveying unconditional positive regard requires a high degree of self-reflectivity, particularly when patients or families seem to be making choices that have negative health effects.

The respect for other people extends to respect for their personal contexts and the way our society shapes people's health status. Your goal is not to make your patients dependent on you but to facilitate their capacity to manage their health. You are working toward promoting their growth. Pay attention to the cues you pick up from patients and families, and follow their lead. Be prepared to think critically about the various contexts that influence people's situations and decisions related to their health.

Empathy

Empathy means viewing the world from another person's inner frame of reference while remaining yourself. Empathy means recognizing and accepting the other person's feelings or actions without criticism; to do this, you must be aware of your own assumptions about the person. Empathy is described as "feeling *with* the person rather than feeling *like* the person." It does not mean you become lost in the other person at the expense of your own self. If this occurred, you would cease to be helpful. Rather, it is to *understand with* the person how he or she understands his or her world.

Active Listening

Listening is not a passive role in the communication process; it is active and demanding. Listening requires your complete attention. You cannot be preoccupied with your own thoughts, preoccupations, needs, or the needs of other patients, or you will miss something important. For the time of an interview, no one is more important than the patient. This person's needs are your sole concern.

Active listening is the route to understanding. You cannot be thinking of what you are going to say as soon as the patient stops for breath. A vast difference exists between listening and simply waiting to speak (Doane & Varcoe, 2005). Listen to *what* the patient says. The story may not come out in the order you would expect or will record it in later. Let the patient talk from his or her own outline; nearly everything that is said will be relevant. Listen to *the way* a patient tells the story, such as difficulty with language, impaired memory, the tone of the patient's voice, and even to what the patient is leaving out (Box 4-1).

Attending to the Physical Setting

Prepare the physical setting. As noted earlier, the setting may be a community health clinic, an outpatient department, a laneway or the street, a hospital room, an examination room an office or clinic, or the patient's home. In any location, optimal conditions are important for the completion of a smooth interview.

BOX 4-1 CLINICAL ILLUSTRATION

Sandra B., 32 years of age, sought care for headaches she had had during the past 3 months, which were unresponsive to aspirin and were interfering with her job. She was interviewed for 30 minutes. Through this time she never mentioned her husband, although they had been married only 5 months earlier. Finally, the examiner asked, "I haven't heard you mention your husband. Tell me about him." It turned out that Sandra's husband had lost his job a few months after they were married because of alcohol-related work errors. Although Sandra related extreme personal stress and worry, she never thought that her headaches might be related to the stressful situation.

Ensure Privacy

Aim for geographical privacy: ideally, a private space. This may involve asking other people who are in that space to step out for a while or finding an alternative unoccupied space. If geographical privacy is not available, "psychological privacy" by curtained partitions may suffice as long as the patient feels sure that no one can overhear the conversation or interrupt.

Refuse Interruptions

Most people resent interruptions except in cases of an emergency. Inform any support staff of your interview, and ask that they not interrupt you during this time. Discourage other health providers from interrupting you with *their* need for access to the patient. You need to concentrate and to establish rapport. An interruption can destroy in seconds what you have spent many minutes building up.

Physical Environment

- Set the room temperature at a comfortable level for the patient.
- Provide sufficient lighting so that you and the patient can see each other clearly. Do not position the patient directly in front of a strong light, in which case the patient must squint as if on stage.
- Reduce noise. Multiple stimuli are confusing. Turn off the television, radio, and any unnecessary equipment.
- Remove distracting objects or equipment. It is appropriate to leave some professional equipment (otoscope/ophthalmoscope, blood pressure manometer) in view. However, clutter, stacks of mail, files of other patients, and your lunch should not be visible. The room should convey the professional nature of the interviewer.
- Make the distance between you and the patient about 1.5 m (twice arm's length). If you place the patient any closer, you may invade his or her private space, which may create anxiety. If you place the patient farther away, you seem distant and aloof.
- Arrange equal-status seating. Both you and the patient should be comfortably seated, at eye level with each other. Avoid facing a patient across a desk or table because that feels like a barrier. Placing the chairs at a 90-degree angle

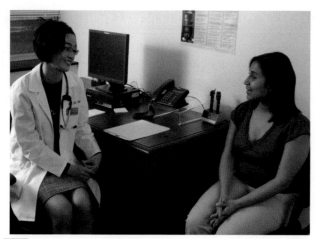

4-1 Equal-status seating.

allows the patient either to face you or to look straight ahead from time to time (Figure 4-1). Of most importance, avoid standing over the patient. Standing creates two negative effects: (a) It communicates your haste, and (b) it communicates your superiority. Standing makes you loom over the patient as an authority figure. When you are sitting, the opportunity to decrease the power differentials becomes more possible and facilitates the patient's sense of comfort and control in the setting.

- Arrange a face-to-face position when you interview a hospitalized, bedridden patient. The patient should not have to stare at the ceiling because this causes him or her to lose the visual message of your communication.

Dress

- The patient should remain in street clothes except in the case of an emergency.
- Your appearance and clothing should be appropriate to the setting and should meet conventional professional standards. Avoid extremes.

Taking Notes

Some use of history forms and note taking may be unavoidable. When you sit down later to record the interview, you cannot rely completely on memory to furnish details of previous hospitalizations or of the review of body systems, for example. Be sure to tell the patient in advance that you will probably take a few notes so that you can better keep track of and remember the information that the patient is conveying. Be aware that taking notes during the interview, however, has disadvantages:

- It breaks eye contact too often.
- It shifts your attention away from the patient, diminishing his or her sense of importance.
- It can interrupt the patient's narrative flow. You may say "Please slow down; I'm not getting it all." Or the patient may see you recording furiously, and in an effort to please you, adjust his or her tempo to your writing. Either way, the patient's natural mode of expression is lost.
- It impedes your observation of the patient's nonverbal behaviour.

- It is threatening to the patient during the discussion of sensitive issues (e.g., amount of alcohol and drug use, number of sexual partners, or incidence of emotional or physical abuse).

Thus keep note taking to a minimum, and try to focus your attention on the patient. Any recording you do should be secondary to the dialogue and should not interfere with the patient's spontaneity. With experience, you will not rely on taking notes as much.

Electronic Clinical Documentation

Technologies such as the electronic health record (EHR) are increasingly being used to record health histories and physical examination findings. EHRs and computer-assisted clinical documentation practices can influence interviewing practice in positive ways if used appropriately. For example, data can be shared more easily among the health care team, which would minimize redundancy (patients being asked the same questions by several members of the health care team). As with handwritten note taking, stay focused on the patient and convey that you are actively listening and interested in the patient's history.

Audio Recording

An audio recording documents everything that is said during the interview. You cannot refer to it as easily as you can to your notes, but the recording is an excellent teaching tool to study your abilities as an interviewer objectively. After listening, other students have made the following comments:

"I never realized how much I talked. I really dominated the patient."
"I need to watch my interrupting. I cut her off that time."
"There. That response really worked. She opened up. I want to be that effective more often."

Audio recordings demonstrate how you can improve your communication. In addition, as you gain experience, the recordings also document your advancing skills. This process can be very helpful.

A video or digital recording takes the teaching-learning tool one step further because you can study both verbal and nonverbal communication at the same time. Initial anxiety is common among students who feel self-conscious on camera, but the video recording can reveal richer detail in nonverbal behaviour.

"I must have crossed and uncrossed my legs 20 times! I never realized I did that. My fidgeting sure made Mr. J. look distracted."
"It was good that I leaned toward her and kept quiet when she paused that time. I think it helped her continue."
"My facial expression conveyed that I was judging her quite negatively when she told me about using street drugs. I really need to reflect critically on how I feel about drug use in pregnancy, so that I don't impose my judgements onto patients or make them feel they have to avoid telling me things."
"I talked for 5 minutes nonstop about how to perform a breast self-examination, without ever letting Mrs. S. ask a question!"

If you use any audio recording, some ethical considerations are necessary. Explain to the patient the purpose of the recording (whether for teaching, supervision, research), exactly who will hear it (you, your supervisor), and that it will then be destroyed. Obtain the patient's consent before you start, with particular attention to the confidentiality agreement that should be outlined in the consent form. Be thoroughly familiar with the equipment; fumbling with the controls is distracting. Arrange the microphone between you and the patient and place the rest of the recording equipment out of sight. It is likely that after a few moments, neither of you will be aware of the recording.

TECHNIQUES OF COMMUNICATION

Introducing the Interview

The patient is available, and you are ready for the interview. If you are nervous about how to begin, remember to keep the beginning short. The patient is probably nervous, too, and is anxious to start. Address the patient, using his or her surname, and shake hands if that seems comfortable. Introduce yourself, and state your role in the agency (if you are a student, say so). If you are gathering a complete history, give the reason for this interview:

> *"Mrs. Singh, I would like to talk about your illness that caused you to come to the hospital."*
> *"Roberta, I want to ask you some questions about your health so that we can identify what is keeping you healthy and explore any problems."*
> *"Mr. Craig, I want to ask you some questions about your health and your usual daily activities so that we can plan your care here in the hospital."*

If the patient is in the hospital, more than one health care team member may be documenting the history. Patients are apt to feel exasperated because they believe they are repeating the same thing unless you give a reason for this interview. You can also warn hospitalized patients that others will probably seek information from them on a frequent basis, so that they are not surprised by numerous requests for information or multiple attempts to document their history.

After this brief introduction, ask an open-ended question (see the following section), and then let the patient proceed. In some instances, and depending on the context of the patient you are interviewing, you may want to engage in a brief informal exchange as a way of building rapport. However, after a brief exchange, patients typically want to "get on" with discussing their health concerns. You will build rapport best by letting the patient discuss the concern as soon as possible in the interview process. See also the later section Cultural and Social Considerations, p. 59).

The Working Phase

The working phase is the data-gathering phase. Verbal skills for this phase include your questions to the patient and your responses to what the patient has said. Two general types of questions exist: open-ended and closed. Each type has a different place and function in the interview.

Open-Ended Questions

The **open-ended question** asks for narrative information. The topic to be discussed is stated, but only in general terms. Use it to begin the interview, to introduce a new section of questions, and whenever the patient introduces a new topic.

> *"Tell me how I can help you."*
> *"What brings you to the clinic (or hospital)?"*
> *"Tell me why you have come here today."*
> *"How have you been getting along?"*
> *"You mentioned shortness of breath. Tell me more about that."*
> *"How have you been feeling since your last appointment?"*
> *"What has been most challenging?"*
> *"What would you like to be able to do, change, or address?"*
> *"What stands out for you as really important for me to know about your situation?"*

The open-ended question leaves the patient free to answer in any way. This type of question encourages the patient to respond in paragraphs and to give a spontaneous account in any order chosen. It lets the patient express herself or himself fully.

As the patient answers, concentrate on how to *actively listen*. This will involve "listening to" and "listening for" particular things (Doane & Varcoe, 2005). For example, *listening to* involves attending to how people describe their health concerns in the larger context of their lives, observing their nonverbal communication, and understanding their beliefs about health and illness. *Listening for* involves learning what is of particular concern to patients and families, observing the emotions that people convey, and discerning the capacities and strengths that they have (which may be discussed tangentially). Also listen for things that patients may not be saying but seem relevant with regard to the other issues that have been raised or that you have observed.

What usually happens is that the patient answers with a short phrase or sentence, pauses, and then looks at you, expecting to receive some direction of how to go on. What you do next is the key to the interview. If you pose new questions on other topics, you may lose much of the initial story. Instead, respond to the first statement with "Tell me about it" or "Anything else?" or merely look acutely interested. The patient will then elaborate. Often, if you remain silent for several seconds before you respond with subsequent questions or comments, patients will continue to explain their situation. Remaining silent is challenging, inasmuch as most health care providers are socialized to rush to fill whatever silences that naturally occur in conversations.

Closed or Direct Questions

Closed or **direct questions** ask for specific information. They elicit a short one- or two-word answer, a "yes" or "no," or a forced choice. Whereas the open-ended question allows patients to answer in a way that is more appropriate for them, the direct question limits the answer (Table 4-1).

Use the direct questions after the patient's opening narrative to fill in any details that he or she left out. In addition,

TABLE 4-1	**Comparison of Open-Ended and Closed Questions**
Open-Ended	**Direct, Closed**
Used for narrative information	Used for specific information
Calls for longer answers	Calls for short (one- to two-word) answers
Elicits feelings, understandings, opinions, ideas	Elicits facts
Builds and enhances rapport	Limits rapport and leaves interaction neutral

use direct questions when you need many specific facts, such as when asking about past health problems or during the review of systems. Direct questions are also needed when you must complete the interview in a brief time. Asking all open-ended questions can yield unwieldy amounts of data. Be careful, however, not to overuse closed questions. Follow these guidelines:

1. Ask only one direct question at a time. Avoid opening the interview with closed-ended questions or bombarding the patient with long lists: "Have you ever had pain, double vision, watering, or redness in the eyes?" Avoid double-barrelled questions, such as "Do you exercise and follow a well-balanced diet?" The patient will not know which question to answer, and if the patient answers "yes," you will not know which question the patient has answered.

2. Use language that the patient understands. You may need to use regional phrases or colloquial expressions.

Responses: Assisting the Narrative

You have asked the first open-ended question, and the patient answers. As the patient talks, your role is to encourage free expression but not let the patient digress. Your responses help the teller amplify the story.

Some people seek health care for short-term or relatively simple needs. Their history is direct and uncomplicated; for these people, two responses (facilitation and silence) may be all you need to get a complete understanding of their situation. Other people have a complex story, a long history of interrelated chronic conditions, or complex emotional responses. Additional responses help you gather data without cutting them off.

There are nine types of verbal responses in all. The first five responses (facilitation, silence, reflection, empathy, clarification) involve your *reactions* to the facts or feelings the patient has communicated. Your response focuses on the patient's frame of reference. Your own frame of reference does not enter into the response. In the last four responses (confrontation, interpretation, explanation, summary), you start to express your *own* thoughts and feelings. The frame of reference shifts from the patient's perspective to yours. In the first five responses, the patient leads; in the last four responses, you lead.

Facilitation. These responses encourage the patient to say more, to continue with the story. Also called *general leads,*

these responses show the patient that you are interested and will listen further. Examples of verbal facilitation are "Mmm-hmm"; "Go on"; "Please continue"; and "Uh-huh." However, simply maintaining eye contact, shifting forward in your seat with increased attention, nodding affirmatively, or using your hand to gesture "Yes, go on, I'm with you" also encourages the patient to continue talking.

Silence. Silence is golden, so to speak, after open-ended questions. Your silent attentiveness communicates that the patient has time to think, to organize what he or she wishes to say without interruption from you. This "thinking silence" is the one health care providers interrupt most often. The interruption destroys the patient's train of thought. The patient is often interrupted because silence is uncomfortable to novice examiners. They feel responsible for keeping the dialogue going and believe they are at fault if it stops. Silence, however, has advantages. One advantage is letting the patient collect his or her thoughts. Also, silence gives you a chance to observe the patient unobtrusively and to note nonverbal cues. Finally, silence gives you time to plan your next approach.

Reflection. This response echoes the patient's words. Reflection is repeating part of what the patient has just said. In this example, it focuses further attention on a specific phrase and helps the patient continue in his own way:

> Patient: "I'm here because of my water. It was cutting off."
> Response: "It was cutting off?"
> Patient: "Yes, yesterday it took me 30 minutes to pass my water. Finally I got a tiny stream, but then it just closed off."

Reflection also can help express feeling behind a patient's words. The feeling is already in the statement. You focus on it and encourage the patient to elaborate:

> Patient: "It's so hard having to stay on bed rest with this pregnancy. I have two more little ones at home. I'm so worried they are not getting the care or attention they need."
> Response: "That's understandable—you may feel that you're not 'there' for your other children?"

Think of yourself as a mirror reflecting the patient's words or feelings. This encourages the patient to elaborate on the problem.

Empathy. A physical symptom, condition, or illness is often accompanied by specific emotions. Many people have trouble expressing these feelings, perhaps because of confusion or embarrassment. In the preceding reflecting example, the patient already had stated her feeling and you echoed it. In the following example, he has not said it yet. An empathic response relays recognition of a feeling and puts it into words. It names the feeling and allows the expression of it. When the empathic response is used, the patient feels accepted and can deal with the feeling openly:

> Patient [sarcastically]: "This is just great. I have my own business, I direct 20 employees every day and now here in hospital, I am having to call you for every little thing."
> Response: "It must be hard—one day having so much control, and now feeling dependent on someone else."

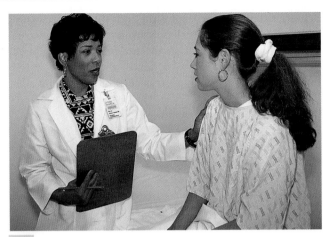

4-2

Your response does not cut off further communication, as would false reassurance ("Oh, you'll be back to work in no time"). Also, it does not deny the feeling and indicate that it is not justified ("Now I don't do *every*thing for you. Why, you are feeding yourself"). An empathic response recognizes the feeling, accepts it, and allows the patient to express it without embarrassment. It strengthens rapport. The patient feels understood, which by itself is therapeutic, because it eases the feelings of isolation brought on by illness. Other empathic responses are "This must be very hard for you"; "I understand"; and just placing your hand on the patient's arm (Figure 4-2).

Clarification. Use this when the patient's word choice is ambiguous or confusing (e.g., "Tell me what you mean by 'tired blood.'"). Clarification also is used to summarize the patient's words, to make them clearer by simplifying them, and then to ensure that you are on the right track. You are asking for agreement, and the patient can confirm or deny your understanding.

> Response: *"Now as I understand you, this heaviness in your chest comes when you shovel snow or climb stairs, and it goes away when you stop doing those things. Is that correct?"*
> Patient: *"Yes, that's pretty much it."*

Confrontation. Recall that in the last four responses (confrontation, interpretation, explanation, summary), the frame of reference shifts from the patient's perspective to yours. These responses now include your own thoughts and feelings. Use the last four responses only when merited by the situation. If you use them too often, you take over at the patient's expense. In the case of confrontation, you have observed a certain action, feeling, or statement, and you now focus the patient's attention on it. You provide your viewpoint about what you see or feel, but in an accepting, nonjudgemental manner. This may focus on a discrepancy ("You say it doesn't hurt, but when I touch you here, you grimace"), or it may focus on the patient's affect ("You *look* sad" or "You *sound* angry").

Interpretation. This statement is based not on direct observation, as is confrontation, but rather on your inference or conclusion. It links events, makes associations, or implies cause: "It seems that every time you feel the stomach pain, you have had some kind of stress in your life." Interpretation also ascribes feelings and helps the patient understand his or her own feelings in relation to the verbal message.

> Patient: *"I have decided I don't want to take any more treatments. But I can't seem to tell my doctor that. Every time she comes in, I tighten up and can't say anything."*
> Response: *"Could it be that you're afraid of her reaction?"*

You do run a risk of making the wrong inference. If this is the case, the patient will correct it. Even if the inference is corrected, however, interpretation helps prompt further discussion of the topic.

Explanation. With these statements, you give the patient information. You share factual and objective data. This information may be for orientation to the agency setting ("Your dinner comes at 5:30 P.M."), or it may be to explain cause ("The reason you cannot eat or drink before your blood test is that the food will affect the test results, and we would like to get as accurate a result as possible").

Summary. This is a final review of your understanding of what the patient has said. In summarizing, you condense the facts and present a survey of how you perceive the health problem or need. It is a type of validation in that the patient can agree with it or correct it. Both you and the patient should participate. When the summary occurs at the end of the interview, it signals that termination of the interview is imminent.

Ten Traps of Interviewing

The verbal skills just discussed are productive and enhance the interview. Now take time to consider nonproductive, defeating verbal messages, or *traps*. It is easy to fall into these traps because you are anxious to help. The danger is that they restrict the patient's response. The following traps are obstacles to obtaining complete data and to establishing rapport.

1. Providing False Assurance or Reassurance

A patient says, "Oh I just know this lump is going to turn out to be cancer." How do you react? The automatic response of many clinicians is to say, "Now don't worry; I'm sure you will be all right." This "courage builder" relieves *your* anxiety and gives you the false sense of having provided comfort. For the patient, however, it actually closes off communication. It trivializes her anxiety and effectively denies any further talk of it. (Also, it promises something that may not happen: that is, she may *not* be "all right"). Consider instead these responses:

> *"You are really worried about the lump, aren't you?"*
> *"It must be hard to wait for the biopsy results."*

These responses acknowledge the emotion and encourage more communication.

A genuine, valid form of reassurance does exist. You *can* reassure patients that you are listening to them, that you understand them, that you have hope for them, and that you will take care of them.

Patient: "I feel so lost here since they transferred me to the medical centre. No one comes to see me. No one here cares what happens to me."

Response: "I care what happens to you. I am here today, and I want you to know that I'll be here all week."

This type of reassurance makes a commitment to the patient, and it can have a powerful effect.

2. Giving Unwanted Advice

Know when to give advice and when to avoid giving it. Often, people seek health care because they want your professional advice and information on the management of a health problem: "My child has chicken pox; how should I take care of him?" This is a straightforward request for information that you have that the parent needs. You respond by giving a health prescription, a therapeutic plan that is based on your knowledge and experience.

In other situations, advice is different; it is based on a hunch or feeling. It is your personal opinion. Consider the woman who has just left a meeting with her consultant physician: "Dr. Kline just told me my only chance of getting pregnant is to have an operation. I just don't know. What would you do?" Does the woman really want your advice? An answer such as "If I were you, I'd…" is a mistake. You are not that woman. If you give this answer, you have shifted the accountability for decision making from her to you. She has not worked out her own solution. She has learned nothing about herself.

Does the woman really want to know what you would do? Probably not. Instead, a better response is reflection:

Response: "He said you should have an operation?"
Woman: "Yes, and I'm terrified of being put to sleep. What if I don't wake up?"

Now you know her *real* concern and can help her deal with it. She has expressed herself in the process and may be better equipped to meet her next decision.

When asked for advice, other preferred responses are as follows:

"What are the pros and cons of [this choice] for you?"
"What concerns do you have?"
"What is holding you back?"

Although it is quicker just to give advice, take the time to involve the patient in a problem-solving process. When a patient participates, he or she is more likely to learn and to change behaviour.

3. Using Authority

"Your doctor/nurse knows best" is a response that promotes dependency and inferiority. The communication pathway looks something like this:

Interviewer:

Patient:

You are talking "down," and little from the patient is going back "up." A better approach is to avoid using authority completely. Although you and the patient may not have equality of professional skill and experience, you do have equally worthy roles in the health process, each respecting the other.

4. Using Avoidance Language

People use euphemisms such as "passed on" to avoid reality or to hide their feelings. They think if they just say the word "died," it might really happen. Thus to "protect" themselves, they evade the issue. Although it seems this will make potentially fearful topics comfortable, it does not. Not talking about the fear does not make it go away; it just suppresses the fear and makes it even worse. Using direct language is the best way to deal with frightening topics.

5. Engaging in Distancing

Distancing is the use of impersonal speech to put space between a threat and the self: "My friend has a problem; she is afraid she…" or "There is a lump in the left breast." By using "the" instead of "my," the woman can deny any association with her diseased breast and not have to deal with it. Health care providers use distancing, too, to soften reality. This does not work because it communicates to the patient that you also are afraid of the procedure. The use of seemingly blunt-sounding specific terms actually is preferable for defusing anxiety.

6. Using Professional Jargon

What is called a *myocardial infarction* in the health care profession is called a *heart attack* by most laypeople. Use of jargon sounds exclusionary and paternalistic. You need to adjust your vocabulary to the patient but avoid sounding condescending.

If a patient uses medical jargon, do not assume he or she always knows the correct meaning. For example, some people think "hypertensive" means that they are very tense. As a result, they take their medication only when feeling stressed and not when they feel relaxed. This misinformation must be corrected. They need to understand that hypertension is a chronic condition that needs consistent medication to avoid side effects. On the other hand, you do not need to feel that it is imperative to correct all misstatements (e.g., when a patient says "prostrate" for "prostate gland").

7. Using Leading or Biased Questions

Asking a man "You don't smoke, do you?" implies that one answer is "better" than another. If the patient wants to please you, either he is forced to answer in a way corresponding to your values or he feels guilty when he must admit the other answer. He risks your judgement and disapproval. If he feels dependent on you for care, he does not want to alienate you.

8. Talking Too Much

Some examiners positively associate helpfulness with verbal productivity. If the air has been thick with their oratory and advice, these examiners leave thinking they have met the patient's needs. Just the opposite is true. Anxious to please the examiner, the patient lets the examiner talk at the expense of his or her need to express himself or herself. A good rule for every interviewer is to *listen more than talk.*

9. Interrupting

Often, when you think you know what the patient will say, you interrupt and cut the patient off. This does not show that you are clever. Rather, it signals that you are impatient or bored with the interview. A related trap is preoccupation with yourself by thinking of your next remark while the patient is talking. The communication pathway looks like this:

Patient: → *Interviewer:* →

As the patient speaks, you are thinking about what to say next. Thus you cannot fully understand what the patient says. You are so preoccupied with your own role as the interviewer that you are not really listening. Aim for a second of silence between the patient's statement and your next response. Ideally, your communication pathway should look like this:

Patient: ↔ *Interviewer:* ↔

with two people talking, and two people listening.

10. Using "Why" Questions

Be careful when using "why" questions. Asking someone "Why were you so late for your appointment?" implies blame and condemnation; it puts the patient on the defensive. Instead, consider reframing your query in a more open-ended manner, such as "I noticed that you were delayed getting here, and I'm wondering how things are going for you?" The latter conveys your intention to inquiry about the circumstances of the person's life, which will provide important contextual information pertinent to the health assessment.

Consider your use of "why" questions in the health care setting; for example, "Why did you take so much medication?" or "Why did you wait so long before coming to the hospital?" The only possible answer to a "why" question is "Because…," and the patient may not know the answer; he or she may not have reasoned it through. You sound accusatory and judgemental. The patient now must produce an excuse to rationalize his or her own behaviour. To avoid this trap, say: "I see you started to have chest pains early in the day. What was happening between the time the pains started and the time you came to the emergency department?"

Nonverbal Skills

Learn to observe with your eyes, as well as with your ears. Nonverbal modes of communication include physical appearance, posture, gestures, facial expression, eye contact, voice, and touch. Nonverbal messages are very important in establishing rapport and in conveying information, especially about feelings. Nonverbal messages provide clues to understanding feelings. When nonverbal and verbal messages are congruent, the verbal message is reinforced. When they are incongruent, the nonverbal message tends to be the true one, because it is under less conscious control.

Physical Appearance

In his classic work *The Stress of Life,* Hans Selye (1956) reported that his interest in the body's total response to stress began when he was a student. Unbiased as yet by medical knowledge, he noted that some patients just "looked sick," even though they did not exhibit the specific characteristic signs that would lead to a precise medical diagnosis. Such people simply felt and looked ill or feverish. The same view can work for you. Inattention to dressing or grooming suggests that the patient is too sick to maintain self-care or has an emotional dysfunction such as depression. Choice of clothing also sends a message, projecting such varied images as role (student, worker, or professional) or attitude (casual, suggestive, or rebellious).

Your own appearance sends a message to the patient. Professional dress varies among agencies and settings. Depending on the setting, the use of a professional uniform may create a positive stereotype (comfort, expertise, or ease of identification) or a negative stereotype (distance, authority, or formality). Whatever your personal choice in clothing or grooming, the aim should be to convey a competent, professional image.

Posture

Note the patient's position. An open position with extension of large muscle groups shows relaxation, physical comfort, and a willingness to share information. A closed position with arms and legs crossed looks defensive and anxious. Note any change in posture. If a patient in a relaxed position suddenly tenses, it suggests discomfort with the new topic.

Your own calm, relaxed posture creates a feeling of warmth and trust and conveys an interest in the patient. Standing and hastily filling out a history form with periodic peeks at your watch communicates that you are busy with many things more important than interviewing the patient. Even when your time is limited, appear calm and unhurried. Sit down, even if it is only for a few minutes, and look as if nothing else matters except the patient.

Gestures

Gestures send messages. For example, nodding or an open turning out of the hand shows acceptance, attention, or agreement. A wringing of the hands often indicates anxiety. Pointing a finger occurs with anger and vehemence. Also, hand gestures can reinforce a patient's description of pain. When a crushing substernal chest pain is described, the patient often holds the hand twisted into a fist in front of the sternum; pain that is intense and sharply localized may be indicated by one finger pointing to the exact spot: "It hurts right here."

Facial Expression

The face reflects a wide variety of relevant emotions and conditions. The expression may look alert, relaxed, and interested, or it may look anxious, angry, and suspicious. Physical conditions such as pain or shortness of breath also show in the expression.

Your own expression should reflect a professional who is attentive, sincere, and interested in the patient. Any expression of boredom, distraction, disgust, criticism, or disbelief is picked up by the other patient, and rapport dissolves.

Eye Contact

Lack of eye contact in some situations or contexts suggests that the patient is shy, withdrawn, confused, bored, intimidated, apathetic, or depressed. This applies to examiners, too. You should aim to maintain eye contact, but do not "stare down" the patient. Maintain not a fixed, penetrating look but rather an easy gaze toward the patient's eyes, with occasional glances away. One exception to this is when you are interviewing someone from a particular ethnocultural group whose members may frequently avoid direct eye contact (see the section Cultural and Social Considerations).

Voice

Besides the spoken words, meaning is expressed through the tone of voice, the intensity and rate of speech, the pitch, and any pauses. These are just as important as words in conveying meaning. For example, the tone of a patient's voice may indicate sarcasm, disbelief, judgement, sympathy, or hostility. An anxious patient often speaks in a loud, fast voice. A soft voice may indicate shyness, fear, or lack of confidence in one's self. A hearing-impaired patient may use a loud voice.

Even the use of pauses conveys meaning. When your question is straightforward, a patient's long, unexpected pause indicates that the patient is taking time to think of an answer. Unusually frequent and long pauses, when combined with speech that is slow and monotonous and a weak, breathy voice, may indicate depression.

Touch

The meaning of physical touch is influenced by the patient's age, gender, family norms, cultural and social backgrounds, past experience, and current setting. The meaning of touch is easily misinterpreted. In most Western cultures, physical touch is reserved for expressions of love and affection or for clearly defined acts of greeting (for example, shaking hands). Do not use touch during the interview unless you know the patient well and are sure how the patient will interpret it. When appropriate, touch communicates effectively, such as a touch of the hand or arm to signal empathy.

In sum, an examiner's nonverbal messages that are productive and enhancing to the relationship are those that show attentiveness and unconditional acceptance. Defeating, nonproductive nonverbal behaviours are those of inattentiveness, authority, and superiority (Table 4-2).

Closing the Interview

The session should end gracefully. An abrupt or awkward closing can destroy rapport and leave the patient with a negative impression of the whole interview. To ease into the closing, ask the patient questions such as the following:

TABLE 4-2	Nonverbal Behaviours of the Interviewer
Positive	**Negative**
Professional appearance is appropriate to the context	Appearance objectionable to patient
Equal-status seating	Standing
Close proximity to patient	Sitting behind desk, far away, turned away
Relaxed open posture	Tense posture
Leaning slightly toward patient	Slouched back
Occasional facilitating gestures	Critical or distracting gestures: pointing finger, clenched fist, finger tapping, foot swinging, looking at watch
Facial animation, interest	Bland expression, yawning, tight mouth
Appropriate smiling	Frowning, lip biting
Appropriate eye contact	Shifty, avoiding eye contact, focusing on notes, computer screen, iPad, etc
Moderate tone of voice	Strident, high-pitched tone
Moderate rate of speech	Rate too slow or too fast
Appropriate use of touch, depending on the context	Too frequent or inappropriate touch

"Is there anything else you would like to mention?"
"Are there any questions you would like to ask?"
"Are there any other areas I should have asked about?"

This gives the patient the final opportunity for self-expression. Then, to indicate that closing is imminent, say something like "Our interview is just about over." No new topic should be introduced now. This is a good time to give your summary or a recapitulation of what you have learned during the interview. The summary is a final statement of what you and the patient agree the health state to be. It should include positive health aspects, any health problems that have been identified, any plans for action, or an explanation of the subsequent physical examination. As you part from patients, thank them for the time spent and for their participation.

DEVELOPMENTAL CONSIDERATIONS

Interviewing Parents

When your patient is a child, you must build rapport with two people: the child and the accompanying parent. Greet both by name, but with a younger child (1 to 6 years old), focus more on the parent. By ignoring the child temporarily, you allow the child to size you up from a safe distance. The child can observe your interaction with the parent, see that the parent accepts and likes you, and relax (Figure 4-3).

Begin by interviewing the parent and child together. If any sensitive topics arise (e.g., the parents' troubled relationship

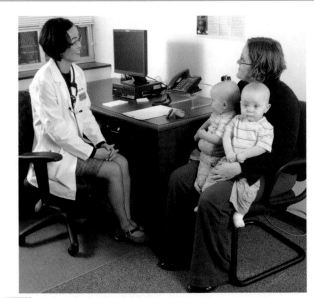

4-3

or the child's problems at school or with peers), explore them with the parent later when he or she is alone. Provide toys to occupy the child as you and the parent talk. This frees the parent to concentrate on the history. Also, the child's play can reveal the level of attention span or independent play. Through the interview, be alert to ways the parent and child interact. The history provides an ideal time to integrate discussion points related to health promotion and prevention, as noted in Chapter 2.

For younger children, the parent will provide all or most of the history. Thus you are collecting the child's health data from the parent's frame of reference. This viewpoint is usually reliable because most parents have the child's well-being as a priority and view cooperation with you as a way to enhance this well-being. The possibilities for parental bias, however, exist. Bias can occur when parents are asked to describe the child's achievements or whenever their own parenting ability seems called into question. For example, saying, "His fever was 39.5 and you did not bring him in?" implies a lack of parenting skill. This puts the parent on the defensive and increases anxiety. Instead, use open-ended questions that increase description and defuse threat, such as "What happened when the fever went up?"

A parent with more than one child has more than one set of data to remember. Be patient as the parent sorts through his or her memory to recall facts of developmental milestones or the history. A comprehensive history may be lacking if the child is accompanied by a family friend or day care provider instead of the parent.

When you collect developmental data, avoid being judgemental about the age at achievement of certain milestones. This can be an opportune time to pose open-ended questions to parents about health promotion and prevention issues, such as "How does Miriam like wearing her bike helmet?" Parents are understandably proud of their child's achievements and are sensitive to inferences that these milestones may occur late. Refer to the child by name, not as "the baby."

Refer to the parent by name and not the label "Mother" or "Dad." Also, be clear when identifying the parents. The mother's current husband may not necessarily be the child's father. Instead of asking about "your husband's" health, ask, "Is Joan's father in good health?"

Although most of your communication is with the parent, do not ignore the child completely. You need to make contact to ease into the physical examination later. Begin by asking about the toys the child is playing with or about a special doll or teddy bear brought from home: "Does your doll have a name?" or "What can your truck do?" Stoop down to meet the child at his or her eye level. Adult size can be threatening to young children and can emphasize their smallness.

Nonverbal communication is even more important to children than it is to adults. Children are quick to pick up feelings, anxiety, or comfort from nonverbal cues. Keep your physical appearance neat and clean, and avoid formal uniforms that distance you. Keep your gestures slow, deliberate, and close to your body. Children are frightened by quick or grandiose gestures. Do not try to maintain constant eye contact; this feels threatening to a small child. Use a quiet, measured voice, and choose simple words in your speech. Considering the child's level of language development is valuable in planning your communication.

Infants

Nonverbal communication is the primary method. Most infants look calm and relaxed when all their needs are met, and they cry when they are frightened, hungry, tired, or uncomfortable. They respond best to firm, gentle handling and a quiet, calm voice. Your calm voice is comforting, even though they do not understand the words. Older infants have anxiety toward strangers. They are more cooperative when the parent is kept in view.

Preschoolers

A 2- to 6-year-old is egocentric. He or she sees the world mostly from his or her own point of view: Everything revolves around him or her. Citing the example of another child's behaviour may not get the child to cooperate; it has no meaning. Only the child's own experience is relevant. Preschoolers' communication is direct, concrete, literal, and set in the present. Avoid figurative expressions such as "climbing the walls" because they are easily misinterpreted by young children. Use short, simple sentences with a concrete explanation. Take time to give a short, simple explanation for any unfamiliar equipment that will be used to examine the child. Preschoolers can have *animistic* thinking about unfamiliar objects. They may imagine that unfamiliar inanimate objects can come alive and have human characteristics (e.g., that a blood pressure cuff can wake up and bite or pinch).

School-Age Children

Children 7 to 12 years old can tolerate and understand others' viewpoints. Such children are more objective and realistic.

They want to know functional aspects: how things work and why things are done.

Children of this age group have the verbal ability to add important data to the history. Interview the parent and child together, but when the child has a presenting symptom or sign, ask the child about it first and then gather data from the parent. For the well child seeking a checkup, pose questions about school, friends, or activities directly to the child.

Adolescents

Adolescents want to be adults, but they do not yet have the cognitive ability to achieve their goal. They are between two stages. Sometimes they are capable of mature actions, and other times they revert to childhood response patterns, especially in times of stress. You cannot treat adolescents as children, but you cannot overcompensate and assume that their communication style, learning ability, and motivation are consistently at an adult level.

Adolescents value their peers. They crave acceptance and sameness with their peers. Most adolescents think no adult can understand them. Because of this, some act with aloof contempt, answering only in monosyllables. Some others make eye contact and tell you what they think you want to hear, but inside they are thinking, "You'll never know the full story about me."

This knowledge about adolescents is apt to paralyze you in communicating with them. However, successful communication is possible and rewarding. The guidelines are simple.

The first consideration is your attitude, which must be one of respect. Respect is the most important thing you can communicate to an adolescent. Adolescents need to feel validated as a human being, accepted, and worthy.

Second, your communication must be totally honest. An adolescent's intuition is highly tuned and can detect phoniness or when information is withheld. Always give them the truth, or you will lose their trust. They will cooperate if they understand your rationale.

Stay in character. Avoid using language or colloquialisms that are not part of your usual way of interacting. It is helpful to understand some of the jargon used by adolescents, but you cannot use those words yourself simply to try to bond with the adolescent. Do not try to be his or her peer. You are not, and the patient will not accept you as such.

Use conversational icebreakers. Focus first on the adolescent, not on the problem. Although an adult often wants to talk about the health concern immediately, the adolescent responds best when the focus is on him or her as a person. Show an interest in the adolescent. Ask open-ended, friendly questions about school, activities, hobbies, friends, and bullying. For example, to explore issues of bullying, you could ask, "You seem to be feeling sick a lot and want to stay home. Tell me a bit more about that." Refrain from asking questions about parents and family for now; these issues can be emotionally charged during adolescence.

Do not assume that adolescents know *anything* about a health interview or a physical examination. Explain every step, and give the rationale for each step. They need direction.

They will cooperate when they know the reason for the questions or actions. Encourage their questions. Adolescents are afraid they will sound "dumb" if they ask a question to which they assume everybody else knows the answer.

Keep your questions short and simple. "Why are you here?" sounds brazen to you, but it is effective with adolescents. Be prepared for the adolescent who does *not* know why he or she is there. Some adolescents are pushed into coming to the examination by a parent.

The communication responses described for adults must be reconsidered in talking with adolescents. Silent periods usually are best avoided. Giving adolescents a little time to collect their thoughts is acceptable, but a silence for other reasons is threatening. Also, avoid reflection. If you use reflection, the adolescent is likely to answer, "What?" They just do not have the cognitive skills to respond to that indirect mode of questioning. Also, adolescents are more sensitive to nonverbal communication than are adults. Be aware of your expressions and gestures. Adolescents are also more sensitive to any comment that can be interpreted as criticism from you and will withdraw.

Later in the interview, after you have developed rapport with the adolescent, you can address the topics that are emotionally charged, including alcohol and drug use, sexual behaviours, suicidal thoughts, and depression. Adolescents assume that health care providers have similar values and standards of behaviour as most of the other authority figures in their lives, and they may be reluctant to share this information. You can assure them that your questions are not intended to be curious or intrusive but cover topics that are important for most teenagers and on which you have relevant health information to share.

If confidential material is uncovered during the interview, consider what can remain confidential and what you feel you must share for the well-being of the adolescent. Provincial and territorial laws vary with regard to confidentiality requirements with minors; several provinces (but not all) observe the "mature minors rule," and health care providers are not required to notify parents about, for example, birth control or treatment for sexually transmitted infections. However, if the adolescent talks about an abusive home situation, state that you must share this information with other health care providers for his or her own protection. Ask the adolescent, "Do you have a problem with that?" and then discuss it. Tell the adolescent, "You will need to trust that I will handle this information professionally and in your best interest."*

Finally, take every opportunity to provide positive reinforcement. Praise every action regarding the health-promoting activities in which they are engaged: "That's great that you aren't smoking cigarettes [or that you've cut down on the number of cigarettes you are smoking]. I realize that's not

---

*As discussed in more detail in Chapter 8 (Interpersonal Violence Assessment), in Canada, all provinces have mandatory requirements for reporting suspected child abuse or other forms of abuse. If you suspect that a child is being maltreated or is at risk of maltreating others, you should involve other members of the health care team. You should be familiar with your legal obligations in the jurisdiction in which you work.

easy, but it's going to have a good impact on your health. And it may save you money as well."

Older Adults

Older adult have the developmental task of reviewing their accomplishments, reflecting on the purpose of their lives, and adjusting to the inevitability of death. Some people have developed comfortable and satisfying answers and greet you with a calm demeanour and self-assurance. Be alert for the occasional patient who sounds hopeless and despairing about life at present and in the future. Symptoms of illness are even more frightening when they mean physical limitation or threaten independence.

Always address the patient by the last name (e.g., "Hello, Mr. Choi"; "Good morning, Mrs. Smith"). Some older adults resent being called by their first name by younger persons, and almost all cringe at the ignominious "Grandma" or "Pop."

The interview usually takes longer with older adults because they have a longer story to tell. You may need to break up the interview into more than one visit, collecting the most important historical data first. Another possibility is for certain portions of the data, such as history or the review of systems, to be provided on a form that is filled out at home, as long as the patient's vision and handwriting are adequate. Take time to review these parts with the patient during the interview.

It is important to adjust the pace of the interview to older patients. Older patients have a great amount of background material to sort through, and this takes some time. Also, some older patients need a greater amount of response time to interpret the question and process their answer. Avoid trying to hurry them along. This approach only affirms their stereotype of younger persons in general and health care providers in particular: that is, people who are merely interested in numbers of patients and filling out forms. Any urge from you to "get on with it" will surely make them retreat. You will lose valuable data, and their needs will not be met (Figure 4-4).

Consider physical limitations when you plan the interview. An older patient may fatigue earlier and may require that the interview be broken up into shorter segments. For the patient

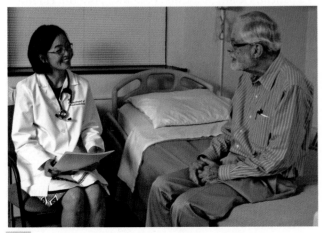

4-4

with impaired hearing, face him or her directly so that your mouth and face are fully visible. Do not shout; it does not help and actually distorts speech.

Touch is a nonverbal skill that is very important to many older patients. Their other senses may be diminished, and touch grounds them in reality. Also, a hand on the arm or shoulder is an empathic message that communicates that you empathize with the patient and want to understand his or her problem (see the section Cultural and Social Considerations for exceptions).

INTERVIEWING IN CHALLENGING SITUATIONS

Patients With Hearing Impairment

Although many patients tell you in advance that they have a hearing deficit, in others it must be recognized from clues, such as staring at your mouth and face, not attending unless looking at you, or speaking in a voice unusually loud or with guttural or garbled sounds. The deaf patient may be familiar with some equipment in the hospital or office setting or may have had previous experience with health care settings. Without full communication, however, the patient with hearing impairment is sure to feel isolated and anxious. Ask his or her preferred way to communicate: by signing, lip-reading, or writing. The use of assistive devices such as PockeTalker may be useful in some situations. The Pocke-Talker is frequently used in Canadian hospitals to foster communication with individuals who have hearing impairment.

A complete health history requires a sign language interpreter. Because most health care providers are not proficient in signing, try to find an interpreter through a social service agency or the patient's own social network. You may use family members, but be aware that they sometimes edit for the patient. Use the same guidelines as for the bilingual interpreter (see the section Working With [and Without] an Interpreter).

If the patient prefers lip-reading, be sure to face him or her squarely and have good lighting on your face. A beard, a moustache, or a foreign accent is less effective with such communication. Do not exaggerate your lip movements because this distorts your words. Similarly, shouting distorts the reception of a hearing aid that a patient may wear. Speak slowly, and supplement your voice with appropriate hand gestures or pantomime. Nonverbal cues are important adjuncts because the lip-reader understands at best only 50% of your speech when relying solely on vision. Be sure that the patient understands your questions. Many people with hearing impairment nod "yes" just to be friendly and cooperative but really do not understand.

Written communication is efficient in sections such as health history or review of systems. For the history of the current illness, writing is very time consuming and laborious. The syntax of the patient's written words is normal if the hearing impairment occurred after speech patterns developed. If the deafness occurred before speech patterns developed, the written syntax follows that of signing, which is different from that of English.

Acutely Ill Patients

An emergency necessitates your prompt action. You must combine interviewing with physical examination skills to determine life-saving actions. Although life support measures may be paramount, try to interview the patient as much as possible nonetheless. Subjective data are crucial for determining the cause and course of the emergency. Abbreviate your questioning. Identify the main area of distress and question about that. Family or friends often can provide important data.

A hospitalized patient with a critical or severe illness is usually too weak, too short of breath, or in too much pain to talk. First attend to the comfort of the patient. Then establish a priority; find out immediately what parts of the history are the most relevant. Explore the first concern the patient mentions. Begin to use closed, direct questions earlier. Finally, ensure that your statements are clear. When a patient is very sick, even the simplest sentence can be misconstrued. The patient will react according to preconceived ideas about what a serious illness means, so anything you say should be direct and precise.

Patients Under the Influence of Alcohol or Drugs

Patients under the influence of alcohol or other mood-altering drugs or substances are commonly admitted to a hospital; all these drugs affect the central nervous system, increasing the risk for accidents and injuries. Also, chronic use creates complex medical problems that necessitate increasingly critical care.

As discussed in Chapter 7, there are various kinds of drugs that people may use, including alcohol, and people may use multiple kinds of substances. A wide range of patient behaviours may be influenced by these substances. Alcohol and the opioids (heroin, meperidine, oxycodone, hydromorphone, dextropropoxyphene) are central nervous system depressants. Stimulants of the central nervous system (cocaine, methamphetamine, amphetamine) can cause an intense high, agitation, and paranoid behaviour. Hallucinogens can cause irrational, erratic, and inappropriate behaviour.

When interviewing a patient currently under the influence of alcohol or illicit drugs, ask simple and direct questions. Take care to make your manner and questions nonthreatening, and convey a nonjudgemental attitude. Avoid confrontation at this time. Furthermore, avoid any display of scolding or negative judgement such as disappointment or disgust, instead, remember that people use substances because of their life contexts, and you may not have a complete picture of the patient's life context. Conveying negative judgements will probably cause the patient to avoid subsequent contact with the health care system. One priority is to find out what time the patient last drank alcohol and how much he or she drank at that episode, or the name and amount of other substances taken. This information helps you assess any withdrawal patterns and needs for support. To ensure safety for your patient, seek assistance from your colleagues as needed to address the patient's issues.

Once the effects of the substances have worn off, a follow-up assessment should be performed to assess the extent of the problem and the meaning of the problem for the patient and family. Initially, the patient may exhibit denial and increased defensiveness; special interview techniques will probably be needed, as discussed in Chapter 7.

Personal Questions

On occasion, patients ask you questions about your personal life or opinions, such as "Are you married?"; "Do you have children?"; or "Do you smoke?" You do not need to answer every question. You may supply brief information when you feel it is appropriate, but be sensitive to the possibility that there may be a motive behind the personal questions such as loneliness or anxiety. Try directing your response back to the patient's frame of reference. You might say something like "No, I don't have children; I wonder if your question is related to how I can help you care for little Jamie?"

Dealing With Sexual Advances

On some occasions, personal questions extend to flirtatious compliments, seductive innuendo, or advances. Your response must make it clear that you are a health care provider who can best care for the patient by maintaining a professional relationship. At the same time, you should communicate that you accept the patient and you understand the patient's need to be self-assertive but that you cannot tolerate sexual advances. This may be difficult, considering that the patient's words or gestures may have left you surprised, embarrassed, or angry. Your feelings are normal. You need to set appropriate verbal boundaries by saying, "I am uncomfortable when you talk to me that way; please don't." A further response that would open communication is "I wonder if the way you're feeling now relates to your illness or to being in the hospital?"

Crying

A novice examiner usually feels very concerned when a patient starts crying. Crying, however, is actually a big relief to a patient. Health problems come with powerful emotions. Keeping worries about illness, death, or loss bottled up inside takes a great amount of energy. When you say something that "makes the patient cry," do not presume that you have hurt the patient. You have just addressed a topic that is important. Do not go on to a new topic. Just let the patient cry and express his or her feelings fully. You can offer a tissue and wait until the crying subsides to talk. The patient will regain control soon.

Sometimes your patient looks as if he or she is on the verge of tears but is trying hard to suppress them. Again, instead of moving on to something new, acknowledge the expression by saying, "You look sad." Do not worry that you will open an uncontrollable floodgate. The patient may cry but will be relieved, and you will have gained insight to a serious concern (Box 4-2).

BOX 4-2 CLINICAL ILLUSTRATION

Alice P., a 49-year-old woman, has a history of long-term problematic alcohol use. Her skin colour is jaundiced and she has entered a substance use treatment facility. Today, she is seeing you for a pelvic examination and Papanicolaou (Pap) smear.

Alice: "I haven't had a pelvic exam in 5 years. I had a hysterectomy 18 years ago. They said I had 'preinvasive' cancer cells." [At this, Alice's lips fold in, her eyes squeeze shut; she puts hand to mouth, and breathes in audibly in jerks.]

Response: "Alice, you look sad." [Examiner puts hand on Alice's upper arm.]

Alice: [crying freely now]: "What if you find more cancer now? They can't operate on me with my liver so big. I'd never survive the anaesthesia. And my father died of cancer. He had cirrhosis too, and they opened him up and he was full of cancer. He never woke up from surgery, and he died 2 weeks later."

Response: "I understand how worried you are. I think you have done the right thing to come in to this treatment centre. That took courage. As for today, let's take one step at a time. Today we need to do the pelvic exam and Pap smear. There is no reason today to assume you need an operation. I'll do your exam today, and I'll be here all week. We'll work together to help you get through this."

Alice: [breathing deeply, sitting up straight, arms down and open at sides, making eye contact]: "All right. I'm better now. Let's go ahead."

Anger

On occasion, you will try to interview a patient who is already angry. Try not to personalize this anger; usually it does not relate to you. The patient is showing aggression as a response to his or her own feelings of anxiety or helplessness. Do ask about the anger and hear the patient out. Deal with the angry feelings before you ask anything else. An angry patient cannot be an effective participant in a health interview.

Maybe, because of an unrelated incident, *you* are angry when you come into an interview. When you are angry, say so and tell the patient that you are angry at something or someone else. Otherwise the patient, unusually vulnerable and dependent on you, thinks you are angry at him or her.

Threat of Violence

The health care setting is not immune to violent behaviour. An individual may act with such angry gestures that you feel a threat to your personal safety. Other troubling behaviours of a potentially disruptive patient include fist clenching, pacing back and forth, a vacant stare, confusion, statements indicating that the patient is out of touch with reality, statements that do not make sense, a history of recent substance use (alcohol, hallucinogen, cocaine), or perhaps even a recent

history of intense bereavement (loss of spouse, loss of job). Trust your instincts. If you sense any suspect or threatening behaviour, act immediately to defuse the situation. Leave the examining room door open and position yourself between the patient and the door. Many departments have a prearranged sign or signal so that a coworker can call 911 and the security department to send help to the setting. Do not raise your own voice or try to argue with a threatening patient. Act quite calm, and talk to the patient in a soft voice. Convey respect for the patient, even if he or she is agitated or expressing frustration toward you. Act interested in what the patient is saying, and behave in an unhurried way. Your most important goal is safety; avoid taking any risks.

Anxiety

Finally, take it for granted that nearly all sick people have some anxiety. This is a normal response to being sick. It makes some people aggressive and others dependent. Remember that the patient is not reacting as typically as when he or she is healthy. When people are anxious, it is important for you to convey acceptance and patience.

CULTURAL AND SOCIAL CONSIDERATIONS

COMMUNICATING ACROSS CULTURES

When people attempting to communicate are from different cultural and social backgrounds, the probability of miscommunication can increase. Verbal and nonverbal communications are influenced by the cultural, social, and family backgrounds of both the health care provider and the patient. Cross-cultural or intercultural communication refers to the communication process occurring between a health care provider and a patient, each with different cultural, social, and historical backgrounds, in which both attempt to understand the other's point of view (Figure 4-5).

Relational practice requires that you connect across differences by relating with people as they are and where they are, no matter what their context, decisions, or life history (Doane & Varcoe, 2005). Nonetheless, you may sometimes find it challenging to relate to or communicate with patients or family members for a variety of reasons. Some people may be living with problematic substance use issues, or they may be harming themselves or others through violence, abuse, or neglect. Communicating with people whose primary language is different from yours may be challenging. In all situations, you need to be highly reflective about your reactions, assumptions, biases, and judgements so that you can be conscious of how you are relating to people, rather than reacting on the basis of habit.

It is particularly important to establish effective communication with people whose primary language is different from yours. Unfortunately, the current patchwork of interpreter services and different levels of understanding about the importance of effective communication in health care have led to inconsistencies in how language barriers are addressed in health care settings (Hoen, Nielsen, & Sasso, 2006). Studies

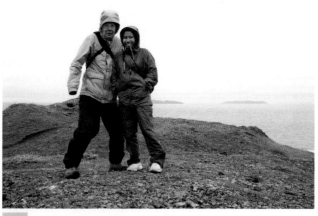

4-5

have repeatedly shown that access to health care and the quality of health services are seriously compromised without interpretation services for patients who need them. For example, nursing and medical errors such as misdiagnosis and inappropriate treatment, inadequate patient comprehension, and higher rates of readmission and emergency room visits can result from poor communication (Anderson et al., 2003; Hoen et al., 2006; Tang, 1999).

As discussed in Chapter 3, people whose proficiency in English and French is limited and who therefore speak one or more languages other than English or French should, ideally, be offered an interpreter who is *not* a family member or friend. In some contexts and urgent situations, an interpreter may not be available, and family or friends or members of the health care team may need to translate. In either case, it is essential to determine and document whether the patient (and the family) fully understand what is happening; what the diagnosis and the implications of this diagnosis are; what procedures, diagnostic and therapeutic, are going to be performed, how the procedures will be performed, and what they mean; how medications are to be taken and when; and the prognosis derived from the given problems. Strategies for working effectively with (and without) an interpreter are discussed later in this chapter.

Perspectives on Professional Interactions

The way you interact with patients and families will vary relationally, depending on their and your social, ethnocultural, and historical contexts. Some patients may nod their head in the affirmative or smile a lot to fulfill their assumptions about what is required of "good patients." In this situation, you may need to invite the patient to respond frankly to your suggestions or by giving the patient "permission" to disagree.

Etiquette

Etiquette refers to the diverse patterns of interaction that are considered to be appropriate in some (although certainly not all) social, familial, or ethnocultural contexts. For example, some people expect you to engage in conversation of a

personal or social nature before they feel comfortable entering into the more personal and intimate aspects of the health history and physical examination. Some people place a high value on developing interpersonal relationships and getting to know about a patient's family, personal concerns, and interests before they allow you to interact therapeutically.

Recognizing that time constraints frequently affect the social interchange expected by some individuals and from some cultures, you should strive to incorporate the patient's interactional style and needs with the health history data categories. For example, using a conversational tone of voice, you might begin the health history by inquiring about the patient's family members and their health.

You should be prepared for the converse; that is, some people may want to interview *you.* They may ask questions about your family, marital status, salary, home address, telephone number, and so forth. You need to determine your level of comfort in responding to these questions, but it is respectful to reply to some of the patient's questions. Remember that you are not obligated to answer questions that you deem too personal, and you always have a right to protect your personal safety. For example, you must *never* provide your home address, e-mail address, or telephone number. Rather, you should provide the patient with the business number of the hospital, clinic, or agency. If you want the patient to be able to contact you while you are at home, you should ask a secretary or other third party at the health care facility to call your home number. You may want to consider in advance which categories of questions you are willing to discuss and which ones you will politely decline to discuss. The manner in which you reply to personal inquiries should be carefully worded, sensitive to the needs of the patient, and congruent with your own needs and comfort level.

When you meet a patient for the first time, it is best to be relatively formal, respectful, and polite. Unless a physical disability or handicap prevents you from doing so, you should be standing when you first greet the patient and those accompanying him or her. Another aspect of etiquette concerns the use of names and titles. To establish a mutually respectful relationship, you should introduce yourself and indicate to the patient how you prefer to be called: that is, by first name, last name, and title. You should elicit the same information from the patient because this enables you to address the patient in a manner that is socially and culturally appropriate and could actually spare you considerable embarrassment. Most people prefer to be called by their correct name. You must be certain that you know your patients' names and pronounce them correctly. Follow cultural conventions concerning the use of titles. Avoid being unduly casual or familiar. For example, refrain from routinely using the patient's first name before you have been invited to do so. The same guidelines should be followed when you address the family members and other visitors. It is suggested to greet the patient with "Hello, Mr. or Mrs. or Ms. [last name], my name is" and to use your last name. The common use of "you guys" and other colloquialisms must be avoided when you talk to patients and family members.

There are ways to establish rapport at the beginning of the interview, as discussed in the earlier section Introducing the Interview (p. 49). For example, when you work in settings in which a high proportion of people self-identify as Aboriginal, you may begin by asking, "Where are you from?" This can convey interest in their personal history. For people from immigrant groups or who are members of visible minority groups (see Chapter 3, page 30, for a definition), this same question is often *inappropriate* and should be avoided because it can signal a questioning of whether they are part of "Canadian" society. You must adapt your opening statements to the context of the patient.

Space and Distance

Both the patient's and your own sense of spatial distance are significant throughout the interview and physical examination, with culturally appropriate distance zones varying widely. For example, you may find yourself backing away from people who seem to be different from you, or wanting to touch people in ways that convey concern or comfort. In all cases, pay close attention to the patient's verbal and nonverbal cues and ask them what they prefer before you make decisions about how to use space and distance.

Considerations Related to Gender

Lack of attention to ethnocultural or family norms with regard to appropriate male–female relationships may jeopardize your professional relationship with many patients. Among some Arab Canadian families, you may find that a man is rarely alone with a woman (except his wife) and is generally accompanied by one or more other men when interacting with women. This is socioculturally very significant; failure to respect norms of behaviour can be viewed as a serious transgression. The best way to ensure that particular norms have been considered is to ask the patient about relevant aspects of male–female relationships, preferably at the beginning of the interview. When you have determined that gender differences are important to the patient, you might try strategies such as offering to have a third person present when this is feasible. If a family member or friend has accompanied the patient, you might inquire whether the patient would like that person to be in the examination room during the history or physical examination, or both. It is not unusual for a female patient to refuse to be examined by a male clinician and for a male patient to refuse to be examined by a woman. Modesty is another issue, and it is imperative to ensure that all patients are carefully draped at all times and that privacy is maintained by closing the door or curtains when possible. You must not enter a room without knocking first and announcing yourself.

Among some ethnocultural groups, it is considered an acceptable expression of friendship and affection to openly and publicly hold hands with or embrace members of the same gender, and no sexual connotation is associated with the behaviour. For example, you may notice that some women hold hands with female relatives and friends while walking with them.

Considerations Related to Sexual Orientation

In interviewing lesbian, gay, bisexual, or transgendered individuals, you should be aware of heterosexist biases and the communication of these biases during the interview and physical examination. *Heterosexism* is the institutionalized belief that heterosexuality is the only natural choice and that it is the norm. For example, most health histories include a question concerning marital status. Although many same-sex couples are in committed, long-term monogamous relationships, seldom is there a category on the standard form that acknowledges this type of relationship. Although technically and legally the patient may be "single," this trivializes the relationship with his or her significant other. This designation may also have family and decision-making implications related to caregiving roles.

OVERCOMING COMMUNICATION BARRIERS

Health care providers tend to have stereotypical expectations of a patient's behaviour during the interview and physical examination. In general, they expect behaviour to consist of undemanding obedience, an attitude of respect toward the health care provider, and cooperation with requests throughout the examination. Although patients may ask a few questions for the purpose of clarification, health care providers generally expect to take the lead in directing the conversation. Some people, however, may have significantly different perceptions about the appropriate role of the patient and his or her family when seeking health care. If you find yourself (a) becoming annoyed that a patient is asking too many questions, (b) assuming a defensive posture, or (c) otherwise feeling uncomfortable, you should pause to reflect critically on the source of the patient's concerns. Consider that some patients who have experienced health care inequities through discrimination or racialization may be concerned that their health concerns will be dismissed or that they will not be treated respectfully because of past experiences with the health care system. In these situations, it is particularly important to convey unconditional positive regard, empathy, and active listening. Remaining reflective will create opportunities for you to make conscious and intentional choices about how best to respond.

Working With (and Without) an Interpreter

Of the people living in Canada in 2006, 20% were born outside of Canada, which was the highest proportion in 75 years (Statistics Canada, 2012). Allophones (people whose mother tongue is neither English nor French) constituted one fifth of the population of Canada. This means that you will have the opportunity to work with a number of patients and family members whose primary language is different from yours. It is helpful to recognize that language is not only a means of communication; language also connects people

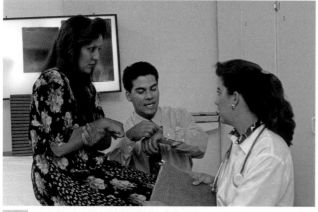

4-6

to their social, emotional, familial, and spiritual vitality (Statistics Canada, 2008). For these reasons, it is important to develop ways of communicating effectively with people so that you can provide the best care possible.

After English and French, the most common mother tongues spoken in Canada in 2006 were the Chinese languages (e.g., Cantonese, Mandarin; Statistics Canada, 2007). Italian was the fourth most common mother tongue, German fifth, and Punjabi sixth, followed by Spanish, Arabic, Tagalog (the national language of the Philippines), and Portuguese. One of the greatest challenges in cross-cultural communication arises when you and the patient speak different languages (Figure 4-6). After assessing the language skills of people who have limited English or French proficiency, you may find yourself in one of two situations: trying to communicate effectively through an interpreter or trying to communicate effectively when no interpreter is present.

Interviewing a patient who speaks neither English nor French requires a bilingual interpreter for full communication. Even the patient from another country who has a basic command of English or French (those for whom English or French is a second language) may need an interpreter when faced with the anxiety-provoking situation of entering a hospital, describing a strange symptom, or discussing sensitive topics such as those related to reproductive or urological concerns.

Interpreters are employed in many health care agencies and hospitals in Canada; however, research demonstrates that nurses and physicians tend not to use interpreter services adequately (Anderson et al., 2003; Hoen et al., 2006; Lynam et al., 2003). Although Canada has a universal health care system, no legislative provisions or court precedents effectively require the availability of interpretation services for patients who need them (Hoen et al., 2006). Only the deaf community in Canada has had success in the courts in obtaining the right to access interpreter services in health care settings.

Whenever possible, work with an interpreter who is trained in interpreting in health care settings. Trained interpreters typically know interpreting techniques, have a health care background, and understand patients' rights. The trained interpreter also is knowledgeable about culturally specific meanings and practices about health, healing, and illness. Such people can help you bridge the cultural communication gap that may exist and can advise you concerning the cultural appropriateness of your recommendations. Learn whether your institution offers training in how to work with interpreters; enhancing your skills will improve the quality of communication (Tang, 1999).

Although interpreters are trained to remain neutral, they can influence both the content of information exchanged and the nature of the interaction. Many trained medical interpreters are members of the linguistic community that they serve. Although this is largely beneficial, it has limitations. For example, interpreters often know patients and details of their circumstances before the interview begins. This is a significant risk in smaller, rural, or northern towns and communities. In these contexts, the choice of an interpreter must be judicious. Although acceptance of a code of ethics governing confidentiality and conflicts of interest is part of the training interpreters receive, discord may arise when they relate information that the patient has not volunteered to the examiner.

Moreover, being bilingual does not necessarily mean an interpreter is able to communicate with the patient. Aboriginal languages, for example, are so diverse that an Aboriginal interpreter from one region of a province or territory may not necessarily understand the language or cultural practices of an Aboriginal patient from another region of the same province or territory. Even when an interpreter and patient are from similar ethnocultural backgrounds, trained interpreters may live in urban areas and in an entirely different social context and may be unaware of particular meanings, practices, or beliefs that are important to the patient for whom they interpret.

As mentioned earlier, in some institutions, access to trained interpreters is not available. As a first preference, language services should include the availability of a bilingual staff member who can communicate directly with patients in their preferred language and dialect. If necessary, enlist the aid of a bilingual staff member at your agency who can interpret. For convenience, it is tempting to ask the patient's relative, friend, or even another patient to interpret because such people are readily available and probably would like to help. This is disadvantageous, however, because it violates confidentiality for the patient, who may not want personal information shared with another person. Furthermore, the friend or relative, although fluent in ordinary language usage, is likely to be unfamiliar with medical terminology, hospital or clinic procedures, consent, or health care ethics.

When it is not possible for a staff member to interpret, or in an immediate emergency situation, a patient's family or friend may need to interpret. This is not desirable, and errors made in translation can be fatal. In the United States, this issue is serious enough to warrant development of bills in some states (e.g., California) prohibiting children younger than 15 years to serve as interpreters, and several states such as Massachusetts and New York are legislating the use of interpreters. In all cases, it is your responsibility to

TABLE 4-3	Use of an Interpreter

CHOOSING AN INTERPRETER

- Before locating an interpreter, identify the language the patient speaks at home. Be aware that it may differ from the language spoken publicly.
- Whenever possible, use a *trained* interpreter, preferably one who knows medical terminology.
- Be aware of gender differences between interpreter and patient. In general, an interpreter of the same gender as the patient is preferred.
- Be aware of age differences between interpreter and patient. In general, an older, more mature interpreter is preferred to a younger, less experienced one.
- Be aware of socioeconomic differences between interpreter and patient.

STRATEGIES FOR EFFECTIVE USE OF AN INTERPRETER'S SERVICES

- Plan what you want to say ahead of time. Meet privately with the interpreter before the interview. Avoid confusing the interpreter by backing up, hesitating, or inserting a proviso.
- Ask the interpreter to provide a line-by-line verbatim account of the conversation. Ask for a detailed interpretation when you are provided with brief summaries of longer exchanges between interpreter and patient.
- Be patient. When an interpreter is involved, interviews often take two to three times longer than usual.
- Longer-than-expected explanatory exchanges are often needed to convey the meaning of words such as *stress, depression, allergy, preventive health care,* and *physical therapy* because comparable terms may not exist in the language that the patient understands.
- When you discuss diagnostic tests such as mammography, magnetic resonance imaging, and computed tomography, or those involving body fluids such as blood, urine, stool, spinal fluid, or saliva, be sure to clarify the nature of the test to the interpreter. Indicate the purpose of the test, exactly what will happen to the patient, approximately how long the test will take, whether the procedure is invasive or noninvasive, and what part or parts of the body will be tested.
- Be aware that the interpreter may modify or edit some aspects of the conversation, especially if he or she thinks you might not understand the cultural, social, or family context of the patient's response (e.g., specific practices or beliefs related to health and healing).
- Avoid ambiguous statements and questions. Refrain from using conditional or indefinite phrasing such as "if," "would," and "could," especially for target languages, such as Khmer (Cambodia), that lack nuances of conditionality or distinctions of time other than actual past and present. Conditional statements may be mistaken for actual agreement or approval of a course of action.
- Avoid abstract expressions, idioms, similes, metaphors, and medical jargon.
- To ensure confidentiality and privacy, avoid relying on children or strangers who may be visiting other patients as interpreters.

RECOMMENDATIONS FOR INSTITUTIONS

- Maintain a current database list of interpreters who may be contacted as needed.
- Network with local community health care centres, hospitals, colleges, universities, and other organizations that may serve as resources.
- Some private companies, and phone companies, offer over-the-phone interpretation for a fee. Some institutions may consider paying for these services if no other interpretation service is available.

ensure that your patients (and, in some situations, their family members) are fully informed of what you are telling them, particularly in relation to informed consent for procedures, treatments, and discharge or follow-up plans (Abraham & Rahman, 2008).

Working With Trained Interpreters

When working with trained interpreters, you are in charge of the focus and flow of the interview, and you should view yourself and the interpreter as a team. Ask the interpreter to meet the patient beforehand to establish rapport and to garner information about the patient's social, cultural, educational, and family contexts. This enables the interpreter to communicate on the patient's level. Allow more time for interviews in such situations. Because the third person is repeating everything, the interview can take considerably longer than interviews with English-speaking patients. You need to focus on priority data.

There are two styles of interpreting: line by line and summarizing. Translating line by line takes more time, but it ensures accuracy. Use this style for most of the interview. Both you and the patient should speak only a sentence or two

and then allow the interpreter some time. Use simple language yourself, not medical jargon that the interpreter must simplify before it can be translated. Summary translation progresses faster and is useful for teaching relatively simple health care techniques with which the interpreter is already familiar. Be alert for nonverbal cues as the patient talks. These cues can give valuable data. A good interpreter also notes nonverbal messages and passes them on to you. Summarized in Table 4-3 are suggestions for the selection and use of an interpreter's services.

Although use of an interpreter is the ideal, you may find yourself in a situation with a patient who speaks no English or French but no interpreter is available. Table 4-4 summarizes some suggestions for overcoming language barriers when no trained interpreter is present. Communicating with these patients may require that you combine verbal and nonverbal communication.

Nonverbal Communication

Basically, five types of nonverbal behaviours convey information about the patient: (a) *vocal cues,* such as pitch, tone, and

TABLE 4-4	Overcoming Language Barriers: How to Communicate When No Interpreter Is Available

1. Be polite and formal. Be sure to convey unconditional positive regard through nonverbal communication such as facial expressions, body positions, and tone of voice.
2. Pronounce the patient's name correctly. Use proper titles of respect, such as "Mr.," "Mrs.," "Ms.," and "Dr." Greet the patient with the last or complete name. Gesture to yourself and say your name. Offer a handshake or nod. Smile.
3. Proceed in an unhurried manner. Pay attention to any effort by the patient or family to communicate.
4. Speak in a low, moderate voice. Avoid talking loudly. Remember that there is a tendency to raise the volume and pitch of your voice when the listener appears not to understand. The listener may perceive that you are shouting or angry.
5. Use any words in the patient's language that you might know. This indicates that you are aware of and respect his or her culture.
6. Use simple words, such as "pain" instead of "discomfort." Avoid medical jargon, idioms, and slang. Avoid using contractions (e.g., "don't," "can't," "won't"). Use nouns repeatedly instead of pronouns.
    Example:
    Do not say: "He has been taking his medicine, hasn't he?"
    Do say: "Does Juan take medicine?"
7. Pantomime words and simple actions while you verbalize them.
8. Give instructions in the proper sequence.
    Example:
    Do not say: "Before you rinse the bottle, sterilize it."
    Do say: "First wash the bottle. Second, rinse the bottle."
9. Discuss one topic at a time. Avoid using conjunctions.
    Example:
    Do not say: "Are you cold and in pain?"
    Do say: "Are you cold (*while pantomiming*)? Are you in pain?"
10. Validate whether the patient understands by having him or her repeat instructions, demonstrate the procedure, or act out the meaning.
11. Write out several short sentences in English and determine the patient's ability to read them.
12. Try a third language. Many Indochinese speak French. Many Europeans know two or more languages. Try Latin words or phrases.
13. Ask who among the patient's family and friends could serve as an interpreter.
14. Obtain phrase books from a library or bookstore, make or purchase flash cards, contact community health care centres or hospitals for a list of interpreters, and use both a formal network and an informal network to locate a suitable interpreter.

quality of voice, including moaning, crying, and groaning; (b) *action cues,* such as posture, facial expression, and gestures; (c) *object cues,* such as clothes, jewellery, and hairstyles; (d) *use of personal and territorial space* in interpersonal transactions and care of belongings; and (e) *touch,* which involves the use of personal space and action (Lapierre & Padgett, 1991).

Unless you make an effort to understand the patient's nonverbal behaviour, you may overlook important information such as that conveyed by facial expressions, silence, eye contact, touch, and other body language. Communication patterns vary widely across families, cultural groups, and social groups, even for such conventional social behaviours as smiling and handshaking.

Wide cultural variation exists in interpreting **silence.** Some individuals find silence extremely uncomfortable and make every effort to fill conversational lags with words. Conversely, many Aboriginal people consider silence essential to understanding and respecting the other person. A pause after your question can signify that what has been asked is important enough to be given thoughtful consideration. For some people from various ethnocultural groups, silence may mean that the speaker wishes the listener to consider the content of what has been said before continuing. For others, silence may be used out of respect for another's privacy or to demonstrate respect for older persons. It is important to remember that there are no "prescriptions" for how to behave when communicating with people whose background may be different from yours. Rather, what is needed is a high degree of

reflectivity, self-observation, an awareness of people's unique contexts and histories, and the intention to ensure that you and the patient (and the family members) are communicating effectively.

Eye contact is perhaps among the most culturally variable nonverbal behaviours. Although you probably have been taught to maintain eye contact when speaking with others, people from some ethnocultural backgrounds may use eye contact in other ways. For example, some people may avert their eyes when talking with you in an effort to convey respect to people in positions of authority. Some First Nations people may look downward during conversations to indicate that the listener is paying close attention to the speaker. In some Inuit communities, people raise their eyebrows as a way to signal an affirmative response to a question, or to signal agreement, rather than nodding.

Bodily Exposure and Touch

For all people, modesty in relation to bodily exposure (e.g., removing clothing for physical examinations) is particularly important in showing respect. For some people, because of past negative experiences, family norms, or culturally specific norms, it is entirely inappropriate for a male examiner to view a woman's body unless she is fully clothed. You need to remain attuned to the verbal and nonverbal cues conveyed by patients or their families as you proceed. In all cases, provide a clear explanation of why you are asking someone to remove part of his or her clothing for the purpose of examination, and be prepared to make adaptations or forgo bodily exposure in some cases.

Without doubt, touching the patient is a necessary component of a comprehensive assessment. From a cultural perspective, however, you are urged to give careful consideration to issues concerning **touch**. Although the benefits in establishing rapport with patients through touch have been reported, physical contact with patients can convey various meanings cross-culturally. For some people, depending on their social, cultural, and historical contexts, male health care providers may be prohibited from touching or examining either all or certain parts of the female body. Adolescent girls often prefer female health care providers or refuse to be examined by a man. You should be aware that the patient's significant others also may exert pressure on nurses by enforcing these culturally meaningful norms in the health care setting.

Touching children also may have associated meaning in some ethnocultural groups. People from some areas of Asia believe that one's strength resides in the head and that touching the head is a sign of disrespect. The clinical significance of this is that you need to be aware that patting a child on the head or examining the fontanelle may need to be avoided or done only with parental permission. Whenever possible, you should explore alternative ways to express affection or to obtain information necessary for assessment of the patient's condition (e.g., hold the child on the lap, observe for other manifestations of increased intracranial pressure or signs of premature fontanelle closure, or place one's hand over the mother's while asking for a description of what she feels).

REFERENCES

Abraham, D., & Rahman, S. (2008). The community interpreter: A critical link between clients and service providers. In S. Guruge & E. Collins (Eds.), *Working with immigrant women: Issues and strategies for mental health professionals* (pp. 103–118). Toronto: Canadian Centre for Addiction and Mental Health.

Anderson, J., Perry, J., Blue, C., Browne, A., Henderson, A., Khan, K., ... Smye, V. (2003). "Rewriting" cultural safety within the postcolonial and postnational feminist project. *Advances in Nursing Science 26*, 196–214.

Browne, A. J., Doane, G. H., Reimer, J., MacLeod, M. L. P., & McLellan, E. (2010). Public health nursing practice with "high priority" families: The significance of contextualizing "risk." *Nursing Inquiry, 17*(1), 27–38. doi:10.1111/j.1440-1800.2009.00478.x

Doane, G. H., & Varcoe, C. (2005). *Family nursing as relational inquiry: Developing health-promoting practice*. Philadelphia: Lippincott Williams & Wilkins.

Hoen, B., Nielsen K., & Sasso, A. (2006). *Health care interpreter services: Strengthening access to primary health care. National report*. Toronto: Access Alliance, Multicultural Community Health Centre.

Lapierre, E. D., & Padgett, J. (1991). How can we become more aware of culturally specific body language and use this awareness therapeutically? *Journal of Psychosocial Nursing and Mental Health Services, 29*(11), 38–41.

Lynam, M. J., Henderson, A., Browne, A., Smye, V., Semeniuk, P., Blue, C., ... Anderson, J. (2003). Healthcare restructuring with a view to equity and efficiency: Reflections on unintended consequences. *Nursing Leadership (Toronto, Ont.), 16*(1), 112–140.

Selye, H. (1956). *The stress of life*. New York: McGraw-Hill.

Statistics Canada. (2008). *Aboriginal peoples in Canada in 2006: Inuit, Métis and First Nations, 2006 census*. Retrieved from *http://www12.statcan.ca/english/census06/analysis/aboriginal/pdf/97-558-XIE2006001.pdf*.

Statistics Canada. (2007). *Immigration in Canada: A portrait of the foreign-born population, 2006 Census: Immigration: Driver of population growth*. Retrieved from *http://www12.statcan.ca/census-recensement/2006/as-sa/97-557/p2-eng.cfm*.

Tang, S. Y. S. (1999). Interpreter services in healthcare: Policy recommendations for healthcare agencies. *JONA: The Journal of Nursing Administration, 29*(6), 23–29.

Web Sites of Interest

Canadian Association for the Deaf: *http://www.cad.ca/*
Canadian Health Network: *http://www.canadian-health-network.ca/*
I Love Languages: *http://www.ilovelanguages.com/index/php*
Statistics Canada: *http://cansim2.statcan.ca*

The Complete Health History

Written by Carolyn Jarvis, PhD, APN, CNP
Adapted by Annette J. Browne, PhD, RN

⊖volve WEBSITE

http://evolve.elsevier.com/Canada/Jarvis/examination/
- Appendices
- Comprehensive Older Person's Evaluation

- Examination Review Questions
- Key Points

OUTLINE

The purpose of the health history is to collect **subjective data:** what the patient says about himself or herself. The history is combined with the **objective data** from the physical examination and with laboratory studies to form the database. The database is used to make a judgement or a diagnosis about the health status of the individual. As noted in Chapter 1, electronic health records are in widespread use in Canada. Nurses can expect to use such records in documenting and managing information collected for the complete health history (Figure 5-1).

The following health history provides a complete picture of the patient's past and current health. It describes the patient as a whole and how he or she interacts with the environment. It is a record of health strengths and coping skills. In documenting the history, the nurse should recognize and affirm what the patient is *doing right:* what he or she is doing to help stay well. For the well patient, the history is used to assess his or her overall health status, health maintenance goals, and health-promoting practices, such as exercise pattern, diet, risk reduction, and preventive behaviours such as immunization status, age-appropriate health screening, or helmet use during sports activities.

For the ill patient, the health history includes a detailed and chronological record of the health problem. For all patients, the health history is a screening tool for abnormal symptoms, health problems, and concerns, and it records ways of responding to the health problems. In many settings, the patient fills out a printed history form or checklist. This allows the patient ample time to recall and consider such items as dates of health landmarks and relevant family history.

The interview is then used to validate the written data and to collect more data on lifestyle management and current health problems.

Although history forms vary, most contain information in this sequence of categories:
1. Biographical data
2. Reason for seeking care
3. Current health or history of current illness
4. Past history
5. Family history
6. Review of systems
7. Functional assessment or assessment of activities of daily living (ADLs)

The health history outlined in the following section follows this format and constitutes a generic database for all practitioners. Nurses in clinical settings may use all of it, whereas those in a hospital may focus primarily on the history of current illness and the functional, or patterns of living, data.

HEALTH HISTORY: ADULTS

Biographical Data

Include the patient's name, address and phone number, age and birthdate, birthplace, gender, marital status, ethnocultural background, and usual and current occupation (an illness or disability may have prompted a change in occupation). Note that in some health care agencies and institutions, the primary language spoken by the patient is recorded. Therefore, the patient's primary language and authorized

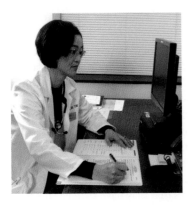

5-1

representative, if any, should be recorded here. This is in response to research showing that differences in language and culture may have an effect on the quality and safety of care (Joint Commission, 2007).

Source of History

1. Record who provides the information: usually the patient herself or himself, a parent, or, in some cases, a relative or friend.
2. Judge how reliable the informant seems and how willing he or she is to communicate. A reliable patient always gives the same answers, even when questions are rephrased or are repeated later in the interview.
3. Note any special circumstances, such as the use of an interpreter. Sample statements are as follows:

> *"Patient herself, who seems reliable."*
> *"Patient's son, John Ramirez, who seems reliable."*
> *"Mrs. R. Fuentes, interpreter for Theresa Castillo, who does not speak English."*

Reason for Seeking Care*

The reason for seeking care is a brief, spontaneous statement in the patient's own words that describes the reason for the visit. Think of it as the "title" for the story to follow. It states one (possibly two) symptoms or signs and their duration. A **symptom** is a subjective sensation that the patient feels from the disorder. A **sign** is an objective abnormality that you as the examiner could detect on physical examination or in laboratory reports. Whatever the patient says is the reason for seeking care is recorded, enclosed in quotation marks to indicate the patient's exact words:

> *"Chest pain" for 2 hours.*
> *"My child has an earache and was fussy all night."*
> *"I need a yearly physical examination for work."*
> *"I want to start jogging, and I need a checkup."*
> *"I would like to cut down the amount of cigarettes I smoke."*

---

*In the past, this statement was called the "chief complaint" (CC). This description is avoided now because it implies that the patient "complains" and, of more importance, does not include health maintenance, health promotion, or wellness needs.

The patient's reason for seeking care should not be used for diagnosis. Avoid translating the patient's statement into the terms of a medical diagnosis. For example, a man enters with shortness of breath, and you ponder writing "emphysema." Even if he is known to have emphysema from previous visits, it is not the chronic emphysema that prompted *this* visit, but rather the "increasing shortness of breath" for 4 hours.

Some people attempt to self-diagnose on the basis of certain information: that obtained from the Internet, which may or may not be accurate; similar signs and symptoms in their relatives or friends; or conditions they know they have. For example, rather than record a woman's statement that she has "strep throat," ask her what symptoms she has that make her think this is present, and record those symptoms.

On occasion, a patient may list *many* reasons for seeking care. The most important reason to the patient may not necessarily be the one stated first. Try to focus on which is the most pressing concern by asking the patient which one prompted him or her to seek help *now*.

Current Health or History of Current Illness

For the well patient, current health is a short statement about the general state of health.

For the ill patient, this section is a chronological record of the reason for seeking care, from the time the symptom first started until now. Isolate each reason for care identified by the patient and say, for example, "Please tell me all about your headache, from the time it started until the time you came to the hospital." If the concern started months or years ago, record what occurred during that time and find out why the patient is seeking care *now*.

As the patient talks, do not jump to conclusions and bias the story by adding your opinion. Collect all the data first. Although you want the patient to respond in a narrative format without interruption from you, your final summary of any symptom the patient has should include the following eight critical characteristics.

Location. Be specific; ask the patient to point to the location. If the problem is pain, note the precise site. "Head pain" is vague, whereas descriptions such as "pain behind the eyes," "jaw pain," and "occipital pain" are more precise and are diagnostically significant. Is the pain localized to this site or radiating? Is the pain superficial or deep?

Character or Quality. This calls for specific descriptive terms such as *burning, sharp, dull, aching, gnawing, throbbing, shooting,* and *viselike.* Use similes: Does blood in the stool look like sticky tar? Does blood in vomitus look like coffee grounds?

Quantity or Severity. Attempt to quantify the sign or symptom, such as "profuse menstrual flow, soaking five pads per hour." The symptom of pain is difficult to quantify because of individual interpretation. What one patient may identify as "terrible pain," another may describe as "not too bad." With pain, avoid adjectives and ask how it affects daily activities. Then the patient might say, "I was so sick I was doubled up and couldn't move" or "I was able to go to work, but then I came home and went to bed."

Timing (Onset, Duration, Frequency). When did the symptom first appear? Give the specific date and time, or state specifically how long ago the symptom started "prior to arrival" (PTA)*.

"The pain started yesterday" will not mean much when you return to read the record in the future. The report must include such information as how long the symptom lasted (duration); whether it was steady (constant) or whether it would come and go during that time (intermittent); and whether it resolved completely and reappeared days or weeks later (cycle of remission and exacerbation).

Setting. Where was the patient or what was the patient doing when the symptom started? What triggers the symptom? For example, you can ask, "Did you notice the chest pain after shovelling snow, or did the pain start by itself?"

Aggravating or Relieving Factors. What makes the pain worse? Is it aggravated by weather, activity, food, medication, bending over, fatigue, time of day, or season? What relieves it (e.g., rest, medication, or ice pack)? What is the effect of any treatment? Ask, "What have you tried?" or "What seems to help?"

Associated Factors. Is the primary symptom associated with any others (e.g., urinary frequency and burning sensation in association with fever and chills)? Review the body system related to this symptom now rather than wait for the review of systems.

Patient's Perception. Find out the meaning of the symptom by asking how it affects daily activities. Also ask directly, "What do you think it means?" This is crucial because it alerts you to potential anxiety if the patient thinks the symptom may be ominous. You may find it helpful to organize this same question sequence into the mnemonic **PQRSTU** to help remember all the points. Note that you still need to address the patient's perception of the problem:

P (**provocative** or **palliative**): "What brings it on? What were you doing when you first noticed it? What makes it better? Worse?"

Q (**quality** or **quantity**): "How does it look, feel, sound? How intense or severe is it?"

R (**region** or **radiation**): "Where is it? Does it spread anywhere?"

S (**severity**): "How bad is it (on a scale of 1 to 10)? Is it getting better, getting worse, or staying the same?"

T (**timing**): "Exactly when did it first occur?" (onset); "How long did it last?" (duration); "How often does it occur?" (frequency).

U (**understand** patient's perception of the problem): "What do you think it means?"

---

*"Prior to arrival" (PTA) is frequently used in primary care and in emergency department settings, when it is clear that the patient arrived for health care at a particular time. For example, for a patient being assessed in an emergency department for abdominal pain, the documentation might read "gradual onset of left lower quadrant abdominal that started 4 hours PTA."

Past Health

Past health events may have residual effects on the current health state. Also, the previous experience with illness may give clues as to how patients respond to illness and to the significance of illness for them.

Childhood Illnesses. Document a history of measles, mumps, rubella, chicken pox, pertussis, and streptococcal infection ("strep throat"). Avoid the wording "usual childhood illnesses" because an illness common in the patient's childhood (e.g., measles) may be unusual today. Ask about serious illnesses that may have sequelae for the patient in later years (e.g., rheumatic fever, scarlet fever, and poliomyelitis).

Accidents or Injuries. Document a history of auto accidents, fractures, penetrating wounds, head injuries (especially if associated with unconsciousness), and burns.

Serious or Chronic Illnesses. Document whether the patient has diabetes, hypertension, heart disease, sickle cell disease, cancer, and seizure disorder.

Hospitalizations. Record cause, name of the hospital, how the condition was treated, how long the patient was hospitalized, and name of the treating physician.

Operations. Document type of surgery, date of surgery, name of the surgeon, name of the hospital, and how the patient recovered.

Obstetrical History. Record the number of pregnancies (gravidity, or *grav*), number of deliveries in which the fetus reached full term (*term*), number of preterm deliveries (*preterm*), number of incomplete pregnancies (abortions, or *ab*), and number of children living (*living*). This information is recorded thus: "Grav _____ Term _____ Preterm _____ Ab _____ Living _____." For each complete pregnancy, note the course of pregnancy; the course of labour and delivery; sex, weight, and condition of each infant; and postpartum course. For any incomplete pregnancies, record the duration and whether the pregnancy resulted in spontaneous (*S*) or induced (*I*) abortion.

Immunizations. Depending on the patient's age group, ask whether the patient has received, for example, measles-mumps-rubella, polio, diphtheria-pertussis-tetanus, hepatitis B, human papillomavirus, *Haemophilus influenzae* type b, and pneumococcal vaccine. Note the dates of the most recent tetanus immunization, most recent tuberculosis skin test, and most recent influenza shot. Consult the latest immunization guidelines used in your province or territory.

Most Recent Examination Date. Document the dates of the most recent physical, dental, vision, hearing, electrocardiographic, and chest radiographic examinations.

Allergies. Note both the allergen (medication, food, or contact agent, such as fabric or environmental agent) and the reaction (rash, itching, runny nose, watery eyes, difficulty breathing). When a drug is involved, determine whether the symptom is a true allergic reaction, rather than a side effect.

Current Medications. Note all prescription and over-the-counter medications. Ask specifically about vitamins and other supplements, birth control pills, aspirin, and antacids, because many people do not consider these medications. For each medication, note the name, dose, and schedule, and ask,

"How often do you take it each day?"; "What is it for?"; and "How long have you been taking it?" Finally, note use of complementary therapies, such as homeopathic or herbal remedies.

Family History

Ask about the ages and health, or the ages at and cause of death, of blood relatives, such as parents, grandparents, and siblings. These data may have genetic significance for the patient. Also ask about close family members, such as spouse and children. You need to know about the patient's prolonged contact with any communicable disease or the effect of a family member's illness on the patient.

Specifically ask for any family history of heart disease, high blood pressure, stroke, diabetes, blood disorders, cancer, sickle cell disease, arthritis, allergies, obesity, alcoholism, mental health issues or illness, seizure disorder, kidney disease, and tuberculosis. Construct an accurate family tree, or genogram, to show this information clearly and concisely (Figure 5-2; Box 5-1).

 CULTURAL AND SOCIAL CONSIDERATIONS

Add several questions to the complete health history for people who are new immigrants:
- Biographical data: When did the patient come to Canada and from what country? If the patient is a refugee, what were the conditions under which he or she came here? Did he or she undergo particularly challenging experiences?
- The older patient may have come to this country after World War II and may be a Holocaust survivor. Questions regarding family and past history may evoke painful memories and must be asked carefully.
- Spiritual resources and religion: Assess whether certain procedures need to be considered in view of the patient's spirituality or religion. For example, people who are members of Jehovah's Witnesses may refuse blood transfusions and may need additional decision-making supports.

BOX 5-1 DRAWING YOUR FAMILY TREE

- Make a list of all of your family members.
- Use this sample family tree as a guide to draw your own family tree.
- Write your name at the top of your paper and date you drew your family tree.
- In place of the words father, mother, etc., write the names of your family members.
- When possible, draw your brothers and sisters and your parents' brothers and sisters starting from oldest to the youngest, going from left to right across the paper.
- If dates of birth or ages are not known, then estimate or guess ("50s," "late 60s").

- Past health: What immunizations were given in the patient's country of origin? For example, was the patient given *bacille Calmette-Guérin* (BCG)? This vaccine is used in many countries to prevent tuberculosis. If the patient has had BCG, the result of the tuberculin test will be positive, and further diagnostic procedures must be performed, including a sputum test and chest radiography.
- Health perception: How does the patient describe health and illness, and what does the patient view as the problem he or she is now experiencing?
- Nutritional: What foods and food combinations are taboo?

Review of Systems

The purposes of this section are (a) to evaluate the past and current health state of each body system, (b) to double-check in case any significant data were omitted in the current illness section, and (c) to evaluate health promotion practices. The order of the examination of body systems is approximately head to toe. The items within each system are not inclusive, and only the most common symptoms are listed. If the section on current illness covered one body system, you do not need to repeat all the data in this section. For example, if the reason for seeking care is earache, the section on current illness contains data about most of the symptoms listed for the auditory system. Just ask now what was not asked in that section.

Medical terms are listed in this section, but they need to be translated for the patient. (Note that symptoms and health promotion activities are merely listed here. These terms are repeated and expanded in each related physical examination chapter, along with suggested ways to pose questions and a rationale for each question.)

When recording information, avoid writing "negative" after the system heading. You need to record the *presence* or *absence* of all symptoms; otherwise the reader does not know about which factors you asked.

A common mistake made by novice practitioners is to record some physical finding or objective data here, such as "skin warm and dry." Remember that the history should be limited to the patient's statements, or subjective data: factors that the patient *says* were or were not present.

General Overall Health State. Ask how the patient feels overall (i.e., "How do you feel overall? Have you experienced any recent changes to your overall health status?"). Current weight (gain or loss, period of time, by diet or other factors). Note any fatigue, weakness or malaise, fever, chills, sweats, or night sweats.

Skin, Hair, and Nails. Record any history of skin disease (eczema, psoriasis, hives), pigment or colour change, change in mole, excessive dryness or moisture, pruritus, excessive bruising, rash, or lesion. Document recent loss and change in texture. For nails, note change in shape, colour, or brittleness.

Health Promotion. Ask what the patient is doing to stay healthy and for prevention. Depending on the patient's age, geographical location, and social–personal circumstances, ask, for example, about the amount of sun exposure and use

Drawing Your Family Tree
- Make a list of all of your family members.
- Use this sample family tree as a guide to draw your own family tree.
- Write your name at the top of your paper and the date you drew your family tree.
- In place of the words *father, mother* etc., write the names of your family members.
- When possible, draw your brothers and sisters and your parents' brothers and sisters starting from oldest to youngest, going from left to right across the paper.
- If dates of birth or ages are not known, then estimate or guess ("50s," "late 60s").

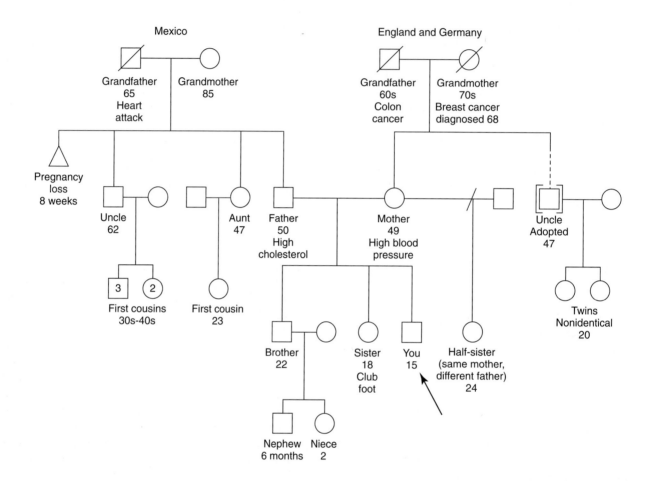

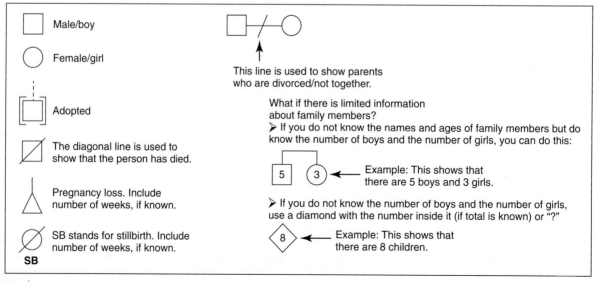

5-2   Genogram or family tree.

of sunscreen and use of appropriate footwear to prevent foot sores (for a patient with diabetes).

Head. Ask whether the patient has had any unusually frequent or severe headache, any head injury, dizziness (syncope), or vertigo.

Health Promotion. Depending on the patient's age, geographical location, and social–personal circumstances, ask, for example, about use of protective gear during sports activities.

Eyes. Document any difficulty with vision (decreased acuity, blurring, blind spots), eye pain, diplopia (double vision), redness or swelling, watering or discharge, glaucoma, or cataracts.

Health Promotion. Ask about the most recent eye examination. As discussed in Chapter 15, Canadians between the ages of 19 and 64 must rely on private (third-party) insurance or out-of-pocket payment to see an eye specialist for routine vision screening (Clinical Practice Guideline Expert Committee, 2007). Many adults cannot afford the cost of vision tests or corrective lenses. You need to know which community agencies provide such services free of charge or at a reduced cost so that you can refer patients accordingly.

Health Promotion. Document whether the patient wears glasses or contact lenses; the most recent vision check or glaucoma test; and how the patient copes with loss of vision, if any.

Ears. Record the presence of earaches, infections, discharge and its characteristics, tinnitus, or vertigo.

Health Promotion. Note any hearing loss, hearing aid use, how loss affects daily life, any exposure to environmental noise, use of earplugs or other noise-reducing devices, and method of cleaning ears.

Nose and Sinuses. Record discharge and its characteristics, any unusually frequent or severe colds, sinus pain, nasal obstruction, nosebleeds, allergies or hay fever, or change in sense of smell.

Mouth and Throat. Document mouth pain, frequent sore throat, bleeding gums, toothache, lesion in mouth or on tongue, dysphagia, hoarseness or voice change, tonsillectomy, or altered taste.

Health Promotion. Ask about the patient's pattern of daily dental care, use of prostheses (dentures, bridge), and most recent dental checkup. Be aware that dental examinations and care may require out-of-pocket payments, which many patients and families cannot afford. You need to know which community health agencies offer dental care for a reduced cost or, in some cases, free of charge, and refer patients accordingly.

Neck. Note pain, limitation of motion, lumps or swelling, enlarged or tender nodes, and goitre.

Breast. Document any pain, lump, nipple discharge, rash, history of breast disease, and any surgery on the breasts.

Health Promotion. Ask about the date of most recent mammogram. Inquire as to whether the patient performs breast self-examination (see Chapter 18 for revised recommendations regarding breast self-examination).

Axilla. Note tenderness, lump or swelling, and rash.

Respiratory System. Document history of lung diseases (asthma, emphysema, bronchitis, pneumonia, tuberculosis), chest pain with breathing, wheezing or noisy breathing, shortness of breath, how much activity produces shortness of breath, cough, sputum (colour, amount), hemoptysis, and toxin or pollution exposure.

Health Promotion. Ask the date of the most recent chest x-ray study.

Cardiovascular System. Note precordial or retrosternal pain, palpitation, cyanosis, dyspnea on exertion (specify amount of exertion that triggers dyspnea, such as walking one flight of stairs, walking from chair to bath, or just talking), orthopnea, paroxysmal nocturnal dyspnea, nocturia, edema, history of heart murmur, hypertension, coronary artery disease, and anemia.

Health Promotion. Ask the patient about the date of most recent electrocardiogram or other tests of heart function.

Peripheral Vascular System. Document coldness, numbness and tingling, swelling of legs (time of day, activity), discoloration in hands or feet (bluish red, pallor, mottling, associated with position, especially around feet and ankles), varicose veins or complications, intermittent claudication, thrombophlebitis, and ulcers.

Health Promotion. Does the patient's work involve long-term sitting or standing? Patients with vascular system issues should be advised to avoid crossing legs at the knees and to wear support hose.

Gastrointestinal System. Note appetite, food intolerance, dysphagia, heartburn, indigestion, pain (associated with eating), other abdominal pain, pyrosis (esophageal and stomach burning sensation with sour eructation), nausea and vomiting (character), vomiting blood, history of abdominal disease (ulcer, liver or gallbladder, jaundice, appendicitis, colitis), flatulence, frequency of bowel movement, any recent change, stool characteristics, constipation or diarrhea, black stools, rectal bleeding, and rectal conditions (hemorrhoids, fistula).

Health Promotion. Document the patient's use of antacids or laxatives. (Alternatively, diet history can be described in this section.)

Urinary System. Record frequency, urgency, nocturia (the number of times the patient awakens at night to urinate; recent change), dysuria, polyuria or oliguria, hesitancy or straining, narrowed stream, urine colour (cloudy or presence of hematuria), incontinence, history of urinary disease (kidney disease, kidney stones, urinary tract infections, prostate), and pain in flank, groin, suprapubic region, or lower back.

Health Promotion. Advise the patient about measures to avoid or treat urinary tract infections and the use of Kegel exercises after childbirth.

Male Genital System. Note penis or testicular pain, sores or lesions, penile discharge, lumps, and hernia.

Health Promotion. Ask whether the patient performs testicular self-examination and how frequently.

Female Genital System. Document menstrual history (age at menarche, most recent menstrual period, cycle and duration, any amenorrhea or menorrhagia, premenstrual pain or dysmenorrhea, intermenstrual spotting), vaginal itching, discharge and its characteristics, age at menopause, menopausal signs or symptoms, and postmenopausal bleeding.

Health Promotion. Ask for the date of the most recent gynecological checkup and most recent Papanicolaou (Pap) test.

Sexual Health. Ask whether the patient is currently in a relationship involving intercourse. Are the aspects of sex satisfactory to the patient and partner? Note any dyspareunia (for a female patient), any changes in erection or ejaculation (for a male patient), and use of contraceptive. Is the contraceptive method satisfactory? Is the patient aware of contact with a partner who has any sexually transmitted infection (STI; e.g., gonorrhea, herpes, chlamydia, venereal warts, human immunodeficiency virus [HIV] infection or acquired immune deficiency syndrome [AIDS], or syphilis)?

Musculoskeletal System. Document any history of arthritis or gout. In the joints, note pain, stiffness, swelling (location, migratory nature), deformity, limitation of motion, and noise with joint motion. In the muscles, note any pain, cramps, weakness, gait problems, or problems with coordinated activities. In the back, note any pain (location and radiation to extremities), stiffness, limitation of motion, or history of back pain or disc disease.

Health Promotion. How much walking does the patient do per day? What is the effect of limited range of motion on daily activities, such as on grooming, eating, toileting, dressing? Are any mobility aids used? For older adults, ask about fall prevention strategies, such as not using throw rugs on floors but using rubberized bath mats.

Neurological System. Document any history of seizure disorder, stroke, fainting, and blackouts. In motor function, note weakness, tic or tremor, paralysis, or coordination problems. In sensory function, note numbness and tingling (paraesthesia). In cognitive function, note memory disorder (recent or distant, disorientation). In mental status, note any nervousness, mood change, depression, or any history of mental health dysfunction or hallucinations. See Chapter 6 for mental health assessment guidelines.

Health Promotion. Data about interpersonal relationships and coping patterns can be placed in this section.

Hematological System. Document any bleeding tendency of skin or mucous membranes, excessive bruising, lymph node swelling, exposure to toxic agents or radiation, blood transfusion, and reactions.

Endocrine System. Record any history of diabetes or diabetic symptoms (polyuria, polydipsia, polyphagia), history of thyroid disease, intolerance to heat and cold, change in skin pigmentation or texture, excessive sweating, relationship between appetite and weight, abnormal hair distribution, nervousness, tremors, and need for hormone therapy.

Health Promotion. Depending on a diabetic patient's health history, ask about use of appropriate footwear to prevent foot sores or ulcers.

Functional Assessment (Including Activities of Daily Living)

In a functional assessment, you measure a patient's self-care ability in the areas of general physical health or absence of illness; ADLs, such as bathing, dressing, toileting, eating, and walking; instrumental activities of daily living (IADLs), which are activities needed for independent living, such as housekeeping, shopping, cooking, doing laundry, using the telephone, and managing finances; nutrition; social relationships and resources; self-concept and coping; and home environment.

Functional assessment may mean organizing the entire assessment around "functional health pattern areas" (Gordon, 2012). Instruments that emphasize functional categories may help in establishing a nursing diagnosis.

Functional assessment may also mean that the health history is supplemented by a standardized instrument on functional assessment. Instruments such as the Katz Index of Activities of Daily Living (see Figure 31-2) and the Lawton Instrumental Activities of Daily Living Scale (see Figure 31-3) are used to objectively measure a patient's current functional status and to monitor any changes over time (Granger, Ottenbacher, Baker, & Ashok, 1995; Mahoney & Barthel, 1965; Pearlman, 1987).

Regardless of whether you use any of these formalized instruments, functional assessment questions such as those listed in the following sections should be included in the standard health history. These questions provide data on the lifestyle and type of living environment to which the patient is accustomed. Because some of the data may be judged private by the individual, the questions are best asked at a later point in the interview, after you have had time to establish rapport.

Self-Concept, Self-Esteem. Ask about the patient's education level (last grade completed, other significant training), financial status (income adequate and health or social concerns), and value–belief system (religious practices and perception of personal strengths).

Activity and Mobility. Obtain a daily profile that reflects usual daily activities. Ask, "Tell me how you spend a typical day." Note ability to perform ADLs: whether the patient is independent or needs assistance with feeding, bathing, hygiene, dressing, toileting, bed-to-chair transfer, walking, standing, or climbing stairs. Document any use of wheelchair, prostheses, or mobility aids. Record leisure activities enjoyed and the exercise pattern (type, amount per day or week, method of warm-up session, method of monitoring the body's response to exercise).

Sleep and Rest. Record sleep patterns, daytime naps, any sleep aids used.

Nutrition and Elimination. Record the diet by a recall of all food and beverages taken over the last 24 hours (see Chapter 12 for suggested method of inquiry). Ask the patient, "Is that menu typical of most days?" Describe eating habits and current appetite. Ask, "Who buys food and prepares food?"; "Are your finances adequate for food?"; and "Who is present at mealtimes?" Indicate any food allergy or intolerance. Record daily intake of caffeine (coffee, tea, cola drinks). Ask about usual pattern of bowel elimination and urinating, including problems with mobility or transfer in toileting, continence, and use of laxatives.

Interpersonal Relationships and Resources. Ask about social roles: "How would you describe your role in the family?" and "How would you say you get along with family, friends, and coworkers?" Ask about support systems composed of family and significant others: "To whom could you go for support with a problem at work, a health problem, or a personal problem?" Include contact with spouse, siblings, parents, children, friends, organizations, and the workplace: "Is time spent alone pleasurable and relaxing, or is it isolating?"

Spiritual Resources. Many people believe in a relationship between spirituality and health, and they may wish to have spiritual matters addressed in the traditional health care setting (Taylor, 2011). One approach to assess the role of spirituality in a patient's life is to use the faith, influence, community, and address (FICA) questions to incorporate the patient's spiritual values into the health history (Post, Puchalski, & Larson, 2000): For *faith,* "Does religious faith or spirituality play an important part in your life? Do you consider yourself to be a religious or spiritual person?" For *influence,* "How does your religious faith or spirituality influence the way you think about your health or the way you care for yourself?" For *community,* "Are you a part of any religious or spiritual community or congregation?" For *address,* "Would you like me to address any religious or spiritual issues or concerns with you?"

Coping and Stress Management. Document kinds of stresses in life, especially in the past year; any change in living situation or any current stress; and methods for dealing with stress and whether these have been helpful. For children and adolescents, ask about bullying, as discussed in Chapter 1.

Smoking History. Strategies for asking about smoking patterns are included in Chapter 7: "Do you smoke cigarettes or a pipe, or do you use chewing tobacco?"; "At what age did you start?"; "How many packs do you smoke per day?"; and "How many years have you smoked?" Record the number of cigarettes or packs smoked per day (based on 20 cigarettes per package) and duration. For example, 10 cigarettes per day × 5 years, or 1 pack per day (20 cigarettes/pack) × 5 years. Then ask, "Have you ever tried to quit?" and "How did it go?" to introduce plans about smoking cessation.

Alcohol. Health care providers often fail to question about alcohol or substance use despite the effect of these activities on health, quality of life, and social relationships. Asking about alcohol use can begin with asking whether the patient drinks alcohol. If the patient replies in the affirmative, you can explain that you would like to follow up with additional questions to better assess his or her health status. Chapter 7 contains in-depth guidelines about how to discuss alcohol and substance use and how to assess the effects on health and well-being. In some cases, and in some agencies, it may be appropriate to use a screening questionnaire to identify when alcohol or other substance use is presenting problems in relation to the patient's functional status, relationships, employment, economic status, and other areas in

life. Common screening tools are discussed in Chapter 7. As explained in Chapter 7, it is imperative to convey acceptance and a nonjudgemental attitude when you discuss alcohol or substance use patterns. To do otherwise can have detrimental effects. For example, if the patient believes that you are negatively judging him or her, the patient may not return for follow-up or may avoid seeking care altogether.

Substance Use. Chapter 7 provides an overview of how to ask about substance use in a nonjudgemental manner. As noted previously, refer to Chapter 7 for guidelines about how to inquire about substance use (including alcohol and drugs) in effective, respectful ways. Depending on the patient's personal context, you may ask specifically about marijuana, cocaine, crack cocaine, amphetamines, heroin, methadone, benzodiazepines, barbiturates, crystal methamphetamine, 3,4-methylenedioxymethamphetamine (Ecstasy), phencyclidine (PCP), and other drugs. Indicate frequency of use and how usage has affected the patient's work, relationships, family, or economic circumstances.

Environmental Hazards. Describe the patient's housing and neighbourhood (living alone, knowledge of neighbours), safety of area, adequacy of heat and utilities, access to transportation, and involvement in community services. Note environmental health, including hazards in the workplace, hazards at home, use of seatbelts, geographical or occupational exposures, and travel or residence in other countries, such as time spent abroad during military service.

Intimate Partner Violence. Begin with open-ended questions. Convey openness and acceptance, and listen in a nonjudgemental manner: "How are things going at home (or at school or work)?" "How are things at home affecting your health?" "Is your home (or work or school) environment safe?" These are valuable questions for all patients. Specifically, in relation to intimate partner violence, patients may not recognize their situation as abusive, or they may be reluctant to discuss their situation because of guilt, fear, or shame. Follow each patient's lead to inquire more specifically. If you sense that violence is an issue, use the strategies discussed in Chapter 8.

Occupational Health. Ask the patient to describe his or her employment situation; he or she may or may not have a clearly identifiable job. Ask whether the patient has ever worked with any health hazard, such as asbestos, inhalants, chemicals, and repetitive motion. Did the patient wear any protective equipment? Are any work programs in place in which exposure is monitored? Is the patient aware of any health problems now that may be related to work exposure?

Note the timing of the reason for seeking care and whether it may be related to work or home activities, job titles, or exposure history. Carefully document a smoking history, which may contribute to occupational hazards. Finally, ask the patient what he or she likes or dislikes about the job.

Perception of Health

Ask the patient questions such as "What does it mean to you to be healthy? How do you define health?"; "How do you view your situation now?"; "What are your concerns?"; "What do you think will happen in the future?"; "What are your health goals?"; and "What do you expect from us as nurses, nurse practitioners, physicians, or other health care providers?"

✤ DEVELOPMENTAL CONSIDERATIONS

HEALTH HISTORY: CHILDREN

The health history is adapted to include information specific for the age and developmental stage of the child (e.g., the mother's health during pregnancy, the course of labour and delivery, and the perinatal period; Figure 5-3). Note that the developmental history and nutritional data are listed in separate sections because of their importance for current health.

Depending on where you are working, developmental assessment tools such as the Nipissing District Developmental Screen, the Rourke Baby Record, or the Ages and Stages Questionnaires are routinely used in documenting the health history. These assessment tools, which are discussed in Chapter 2, provide an excellent way to frame discussions about the importance of health promotion and disease prevention activities.

Biographical Data

Include the child's name, nickname, address, and phone number; parents' names and work numbers; child's age and birthdate, birthplace, gender, race, and ethnic origin; and information about other children and family members at home.

Source of History

Document the sources of historical information:
1. The person providing information and relation to the child

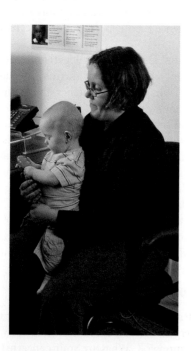

5-3

2. Your impression of reliability of information
3. Any special circumstances, such as the use of an interpreter

Reason for Seeking Care

Record the parent's or caregiver's spontaneous statement. The reason for seeking care may be be identified or initiated by the child, the parent or caregiver, or by a third party such as a classroom teacher.

Sometimes the reason stated may not be the real reason for the visit. A parent may have a "hidden agenda," such as the mother who brought her 4-year-old child in because "she looked pale." Further questioning revealed that the mother had heard recently from a former college friend whose own 4-year-old child had just received a diagnosis of leukemia.

Current Health or History of Current Illness

If the parent or child seeks routine health care, include a statement about the usual health of the child and any common health problems or major health concerns. Using the same format as for the adult, describe any presenting symptom or sign. Some additional considerations are as follows:
- Severity of pain: "How do you know the child is in pain?" (e.g., pulling at ears alerts parent to ear pain). Note effect of pain on usual behaviour (e.g., whether it stops the child from playing).
- Associated factors, such as relation to activity, eating, and body position.
- The parent's intuitive sense of a problem. As the constant caregiver, the parent has an intuitive sense that is often very accurate. Even if findings prove otherwise, this sense gives you an idea of the parent's area of concern.
- Parent's coping ability and reaction of other family members to child's symptoms or illness.

Past Health

Prenatal Status. Ask the mother how this pregnancy was spaced in relation to other children. Was it planned? What was the mother's attitude toward the pregnancy? What was the father's attitude? Was the mother under medical supervision? At what month was the supervision started? What was the mother's health during pregnancy? Were there any complications, such as bleeding, excessive nausea and vomiting, unusual weight gain, high blood pressure, swelling of hands and feet, infections (rubella or STIs), or falls? During what month was a diet prescribed? During what month were medications prescribed or taken during pregnancy (dose and duration)? Using sensitivity in posing questions, ask about the mother's use of alcohol, drugs, or cigarettes and any radiographs taken during pregnancy. Chapter 7 describes strategies for asking about substance use during pregnancy in ways that convey acceptance and will minimize the risk that the woman will feel negatively judged and avoid care.

Start with an open-ended question: "Tell me about your pregnancy." If she questions the relevancy of the statement, mention that these questions are important for obtaining a complete overview of the child's health.

Labour and Delivery. Record parity of the mother, duration of the pregnancy, name of the hospital, course and duration of labour, use of anaesthetics, type of delivery (vertex, breech, Caesarean section), birth weight, Apgar scores, onset of breathing, any cyanosis, need for resuscitation, and use of special equipment or procedures.

Postnatal Status. Note any problems in the neonatal nursery, length of hospital stay, neonatal jaundice, whether the baby was discharged with the mother, whether the baby was breastfed or formula-fed, weight gain, any feeding problems, "blue spells," colic, diarrhea, patterns of crying and sleeping, the mother's postpartum health, and the mother's reaction to the baby.

Childhood Illnesses. Document age at onset and any complications of measles, mumps, rubella, chicken pox, whooping cough, streptococcal infection ("strep throat"), and frequent ear infections. Also note any recent exposure to illness.

Serious Accidents or Injuries. Record age at occurrence, extent of injury, how the child was medically treated, and complications of auto accidents, falls, head injuries, fractures, burns, and poisonings.

Serious or Chronic Illnesses. Document age at onset, how the child was medically treated, and complications of meningitis or encephalitis; seizure disorders; asthma, pneumonia, and other chronic lung conditions; rheumatic fever; scarlet fever; diabetes; kidney problems; sickle cell disease; high blood pressure; and allergies.

Operations or Hospitalizations. Note reason for care, age at admission, name of surgeon or health care provider, name of hospital, duration of stay, how the child reacted to hospitalization, and any complications. (If child reacted poorly, he or she may be frightened now and will need special preparation for the examination that is to follow.)

Immunizations. Document age when immunizations were administered, date administered, and any reactions after immunizations. Appendix A on the Evolve Web site lists suggested immunization schedules.

Allergies. Record any drugs, foods, contact agents, and environmental agents to which the child is allergic and the reaction to allergens. Note allergic reactions particularly common in childhood, such as allergic rhinitis, insect hypersensitivity, eczema, and urticaria.

Medications. Document any prescription and over-the-counter medications (or vitamins and other supplements) the child takes, including the dose, daily schedule, why the medication is given, and any problems.

Developmental History

Growth. Record the height and weight at birth and at 1, 2, 5, and 10 years; any periods of rapid growth or weight loss; and process of dentition (age at tooth eruption and pattern of loss).

Milestones. Document the age when the child first held the head erect, rolled over, sat alone, walked alone, developed the first tooth, said his or her first words with meaning, spoke in sentences, was toilet trained, tied shoes, and dressed without help. Does the parent believe this development has been normal? How does this child's development compare with that of siblings or peers?

Current Development

Children Aged 1 Month Through Preschool Age. Record current gross motor skills (rolling over, sitting alone, walking alone, skipping, climbing), fine motor skills (inspecting hands, bringing hands to mouth, pincer grasp, stacking blocks, feeding self, using crayon to draw, using scissors), language skills (vocalizing, first words with meaning, sentences, persistence of baby talk, speech problems), and personal–social skills (smiling, tracking movement with eyes to midline and past midline, attending to sound by turning head, recognizing own name). If the child is undergoing toilet training, indicate the method used, age at which bladder and bowel are controlled, parents' attitude toward toilet training, and terms used for toileting.

School-Age Children. Document current gross motor skills (running, jumping, climbing, riding bicycle, general coordination), fine motor skills (tying shoelaces, using scissors, writing name and numbers, drawing pictures), and language skills (vocabulary, verbal ability, ability to tell time, reading level).

Nutritional History

The amount of nutritional information needed depends on the child's age; the younger the child is, the more detailed and specific the data should be. For infants, record whether breast milk or formula is used. If the child is breastfed, record nursing frequency and duration, any supplements (vitamin, iron, fluoride, formula), family support for nursing, and age at and method of weaning. If the child is formula-fed, record type of formula used, frequency and amount, any problems with feeding (spitting up, colic, diarrhea), supplements used, and any bottle propping. Record introduction of solid foods (age when the child began eating solids, which foods, whether foods are home or commercially made, amount given, child's reaction to new food, parent's reaction to feeding).

For preschool- and school-age children and adolescents, record the child's appetite, 24-hour diet recall (meals, snacks, amounts), vitamins taken, how much junk food is eaten, who eats with the child, food likes and dislikes, and parent's perception of child's nutrition. A week-long diary of food intake may be more accurate than a spot 24-hour recall. Also, consider cultural practices in assessing child's diet.

Family History

As with the adult, diagram a family tree for the child, including siblings, parents, and grandparents. For each, record the age and health or the age at and cause of death. Ask specifically for the family history of heart disease, high blood pressure, diabetes, blood disorders, cancer, sickle cell disease, arthritis, allergies, obesity, cystic fibrosis, alcoholism, mental health problems or illness, seizure disorder, kidney disease, intellectual disability, learning disabilities, birth defects, and sudden infant death. (When interviewing the mother, ask about the "child's father," not "your husband," in case the child's biological father is not present.)

Review of Systems

General. Document significant gain or loss of weight, failure to gain weight appropriate for age, frequent colds, ear infections, illnesses, energy level, fatigue, overactivity, and behaviour change (irritability, increased crying, nervousness).

Skin. Note birthmarks, skin disease, pigment or colour change, mottling, change in mole, pruritus, rash, lesion, acne, easy bruising or petechiae, easy bleeding, and changes in hair or nails.

Head. Ask whether the patient suffers from headache or dizziness and whether the patient has had a head injury.

Eyes. Note strabismus, diplopia, pain, redness, discharge, cataracts, vision changes, and reading problems. Is the child able to see the board at school? Does the child sit too close to the television?

Health Promotion. Document use of eyeglasses and date of most recent vision screening.

Ears. Note earaches, frequency of ear infections, the presence of myringotomy tubes in the ears, discharge (characteristics), cerumen, sensation of ringing or crackling, and whether the parent perceives any hearing problems.

Health Promotion. Note how the child cleans his or her ears.

Nose and Sinuses. Record discharge and its characteristics, frequency of colds, nasal stuffiness, nosebleeds, and allergies.

Mouth and Throat. Document any history of cleft lip or palate, frequency of sore throats, toothache, caries, sores in the mouth or tongue, presence of tonsils, mouth breathing, difficulty chewing, difficulty swallowing, and hoarseness or voice change.

Health Promotion. Record the child's pattern of brushing teeth and the date of the most recent dental checkup.

Neck. Note swollen or tender glands, limitation of movement, or stiffness.

Breast. For preadolescent and adolescent girls, ask when they noticed that their breasts were changing. What is the girl's self-perception of development? Does the older adolescent girl perform breast self-examination? (See Chapter 18 for suggested phrasing of questions.)

Respiratory System. Document croup or asthma, wheezing or noisy breathing, shortness of breath, and chronic cough.

Cardiovascular System. Document congenital heart problems, history of murmur, and cyanosis (what prompts this condition). Is activity limited, or can the child keep up with peers? Does the child have any dyspnea on exertion, palpitations, high blood pressure, or coldness in the extremities?

Gastrointestinal System. Note abdominal pain, nausea and vomiting, history of ulcer, frequency of bowel movements, stool colour and characteristics, diarrhea, constipation or stool-holding, rectal bleeding, anal itching, history of pinworms, and use of laxatives.

Urinary System. Note painful urination, polyuria or oliguria, narrowed stream, urine colour (cloudy, dark), history of urinary tract infection, whether the child is toilet trained, when toilet training was planned, any toilet training problems, and bedwetting (when the child started, frequency, association with stress, how child feels about it).

Male Genital System. Record penis or testicular pain, whether the parent was told that testes are descended, any sores or lesions, discharge, hernia or hydrocele, or swelling in scrotum during crying. Has the preadolescent or adolescent boy noticed any change in the penis and scrotum? Is the boy familiar with normal growth patterns, nocturnal emissions, and sex education? Screening for sexual abuse is not normally part of the routine review of systems. (See Chapter 8 for rationale.)

Female Genital System. Has the girl noted any genital itching, rash, or vaginal discharge? For the preadolescent and adolescent girl, document when menstruation started. Was she prepared? Screening for sexual abuse is not normally part of the routine review of systems. (See Chapter 8 for rationale.)

Sexual Health. What is the child's attitude toward the opposite sex? Who provides sex education? How does the family deal with sex education, masturbation, dating patterns? Is the adolescent in a relationship involving intercourse? Does he or she have information on birth control and STIs? (See Chapters 26 and 27 for suggested phrasing of questions.)

Musculoskeletal System. For bones and joints, document arthritis, joint pain, stiffness, swelling, limitation of movement, gait strength, and coordination. For muscles, document pain, cramps, and weakness. For the back, document pain, posture, spinal curvature, and any treatment.

Neurological System. Note numbness and tingling sensation. (Behaviour and cognitive issues are covered in the sections on development and interpersonal relationships.)

Hematological Systems. Record excessive bruising, lymph node swelling, and exposure to toxic agents or radiation.

Endocrine System. Record a history of diabetes or thyroid disease; excessive hunger, thirst, or urinating; abnormal hair distribution; and precocious or delayed puberty.

Functional Assessment (Including Activities of Daily Living)

Interpersonal Relationships. Record the child's position within the family constellation; whether the child is adopted; who lives with the child; who is the primary caretaker; who is the caretaker if both parents work outside the home; any support from relatives, neighbours, or friends; and the ethnic or cultural milieu.

Indicate family cohesion. Does the family enjoy activities as a unit? Has there been a recent family change or crisis (death, divorce, move)? Record information about the child's self-image and level of independence. Does the child use a security blanket or toy? Is there any repetitive behaviour (bed rocking, head banging), pica, thumb sucking, or nail biting? Note method of discipline used. Indicate type used at home. How effective is it? Who disciplines the child? Is there any occurrence of negativism, temper tantrums, withdrawal, or aggressive behaviour?

Provide information on the child's friends: whether the child makes friends easily. How does the child get along with friends? Does he or she play with same-age or older or younger children?

Activity and Rest. Record the child's play activities. Indicate amount of active and quiet play, outdoor play, time watching television, and special hobbies or activities. Record sleep and rest. Indicate pattern and number of hours at night and during the day and the child's routine at bedtime. Is the child a sound sleeper, or is he or she wakeful? Does the child have nightmares, night terrors, or somnambulation? How does the parent respond? Does the child have naps during the day?

Record school attendance. Has the child had any experience with day care or nursery school? In what grade is the child in school? Has the child ever skipped a grade or been held back? Does the child seem to like school? What is his or her school performance? Are the parent and child satisfied with the performance? Were days missed in school? Provide a reason for the absence. (Answers to these questions provide an important index to the child's functioning outside the home.)

Economic Status. Ask about either or both parents' or caregivers' occupations. Indicate the number of hours each parent or caregiver is away from home. Do parents perceive their income as adequate? What is the effect of the child's illness on financial status?

Home Environment. Where does the family live (house, apartment)? Is the size of the home adequate? Is an outdoor play area accessible? Does the child share a room, have his or her own bed, and have toys appropriate for his or her age?

Environmental Hazards. Inquire about home safety (precautions for poisons, medications, household products, presence of gates for stairways, and safe yard equipment). Provide information on the child's residence (adequate heating, ventilation, bathroom facilities), neighbourhood (residential or industrial, age of neighbours, safety of play areas, availability of playmates, distance to school, amount of traffic, whether area is remote or congested and overcrowded, whether crime is widespread, presence of air or water pollution), and automobile (child safety seat, seatbelts).

Coping and Stress Management. Does the child have the ability to adapt to new situations? Record recent stressful experiences (death, divorce, move, loss of special friend). How does the child cope with stress? Has there been any recent change in behaviour or mood? Has counselling ever been sought?

Alcohol and Substance Use. Has the child ever tried cigarette smoking? How much did he or she smoke? Has the child ever tried alcohol? How much alcohol did he or she drink weekly or daily? Has the child ever tried other drugs (marijuana, cocaine, amphetamines, barbiturates)?

Health Promotion. Ask the parent or caregiver to identify their primary health care provider, such as a physician or nurse practitioner. When was the child's most recent checkup? Who is the dental care provider, and when was the most recent dental checkup? Provide date and result of screening for vision, hearing, urinalysis, phenylketonuria, hematocrit, tuberculosis skin test, sickle cell trait, blood lead, and other tests specific to high-risk populations.

HEALTH HISTORY: ADOLESCENTS

Chapter 6 discusses approaches to psychosocial and mental health assessment among adolescents and young adults. This section presents a psychosocial review of symptoms intended to maximize communication with youth. The **HEEADSSS** method of interviewing focuses on assessment of the *home* environment, *e*ducation and employment, *e*ating, peer-related *a*ctivities, *s*ubstance use, *s*exuality, *s*uicide or depression, and *s*afety from injury and violence (Figure 5-4). The tool minimizes adolescent stress because it moves from expected and less threatening questions to those that are more personal. The tool presents the questions in three colours: Those in green are considered essential to explore with every adolescent; those in blue are important to ask if time permits; and red questions delve more deeply and are asked if they are appropriate to the context or situation (Goldenring & Rosen, 2004). Interview the youth alone, while the parent waits outside and fills out questionnaires about past health.

It is important to review Chapters 6, 7, and 8 before asking about mental health, substance use, and interpersonal violence issues, so that those areas are explored respectfully and in ways that convey openness and acceptance. It is imperative that you follow the adolescent's lead when exploring these areas.

HEALTH HISTORY: OLDER ADULTS

The health history for an older adult includes the same format as that described for a younger adult, as well as some additional questions. These questions address ways in which the ADLs may have been affected by normal aging processes or by the effects of chronic illness or disability. There is no specific age at which to ask these additional questions. Use them when it seems appropriate to the patient's life context. Please review Chapter 31 for completed guidelines on assessing older adults.

It is important for you to recognize positive health measures: what the patient has been doing to help himself or herself stay well and to live to an older age. Many older people have spent a lifetime obtaining care from traditional health care systems that focus on pathological processes, medical problems, and what is wrong with their health. It may be a pleasant and welcome surprise to have a health care provider affirm the things that they are "doing well" and to note health strengths, social supports, and capabilities. As you study the following, keep in mind the format for younger adults. Only *additional* questions or those of a varying focus are addressed in this section.

The HEEADSSS psychosocial interview for adolescents

Home

Who lives with you? Where do you live? Do you have your own room?
What are relationships like at home?
To whom are you closest at home?
To whom can you talk at home?
Is there anyone new at home? Has someone left recently?
Have you moved recently?
Have you ever had to live away from home? (Why?)
Have you ever run away? (Why?)
Is there any physical violence at home?

Education and employment

What are your favourite subjects at school? Your least favourite subjects?
How are your grades? Any recent changes? Any dramatic changes in the past?
Have you changed schools in the past few years?
What are your future education and employment plans and goals?
Are you working? Where? How much?
Tell me about your friends at school.
Is your school a safe place? (Why?)
Have you ever had to repeat a class? Have you ever had to repeat a grade?
Have you ever been suspended? Expelled? Have you ever considered dropping out?
How well do you get along with the people at school? Work?
Have your responsibilities at work increased?
Do you feel connected to your school? Do you feel as if you belong?
Are there adults at school you feel you could talk to about something important? (Who?)

Eating

What do you like and not like about your body?
Have there been any recent changes in your weight?
Have you dieted in the last year? How? How often?
Have you done anything else to try to manage your weight?
How much exercise do you get in an average day? Week?
What do you think would be a healthy diet? How does that compare to your current eating patterns?
Do you worry about your weight? How often?
Do you eat in front of the TV? Computer?
Does it ever seem as though your eating is out of control?
Have you ever made yourself throw up on purpose to control your weight?
Have you ever taken diet pills?
What would it be like if you gained (lost) 10 pounds*?

Activities

What do you and your *friends* do for fun? (With whom, where, and when?)
What do you and your *family* do for fun? (With whom, where, and when?)
Do you participate in any sports or other activities?
Do you regularly attend a church group, club, or other organized activity?
Do you have any hobbies?
Do you read for fun? (What?)
How much TV do you watch in a week? How about video games?
What music do you like to listen to?

Drug Use (Substance Use)†

Do any of your friends use tobacco? Alcohol? Other drugs?
Does anyone in your family use tobacco? Alcohol? Other drugs?
Do you use tobacco? Alcohol? Other drugs?
Is there any history of alcohol or drug problems in your family?
Do you ever drink or use drugs when you're alone?
(Assess frequency, intensity, patterns of use or abuse, and how youth obtains or pays for drugs, alcohol, or tobacco.)

Sexuality

Have you ever been in a romantic relationship?
Tell me about the people that you've dated. *OR* Tell me about your sex life.
Have any of your relationships ever been sexual relationships?
Are your sexual activities enjoyable?
What does the term "safer sex" mean to you?
Are you interested in boys? Girls? Both?
Have you ever been forced or pressured into doing something sexual that you didn't want to do?
Have you ever been touched sexually in a way that you didn't want?
Have you ever been raped‡, on a date or any other time?
How many sexual partners have you had altogether?
Have you ever been pregnant or worried that you might be pregnant? (females)
Have you ever impregnated someone or worried that that might have happened? (males)
What are you using for birth control? Are you satisfied with your method?
Do you use condoms every time you have intercourse?
Does anything ever get in the way of always using a condom?
Have you ever had an STI or worried that you had an STI?

Suicide and depression

Do you feel sad or down more than usual? Do you find yourself crying more than usual?
Are you "bored" all the time?
Are you having trouble getting to sleep?
Have you thought a lot about hurting yourself or someone else?
Does it seem that you've lost interest in things that you used to really enjoy?
Do you find yourself spending less and less time with friends?
Would you rather just be by yourself most of the time?
Have you ever tried to kill yourself?
Have you ever had to hurt yourself (by cutting yourself, for example) to calm down or feel better?
Have you started using alcohol or drugs to help you relax, calm down, or feel better?

Safety

Have you ever been seriously injured? (How?) How about anyone else you know?
Do you always wear a seatbelt in the car?
Have you ever ridden with a driver who was drunk or high? When? How often?
Do you use safety equipment for sports and other physical activities (e.g., helmets for biking or skateboarding)?
Is there any violence in your home? Does the violence ever get physical?
Is there a lot of violence at your school? In your neighbourhood? Among your friends?
Have you ever been physically or sexually abused? Have you ever been raped, on a date or at any other time? (If not asked previously)
Have you ever been in a car or motorcycle accident? (What happened?)
Have you ever been picked on or bullied? Is that still a problem?
Have you participated in physical fights in school or your neighbourhood? Are you still getting into fights?
Have you ever felt that you had to carry a knife, gun, or other weapon to protect yourself? Do you still feel that way?

Green = essential questions
Blue = as time permits
Red = optional or when situation requires

---

*5 kilograms.

†Please see Chapter 7 for the correct terms used to describe substance use (including alcohol, drug and other substance use). The terms listed in this Figure reflect terms that will soon be outdated given the release of the new *Diagnostic and Statistical Manual of Mental Disorders (DSM-V)* and the new terms used to describe peoples' use of substances.

‡The more commonly accepted term in Canada is "sexually assaulted."

5-4 The HEEADSSS psychosocial interview for adolescents. *Green* represents essential questions; *blue* represents those to be asked as time permits; *red* represents optional questions or those to be asked as the situation requires. *STI*, sexually transmitted infection.

Reason for Seeking Care

It may take time to figure out the reason why an older patient has come in for an examination. An older patient may shrug off a symptom as evidence of growing old and may be unsure whether it is "worth mentioning." Also, some older people have a conservative philosophy toward their health status: "If it isn't broken, don't fix it." These people come for care only when something is blatantly wrong.

An older patient may have many chronic problems, such as diabetes, hypertension, or constipation. It is challenging to filter out what brought the patient in this time. The final statement should be the *patient's* reason for seeking care, not your assumption of what the problem is.

Past Health

General Health. Document the health state over the past 5 years.

Accidents or Injuries, Serious or Chronic Illnesses, Hospitalizations, Operations. These areas may produce lengthy responses, and the patient may not relate them in chronological order. Let the patient talk freely; you can reorder the events later when you prepare the write-up. The amount of data included here can indicate the amount of stress the patient has faced during his or her lifetime. This section of the history can be filled out at home or before the interview if the patient's vision and writing ability are adequate. Then you can concentrate the remaining time of the interview on reviewing pertinent data and on the current health of the patient.

Most Recent Examination. Document the results of the most recent mammography, colonoscopy, and tonometry.

Obstetrical Status. It is *not* necessary to collect a detailed account of each pregnancy and delivery if the woman has passed menopause and has no gynecological symptoms. Merely record the number of pregnancies and the health of each newborn.

Current Medications

For each medication, record the name, purpose, and daily schedule. Does the patient have a system in place to remember to take the medicine? Does the medicine seem to work? Are there any side effects? If so, does the patient feel like skipping the medicine because of them? Also consider the following issues:

- Some older patients take a large number of drugs, prescribed by different physicians.
- The patient may not know a drug name or purpose. When this is the case, ask the patient to bring in the drug (in their prescription containers) to be identified.
- Is cost a problem? When a patient is unable to afford a drug, he or she may decrease the dosage, take one pill instead of two, or not refill the empty bottle immediately. Many patients cannot afford the costs of drugs; be prepared to obtain input from a social worker or other team member to connect patients to agencies or services that can provide assistance with the cost of prescription and over-the-counter drugs.
- Is travelling to the pharmacy to refill a prescription a problem?
- Is the patient taking any over-the-counter medications? Some people take advice from a local pharmacist or recommendations from family or friends for self-treatment.
- Has the patient ever shared medications with neighbours or friends? Some people establish "lay referral" networks by comparing symptoms and thus medications.

Family History

Family history is not as useful in predicting which familial diseases the patient may contract because most of those occur at an earlier age. These data, however, are useful to assess which diseases have occurred or to assess causes of death of relatives. These data also describe the patient's existing social network.

Review of Systems

Remember that these are *additional* items to question for the older adult. Refer to the format for younger adults for the basic list.

General. Note current weight and what the patient would like to weigh (gives idea of body image).

Skin. Document change in sensation of pain, heat, or cold.

Eyes. Record use of bifocal glasses and any trouble adjusting to far vision (e.g., problems with climbing stairs).

Ears. Document increased sensitivity to background noise and whether conversation sounds garbled or distorted.

Mouth. Note use of dentures, when the patient wears them (always, all day, only at meals, only at social occasions, or never), method of cleaning, any difficulty wearing the dentures (looseness, pain, making whistling or clicking noise), and cracks at the corners of the mouth.

Respiratory System. Document shortness of breath and level of activity that produces it. Shortness of breath is often an early sign of cardiac dysfunction, but many older people dismiss it as "a cold" or getting "winded" because of old age.

Cardiovascular System. If chest pain occurs, an older adult may not feel it as intensely as a younger person. Instead, the patient may feel dyspnea on exertion.

Peripheral Vascular System. Record whether the patient wears constrictive clothing or garters, or whether stockings are rolled at the knees. Also record any colour change at the feet or ankles.

Urinary System. Document urinary retention, incomplete emptying, straining to urinate, and change in force of stream. If the stream becomes weaker, men may note the need to stand closer to the toilet. Women may note incontinence when coughing, laughing, or sneezing.

Sexual Health. Ask about any changes in the sexual relationship the patient has experienced. Note that for older men it is normal for an erection to develop more slowly. (See Chapter 26.) For women, note any comments about vaginal dryness or pain with intercourse. Note for all whether aspects of sex are satisfactory and whether privacy for a sexual relationship is adequate.

Musculoskeletal System. Record gait change (balance, weakness, difficulty with stairs, fear of falling) and use of any assistive device (cane, walker). Does the patient have any joint stiffness? During what part of the day does the stiffness occur? Does pain or stiffness occur with activity or rest?

Neurological System. Does the patient have any problem with memory (recent or remote) or disorientation (time of day, in what settings)?

Functional Assessment (Including Activities of Daily Living)

In functional assessment, you measure how a patient manages day-to-day activities. For older patients, the meaning of health refers to the activities that they can or cannot perform. The *effect* of a disease on their daily activities and overall quality of life (called the *disease burden*) is more important to older people than the actual disease diagnosis or pathological features. Thus the functional assessment—because it emphasizes function—is very important in the evaluation of older patients (see Chapter 31: Functional Assessment of the Older Adult).

Many functional assessment instruments are available for objectively measuring a patient's current functional status and monitoring any changes over time. Most instruments are used to measure the performance of specific tasks such as the ADLs and IADLs (for examples, see Figures 31-2 and 31-3). The Comprehensive Older Person's Evaluation (see Table 31-2) is particularly useful because it contains the basic ADL and IADL functional assessment and addresses physical, social, psychological, demographic, financial, and legal issues.

Regardless of whether a standardized instrument is used, the following functional assessment questions are important additions to an older adult's health history.

Self-Concept, Self-Esteem. When the older patient was an adolescent, educational opportunities were not as available as they are today, nor were they equally available for women. An older patient may be sensitive about having achieved only the level of elementary school education or less.

Occupation. Document past positions, volunteer activities, and community activities. Many people continue to work past the age of 65; they grew up with a strong work ethic and are proud to continue. If the patient is retired, how has he or she adjusted to the change in role? It may mean loss of social role or social status, loss of personal relationships formed at work, and reduced income.

Activity and Mobility. How does the patient spend a typical day in work, hobbies, and leisure activities? Is there any day this routine changes (e.g., Sunday because of visits from family)? Note that the patient suffering from chronic illness or disability may have a self-care deficit, musculoskeletal changes such as arthritis, and mental confusion.

List significant leisure activities, hobbies, sports, and community activities. Is a community centre available to older

adults for nutrition, social networking, and screening of health status? What are the type, amount, and frequency of exercise? Is a warm-up included? How does the patient's body respond?

Sleep and Rest. Note the usual sleep pattern: Does the patient feel rested during the day? Is energy sufficient to carry out daily activities? Does the patient need naps? Is there a problem with night awakenings, such as nocturia, shortness of breath, light sleep, or insomnia (difficulty falling asleep, awakening during the night, early morning awakening)? If the patient has no routine, does he or she tend to nap all afternoon? Does insomnia worsen with lack of a daily schedule?

Nutrition and Elimination. Record a 24-hour recall of the diet. Is this diet typical of most days? (Nutrition may vary greatly. Ask the patient to keep a weekly log to bring in.) What are the meal patterns? Are there three full meals or five to six smaller meals per day? How many convenience foods and soft foods are eaten? Who prepares meals? Does the patient eat alone? Who shops for food? How are groceries transported home? Is the income adequate for groceries? Does the patient have a problem preparing meals (adequate vision, motor deficit, adequate energy)? Are the appliances, water, and utilities adequate for meal preparation? Does the patient have any difficulty chewing or swallowing? What are the food preferences? (Older adults often eat high amounts of carbohydrates because these foods are cheaper, easier to make, and easier to chew.)

Interpersonal Relationships and Resources. Who else is at home with the patient? Does the patient live alone? Is this living arrangement satisfactory? Does the patient have a pet? How close are family or friends? How often does the patient see family or friends? If visits are infrequent, is this experienced as a loss?

Does the patient live with family, such as a spouse, children, or a sibling? Is this arrangement satisfactory? What is the role in family for preparation of meals, housework, and other activities? Are there any conflicts? Is the family caregiver experiencing any financial, physical, or social strain (see Figure 31-4)?

Does the patient rely on any formal support programs such as social welfare or home health care? Does the patient utilize any semiformal supports such as church societies or senior centres?

On whom does the patient depend for emotional support? For help with problems? Who meets affection needs?

Coping and Stress Management. Has the patient experienced a recent change in living conditions or social circumstances, such as loss of occupation, spouse, or friends; a move from home; illness of self or family member; or decrease in income? How does the patient deal with stress? If a loved one has died, how is the patient responding to the loss? Ask, "How do you feel about being 'alone' and having to take on unfamiliar responsibilities now?"

Environmental Hazards. Record home safety: Does the home have one floor or are there stairs? What is the state of repair? Is money adequate to maintain the home? Are there exits for fire? Are heating and utilities adequate? How long has the patient lived in the current home?

Note transportation: Does the patient own his or her own automobile? When was the most recent driver's test? Does the patient consider himself or herself a safe driver? Is income adequate for maintenance? Is public transportation accessible? Does the patient receive drives from community resources or friends?

Document aspects of the neighbourhood: Does the patient feel secure in personal safety at day or night? Is there danger of loss of possessions? What is the amount of noise and pollution? Does the patient have access to family and friends, a grocery store, a drug store, laundry, religious communities (church, temple, mosque), and health care facilities?

REFERENCES

Clinical Practice Guideline Expert Committee. (2007). Canadian Ophthalmological Society evidence-based clinical practice guidelines for the periodic eye examination in adults in Canada. *Canadian Journal of Ophthalmology, 42,* 39–45.

Goldenring, J. M., & Rosen, D. S. (2004). Getting into adolescent heads: An essential update. *Contemporary Pediatrics, 21*(1), 64–75.

Gordon, M. (2012). *Manual of nursing diagnosis* (12th ed.). Sudbury, MA: Jones & Bartlett.

Granger, C. V., Ottenbacher, K. J., Baker, J. G., & Ashok, S. (1995). Reliability of a brief outpatient functional outcome assessment measure. *American Journal of Physical Medicine, 74,* 469–475.

Joint Commission. (2007). *Hospitals, language, and culture.* Retrieved from *http://www.jointcommission.org/PatientSafety/HLC/.*

Mahoney, F. I., & Barthel, D. W. (1965). Functional evaluation: The Barthel Index. *Maryland State Medical Journal, 14,* 61–65.

Pearlman, R. (1987). Development of a functional assessment questionnaire for geriatric patients: The Comprehensive Older Person's Evaluation (COPE). *Journal of Chronic Disease, 40,* 85S–94S.

Post, S. G., Puchalski, C. M., & Larson, D. B. (2000). Physician and patient spirituality: Professional boundaries, competency, and ethics. *Annals of Internal Medicine, 132,* 578–583.

Taylor, E. J. (2011). Religion and patient care. In M. Fowler, S. Reimer Kirkham, R. Sawatzky, & E. J. Taylor (Eds.), *Religion, religious ethics, and nursing* (pp. 313–358). New York: Springer.

Written by Kathryn Weaver, PhD, RN

evolve WEBSITE

OUTLINE

SIGNIFICANCE OF MENTAL HEALTH ASSESSMENT FOR CANADIANS

The World Health Organization (2008) estimates that mental disorders such as depression, alcohol use disorders, and psychoses (e.g., bipolar disorder and schizophrenia) are among the leading causes of disability globally. Of all Canadians, 20% personally experience a diagnosed mental illness during their lifetime (Health Canada, 2006), and one per three are expected to experience a mental health problem at some point in their life (Public Health Agency of Canada [PHAC], 2011); thus mental illness is not only a global health issue but also a major public health concern for this country.

A variety of factors influence a person's mental health. Some are internal, such as emotional problems; some come from within the person's social network and include the development of values, self-knowledge, self-control, and common sense (which helps us to learn from experience and plan for the future); and others are related to the person's broader community. This "broader community" extends to the health care and mental health care systems and also to other sectors such as employment, education, and housing. No single circumstance influences mental health; rather, people are affected by a complex series of interacting factors. Strategies to improve the mental health of Canadians therefore require active involvement from all community sectors.

In addition to internal, familial, and community influences, larger social issues such as poverty, racism, and other forms of discrimination influence mental health. Canada's population includes many immigrant groups, as well as a large number of Aboriginal groups. People who are members of these groups often face unique challenges in maintaining cultural, social, and economic integrity. Without adequate social resources or access to needed services, the stressors experienced by some ethnocultural and social groups in Canada can lead to increases in mental illnesses and suicide. For example, although there are great variations across communities, bands, and nations, the suicide rate among First Nations communities is at least twice as high as that of the general population, and the rate among Inuit is 6 to 11 times higher than that of the general population (Kirmayer, Bass, Holton, Paul, Simpson, & Tait, 2007; PHAC, 2006). These disturbingly high rates stem from the complex interplay of social determinants of health, intergenerational and historical traumas, and ongoing discrimination.

Defining Mental Health and Mental Illness

Mental health is a crucial dimension of overall health and an essential resource for everyday living. Broadly defined, **mental health** is the capacity to feel, think, express emotions, and behave in ways that enhance personal capacity to manage challenges, adapt successfully to a range of demands, and enjoy life (PHAC, 2011). The World Health Organization (2007) described mental health as a relative and ongoing state of well-being in which individuals realize their abilities, cope with the normal stresses of life, work productively, and contribute meaningfully to the community. Characteristics indicative of mental health include finding balance in all aspects of life—social, physical, spiritual, economic, and mental— and developing resilience, flexibility, and self-actualization (Canadian Mental Health Association, 2008). Some individuals are more mentally healthy than others, and, depending on life circumstances, mental health even for the same individual can vary over time across a continuum of optimal and minimal mental health described by Epp (1986). Optimal mental health entails satisfaction within work, caring relationships, and the self; it draws on a learning process in which individuals can greatly benefit from developing positive coping, assertiveness, interpersonal, and time management skills.

Mental disorder is the medical term for **mental illness** and is defined and diagnosed in Canada according to criteria specified in the *Diagnostic and Statistical Manual of Mental Disorders,* Fifth Edition, Text Revision (*DSM-V*)* by the American Psychiatric Association (APA; 2000). Mental disorders are depicted as constellations of co-occurring symptoms that may involve alterations in thought, experience, and emotion that are serious enough to cause distress and impair functioning, cause difficulties in sustaining interpersonal relationships and performing jobs, and sometimes lead to self-destructive behaviour and suicide (Perring, 2010; PHAC, 2011). Multiple factors—including the physical environment, genetics, biology, personality, culture, socioeconomic status, and life events—may contribute to the development of a mental disorder. Men and women, young and old, and people of all ethnic groups and economic brackets may be affected. Mental illnesses account for a large percentage of hospital stays every year, causing as many lost days of work as physical problems such as cancer, heart attack, or back pain.

Mental disorder is not positioned on the same continuum as mental health. Rather, mental disorder is represented as a level of impairment and distress ranging from absence of a disorder to maximal illness (Epp, 1988). When mental health and mental illness were assigned to two disparate continua, the intent was to highlight the importance of each. Indeed, a person with mental illness can experience optimal mental health and a person without mental illness can experience minimal mental health (Healey-Ogdon, 2010).

A major detriment for persons with a mental illness is stigma and its associated cycle of alienation and discrimination, which affect the abilities to seek and obtain help and support in the community (Canadian Alliance on Mental Illness and Mental Health, 2007; Canadian Medical Association, 2008). Reducing stigma is a responsibility shared by health professionals, communities, and people with mental illness. As a nurse working within this population, you need to self-monitor for stigmatizing behaviours and beliefs.

MENTAL HEALTH NURSING ASSESSMENT

The nurse–patient relationship is directed toward advancing the best interest and best health outcome of the patient (Canadian Nurses Association, 2012). To this end, the purpose of the mental health nursing assessment is to understand the patient's health and illness experiences, problems and deficits in daily living, and strengths and resources in relation to mental health. Nurses accordingly partner with patients to assess the full scope of the patient's mental health, patient interactions with service providers and other professionals, any risk of violence posed by the patient, the patient's needs, and needed intervention. Because there is a lack of peer-reviewed publications describing what and how information should be collected as part of a comprehensive mental health nursing assessment, gaps exist, particularly in the areas of social and physical health (Coombs, Curtis, & Crookes, 2011). Barratt (1989) found that mental health nursing assessment in practice means different things to different nurses. In addition, the assessment skills of nurses are often developed in settings in which mental illness has already been identified by the psychiatrist and heavily influenced by the medical judgement, which may focus on "the 'cure' of patients…potentially discount[ing] their experiences" (Hamilton, Manias, Maude, Marjoribanks, & Cook, 2004, p. 686).

Methods and Components

To provide comprehensive mental health nursing assessment, you will integrate close observations and routine social interactions into the collection of information about the patient's circumstances. You will combine (a) observation, (b) interview, (c) examination, (d) physical assessment, and (e) collaboration with others. Observing the patient at different times of the day and in differing situations provides information about hygiene, grooming, attire, facial expressions, gestures, and interactions with others. Identify disturbances in perception and thought and any inconsistencies between what the patient states and what you notice. Analyze findings from physical, mental, cognitive, and diagnostic examinations to reveal symptoms and potential problems in self-care. Through interviewing, you will build rapport with the patient, clarify the patient's perceptions and meanings, and gather factual knowledge. Collaborate with the patient's family and with other members of the health care team to develop and

---

*The *DMS IV-TR* was updated and replaced by the *DSM-V* in May 2013.

TABLE 6-1	Elements of a Mental Health History
Assessment Method	**Components**
Interview	Complete health history • Source of information • Identification/biographic information • Reason for seeking care (verbatim, psychiatric diagnoses (*DSM-V*)) • Past health (past illness, injury, hospitalization; chronic illnesses) • Family health history • Developmental considerations • Present health (allergies, immunization/HIV/hepatitis status; current medications)
Observation, may include examination	Mental status examination • Appearance • Behaviour (mood and affect, speech) • Cognitive function (level of consciousness; orientation to time, place, person, self; memory; attention and concentration; comprehension and abstract reasoning), • Thought (perception, content, process, judgement, and insight)
Examination	Supplemental Mental Status Examination (if warranted)
Interview, with added physical assessment	Functional assessment of activities of daily living: nutrition patterns; sleep/rest changes; activity/mobility; elimination; interpersonal relationships and resources; self-esteem/self-concept; ethnicity/culture; spirituality; coping and stress management; smoking, alcohol and drug use, and problem gambling; home environmental hazards)
Collaboration with health care team	Risk assessment (suicide, assaultive or homicidal ideation, elopement) Treatment plan (Global Assessment of Function)

HIV, human immunodeficiency virus.

evaluate treatment plans and risk of harm. The development of trust within the therapeutic relationship is crucial (O'Brien, 1999); trust builds through making yourself available, expressing interest in the patient as a person, and being accountable. Mental health nursing assessment may include the methods and components described in the following sections (Table 6-1).

Sources of Information

Patient information can be *subjective* (symptoms reported that are not directly observable or measurable) and *objective* (signs directly observed and measured, such as diagnostic test results). Although the patient is ideally the primary provider of information, collaboration with secondary sources (including family, health care providers, and patient records) is needed for children and when the patient is at risk of harm to self or others.

Indication for Comprehensive Mental Health Nursing Assessment

The full comprehensive mental health examination with its accompanying components for mental status assessment, as outlined previously, rarely needs to be performed in its entirety. Usually, you can assess mental health through the context of the health history interview; hence, the mental health nursing assessment follows the major subjects of the complete health history (see Chapter 5), and this approach is recommended for most situations. You will collect ample data to be able to assess mental health strengths and coping skills and to screen for any dysfunction.

A distinguishing component of the mental health assessment is the **mental status examination** (Box 6-1). **Mental status** is an aspect of mental health that involves emotional and cognitive functioning. Mental status assessment is a structured way of observing and describing a person's current state of mind, under the domains of appearance, behaviour, cognition, and thought processes. It is beneficial to assess mental status when you sense that something is "not quite right." If, for instance, you see a person whose speech is slow and unclear, whose eyes do not focus, whose clothes are soiled and dishevelled, and whose thoughts are confused, you suspect that something is wrong. If the person smells of alcohol, then you begin to form an opinion about the cause of the abnormal mental status. On the other hand, if there is no such odour, you eliminate it from the wide range of other possible causes of the person's behaviour. As additional symptoms are identified, it is possible to more fully understand the impairment and subsequently design support/intervention.

It is necessary to perform the mental health assessment when you discover any abnormality in mood or behaviour and in the following situations:

• Family members are concerned about a person's behavioural changes, such as memory loss or inappropriate social interaction.
• Brain lesions (trauma, tumour, stroke): A mental health assessment documents any emotional, cognitive, or behavioural change associated with the lesion. Not recognizing these changes hinders care planning and creates problems with social readjustment.
• Aphasia (the impairment of language ability secondary to brain damage): A mental health assessment documents

BOX 6-1 MENTAL STATUS EXAMINATION

I. Appearance
General presentation to others.

II. Behaviour
Mood and affect: Expressing the prevailing feelings through mood (a sustained emotion that the patient is experiencing) and affect (a display of feelings or state of mind).

Speech: Using language and the voice to communicate one's thoughts and feelings. Because this is a basic tool of humans, its loss has a devastating social effect on the individual.

III. Cognition
Consciousness: Being aware of one's feelings, thoughts, and environment. This is the most elementary of mental health functions.

Orientation: Awareness of the objective world in relation to the self.

Memory: The ability to set down and store experiences and perceptions for later recall; *immediate* memory involves on-the-spot recall, *recent* memory evokes day-to-day events, and *remote* memory includes years' worth of experiences.

Attention and concentration: The power to direct thinking toward an object or topic with the ability to focus on one specific thing without being distracted by other competing stimuli.

Comprehension and abstract reasoning: Pondering a deeper meaning beyond the concrete and literal.

IV. Thinking
Perception: An awareness of objects through the five senses.

Content: What the person thinks: specific ideas, beliefs, the use of words.

Process: The *way* a person thinks; the logical train of thought.

Insight: Awareness of the reality of the situation.

Judgement: Ability to choose a logical course of action.

---

language function, as well as any associated emotional problems such as depression or agitation.

- Symptoms (e.g., extreme worrying and avoidance) of psychiatric mental illness, especially with acute onset, are evident.

In every mental health assessment, note the following factors that could affect your interpretation:

- Any known illnesses or health problems, such as alcoholism or chronic renal disease.
- Current medications, the adverse effects of which may cause confusion or depression.
- The usual educational and behavioural level; note that factor as the normal baseline, and do not expect performance on the mental health assessment to exceed it.
- Responses to personal history questions, indicating current stress, social interaction patterns, sleep habits, drug and alcohol use.

 DEVELOPMENTAL CONSIDERATIONS

Children and Adolescents

The maturation of emotional and cognitive functioning is described in the Evolve Online materials for this book. All aspects of mental health are interdependent. For example, the concept of language as a social tool of communication occurs around 3 to 5 years of age, coincident with the child's readiness to play cooperatively with other children. School readiness coincides with the development of the thought process; around age 7, thinking becomes more logical and systematic, and the child is able to reason and understand. Progression through developmental stages toward independence and the full range of health determinants affects the experience of adolescence (Kidder & Rogers, 2004; World Health Organization, 2007). At this time, multiple cellular, molecular, and anatomical modifications contribute to pronounced changes in cognition, behaviour, and temperament; risk taking and novelty seeking are perhaps the greatest changes (Kelley, Schochet, & Landry, 2004). Abstract thinking—the ability to consider a hypothetical situation—usually develops between ages 12 and 15, although a few adolescents never achieve it.

The leading cause of mortality among youth in Canada is unintentional injuries, at a rate of 21.3 per 100,000 population (Statistics Canada, 2010). For adolescents aged 15 to 19 years, suicide (intentional self-harm) is the second leading cause of death. Another increasing trend is homicide; in fact, the rate of mortality from firearms among Canadians younger than 15 years is one of the highest in the world, with Canada ranking fifth, behind the United States, Finland, Northern Ireland, and Israel (Adolescent Health Committee, Canadian Paediatric Society, 2005).

The most common mental health disorders among adolescents include depression, anxiety disorders, attention-deficit/hyperactivity disorder, and substance use disorder; half of diagnosable mental health disorders over the lifetime begin by age 14 (Knopf, Park, & Mulye, 2008; PHAC, 2011). Eating disorders represent the third most common chronic illness among Canadian female adolescents (National Eating Disorder Information Centre, 2005); 34% of adolescent girls in grades 6 to 10 described themselves as too fat, whereas only 15% of those grade 10 girls were actually overweight, according to their self-reported heights and weights (PHAC, 2008). Adolescent girls tend to have poorer self-confidence (a measure of mental health), and higher rates of depression and experience more sexual harassment than do adolescent boys (Ge, Conger, & Elder, 2001; PHAC, 2008). Youth who are Aboriginal, immigrant, homeless, and within a sexual minority (those who identified as lesbian, gay, bisexual, transgender, or questioning) in Canada were more likely to experience discrimination, stigmatization, harassment, bullying, less sense of belonging to their school community, and a lack of appropriate education, services, and protective measures and policies—all of which increase their risk for mental health problems (Birkett, Espelage, & Koenig, 2009; Evenson & Barr, 2009; Mental Health Commission of Canada, 2012; Statistics Canada, 2009; Taylor et al., 2008).

Young Adults

A task of young adulthood is adopting health behaviours while facing different types of health challenges, which may include experiencing social isolation (Cacioppo et al., 2006) and adjusting to disabilities and academic stressors during postsecondary education programs. Of all Canadians aged 15 years and older, young adults report the highest percentage of smoking and the highest incidence of depression. By age 34, 75% of mental health disorders diagnosable over the lifetime have begun (Knopf et al., 2008; PHAC, 2011). Many young adults also begin their working lives in debt from their years in postsecondary education. In 2009, 45% of college graduates owed on average $13,600, and 60% of university graduates owed twice as much (Berger, 2009; Canadian Council on Learning, 2010).

Middle-Aged Adults

People in their 40s, 50s, and early 60s commonly process information more slowly and are more vulnerable to distraction than in their youth. They use experience to compensate for age-related deficiencies in memory and reaction time. There is evidence that the brain can remain strong and even improve its performance well through the middle-age years, a period of maximum performance for some of the more complex, higher order mental abilities, such as inductive reasoning, spatial orientation, and vocabulary (Schaie & Willis, 2011). Moreover, middle age may also bring more confidence, more skill at quick assessment, and adaptability. Men reach their peak performance in these abilities in their 50s and women in their early 60s.

Challenges during middle age require skills in organizing, problem solving, and multitasking. For example, family obligations peak for middle-aged adults who have good health and numerous elderly relatives and whose children are just moving out and establishing their own families. The effect of being "caught in the middle," albeit not a typical experience for most Canadian adults, may be severe (Rosenthal, Matthews, & Matthews, 1996).

High demands and low social support within the workforce can cause the development of depressive symptoms among middle-aged workers. Job losses caused by firings or layoffs reduce health, self-esteem, and the sense of control (Clark, 2005). Concurrently, daily stressors directly affect emotional and physical functioning, and the accumulation of persistent irritations and overloads may result in more serious stress reactions such as anxiety and depression. Middle-aged adults with high mastery (e.g., successful problem-solving skills) reported less emotional reactivity to stressors (Neupert, Almeida, & Charles, 2007).

Biological changes related to menopause or late onset male hypogonadism may influence cognition and well-being. Middle-aged people tend to reassess their achievements in terms of ideals and may subsequently make significant changes in day-to-day life or situations, such as career, work–life balance, marriage, romantic relationships, large expenditures, or physical appearance (Lachman, 2004).

Older Adults

The aging process leaves the parameters of mental health mostly intact. There is no decrease in general knowledge and little or no loss in vocabulary. Because it takes a bit longer for the brain to process information and react to it, performance on timed intelligence tests may be poorer for older adults. The slower response time affects new learning; older adults have difficulty responding to a rapidly paced new presentation (Birren & Schaie, 2005). Recent memory, which requires some processing (e.g., medication instructions, 24-hour diet recall), decreases somewhat with aging. Intelligence and remote memory are not affected.

Age-related changes in sensory perception can affect mental functioning. For example, vision loss (as detailed in Chapter 15) may result in apathy, social isolation, and depression. Hearing changes are common (see the discussion of presbycusis in Chapter 16). Age-related hearing loss involves sounds of high frequencies. Consonants are high-frequency sounds, and so older adults who have difficulty hearing them have problems with normal conversation. This problem produces frustration, suspicion, and social withdrawal, and it makes the person look confused. Data analyzed from a large Canadian study suggested that older adults with overall functional impairment (e.g., inability to perform housework) exhibited more cognitive impairment 5 years later than did those without functional impairment (Tuokko, Morris, & Ebert, 2005).

Meanwhile, the era of older adulthood contains much potential for loss of loved ones, job status and prestige income, energy, and resilience of the body. The grief and despair surrounding these losses can affect mental health and result in disorientation, disability, or depression.

SCREENING

In 2005 the Canadian Task Force on Preventative Health Care concluded that there is fair evidence to support routine screening for depression in primary care settings as a way of improving detection rates (MacMillan, Patterson, & Wathen, 2005). Screening is effective if it successfully identifies depressed patients who are not already identified and treated and if the number of people incorrectly labelled as possibly depressed is minimized (Thombs et al., 2012). In studies in which the screening process was linked to an integrated system of treatment and follow-up, patient outcomes improved. More extensive patient education about depression, alertness and response to symptoms of depression, and targeting of specific at-risk groups, including older individuals, is recommended (National Collaborating Centre for Mental Health, 2010; O'Connor, Whitlock, Gaynes, & Beil, 2009).

A number of screening tools are available; however, Dowrick (2004) cautioned that the use of screening instruments may encourage practitioners to take a reductionist, biomedical approach, which would divert attention from a broader biopsychosocial approach to identifying depression.

MENTAL HEALTH ASSESSMENT: ADULTS

Patients can perceive the mental health assessment as threatening even though their cooperation is necessary for its success. Although many nurses find it desirable to establish some degree of rapport first and thereby place the patient at ease, some nurses assess mental health before working with the patient so that the findings can serve as a template against which to measure the accuracy of the rest of the health history. The successful clinician must develop a style in which much of the mental health assessment is performed through relatively unstructured observations made during history taking and physical examination. The way in which patients relate the history of the current situation and interact in the clinical setting reveals much about their mental health.

Identification/Biographical Information

Note the primary language spoken by the patient, the name the patient prefers to be called, legal name, address, telephone numbers, birthdate and birthplace, gender, relationship status, ethnicity, education, and employment. Usually questions about this information are nonthreatening and thus a safe way to begin.

Reason for Seeking Care

Record the patient's explanation verbatim to describe the reason for the visit. Be knowledgeable of the psychiatric diagnoses (*DSM-V*) provided by the attending physician/psychiatrist. Ask what the patient understands about the need to visit your agency.

Past Health

Past Illness, Injury, Hospitalization

Note childhood diseases, surgeries, and trauma (especially if any resulted in concussion or loss of consciousness). Ask about parental use of alcohol and drugs, birth trauma, any pattern of injury suggestive of childhood abuse or neglect, and any obstetrical history. Ask specifically, "Have you ever experienced or witnessed anything that threatened your life or safety or the life and safety of a loved one?" If the answer is "yes," ask for details, keeping in mind that psychological trauma is associated with many mental disorders (e.g., anxiety and depression).

Chronic Illnesses

The stress of chronic illnesses, even when well managed, may affect mental health.

Family Health History

Ask the age and current health of close relatives (e.g., partner, children, parents, siblings, grandparents, aunts, and uncles). If the patient reports a family member's death, ask for the date, the cause, and the effect on the patient. Ask about any illnesses that "run in the family" because many mental disorders are genetically linked and family health history provides information about the patient's risk factors. Ask about any history of postpartum depression because this can induce maternal physical, marital, social, and vocational difficulties; impair maternal–infant interactions; and affect an infant's cognitive and emotional development (Poobalan et al., 2007). Assessing family health identifies sources of social support, family stress, coping ability, and resources.

 DEVELOPMENTAL CONSIDERATIONS

Ask about the achievement of educational and developmentally appropriate tasks and milestones that may indicate attention, interpersonal, or behavioural problems. Ask specifically about parental death or separation at an early age because these are often associated with issues of attachment and later relationships. The past Canadian government practice of sending Aboriginal children to residential schools perpetuated social and psychological trauma among First Nations people.

Current Health

Using a systematic approach to ensure comprehensiveness, sort and cluster information about conditions that affect patient mental health, overall functioning, and quality of life. In addition to asking the patient to describe the critical characteristics of specific concerns outlined in Chapter 5, note the following:

1. Known allergies, type of reaction, and usual treatment and relief measures.
2. Status of immunizations, human immunodeficiency virus (HIV), infection, and hepatitis infection. Persons experiencing mental illness may often dwell in poverty, lack knowledge and supports for health promotion, and have lifestyles that put them at risk for communicable diseases.
3. Current medications. Specify the name of the medication, purpose, usual dose, frequency, effectiveness, side effects, name of prescriber, duration of taking the medication, and any over-the-counter and herbal preparations. This information helps identify health maintenance behaviours, drug interactions, and potential knowledge deficits.

DETAILED MENTAL STATUS EXAMINATION

The mental status examination, an integral subset of the comprehensive mental health nursing assessment, involves a sequence of steps that form a *hierarchy* in which the most basic functions (consciousness, language) are assessed first. Accurate assessment of the first steps ensures validity for the steps that follow; that is, if consciousness is clouded, then the patient cannot be expected to have full attention and cooperate with new learning. If language is impaired, subsequent assessment of new learning or abstract reasoning (which requires language functioning) can yield erroneous conclusions. Strive to ask questions that can be corroborated, to enhance reliability.

PREPARATION

Record the exact time and date of the mental status examination because the mental status can change quickly, as in delirium.

EQUIPMENT NEEDED

Pencil, paper, reading material (occasionally)

Normal Range of Findings	Abnormal Findings

Appearance

Posture. *Posture* is erect, and *position* is relaxed.

Sitting on edge of chair or curled in bed, tense muscles, frowning, darting eyes, and restless pacing occur with anxiety and hyperthyroidism. Sitting slumped in chair, walking slowly, and dragging feet occur with depression and some organic brain diseases.

Body Movements. *Body movements* are voluntary, deliberate, coordinated, smooth, and even.

Restless, fidgety movements may occur with anxiety.

Apathy and psychomotor slowing may occur with depression and organic brain disease.

Abnormal posturing and bizarre gestures may occur with schizophrenia.

Facial grimaces may be associated with such conditions as cerebral palsy, chorea, hypocalcemia, tetanus, pain, tardive dyskinesia, tic disorder, and Tourette's syndrome.

Dress. *Dress* is appropriate for setting, season, age, gender, and social group. Clothing fits and is put on appropriately.

Dress can be inappropriate with organic brain syndrome. Eccentric dress combination and bizarre makeup may occur with schizophrenia or manic syndrome.

Grooming and Hygiene. The patient is clean and well-groomed; hair is neat and clean; women have moderate or no makeup; men are shaved, or beard or moustache is well-groomed. Nails are clean (though some jobs leave nails chronically dirty). Use care in interpreting clothing that is dishevelled, bizarre, or in poor repair; piercings; and tattoos, because these sometimes reflect the person's economic status or a deliberate fashion trend (especially among adolescents).

Unilateral neglect (total inattention to one side of body) may occur after stroke. Inappropriate dress, poor hygiene, and lack of concern with appearance occur with depression and severe Alzheimer's disease. Meticulously dressed and groomed appearance and fastidious manner may occur with obsessive–compulsive disorders.

Note: A dishevelled appearance in a previously well-groomed patient is significant.

Behaviour

Level of Consciousness. The patient is awake, alert, and aware of stimuli from the environment and within the self and responds appropriately to stimuli.

Altered levels of consciousness may include coma (unresponsiveness); stupor (responsiveness to pain), and lethargy (drowsiness; Table 6-2 on page 98).

Facial Expression. The expression is appropriate to the situation and changes appropriately with the topic. There is comfortable eye contact unless precluded by cultural norm, e.g., for members of some Aboriginal cultures.

Expression may be flat and masklike with parkinsonism and depression.

Speech. Judge the quality of speech by noting that the patient makes laryngeal sounds effortlessly and makes conversation appropriately. Note whether the voice is raised or muffled, whether the replies to questions are one-word or elaborative, and how fast or slow the patient speaks.

Normally, the pace of the conversation is moderate, and stream of talking is fluent.

Dysphonia is abnormal volume and pitch. Patient may monopolize the interview or may remain silent, secretive, or uncommunicative.

Speech may be slow and monotonous with parkinsonism and depression. Speech may be rapid-fire, pressured, and loud with manic syndrome.

Normal Range of Findings	**Abnormal Findings**

Articulation (ability to form words) is clear and understandable.

Word choice is effortless and appropriate to educational level. The patient completes sentences, occasionally pausing to think.

Mood and Affect. Judge this by body language and facial expression and by the answer to the direct question "How do you feel today?" or "How do you feel most days?" Ask about the length of a particular mood, whether the mood has been reactive or not, and whether the mood has been stable or unstable. The affect (expression) should be appropriate to the mood and change appropriately with topics.

Cognitive Functions

Orientation. You can discern orientation through the course of the interview, or you may ask for it directly but tactfully: "Some people have trouble keeping up with the dates while in the hospital. Do you know today's date?" Assess the patient's orientation:

Time: day of week, date, year, season
Place: where person lives, present location, type of building, names of city and
 province
Person: who examiner is, type of worker
Self: person's own name, age

Many hospitalized patients normally have trouble with the exact date but are fully oriented on the remaining items.

Attention Span. Check ability to concentrate by noting whether the patient completes a thought without wandering. Note any distractibility or difficulty attending to you. An alternative approach is to give a series of directions to follow in a correct sequence of behaviours, such as "Please put this label on your keys, place the keys into the brown envelope, and give the envelope to the clerk for safe keeping during your admission."

Immediate Memory. Immediate memory enables making sense of what is going on. For example, it is used during reading to recall what happens sentence by sentence. Assess by asking the patient to recall a statement you just made.

Recent Memory. Assess recent memory in the context of the interview by the 24-hour diet recall or by asking what time the patient arrived at the agency. Ask verifiable questions to screen for the occasional person who confabulates (makes up) answers to fill in the gaps of memory loss.

Remote Memory. In the context of the interview, ask the patient about verifiable past events; for example, ask to describe historical events that are relevant for the patient.

Abnormal Findings

Dysarthria is distorted speech. Misuse of words; omitting letters, syllables, or words; and transposing words occur with aphasia.

Unduly long word-finding or failure in word search occurs with aphasia.

Table 6-3 lists mood and affect abnormalities. Wide mood swings occur with manic syndrome. Altered mood states are apparent in schizophrenia. Heightened emotional activity and severely limited emotional or elicited responses (e.g., "OK," "Rough," and "Don't know") necessitate further questioning for clarification of mood.

Disorientation occurs with organic brain disorders, such as delirium and dementia. Orientation is usually lost in this order: first to time, then to place, and rarely to person and self. Disorientation to personal identity is associated with post-epileptic seizure states, other dissociative disorders, and agnosia (loss of the ability to recognize sensory inputs).

Attention span is commonly impaired in persons who experience anxiety, fatigue, drug intoxication, or attention-deficit/hyperactivity disorder. Impairment is conveyed as confusion, negativism, digression from initial thought, irrelevant replies to questions, or being "stimulus bound" (i.e., any new stimulus quickly draws attention).

Head injury, fatigue, anxiety, and strong emotions can affect immediate memory.

The individual affected may demonstrate repetition (e.g., asking the same question) and difficulty finding words during conversation which may lead to frustration.

Recent memory deficit occurs with organic disorders, such as delirium, dementia, amnesia, or, in chronic alcoholism, Korsakoff's syndrome.

Remote memory is lost when the cortical storage area for that memory is damaged, as in Alzheimer's dementia or any disease that damages the cerebral cortex.

Normal Range of Findings	Abnormal Findings

New Learning: The Four Unrelated Words Test. This tests the patient's ability to acquire new memories. It is a highly sensitive and valid memory test that avoids the danger of unverifiable material.

Say to the patient, "I am going to say four words. I want you to remember them. In a few minutes I will ask you to recall them." To be sure that the patient has understood, repeat the words. Pick four words with semantic and phonetic diversity:

1. brown	1. fun
2. honesty	2. carrot
3. tulip	3. ankle
4. eyedropper	4. loyalty

After 5 minutes, ask the patient to recall the four words. To test the duration of memory, ask for a recall at 10 minutes and at 30 minutes. The normal response for persons younger than 60 years is an accurate three- or four-word recall after a 5-, 10-, and 30-minute delay (Osaka & Logie, 2007).

People with Alzheimer's dementia score a zero- or one-word recall. Ability for new learning is also impaired with anxiety (because of inattention and distractibility) and depression (because of a lack of interest or motivation).

Additional Testing for Patients With Aphasia

Word Comprehension. Point to articles in the room, and ask the patient to name them.

Aphasia is the loss of ability to speak or to understand speech, as a result of a stroke.

Speech and language dyslexia, a neurological disorder or learning disability, may create difficulty understanding what other people say (developmental receptive language disorder) or difficulty using spoken language to communicate (developmental expressive language disorder).

Aphasia may limit ability to understand written words. Speech and language dyslexia may create difficulty producing speech sounds (developmental articulation disorder). The individual might mispronounce certain letters or letter combinations. With academic learning dyslexia, the individual cannot identify different word sounds.

Reading. An awareness of a patient's reading and writing impairment is important in planning health teaching and rehabilitation. To assess reading, ask the patient to read available print, being careful not to test just literacy.

Writing. Ask the patient to compose and write a sentence. Note coherence, spelling, and parts of speech (the sentence should have a subject and verb).

Aphasia may limit ability to write coherently. Dyslexia may affect writing abilities, and performance in written language exams will be very poor. With developmental writing disorder, or dysgraphia, the individual has problems with handwriting or with creating sentences that make sense to others.

Higher Intellectual Function

Tests of higher intellectual functioning measure problem-solving and reasoning abilities. Results correspond closely to the patient's general intelligence and must be assessed in view of educational and cultural backgrounds. These tests have been widely used to distinguish between organic brain disease and psychiatric disorders; however, there is little evidence that most of these tests validly detect organic dysfunction or have relevance for daily clinical care. Thus, many time-honoured, standard tests of higher intellectual function (such as proverb interpretation) are not discussed here.

Many mental illnesses are associated with varying levels of insight. For example, people with obsessive–compulsive disorder (OCD) often have relatively good insight that they have a problem and that their thoughts and actions are unreasonable, but they are nonetheless compelled to carry out the thoughts and actions (Marková, Jaafari, & Berrios, 2009).

Normal Range of Findings	Abnormal Findings

Insight and Judgement

Insight is the ability to recognize one's own illness, need for treatment, and consequences of one's behaviour as stemming from an illness.

Patients exercise judgement when they compare and evaluate the alternatives in a situation and reach an appropriate course of action. To assess judgement in the context of the interview, note what the patient says about job plans and social or family obligations; plans for the future; and capacity for violent or suicidal behaviour. Job and future plans should be realistic, in view of the patient's health situation. To assess insight into illness, ask whether patients believe they need help or whether they believe their feelings or conditions are normal.

Further assess insight by asking patients to describe their rationale for personal health care and how they decided about whether to comply with prescribed health regimens. The patient's actions and decisions should be realistic.

Persons with Alzheimer's disease, schizophrenia, or various psychotic conditions tend to have poor awareness that anything is wrong with them (Marková, Berrios, & Hodges, 2004). Judgement is impaired (unrealistic or impulsive decisions) with intellectual disability, emotional dysfunction, schizophrenia, and organic brain disease.

Thought Processes, Thought Content, and Perceptions

Thought Processes. Ask yourself, "Does this person make sense? Can I follow what the person is saying?" Note whether the patient responds directly to the questions or deviates from the subject at hand and has to be guided back to the topic more than once.

The *way* a patient thinks should be logical, goal directed, coherent, and relevant. The patient should complete a thought.

Thought Content. *What* the patient says should be consistent and logical. To identify any obsessions or compulsions, ask such questions as these:

"How often do you wash your hands or count things over and over?"
"Do you perform specific actions to reduce certain thoughts?"

Explore ritualistic behaviours further to determine the severity of the obsession or compulsion.

To identify any fears that cause the patient to avoid certain situations, ask if he or she has any fears, such as fear of animals, needles, heights, snakes, public speaking, or crowds.

Table 6-4 lists examples of abnormal thought processes.

Persons with OCD often demonstrate both obsessions (obsessive thoughts, ideas, or fears) and compulsions (repetitive rituals to reduce anxiety and stress in response to obsessions). Obsessions are annoying, fearful, at times harmful, and driven by different motives (e.g., fear of being hurt or hurting others, fear of infections or contamination, and need to make everything clean and orderly). Obsessions may have a religious, medical, sexual, or sadistic underpinning. Compulsions bring temporary relief but do not eliminate the obsessions. For example, if a person is afraid of germs and washes hands again and again, every washing does not make the person believe that hands are already clean enough and that there is no danger of receiving germs anymore; thus repeated washing continues. Table 6-5 lists examples of disordered thought content.

To determine whether a person is having delusions, ask, "Do you have any thoughts that other people think are strange?" or "Do you have any special powers or abilities?"

Delusions are false beliefs that occur when abnormal significance is attached to a genuine perception without rational or emotional justification. Types of delusions include grandiose (delusions of grandeur, entitlement), religious (belief that one *is* a [or the] deity), persecution (belief that someone wants to cause the patient harm), erotomanic (belief that someone famous is in love with the patient), jealousy (belief that everyone wants what the patient has), thought insertion (belief that someone is putting ideas into the patient's mind), and ideas of reference (belief that everything refers to the patient).

Normal Range of Findings	Abnormal Findings

Perceptions. The patient should be consistently aware of reality, and his or her perceptions should be congruent with yours. Ask the following:

- "How do people treat you?"
- "Do you feel as if you are being watched, followed, or controlled?"
- "Is your imagination very active?"
- "Have you heard your name when you're alone?"

If the responses to these questions suggest that a person is experiencing hallucinations, ask some of the following questions: "Do you ever hear voices when no one else is around?" "Can you sometimes see things that no one else can see?" "Do you have other unexplained sensations such as smells, sounds, or feelings?"

If command-type hallucinations are experienced, always ask what the person will do in response. For example, "When the voices tell you to do something, do you obey their instructions or ignore them?"

Illusions (misinterpretation of a true optical, auditory, tactile, or olfactory sensation). For example, a brown sock on the floor appears to be a mouse.

Hallucinations (perceptions occurring while the patient is awake and conscious and in the absence of external stimuli): Auditory and visual hallucinations occur with psychiatric and organic brain disease and with ingestion of psychedelic drugs. Tactile hallucinations occur with alcohol withdrawal.

SUPPLEMENTAL MENTAL STATUS EXAMINATION

The Montreal Cognitive Assessment (MoCA; Nasreddine et al., 2005) is quick, includes standard sets of questions, has standardized administration methods, requires only 10 to 15 minutes to administer, and is free for nonprofit use (Figure 6-1). The MoCA is useful for initial and serial measurements, and so you can use it to demonstrate worsening or improving cognition over time and with treatment. The MoCA includes a clock-drawing test (also see p. 93).

With its sensitivity of 90% for detecting mild cognitive impairment and specificity of 87% (Nasreddine et al., 2005),

the MoCA is considered a good screening tool to detect dementia and delirium and to differentiate these from psychiatric mental illness. The MoCA demonstrated adequate psychometric properties as a screening instrument for the detection of mild cognitive impairment or dementia in Parkinson's disease (Hoops et al., 2009; Zadikoff et al., 2008), in transient ischemic attack and stroke (Pendlebury, Cuthbertson, Welch, Mehta, & Rothwell, 2010), and in psychiatric rehabilitation (Aggarwal & Kean, 2010). The validity of the MoCA has been established in memory clinic settings (Smith, Gildeh, & Holmes, 2007).

Normal Range of Findings	Abnormal Findings

The maximum score on the MoCA is 30; scores above 26 indicate no cognitive impairment.

Scores that occur with dementia and delirium are classified as follows:
18 to 23 = mild cognitive impairment
0 to 7 = severe cognitive impairment

FUNCTIONAL ASSESSMENT (INCLUDING ACTIVITIES OF DAILY LIVING)

Record the dates of the most recent medical examination, eye examination, and dental examination. Ask the patient to describe a typical day and what the patient does on a daily, weekly, and annual basis to promote and maintain health. Assess self-care abilities, including activities of daily living such as bathing, hygiene, dressing, toileting, eating, walking, housekeeping, shopping, cooking, communicating with others, social relationships, finances, and coping. In particular, note the following:

Nutritional Patterns. Record the dietary intake recalled by the patient over the past 24 hours (Chapter 12). Ask whether any recent dietary changes have occurred. Note any dissatisfaction with body size, weight, or shape, as well as practices directed at weight loss, particularly if the patient is

female, an elite athlete, or engaged in an occupation that emphasizes physical appearance, inasmuch as these factors contribute to eating disorders.

Sleep/Rest Changes. Ask about sleep onset (how much time it takes to fall asleep), sleep maintenance (frequency of wakening and returning to sleep), early awakening (before the patient needs to be awake), sleep hygiene (measures to promote sleep, such as avoiding caffeine at bedtime), and sleep satisfaction (feeling rested and refreshed). Alterations in sleep are common in many mental disorders (e.g., mania, depression, schizophrenia).

Activity/Mobility. Withdrawal from usual activities may signal illness. Avolition (lack of motivational drive and energy) is a symptom of depression, schizophrenia, and chronic marijuana use. Excessive pursuit of physical activity may be associated with mania and eating disorders.

MONTREAL COGNITIVE ASSESSMENT (MOCA)
Version 7.1 Original Version

NAME :
Education :   Date of birth :
Sex :   DATE :

VISUOSPATIAL / EXECUTIVE

Copy cube

Draw CLOCK (Ten past eleven)
(3 points)

POINTS

[ ]   [ ]   [   ]   [   ]   [   ]   __/5
                         Contour   Numbers   Hands

NAMING

[ ]   [ ]   [ ]   __/3

MEMORY
Read list of words, subject must repeat them. Do 2 trials, even if 1st trial is successful. Do a recall after 5 minutes.

	FACE	VELVET	CHURCH	DAISY	RED
1st trial					
2nd trial					

No points

ATTENTION
Read list of digits (1 digit/ sec.).

Subject has to repeat them in the forward order   [ ] 2 1 8 5 4

Subject has to repeat them in the backward order   [ ] 7 4 2

__/2

Read list of letters. The subject must tap with his hand at each letter A. No points if ≥ 2 errors

[ ]   F B A C M N A A J K L B A F A K D E A A A J A M O F A A B

__/1

Serial 7 subtraction starting at 100   [ ] 93   [ ] 86   [ ] 79   [ ] 72   [ ] 65

4 or 5 correct subtractions: **3 pts**, 2 or 3 correct: **2 pts**, 1 correct: **1 pt**, 0 correct: **0 pt**

__/3

LANGUAGE
Repeat : I only know that John is the one to help today. [ ]
The cat always hid under the couch when dogs were in the room. [ ]

__/2

Fluency / Name maximum number of words in one minute that begin with the letter F   [ ] _____ (N ≥ 11 words)

__/1

ABSTRACTION
Similarity between e.g. banana - orange = fruit   [ ] train – bicycle   [ ] watch - ruler

__/2

DELAYED RECALL

	FACE	VELVET	CHURCH	DAISY	RED	Points for UNCUED recall only
Has to recall words **WITH NO CUE**	[ ]	[ ]	[ ]	[ ]	[ ]	
Optional Category cue						
Multiple choice cue						

__/5

ORIENTATION
[ ] Date   [ ] Month   [ ] Year   [ ] Day   [ ] Place   [ ] City

__/6

© Z.Nasreddine MD   www.mocatest.org   Normal ≥ 26 / 30   TOTAL   __/30

Administered by: _____   Add 1 point if ≤ 12 yr edu

6-1 Montreal Cognitive Assessment. *Source: Copyright Z. Nasreddine, MD. Reproduced with permission. Copies are available at* www.mocatest.org.

Elimination. Psychotropic medications may lead to constipation and urinary retention. People may misuse laxatives and diuretics in an attempt to lose weight.

Interpersonal Relationships and Resources. Assess the patient's role in family and social networks to identify sources of stress and support. Any withdrawal from usual relationships could indicate declining mental health.

Self-Esteem/Self-Concept. Ask the patient to rate self on a scale from 0 to 10, on which 10 represents the best possible way to feel about self. Ask about values, beliefs, practices, and accomplishments that are most important to the patient.

Spirituality. Ask questions to understand the meaning of faith, spirituality, and religion:

> *"What is it that gives your life meaning? What gives you joy?"*
> *"What, if any, religious activities do you participate in?"*
> *"Do you feel connected with the world?"*
> *"Do you believe in God or a higher power?"*

Coping and Stress Management. Ask about major stressors to understand and evaluate current coping behaviours.

Smoking, Alcohol/Drug Use, and Problem Gambling. Inquire about usual patterns of alcohol use, drug use, and gambling and about any recent changes to those patterns. Ask whether persons close to the patient would believe that alcohol, drug use, or gambling is a problem in the patient's life.

Home and Environmental Hazards. Ask about safety issues associated with meal preparation, bathing, walking in the home and community, lighting, home heating, transportation to health care clinics, social and commercial services, and social events.

RISK ASSESSMENT

Screen for Suicidal Thoughts

It is difficult to question patients about possible suicidal wishes, especially for novice examiners who may fear invading privacy and may have their own normal discomfort with death and suicide. However, the risk is far greater if you skip these questions; you may be the only health care provider to detect clues of suicide risk.

When the patient expresses sadness, hopelessness, despair, or grief, assess any possible risk that the patient will cause physical harm to himself or herself. Begin with more general questions; if you hear affirmative answers, continue with more specific questions:

> *"Have you ever felt so blue you thought of hurting yourself?"*
> *"Do you feel like hurting yourself now?"*
> *"Do you have a plan to hurt yourself?"*
> *"What would happen if you were dead?"*
> *"How would other people react if you were dead?"*

Inquire directly about specific plans, suicide notes, family history (anniversary reaction), and impulse control. Use a matter-of-fact tone of voice and open posture, and attend with interest (e.g., lean toward the person). If you are unsure whether the patient is at high risk for suicide, get help from an experienced health care team leader.

Important clues and warning signs of suicide are as follows:
- A precise suicide plan to take place in the next 24 to 48 hours with the use of a lethal method (constitutes high risk)
- Prior suicide attempts
- Depression, hopelessness
- Social withdrawal, running away
- Self-mutilation
- Hypersomnia or insomnia
- Slowed psychomotor activity
- Anorexia
- Verbal suicide messages (defeat, failure, worthlessness, loss, giving up, desire to kill self)
- Death themes in art, jokes, writing, behaviours
- Saying goodbye (giving away prized possessions)

You are responsible for encouraging the patient to talk about suicidal thoughts and for obtaining immediate help. Determine whether the patient will agree to make a commitment to treatment and living and to contract for safety by agreeing to implement a plan such as calling a crisis hot line or going to the emergency department.

Although you cannot always prevent a suicide, you can often buy time so that the patient can be helped to find an alternative solution to problems. As soon as possible, share with the health care team any concerns you have about a person's suicide ideation.

Screen for Assaultive or Homicidal Ideation

In addition to assessing suicide threat, inquire about past acts of self-harm or violence:

> *"Do you have any thoughts of wanting to hurt anyone?"*
> *"Do you have any feelings or thoughts that you wish someone were dead?"*

If the reply to either question is positive, ask about any specific plans to injure someone and how the patient plans to control these feelings if they occur again.

Screen for Elopement Risk

Elopement from psychiatric facilities increases risk of injury for patients and others in the community and increases the potential for litigation against the facility (Jayaram, 2009). To reduce risk, check the following:
- Are the doors locked? Are they unlocked manually (not electronically) so that the patient does not slip out with visitors?
- Is the patient restricted to the unit, or does the patient have off-unit privileges?
- Does the patient have an adequate understanding of the need for hospitalization?
- Does the family have adequate knowledge of the risk of elopement?

- Should the patient be placed in hospital clothing, with street clothing and shoes removed, to discourage elopement?
- Has the patient been placed on increased observation status?

GLOBAL ASSESSMENT OF FUNCTIONING

Global assessment of functioning is performed by the psychiatrist or qualified clinician. It is used to estimate overall psychological, social, and occupational functioning within any limitations imposed by patient physical and environmental factors. The findings are scored from low functioning (0 to 10) to high functioning (91 to 100); the scores change over time, and scoring is calculated at the start of treatment, during treatment, at discharge, and at any time after (Table 6-6).

Additional content on mental disorders is listed in Tables 6-7 (delirium and dementia), 6-8 (schizophrenia), 6-9 (mood disorders), and 6-10 (anxiety disorders).

ASSESSING PATIENT ATTITUDE TOWARD THE EXAMINER/ASSESSMENT

Record whether the patient appears hostile, defensive, guarded, or uncomfortable. Often, the patient is willing to cooperate and appears interested, friendly, relaxed, or perhaps bored with the interview process.

 DEVELOPMENTAL CONSIDERATIONS

Normal Range of Findings	Abnormal Findings
Children and Adolescents Essentially, you will follow the same guidelines (assessing appearance, behaviour, cognition, and thought processes) as for adults, with an emphasis on developmental milestones. Thorough knowledge of developmental milestones, as presented in the online Evolve resources accompanying this book, is critical. Although not exclusive to mental health assessment, the Nipissing District Developmental Screen (see Chapter 2) is a screening tool designed to help parents and caregivers monitor children's development from birth to 6 years of age. Areas assessed include vision, hearing, communication, gross motor, fine motor, cognitive, social–emotional, and self-help skills. Other reliable screening instruments (e.g., the Pediatric Symptom Checklist-17) can be given to the parent to assess emotional and behavioural wellness of children aged 4 to 18 years (Gardner, Lucas, Kolko, & Campo, 2007). For adolescents, continue to follow the same guidelines as described for adults. In consideration of adolescent development patterns, specifically evaluate weight in the appearance assessment; regulation (e.g., self-soothing capacity and anger management skills) in the behaviour assessment; and sleep patterns, eating patterns, interpersonal behaviours (with parents, teachers, and examiner), risk (to self and others), high-risk behaviours (e.g., bullying/fire setting/running away/ high-risk sexual activity/cruelty/breaking curfew/lying/stealing/truancy), academic performance (grade, least and most favourite subjects), and substance use with the cognition and thought processes assessments (Canadian School Health Community, 2010).	Abnormalities are often problems of *omission;* the child does not achieve an expected milestone. Trust is a particular challenge in working with adolescents. Responses to questions in areas of behaviour risk and personal safety are apt to be guarded unless the examiner has developed rapport with the adolescent. When possible, it is preferred that you interview the adolescent first, before meeting with parents/guardians.
Adults and Older Adults Always conduct even a brief examination of all older people. Check sensory status before assessing their mental health. It is recommended that you take time, reduce distractions, and minimize sensory impairments to help older people maintain their dignity and perform at their actual level of ability. Age is the greatest risk factor for Alzheimer's disease: 10% of people older than 65 and almost 50% of those older than 85 receive a diagnosis of Alzheimer's disease (Alzheimer's Association, 2011). By 2015, Canada will have more people aged 65 and older than people younger than 15 (Canadian Institutes of Health Research, 2007). Follow the guidelines as described for adults with the *additional* considerations listed in the Older Adult Mental Health Assessment (see next description).	More than 33% of older adults admitted to acute care medical and surgical services show varying degrees of confusion.

OLDER ADULT MENTAL HEALTH ASSESSMENT

Normal Range of Findings	Abnormal Findings

Behaviour

Level of Consciousness. Scales such as the Glasgow Coma Scale (see Chapter 25) that give a numerical value to the person's response avoid ambiguity when numerous examiners care for the same person.

Patients with altered levels of consciousness were found to present with stroke or transient ischemic attack (TIA), diabetes, alcohol use, substance abuse and seizures (Durant & Sporer, 2011).

Cognitive Functions

Orientation. Older adults may not provide the precise date or complete name of the clinic or setting. You may consider older adults oriented to time if the year and month are correctly stated. Orientation to place is considered acceptable if the patient correctly identifies the type of setting (e.g., the hospital) and the name of the town.

Confusion or inability to correctly identify season, name of hometown, name of family members.

New Learning. In people of normal cognitive function, an age-related decline occurs in performance in the Four Unrelated Words Test described on p. 90. Persons in the eighth decade average two of four words recalled over 5 minutes. Their performance improves at 10 and 30 minutes after being reminded by verbal cues (e.g., "one word was a colour; a common flower in Holland is _____").

In people with Alzheimer's dementia, performance does not improve on subsequent trials.

Supplemental Mental Status Examination

Set Test. The Set Test was developed specifically for use with older adults. In the original study (Isaacs & Kennie, 1973), people 65 to 85 years of age were tested. It is a quantifiable test, designed to screen for dementia. The test is easy to administer and takes less than 5 minutes. Ask the patient to name 10 items in each of four categories or sets: fruits, animals, colours, and towns (FACT). Do not coach, prompt, or hurry the person. Each correct answer is scored one point. The maximum total score is 40. No one with a score over 25 has been found to have dementia. (Note: Because this is a verbal test, do not use it with persons with hearing impairments or aphasia.)

Set Test scores lower than 15 indicate dementia. Scores between 15 and 24 show less association with dementia and should be evaluated carefully.

The Set Test assesses mental function as a whole instead of examining individual parts of cognitive function. By asking the person to categorize, name, remember, and count the items in the test, you are really assessing this person's alertness, motivation, concentration, short-term memory, and problem-solving ability.

Clock Test. The patient is asked to draw a clock face to depict a specific time, which requires a variety of cognitive functions, including long-term memory, auditory processing, visual–spatial acuity, concentration, numerical knowledge, and abstract thinking. The advantages to this type of screening tool are the short time it takes to administer (approximately 2 minutes), its ability to be used by individuals with little or no experience in cognitive assessment and minimal training in test administration, and its excellent interrater reliability and sensitivity for differentiating patients with mild Alzheimer's disease from patients without Alzheimer's disease when scored by clinicians with expertise in dementia (Nair et al., 2010). Clock-drawing tests are not recommended for use as the sole screening tools for dementia because the results are influenced by the severity of the cognitive impairment, limited education, and advanced age (Lorentz, Scanlan, & Borson, 2002).

Someone with a delirium might exhibit disorganized thinking, poor planning and reasoning ability; poor visuospatial ability; and distractibility while attempting to focus on the task.

DOCUMENTATION AND CRITICAL THINKING

Sample Charting

Appearance. Posture is erect, with no involuntary body movements. Dress and grooming are appropriate for season and setting.

Behaviour. Alert, with appropriate facial expression and fluent, understandable speech. Affect and verbal responses are appropriate.

Cognitive Functions. Oriented to time, place, person, and self. Able to attend cooperatively with examiner. Recent and remote memory intact. Can recall four unrelated words at 5-, 10-, and 30-minute intervals. Future plans include returning to home and to local university once individual therapy is established and medication is adjusted.

Thought Processes. Perceptions and thought processes are logical and coherent. No suicide ideation.

Focused Assessment: Clinical Case Study

SUBJECTIVE

Mrs. Lola P. is a 79-year-old married woman, recently hospitalized for evaluation of increasing memory loss, confusion, and socially inappropriate behaviour. Her daughter, who visits daily, reports that Mrs. P.'s hygiene and grooming have decreased; Mrs. P. eats very little, has lost weight, does not sleep through the night, displays angry emotional outbursts that are unlike her former demeanour, and does not recognize her younger grandchildren. According to her husband, Mrs. P. has drifted away from the stove while cooking, allowing food to burn on the stovetop. He has found her wandering through the house in the middle of the night, unsure of where she is. She used to "talk on the phone for hours" but now he has to force her into conversations.

OBJECTIVE

During this hospitalization, Mrs. P. has undergone a series of medical tests, including a lumbar puncture, electroencephalography, and computed tomography of the head, all of which yielded normal findings. Her physician suggests a diagnosis of senile dementia of the Alzheimer's type.

Appearance. Mrs. P. is sitting quietly, somewhat slumped, picking at loose threads on her dress. A hooded, zippered sweatshirt top is worn over her dress. Her hair is gathered in a loose ponytail with stray wisps. She wears no makeup.

Behaviour. Mrs. P. is awake and gazing at her hands and lap. Her expression is flat and vacant. She makes eye contact when called by name, although her gaze quickly shifts back to her lap. Her speech is a bit slow but articulate; she has some trouble with word choice.

Cognitive Functions. Mrs. P. is oriented to person and place. She can state the season but not the day of the week or the year. She is not able to repeat the correct sequence of complex directions involving lifting and shifting a glass of water to the other hand. She scores a one-word recall on the Four Unrelated Words Test. She cannot tell the examiner how she would plan a grocery-shopping trip.

Thought Processes. Mrs. P. experiences blocking in train of thought. Her thought content is logical. She acts cranky and suspicious with family members. She reports no suicide ideation.

Her MoCA score is 16.

ASSESSMENT

Confusion
Impaired social interaction
Impaired memory
Wandering

Nursing Diagnoses That May Be Relevant to Mrs. P.

Impaired verbal communication related to cerebral impairment, as demonstrated by altered memory and judgement.

Bathing self-care deficit, feeding self-care deficit, and toileting self-care deficit related to cognitive impairment, as demonstrated by inattention to hygiene, nutrition, and sleep needs.

Altered nutrition: less than body requirements as evidenced by reduced intake and weight loss.

Impaired social interaction related to cognitive impairment and withdrawal from others.

Risk for injury related to cognitive impairment, unsupervised cooking, and wandering behaviour.

Risk for self-directed violence and risk for other-directed related to angry outbursts.

All nursing diagnoses can be found on the Evolve Web site at *http://evolve.elsevier.com/Canada/Jarvis/examination/*.

Overall Goals

Help Mrs. P achieve her highest level of safety and independence in such areas as nutrition, activities of daily living, grooming, and social interaction.

Sample Interventions

Ensure that any aids for vision and hearing are positioned correctly and in good working order. Each time you begin a conversation with Mrs. P., make eye contact, identify yourself, and call her by name. Communicate slowly and clearly through short conversations, single-step instructions, and repetition; reduce background distractions such as television.

Allow Mrs. P. enough time to process questions and formulate responses. Observe her verbal and nonverbal communications, and show interest in what she is communicating. Do not interrupt when she is trying to communicate an idea because this may distract her and cause her to lose her train of thought. Unless you are conducting a supplemental mental status assessment, it may be helpful to supply a word that she is struggling to find. Speak in a low-pitched voice while maintaining an open, calm and friendly communication manner.

It is important to remember to break down tasks into very basic steps (e.g., [1] Pick up hairbrush, [2] brush front of hair, [3] brush back of hair, [4] put hair brush down).

Evaluation and Reassessment

Evaluate mental health at least partially during every shift and reassess in full when a change in status is observed.

ABNORMAL FINDINGS

TABLE 6-2	Levels of Consciousness

The terms below are commonly used in clinical practice. To increase clarity, record also:

1. The level of stimulus used, ranging progressively from
   - Name called in normal tone of voice
   - Name called in loud voice
   - Light touch on person's arm
   - Vigorous shake of shoulder
   - Pain applied
2. The patient's response
   - Amount and quality of movement
   - Presence and coherence of speech
   - Opening of eyes and making eye contact
3. What the patient does on cessation of your stimulus

Alert

Awake or readily aroused, oriented, fully aware of external and internal stimuli and responds appropriately, conducts meaningful interpersonal interactions

Lethargic (or Somnolent)

Not fully alert, drifts off to sleep when not stimulated, can be aroused to name when called in normal voice but looks drowsy, responds appropriately to questions or commands but thinking seems slow and fuzzy, inattentive, loses train of thought, spontaneous movements are decreased

Obtunded

(Transitional state between lethargy and stupor)

Sleeps most of time, difficult to arouse: needs loud shout or vigorous shake, acts confused when is aroused, converses in monosyllables, speech may be mumbled and incoherent, requires constant stimulation for even marginal cooperation

Stupor or Semicoma

Spontaneously unconscious, responds only to persistent and vigorous shake or pain; has appropriate motor response (i.e., withdraws hand to avoid pain); otherwise can only groan, mumble, or move restlessly; reflex activity persists

TABLE 6-2	Levels of Consciousness—cont'd

Coma

Completely unconscious, no response to pain or to any external or internal stimuli (e.g., when suctioned, does not try to push the catheter away); in light coma, has some reflex activity but no purposeful movement; in deep coma, has no motor response

Acute Confusional State (Delirium)

Clouding of consciousness (dulled cognition, impaired alertness); inattentive; incoherent conversation; impaired recent memory and confabulatory for recent events; often agitated and having visual hallucinations; disoriented, with confusion worse at night when environmental stimuli are decreased.

Source: Adapted from Porth, C. (2007). *Essentials of pathophysiology: Concepts of altered health states* (p. 835). Hagerstown, MD: Lippincott Williams & Wilkins.

TABLE 6-3	Abnormalities of Mood and Affect

Type of Mood or Affect	Definition	Clinical Example
Flat affect (blunted affect)	Lack of emotional response; no expression of feelings; voice monotonous and face immobile	Topic varies, expression does not
Depression	Sad, gloomy, dejected; symptoms may occur with rainy weather, after a holiday, or with an illness; if the situation is temporary, symptoms fade quickly	Saying, "I've got the blues."
Depersonalization (lack of ego boundaries)	Loss of identity, feeling estranged, perplexed about own identity and meaning of existence	Saying, "I don't feel real" or "I feel as if I'm not really here."
Elation	Joy and optimism, overconfidence, increased motor activity, not necessarily pathological	Saying, "I'm feeling very happy."
Euphoria	Excessive well-being, unusually cheerful or elated, that is inappropriate considering physical and mental condition, implies a pathological mood	Saying, "I am high"; "I feel like I'm flying"; or "I feel on top of the world"
Anxiety	Worried, uneasy, apprehensive from the anticipation of a danger whose source is unknown	Saying, "I feel nervous and high strung"; "I worry all the time"; or "I can't seem to make up my mind"
Fear	Worried, uneasy, apprehensive; external danger is known and identified	Fear of flying in airplanes
Irritability	Annoyed, easily provoked, impatient	Internalizing a feeling of tension, so that a seemingly mild stimulus "sets off" the patient
Rage	Furious, loss of control	Expressing violent behaviour toward self or others
Ambivalence	The existence of opposing emotions toward an idea, object, person	Feeling love and hate toward another person at the same time
Lability	Rapid shift of emotions	Person expresses euphoric, tearful, angry feelings in rapid succession
Inappropriate affect	Affect that is clearly discordant with the content of the person's speech	Laughing while discussing admission for liver biopsy

SPECIAL CONSIDERATIONS FOR ADVANCED PRACTICE

TABLE 6-4	Examples of Abnormalities of Thought Process	
Type of Process	Definition	Clinical Example
Blocking	Sudden interruption in train of thought, seems related to strong emotion	Unable to complete sentence, saying, "Forgot what I was going to say."
Confabulation	Fabricating events to fill in memory gaps	Giving detailed description of a long walk around the hospital although the patient is known to have remained in his or her room all afternoon
Neologism	Coining a new word; invented word has no real meaning except for the patient; several words may be condensed	Saying, "I'll have to turn on my thinkilator."
Circumlocution	Roundabout expression, substituting a phrase when patient cannot think of name of object	Saying, "the thing you open the door with" instead of "key."
Circumstantiality	Talking with excessive and unnecessary detail, delay in reaching point; sentences have a meaningful connection but are irrelevant (this occurs normally in some people)	Saying, "When was my surgery? Well I was 28, I was living with my aunt, she's the one with psoriasis, she had it bad that year because of the heat, the heat was worse then than it was the summer of '92...."
Loosening associations	Shifting from one topic to an unrelated topic; person seems unaware that topics are unconnected	Saying, "My boss is angry with me and it wasn't even my fault. [pause] I saw that movie, too, Lassie. I felt really bad about it. But she kept trying to land the airplane and she never knew what was going on."
Flight of ideas	Abrupt change, rapid skipping from topic to topic, practically continuous flow of accelerated speech; topics usually have recognizable associations or are plays on words	Saying, "Take this pill? The pill is blue. I feel blue. [sings] She wore blue velvet."
Word salad	Incoherent mixture of words, phrases, and sentences; illogical, disconnected, includes neologisms	Saying, "Beauty, red based five, pigeon, the street corner, sort of."
Perseveration	Persistent repeating of verbal or motor response, even with varied stimuli	Saying, "I'm going to lock the door, lock the door. I walk every day and I lock the door. I usually take the dog and I lock the door."
Echolalia	Imitation, repeats others' words or phrases, often with a mumbling, mocking, or mechanical tone	[In response to the nurse's request to take a pill] Saying mockingly, "Take your pill. Take your pill."
Clanging	Word choice based on sound, not meaning; includes nonsense rhymes and puns	Saying, "My feet are cold. Cold, bold, told. The bell tolled for me."

TABLE 6-5	Abnormalities of Thought Content	
Type of Content	Definition	Clinical Example
Phobia	Strong, persistent, irrational fear of an object or situation; feeling driven to avoid it	Cats, dogs, heights, enclosed spaces
Hypochondriasis	Morbid worrying about own health; feeling sick with no actual basis for that assumption	Preoccupation with the possibility of having cancer; belief that any symptom or physical sign means cancer
Obsession	Unwanted, persistent thoughts or impulses experienced as intrusive and senseless; logic does not purge them from consciousness	Violence (parent having repeated impulse to kill a loved child); contamination (becoming infected by shaking hands)
Compulsion	Unwanted repetitive act thought to neutralize or prevent discomfort or some dreaded event	Handwashing, counting, checking and rechecking, touching
Delusions	Fixed, false beliefs; irrational beliefs; clinging to delusion despite objective evidence to contrary	Grandiose delusion: belief that one is God, a famous person, a historical figure, a sports figure, or another well-known person
Persecution: saying, "They are out to get me."

TABLE 6-6	Global Assessment of Functioning Scale

Consider psychological, social, and occupational functioning on a hypothetical continuum of mental health illness. Do not include impairment in functioning caused by physical (or environmental) limitations.

Scoring Range	Description of Level of Functioning
100-91	Superior functioning in a wide range of activities; life's problems never seem to get out of hand; person is sought out by others because of his or her many positive qualities. No symptoms.
90-81	Absent or minimal symptoms (e.g., mild anxiety before an examination); good functioning in all areas; interested and involved in a wide range of activities; socially effective; generally satisfied with life; no more than everyday problems or concerns (e.g., an occasional argument with family members).
80-71	If symptoms are present, they are transient and expectable reactions to psychosocial stressors (e.g., difficulty concentration after family argument); no more than slight impairment in social, occupational, or school functioning (e.g., temporarily falling behind in school work).
70-61	Some mild symptoms (e.g., depressed mood and mild insomnia) *or* some difficulty in social, occupational, or school functioning (e.g., occasional truancy, or theft within the household), but generally functioning pretty well, has some meaningful interpersonal relationships.
60-51	Moderate symptoms (e.g., flat and circumstantial speech, occasional panic attacks) *or* moderate difficulty in social occupational, or social functioning (e.g., few friends, conflicts with coworkers).
50-41	Serious symptoms (e.g., suicidal ideation, severe obsessional rituals, frequent shoplifting) *or* any serious impairment in social, occupational, or school functioning (e.g., no friends, unable to keep a job).
40-31	Some impairment in reality testing or communication (e.g., speech is at times illogical, obscure, or irrelevant) *or* major impairment in several areas, such as work or school, family relations, judgement, thinking, or mood (e.g., depressed man avoids friends, neglects family, and is unable to work; child frequently beats up younger children, is defiant at home, and is failing at school).
30-21	Behaviour is considerably influenced by delusions or hallucinations *or* serious impairment in communication or judgement (e.g., sometimes incoherent, acts grossly inappropriately, suicidal preoccupation) *or* inability to function in almost all areas (e.g., stays in bed all day; has no job, home, or friends).
20-11	Some danger of hurting self or others (e.g., suicide attempts without clear expectation of death; frequently violent; manic excitement) *or* occasionally fails to maintain minimal personal hygiene (e.g., smears feces) *or* gross impairment in communication (e.g., largely incoherent or mute).
10-1	Persistent danger of severely hurting self or others (e.g., recurrent violence) *or* persistent inability to maintain minimal personal hygiene *or* serious suicidal act with clear expectation of death.
0	Inadequate information.

Source: From Access Behavioral Health. (n.d.). *Global assessment of function.* Retrieved from *http://www.omh.ny.gov/omhweb/childservice/mrt/global_assessment_functioning.pdf.*

TABLE 6-7	Comparison of Characteristics of Delirium and Dementia

Characteristic	Delirium	Dementia
Onset	Sudden; hours to days	Progressive; months to years
Course	Acute; temporary; considered reversible	Chronic, with deterioration over time
Prevalence	Present in 10%-30% of hospitalized older adults	Estimated to affect >30% of people older than 85
Distinguishing feature	Presence of an underlying medical disorder (e.g., urinary tract infection, hypoxia)	Age-associated illness with decline in multiple areas of cognitive function, eventually leading to a significant inability to maintain occupational and social performance
Self-awareness	May be aware of changes in cognition; fluctuates	Likely to hide or be unaware of cognitive deficits
Activities of daily living	May be intact or impaired	May be intact early, impaired as disease progresses
Consequences	Contributes to outcomes of longer hospitalization, higher rates of nursing home placement, and possibly higher mortality rate	Major cause of disability, self-neglect, nutrition problems, incontinence, falls, communication difficulties, financial stress from job loss, and caregiver burden and depression

Sources: Data from Gagliardi, G. P. (2008). Differentiating among depression, delirium, and dementia in elderly patients. *American Medical Association Journal of Ethics Virtual Mentor, 10*(6), 383-388; and from Mental health: Dementia. (n.d.). *Clinical Knowledge Summaries, NHS Evidence.* Retrieved from *http://www.cks.nhs.uk/dementia/background_information/consequences_of_dementia.*

TABLE 6-8	Diagnostic Criteria for Schizophrenia*

DSM-IV-TR	ICD-10
At Least One of the Following: • Bizarre delusions or • Third-person auditory hallucinations with running commentary (voice/voices continuously comment about the person's behaviour or thought)	• Thought echo, thought insertion/withdrawal/broadcast • Passivity, delusional perception • Third-person auditory hallucination with running commentary • Persistent bizarre delusions
OR **Two or More of the Following:** • Delusions • Hallucinations • Disorganized speech • Grossly disorganized behaviour • Negative symptoms (e.g., flat affect, avolition)	• Persistent hallucinations • Thought disorder • Catatonic behaviour • Negative symptoms • Significant behaviour change
AND **At Least One of the Following:** • Social dysfunctioning (e.g. relationships, ability for self-care) • Occupational dysfunctioning (e.g., work)	
Duration 1 month of characteristic symptoms with 6 months of social/occupational dysfunction	More than 1 month

Source: From Wing, J. K., & Agrawal, N. (2007). Concepts and classification of schizophrenia. In S. R. Hirsch & D. R. Weinberger (Eds.), *Schizophrenia* (2nd ed.). Oxford, UK: Blackwell Science Ltd. (doi:10.1002/9780470987353).
*The reader is encouraged to check out the primary sources of the *DSM-V* (APA, 2013) and *ICN-10*.
DSM-IV, Diagnostic and Statistical Manual of Mental Disorders, Fourth Edition; *ICD-10*, International Statistical Classification of Diseases and Related Health Problems.

TABLE 6-9	Mood Disorders*

The definitions of mood disorders and their primary symptoms can be found in *DSM-V* (APA, 2013). Please refer to the source document for a complete description of the disorders below:

	Major Depressive Disorder (APA, 2013, pp. 160-162)
300.4	Persistent Depressive Disorder (Dysthymia) (APA, 2013, pp. 168-171)
	Bipolar 1 Disorder (APA, 2013, pp. 123-132)
296.89	Bipolar II Disorder (APA, 2013, pp. 132-139)

Source: *The reader is referred to the original source listing these disorders (American Psychiatric Association, 2013) or to a psychiatry textbook for further details and categories of anxiety disorders.

Special Considerations for Advanced Practice

TABLE 6-10	Anxiety Disorders*

Anxiety disorders encompass a multitude of disorders whose primary feature is abnormal or inappropriate anxiety. Patients with anxiety experience an increased heart rate, tensed muscles, and other "fight or flight" processes; these symptoms become a problem when they occur without any recognizable stimulus or when the stimulus does not warrant the reaction.

Anxiety disorders as listed in the *DSM-V* (American Psychiatric Association, 2013) include the following:

308.3	Acute stress disorder
300.22	Agoraphobia (with or without a history of panic disorder)
300.02	Generalized anxiety disorder [GAD]
300.3	Obsessive–compulsive disorder [OCD]
300.01	Panic disorder (with or without agoraphobia)
300.23	Social anxiety disorder (social phobia)
309.81	Post-traumatic stress disorder [PTSD]

*See *http://allpsych.com/disorders/disorders_alpha.html*. The reader is referred to the original source listing these disorders (American Psychiatric Association, 2013) or to a psychiatry textbook for further details and categories of anxiety disorders.

Summary Checklist: Mental Health Assessment

For a downloadable version, go to *http://evolve.elsevier.com/Canada/Jarvis/examination/*.

1. Health history
   Source of information
   Identification/biographic information
   Reason for seeking care (patient's verbatim reason; psychiatric diagnoses [*DSM-V*])
   Past health (past illness, injury, hospitalization; chronic illnesses)
   Family health history
   Developmental considerations
   Present health (allergies, immunization/HIV/hepatitis status; current medications)
2. Mental status examination
   Appearance
   Behaviour (mood and affect, speech)

   Cognitive function (level of consciousness; orientation to time, place, person, self; memory; attention and concentration; comprehension and abstract reasoning)
   Thought (perception, content, process, judgement, and insight)
3. Supplemental mental status examination (if warranted)
   Montreal Cognitive Assessment
4. Functional assessment of activities of daily living
   Nutrition patterns
   Sleep/rest changes
   Activity/mobility
   Elimination

   Interpersonal relationships and resources
   Self-esteem/self-concept
   Ethnicity/culture
   Spirituality
   Coping and stress management
   Smoking, alcohol and drug use, problem gambling
   Home environmental hazards
5. Screen for suicidal thoughts, assaultive or homicidal ideation, and elopement risk (when indicated)
6. Treatment plan (global assessment of function)
7. Teaching and health promotion

DSM-V, Diagnostic and statistical manual of mental health disorders (5th ed.). (APA, 2013); *HIV,* human immunodeficiency virus.

REFERENCES

Adolescent Health Committee, Canadian Paediatric Society (CPS). (2005). Youth and firearms in Canada. *Paediatric Child Health*, *10*(8), 473–477. (Reference No. AH05-02, formerly AM95-01; reaffirmed 2011).

Aggarwal, A., & Kean, K. (2010). Comparison of the Folstein Mini Mental State Examination (MMSE) to the Montreal Cognitive Assessment (MoCA) as a cognitive screening tool in an inpatient rehabilitation setting. *Neuroscience & Medicine*, *1*(2), 39–42. doi:10.4236/nm.2010.12006

Alzheimer's Association. (2011). *Alzheimer's disease: Facts and figures.* Retrieved from *http://www.alz.org/downloads/facts_figures_2011.pdf.*

American Psychiatric Association. (2000). *Diagnostic and statistical manual of mental disorders* (4th ed., Rev. ed.). Washington, DC: Author.

American Psychiatric Association. (2012). DSM-5: *The Future of Psychiatric Diagnosis.* Retrieved from *http://www.dsm5.org/Pages/Default.aspx.*

American Psychiatric Association. (2013). *Diagnostic and statistical manual of mental disorders* (5th ed.). Washington, DC: Author.

Barratt, E. (1989). Community psychiatric nurses: Their self-perceived roles. *Journal of Advanced Nursing, 14*, 42–48.

Berger, J. (2009). Student debt in Canada. In J. Berger, A. Motte, & A. Parkin (Eds.), *The price of knowledge: Access and student finance in Canada* (4th ed., pp. 181–206). Montreal: Millennium Scholarship Foundation.

Birkett, M., Espelage, D. L., & Koenig, B. (2009). LGB and questioning students in schools: The moderating effects of homophobic bullying and school climate on negative outcomes. *Journal of Youth and Adolescence, 38*(7), 989–1000.

Birren, J. E., & Schaie, K. W. (Eds.). (2005). *Handbook of the psychology of aging* (6th ed.). San Diego, CA: Academic Press.

Cacioppo, J. T., Hawkley, L. C., Ernst, J. M., Burleson, M., Berntson, G. G., Nouriani, B., & Spiegel, D. (2006). Loneliness within a nomological net: An evolutionary perspective. *Journal of Research in Personality, 40*(6), 1054–1085.

Canadian Alliance on Mental Illness and Mental Health. (2007). *Mental health literacy in Canada: Phase 1 draft report. Mental Health Literacy Project.* Retrieved from *http://www.camimh.ca/files/literacy/MHL_REPORT_FINAL.pdf.*

Canadian Council on Learning. (2010). Tallying the costs of post-secondary education: The challenge of managing student debt and loan repayment in Canada. *Challenges in Canadian Post-secondary Education* (Monograph 3). Retrieved from *http://www.ccl-cca.ca/pdfs/PSE/2010/PSEChallengesMonograph3_EN.pdf.*

Canadian Institutes of Health Research. (2007). *The future is aging. CIHR Institute of Aging strategic plan 2007 to 2012.* Ottawa: Author. Retrieved from *http://www.cihr-irsc.gc.ca/e/34013.html.*

Canadian Medical Association. (2008). *8th Annual national report on health care.* Retrieved from *http://www.cma.ca/multimedia/CMA/Content_Images/Inside_cma/Annual_Meeting/2008/GC_Bulletin/National_Report_Card_EN.pdf.*

Canadian Mental Health Association. (2008). *Your mental health.* Retrieved from *http://www.cmha.ca/bins/content_page.asp?cid=2-267-1319&lang=1.*

Canadian Nurses Association. (2012). *Professional practice: Canadian Registered Nurse Examination competencies, June 2010–May 2015.* Retrieved from *http://www.cna-aiic.ca/CNA/nursing/rnexam/competencies/default_e.aspx.*

Canadian School Health Community. (2010). *The mental health status & prevalence of MH problems in Canadian children & adolescents.* Retrieved from *http://www.canadianschoolhealth.ca/page/The+Mental+Health+Status+%26+Prevalence+of+MH+Problems+in+Canadian+Children+%26+Adolescents.*

Clark, C. M. (2005). *Relations between social support and physical health.* Retrieved from *http://www.personalityresearch.org/papers/clark.html.*

Coombs, T., Curtis, J., & Crookes, P. (2011). What is a comprehensive mental health nursing assessment? A review of the literature. *International Journal of Mental Health Nursing, 20*, 364–370. doi:10.1111/j.1447-0349.2011.00742.x

Dowrick, C. (2004). *Beyond depression: A new approach to understanding and management.* Oxford, UK: Oxford University Press.

Durant, E., & Sporer, K. A. (2011). Characteristics of Patients with an Abnormal Glasgow Coma Scale Score in the Prehospital Setting. *Western Journal of Emergency Medicine, 12*(1), 30–36. Retrieved from: *http://www.ncbi.nlm.nih.gov/pmc/articles/PMC3088371/*

Epp, J. (1986). Achieving health for all: A framework for health promotion. *Health Promotion, 1*(4), 419–428.

Epp, J. (1988). *Mental health for Canadians: Striking a balance.* Retrieved from *http://www.hc-sc.gc.ca/hcs-sss/pubs/system-regime/1986-frame-plan-promotion/index-eng.php.*

Evenson, J., & Barr, C. (2009). *Youth homelessness in Canada: The road to solutions.* Toronto: Raise the Roof Foundation. Retrieved from *http://www.raisingtheroof.org/RaisingTheRoof/.../RaisingTheRoofMedia/...*

Gardner, W., Lucas, A., Kolko, D. J., & Campo, J. V. (2007). Comparison of the PSC-17 and alternative mental health screens in an at-risk primary care sample. *Journal of the American Academy of Child and Adolescent Psychiatry, 46*(5), 611–618.

Ge, X., Conger, R., & Elder, G., (2001). Pubertal transition, stressful life events, and the emergence of gender differences in adolescent depressive symptoms. *Developmental Psychology, 37*(3), 404–417. doi:10.1037//0012-1649.37.3.404

Hamilton, B., Manias, E., Maude, P., Marjoribanks, T., & Cook, K. (2004). Perspectives of a nurse, a social worker and a psychiatrist regarding patient assessment in acute inpatient psychiatry settings: A case study approach. *Journal of Psychiatric and Mental Health Nursing, 11*, 683–689.

Healey-Ogdon, M. J. (2010). Mental health and mental illness. In W. Austin & M. A. Boyd (Eds.), *Psychiatric & mental health nursing for Canadian practice* (2nd ed., pp. 19–29). Philadelphia: Lippincott Williams & Wilkins.

Health Canada. (2006). *Mental health—mental illness.* Ottawa: Author. Retrieved from *http://www.hc-sc.gc.ca/hl-vs/iyh-vsv/diseases-maladies/mental-eng.php.*

Hoops, S., Nazem, S., Siderowf, A. D., Duda, J. E., Xie, S. X., Stern, M. B., & Weintraub, D. (2009). Validity of the MoCA and MMSE in the detection of MCI and dementia in Parkinson disease. *Neurology, 73*(21), 1738–1745. doi:10.1212/WNL.0b013e3181c34b47

Isaacs, B., & Kennie, A. (1973). The set test as an aid to the detection of dementia in old people. *British Journal of Psychiatry, 123*, 467–470.

Jayaram, G. (2009). Elopement: A primer on safety and prevention. In G. Jayaram & A. Herzog (Eds.), *SAFE MD: Practical applications and approaches to safe psychiatric practice* (pp. 16–18). Retrieved from *http://suicidepreventioncommunity.files.wordpress.com/2009/01/apa-patientsafety-suicideexcerpt.pdf.*

Kelley, A. E., Schochet, T., & Landry, C. F. (2004). Risk taking and novelty seeking in adolescence. *Annals of The New York Academy of Sciences, 1021*, 27–32. doi:10.1196/annals.1308.003

Kidder, K., & Rogers, D. (2004). *Why Canada needs a national youth policy agenda.* Washington, DC: National Children's Alliance. Retrieved from *http://www.nationalchildrensalliance.com/nca/pubs/2004/youthpolicypaper.htm.*

Kirmayer, L., Bass, G., Holton, T., Paul, K., Simpson, C., & Tait, C. (2007). *Suicide among Aboriginal people in Canada.* Ottawa: Aboriginal Healing Foundation.

Knopf, D., Park, M. J., & Mulye, T. P. (2008). *The mental health of adolescents: A national profile, 2008.* San Francisco: National Adolescent Health Information Center, University of California, San Francisco.

Lachman, M. E. (2004). Development in midlife. *Annual Review of Psychology, 55,* 305–331. doi:10.1146/annurev.psych.55.090902.141521

Lorentz, W., Scanlan, J. M., & Borson, S. (2002). Brief screening tests for dementia. *Canadian Journal of Psychiatry, 47,* 723–733.

MacMillan, H. L., Patterson, C. J. S., & Wathen, C. N. (2005). Screening for depression in primary care: Recommendation statement from the Canadian Task Force on Preventive Health Care. *Canadian Medical Association Journal, 172*(1), 33–35.

Marková, I. S., Berrios, G. E., & Hodges, J. H. (2004). Insight into memory function. *Neurology, Psychiatry & Brain Research, 11,* 115–126.

Marková, I. S., Jaafari, N., & Berrios, G. E. (2009). Insight and obsessive-compulsive disorder: A conceptual analysis. *Psychopathology, 42,* 277–282

Mental Health Commission of Canada. (2012). *Changing directions, changing lives: The mental health strategy for Canada.* Calgary: Author. Retrieved from *http:// www.mentalhealthcommission.ca/English/Pages/Strategy.aspx.*

Nair, A. K., Gavett, B. E., Damman, M., Dekker, W., Green, R. C., Mandel, A., ... Stern, R. A. (2010). Clock drawing test ratings by dementia specialists: Interrater reliability and diagnostic accuracy. *Journal of Neuropsychiatry and Clinical Neurosciences, 22,* 85–92.

Nasreddine, Z. S., Phillips, N. A., Bédirian, V., Charbonneau, S., Whitehead, V., Collin, I., ... Chertkow, H. (2005). The Montreal Cognitive Assessment (MoCA): A brief screening tool for mild cognitive impairment. *Journal of American Geriatric Society, 53,* 695–699.

National Collaborating Centre for Mental Health. (2010). *Depression: The NICE guideline on the treatment and management of depression in adults (Updated Edition)* (National Clinical Practice Guideline 90). Leicester and London, UK: The British Psychological Society and The Royal College of Psychiatrists. Retrieved from *http://www.nice.org.uk/nicemedia/ live/12329/45896/45896.pdf.*

National Eating Disorder Information Centre. (2005). *Statistics: Understanding statistics on eating disorders.* Retrieved from *http://www.nedic.ca/knowthefacts/statistics.shtml.*

Neupert, S. D., Almeida, D. M., & Charles, S. T. (2007). Age differences in reactivity to daily stressors: The role of personal control. *Journal of Gerontology: Psychological Sciences, 62B*(4), 216–225.

O'Brien, A. J. (1999). Negotiating the relationship: Mental health nurses' perceptions of their practice. *Australian and New Zealand Journal of Mental Health Nursing, 8,* 153–161.

O'Connor, E. A., Whitlock, E. P., Gaynes, B., & Beil, T. L. (2009). *Screening for depression in adults and older adults in primary care: An updated systematic review* (Report No.: 10-05143-EF-1). Rockville, MD: Agency for Healthcare Research and Quality.

Osaka, N., & Logie, R. H. (2007). *The cognitive neuroscience of working memory.* Oxford, UK: Oxford University Press.

Pendlebury, S. T., Cuthbertson, F. C., Welch, S. J. V., Mehta, Z., & Rothwell, P. M. (2010). Underestimation of cognitive impairment by Mini-Mental State Examination versus the Montreal Cognitive Assessment in patients with Transient Ischemic Attack and Stroke: A population-based study. *Stroke, 41,* 1290–1293. doi:10.1161/STROKEAHA.110.579888

Perring, C. (2010). Mental illness. In E. N. Zalta (Ed.), *The Stanford encyclopedia of philosophy* (Spring 2010 ed.). Retrieved from *http://plato.stanford.edu/archives/spr2010/entries/ mental-illness/.*

Poobalan, A. S., Aucott, L. S., Ross, L., Cairns, W., Smith, S., Helms, P. J., & Williams, J. H. G. (2007). Effects of treating postnatal depression on mother-infant interaction and child development: Systematic review. *British Journal of Psychiatry, 191,* 378–386. doi:10.1192/bjp.bp.106.032789

Public Health Agency of Canada. (2006). *The human face of mental health and mental illness in Canada.* Ottawa: Minister of Public Works and Government Services Canada.

Public Health Agency of Canada. (2008). *Healthy settings for young people in Canada.* Retrieved from *http://www.phac-aspc.gc.ca/ hp-ps/dca-dea/publications/yjc/index-eng.php.*

Public Health Agency of Canada. (2011). The mental health status & prevalence of MH problems in Canadian children & adolescents. In *The Chief Public Health Officer's report on the state of public health in Canada, 2011.* Retrieved from *http://www.canadianschoolhealth.ca/page/ The+Mental+Health+Status+%26+Prevalence+of+MH+ Problems+in+Canadian+Children+%26+Adolescents.*

Rosenthal, C. J., Matthews, A. M., & Matthews, S. H. (1996). Caught in the middle? Occupancy in multiple roles and help to parents in a national probability sample of Canadian adults. *IESOP Research Paper No. 4.* Retrieved from *http:// socserv.mcmaster.ca/iesop/papers/iesop_04.pdf.*

Schaie, K. W., & Willis, S. L. (2011). *Handbook of the psychology of aging* (7th ed.). Burlingham, MA: Elsevier.

Smith, T., Gildeh, N., & Holmes, C. (2007). The Montreal Cognitive Assessment: Validity and utility in a memory clinic setting. *Canadian Journal of Psychiatry, 52,* 329–332.

Statistics Canada. (2009). *Canadian Community Health Survey, 2009: Annual* [Share Microdata File]. Ottawa: Author.

Statistics Canada. (2010). *Table 5.7: Leading causes of death of children and youth, by age group, 2003 to 2005.* Ottawa: Author. Retrieved from *http://www41.statcan.ca/2009/20000/tbl/ cybac20000_2009_000_t07-eng.htm.*

Taylor, C., Peter, T., Schachter, K., Paquin, S., Beldom, S., Gross, Z., & McMinn, T. L. (2008). *Youth speak up about homophobia and transphobia: The first national climate survey on homophobia in Canadian schools. Phase one report.* Toronto: Eagle Canada Human Rights Trust.

Thombs, B. D., Coyne, J. C., Cuijpers, P., de Jonge, P., Gilbody, S., Ioannidis, J. P., ... Ziegelstein, R. C. (2012). Rethinking recommendations for screening for depression in primary care. *Canadian Medical Association Journal, 184*(4), 413–418.

Tuokko, H., Morris, C., & Ebert, P. (2005). Mild cognitive impairment and everyday functioning in older adults. *Neurocase: The Neural Basis of Cognition, 11*(1), 40–47. doi: 10.1080/13554790490896802

World Health Organization. (2007). *Mental health: Strengthening mental health promotion.* Geneva, Switzerland: Author.

World Health Organization. (2008). *Investing in mental health.* Department of Mental Health and Substance Dependence, Noncommunicable Diseases and Mental Health. Geneva. ISBN 92 4 156257 9. Retrieved from: *http://www.who.int/mental_ health/media/investing_mnh.pdf.*

Zadikoff, C., Fox, S. H., Tang-Wai, D. F., Thomsen, T., de Bie, R. M., Wadia, P., ... Marras, C. (2008). A comparison of the Mini Mental State Exam to the Montreal Cognitive Assessment in identifying cognitive deficits in Parkinson's disease. *Movement Disorders, 23,* 297–299.

Web Sites of Interest

Aboriginal Healing Foundation: *http://www.ahf.ca/*
Alzheimer Society: *http://www.alzheimer.ca/*
Canadian Alliance on Mental Illness and Mental Health: *http:// camimh.ca/*
Canadian Coalition for Seniors' Mental Health: *http:// www.ccsmh.ca/*

Canadian Collaborative Mental Health Initiative: *http://www.iccsm.ca/en/who/index.html*

Canadian Institute for Health Information: *http://www.cihi.ca*

Canadian Mental Health Association: *http://www.cmha.ca/bins/index.asp*

Centre for Addiction and Mental Health: *http://www.camh.net/*

Mental Health Commission of Canada: *http://www.mentalhealthcommission.ca/mhcc.html*

Mental Health Glossary, Royal Ottawa Health Care Group: *http://www.rohcg.on.ca/resources/glossary-e.cfm*

Mood Disorder Society of Canada: *http://www.mooddisorderscanada.ca/*

National Eating Disorder Information Centre: *http://www.nedic.ca/*

Psychosocial Rehabilitation Canada: *http://www.psrrpscanada.ca/*

Schizophrenia Society of Canada: *http://www.schizophrenia.ca/*

Seniors Mental Health Web site created to facilitate activities related to supporting seniors' mental health: *http://www.seniorsmentalhealth.ca/index.html*

Substance Use in the Context of Health Assessment

Written by Colleen Varcoe, PhD, RN, Annette J. Browne, PhD, RN, and Laraine Michalson, MSN, RN

⊖volve WEBSITE

http://evolve.elsevier.com/Canada/Jarvis/examination/
- Animations
- Examination Review Questions
- Key Points

OUTLINE

The purpose of this chapter is to provide nurse clinicians with knowledge regarding substance use that can be integrated into health assessment across a range of practice contexts with patients of all ages. To help prevent and minimize the harmful effects of **substance use,** and to develop health-promoting nursing practice that accounts for a range of substance use practices, nurses must understand the dynamics of substance use, the social and health effects of substance use, and the root causes of substance use. This is relevant to assessment of *every* patient, regardless of whether they appear to have problems with substance use. People from all walks of life can experience substance use problems; conversely, people who are disadvantaged in multiple ways cannot be assumed to have such problems. The risks of disclosure of **problematic substance use,** such as job loss, removal of children by protective agency, and relationship damage, are significant, regardless of social location. This knowledge is necessary for conducting thorough, respectful, and useful health assessments.

SUBSTANCE USE, ADDICTION, AND DEPENDENCE

Substance use is widespread in Canada; levels of use and acceptability vary according to the type of substance and the community. Judgements as to whether substance use is "misuse," "abuse," or "problematic use" are variable, again depending on the substance and community. The terms substance use, substance abuse, addiction, and dependence are sometimes used interchangeably, which is erroneous. Some of these terms are more pejorative than others; the term *addiction* carries the greatest stigma and is perhaps the most overused. **Addiction** generally implies compulsion and dependence. However, there is considerable disagreement regarding the meaning and usefulness of these terms. This has led the American Psychiatric Association work group to propose that the current *Diagnostic and Statistical Manual of Mental Disorders (DSM-IV)** categories of substance abuse and substance dependence be replaced with the category of "substance use disorder" in the new *DSM-V*, which states that "addiction" is not a proposed disorder for *DSM-V* (American Psychiatric Association, 2012a). Further, people diagnosed under the current category of "substance abusers" in the *DSM-IV* will not be categorized as "addicts." Rather, in the *DSM-V*, they receive a diagnosis of mild, moderate, or severe substance use disorder. Additionally,

> *In the current proposal for DSM-5, substance use disorder would strengthen the diagnosis by increasing the number of symptoms required for a mild diagnosis to two symptoms (DSM-IV required one). Additionally, the DSM-5 draft criteria require that symptoms lead to clinically significant impairment or distress …. There is no intent or proposal to include a "catchall category" for other behaviors. … The only behavioral disorder (non substance diagnosis) proposed is*

*The DMS IV-TR was updated and replaced by the *DSM-V* in May 2013.

gambling disorder. Gambling disorder has been included in previous editions of the DSM as pathological gambling.

(American Psychiatric Association, 2012a)

By shifting away from erroneous assumptions about "addiction," the aim is to "avoid patients with normal tolerance and withdrawal being labeled as 'addicts'" (O'Brien, 2010, p. 106). Most importantly,

> *the major reason given for the under-treatment of pain with opioids has been the fear that the physician will create an addiction when, in reality, addiction in the course of pain treatment is relatively uncommon. Thus patients have been made to suffer by receiving inadequate pain medication doses when there is evidence of tolerance or withdrawal symptoms. In order to address these problems, the proposed changes for DSM-V include some changes in terminology.*
>
> (O'Brien, 2010, p. 106).

It is essential to be clear about the definition of dependence. Dependence as a label for compulsive, out-of-control drug use has been problematic. It has been confusing to physicians and has resulted in patients with normal tolerance and withdrawal being labelled as "addicts." Accordingly, the term **dependence** is now limited to physiological dependence, which is a normal response to repeated doses of many medications including beta-blockers, antidepressants, opioids, anti-anxiety agents and other drugs. Dependence is characterized by tolerance (needing more amounts of the medication or substance to produce the desired effect) and withdrawal (physiological symptoms that occur when the medication or drug is withdrawn). However, the presence of tolerance and withdrawal symptoms are not counted as symptoms to be counted for the diagnosis of "substance use disorder" in the *DSM-IV* when occurring in the context of appropriate medical treatment with prescribed medications (O'Brien, 2010).

In contrast, consider the argument that Alexander (2001) made to the Canadian House of Parliament. His brief, entitled *The Myth of Drug-Induced Addiction*, opens as follows:

> *Most Canadians believe that certain drugs cause catastrophic addictions in people who use them. This conventional belief is reflected in such familiar phrases as "Crack cocaine is instantly addictive" or "Heroin is so good, don't even try it once." It is also implied in the professional literature which routinely describes certain drugs as "addictive," "dependency producing," or "habit forming." The belief that drugs can induce addiction has shaped drug policy for more than a century.*
>
> *However, the only actual evidence for the belief in drug-induced addiction comes 1) from the testimonials of some addicted people who believe that exposure to a drug caused them to "lose control" and 2) from some highly technical research on laboratory animals. These bits of evidence have been embellished in the news media to the point where the belief in drug-induced addiction has acquired the status of an obvious truth that requires no further testing. But the widespread acceptance of this belief is a better demonstration of the power of repetition than of the influence of empirical research, because the great bulk of empirical evidence runs against it. Belief in drug-induced addiction may have deep cultural roots as well, since it is a pharmacological version of the belief in "demon possession" that has entranced Western culture for centuries.*
>
> (Alexander, 2001)

Throughout this chapter, the term *substance use* is used in recognition of the controversial, variable, and socially constructed nature of more pejorative terms, including addiction, dependence, and misuse. Clinicians are urged to do the same: Use the term *substance use,* and specify the physiological and social effects of such use as they are experienced by individuals.

THE CANADIAN CONTEXT OF SUBSTANCE USE

Like most societies, Canadian society has its particular set of values, beliefs, laws, policies, and practices related to substance use, many of which are contradictory to one another. Awareness of these values, laws, and policies provides clinicians with a "bigger picture" perspective on substance use.

In Canada, certain substances, such as alcohol and tobacco, are legal and are the source of government tax revenue, and their use is socially acceptable in many communities. Other substances, such as crack or heroin, are illegal, are the sources of illegal profit-making, and are considered in popular thinking to be extremely dangerous, and their use is generally deemed socially reprehensible. Still others, such as marijuana, are formally illegal but their use is more socially tolerated, and they are very lucrative financially for those producing and selling them. Finally, some substances, such as solvents and prescription drugs, have legal purposes but are used in ways other than formally intended. The use of substances has intertwined social and health effects that arise not only from the physiological effects of the substance (e.g., reduced or increased anxiety) but also from the social acceptability (e.g., inclusion) and legal consequences of using the substance (e.g., incarceration, impoverishment).

The social, economic, legal, and policy context of substance use in Canada is continually in flux. For example, because of a rapid rise in illegal drug use, Canadian policy at a federal level has followed that of the United States, moving to an American-style criminalization approach over time. In 1987, the federal government launched its National Drug Strategy, which became Canada's Drug Strategy in 1992 (Collin, 2006), when cabinet regrouped the National Strategy to Reduce Impaired Driving and the National Drug Strategy under one initiative. Funding was significantly cut through the 1990s, but the cornerstone of policy remained the long-term goal of reducing the harms associated with the use of alcohol, tobacco, and other substances to individuals, families, and communities. However, from 2002 to the 2008 Anti-Drug Strategy (which remains in effect), harm reduction*

---

*Harm-reduction strategies include policy and public health efforts to reduce the harm associated with using alcohol and other legal drugs, driving cars, riding bicycles, and sexual practices, by encouraging the use of safe drinking guidelines, seatbelts, helmets, and condoms, respectively (Canadian Nurses Association, 2011). In relation to substance use, the International Harm Reduction Association (2010) defined harm reduction as the "policies, programmes and practices that aim primarily to reduce the adverse health, social and economic consequences of the use of legal and illegal psychoactive drugs without necessarily reducing drug consumption. Harm reduction benefits people who use drugs, their families and the community" (p. 1).

was increasingly washed out of federal policy, with resources funnelled more to enforcement and less to prevention and treatment. Indeed, the Anti-Drug Strategy includes three action plans—preventing illicit drug use; treating patients with dependencies on illicit drugs; and combating the production and distribution of illicit drugs—with no mention of harm reduction.

Social attitudes toward substance use in general and toward specific substances have shifted along with legal, economic, and policy changes. For example, attitudes toward tobacco use have grown increasingly less tolerant. In contrast, in most communities in Canada, alcohol use has become increasingly acceptable (Giesbrecht, Ialomiteanu, Anglin, & Adlaf, 2007), with evidence that perception of norms influences use in some populations (Arbour-Nicitopoulos, Kwan, Lowe, Taman, & Faulkner, 2010).

You need to be aware of these trends so that you can conduct assessments in ways that are respectful, that encourage (rather than inhibit) discussions related to the health effects of substance use, and that encourage health care access rather than alienation through shame and stigma.

SUBSTANCE USE IN CANADA

The Canadian Addiction Survey was completed in 2004 and provides the most recent and comprehensive national view of substance use in Canada. Most Canadians are moderate drinkers, and cannabis is the most commonly used illegal drug (Box 7-1). Both high-risk drinking and levels of drug use are higher among men and among youth. Tobacco use has declined overall for those aged 15 years and older, from 25% in 1999 to 17% in 2010 (see the section Web Sites of Interest at the end of this chapter). In Canada, general population trends show a decline in problematic substance use (in comparisons of 2004 and 2008 rates) but increase in harm for certain subgroups, including people in prisons, Aboriginal people, and youth.

CAUSES AND FACTORS INFLUENCING SUBSTANCE USE

What influences substance use? Do different factors influence "problematic" substance use? The answers to such questions are not simple.

First, social practices and acceptability are the most influential determinants of substance use patterns. In much of Canada, for example, alcohol use is legal, and certain levels of use are socially accepted; daily consumption of wine with meals is acceptable in many communities. However, for other communities, such as certain Christian and Muslim communities, any consumption of alcohol is considered unacceptable. Thus what is considered "problematic" varies considerably.

Second, affordability is an important determinant of both levels of substance use and types of substances consumed. The importance of affordability has led to the use of pricing as a major policy tool in trying to curb levels of substance use (Bader, Boisclair, & Ferrence, 2011; Giesbrecht, 2008).

BOX 7-1   KEY FINDINGS FROM THE CANADIAN ADDICTION SURVEY*

Alcohol Use
- Nearly 80% of Canadians aged 15 years and older drink; most drink in moderation and without harm.
- Of drinkers in the year prior to the survey, 17% were considered to be at high risk for alcoholism, according to the World Health Organization's Alcohol Use Disorders Identification Test (AUDIT).
- High-risk drinkers were predominantly men and younger than 25.

Cannabis and Other Drug Use
- Of all Canadians, 14% reported using cannabis in the past year prior to the survey, nearly double the rate reported in 1994 (7.4%); however, almost 46% of these people had not used cannabis or had used it only once or twice in the 3 months preceding the survey.
- Although about 1 per 6 Canadians had used an illicit drug other than cannabis in their lifetime, few used these drugs during the past year prior to the survey. The rates for the past year prior to the survey were generally 1% or less.
- Both lifetime and past year prior to the survey, use of illicit substances other than cannabis was highest among men and people aged 18 to 24.

Source: Modified from Canadian Centre on Substance Abuse. (2011). *Canadian addiction survey.* Ottawa: Author. Retrieved from *http://www.ccsa.ca/eng/priorities/research/canadianaddiction/pages/default.aspx.*
*The Canadian Addictions Survey (Adlaf, Begin, & Sawka, 2005) is one of the most detailed and extensive surveys ever conducted on how Canadians aged 15 years and older use alcohol, cannabis, and other drugs, and the impact that use has on their physical, mental, and social well-being.

Third, however, regardless of how problematic substance use is defined, substance use with profoundly negative effects on people's health and social well-being has been repeatedly linked to the intertwined issues of trauma, violence, and chronic pain (Walsh, Jamieson, MacMillan, & Boyle, 2007; Wuest et al., 2008).

Finally, mental health and substance use are consistently linked (e.g., Gilchrist, Hegarty, Chondros, Herrman, & Gunn, 2010; McLaughlin et al., 2010; Schneider, Burnette, Ilgen, & Timko, 2009); therefore, substance use, violence, and mental health cannot be considered separately. Nurses must understand that histories of trauma are common among people who have problems with substance use and among people with mental health problems such as post-traumatic stress disorder and depression.

VIOLENCE, TRAUMA, MENTAL HEALTH, AND SUBSTANCE USE

All forms of interpersonal violence—including intimate partner violence (IPV), child abuse, and sexual assault—consistently have been shown to be related to substance use

BOX 7-2 LIFETIME VIOLENCE, MENTAL HEALTH, AND SUBSTANCE USE

Hedtke and associates (2008) assessed lifetime violence history (sexual assault, physical assault, witnessed serious injury or violent death), mental health functioning in the year before the baseline interview (post-traumatic stress disorder [PTSD], depression, and substance use problems), and instances of violence that occurred after the baseline interview in a household probability sample of 4008 women (18 to 89 years of age). Lifetime violence exposure was associated with increased risk of PTSD, depression, and substance use problems; symptoms of PTSD and depression, and the occurrence of substance use problems increased incrementally with the number of different types of violence experienced; and incidents of violence between the baseline and follow-up interviews over 2 years were associated with heightened risk of PTSD and substance use problems.

problems and mental health problems (Box 7-2). For example, Fowler (2007) found that IPV and substance use problems were estimated to co-occur at rates of 38% to 85% in various samples of women. Carbone-López, Kruttschnitt, and Mac-Millan (2006) found that women who had experienced IPV had significantly higher odds of having serious depression and mental health disability and, in comparison with women with no history of IPV, were more than twice as likely to use tranquillizers, sleeping pills, or sedatives and to report drinking alcohol "every day." However, the health effects of violence such as substance abuse must be understood in the context of cumulative lifetime abuse rather than as a consequence of one type of violence (Scott-Storey, 2011). Thus, more recent research has focused on the relationship between (a) cumulative experiences of various types of violence and (b) mental health and substance use (e.g., Engstrom, El-Bassel, Go, & Gilbert, 2008; Hedtke et al., 2008). These findings, as well as those of research that suggest that violence during childhood or adolescence has more profound effects than violence at later stages of life (Green et al., 2010; Kaukinen & Demaris, 2005; McLaughlin et al., 2010; Smith, Elwyn, Ireland, & Thornberry, 2010), emphasize the importance of considering experiences of multiple forms and patterns of lifetime violence in relation to substance use. Clinicians must consider substance use within a broader patient history. Therefore, clinicians must ensure that their approach to health assessment is "trauma and violence informed," as discussed in the following sections.

SUBSTANCE USE AND INEQUITIES

Understanding the relationships among trauma, violence, and substance use helps care providers understand why certain populations are more likely to experience higher levels of and more problematic substance use. Besides gender and age differences, other differences come into play, so that inequities (unfair differences that can be modified) intersect to influence rates of substance use and problems. For example, tobacco use is declining dramatically in Canada, except among low-income populations, among whom rates are increasing (Frohlich & Poland, 2007). This fact reflects the stress of living in poverty, limited options for dealing with stress, limited access to tobacco reduction supports, and health education strategies related to tobacco cessation that are not appropriate or relevant to this population. Similar dynamics have been shown in Canada among women who experience violence (Poole, Greaves, Jategaonkar, McCullough, & Chabot, 2008). Likewise, Bottorff and colleagues (2009) showed how the economy in isolated, rural First Nation communities influenced tobacco use and second-hand smoke exposure to make it difficult for young Aboriginal women to reduce tobacco exposure for themselves and their children. Understanding how inequities influence substance use can also help health care providers identify potentially successful approaches (Browne, Varcoe, & Fridkin, 2011). For example, Aboriginal people in Canada who have gained considerable political power and economic control over their circumstances were consuming less alcohol per capita than the general population (British Columbia Provincial Health Officer, 2002).

Health care providers should know that substance use varies within historical and economic contexts. Which drugs are used, how much is used, and how problematic such use is depend on geography (including the local history, what substances are available, and local norms) and on income (what is affordable and what is profitable). Clinicians should learn about the particular context in which they are providing care, including the histories of trauma and violence and the economic conditions.

THE EFFECTS OF SUBSTANCE USE VARY BY GENDER, CLASS, AGE

Numerous negative individual, family, and societal outcomes result from high levels of substance use. Social harm arises not only from the behaviours of the individual but also from the legal and social ramifications of use, such as incarceration, illegal activities, and child apprehension by the state, and from the different levels of stigma that people face, depending on their social positions. For example, women with high levels of substance use are at increased risk for incarceration, economic deprivation, diseases such as human immunodeficiency virus (HIV) infection and acquired immune deficiency syndrome (AIDS), dual diagnosis, and psychological disorders such as depression and post-traumatic stress disorder, as well as for loss of child custody and subsequent risk of victimization, including IPV (Golinelli, Longshore, & Wenzel, 2009; Gutierres & Van Puymbroeck, 2006; Salomon, Bassuk, & Huntington, 2002; Schneider et al., 2009). Furthermore, "women do worse, relative to men, in substance misuse treatment programs, and . . . rates of women's entry into treatment, retention in treatment and successful completion of treatment are significantly lower than those for men" (Gutierres & Van Puymbroeck, 2006, p. 498). For example, prescribing narcotics to Aboriginal people has become common and widespread practice by physicians (Salmon, 2006). In our research, a 29-year-old Aboriginal woman with a history of violent victimization had suffered persistent abdominal pain since the age of 12, for which she had been prescribed acetaminophen (Tylenol) with codeine. Her pain issues were not actually investigated, however, until she was 28 years old. Like many other Aboriginal patients in the study, she described how difficult it was for her to not use substances.

These effects vary with intersecting aspects of social position, such as gender, income, age, and ethnicity. Economic and social influences mean that the substance use practices of certain populations are more visible and open to scrutiny. For example, consider two people who use alcohol to the point of being visibly impaired. If one person lives on the street, is homeless, and is unemployed and the other person owns a home and has steady employment, the visibility of their alcohol use will be different and will have different consequences (Robertson & Culhane, 2005).

People are subject to different forms of stigma and discrimination related to substance use. For example, women who use substances are perceived differently from their male counterparts in society, the legal system, and the health care system. Women who use substances are often perceived as more out of control, deviant, pathological, unfit to parent, and more sexually promiscuous than are their male counterparts, whereas men are judged less harshly, and their parenting and responsibility to family are less scrutinized (Boyd, 1999, 2004). According to Boyd, women receive harsher sentences than men for drug-related convictions and often lose custody of their children when in prison.

Substance use is often viewed as a recreational, indulgent activity in which the participants seek a "high" to enjoy themselves. This limited interpretation can hinder the nurse's understanding of other reasons why people use substances. Many people use substances to feel numb; to stop pain (physical or emotional); or to control anxiety, nightmares, or sadness associated with past, current, and ongoing trauma. Sometimes people use substances to "feel normal" when prescribed therapies have failed. For example, most people using substances on the streets of the Downtown Eastside of Vancouver do not see themselves as "having fun" or enjoying being "high." In that context, a former drug user said, "Drugs make life bearable. Reality is too frightening without drugs" (Robertson & Culhane, 2005).

Understanding the relationship between patterns of violence across the lifespan, social inequities, and substance use helps health care providers understand substance use as a consequence of multiple influences. Understanding these patterns for both men and women, including different levels of scrutiny and judgement, is critical for improving health care, health policies, ways of approaching health assessment, and, ultimately, health.

As demonstrated by the statistics on substance use in Canada, there is considerable variability with age in relation to the use of particular substances. Furthermore, although substance use occurs throughout the lifespan, some issues are particularly salient for different age groups. For example, for

children, the prescription of medications such as Ritalin (methylphenidate) for behaviour problems has become a widespread concern, with controversy regarding the medical diagnoses leading to such prescription (Visser & Jehan, 2009). For young people, drinking, and sometime binge drinking, has increasingly become a rite of passage to adulthood. When pregnant, women who consume substances are more intensely scrutinized. Many older adults take multiple medications and are overmedicated with prescription drugs. Health care providers need to have an awareness of the most common problems facing each age group, without making assumptions about particular individuals, in order to tailor their health assessments most effectively.

UNDERSTANDING SUBSTANCE USE IN THE CONTEXT OF HEALTH CARE

Health care is supposed to be aimed at the promotion of health. However, in relation to substance use, health promotion objectives are often at odds with policies that focus on criminalizing substance use and targeting substance use–related behaviours rather than addressing the causes and factors influencing such use. Health care objectives may be subverted within health care settings by objectives of criminal justice, child welfare, or other organizations. For example, health care providers may participate in the surveillance and monitoring of people's drug use through observed urine tests; such practices may challenge the trust needed for an effective provider–patient relationship. It is critical that nurses remain focused on health promotion, not law enforcement.

In understanding the links between violence, trauma, pain, mental health, and substance use, and in understanding the influence of broader social and policy influences, health care providers can approach health assessments and practice from a comprehensive base. Health care providers must avoid viewing substance use as a primary problem to be targeted, rather than as a symptom of other preexisting problems and circumstances. Viewing substance use not solely or narrowly as a criminal or health problem but rather as a consequence of other social problems means that nurses should assess substance use in the context of a comprehensive health history, including violence, trauma, and mental health histories, and in the contexts of income, housing, employment, food security, and access to services such as counselling. This broader assessment provides the basis for meaningful interventions to support people in successfully addressing their substance use issues.

INCORPORATING KNOWLEDGE OF SUBSTANCE USE IN HEALTH ASSESSMENT

The understanding of substance use just described suggests that health assessment be based on the following principles:
- *It should be health promoting.* Assessments that involve negative judgements, are intrusive, or are punitive will deter patients from accessing care and, through shame, will increase secrecy and failure to access care, thereby increasing harm to health.

- *It should take the patient's and population's context into account.* Understanding the history, economics, and social conditions (e.g., those of a group of refugees from a war-torn country) will lead practitioners to convey understanding and to focus on salient issues during health assessment.
- *It should be trauma- and violence-informed.* Trauma-informed care, according to relational–cultural theory, addiction theory, and trauma theory, is care that takes into account how histories of various forms of abuse shape experiences of substance use (Chung, Domino, & Morrissey, 2009; Covington, 2008). Violence-informed care further accounts for the dynamics of ongoing violence. Patients' substance use patterns are shaped by their histories of abuse and are difficult to change when those histories are not addressed and when the patients are facing ongoing violence.
- *It should minimize harm.* Harm reduction in relation to substance use often focuses narrowly on reducing the harms of drug use, such as by reducing overdoses or infections for people who are injecting drugs. A broader understanding of harm reduction recognizes that harms arise from the social, economic, political, and legal context of substance use. Harm reduction also aims to address these contexts by attempting to minimize homelessness, violence and poverty (Pauly, 2008a; Box 7-3).

To develop the skills to put these principles into action, we suggest a process of five elements (Box 7-4). Integrating knowledge requires that you develop your knowledge base widely. Accurate, current, evidence-informed knowledge about the pharmacological actions and physiological effects of different substances is required. For example, knowing Health Canada's guidelines regarding low-risk alcohol use (Box 7-5) allows you to provide guidance about drinking.

Knowledge about the effects of various prescription drugs, illegal drugs, and alcohol is continuously developing.

Providers must critically analyze scientific evidence. As argued previously, health care providers also require knowledge about the root causes and social factors affecting substance use and problems. Developing such knowledge requires identifying, questioning, and testing assumptions and stereotypes.

In the process of conducting health assessments, you must be aware of prevalent stereotypes and assumptions related to

---

BOX 7-4 5 As FOR INTEGRATING KNOWLEDGE OF SUBSTANCE USE IN HEALTH ASSESSMENT

1. **A**cquire knowledge; replace erroneous assumptions. Know yourself: your assumptions, attitudes, values, beliefs.

   Do assume that the majority of your patients use substances and that most feel embarrassed and stigmatized.

   Do not assume that substance use is a simple choice.

   Do assume that many people who experience problematic substance use also have significant histories of trauma.

2. **A**nticipate harm that may be caused by your practices, reactions, judgements (e.g., deterring patients from accessing the health care system); harm that may be linked to substance use, such as the social, legal, and economic contexts of use; and harm that may be caused by the substances used.

3. **A**void social judgement about substance use, such as seeing a person as "bad," deviant, or morally weak.

4. **A**nalyze organizational practices (e.g., clinical assessment tools) and resources.

5. **A**pproach patients respectfully.

BOX 7-3 PRINCIPLES OF HARM REDUCTION

According to the Canadian Nurses Association (2011, pp. 13–14), harm reduction

- Focuses on reducing the harm associated with a broad range of substances
- Does not require abstinence or discontinuation of use
- Is complementary to prevention and treatment approaches
- Empowers people who use drugs to make informed decisions
- Emphasizes humanistic values, including dignity, compassion, and nonjudgemental acceptance of people who use drugs
- Is cost effective and evidence informed
- Requires that people who use drugs participate in policymaking and program development
- Challenges policies and programs that maximize harm

BOX 7-5 HEALTH CANADA'S LOW-RISK ALCOHOL DRINKING GUIDELINES

Low-Risk Drinking Guideline 1

Chronic: Within this guideline, women must drink no more than 10 drinks a week, with no more than 2 drinks a day most days, and men must drink no more than 15 drinks a week, with no more than 3 drinks a day most days. Plan nondrinking days every week to avoid developing a habit.

Low-Risk Drinking Guideline 2

Acute: Within this guideline, women must drink no more than 3 drinks on any single occasion, and men must drink no more than 4 drinks on any single occasion. Plan to drink in a safe environment. Stay within the weekly limits outlined in guideline 1.

Source: Modified from Canadian Centre on Substance Abuse. (2012). *Canada's low-risk alcohol drinking guidelines.* Ottawa: Author. Retrieved from *http://www.ccsa.ca/Eng/Priorities/Alcohol/Canada-Low-Risk-Alcohol-Drinking-Guidelines/Pages/default.aspx.*

BOX 7-6 EXAMINING YOUR OWN ATTITUDES

Reflect on your own attitudes, beliefs, and values related to substance use. Ask yourself these questions:

- What were your own family's values and attitudes toward substance use?
- How have your values changed over time?
- What social issues do you view as influencing people's substance use patterns?
- How do you feel about working with people whose substances use has become problematic?
- What judgements arise when you provide health care to people who use substances?
- In what situation might you find it most challenging to be respectful?
- How do you feel about women who use substances during pregnancy or when they are mothers?

TABLE 7-1   Sample Screening Tool

The TWEAK questions (Russell, Materier, & Sokol, 1994) help identify at-risk drinking in women, especially pregnant women. Each question is scored on a 7-point scale. A woman who has a total score of 2 or more points is likely to be an at-risk drinker (Carson et al., 2010, p. S16).

- **T**olerance: How many drinks does it take to make you feel the first effect?
- **W**orry: Have close friends or relatives worried or complained about your drinking in the past year?
- **E**ye-opener: Do you sometimes take a drink in the morning when you first get up?
- **A**mnesia: Has a friend or family member ever told you about things you said or did that you could not remember?
- **K(C)**ut down: Do you sometimes feel the need to cut down on your drinking?

SCORING:

Taking ≥3 drinks to feel high = tolerance.
Score 2 points each for tolerance and worry.
Score 1 point each for the rest.
A low-risk response is ≤1 point.
≥2 points = a likely drinking problem.

substance use. To approach assessments related to substance use in a nonjudgemental way, you must engage in critical self-reflection (Box 7-6). People who experience persistent, negative social and health effects of substance use are highly sensitive to the attitudes of clinicians. For these reasons and as discussed in Chapter 5, you must be aware of how your attitudes are conveyed through tone of voice, types of questions, and nonverbal behaviours such as facial expressions.

Challenging the Idea of "Choice"

One key assumption that must be challenged is that substance use is simply a matter of individual "choice." Canada has increasingly imported ideas of individualism (that each person is autonomous, making decisions independent of his or her circumstances), martial language (such "the war on drugs"), and criminalizing approaches to dealing with substance use. This results in pervasive and popularized assumptions that problematic substance use primarily reflects individual choice and in a shift away from an illness model to an individual choice model (Pauly, 2008b). Understanding drug use as "choice" draws attention away from the underlying causes and factors influencing substance use and increases the likelihood of blaming and stigmatizing people who use substances beyond dominant social norms. Health care providers can (often unwittingly) communicate blame and shame if they consciously or unconsciously hold assumptions that people "ought to know better" or "should pull up their socks and just say no" or are morally weak because they rely on alcohol or drugs. Furthermore, commonly held assumptions that people in particular ethnocultural or social groups use alcohol or drugs more than do people in others—despite the evidence to the contrary—can, unless challenged, lead to damaging health care encounters. As discussed in Chapter 4, this in turn can lead to errors in clinical judgement with serious consequences.

Putting Principles Into Action

What does it mean to be respectful? How can you gather the information you need in the least invasive, least harmful way?

1. Learn about the context and population you serve. What are the most common substance use issues? What are the common histories? What substances are being used? What are the differential effects on particular populations within the communities served? What resources are available? Health care providers who work specifically with people who use substances usually wish to help clinicians who work in more generalist areas acquire new knowledge and skill related to substance use.

2. Be clear about why you are gathering information, and convey your reasons to patients you are assessing. For example, if an alcohol screening tool is used in your institution (e.g., the TWEAK screening tool shown here, or the CAGE screening tool described in the footnote on p. 114. Table 7-1), you might introduce it by saying, "We know that many people use alcohol, but we ask everyone about their alcohol use so that we can provide better pain management and anticipate reactions to medications and other problems."

3. Do not gather information that is not needed or will not be used. When people understand the rationale for being asked about substance use and trust that the information will be used for health reasons, they are more likely to disclose accurate information.

4. Assess individuals in context. If you have begun to learn about the context of people's lives in the populations you are serving, you will be better able to listen for and understand individuals' histories. Although you should anticipate that most people use substances of some sort, you should be especially alert when people present with a history of violent victimization or perpetration or with mental health problems.

5. Start history-taking with the least intrusive questions. Because alcohol is legal and its use is generally more acceptable than use of other substances, a person may be more amenable to disclosing information about alcohol use than about other substances. Once you have established a relationship of trust and openness, this may be a good entry point to discussing illicit substance use or prescription drug use. Because many people use multiple substances, this is a logical progression. For example, you may say, "Many people who use alcohol also use cocaine/speed/marijuana and so on to counteract the effects or to enhance the effects. Is that something you have tried?" Ask progressively more detailed questions to assess

- Substances used?
- Amount of substances used? If you don't understand the terms patients use (e.g., "points of heroin"), ask the patient for clarification.
- How often?
- By what route ("how do you take that particular drug")?
- For how long have you used these substances?
- When was the last time you used?

This information will guide you in knowing what other tests or assessments are indicated.

Regardless of whether you are using a particular assessment tool, make your questions specific. For example, with regard to alcohol, ask, "How much do you drink each week [or each day]?" rather than "How much do you drink?" (which is too general). Pose your questions in a way that conveys your knowledge about a given drug. For example, with regard to drugs such as crack, cocaine, or speed, ask "How do you use the drug? Do you smoke it? Inject with needles? Snort?"

If using a standardized assessment tool, you may have to "translate" the wording. For example, for the question "Do you ever have an eye-opener?" a patient might answer, "No" without understanding the meaning of the question. A clearer question, such as "Do you ever have a drink when you wake up, to get you going?" will elicit a more useful answer.

Although it is important to obtain a complete history of substance use, many patients do not trust the clinician adequately to disclose fully. Consider a lack of disclosure a protective mechanism, and assume that developing trust is your responsibility. If the setting allows, obtain as much information as the patient is willing to share, and then complete the assessment at a later time when you have had time to develop a more trusting relationship.

6. Use assessment as an opportunity to promote health and offer suggestions for harm reduction. Discussing the patient's substance use will provide insight into whether the patient views it as problematic. Performing an assessment is also an opportunity to provide brief factual information. Again, start with the least invasive topic; for example, "Cigarette smokers who also use marijuana can decrease the harmful effects of tobacco by not smoking a cigarette while still under the effects of marijuana; the marijuana dilates the lung bed and opens it up more to the toxins from the cigarettes."

Linking your assessment to the person's health emphasizes why you are asking the questions and provides ongoing opportunities to remain focused on promoting health. Explain to the patient that the questions you are asking are important so that appropriate and specific care and testing can be provided: for example, liver function tests for people who use alcohol, skin care/wound care for people who use needles, and testing for infections, and respiratory assessment for people who inhale substances. Examples of such explanations are as follows:

"People who smoke or snort drugs sometimes have wheezing, or productive coughs, or ulcerations in the nose. Has this been a problem for you?"

"If you have ever used needles, then I can offer you blood testing for some infections such as hepatitis C, hepatitis B, and HIV."

Most people are relieved to be offered testing.

7. Throughout the assessment, avoid making assumptions and being influenced by popularized stereotypes about people who use drugs or alcohol. This is also crucial during the physical examination. For example, if during a physical examination you notice that a person has needle marks on his or her arms, do not assume that they are signs of injecting drugs! Many people, including illicit substance users, undergo blood tests for medical reasons. Instead, you might frame your observation neutrally: "I see you've had a needle." If the patient is using needles to inject substances, teaching about hygienic and safer injection techniques, as well as never injecting when alone, can reduce harm. At the same time, this is an opportunity to discuss whether the patient has thought of quitting or cutting down and what supports he or she might need in order to do so.

Helping the patient feel accepted and worthy of care, even if he or she is using illicit substances, is key to building trust. Remember that if a person is not able to tell you about his or her substance use, it is a reflection on your skill at building trust and conveying a nonjudgemental attitude. When a nurse thinks that a patient "lied" about something such as drug use, medications, or diet, the nurse ought to ask, "What did I do to make the patient fear a punitive response if they told the truth?"

The following case example is illustrative:

I was doing research in an emergency unit, following nurses as they did assessments. The nurse I was following was assigned to a man with chest pain. He was in "bed 1," the first monitor unit nearest the nursing desk reserved for possible myocardial infarction. She took his history: when his symptoms had begun, the nature of the pain, and how had it changed. In the process, she asked him the questions on the CAGE questionnaire.*

***The CAGE questionnaire** (cutdown, annoyed, guilty, eye-opener) takes less than 1 minute to complete and has four straightforward "yes"/"no" questions. The CAGE tests for lifetime alcohol abuse and dependence but does not distinguish past problem drinking from active present drinking (Bush, Kivlahan, McDonell, Fihn, & Bradley, 1998).

The man looked distraught but almost relieved as she asked the questions. Yes, he felt he should cut down. Yes, his wife was constantly worrying. Yes, he felt terrible about his drinking. He was up to drinking "a 26er" a day. He wanted to quit.

The nurse ticked the boxes but then hurriedly left the stretcher to get an electrocardiogram on another patient, as the emergency unit filled past capacity. She was darting between about six different stretchers, another patient was vomiting, and I was caught up helping. Twenty minutes later, I noticed bed 1 was empty and asked what happened. "Oh," she replied, "it was just muscle strain, no cardiac problems." "What about the alcohol?" I asked. "We just ask about that in case they are admitted, in case of DTs," she said.

Screening tools (such as the TWEAK or CAGE described on pp. 113 and 114) may be required by your clinical setting and may provide useful ways to initiate a conversation about substance use. However, how such tools are implemented may be harmful. With regard to the case example just mentioned.

- What are the practice conditions that might influence how effectively such a tool may be used?
- What do you think is required to use such tools in a way that promotes health?
- What do you think is the most important goal of such a tool?

Similarly, when biochemical assays such as urine samples are used as part of the physical assessment to screen for particular drugs, collection should be performed in a way that optimizes trust, harm reduction, and health promotion. For example, a urine screen to detect the use of specific substances such as cocaine is often required as part of "conditions" for care contracts or child custody and visitation. The principles discussed previously apply directly to the collection of biochemical assays. Treating patients respectfully while they are subject to such surveillance is challenging but can build trust toward a more effective provider–patient relationship.

We believe that the conditions of practice should allow nurses to use tools in a health-promoting way. Some of these conditions include taking time to pay attention to patients' answers, listening respectfully, following up appropriately, and having resources to offer patients (educational, clinical, and community resources).

Assessing for Withdrawal

Often when patients are admitted to the hospital, their usual patterns of substance use are interrupted. If documentation of the history includes substance use, your health assessment increases the likelihood that you will be alert to the need to assess for and manage withdrawal. Table 7-2 lists the signs and symptoms of intoxication and withdrawal with selected substances.

THE SPECIAL CASE: SUBSTANCE USE ASSESSMENT IN PREGNANCY

During pregnancy, women face intense scrutiny related to substance use, including smoking, alcohol use, and use of illegal substances. Societal attitudes can create significant barriers that prevent women from receiving adequate prenatal care. Some women may hide the fact that they are drinking an occasional glass of wine, for example, whereas others may avoid health care altogether, fearing judgement, punitive treatment, or the threat of having their babies removed from their care at birth. Nurses must understand that the fear of punishment is a major concern for many women. In many jurisdictions, because of the belief that use of illicit substances means that a woman is not a fit mother, a positive result of a drug test (in the mother or her newborn) can lead to an apprehension of the child because of "neglect" or "abuse" (Boyd, 2004, p. 135).

A woman who fears that her child may be removed from her care may not seek or may avoid prenatal or other medical or social care. Paradoxically, policies intended to promote healthy pregnancies, births, and children may do the opposite. For example, inadequate nutrition and stress (from poverty, violence, homelessness, and so on) may contribute more to poor obstetrical outcomes than does substance use in pregnancy (Boyd, 2004). Furthermore, good nutrition in pregnancy helps mitigate some of the harmful effects of substance use. However, women avoiding care may miss out on support for nutrition and housing.

Although all health care providers have a duty to report suspected child abuse (as discussed in Chapter 8), in Canada, a fetus is not legally considered a child, and therefore this duty does not apply, despite attempts by lobby groups to define substance use by pregnant women as child abuse. Involvement of child protection services when women are using substances during pregnancy is not appropriate. If a patient discloses substance use and has children in his or her care, the children are not necessarily at risk for harm. It is appropriate to ask about the safety plan for the children when the patient is using substances. Substance use can be compatible with safe parenting.

Sometimes, with full agreement of the pregnant patient, an early referral to child protection services can be beneficial if supportive services are available to assist the pregnant woman in preparing for birth. When the woman has a history with child protection services (e.g., a child removed from her care in the past), it may be beneficial for her to meet with a child protection worker to demonstrate how well she is doing, what positive changes she has made, and what her plans are for providing a safe environment. This might prevent a removal at birth, in contrast to when decisions are based solely on the woman's history. Some jurisdictions are not adequately staffed to carry out investigations before the birth or to provide prenatal support.

Health care providers must have up-to-date and factual information regarding specific substances and their effects on the fetus. Alcohol and tobacco, both legal substances, are known to put the health of the fetus at risk. However, it is important to reassure women that moderate social drinking before confirmation of pregnancy has not been shown to cause birth defects.

Considerable misinformation regarding the effects of illegal substances, particularly the effects of drugs such as cocaine on the fetus, has been popularized. For example, a

TABLE 7-2	Signs and Symptoms of Intoxication and Withdrawal* With Selected Substances	
Substance	Intoxication	Withdrawal
Alcohol	Appearance: unsteady gait, incoordination, nystagmus, flushed face Behaviour: sedation, relief of anxiety, dulled concentration, impaired judgement, expansive, uninhibited behaviour, talkativeness, slurred speech, impaired memory, irritability, depression, emotional lability	Uncomplicated (shortly after cessation of drinking, peaks at second day, improves by fourth to fifth day): coarse tremor of hands, tongue, eyelids; anorexia; nausea and vomiting; malaise; autonomic hyperactivity (tachycardia, sweating, elevated blood pressure); headache; insomnia; anxiety; depression or irritability; transient hallucinations or illusions Withdrawal delirium, "delirium tremens" (much less common than uncomplicated, occurs within 1 week of cessation): coarse, irregular tremor; marked autonomic hyperactivity (tachycardia, sweating); vivid hallucinations; delusions; agitated behaviour; fever
Sedatives, hypnotics	Similar to alcohol Appearance: unsteady gait, incoordination Behaviour: talkativeness, slurred speech, inattention, impaired memory, irritability, emotional lability, sexual aggressiveness, impaired judgement, impaired social or occupational functioning	Anxiety or irritability; nausea or vomiting; malaise; autonomic hyperactivity (tachycardia, sweating); orthostatic hypotension; coarse tremor of hands, tongue, and eyelids; marked insomnia; grand mal seizures
Nicotine	Appearance: highly alert increased systolic blood pressure, increased heart rate, vasoconstriction Behaviour: nausea, vomiting, indigestion (first use); loss of appetite, head rush, dizziness, jittery feeling, mild stimulation	Vasodilation, headaches; anger, irritability, frustration, anxiety, nervousness, awakening at night, difficulty concentrating, depression, hunger, impatience or restlessness
Cannabis (marijuana)	Appearance: injected (reddened) conjunctivae, tachycardia, dry mouth, increased appetite, especially for "junk" food Behaviour: euphoria, anxiety, perception of slowed time, increased sense of perception, impaired judgement, social withdrawal, suspiciousness or paranoid ideation	
Cocaine	Appearance: pupillary dilation, tachycardia or bradycardia, elevated or lowered blood pressure, sweating, chills, nausea, vomiting, weight loss Behaviour: euphoria, talkativeness, hypervigilance, pacing, psychomotor agitation, impaired social or occupational functioning, fighting, grandiosity, visual or tactile hallucinations	Dysphoric mood (anxiety, depression, irritability), fatigue, insomnia or hypersomnia, psychomotor agitation
Amphetamines	Similar to cocaine Appearance: pupillary dilation, tachycardia or bradycardia, elevated or lowered blood pressure, sweating or chills, nausea and vomiting, weight loss Behaviour: elation, talkativeness, hypervigilance, psychomotor agitation, fighting, grandiosity, impaired judgement, impaired social and occupational functioning	Dysphoric mood (anxiety, depression, irritability), fatigue, insomnia or hypersomnia, psychomotor agitation
Opiates (morphine, heroin, meperidine)	Appearance: pinpoint pupils; decreased blood pressure, pulse, respirations, and temperature Behaviour: lethargy; somnolence; slurred speech; initial euphoria followed by apathy, dysphoria, and psychomotor retardation; inattention; impaired memory; impaired judgement; impaired social or occupational functioning	Dilated pupils, lacrimation, runny nose, tachycardia, fever, elevated blood pressure, piloerection, sweating, diarrhea, yawning, insomnia, restlessness, irritability, depression, nausea, vomiting, malaise, tremor, muscle and joint pains; symptoms are remarkably similar to clinical picture of influenza

*Intoxication refers to behavioural and physiological changes resulting from the effects of substances on the central nervous system. Withdrawal refers to the physiological symptoms that are produced when use of the substance is discontinued.

large-scale longitudinal study of the effects on children of maternal substance use in pregnancy revealed that "infant prenatal exposure to cocaine and to opiates was not associated with mental, motor, or behavioural deficits after controlling for birth weight and environmental risks" (Messinger, 2004, p. 1677). Heroin, in its pure form, is not teratogenic; however, as with all other illicit drugs, the safety of this substance cannot be verified.

Life circumstances that accompany illicit drug use are as detrimental to health as the substances: stigma, poverty, poor nutrition, needle use or sharing, smoking, lung irritants, survival sex work and the illegal activities necessary to obtain enough money to buy drugs, and associated exposure to sexually transmitted infections and violence.

You must recognize the stigma faced by women who use substances while pregnant, and you should provide nonjudgemental, supportive care. Stigma, judgement, and punitive treatment cause harm to the patient. In order to engage with patients successfully, nurses must actively work to counter such stigma and assure women of confidentiality (Radcliffe, 2011). Nurses can work to eliminate barriers to care by welcoming the patient and reassuring her that her well-being is the primary goal. By caring for the mother, you are caring for the fetus and infant. For example, some infants prenatally exposed to substances such as opiates, antidepressants, and certain prescription medications may exhibit symptoms of withdrawal in the first hours to days of life; however, when carefully monitored and managed with rooming-in with the mother, skin-to-skin contact, and breastfeeding, most such infants do not require medical treatment for withdrawal (Abrahams et al., 2007, 2010). There is increasing evidence that people who use illicit drugs can be adequate parents (Boyd, 1999, pp. 14–17). Most women share concern for the safety of the fetus, and so discussing this with the woman in a nonthreatening way can provide you with the opportunity to offer information about supports in the community (such as prenatal nutrition programs, housing advocates, food banks, etc.).

DOCUMENTATION

Charting about substance use, like all other aspects of care, should be aimed at promoting the health of the patient. Charting should be factual and nonjudgemental, and nonstigmatizing phrasing should be used. Document as accurately as possible the type of drugs used, the amount, the route, and the results of your history and physical assessment.

Nurses and other clinical staff may wonder whether illegal drug use discussed during the process of assessment should be reported to "authorities" (e.g., to police, security officers, supervisors); however, there is no legal requirement to report, and doing so would be a breach of confidentiality if it is done for nonmedical reasons.

Often, efforts must be made to avoid using stigmatizing language and phrasing. For example, avoid labels such as "drug user," which tends to focus on a narrow aspect of a patient's life. Of importance is that the term *addict* not be used, unless to record a patient's statement that he or she thinks or has been told that he or she has "an addiction." As discussed earlier, the term *addiction* has a very specific meaning, and it serves as a diagnosis that nurses are not qualified to make. Furthermore, people who use alcohol or drugs frequently resume and discontinue substance use as their life circumstances change. An example of less deterministic phrasing is "Uses heroin 2 to 4 times per week for the past year via injection into arm veins. For past year, has been using sterile needles obtained through the local needle-exchange unit."

In some cases, documentation of substance use by women who are pregnant and under surveillance by child welfare authorities can increase the risk that their newborns will be removed from their care or the risk that children who are currently in their custody will be removed from their care (Cory, Ruebsaat, Hankivsky, & Dechief, 2003; Greaves et al., 2004). As with the overall approaches to documentation, it is essential to chart only aspects of the history and physical examination that are directly relevant to assessment of the woman's health status. Pay extra attention to avoiding judgemental phrasing when you chart, in view of the extent to which pregnant women who use alcohol or substances are stigmatized in society.

REFERENCES

Abrahams, R. R., Kelly, A., Payne, S., Thiessen, P. N., Mackintosh, J., & Janssen, P. A. (2007). Rooming-in compared with standard care for newborns of mothers using methadone or heroin. *Canadian Family Physician, 53*, 1722–1730.

Abrahams, R. R., MacKay-Dunn, M. H., Nevmerjitskaia, V., MacRae, G. S., Payne, S. P., & Hodgson, Z. G. (2010). An evaluation of rooming-in among substance-exposed newborns in British Columbia. *Journal of Obstetrics and Gynaecology Canada, 32*(9), 866–871.

Adlaf, E.M., Begin, P., & Sawka, E. (Eds.). (2005). Canadian Addiction Survey (CAS): A national survey of Canadians' use of alcohol and other drugs: Prevalence of use and related harms: Detailed report. Ottawa: Canadian Centre on Substance Abuse. Retrieved from *http://www.ccsa.ca/2005%20CCSA%20 Documents/ccsa-004028-2005.pdf*.

Alexander, B. K. (2001). *The myth of drug-induced addiction*. Presentation to the Canadian Senate on Special Committee on Illegal Drugs. Retrieved from *http://www.parl.gc.ca/Content/ SEN/Committee/371/ille/presentation/alexender-e.htm*.

American Psychiatric Association. (2012a). *APA corrects New York Times Article on changes to DSM-5's substance use disorders*. Retrieved from *http://dsmfacts.org/issue-accuracy/ apa-corrects-new-york-times-article-on-changes-to-dsm-5s- substance-use-disorders/*.

American Psychiatric Association. (2012b). *DSM-5: The Future of Psychiatric Diagnosis*. Retrieved from *http://www.dsm5.org/ Pages/Default.aspx*.

Arbour-Nicitopoulos, K. P., Kwan, M. Y. W., Lowe, D., Taman, S., & Faulkner, G. E. J. (2010). Social norms of alcohol, smoking, and marijuana use within a Canadian university setting. *Journal of American College Health, 59*(3), 191–196.

Bader, P., Boisclair, D., & Ferrence, R. (2011). Effects of tobacco taxation and pricing on smoking behavior in high risk populations: A knowledge synthesis. *International Journal of Environmental Research and Public Health, 8*(11), 4118–4139. doi:10.3390/ijerph8114118

Bottorff, J. L., Carey, J., Mowatt, R., Varcoe, C., Johnson, J. L., Hutchinson, P., … Wardman, D. (2009). Bingo halls and smoking: Perspectives of First Nations women. *Health & Place, 15*(4), 1014–1021. doi:10.1016/j.healthplace.2009.04.005

Boyd, S. C. (1999). *Mothers and illicit drugs: Transcending the myths*. Toronto: University of Toronto Press.

Boyd, S. C. (2004). *From witches to crack moms: Women, drug law and policy*. Durham, NC: Carolina Academic Press.

British Columbia Provincial Health Officer. (2002). *Report on the health of British Columbians: Provincial health officer's annual report 2001: The health and well-being of Aboriginal people in British Columbia.* Victoria, BC: Ministry of Health Planning.

Browne, A., Varcoe, C., & Fridkin, A. (2011). Addressing trauma, violence and pain: Research on health services for women at the intersections of history and economics. In O. Hankivsky (Ed.), *Health inequities in Canada: Intersectional frameworks and practices* (pp. 295–311). Vancouver: University of British Columbia Press.

Bush, K., Kivlahan, D. R., McDonell, M. B., Fihn, S. D., & Bradley, K. A., for the Ambulatory Care Quality Improvement Project. (1998). The AUDIT alcohol consumption questions. *Archives of Internal Medicine, 158*(16), 1789–1795.

Canadian Nurses Association. (2011). *Harm reduction and currently illegal drugs: Implications for nursing policy, practice, education and research.* Retrieved from *http://www2.cna-aiic.ca/CNA/documents/pdf/publications/Harm_Reduction_2011_e.pdf.*

Carbone-López, K., Kruttschnitt, C., & MacMillan, R. (2006). Patterns of intimate partner violence and their associations with physical health, psychological distress, and substance use. *Public Health Reports, 121*(4), 382–392.

Carson, G., Cox, L., Crane, J., Croteau, P., Graves, L., Kluka, S., … Wood, R. (2010). Alcohol use and pregnancy consensus clinical guidelines [Whole issue]. *Journal of Obstetrics and Gynaecology Canada, 32*(8, Suppl. 3), S1–S31. Retrieved from *http://www.sogc.org/guidelines/documents/gui245CPG1008E.pdf.*

Chung, S., Domino, M. E., & Morrissey, J. P. (2009). Changes in treatment content of services during trauma-informed integrated services for women with co-occurring disorders. *Community Mental Health Journal, 45*(5), 375–384. doi:10.1007/s10597-009-9192-9

Collin, C. (2006). *Substance use issues and public policy in Canada: II Parliamentary action (1987-2005).* Ottawa: Political and Social Affairs Division, Library of Parliament, Canada.

Cory, J., Ruebsaat, G., Hankivsky, O., & Dechief, L. (2003). *Reasonable doubt: The use of health records in criminal and civil cases of violence against women in relationships.* Retrieved from *http://www.bccewh.bc.ca/publications-resources/documents/reasonabledoubt.pdf.*

Covington, S. S. (2008). Women and addiction: A trauma-informed approach. *Journal of Psychoactive Drugs,* (Suppl 5), 377–385.

Engstrom, M., El-Bassel, N., Go, H., & Gilbert, L. (2008). Childhood sexual abuse and intimate partner violence among women in methadone treatment: A direct or mediated relationship? *Journal of Family Violence, 23*(7), 605–617.

Fowler, D. (2007). The extent of substance use problems among women partner abuse survivors residing in a domestic violence shelter. *Family and Community Health, 30,* S106–S108.

Frohlich, K. L., & Poland, B. (2007). Points of intervention in health promotion practice. In M. O'Neill, A. Pederson, S. Dupere, & I. Rootman (Eds.), *Health promotion in Canada: Critical perspectives* (2nd ed., pp. 46–60). Toronto: Canadian Scholars' Press Inc.

Giesbrecht, N. (2008). Recent developments in overall alcohol consumption and high risk drinking: A case for effective population level interventions in Canada. *Adicciones, 20*(3), 207–219.

Giesbrecht, N., Ialomiteanu, A., Anglin, L., & Adlaf, E. (2007). Alcohol marketing and retailing: Public opinion and recent policy developments in Canada. *Journal of Substance Use, 12*(6), 389–404.

Gilchrist, G., Hegarty, K., Chondros, P., Herrman, H., & Gunn, J. (2010). The association between intimate partner violence, alcohol and depression in family practice. *BMC Family Practice, 11,* 72–81.

Golinelli, D., Longshore, D., & Wenzel, S. L. (2009). Substance use and intimate partner violence: Clarifying the relevance of women's use and partners' use. *Journal of Behavioral Health Services & Research, 36,* 199–211.

Greaves, L., Pederson, A., Varcoe, C., Poole, N., Morrow, M., Johnson, J. L., & Irwin, L. (2004). Mothering under duress: Women caught in a web of discourses. *Journal of the Association for Research on Mothering, 6*(1), 16–27.

Green, J. G., McLaughlin, K. A., Berglund, P. A., Gruber, M. J., Sampson, N. A., Zaslavsky, A. M, … Kessler, R. C. (2010). Childhood adversities and adult psychiatric disorders in the National Comorbidity Survey Replication I: Associations with first onset of *DSM-IV* disorders. *Archives of General Psychiatry, 67*(2), 113–123.

Gutierres, S. E., & Van Puymbroeck, C. (2006). Childhood and adult violence in the lives of women who misuse substances. *Aggression & Violent Behavior, 11*(5), 497–513.

Hedtke, K. A., Ruggiero, K. J., Fitzgerald, M. M., Zinzow, H. M., Saunders, B. E., Resnick, H. S., & Kilpatrick, D. G. (2008). A longitudinal investigation of interpersonal violence in relation to mental health and substance use. *Journal of Consulting and Clinical Psychology, 76*(4), 633–647.

International Harm Reduction Association. (2010). *What is harm reduction? Position statement.* London: Author.

Kaukinen, C., & Demaris, A. (2005). Age at first sexual assault and current substance use and depression. *Journal of Interpersonal Violence, 20,* 1244–1270.

McLaughlin, K. A., Green, J. G., Gruber, M. J., Sampson, N. A., Zaslavsky, A. M., & Kessler, R. C. (2010). Childhood adversities and adult psychiatric disorders in the National Comorbidity Survey Replication II: Associations with persistence of *DSM-IV* disorders. *Archives of General Psychiatry, 67*(2), 124–132.

Messinger, D. S. (2004). The Maternal Lifestyle Study: Cognitive, motor, and behavioral outcomes of cocaine-exposed and opiate-exposed infants through three years of age. *Pediatrics, 113*(6), 1677–1685.

O'Brien, C. (2010). Addiction and dependence in DSM-V. *Addiction, 106*(5), 866–867. doi:10.1111/j.1360-0443.2010.03144.x

Pauly, B. (2008a). Harm reduction through a social justice lens. *International Journal of Drug Policy, 19*(1), 4–10.

Pauly, B. (2008b). Shifting moral values to enhance access to health care: Harm reduction as a context for ethical nursing practice. *International Journal of Drug Policy, 19,* 195–204.

Poole, N., Greaves, L., Jategaonkar, N., McCullough, L., & Chabot, C. (2008). Substance use by women using domestic violence shelters. *Substance Use & Misuse, 43*(8/9), 1129–1150.

Radcliffe, P. (2011). Substance-misusing women: Stigma in the maternity setting. *British Journal of Midwifery, 19*(8), 497–506.

Robertson, L. A., & Culhane, D. (2005). *In plain sight: Reflections on life in Downtown Eastside Vancouver.* Vancouver: Talonbooks.

Russell, M., Materier, S. S., & Sokol, R. J. (1994). Screening for pregnancy risk drinking. *Alcoholism: Clinical and Experimental Research, 18*(5), 1156–1161.

Salmon, A. (2006). Dangerous prescriptions? Benzodiazepine use among Aboriginal senior women [Bulletin]. *Boltan-e-Pizhuhishi, 5*(1), 6–8.

Salomon, A., Bassuk, S. S., & Huntington, N. (2002). The relationship between intimate partner violence and the use of addictive substances in poor and homeless single mothers. *Violence Against Women, 8*(7), 785–815.

Schneider, R., Burnette, M. L., Ilgen, M. A., & Timko, C. (2009). Prevalence and correlates of intimate partner violence victimization among men and women entering substance use disorder treatment. *Violence and Victims, 24*(6), 744–756.

Scott-Storey, K. (2011). Cumulative abuse: Do things add up? An evaluation of the conceptualization, operationalization, and methodological approaches in the study of the phenomenon of cumulative abuse. *Trauma, Violence & Abuse, 12*(3), 135–150. doi:10.1177/1524838011404253

Smith, C. A., Elwyn, L. J., Ireland, T. O., & Thornberry, T. P. (2010). Impact of adolescent exposure to intimate partner violence on substance use in early adulthood. *Journal of Studies on Alcohol & Drugs, 71,* 219–230.

Visser, J., & Jehan, Z. (2009). ADHD: A scientific fact or a factual opinion? A critique of the veracity of attention deficit hyperactivity disorder. *Emotional & Behavioural Difficulties, 14*(2), 127–140. doi:10.1080/13632750902921930

Walsh, C. A., Jamieson, E., MacMillan, H., & Boyle, M. (2007). Child abuse and chronic pain in a community survey of women. *Journal of Interpersonal Violence, 22*(12), 1536–1554.

Wuest, J., Merritt-Gray, M., Ford-Gilboe, M., Lent, B., Varcoe, C., & Campbell, J. C. (2008). Chronic pain in women survivors of intimate partner violence. *Journal of Pain, 9*(11), 1049–1057.

Additional Resources

Action on Women's Addictions—Research & Education (AWARE): *http://www.aware.on.ca/resources/resources-service-providers*

Alberta Alcohol & Drug Abuse Commission: *http://aadac.com/*

Bevel Up: National Film Board of Canada: *http://www.bccdc.ca/SexualHealth/Programs/StreetOutreachNurseProgram/BevelUp.htm*

B.C. Mental Health & Addictions Services: *http://www.bcmhas.ca/default.htm*

Canadian Addiction Survey: *http://www.hc-sc.gc.ca/hc-ps/tobac-tabac/research-recherche/stat/index-eng.php*

Canadian Centre on Substance Use (CCSU): *http://www.ccsa.ca/Pages/Home.aspx*

Centre for Addiction & Mental Health: *http://www.camh.net/*

Centre for Addictions Research of B.C. (CAR-BC): *http://www.carbc.uvic.ca/*

Coalescing on Women and Substance Use: *http://www.bccewh.bc.ca/bccewh-initiatives/coalescing-on-women-and-substance-use.htm*

Pregnancy-Related Issues in the Management of Addictions (PRIMA): A Reference for Care Providers (2008): *http://www.addictionpregnancy.ca*

Substance Abuse & Mental Health Services Administration (SAMHSA): *http://www.samhsa.gov/*

University of Washington, Alcohol and Drug Abuse Institute: *http://depts.washington.edu/adai/*

8

Interpersonal Violence Assessment

Written by Colleen Varcoe, PhD, RN

With contributions from the original chapter by Daniel J. Sheridan, PhD, RN, FAAN, and Shawna S. Mudd, MSN, CRNP

⊖volve WEBSITE

OUTLINE

Interpersonal violence—including intimate partner violence, sexual assault, child abuse, and elder abuse—is a serious problem that health care providers must recognize, assess, and address. In Canada, all provinces have mandatory requirements for reporting child abuse, and some provinces have general mandatory reporting requirements within adult legislation that apply to some forms of elder abuse or abuse of people with developmental disabilities. Beyond these legal requirements, all forms of interpersonal violence have significant, long-lasting health consequences and require a meaningful response by health care providers.

INTIMATE PARTNER VIOLENCE DEFINED

Intimate partner violence (IPV) encompasses spousal violence and violence committed by current or former dating partners (Johnson, 2006). **Spousal abuse** is physical or sexual violence, psychological violence, or financial abuse within current or former marital or common-law relationships, including same-sex spousal relationships. Behaviours used to dominate another person in the context of an intimate relationship may include physical or sexual assault and acts such as verbal abuse, imprisonment, humiliation, stalking, and denial of access to financial resources, shelter, or services (Tjaden & Thoennes, 2000). Gender is a key risk factor for

IPV: "Men's and boys' experiences of violence are different than women's and girls' in important ways. While men are more likely to be injured by strangers in a public or social venue, women are in greater danger of experiencing violence from intimate partners in their own homes. Women are also at greater risk of sexual violence" (Johnson, 2006, p. 1). For example, in 2009, women who reported spousal violence were about three times more likely than men (34% versus 10%) to report that they had been sexually assaulted, beaten, choked, or threatened with a gun or a knife by their partner or ex-partner in the previous 5 years (Statistics Canada, 2011). For women, IPV is acknowledged to be a pattern of physical, sexual, or emotional violence (or all three) in the context of coercive control (Cherniak, Grant, Mason, Moore, & Pellizzari, 2005; Tjaden & Thoennes, 2000).

SEXUAL ASSAULT DEFINED

Sexual assault usually occurs either within the context of a partner relationship or by a known assailant but may also be perpetrated by a stranger. The Canadian *Criminal Code* identifies both sexual assault and sexual touching as crimes. There are four levels of **sexual assault:** (1) sexual assault that is forced sexual activity without physical injury, (2) sexual assault with a weapon or verbal threats to a third party, (3) sexual assault causing bodily harm, and (4) aggravated sexual assault, which is forced sexual activity where the attacker seriously injures, wounds, maims, disfigures, or endangers life.

CHILD ABUSE AND NEGLECT DEFINED

In Canada, child abuse and exploitation are prohibited by the *Criminal Code* (Department of Justice Canada, 1985). Most provinces and territories have child welfare laws that require the public, including health care providers, to report suspected child abuse. The Department of Justice Canada (1985) defined **child abuse** as "the violence, mistreatment or

neglect that a child or adolescent may experience while in the care of someone they either trust or depend on, such as a parent, sibling, other relative, caregiver or guardian. Abuse may take place anywhere and may occur, for example, within the child's home or that of someone known to the child. There are many different forms of abuse and a child may be subjected to more than one form." Child abuse and IPV against women often overlap, with estimates that in up to 70% of families in which women are abused, children are also abused (Edleson, 1999; Folsom, Christensen, Avery, & Moore, 2003). Box 8-1 lists Department of Justice Canada's definitions that are consistent with those used in most provincial and territorial laws.

BOX 8-1 TYPES OF CHILD ABUSE

Physical Abuse

Physical abuse is the intentional use of force against a child. It can cause physical pain, injury, or injury that may last a lifetime. This type of abuse includes:
- pushing or shoving
- hitting, slapping, or kicking
- strangling or choking
- pinching or punching
- biting
- burning
- throwing an object at a child, and
- excessive or violent shaking.
  All of these acts are crimes in Canada.

Sexual Abuse

Child sexual abuse happens when a person takes advantage of a child for sexual purposes. It does not always involve physical contact with a child. For example, it could happen when an adult:
- makes sexual comments to a child, or
- secretly watches or films a child for sexual purposes.
  Sexual abuse of a child includes:
- any sexual contact between an adult and a child under 16
- any sexual contact with a child between the age of 16 and 18 without consent, or
- any sexual contact that exploits a child under 18.

Any sexual contact between an adult and a child under 16 is a crime. In Canada, the age of consent for sexual activity is 16, but there are some exceptions if the other person is close in age to the child. For more information on the age of consent and teenage relationships, visit the Department of Justice links found in "Who Can Help?" [at] http://www.justice.gc.ca/eng/pi/fv-vf/pub/caw-mei/p14.html.

In addition, children under 18 cannot legally give their consent to sexual activity that exploits them. Sexual activities that exploit a child include prostitution and pornography. They also include situations where someone in a position of authority or trust, or someone the child depends

on, has any kind of sexual activity with the child. A person of authority or trust could be a step-parent, a babysitter or a coach.

Neglect

Neglect happens when a parent or guardian fails to meet a child's basic needs. Sometimes parents neglect their children on purpose. Sometimes parents don't mean to neglect their children, but they have so many problems themselves that they can't look after their children properly. Neglect can include:
- not giving a child proper food or warm clothing
- not providing a child with a safe and warm place to live
- not making sure a child washes regularly
- not providing enough health care or medicine
- not paying any attention to a child's emotional needs
- not preventing physical harm, and
- not making sure a child is supervised properly.
  Sometimes, neglect can hurt just as much as physical abuse.

Some forms of neglect are crimes in Canada. For example, failing to provide the necessaries of life (http://www.justice.gc.ca/eng/pi/fv-vf/pub/caw-mei/p15.html#n7) and child abandonment (http://www.justice.gc.ca/eng/pi/fv-vf/pub/caw-mei/p15.html#n3) are crimes. The provinces and territories also have laws to protect children from neglect. These laws protect children even if the type of abuse is not a crime.

Emotional Abuse

Emotional abuse happens when a person uses words or actions to control, frighten, isolate, or take away a child's self-respect and sense of worth. Emotional abuse is sometimes called psychological abuse. It can include:
- putting a child down or humiliating a child
- constantly criticizing a child
- constantly yelling at a child
- threatening to harm a child or others
- keeping a child from seeing their family or friends without good reason, or
- threatening to move a child out of their home

Source: Department of Justice Canada. (2007). *Child Abuse: Fact Sheet.* Retrieved from http://publications.gc.ca/collections/Collection/J2-295-2002E.pdf. Reproduced with the permission of the Minister of Public Works and Government Services Canada, 2013.

Abuse is a misuse of power and a violation of trust. Children who are being abused are usually in a position of dependence on the person who is abusing them. An abuser may use a number of different tactics to gain access to a child, exert power and control over the child, and prevent the child from telling anyone about the abuse or seeking support. The abuse may happen once or in a repeated and escalating pattern over a period of months or years, and it may change form over time.

ELDER ABUSE AND NEGLECT DEFINED

Elder abuse and neglect are forms of IPV that continue into older adulthood or arise as persons become more vulnerable with age. Spousal abuse may continue as people age, or may begin later in life, or new forms of abuse may arise with increasing vulnerability. Between 1994 and 2003, police reported a history of family violence among 32% of family-related homicides against older adults (Turcotte & Schellenberg, 2007). As with any form of IPV, gender is a risk factor in older adults, too: that is, older women are at higher risk than are older men. For example, in 2009, 41% of all victimizations of family members were against older women, in comparison with 23% against older men (Statistics Canada, 2011). Seniors Canada (2011) describes the abuse of seniors as including mistreatment or violence, or even neglect. "Abuse can be at the hands of a spouse, an adult child or other family member. Abuse can be inflicted by a caregiver, a service provider, or other person in a situation of power or trust. Abuse can happen when a senior is living in an institution or a private residence." Elder abuse and neglect include violence in the home, violence in institutions, and even self-neglect (McDonald & Collins, 2000). McDonald and associates (2012) noted that research has tended to focus on violence in the home and overlook institutional abuse. Older adults who become frail and require medical or other health-related services may experience abuse in the form of failure to facilitate their access to medical or health services, failure to provide medical attention appropriate for age, or conducting a procedure or treatment without the informed consent of the patient or the patient's recognized substitute decision maker. The Department of Justice Canada (2007) identified many forms of elder abuse and neglect, including psychological, financial, physical, sexual, and spiritual abuses and neglect (see Box 31-2 for definitions of types of elder abuse). Although age and gender can increase vulnerability, it is important to note that other factors, such as economic dependence, disabilities (e.g., intellectual and physical disabilities), and rural isolation also increase vulnerability to violence. For more information on elder abuse, see Chapter 31.

EFFECTS OF VIOLENCE ON HEALTH

IPV, child abuse, and elder abuse remain significant problems globally and in Canada, although all estimates are widely acknowledged to be underestimates. According to the most conservative estimates in the 2009 Canadian General Social Survey, 7% of women and 6% of men in current or previous spousal relationships reported having experienced some form of spousal violence during the previous 5 years, but violence against women tended to be much more severe (Statistics Canada, 2011). Between 2000 and 2009, there were 738 spousal homicides, representing 16% of all solved homicides and nearly half (47%) of all family-related homicides. Women continue to be more likely than men to be victims of spousal homicide. In 2009, the rate of spousal homicide against women was about three times higher than that for men (Statistics Canada, 2011). Prevalence studies in Canada have been criticized as gross underestimates; according to more accurate estimates, up to 23% of women experience IPV each year (Clark & Du Mont, 2003).

Lifetime rates of physical assault by an intimate partner have been estimated at 25% to 30% in Canada and the United States (Johnson & Sacco, 1995; Jones et al., 1999). Physical assault is often accompanied by sexual violence or emotional abuse, and many women experience IPV in more than one relationship over their lifetime (Johnson, 1996).

As of 2012, the most detailed information on sexual assault is available from the 1993 National Violence Against Women Survey (Johnson, 1996). At that time, 39% of Canadian women reported having experienced at least one sexual assault since the age of 16. In 2000, women made up the vast majority of victims of sexual assault (86%) and other types of sexual offences (78%) (Statistics Canada, 2001). In 2010, 22,000 sexual assaults were reported to police in Canada, a number that is estimated to be extremely conservative because close to 90% of sexual assaults are not brought to the attention of the police (Perreault & Brennan, 2010).

The incidence of child abuse is also difficult to estimate and often based on only *reported* cases. With data from child welfare authorities, the Canadian Incidence Study of Reported Child Abuse and Neglect estimated a rate of 21.52 investigations of child abuse per 1000 children (Public Health Agency of Canada, 2001). The highest proportion of reported and substantiated child abuse cases involved **neglect** (Table 8-1). Analyses of this report support the growing concern that insufficient attention has been paid to neglect in comparison with sexual abuse, partly because sexual abuse is a more sensational issue (McLean, 2001). Emphasis has been on risk

TABLE 8-1	Investigations of Types of Child Maltreatment	
Types of Abuse	Percentage of Investigations	Percentage Substantiated
Physical abuse	31	34
Sexual abuse	10	38
Neglect	40	43
Emotional maltreatment	19	54

Source: From Public Health Agency of Canada. (2001). *The Canadian incidence study of reported child abuse and neglect: Highlights.* Retrieved from *http://www.phac-aspc.gc.ca/cm-vee/cishl01/.*

assessment and urgent intervention for abuse but not on the more frequent cases of neglect. Because they found that 96% of substantiated cases did not involve severe physical harm (harm severe enough to warrant medical attention in about 4% of substantiated cases), Trocmé, MacMillan, Fallon, and De Marco (2003) argued that assessment and investigation priorities need to be revised and to include consideration of long-term needs for housing, income, child care, and so on. Of importance is that socioeconomic status has been consistently shown to be related to parenting effectiveness (Wekerle, Wall, Leung, & Trocmé, 2007), which also suggests that health care providers should assess for longer term and broader social support.

The extent of elder abuse is also difficult to determine. Walsh and Yon (2012) noted that although the first and only national population survey was conducted in 1989, Canadian prevalence data on elder abuse in the community are consistent with international rates, ranging from 4% to 10%, of older persons experiencing some form of abuse. Poole and Rietschlin (2012) analyzed the Canadian General Social Survey and estimated that the 5-year prevalence of abuse by a current or former spouse/partner was 6.8% among persons aged 60 and over. The most common type was emotional abuse (prevalence, 6.3%), in comparison with financial abuse (prevalence, 1.2%) and physical abuse (prevalence, 0.9%). In 2001, Statistics Canada reported that in the 1999 General Social Survey on Victimization (as of 2012, the most recent source of data on broader forms of adult victimization), approximately 7% of the sample of more than 4000 adults older than 65 years reported that they had experienced some form of emotional or financial abuse by an adult child, spouse, or caregiver in the 5 years before the survey; the vast majority of cases were committed by spouses. Emotional abuse was more frequently reported (7%) than financial abuse (1%). The two most common forms of emotional abuse reported were snubbing or name-calling and limiting contact with family and friends. Only a small proportion of older adults (1%) reported experiencing physical or sexual abuse. Almost 2% of older Canadians indicated that they had experienced more than one type of abuse (Canadian Centre for Justice Statistics, 2002). These statistics likely underrepresent those most vulnerable and institutionalized.

All forms of violence have significant effects on health, and because individuals may experience multiple forms of violence and multiple incidents of violence, the health effects are likely to be cumulative (Scott-Storey, 2011). The health consequences of IPV result not only from physical assault but also from sexual assault (Campbell & Soeken, 1999) and from emotional abuse (Carlson, 2005). A persuasive body of knowledge accumulated since the 1990s has established that violent experiences have significant effects on women's health. The health consequences of IPV include the following:

- **Direct effects of physical injuries,** such as bruises and fractures (Muellman, Lenaghan, & Pakieser, 1996; Wuest et al., 2009)
- **Chronic physical health problems,** such as chronic pain and arthritis; frequent headaches and migraines; visual

problems; unexplained dizziness and fainting; sexually transmitted infections (STIs); unwanted pregnancies; gynecological symptoms; hypertension; viral infections such as colds and flu; peptic ulcers; and functional or irritable bowel disease (Campbell & Lewandowski, 1997; Kendall-Tackett, Marshall, & Ness, 2003; Leserman & Drossman, 2007; Wuest et al., 2007)
- **Mental health problems,** including clinical depression; acute and chronic symptoms of anxiety; serious sleep disturbances; symptoms consistent with post-traumatic stress disorder (PTSD); substance abuse and dependence; and thoughts of suicide, which are significantly more prevalent among women who have been abused than among those not abused (Campbell, 2002; Gilchrist, Hegarty, Chondros, Herrman, & Gunn, 2010; Hill, Schroeder, Bradley, Kaplan, & Angel, 2009).

The most obvious health care problem in abused women is injury; approximately 52% reported that they were injured seriously enough in an abusive incident to need medical attention (Bachman & Saltzman, 1995). Such injuries have particular patterns that can be recognized. Head and neck injuries and musculoskeletal injuries such as sprains and fractures are common (Bhandari, Dosanjh, Tornetta, & Matthews, 2006).

Chronic health problems are less obviously linked to IPV but are very significant clinically. In many controlled investigations of women in a variety of health care settings, abused women have been found to have significantly more chronic health problems, including more neurological, gastrointestinal, and gynecological symptoms and chronic pain (Campbell, 2002; Campbell, Sharps, & Glass, 2001; Coker, Smith, McKeown, & King, 2000; Leserman & Drossman, 2007; Plichta, 1996; Wuest et al., 2007). Abused women also visit health care providers more often than do women not battered and incur higher health care costs (Coker, Fadden, Reeder, & Smith, 2004; Rivara et al., 2007a; Schollenberger et al., 2003; Snow Jones et al., 2006; Varcoe et al., 2011), with potential long-term costs both for themselves and employers (Reeves & O'Leary-Kelly, 2007). In terms of mental health, abused women also experienced significantly more depression, suicidal thoughts and attempts, and symptoms of PTSD, as well as substance abuse (Carbone-López, Kruttschnitt, & MacMillan, 2006; Hill et al., 2009; Mechanic, Weaver, & Resick, 2008). The forced sex that accompanies physical abuse in 40% to 45% of the cases contributes to a host of gynecological health problems, including chronic pelvic pain, unintended pregnancy, STIs (including human immunodeficiency virus [HIV] infection), and urinary tract infections (Campbell & Soeken, 1999; Maman, Campbell, Sweat, & Gielen, 2000). Abuse during pregnancy is also a significant health issue, with serious consequences for both the pregnant woman (e.g., antepartum hemorrhage, death, depression, substance abuse) and the infant (low birth weight, increased risk for child abuse (Janssen, Holt, Sugg, Emanuel, Critchlow, & Henderson, 2003; Murphy, Schei, Myhr, & Du Mont, 2001; Tiwari et al., 2008).

Although more than 50% of abused women say they have been injured, only 25% to 30% say they have actually sought health care for one of the injuries (Du Mont, Forte, Cohen, Hyman, & Romans, 2005; Plichta, 1996). Even so, the majority of abused women (80%) say they have been in a health care setting for some reason, either for regular checkups or for one of the chronic health problems described previously. Because many abused women may not be ready to seek help from a shelter or from the criminal justice system (Landenburger, 1998) or are reluctant to do so (Beaulaurier, Seff, Newman, & Dunlop, 2007; Fugate, Landis, Riordan, Naureckas, & Engel, 2005), the health care system can be an extremely important early point of contact. It is hoped that dealing effectively with abuse in its early stages can stop the pattern of violence and prevent or minimize chronic health problems.

Health care providers need to be alert for the conditions particularly associated with IPV, including gynecological problems (especially STIs, pelvic pain, and complaints of sexual dysfunction), chronic irritable bowel syndrome, back pain, depression, and the presenting symptoms of PTSD (especially problems sleeping and "panic" attacks or problems with "nerves"). When these problems occur, and especially when they persist, a thorough and repeated assessment of interpersonal violence is needed. In this case, an instrument such as the Women's Experience of Battering Scale (Coker et al., 2000) might be used, or gentle indirect queries (e.g., "I am concerned about your health conditions; is there any chance that stress at home is contributing to these problems?") may be used. The health effects of violence on a woman and the associated social and economic costs also extend to the woman's children (Bogat, DeJonghe, Levendosky, Davidson, & von Eye, 2006; Rivara et al., 2007b), partly as a result of witnessing abuse (Carlson, 2000).

The health effects of elder abuse are not nearly as well studied, but the consequences of IPV can be presumed similar for older people. Complications from intentional injury can range from minor pain and discomfort to life-threatening injuries. Bleeding from intentional trauma can cause significant changes in circulatory homeostasis, leading to marked fluctuations in blood pressure and pulse, shock, and ultimately death. Localized infections can progress to generalized sepsis, even death, in older patients who are immunocompromised. The actual assault or the stress leading up to or after an assault can contribute to cardiac complications. All of the STIs and related complications that are sequelae of abuse in younger women are also present in older women who have been sexually assaulted. In addition, postmenopausal women have more friable vaginal mucosal tissue as a result of estrogen loss, which increases their risk for STIs and vaginal trauma.

Abuse of older adults often is coupled with neglect. Neglect can manifest as symptoms of dehydration and malnutrition. Neglect can be intentional or nonintentional. Some family members or caregivers working with older persons consciously, and with malice, withhold food, water, medication, and appropriate necessities, often concurrently stealing the financial assets of the older, dependent person. This type of neglect is often, by definition, criminal in nature.

Some family members or caregivers working with an older person struggle with their own severe physical and cognitive

health challenges. All caregivers should be assessed for caregiver burden (see Modified Caregiver Strain Questionnaire in Figure 31-4). In spite of the caregiver's good intentions, the older patient may experience profound unintentional neglect. Unintentional neglect is usually not viewed as a crime, but it must be addressed. Finally, self-neglect raises often unanswerable questions about one's right to live autonomously versus society's obligation to care for a person who is not able to care for herself or himself.

Older women face specific barriers to getting help. They may be more vulnerable because of economic dependence, physical and cognitive health challenges, and isolation. Services may not be appropriate for their needs in dealing with IPV. Leaving their partners may not be possible, but services and social expectations are not oriented to the fact that leaving poses special challenges to older women (Beaulaurier et al., 2007). Thus assessment must include a broad understanding of the patient's life circumstances.

Child maltreatment has many possible long-term physical and psychological effects. The immediate consequences can include a spectrum of physical injuries such as bruises, fractures, and lacerations and can involve more severe injury such as head trauma. More severe forms of maltreatment can lead to death or long-term problems such as intellectual disability, blindness, and physical disability.

Child maltreatment can have effects on a child's development by disrupting the bond between child and caregiver (Hagele, 2005). Ongoing child maltreatment can lead to changes in brain structure and chemistry, which may lead to long-term physical, psychological, emotional, social, and cognitive dysfunctions in adulthood (Hagele, 2005). Although physical harm is one form of child abuse, other forms of abuse often co-occur and also have long-term adverse effects. For example, an analysis of 554 youth found that verbal aggression was associated with moderate to large effects on psychiatric symptoms, comparable with the effects of witnessing IPV or nonfamilial sexual abuse and larger than those associated with familial physical abuse (Teicher, Samson, Polcari, & McGreenery, 2006). Childhood abuse puts children at risk for depression and PTSD, participating in harmful activities, having difficulties in relationships, and having negative beliefs and attitudes toward others. Each of these increases the likelihood of health problems, and they are closely related to each other (Kendall-Tackett, 2002). Child abuse is related to substance use, eating disorders, suicide, high-risk sexual behaviour, and sleep disorders (McLaughlin, et al., 2010; Wekerle et al., 2007). Child abuse may also increase vulnerability to later victimization and homelessness. The idea that people who are abused as children are more likely to abuse their children is popular, but evidence of this is inconclusive (Ozturk Ertem, Leventhal, & Dobbs, 2000; Renner & Slack, 2006).

Department of Justice Canada (2007) noted that

there is no single, definitive cause of child abuse, and any child—regardless of age, gender, race, ethnicity, cultural identity, socioeconomic status, spirituality, sexual orientation, physical or mental abilities or personality—may be vulnerable to being abused .... Many experts believe that

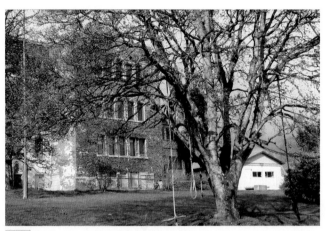

8-1 For many generations, children from communities along the coast of British Columbia were taken from their families and sent to residential schools, including this one in Alert Bay, where they experienced multiple forms of abuse.

child abuse is linked to inequalities among people in our society and the power imbalance between adults and children. A child is usually in a position of dependence on his or her abuser, and has little or no power compared to the abuser. There is increasing understanding that a child's vulnerability to abuse may be increased by factors such as dislocation, colonization, racism, sexism, homophobia, poverty and social isolation. For example, in the past, many children sent to institutions experienced abuse [Figure 8-1]. Most of these children were from marginalized groups in our society including, among others, children with disabilities, children from racial and ethnic minorities, Aboriginal children and children living in poverty. There are also factors that may increase a child's vulnerability to being abused—or compound the effects of abuse. For example, a child's caregivers may experience barriers that prevent them from acquiring the necessary skills, resources and supports to prevent abuse, or they may lack access to the services and supports they need to address it.

Risk factors for child maltreatment are identifiable; however, in a study of missed cases of abusive head trauma, Jenny, Hymel, Ritzen, Reinert, and Hay (1999) found that cases of abusive head injury were missed more often in White children than children in racialized groups, in children living with both parents, in younger children, and in children with less severe presenting symptoms. These dynamics may reflect stereotypical thinking regarding who is abused. For example, in one Canadian study, nurses tended to anticipate IPV among poor and racialized people and to anticipate child abuse in Aboriginal families (Varcoe, 2001). Such attitudes may contribute to the fact that Aboriginal families are more often investigated for neglect. Blackstock, Trocmé, and Bennett (2004) analyzed the Canadian investigations of child abuse and found that at every decision point in the cases, Aboriginal children are overrepresented: Investigations were more likely to be substantiated, cases were more likely to be kept open for ongoing services, and children were more likely to be placed in out-of-home care.

HEALTH CARE PROVIDERS' RESPONSES TO INTIMATE PARTNER VIOLENCE

To date, the health care response to IPV has been inadequate at best. Research has consistently shown that health care providers fail to identify when their patients are abused. The main recommendation for health care providers has been to routinely screen for violence. However, evidence regarding whether this is effective is, to date, inconclusive (Coker, 2006). In a systematic review of available literature published in English, Ramsey, Richardson, Carter, Davidson, and Feder (2002) found that in most studies, greater numbers of abused women were detected with screening than without screening. However, detecting abuse does not necessarily lead to meaningful responses. In intervention studies, researchers used weak study designs and produced inconsistent results. In no studies did researchers measure quality of life, mental health outcomes, or potential harm to women from screening programs. Ramsey and colleagues (2002) concluded that other than an increase in referrals to outside agencies, little evidence exists that screening leads to changes in important outcomes such as decreased exposure to violence. Nelson, Nygren, McInerney, and Klein (2004) conducted a systematic review and found no studies that directly addressed the effectiveness of screening in a health care setting in reducing harm from family and intimate partner violence or the adverse effects of screening and interventions. In Canada, MacMillan and colleagues (2009) found that evidence of benefit was insufficient to justify implementation of screening programs. More recently, Klevens and colleagues (2012) found no significant benefits from screening for IPV.

Some of the challenges to screening for abuse include the following:

- People who are experiencing violence may not identify their experiences as abuse.
- People who are experiencing violence may be ashamed or anticipate judgement by service providers.
- Privacy for disclosure may not be available in health care settings.
- Women may fear the responses from health care providers, including acts that will increase their risks, such as those that increase danger for themselves or family members or increase the risk that their children will be apprehended.
- Health care providers may ask screening questions more often of racialized or poor women, further perpetuating stereotypes of abuse and underinvestigating the abusive experiences of middle-class and Euro-Canadian women (Cory & Dechief, 2007).

Even when the abuse is recognized, women's experiences with health care providers tend to be negative (Bacchus, Mezey, & Bewley, 2003; Gerbert et al., 1999; Humphreys & Campbell, 2010; McCloskey & Grigsby, 2005). Research has shown that women often find professional responses to abuse unsympathetic, disempowering, victim-blaming, and focused on physical consequences of violence rather than on the wider effects and the context of women's lives (Gerbert et al., 1996; Tower, 2007). Health care providers often provide inappropriate or even harmful treatment. A Canadian study of

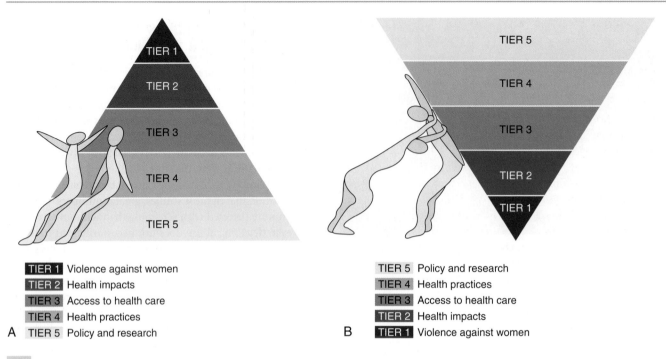

TIER 1 Violence against women
TIER 2 Health impacts
TIER 3 Access to health care
TIER 4 Health practices
A   TIER 5 Policy and research

TIER 5 Policy and research
TIER 4 Health practices
TIER 3 Access to health care
TIER 2 Health impacts
B   TIER 1 Violence against women

8-2   **A,** Safety and Health Enhancement (SHE) model. **B,** Compounding Harms model.

emergency department responses to violence against women showed that nurses' responses were shaped by stereotypical thinking about violence as a problem primarily of poor and racialized people, by judgements of the extent to which women "deserved" help, and by the patterns of practice that required nurses to process cases as quickly as possible (Varcoe, 2001). Health care providers often lack knowledge about IPV, have attitudes and values that inhibit an effective response, and think they have only minimal time to respond (Tower, 2007).

Assessing for IPV should be seen as part of a larger response to violence. The British Columbia Women's Hospital Woman Abuse Response Team has developed the Safety and Health Enhancement (SHE) model (Figure 8-2; Cory & Dechief, 2007), which guides health care providers to develop more effective responses, beginning with effective policy and research driving the process, rather than violence driving the process, as depicted in the Compounding Harms model (see Figure 8-2). Key features of the approach include the following:

- Putting safety first: always beginning with attention to the patients' and your emotional, cultural, and physical safety
- Making connections: knowing and connecting with a range of resources and services so that you can facilitate access for patients
- Offering more than quick-fix solutions: shifting from a focus on disclosure of abuse to responsiveness to an individual's needs
- Doing no harm: ensuring that health care responses do not disempower, demean, or increase danger
- Seeing the "big picture": keeping the wider context of women's lives in mind and viewing violence as a widespread social problem rather than an individual aberration

Assessing for Intimate Partner Violence

Even if it is not known whether screening is useful, health care providers cannot ignore the problem of violence (Coker, 2006). Although the idea of screening may imply that health care providers need to know a person's history of abuse to complete a thorough assessment or provide adequate care, this is not true. Furthermore, research has revealed that women are prepared to disclose IPV to health care providers when they feel confident and safe enough to do so (Bacchus et al., 2003; Gerbert et al., 1999). All care should be "trauma- and violence-informed"; that is, all care, including assessment, should be informed by knowledge about the dynamics of violence and the effect of violence (Covington, 2008; Hopper, Bassuk, & Oliver, 2010). Health care providers can take the following steps:

- Assume that a majority of patients will have a history of abuse of some form.
- Assume that any patient may be currently experiencing abuse.
- Provide care that is appropriate for people who have histories of, or are experiencing, abuse, *regardless* of whether abuse has been disclosed.
- Routinely inquire about how a patient's home life and work life are affecting his or her health.

On the basis of awareness that abuse may be part of any patient's history, and with the use of a relational approach as described in earlier chapters, assessment should routinely include the following:

- **Listening** in a nonjudgemental and accepting manner
- Having a **high index of suspicion** for abuse (MacMillan & Wathen, 2003) when patients present with direct injuries consistent with abuse, chronic health problems associated with abuse (e.g., chronic pain), mental health

problems consistent with abuse, or factors known to increase vulnerability (e.g., disabilities, economic dependence, isolation)

- Assessing and intervening collaboratively

Listening

Because women report that they feel judged and disbelieved by health care providers, it is vital to begin by examining your own knowledge and beliefs about IPV. If a health care provider thinks that women should "just leave" their partners or that they are responsible for the abuse they experience, these ideas will be conveyed to patients and discourage them from seeking further help or from disclosure.

Listening nonjudgementally requires health care providers to evaluate social judgements that are commonly made about women who are abused and to acquire sufficient knowledge to counter those negative judgements. You might ask yourself the following questions:

- What do I know about IPV? Whom do I hold responsible for IPV? What do I think are the causes of IPV?
- What are my own personal experiences of violence, and how do they shape my understanding?
- What groups do I view as most vulnerable to IPV?
- How might my beliefs about IPV be conveyed to patients in ways that are judgemental or affirming?

Your practice environment also shapes your ability to listen effectively to and assess your patients. Hollingsworth and Ford-Gilboe (2006) studied emergency nurses in Ontario and found that those who believed that it was futile to assess and respond to women who have experienced abuse were less likely to engage in appropriate clinical practices, whereas those who had more positive beliefs about the benefits of assessing and responding to abuse were more likely to engage in appropriate clinical practices. In contrast to literature portraying health providers as unsympathetic and uninterested in providing care to women who have experienced abuse, Hollingsworth and Ford-Gilboe found that the nurses had relatively high levels of positive expectations regarding outcomes. Because *any* of your patients may have a history of abuse, it is critical to listen to *all* patients with that in mind and be confident that you can make a positive difference in their lives. This means using professional interpreters routinely with all patients who speak a different language from you. Questions to ask yourself about your work environment include the following:

- How is "listening" to patients valued (by colleagues, managers, work expectations)? How much time is available for listening?
- How much privacy is afforded when patients are assessed?
- What is the workplace cultural norm with regard to attitudes toward patients in general (whether you are encouraged to view yourself as the expert), toward women, and toward people who experience violence?
- How do these factors shape your practice? How might you optimize the environment?

Your listening in a nonjudgemental manner can be very reassuring for someone who previously may have encountered disbelief, blame, or judgement from friends or health care providers (Lempert, 1997; Tower, 2007) and will contribute to building trust so that the person may feel confident enough to disclose abuse. Both women who have experienced abuse and health care providers with experience responding to abuse assert that validation of the woman's worth as a human being and of abuse as undeserved are the most important aspects of an effective response and the foundation for a trusting relationship (Gerbert et al., 1999, 2000). Expressing interest in the conditions of people's lives beyond the immediate presenting health problem can be a way of conveying openness. For example, with any patient, simple questions such as "How are your work and your home life affecting your health?" can convey interest and acceptance. Furthermore, if a person "hints" at or discloses abuse, conveying belief in the person's narrative by continuing to be nonjudgemental can also be empowering. Sometimes women who are experiencing IPV offer explanations for illnesses or injuries that downplay, overlook, or deny abuse—perhaps because of shame, fear of judgement, or fear of the consequences of disclosure, or because it has not occurred to the woman that her health problems are connected to abuse. Openly indicating a possible connection to abuse—if done in a nonjudgemental, validating manner—can invite a direct conversation about IPV.

Anticipating Abuse

According to the available statistics, up to half your female patients will have experienced at least one incident of physical or sexual assault in their lifetime. Because statistics suggest that about 7% of Canadian women currently in relationships have experienced violence in the past 5 years, violence is a relevant issue to many. Some patients, however, are more vulnerable to abuse: those who are isolated, economically dependent on others (e.g., immigrants sponsored as spouses), or dependent on others for care (e.g., those with disabilities). Furthermore, as noted previously, IPV is often associated with specific injuries, such as fractures, bruises, and sprains; with many chronic health challenges; and with many mental health issues. Thinking about IPV as a possible contributing factor is important in relation to diverse health issues ranging from substance abuse to vaginal bleeding to migraines. In view of the high association of chronic pain with histories of abuse (Campbell, 2002; Kendall-Tackett et al., 2003; Walsh, Jamieson, MacMillan, & Boyle, 2007), you should have a high index of suspicion for abuse of any person experiencing chronic pain or substance use, and you should identify the factors related to abuse that are most relevant in your specific clinical area.

Assessing Collaboratively

Because research has repeatedly shown that women feel disempowered by health care providers, which echoes their experiences of abuse, it is crucial to foster women's sense of control in decision making (Ford-Gilboe, Wuest, & Merritt-Gray, 2005; Wuest, Merritt-Gray, & Berman, 2003), which includes helping them identify the risks and benefits of seeking help (Ford-Gilboe, Wuest, Varcoe, & Merritt-Gray, 2006). When beginning most assessments, you do not know patients' abuse histories. On the basis of the relational approach introduced in Chapters 1 and 3 (Doane & Varcoe, 2005), a collaborative approach to assessment involves several elements:

- Following the lead of the patient: conveying a willingness to listen and trustworthiness, allowing the patient to take the lead in disclosing (or not), and drawing on the patient's knowledge to assess the levels of danger and options
- Listening to and for cues that might suggest abuse
- Self-observation: paying attention to how your assumptions and biases may shape your interactions and how you are reacting
- Pattern recognition: attending to patterns of physical symptoms (e.g., injuries, chronic pain) and health problems (e.g., substance abuse, sleep problems)
- Collaboratively developing knowledge: for example, helping an individual recognize the connection between health problems and abuse, and helping the patient evaluate levels of danger
- Naming and supporting capacity: focusing on strengths and capacities; for example, you might say, "It sounds as though you have been through a lot—you are doing a great job of …"

Assessment for abuse is much broader than screening. However, it may be useful to adapt questions designed for screening purposes in your assessments in order to follow the lead of the patient; you may suggest that his or her intimate relationships may be negatively affecting health, or you may ask about health problems or circumstances that warrant a high index of suspicion for abuse. For example, an 80-year-old woman presenting with tachycardia replied to the nurse's observation that her relationship did not seem to be helping her health, with the disclosure that "this [tachycardia] happens every time he gets like that." The nurse was able to clarify the woman's meaning: that the woman's husband battered her frequently.

Inquiring about a person's relationships and their effect on health should be included in the assessment of any person (e.g., "How do the people in your life affect your health?") because the answers provide important information beyond what might be classified as violence or abuse.

Even when a person describes abuse, he or she may downplay it, saying it is "only emotional" or "not that bad" or "we just fight a lot." More abuse may be revealed as you listen. The downplaying is not "denial" but rather the normal minimization that often accompanies trauma from violence. It is important to reinforce that emotional abuse is of concern: for example, you can say, "The stress associated with being treated that way can be just as bad for your physical and mental health as if someone were hitting you."

It is appropriate for you to show that you are concerned and even distressed about the degree of violence. One message that needs to be conveyed during the assessment is that the abuse is not the patient's fault; you can state this several times. Another important message is that you are concerned and that help is available: "I am really concerned about your health and the danger you are in, and I would like to help you make a plan for you to be as safe as possible." Still another is

that several health problems can occur because of violence: "I am really worried about the amount of pain you are having and the stress you are under. This is very damaging to your health … . [add specifics particular to the patient]." In fact, in a survey of 265 abused women who accepted a referral to a social worker, 59% said they accepted the referral because the medical provider expressed concern that their presenting health problem was related to IPV (McCaw, Berman, Syme, & Hunkeler, 2002).

Specific clinical contexts have assessment approaches that integrate attention to violence. For example, in the perinatal context, in contrast to the usual assumption that pregnancy is a positive event, it is important to be amenable to the possibility that being in an abusive relationship may be a challenge for a pregnant woman.

Humphreys and Campbell (2010) proposed that when abuse of a woman is suspected or confirmed, the following clinical responses are appropriate:

- Assessing the woman's level of risk and developing a safety plan
- Conducting a thorough health assessment
- Identifying personal strengths and support systems
- Identifying appropriate goals with the woman in collaboration with other health care providers

Assessment related to sexual assault should be based on the same principles as assessment for IPV. The emotional, cultural, and physical safety of the patient should come first, and a validating, nonjudgemental response is essential. It is important that the patient remain in control of care as much as possible, including the decision to call the police and to have forensic evidence collected. Sexual assault victims may be male or female, and assault may occur within the context of an intimate relationship (e.g., a spousal or dating relationship) or in a nonintimate relationship (with a client of a sex worker, or with others such as coworkers, employers, and health care providers). Assault by unknown assailants is much less common. McConkey, Sole, and Holcomb (2001) noted that a survivor may seek treatment immediately, within days, or weeks after the assault. Survivors may go to a primary care setting to receive treatment for prevention of pregnancy or STIs.

Many survivors are embarrassed and fear being dismissed as undeserving of care, especially those who are victims of date rape, those who use alcohol or drugs, and those for whom the assault is associated with sex work. In cases in which the assailant is known, the survivor may be fearful of repercussions from seeking treatment (McConkey et al., 2001).

HEALTH CARE PROVIDERS' RESPONSES TO ELDER AND VULNERABLE PERSON ABUSE AND NEGLECT

Assessing possible elder abuse and neglect can be more complicated than assessments for other forms of IPV if an older person presents for health care with multiple health, physical, and cognitive challenges. Although some older women have been in abusive relationships for decades, others are experiencing for the first time physical and sexual violence from previously nonabusive partners who themselves may be afflicted with behaviour-altering neurological illnesses (Alzheimer's disease, organic brain syndromes). An older woman in a long-term abusive relationship may be trying to outlive the abuser, whereas the newly abused older woman may be reluctant to disclose abuse because of embarrassment, shame, and fears that her partner will be institutionalized. Older men and women may be more vulnerable financially, dependent on other people for care, and fearful of retribution. Physical findings that are inconsistent with the history provided by the patient, family member, or caregiver are significant clues to possible abuse and neglect. The Ontario Network for the Prevention of Elder Abuse (ONPEA) outlines indicators for recognizing older adult abuse (see the section Web Sites of Interest at the end of this chapter), and the Canadian Medical Association suggests eight screening questions that can be used to help identify potential abuse (see Box 31-3).

Mandatory Reporting of Abuse of Older or Vulnerable Persons

In some provinces, such as Nova Scotia and Newfoundland, adult protection legislation includes general mandatory reporting requirements that cover different forms of abuse. The effectiveness of such laws is controversial. The Canadian Network for the Prevention of Elder Abuse has a good summary of the arguments for and against mandatory reporting (see the section Web Sites of Interest at the end of this chapter). You should be familiar with your legal obligations. The Canadian Centre for Elder Law updated its guide to elder abuse law and neglect in 2011, including a summary of the laws in each province and territory (see the section Web Sites of Interest at the end of this chapter). As with other obligations, however, legal obligations are the minimum standard. Health care providers have an ethical obligation to provide a meaningful, health-promoting response whenever abuse is suspected.

HEALTH CARE PROVIDERS' RESPONSES TO CHILD ABUSE

In Canada, screening for child abuse is not recommended. Because of the high rate of false-positive results of screening tests and the potential for incorrectly labelling individuals as child abusers, the possible harm associated with screening outweighs the benefits (MacMillan, 2000). Although screening is not recommended, reporting suspected child abuse is mandatory in most provinces and territories, which means that the identification of child abuse relies on careful assessment by health care providers.

It is important that approaches to child abuse be similar to those recommended for IPV but modified (a) to take into account that children are even more vulnerable to family members and (b) to accommodate the developmental stage of each child. Keep in mind the following information:

- Race and class stereotypes are widely perpetuated and must be actively countered so that they do not inappropriately influence your assessment. Any child may be at risk of some form of abuse, regardless of the ethnicity or income of the family; conversely, no ethnic group is at "greater risk" of perpetrating child abuse.
- Neglect and emotional abuse are the most common forms of abuse and are harmful; thus if you rely only on obvious indicators of physical abuse or look only for cues of sexual abuse, you may overlook significant damage.
- Parents are not the only possible perpetrators of child abuse.
- Many allegations of suspected child abuse are unsubstantiated.
- Although some situations warrant removal of children from their parents, this step also is stressful for children, and in most cases the children remain in contact with their parents for life.
- Assessments for child abuse are evaluations of parenting and often focus uncritically on evaluating mothers against culturally specific dominant stereotypes of mothering even when the mother is not the perpetrator (Einboden, Rudge, & Varcoe, 2011; Tanner & Turney, 2000).
- Ethically, as a health care provider, you are obligated to provide "good" care to all, including a child's parents.
- Although you must intervene and report suspected child abuse, your role as a health care provider is not to "rescue" the child at the expense of your relationship with the parents or of the relationship between the child and the parents.

Again, your assumptions and beliefs will be conveyed to children and parents. It is crucial to reflect on your own ideas and experiences so that you can work toward the short- and long-term well-being of all parties. Assessment and intervention for suspected child abuse are possible without alienation of the parents, regardless of whether the parents are suspected of perpetrating the abuse.

Assessing for Child Abuse

Assessing for child abuse means integrating awareness of the possibility of child abuse into every assessment. It is important to be alert for signs of physical abuse and intentional injury. However, it is crucial to carefully evaluate any physical injury within the context of a child's age and developmental stage. Is the injury that is being reported in line with the child's developmental level? For example, the explanation that a 3-week-old child was injured rolling off a bed is not developmentally plausible. Because the nurse may not be able to directly observe the child's motor and cognitive milestones while documenting the history, it is important to ask the caregivers directly whether the child is crawling, pulling up to stand, or walking and what other developmental issues are currently being faced at home (e.g., tantrums, toilet training). It is also important to be aware of the possible indicators of neglect and emotional and sexual abuse because determining these is much more challenging. Tanner and Turney (2000) recommended repeated observations of parenting and

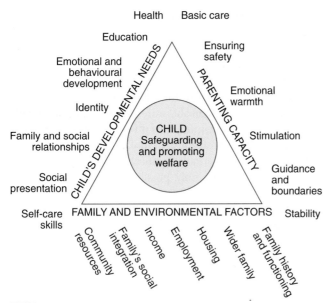

8-3 Framework for the Assessment of Children in Need and Their Families in Cases of Child Neglect.

critical reflection on the part of health care providers to account for biases that arise from stereotypical and dominant assumptions in the providers' own cultural context. Horwath (2002) described the Framework for the Assessment of Children in Need and Their Families in Cases of Child Neglect, which can help health care providers focus on broader issues rather than on dramatic situations of severe physical abuse. The framework features an assessment triangle with three interrelated systems or domains: the child's developmental needs, parenting capacity, and family and environmental factors (Figure 8-3). The framework attends to the complexity of responding to child neglect, but Horwath cautioned that the tensions among these domains must be taken into account to avoid losing focus on the child in question.

Responses to known child abuse are much more comprehensive than the well-publicized interventions of placing children in out-of-home care. There has been some evidence of the successful support of parents. For example, three randomized controlled trials have shown a reduction in the incidence of child abuse or outcomes related to physical abuse and neglect among first-time disadvantaged mothers and their infants who received a program of home visitation by nurses from the perinatal period through the children's infancy (Gonzalez, & MacMillan, 2008; MacMillan, 2000; Olds et al., 2010).

Mandatory Reporting of Child Abuse

In Canada, provincial and territorial jurisdictions have the legislative responsibility for child and family services (child welfare). One exception is the federal responsibility for Aboriginal peoples with status under the *Indian Act* (Canada). Each province and territory has specific legislation providing protection for neglected and abused children. Most provinces and territories have legislation that makes it mandatory for

the public, including health care providers, to report child abuse. If you are working with children, you should review the specific requirements for the jurisdiction in which you are working. The Canadian Child Welfare Research Portal has a comprehensive description of policies across Canada, research reports, and contact information for each province and territory (see the section Web Sites of Interest at the end of this chapter). If you suspect that a child is being maltreated, you should involve other members of the health care team. Most health care settings have access to social workers who are specifically trained in dealing with child abuse. They are often the first point of contact for reporting suspected abuse.

HISTORY

It is important also to assess and document prior abuse, including prior IPV, childhood physical and sexual abuse, and prior rapes of all kinds (stranger, acquaintance, date, intimate partner). Cumulative abuse has been shown to be associated with more severe mental and physical health problems (Elliott, Alexander, Pierce, Aspelmeier, & Richmond, 2009; Gustafsson, Nilsson, & Svedin, 2009). Also, determine the history of traumatic injuries because these may have an effect on the current health condition. For instance, a woman may have experienced prior episodes of head trauma and strangulation, both of which may be related to chronic but subtle neurological symptoms and problems. A mental status examination is also important, both for potential head trauma and neurological symptoms and for mental health problems. Pay particular attention to the most frequent mental health problems associated with violence: depression, suicidal thoughts and attempts, PTSD, substance abuse, and anxiety. Chapters 6 and 7, on mental health and substance use, respectively, give direction for conducting this part of the history.

If child abuse is suspected and if the child is verbal, a history should be obtained from the child separately from the caregivers through open-ended questions or spontaneous statements. It is important to remember that children may have suffered significant trauma but may respond only minimally to open-ended questions (Myers et al., 2002). Keeping the questions short and using age-appropriate language and familiar words can help to enrich the documentation of the history. Children older than 11 years can generally be expected to provide a history at the level of most adults (Myers et al., 2002).

The medical history is also an important part of your evaluation. Has the child had previous hospitalizations or injuries, or does he or she suffer from any chronic medical conditions? Does the child take any medication that may cause easy bruising? Does the child have a history of repeated visits to the hospital? Was there a delay in seeking care for anything other than a minor injury?

PHYSICAL EXAMINATION

Important components of the physical examination of a patient known to have survived IPV or elder abuse include a complete head-to-toe visual examination, especially if the patient is receiving health care services secondary to reported abuse. When the examination reveals physical findings, accurate use of medical terminology to describe injuries is essential. In Canada, it is controversial whether forensic evidence is supportive of women who experience IPV; for example, a study in British Columbia revealed that health records were inaccurate reflections of the woman's experience and were most often used to undermine the woman and her legal claims (Cory, Ruebsaat, & Hankivsky, 2003). However, there is some evidence that forensic examinations do lead to a higher probability of charges and conviction rates in sexual assault cases (Du Mont, McGregor, Myhr, & Miller, 2000; McGregor, Du Mont, & Myhr, 2002).

There is no scientific evidence of the accuracy of dating injuries on the basis of the colour of contusions (Langlois & Greshman, 2001). However, a new bruise is usually red and often turns purple or purple-blue 12 to 36 hours after blunt-force trauma. The colour of bruises (and ecchymoses) generally progresses from purple-blue to bluish green to greenish brown to brownish yellow before the bruise fades away.

Physical assessment after sexual assault can also include the collection of forensic evidence: that is, evidence that can be admitted in court. Such collection usually requires the expert skills of a nurse examiner or physician specially trained in evaluating sexual assault. The details of collection of such evidence are beyond the scope of this chapter, but you should be familiar with the protocols and resources available in your area.

Bruising is an important sign of elder abuse. There are multiple factors that can contribute to bruising more readily or more severely in older adults than in younger people. Medications and abnormal blood values related to their side effects, as well as underlying hematological disorders, can affect ease of bruising or the formation of ecchymoses. Common medications that increase risk for bruising or bleeding complications include but are not limited to aspirin, ibuprofen, any of the nonsteroidal anti-inflammatory drugs, warfarin, heparin, valproic acid, prednisone, and clopidogrel. Mosqueda, Burnight, and Liao (2005) studied older adults who had accidental bruises and found that nearly 90% of their bruises were on their extremities, and no accidental bruises were found on the neck, ears, genitalia, buttocks, or soles of the feet; hence, injuries in the latter area are suspect for abuse.

Any health evaluation for known or suspected elder abuse and neglect should include baseline laboratory tests, including, at a minimum, a complete blood cell count with platelet measurement, basic blood chemistry profiles (including blood urea nitrogen, creatinine, protein, and albumin measurements), serum liver function tests, a coagulation panel, and a urinalysis (Geroff & Olshaker, 2001). For more information on elder abuse, see Chapter 31.

Physical Examination of Children

A visual inspection from head to toe is important in any physical examination of a child. Significant injuries can be hidden under clothing, diapers, socks, and long hair. The American Academy of Pediatrics (2002) defined significant trauma as any injury more severe than temporary redness of the skin. Accidental bruising in healthy, active children is common, but the presence of bruises in babies has significance in evaluating for abuse. Children who are walking with support but not yet independently—"cruising"—typically should not have bruises (Sugar, Taylor, & Feldman, 1999). Bruising in infants who are not yet cruising, usually infants younger than 9 months, should alert you to possible abusive mechanisms underlying the injury or an underlying medical illness.

Once children begin to walk, bruising, particularly on the bony prominences, is common (Sugar et al., 1999). Reece and Ludwig (2001) found that in children who were walking, 40% to 50% had bruises over the bony prominences of the front of their bodies. Sugar and colleagues (1999) found that bruising in "atypical" places such as the buttocks, hands, feet, and abdomen was exceedingly rare and should arouse concerns. Furthermore, any bruise that takes the shape of an object should be considered highly specific for abuse. Bruising found in nonmobile children should raise concerns about other injuries, including fractures and intracranial injury (Barber & Sibert, 2000).

The Canadian Paediatric Society (2007) provided comprehensive guidelines to health care providers regarding abusive head trauma, including what was previously known as "shaken baby syndrome." The guidelines advises that abusive head trauma always be considered in infants without a definite diagnosis. Symptoms can include lethargy, decreased feeding, irritability, vomiting, respiratory distress, apnea, seizures, and an altered level of consciousness. The guidelines stress that the accompanying caregiver may not know the cause of the child's symptoms or may not give a complete and accurate history. The guidelines state that a full assessment for suspected abusive head trauma should be considered in infants and young children with any of the following signs:

- An acute or chronic injury that has inadequate, inconsistent, evolving, or no explanation
- A severe head injury alleged to be the result of a short fall or minor trauma
- An unexplained symptomatic head injury in a child who was well when last seen
- Subdural hemorrhage, retinal hemorrhage, or rib, skull, or metaphyseal fractures

DOCUMENTATION

Documentation of IPV and elder abuse must include objective progress notes, written in unbiased language. Injury maps and photographic documentation may be useful. Examples of photographic documentation of patients are included in this chapter (Figures 8-4 through 8-6*).

Histories of IPV and elder abuse need to be recorded directly from the patients within reason. It is clinically unrealistic to document verbatim every statement made by a

---

*Many of these photos were first published by Sheridan (2001). Reprinted here with the author's permission.

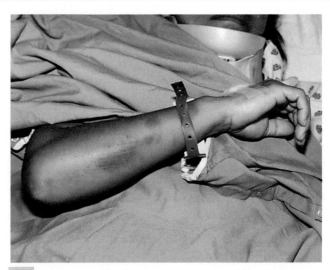

8-4 Patterned, fingernail-like scratch abrasions to the left lateral aspect of the neck caused by manual strangulation.

8-5 Patterned, defensive posture–like bruises to the right forearm.

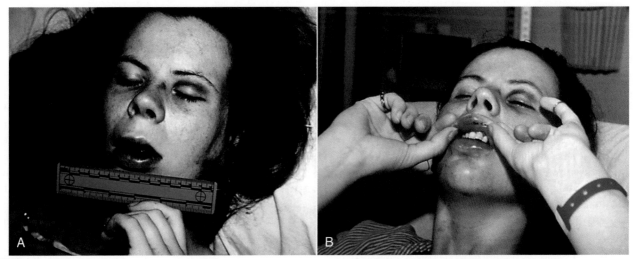

8-6 Examples of how photographs can be used to demonstrate mechanisms of injuries. **A,** Victim has obvious facial trauma to her left eyelid, left lateral aspect of the nose, and mouth. The nose contusion was caused when the nose piece of her glasses was forcefully pushed into her skin from a punch to the left eye. The patient's glasses absorbed much of the punch force and were broken (not shown). A second punch produced the mouth trauma. **B,** The force of the mouth punch caused the upper teeth to leave a patterned contusion, abrasion, and minor laceration to the oral mucosa of the upper lip.

patient. However, it is critical to document exceptionally poignant statements made by the victim that identify the reported perpetrator and severe threats of harm made by the reported perpetrator. Other aspects of the abuse history, including reports of past abusive incidents, can be paraphrased with the use of partial direct quotations.

When quoting or paraphrasing the history, you should not sanitize words reportedly heard by the victim. Verbatim documentation of the reported perpetrator's threats interlaced with curses and expletives may be useful in future court proceedings. Also, be careful to use the exact terms an abused patient may use to describe sexual organs or sexually assaultive behaviours.

Photographic documentation in the medical record can be invaluable. Prior written consent to take photographs should be obtained from all cognitively intact, competent adults. Most health care facilities have standardized consent-to-photograph forms. If a patient is unconscious or cognitively impaired, taking photographs without consent is generally viewed as ethically sound, inasmuch as it is a noninvasive, painless intervention that may help a suspected abuse victim.

When documenting the history and physical findings of child abuse and neglect, use the words of the child to describe how his or her injury occurred. Remember the possibility that the abuser may be accompanying the child. If the child is nonverbal, use statements from caregivers. It is important to know your employer's or institution's protocol for obtaining history in cases of suspected child maltreatment. Some protocols may delay a full interview until it can be conducted by a forensically trained interviewer.

ASSESSING FOR RISK OF HOMICIDE

Women in both the United States and Canada have been killed more often by a husband, a boyfriend, or an ex-husband than by anyone else, and about 75% of these women had been abused by the man who subsequently killed them (Campbell et al., 2001; Statistics Canada, 2005). Since 1980, the rate of spousal homicides of women in Canada has consistently been about three to four times higher than that of men (Statistics Canada, 2011). In a study of intimate partner homicide of women in the United States, 42% of the women killed had been seen by someone in the health care system (the emergency department in the majority of cases, but also in primary care, prenatal care, and other settings) for some health issue

in the year before their murder (Sharps, Koziol-McLain, McFarlane, Sachs, & Xu, 2001). These encounters were missed opportunities for health care providers to identify IPV and intervene to decrease the danger.

The same study demonstrated reliability and validity support for the Danger Assessment, a 19-item "yes"/"no" instrument that has been used extensively by nurses in the health care system, as well as by advocates in other settings involving battered women (Campbell et al., 2002; Figure 8-7). The instrument starts with a calendar so that women can more accurately see for themselves how frequent and severe the violence has become over the past year. This is also an excellent tool for the health care provider to assess frequency and severity. Although there are no predetermined

---

DANGER ASSESSMENT
Jacquelyn C. Campbell, Ph.D., R.N.
Copyright 1985, 1988, 2001

Several risk factors have been associated with homicides (murders) of both batterers and battered women in research conducted after the murders have taken place. We cannot predict what will happen in your case, but we would like you to be aware of the danger of homicide in situations of severe battering and for you to see how many of the risk factors apply to your situation.

Using the calendar, please mark the approximate dates during the past year when you were beaten by your husband or partner. Write on that date how bad the incident was according to the following scale:

1. Slapping, pushing; no injuries and/or lasting pain
2. Punching, kicking; bruises, cuts, and/or continuing pain
3. "Beating up"; severe contusions, burns, broken bones
4. Threat to use weapon; head injury, internal injury, permanent injury
5. Use of weapon; wounds from weapon

(If **any** of the descriptions for the higher number apply, use the higher number.)

Mark **Yes** or **No** for each of the following. ("He" refers to your husband, partner, ex-husband, ex-partner, or whoever is currently physically hurting you.)

_____   1. Has the physical violence increased in severity or frequency over the past year?
_____   2. Has he ever used a weapon against you or threatened you with a weapon?
_____   3. Does he ever try to choke you?
_____   4. Does he own a gun?
_____   5. Has he ever forced you to have sex when you did not wish to do so?
_____   6. Does he use drugs? By drugs, I mean "uppers" or amphetamines, speed, angel dust, cocaine, "crack," street drugs or mixtures.
_____   7. Does he threaten to kill you and/or do you believe he is capable of killing you?
_____   8. Is he drunk every day or almost every day? (In terms of quantity of alcohol.)
_____   9. Does he control most or all of your daily activities? For instance: does he tell you who you can be friends with, when you can see your family, how much money you can use, or when you can take the car? (If he tries, but you do not let him, check here: _____)
_____ 10. Have you ever been beaten by him while you were pregnant? (If you have never been pregnant by him, check here: _____)
_____ 11. Is he violently and constantly jealous of you? (For instance, does he say "If I can't have you, no one can"?)
_____ 12. Have you ever threatened or tried to commit suicide?
_____ 13. Has he ever threatened or tried to commit suicide?
_____ 14. Does he threaten to harm your children?
_____ 15. Do you have a child that is not his?
_____ 16. Is he unemployed?
_____ 17. Have you ever left him during the past year? (If you have *never* lived with him, check here: _____)
_____ 18. Do you currently have another (different) intimate partner?
_____ 19. Does he follow or spy on you, leave threatening notes, destroy your property, or call you when you don't want him to?

_____   Total "Yes" Answers

Thank you. Please talk to your nurse, advocate, or counsellor about what the Danger Assessment means in terms of your situation.

8-7 Danger Assessment form.

cutoff scores on the Danger Assessment, the more "yes" answers there are, the more serious is the danger of the woman's situation. In the previously described multicity study (Sharps et al., 2001), abused women who were victims of homicide had an average score of 7.1 on the original 15-item Danger Assessment. The Danger Assessment is copyrighted; therefore, it must be used intact, and users are asked to communicate with Dr. Campbell (Campbell et al., 2002) if they are planning to use it for research purposes. It can also be downloaded from the Internet once you have registered (see the section Web Sites of Interest at the end of this chapter).

CULTURAL AND SOCIAL CONSIDERATIONS

Violence is a widespread sociocultural problem, but in Western societies, there is a tendency to treat interpersonal violence as a problem of individuals. Rather than social prevention and intervention, efforts to deal with violence are targeted toward individuals rather than toward the social context, often leaving victims responsible for dealing with violence. Furthermore, despite the fact that violence is well known to occur across all societies and cultural groups, there is a tendency to associate violence with particular groups. To effectively deal with violence, health care providers must take three steps. First, as argued in earlier chapters, health care providers must evaluate how their own cultural values and beliefs, as well as the dominant values operating in health care, affect the care they provide. Second, health care providers need to consider their own stereotypes and assumptions regarding IPV, sexual assault, child abuse and neglect, and elder abuse and neglect, and they must replace those stereotypes and assumptions with knowledge regarding all forms of violence. Third, health care providers need to take into account how ideas about certain groups of people (e.g., stereotypes about some groups as being more violent or more likely to be abusive toward children) support discrimination in the provision of health care and deter people from seeking health care.

Rather than assessing how experiences of violence are shaped by culture, narrowly defined as ethnicity, it is important to assess how they are shaped by culture in the broader sense. For example, rather than focusing on particular ethnocultural groups, it is more useful to consider how racialization, gender discrimination, experiences of immigration, other discrimination, language barriers, and inequitable access to employment and resources shape experiences of violence and access to social support in response to violence (Hyman, Forte, Du Mont, Romans, & Cohen, 2006; Jiwani, 2000; Varcoe, 2008).

REFERENCES

American Academy of Pediatrics Committee on Child Abuse and Neglect. (2002). When inflicted skin injuries constitute child abuse. *Pediatrics, 110*(3), 644–645.

Bacchus, L., Mezey, G., & Bewley, S. (2003). Experiences of seeking help from health professionals in a sample of women who experienced domestic violence. *Health and Social Care in the Community, 11*(1), 10–18.

Bachman, R., & Saltzman, L. E. (1995). *Violence against women: Estimates from the redesigned survey.* Washington, DC: Bureau of Justice Statistics, National Institute of Justice.

Barber, M. A., & Sibert, J. R. (2000). Diagnosing physical child abuse: The way forward. *Post-Graduate Medical Journal, 76,* 743–749.

Beaulaurier, R., Seff, L., Newman, F., & Dunlop, B. (2007). External barriers to help seeking for older women who experience intimate partner violence. *Journal of Family Violence, 22,* 747–755.

Bhandari, M., Dosanjh, S., Tornetta, P., III, & Matthews, D. (2006). Musculoskeletal manifestations of physical abuse after intimate partner violence. *Journal of Trauma, 61,* 1473–1479.

Blackstock, C., Trocmé, N., & Bennett, M. (2004). Child maltreatment investigations among Aboriginal and non-Aboriginal families in Canada. *Violence Against Women, 10,* 901–916.

Bogat, G. A., DeJonghe, E., Levendosky, A. A., Davidson, W. S., & von Eye, A. (2006). Trauma symptoms among infants exposed to intimate partner violence. *Child Abuse and Neglect, 30*(2), 109–125.

Campbell, J., Jones, A. S., Dienemann, J., Kub, J., Schollenberger, J., O'Campo, P., ... Wynne, C. (2002). Intimate partner violence and physical health consequences. *Archives of Internal Medicine, 162,* 1157–1163.

Campbell, J., & Soeken, K. (1999). Forced sex and intimate partner violence: Effects on women's health. *Violence Against Women, 5,* 1017–1035.

Campbell, J. C. (2002). Health consequences of intimate partner violence. *Lancet, 359*(9314), 1331–1336.

Campbell, J. C., & Lewandowski, L. (1997). Mental and psychical health effects of intimate partner violence on women and children. *Psychiatric Clinics of North America, 20,* 353–374.

Campbell, J. C., Sharps, P., & Glass, N. E. (2001). Risk assessment for intimate partner homicide. In G. F. Pinard & L. Pagani (Eds.), *Clinical assessment of dangerousness: Empirical contributions* (pp. 136–157). New York: Cambridge University Press. doi: 10.1017/CBO9780511500015.009

Canadian Centre for Justice Statistics. (2002). *Family violence in Canada: A statistical profile.* Ottawa: Statistics Canada.

Canadian Paediatric Society. (2007). *Multidisciplinary guidelines on the identification, investigation and management of suspected abusive head trauma.* Retrieved from *http://www.cps.ca/documents/AHT.pdf.*

Carbone-López, K., Kruttschnitt, C., & MacMillan, R. (2006). Patterns of intimate partner violence and their associations with physical health, psychological distress, and substance use. *Public Health Reports, 121*(4), 382–392.

Carlson, B. (2000). Children exposed to intimate partner violence: Research findings and implications for intervention. *Trauma, Violence, and Abuse, 1,* 321–342.

Carlson, B. (2005). The most important things learned about violence and trauma in the past 20 years. *Journal of Interpersonal Violence, 20,* 119–126.

Cherniak, D., Grant, L., Mason, R., Moore, B., & Pellizzari, R. (2005). Intimate partner violence consensus statement. *Journal of Obstetrics and Gynaecology Canada, 157,* 365–388.

Clark, J. P., & Du Mont, J. (2003). Intimate partner violence and health: A critique of Canadian prevalence studies. *Revue canadienne de santé publique, 94*(1), 52–58.

Coker, A. L. (2006). Preventing intimate partner violence: How we will rise to this challenge. *American Journal of Preventive Medicine, 30*(6), 528–529.

Coker, A. L., Fadden, M. K., Reeder, C. E., & Smith, P. H. (2004). Physical partner violence and medicaid utilization and expenditures. *Public Health Reports, 119*, 557–567.

Coker, A. L., Smith, P. H., McKeown, R. E., & King, M. J. (2000). Frequency and correlates of intimate partner violence by type: Physical, sexual, and psychological battering. *American Journal of Public Health, 90*, 553–559.

Cory, J., & Dechief, L. (2007). *SHE framework: Safety and health enhancement for women experiencing abuse.* Retrieved from *http://www.bcwomens.ca/Services/HealthServices/WomanAbuseResponse/Resources.htm*.

Cory, J., Ruebsaat, G., & Hankivsky, O. (2003). *Reasonable doubt: The use of health records in criminal and civil cases of violence against women in relationships.* Retrieved from *http://www.bccewh.bc.ca/publications-resources/documents/reasonabledoubt.pdf*.

Covington, S. S. (2008). Women and addiction: A trauma-informed approach. *Journal of Psychoactive Drugs* (Suppl 5), 377–385.

Department of Justice Canada. (1985). *Criminal Code*, R.S.C. 1985, c. C-46 (Canada), s. 150.1.

Department of Justice Canada. (2007). *Elder abuse fact sheet.* Retrieved from *http://www.justice.gc.ca/en/ps/fm/adultsfs.html#head1*.

Department of Justice Canada. (2012). Child abuse is wrong: What can I do? *http://www.justice.gc.ca/eng/pi/fv-vf/pub/caw-mei/toc-tdm.html*

Doane, G., & Varcoe, C. (2005). *Family nursing as relational inquiry: Developing health-promoting practice.* Philadelphia: Lippincott Williams & Wilkins.

Du Mont, J., Forte, T., Cohen, M. M., Hyman, I., & Romans, S. (2005). Changing help-seeking rates for intimate partner violence in Canada. *Women and Health, 41*(1), 1–19.

Du Mont, J., McGregor, M. J., Myhr, T. L., & Miller, K.-L. (2000). Predicting legal outcomes from medicolegal findings: An examination of sexual assault in two jurisdictions. *Journal of Women's Health and Law, 1*, 219–233.

Edleson, J. L. (1999). The overlap between child maltreatment and woman battering. *Violence Against Women, 5*, 134–154.

Einboden, R., Rudge, T., & Varcoe, C. (2011). Battling the passions: The birth of a conceptual understanding of suspicion for child abuse and neglect. *Aporia—La revue infirmière/The Nursing Journal, 3*(2), 5–14.

Elliott, A. N., Alexander, A. A., Pierce, T. W., Aspelmeier, J. E., & Richmond, J. M. (2009). Childhood victimization, poly-victimization, and adjustment to college in women. *Child Maltreatment, 14*(4), 330–343.

Folsom, W. S., Christensen, M. L., Avery, L., & Moore, C. (2003). The co-occurrence of child abuse and domestic violence: An issue of service delivery for social service professionals. *Child and Adolescent Social Work Journal, 20*, 375–387.

Ford-Gilboe, M., Wuest, J., & Merritt-Gray, M. (2005). Strengthening capacity to limit intrusion: Theorizing family health promotion in the aftermath of woman abuse. *Qualitative Health Research, 15*, 477–501.

Ford-Gilboe, M., Wuest, J., Varcoe, C., & Merritt-Gray, M. (2006). Developing an evidence-based health advocacy intervention to support women who have left abusive partners. *Canadian Journal of Nursing Research, 38*(1), 147–167.

Fugate, M., Landis, L., Riordan, K., Naureckas, S., & Engel, B. (2005). Barriers to domestic violence help seeking: Implications for intervention. *Violence Against Women, 11*, 290–310.

Gerbert, B., Abercrombie, P., Caspers, N., Love, C., & Bronstone, A. (1999). How health care providers help battered women: The survivor's perspective. *Women and Health, 29*, 115–135.

Gerbert, B., Caspers, N., Bronstone, A., Moe, J., & Abercrombie, P. (1999). A qualitative analysis of how physicians with expertise in domestic violence approach the identification of victims. *Annals of Internal Medicine, 131*, 578–584.

Gerbert, B., Caspers, N., Milliken, N., Berlia, M., Bronstone, A., & Mof, J. (2000). Interventions that help victims of domestic violence. *Journal of Family Practice, 49*, 889.

Gerbert, B., Johnston, K., Caspers, N., Bleecker, T., Woods, A., & Rosenbaum, A. (1996). Experiences of battered women in health care settings: A qualitative study. *Women and Health, 24*, 1–17.

Geroff, A. J., & Olshaker, J. S. (2001). Elder abuse. In J. S. Olshaker, M. C. Jackson, & W. S. Smock (Eds.), *Forensic emergency medicine*. Philadelphia: Lippincott Williams & Wilkins.

Gilchrist, G., Hegarty, K., Chondros, P., Herrman, H., & Gunn, J. (2010). The association between intimate partner violence, alcohol and depression in family practice. *BMC Family Practice, 11*, 72–81.

Gonzalez, A., & MacMillan, H. L. (2008). Preventing child maltreatment: An evidence-based update. *Journal of Postgraduate Medicine, 54*(4), 280–286.

Gustafsson, P., Nilsson, D., & Svedin, C. (2009). Polytraumatization and psychological symptoms in children and adolescents. *European Child & Adolescent Psychiatry, 18*, 274–283.

Hagele, D. M. (2005). The impact of maltreatment on the developing child. *NC Medical Journal, 66*, 356–359.

Hill, T. D., Schroeder, R. D., Bradley, C., Kaplan, L. M., & Angel, R. J. (2009). The long-term health consequences of relationship violence in adulthood: An examination of low-income women from Boston, Chicago, and San Antonio. *American Journal of Public Health, 99*(9), 1645–1650.

Hollingsworth, E., & Ford-Gilboe, M. (2006). Registered nurses' self-efficacy for assessing and responding to woman abuse in emergency department settings. *Canadian Journal of Nursing Research, 38*(4), 54–77.

Hopper, E. K., Bassuk, E. L., & Oliver, J. (2010). Shelter from the storm: Trauma-informed care in homelessness services settings. *The Open Health Services and Policy Journal, 3*, 80–100.

Horwath, J. (2002). Maintaining a focus on the child? First impressions of the Framework for the Assessment of Children in Need and Their Families in Cases of Child Neglect. *Child Abuse Review, 11*(4), 195–213.

Humphreys, J., & Campbell, J. C. (2010). *Family violence in nursing practice.* New York: Lippincott Williams & Wilkins.

Hyman, I., Forte, T., Du Mont, J., Romans, S., & Cohen, M. (2006). The association between length of stay in Canada and intimate partner violence among immigrant women. *American Journal of Public Health, 96*, 654–659.

Janssen, P. A., Holt, V. L., Sugg, N. K., Emanuel, I., Critchlow, C. M., & Henderson, A. D. (2003). Intimate partner violence and adverse pregnancy outcomes: A population-based study. *American Journal of Obstetrics and Gynecology, 188*, 1341.

Jenny, C., Hymel, K. P., Ritzen, A., Reinert, S. E., & Hay, T. C. (1999). Analysis of missed cases of abusive head trauma. *Journal of the American Medical Association, 281*, 621–626.

Jiwani, Y. (2000). *Race, gender, violence and health care: Immigrant women of colour who have experienced violence and their encounters with the health care system.* Vancouver: Feminist Research, Education, Development and Action.

Johnson, H. (1996). *Dangerous domains: Violence against women in Canada.* Scarborough, ON: International Thompson Publishing.

Johnson, H. (2006). *Measuring violence against women: Statistical trends.* Ottawa: Statistics Canada.

Johnson, H., & Sacco, V. (1995). Researching violence against women: Statistics Canada's national survey. *Canadian Journal of Criminology, 7*(3), 281–304.

Jones, A. S., Gielen, A. C., Campbell, J. C., Schollenberger, J., Dienemann, J. A., Kub, J., ... Wynne, E. C. (1999). Annual and lifetime prevalence of partner abuse in a sample of female HMO enrollees. *Women's Health Issues, 9,* 295–305.

Kendall-Tackett, K. (2002). The health effects of childhood abuse: Four pathways by which abuse can influence health. *Child Abuse and Neglect, 26,* 715.

Kendall-Tackett, K., Marshall, R., & Ness, K. (2003). Chronic pain syndromes and violence against women. *Women and Therapy, 26,* 45–56.

Klevens, J., Kee, R., Trick, W., Garcia, D., Angulo, F. R., Jones, R., & Sadowski, L. S. (2012). Effect of screening for partner violence on women's quality of life. [Article]. *JAMA: Journal of the American Medical Association, 308*(7), 681–689.

Landenburger, K. (1998). Exploration of women's identity: Clinical approaches with abused women. In J. Campbell (Ed.), *Empowering survivors of abuse: Health care for battered women and their children.* Newbury Park, CA: Sage.

Langlois, N. E. I., & Greshman, G. A. (2001). The aging of bruises: A review and study of the colour changes with time. *Forensic Science International, 50,* 227–238.

Lempert, L. B. (1997). The other side of help: Negative effects in the help-seeking processes of abused women. *Qualitative Sociology, 20,* 289–309.

Leserman, J., & Drossman, D. A. (2007). Relationship of abuse history to functional gastrointestinal disorders and symptoms. *Trauma, Violence & Abuse, 8*(3), 331–343.

MacMillan, H. L. (2000). Preventive health care, 2000 update: Prevention of child maltreatment. *Canadian Medical Association Journal, 163,* 1451–1458.

MacMillan, H. L., & Wathen, C. N. (2003). Violence against women: Integrating the evidence into clinical practice. *Canadian Medical Association Journal, 169,* 570–571.

MacMillan, H. L., Wathen, C., Jamieson, E., Boyle, M., Shannon, H., Ford-Gilboe, M., ... McMaster Violence Against Women Research Group. (2009). Screening for intimate partner violence in health care settings: A randomized trial. *Journal of the American Medical Association, 302*(5), 493–501.

Maman, S., Campbell, J., Sweat, M., & Gielen, A. C. (2000). The intersection of HIV and violence: Directions for future research and interventions. *Social Science and Medicine, 4,* 459–478.

McCaw, B., Berman, W. H., Syme, S. L., & Hunkeler, E. F. (2002). Women referred for on-site domestic violence services in a managed care organization. *Women and Health, 35*(2/3), 23–40.

McCloskey, K., & Grigsby, N. (2005). The ubiquitous clinical problem of adult intimate partner violence: The need for routine assessment. *Professional Psychology: Research and Practice, 36,* 264–275.

McConkey, T. E., Sole, M. L., & Holcomb, L. (2001). Assessing the female sexual assault survivor. *Nurse Practitioner, 26*(7, Pt. 1), 28.

McDonald, L., Beaulieu, M., Harbison, J., Hirst, S., Lowenstein, A., Podnieks, E., & Wahl, J. (2012). Institutional abuse of older adults: What we know, what we need to know. *Journal of Elder Abuse & Neglect, 24*(2), 138–160. doi:10.1080/08946566.2011.646512

McDonald, L., & Collins, A. (2000). *Abuse and neglect of older adults: A discussion paper.* Ottawa: Health Canada.

McGregor, M. J., Du Mont, J., & Myhr, T. L. (2002). Sexual assault forensic medical examination: Is evidence related to successful prosecution? *Annals of Emergency Medicine, 39,* 639–647.

McLaughlin, K. A., Green, J. G., Gruber, M. J., Sampson, N. A., Zaslavsky, A. M., & Kessler, R. C. (2010). Childhood adversities and adult psychiatric disorders in the national comorbidity survey replication II: Associations with persistence of *DSM-IV* disorders. *Archives of General Psychiatry, 67*(2), 124–132.

McLean, C. (2001). Less sensational but more dangerous. *Report/Newsmagazine (National Edition), 28*(22), 44.

Mechanic, M., Weaver, T., & Resick, P. (2008). Mental health consequences of intimate partner abuse: A multidimensional assessment of four different forms of abuse. *Violence Against Women, 14,* 634–654.

Mosqueda, L., Burnight, K., & Liao, S. (2005). The life cycle of bruises in older adults. *Journal of the American Geriatrics Society, 53,* 1339–1343.

Muellman, R. L., Lenaghan, P. A., & Pakieser, R. A. (1996). Battered women: Injury locations and types. *Annals of Emergency Medicine, 28,* 468–492.

Murphy, C. C., Schei, B., Myhr, T. L., & Du Mont, J. (2001). Abuse: A risk factor for low birth weight? A systematic review and metaanalysis. *Canadian Medical Association Journal, 164,* 1567–1572.

Myers, J. E., Berliner, L., Briere, J., Hendrix, C. T., Jenny, C., & Reid, T. A. (2002). *The APSAC handbook on child maltreatment.* Thousand Oaks, CA: Sage.

Nelson, H. D., Nygren, P., McInerney, Y., & Klein, J. (2004). Screening women and elderly adults for family and intimate partner violence: A review of the evidence for the U.S. Preventive Services Task Force. *Annals of Internal Medicine, 140*(5), 387–404.

Olds, D. L., Kitzman, H. J., Cole, R. E., Hanks, C. A., Arcoleo, K. J., Anson, E. A., ... Stevenson, A. J. (2010). Enduring effects of prenatal and infancy home visiting by nurses on maternal life course and government spending: Follow-up of a randomized trial among children at age 12 years. *Archives of Pediatrics & Adolescent Medicine, 164*(5), 419–424.

Ozturk Ertem, I., Leventhal, J. M., & Dobbs, S. (2000). Intergenerational continuity of child physical abuse: How good is the evidence? *Lancet, 356*(9232), 814.

Perreault, S., & Brennan, S. (2010). Criminal victimization in Canada, 2009. *Juristat, 30*(2) (Cat. no. 85-002-X). Ottawa: Author.

Plichta, S. B. (1996). Violence and abuse: Implications for women's health. In M. K. Falik & K. S. Collins (Eds.), *Women's health: The Commonwealth Fund survey.* Baltimore: Johns Hopkins University Press.

Poole, C., & Rietschlin, J. (2012). Intimate partner victimization among adults aged 60 and older: An analysis of the 1999 and 2004 General Social Survey. *Journal of Elder Abuse & Neglect, 24*(2), 120–137. doi:10.1080/08946566.2011.646503

Public Health Agency of Canada. (2001). The Canadian incidence study of reported child abuse and neglect: Highlights. Retrieved from *http://www.phac-aspc.gc.ca/cm-vee/cishl01/.*

Ramsey, J., Richardson, J., Carter, Y. H., Davidson, L. L., & Feder, G. (2002). Should health professionals screen women for domestic violence? Systematic review. *British Medical Journal, 325*(7359), 314–318.

Reece, R. M., & Ludwig, S. (2001). *Child abuse: Medical diagnosis and management* (2nd ed.). Philadelphia: Lippincott Williams & Wilkins.

Reeves, C., & O'Leary-Kelly, A. M. (2007). The effects and costs of intimate partner violence for work organizations. *Journal of Interpersonal Violence, 22,* 327–344.

Renner, L. M., & Slack, K. S. (2006). Intimate partner violence and child maltreatment: Understanding intra- and intergenerational connections. *Child Abuse and Neglect, 30,* 599–617.

Rivara, F. P., Anderson, M. L., Fishman, P., Bonomi, A. E., Reid, R. J., Carrell, D., & Thompson, R. S. (2007a). Healthcare utilization and costs for women with a history of intimate partner violence. *American Journal of Preventive Medicine, 32*(2), 89–96.

Rivara, F. P., Anderson, M. L., Fishman, P., Bonomi, A. E., Reid, R. J., Carrell, D., & Thompson, R. S. (2007b). Intimate partner violence and health care costs and utilization for children living in the home. *Pediatrics, 120,* 1270–1277.

Schollenberger, J., Campbell, J., Sharps, P. W., O'Campo, P., Gielen, A. C., Dienemann, J., & Kub, J. (2003). African American HMO enrollees: Their experiences with partner abuse and its effect on their health and use of medical services. *Violence Against Women, 9,* 599–618.

Scott-Storey, K. (2011). Cumulative abuse: Do things add up? An evaluation of the conceptualization, operationalization, and methodological approaches in the study of the phenomenon of cumulative abuse. *Trauma, Violence & Abuse, 12*(3), 135–150. doi:10.1177/1524838011404253

Seniors Canada. (2011). Facts on the abuse of seniors. Retrieved from *http://www.seniors.gc.ca/c.4nt.2nt@.jsp?lang=eng&geo=106 &cid=155.*

Sharps, P., Koziol-McLain, J., McFarlane, J., Sachs, C., & Xu, X. (2001). Opportunities for prevention of femicide by health care providers. *Preventive Medicine, 33,* 373–380.

Sheridan, D. J. (2001). Treating survivors of intimate partner abuse: Forensic identification and documentation. In J. S. Olshaker, M. C. Jackson, & W. S. Smock (Eds.), *Forensic emergency medicine* (pp. 203–228). Philadelphia: Lippincott Williams & Wilkins.

Snow Jones, A., Dienemann, J., Schollenberger, J., Kub, J., O'Campo, P., Gielen, A. C., & Campbell, J. C. (2006). Long-term costs of intimate partner violence in a sample of female HMO enrollees. *Women's Health Issues, 16,* 252–261.

Statistics Canada. (2001). *Family violence in Canada: A statistical profile 2001.* Ottawa: Canadian Centre for Justice Statistics.

Statistics Canada. (2005). *The Daily: Homicides.* Retrieved from *http://www.statcan.ca/Daily/English/051006/d051006b.htm.*

Statistics Canada. (2011). *Family violence in Canada: A statistical profile 2011.* Ottawa: Canadian Centre for Justice Statistics.

Sugar, N. F., Taylor, J. A., & Feldman, K. W. (1999). Bruises in infants and toddlers: Those who don't cruise rarely bruise. *Archives of Pediatric and Adolescent Medicine, 153,* 399–403.

Tanner, K., & Turney, D. (2000). The role of observation in the assessment of child neglect. *Child Abuse Review, 9,* 337–348.

Teicher, M. H., Samson, J. A., Polcari, A., & McGreenery, C. E. (2006). Sticks, stones, and hurtful words: Relative effects of various forms of childhood maltreatment. *American Journal of Psychiatry, 163,* 993–1000.

Tiwari, A., Chan, K. L., Fong, D., Leung, W. C., Brownridge, D. A., Lam, H., … Ho, P. C. (2008). The impact of psychological abuse by an intimate partner on the mental health of pregnant women. *BJOG: An International Journal of Obstetrics & Gynaecology, 115*(3), 377–384.

Tjaden, P., & Thoennes, N. (2000a). *Extent, nature and consequences of intimate partner violence: Findings from the National Violence Against Women survey.* National Institute of Justice and the Centers for Disease Control and Prevention. Washington, DC: U.S. Department of Justice, Office of Justice Programs, National Institute of Justice.

Tjaden, P., & Thoennes, N. (2000b). *Full report of the prevalence, incidence, and consequences of violence against women* (Report No. NCJ-183781). Washington, DC: National Institute of Justice.

Tower, M. (2007). Intimate partner violence and the health care response: A postmodern critique. *Health Care for Women International, 28,* 438–452.

Trocmé, N., MacMillan, H., Fallon, B., & De Marco, R. (2003). Nature and severity of physical harm caused by child abuse and neglect: Results from the Canadian Incidence Study. *Canadian Medical Association Journal, 169,* 911–915.

Turcotte, M., & Schellenberg, G. (2007). *A portrait of seniors in Canada, 2006.* Ottawa: Statistics Canada.

Varcoe, C. (2001). Abuse obscured: An ethnographic account of emergency nursing in relation to violence against women. *Canadian Journal of Nursing Research, 32*(4), 95–115.

Varcoe, C. (2008). Inequality, violence and women's health. In B. S. Bolaria & H. Dickinson (Eds.), *Health, illness and health care in Canada* (4th ed.). Toronto: Nelson.

Varcoe, C., Hankivsky, O., Ford Gilboe, M., Wuest, J., Wilk, P., Hammerton, J., & Campbell, J. C. (2011). Attributing selected costs to intimate partner violence in a sample of women who have left abusive partners: A social determinants of health approach. *Canadian Public Policy, 37*(3), 359–380.

Walsh, C. A., Jamieson, E., MacMillan, H., & Boyle, M. (2007). Child abuse and chronic pain in a community survey of women. *Journal of Interpersonal Violence, 22,* 1536–1554.

Walsh, C. A., & Yon, Y. (2012). Developing an empirical profile for elder abuse research in Canada. *Journal of Elder Abuse & Neglect, 24*(2), 104–119. doi:10.1080/08946566.2011.644088

Wekerle, C., Wall, A.-M., Leung, E., & Trocmé, N. (2007). Cumulative stress and substantiated maltreatment: The importance of caregiver vulnerability and adult partner violence. *Child Abuse and Neglect, 31,* 427–443.

Wuest, J., Ford-Gilboe, M., Merritt-Gray, M., & Berman, H. (2003). Intrusion: The central problem for health promotion among children and single mothers after leaving an abusive partner. *Qualitative Health Research, 13,* 597–622.

Wuest, J., Merritt-Gray, M., Lent, B., Varcoe, C., Conners, A. J., & Ford-Gilboe, M. (2007). Patterns of medication use among women survivors of intimate partner violence. *Canadian Journal of Public Health, 98,* 460–464.

Wuest, J., Ford-Gilboe, M., Merritt-Gray, M., Varcoe, C., Lent, B., Wilk, P., & Campbell, J. C. (2009). Abuse-related injury and symptoms of posttraumatic stress disorder as mechanisms of chronic pain in survivors of intimate partner violence. *Pain Medicine, 10*(4), 739–747.

Web Sites of Interest

Canadian Centre for Elder Law, *A practical guide to elder abuse and neglect law in Canada: http://www.bcli.org/ccel/projects/ practical-guide-elder-abuse-and-neglect-law-canada*

Canadian Child Welfare Research Portal: *http://www.cecw-cepb.ca*

Canadian Network for the Prevention of Elder Abuse: *http:// www.cnpea.ca/mandatory_reporting.htm*

Danger Assessment: *http://www.dangerassessment.org/* Ontario Network for the Prevention of Elder Abuse (ONPEA): *http://www.onpea.org/english/elderabuse/recognizingabuse.html*

Assessment Techniques and the Clinical Setting

Written by Carolyn Jarvis, PhD, APN, CNP
Adapted by June MacDonald-Jenkins, RN, BScN, MSc

⊖volve WEBSITE

http://evolve.elsevier.com/Canada/Jarvis/examination/
*   Appendices
*   Examination Review Questions
*   Key Points

OUTLINE

The health history described in the preceding chapters provides **subjective data** for health assessment: the individual's *own* perception of the health state. Unit 2 describes **objective data,** which are the signs perceived by the examiner through the physical examination.

Performing a physical examination requires technical skills and a knowledge base. The technical skills are the tools for gathering data. You will relate those data to your knowledge base and to your previous experience. A sturdy knowledge base enables you to look *for,* rather than merely look *at.* Consider a statement by the eighteenth-century poet Goethe: "We see only what we know." To recognize a significant finding, you need to know what to look for.

CULTIVATING YOUR SENSES

You use your senses—sight, smell, touch, and hearing—to gather data during the physical examination. You always have perceived the world through your senses, but now they are focused in a new way. Applying your senses to assess each patient's health state may seem awkward at first, but this skill will be polished with repetition and tutored practice. The skills requisite for the physical examination are inspection, palpation, percussion, and auscultation. The skills are performed one at a time and in this order.

Inspection

Inspection is concentrated watching. It is close, careful scrutiny, first of the individual patient as a whole and then of each body system. Inspection begins the moment you first meet the patient and develop a "general survey." (Specific data to consider for the general survey are described in the following chapter.) Then as you proceed through the examination, start the assessment of each body system with inspection. Inspection is always performed first. Initially you may feel embarrassed "staring" at the patient without also "doing something." However, do not be too eager to touch the patient. A focused inspection takes time and yields a surprising amount of data. Learn to use each patient as his or her own control by comparing the right and left sides of the body. The two sides are nearly symmetrical. Inspection requires good lighting, adequate exposure, and occasional use of certain instruments (otoscope, ophthalmoscope, penlight, nasal and vaginal specula) to enlarge your view.

Palpation

Palpation follows and often confirms points you noted during inspection. In palpation, you apply your sense of touch to assess texture, temperature, moisture, and organ location and size, as well as any swelling, vibration or pulsation, rigidity or spasticity, crepitation, presence of lumps or masses, and presence of tenderness or pain. Different parts of your hands are best suited for assessing different factors:
*   Fingertips: best for fine tactile discrimination (the ability to differentiate information received through the sense of touch) such as skin texture, swelling, pulsation, and determining presence of lumps

- Fingers and thumb: to detect the position, shape, and consistency of an organ or mass through these digits' grasping action
- The dorsa (backs) of hands and fingers: best for determining temperature because the skin is thinner on the dorsa than on the palms
- Base of fingers (metacarpophalangeal joints) or ulnar surface of the hand: best for vibration

Your palpation technique should be slow and systematic. A patient stiffens when touched suddenly, which makes it difficult for you to feel very much. Use a calm, gentle approach. Warm your hands by kneading them together or holding them under warm water. Identify any tender areas, and palpate them last.

Start with light palpation, using the pads of your fingertips to detect surface characteristics and to accustom the patient to being touched. Then perform deeper palpation, perhaps by helping the patient use relaxation techniques such as imagery or deep breathing. Your sense of touch becomes blunted with heavy or continuous pressure. When deep palpation is needed (as for abdominal contents), intermittent pressure is better than one long, continuous palpation. Avoid deep palpation in situations in which it could cause internal injury or pain. Also avoid "digging in" with the ends of your fingers; it will cause pain or discomfort to your patient and may result in increased guarding, by the patient, of the affected areas. Bimanual palpation requires the use of both of your hands to envelop or detect certain body parts or organs—such as the kidneys, uterus, or adnexa—for more precise delimitation (see Chapters 22 and 27).

Percussion

Percussion is tapping the person's skin with short, sharp strokes to assess underlying structures. The strokes yield a palpable vibration and a characteristic sound that depicts the location, size, and density of the underlying organ. Why learn percussion when an x-ray study is so much more accurate? Because your percussing hands are always available, are easily portable, and give instant feedback. Percussion has the following uses:

- Mapping out the *location* and *size* of an organ by exploring where the percussion note changes between the borders of an organ and its neighbours
- Signalling the *density* (air, fluid, or solid) of a structure by a characteristic note
- Detecting an abnormal mass if it is fairly superficial; the percussion vibrations penetrate about 5 cm deep, and so a deeper mass would yield no change in percussion
- Eliciting pain if the underlying structure is inflamed, as with sinus areas or over the kidneys
- Eliciting a deep tendon reflex with the percussion hammer

Two methods of percussion can be used: *direct* (sometimes called *immediate*) and *indirect* (or *mediate*). In direct percussion, the striking hand contacts the body wall directly. This produces a sound and is used in percussing an infant's thorax or an adult's sinus areas. *Indirect* percussion is used more often and involves both hands. The striking hand contacts the

stationary hand, which is fixed on the person's skin. This yields a sound and a subtle vibration. The procedure is as follows:

- The stationary hand: Hyperextend the middle finger (sometimes called the *pleximeter*) of your nondominant hand, and place its distal portion, the phalanx and distal interphalangeal joint, firmly against the patient's skin. Avoid the patient's ribs and scapulae; percussing over a bone yields no data because it always sounds "dull." Lift the rest of the stationary hand off the person's skin (Figure 9-1); otherwise the stationary hand will dampen the produced vibrations, just as a drummer uses a hand to halt a drum roll.
- The striking hand: Use the middle finger of your dominant hand as the *striking finger* (sometimes called the *plexor*; Figure 9-2). Hold your forearm close to the patient's skin surface, with your upper arm and shoulder steady. Scan your muscles to make sure they are steady but not rigid. The action is all in the wrist, and it must be relaxed. Spread your fingers, flick your wrist, and bounce your middle finger off the stationary finger. Aim for just behind the nail bed or at the distal interphalangeal joint; the goal is to hit the portion of the finger that is pushing the hardest into the patient's skin surface. Flex the striking finger so that its tip, not the finger pad, makes contact. It hits directly at right angles to the stationary finger. Percuss two times in this location, using even, staccato blows. Lift the striking finger off quickly; a resting finger dampens

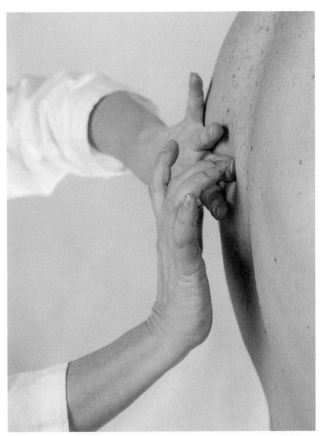

9-1

vibrations. Then move to a new body location and repeat, keeping your technique even. The force of the blow determines the loudness of the note. You do not need a very loud sound; use just enough force to achieve a clear note. The thickness of the patient's body wall affects the clarity of the sound. You need a stronger percussion strike for patients who are obese and for those with very muscular body walls.

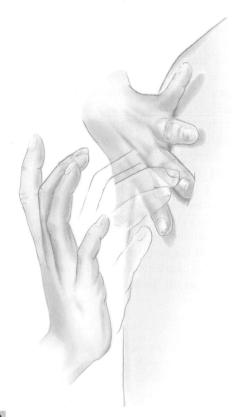

9-2

Percussion can be an awkward technique for beginning examiners. You may feel surprised and embarrassed if your striking finger misses your stationary hand completely. You may wince if the fingernail of your striking finger is too long and painfully gouges your stationary finger. As with all new skills, refinement follows practice. After a few weeks, your hand placement becomes precise and feels natural, and you learn to perceive the subtle difference in percussion notes. It is often useful to practice on a wall at home and percuss for the placement of the studs along the width of the wall. The changes are distinct and easy to discriminate, enabling you to "establish an ear" for subtle changes in sound, when examining a patient's body.

Production of Sound

All sound results from vibration of some structure (Figure 9-3). Percussing over a body structure causes vibrations that produce characteristic waves and are heard as "notes" (Table 9-1). Each of the five percussion notes is differentiated by the following components:

1. **Amplitude** (or intensity): loudness or softness of a sound. The louder the sound, the greater the amplitude. Loudness depends on the force of the blow and the structure's ability to vibrate.
2. **Pitch** (or frequency): the number of vibrations or cycles per second, written as "cps." More rapid vibrations produce a high-pitched tone; slower vibrations yield a low-pitched tone.

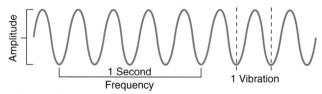

9-3   Sound wave.

TABLE 9-1	Characteristics of Percussion Notes				
Characteristic	Amplitude	Pitch	Quality	Duration	Sample Location
Resonant	Medium-loud	Low	Clear, hollow	Moderate	Over normal lung tissue
Hyperresonant	Louder	Lower	Booming	Longer	Normal finding over child's lung Abnormal finding in an adult over lungs with increased amount of air, as in emphysema
Tympany	Loud	High	Musical and drumlike (like the kettle drum)	Sustained longest	Over air-filled viscus, such as the stomach or the intestine
Dull	Soft	High	Muffled thud	Short	Relatively dense organ, such as liver or spleen
Flat	Very soft	High	An instant stop of sound, absolute dullness	Very short	When no air is present, over thigh muscles, bone, or tumour

3. **Quality** (timbre): a subjective difference in a sound's distinctive overtones. A pure tone is a sound of one frequency. Variations within a sound wave produce overtones. Overtones enable you to distinguish a C note played on a piano from a C note played with vibrato on a violin.

4. **Duration:** the length of time the note lingers. A basic principle is that a structure with relatively more air (such as the lungs) produces a louder, deeper, and longer sound because it vibrates freely, whereas a denser, more solid structure (such as the liver) produces a softer, higher, shorter sound because it does not vibrate as easily.

Although Table 9-1 describes five "normal" percussion notes, variations occur in clinical practice. The "note" you hear depends on the nature of the underlying structure, as well as the thickness of the body wall and your technique. Do not learn these various notes just from written description. Practise on a willing partner.

Auscultation

Auscultation is listening to sounds produced by parts of the body, such as the heart and blood vessels, the lungs, and the abdomen. You have probably already heard certain body sounds with your ear alone: for example, the harsh gurgling of very congested breathing. However, most body sounds are very soft and must be channelled through a **stethoscope** for you to evaluate them. The stethoscope does not magnify sound but does block out extraneous room sounds. Of all the equipment you use, the stethoscope quickly becomes a very personal instrument. Take time to learn its features and to fit one individually to yourself.

The fit and quality of the stethoscope are important. You cannot assess what you cannot hear through a poor-quality instrument. The slope of the earpiece should point forward toward your nose. This matches the natural slope of the normal ear canal and efficiently blocks out environmental sound. If necessary, twist the earpieces to parallel the slope of your ear canals. The earpieces should fit snugly, but if they hurt, they are inserted too far. Adjust the tension, and experiment with different rubber or plastic earplugs to achieve the most comfort. The tubing should be of thick material, with an internal diameter of 4 mm and about 36 to 46 cm long. Longer tubing may distort the sound.

Choose a stethoscope with two endpieces: a diaphragm and a bell (Figure 9-4). You use the **diaphragm** most often because its flat edge is best for hearing high-pitched sounds: breath, bowel, and normal heart sounds. (Because your stethoscope touches many people, clean the endpieces with an alcohol swab to eliminate a possible vector of infection.) Hold the diaphragm against the patient's skin firmly enough to leave a slight ring afterward. The **bell** endpiece has a deep, hollow, cuplike shape. It is best for soft, low-pitched sounds such as extra heart sounds or murmurs. Hold it lightly against the patient's skin, just enough that it forms a perfect seal. Pressing any harder causes the patient's skin to act as a diaphragm, obliterating the low-pitched sounds.

Some newer stethoscopes have one endpiece with a "tunable diaphragm." This enables you to listen to both

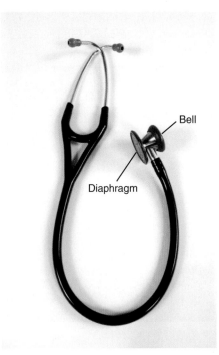

9-4   Stethoscope. The endpieces are the diaphragm (on the left) and the bell (on the right).

low- and high-frequency sounds without rotation of the endpiece. To hear low-frequency sounds (traditional bell mode), hold the endpiece very lightly on the patient's skin; to hear high-frequency sounds (traditional diaphragm mode), press the endpiece firmly on the skin. Before you can evaluate body sounds, it is essential that you eliminate any confusing artifacts:

- Any extra *room noise* can produce a "roaring" in your stethoscope, and so the examination room must be quiet.
- Keep the examination room *warm*. If the patient starts shivering, the involuntary muscle contractions could drown out other sounds.
- *Clean* the stethoscope endpiece with an alcohol wipe, and then warm it by rubbing it against the palm of your hand. Clean the earpieces of your stethoscope as well, especially if it is used by multiple care providers.
- The friction on the endpiece caused by chest hair (on men) causes a crackling sound that mimics an abnormal breath sound called *crackles*. To minimize this problem, wet the hair before auscultating the area.
- *Never* listen through a gown. Reach under a gown to listen, but take care that no clothing rubs on the stethoscope.
- Prevent your own "artifact," such as breathing on the tubing or the thump from bumping the tubing together.

Auscultation is a skill that beginning examiners are eager to learn but is difficult to master. First you must learn the wide range of normal sounds. Once you can recognize normal sounds, you can distinguish the abnormal sounds and extra sounds. Be aware that in some body locations you may hear more than one sound; this can be confusing. You will need to listen selectively to only one thing at a time. As you listen, ask yourself, "What am I *actually hearing?* What *should* I be hearing at this spot?"

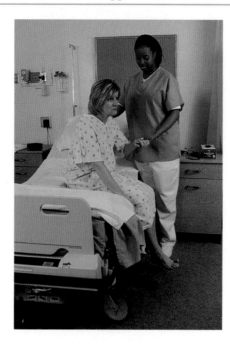

9-5

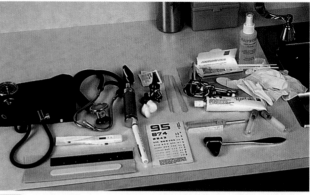

9-6

SETTING: CONTEXT OF CARE

The examination environment should be warm and comfortable, quiet, private, and well-lit. An acute care setting is the first environment that many novice practitioners encounter. The majority of nurses and health practitioners never examine a patient in a clinic setting; many practise in the community in patients' homes and in acute and long-term care facilities. Keep in mind that the suggestions for examination are universal, regardless of whatever setting you are in. When possible, stop any distracting noises—such as humming machinery, radio or television, or people talking—that could make it difficult to hear body sounds. Your time with the individual should be secure from interruptions by other health care personnel. Lighting with natural daylight is best, although it is often not available; artificial light from two sources suffices and prevents shadows. A wall-mounted or gooseneck stand lamp is needed for high-intensity lighting.

Position the patient so that both sides of his or her body are easily accessible (Figure 9-5). The examination or bedside table should be at a height at which you can stand without stooping and should be equipped to raise the person's head up to 45 degrees. A roll-up stool is used for the sections of the examination for which you must be sitting. A bedside stand, table, or flat surface is needed to lay out all your equipment.

EQUIPMENT

During the examination, you should not need to search for equipment or leave the room to find an item. Have all your equipment at easy reach and laid out in an organized manner (Figure 9-6). The following items are usually needed for a screening physical examination:

- Platform scale with height attachment
- Sphygmomanometer (blood pressure monitor)
- Stethoscope with bell and diaphragm endpieces
- Thermometer
- Pulse oximeter (in hospital or clinic setting)
- Flashlight or penlight
- Otoscope/ophthalmoscope
- Nasal speculum (if a short, broad speculum is not included with the otoscope)
- Tongue depressor
- Pocket vision screener
- Skin-marking pen
- Flexible tape measure and ruler marked in centimetres
- Reflex hammer
- Sharp object (split tongue blade)
- Cotton balls
- Clean gloves
- Lubricant

Most of the equipment is described as it comes into use throughout the text. However, consider these introductory comments on the otoscope and ophthalmoscope. The **otoscope** funnels light into the ear canal and onto the tympanic membrane. The base serves both as the handle and the battery power source. To attach the head, press it down onto the "male" adaptor end of the base and turn clockwise until you feel it stop. To turn the light on, press the red button rheostat down and clockwise. (Always turn it off after use to increase the life of the bulb and battery.) Five specula, each a different size, are available to attach to the head (Figure 9-7). (The short, broad speculum is for viewing the nares.) Choose the largest one that will fit comfortably into the patient's ear canal. See Chapter 16 for technique on use of the otoscope.

The **ophthalmoscope** illuminates the internal eye structures. Its system of lenses and mirrors enables you to look through the pupil at the fundus (background) of the eye, much like looking through a keyhole at a room beyond. The ophthalmoscope head attaches to the base "male" adaptor just as the otoscope head does (Figure 9-8). The head has five different parts:

1. Viewing aperture, with five different aperture sizes
2. Aperture selector dial on the front

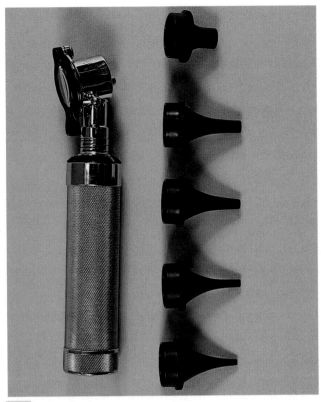

9-7 Otoscope.

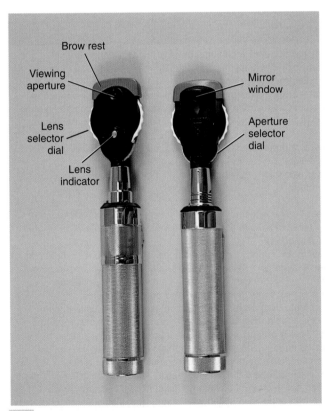

9-8 Ophthalmoscopes.

◯ Large (full spot) for dilated pupils

◯ Small for undilated pupils

◉ Red-free filter — a green beam, used to examine the optic disc for hemorrhage (which looks black) and melanin deposits (which look grey)

⊞ Grid — to determine fixation pattern and to assess size and location of lesions on the fundus

▯ Slit — to examine the anterior portion of the eye and to assess elevation or depression of lesions on the fundus

9-9

3. Mirror window on the front
4. Lens selector dial
5. Lens indicator

Select the aperture to be used (Figure 9-9).

Rotating the lens selector dial brings the object into focus. The lens indicator shows a number, or *dioptre*, that indicates the value of the lens in position. The black numbers indicate a positive lens, from 0 to +40. The red numbers indicate a negative lens, from 0 to −20. The ophthalmoscope can compensate for myopia (nearsightedness) or hyperopia (farsightedness) in the examiner but does not correct for astigmatism. See Chapter 15 for details on how to hold the instrument and what to inspect.

These are excellent tools that are used regularly by health care providers in advanced practice roles. They are occasionally used during basic assessment, along with some other tools that are specific to the patients' needs, such as the goniometer to measure joint range of motion, the Doppler sonometer to augment pulse or blood pressure measurement, the fetoscope for auscultating fetal heart tones, and the pelvimeter to measure pelvic width. For a child, you also need appropriate pediatric-sized endpieces for the stethoscope and otoscope speculae, materials for developmental assessment, age-appropriate toys, or an infant's soother, if available.

A Clean Field

Do not let your stethoscope become a "*Staph*-oscope"! Stethoscopes and other equipment that are frequently used on many patients can become a common vehicle for transmission of infection. Cleaning instruments with an alcohol swab before use in different patients is an effective control of infection.

Designate "clean" and "used" areas for handling of your equipment. In a hospital setting, you may use the overbed table for your clean surface and the bedside stand for the used equipment surface. In a clinic setting, use two separate areas of the pull-up table. Distinguish the clean area by one or two disposable paper towels. On the towels, place all the new, newly cleaned, or newly alcohol-swabbed equipment that you will use on the current patient. Use alcohol swabs to clean all equipment that you carry from patient to patient (e.g., your stethoscope endpieces, the reflex hammer, the ruler). As you proceed through the examination, pick up each piece of equipment from the clean area and, after use on the patient, place it in the used area, or (as in the case of tongue blades and gloves) throw it directly in the trash.

A SAFER ENVIRONMENT

In addition to monitoring the cleanliness of your equipment, take all steps to avoid any possible transmission of infection between patients or between patient and examiner. A **nosocomial infection** (an infection acquired during hospitalization) is a hazard because hospitals have sites that are possible reservoirs for virulent microorganisms. Some microorganisms have become resistant to antibiotics; these include methicillin-resistant *Staphylococcus aureus* (MRSA), vancomycin-resistant *Enterococcus* (VRE), or multidrug-resistant tuberculosis. Other microorganisms include those for which there is currently no known cure, such as the human immunodeficiency virus (HIV).

The most important step to decrease risk of microorganism transmission is to wash your hands promptly and thoroughly. Ensure that you remove all jewellery before washing and that your hands are rinsed under running water; lather the soap and rub your hands together, thoroughly covering all surfaces, for 10 to 15 seconds (longer if hands appear visibly soiled). Rinse and dry thoroughly with a single-use towel or forced-air dryer. Ensure that you turn off the faucets without recontaminating your hands. Hospitals now have dispensers mounted on the wall outside every patient room.

These dispensers contain a waterless, quick-drying, antiseptic solution for handwashing for use on entering and leaving the room. Wear gloves when the potential exists for contact with any body fluids (e.g., blood, mucous membranes, body fluids, drainage, open skin lesions). Wearing gloves is *not* a protective substitute to washing hands, however, because gloves may have undetectable holes or may become torn during use, or hands may become contaminated as gloves are removed. Wear a gown, mask, and protective eyewear when the potential exists for any blood or body fluid spattering (e.g., with suctioning or arterial puncture).

Public Health Agency of Canada's (2007) Laboratory Centre for Disease Control guidelines include the most recent epidemiological information for decreasing transmission of bloodborne and other infections in hospitals. The guidelines include two tiers of precautions. **Routine practices** (Table 9-2) are intended for use with *all* patients regardless of their risk or presumed infection status. Routine practices are designed to reduce the risk of transmission of microorganisms from both recognized and unrecognized sources, and they apply to (a) blood; (b) all body fluids, secretions, and excretions except sweat, regardless of whether they contain visible blood; (c) nonintact skin; and (d) mucous membranes.

The second tier is **transmission-based precautions,** intended for use with patients with documented or suspected transmissible infections. They are designed to be used in addition to routine practices to interrupt transmission in

TABLE 9-2	Routine Practices for Use With All Patients

1. *Wash hands* after touching blood, body fluids, secretions, excretions, and contaminated items, regardless of whether you are wearing gloves. Wash hands immediately after gloves are removed and between patient contacts. You may need to wash hands between procedures on the same patient to prevent cross-contamination of different body sites.
2. *Wear clean gloves* when touching blood, body fluids, secretions, excretions, or items contaminated with these materials; mucous membranes; and nonintact skin. Change gloves between tasks and procedures on the same patient after contact with material that may contain a high concentration of microorganisms. Remove gloves promptly after use, before touching noncontaminated items, and before examining another patient, and wash hands immediately.
3. *Wear a mask and eye protection* to protect your mucous membranes during procedures and during patient care activities that are likely to generate splashes of blood, body fluids, secretions, and excretions.
4. *Wear a gown* (clean, nonsterile, appropriate for activity) to protect your skin and prevent soiling of your clothing during procedures and during patient care activities that are likely to generate splashes of blood, body fluids, secretions, or excretions. Remove a soiled gown promptly, and wash hands.
5. *Place in a private room* any patient who contaminates the environment or who does not or cannot assist in appropriate hygiene or environmental control. Some transmission-based precautions call for providing single accommodations or other negative-pressure–enhanced environments for certain contact and airborne-transmitted pathogens.
6. *Be especially careful with used patient care equipment* if it is soiled with blood, body fluids, secretions, and excretions; handle it in a manner that prevents skin and mucous membrane exposure, contamination of clothing, and transfer of microorganisms to other patients and environments. Do not use the reusable equipment on another patient until it has been cleaned and reprocessed appropriately. Discard single-use items appropriately. Personal care supplies should never be shared between patients.
7. *Prevent injuries by bloodborne pathogens* when you use or handle needles, scalpels, and other sharp instruments. Never recap used needles, manipulate them with both hands, or direct the point of a needle toward any part of your body; rather, use either a one-handed "scoop" technique or an appropriate mechanical device. Do not remove used needles from disposable syringes by hand, and do not otherwise bend, break, or manipulate used needles by hand. Place used disposable syringes, needles, scalpel blades, and other sharp items in appropriate puncture-resistant containers. Use mouthpieces, resuscitation bags, or other ventilation devices instead of mouth-to-mouth resuscitation methods in areas where the need for resuscitation is predictable.
8. *Follow environmental control policies* for the routine care, cleaning, and disinfection of environmental surfaces, beds, bed rails, bedside equipment, and other frequently touched surfaces. Take care with used linen soiled with blood, body fluids, secretions, and excretions; handle, transport, and process this linen in a manner that prevents skin and mucous membrane exposure.

Source: Adapted from Public Health Agency of Canada. (2007). Infection Prevention and Control Best Practices for Long Term Care, Home and Community Care including Health Care Offices and Ambulatory Clinics. Retrieved from *http://www.phac-aspc.gc.ca/amr-ram/ipcbp-pepci/infection-eng.php*.

hospitals. Routes of transmission have been classified as contact (direct, indirect, and droplet), airborne, common vehicle (single contaminated source, such as food), and vectorborne. The two tiers of precautions may be combined for diseases that have multiple routes of transmission, such as varicella (chicken pox) (see Appendix B on the Evolve Web site). Vectorborne transmission by insects of a pathogen such as West Nile virus has been reported in Canada.

THE CLINICAL SETTING

General Approach

Consider your emotional state and that of the patient being examined. The patient is usually anxious because of the anticipation of being examined by a stranger and the unknown outcome of the examination. If anxiety can be reduced, the patient will feel more comfortable and the data gathered will more accurately reflect the patient's natural state. Anxiety can be reduced by an examiner who is confident and self-assured, as well as considerate and unhurried.

Most beginning examiners feel anything *but* self-assured! Most worry about their technical skill, about missing a significant finding, or about forgetting a step. Many are embarrassed about encountering a partially dressed individual. All these fears are natural and common. The best way to minimize them is with a lot of practice on a healthy, willing subject, usually a fellow student. You have to feel comfortable with your motor skills before you can absorb what you are actually seeing or hearing in a real patient. This comfort develops with practice under the guidance of an experienced peer or mentor, in an atmosphere in which it is acceptable to make mistakes and to ask questions. Your subject should "act like a patient" so that you can deal with a "real" situation while still in a safe setting. After you feel comfortable in the laboratory setting, accompany your preceptor or co-assigned nurse as he or she examines an actual patient so that you can observe an experienced examiner in the practice setting.

Hands On

With this preparation, it is possible to interact with your own patient in a confident manner. Begin by measuring the patient's height, weight, blood pressure, temperature, pulse, and respiration (see Chapter 10). If necessary, measure visual acuity at this time, using the Snellen eye chart. All of these are familiar, relatively nonthreatening actions; they gradually accustom the patient to the examination. Then ask the patient to change into an examination gown or other clothing that gives you access, leaving his or her underpants on. The patient will feel more comfortable with underpants, and the underpants can easily be removed just before the genital examination. Unless your assistance is needed, leave the room as the person undresses. Keep in mind that some patients may not wish to disrobe fully or at all, depending on ethnocultural considerations. As you re-enter the room, wash your hands in the person's presence. Not only is this an infection control measure but it also demonstrates a readiness to provide

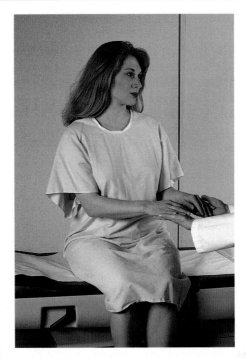

9-10

safe care. Explain each step in the examination and how the patient can cooperate. Encourage the patient to ask questions. Keep your own movements slow, methodical, and deliberate.

Begin by touching the patient's hands, checking skin colour, nail beds, and metacarpophalangeal joints (Figure 9-10). Again, this is a less threatening way to ease a patient into being touched. Most people are used to having relative strangers touch their hands.

As you proceed through the examination, avoid distractions and concentrate on one step at a time. The sequence of the steps may differ, depending on the age of the patient and your own preference. However, you should establish a system that works for you and stick to it to avoid omissions. Organize the steps so that the patient does not change positions too often. Although proper exposure is necessary, use additional drapes to maintain the patient's privacy and to prevent chilling. Consider possible ethnocultural considerations in regard to touch. As you proceed through the examination, ensure that the patient is comfortable with the progression of the assessment.

Do not hesitate to write out the examination sequence and refer to it as you proceed. The patient will accept this as quite natural if you explain you are making brief notations to ensure accuracy. Many agencies use a printed form. You will find that you glance at the form less and less as you obtain experience. Even with a form, you sometimes may forget a step in the examination. When you realize this, perform the manoeuvre in the next logical point in the sequence. (See Chapter 28 for the sequence of steps in the complete physical examination.)

As you proceed through the examination, occasionally offer some brief teaching about the patient's body. For example, you might say, "This tapping on your back (percussion) is a little like playing different drums. The different notes I hear tell me where each organ starts and stops. You probably can hear the difference yourself from within your body." Or you might say, "Everyone has two sounds for each heartbeat, something like this: lub-dup. Your own beats sound normal." Do not do this with every single step, or you will be hard pressed to make a comment when you do come across an abnormality. Some sharing of information, however, builds rapport and increases the patient's confidence in you as an examiner. It also gives the patient a little more control in a situation in which it is easy to feel completely helpless.

At some point, you may want to linger in one anatomical location to concentrate on some complicated findings. To avoid causing anxiety, tell the person, "I always listen to heart sounds on a number of places on the chest. Just because I am listening a long time does not necessarily mean anything is wrong." Sometimes, of course, you *will* discover a possible abnormality, and you want another examiner to double-check. You need to give the patient some information, but you should not alarm the person unnecessarily. Say something like, "I do not have a complete assessment of your heart sounds. I want Ms. Wright to listen to you, too."

At the end of the examination, summarize your findings and share the necessary information with the patient. Thank the patient for the time spent. In a hospital setting, apprise the patient of what is scheduled next. Before you leave a hospitalized patient, lower the bed; make the patient comfortable and safe; and return the bedside table, television, or any equipment to the way it was originally. In a clinic or home care setting, your assessment data provide the basis of information needed to develop a collaborative plan of care with your patient.

✦ DEVELOPMENTAL CONSIDERATIONS

Children are different from adults in many ways. Their difference in size is obvious. Their bodies grow in a predictable pattern that is assessed during the physical examination. However, their behaviour is also different. Behaviour develops and changes through predictable stages, just as the body does. Each examiner needs to know the expected emotional and cognitive features of these stages and to perform the physical examination on the basis of developmental principles (Berk, 2007; Perry, Hockenberry, Lowdermilk, & Wilson, 2010).

With all children, the goal is to increase their comfort in the setting. This approach reveals their natural state as much as possible and will give them a more positive memory of health care providers. Remember that a "routine" examination is anything but routine to children. You can increase their comfort by attending to the developmental principles and approaches discussed in the following sections. The *order* of the developmental stages is more meaningful than the exact chronological age. Each child is an individual, and no child's development fits exactly into one category. For example, if your efforts to "play games" with a preschool-age child are rebuffed, modify your approach to the security measures used with a toddler.

Infants

Erik Erikson defined the major task of infancy as establishing trust. An infant is completely dependent on the parent for his or her basic needs. If these needs are met promptly and consistently, the infant feels secure and learns to trust others.

Position

- A parent always should be present to understand normal growth and development and for the child's feeling of security.
- Place the neonate or young infant supine on a padded examination table (Figure 9-11). The infant also may be held against the parent's chest for some steps.
- Once the baby can sit without support (at approximately 6 months of age), as much of the examination as possible should be performed while the baby is in the parent's lap.
- By ages 9 to 12 months, the baby is acutely aware of the surroundings. Anything outside the infant's range of vision is "lost," and so the parent must be in full view.

Preparation

- Perform the examination 1 to 2 hours after the baby is fed, when the baby is not too drowsy or too hungry.
- Maintain a warm environment. A neonate may require an overhead radiant heater.
- Infants do not object to being nude. Have the parent remove outer clothing, but leave a diaper on a boy.
- Infants do not mind being touched, but make sure your hands and stethoscope endpieces are warm.
- Use a soft, crooning voice during the examination; babies respond more to the feeling in the tone of the voice than to what is actually said.

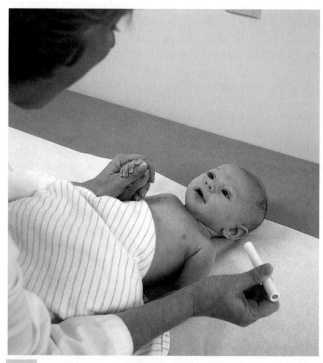

9-11

- Most infants like eye contact; lock your eyes with the baby's from time to time.
- Smile; a baby prefers a smiling face to a frowning one. (Often beginning examiners are so absorbed in their technique that they look serious or stern.) Take time to play.
- Keep movements smooth and deliberate, not jerky.
- Offer the baby a pacifier for crying or during invasive steps.
- Offer brightly coloured toys for a distraction when an infant is fussy.
- Let an older baby touch the stethoscope or tongue blade.

Sequence

- When a baby is sleeping, seize the opportunity to listen to heart, lung, and abdomen sounds first.
- Perform least distressing steps first. (See the sequence in Chapter 28.) Save the invasive steps of examination of the eye, ear, nose, and throat until last.
- Elicit the Moro, or "startle," reflex at the end of the examination because it may cause the baby to cry.

Toddlers

Toddlers are at Erikson's stage of developing autonomy. However, the need to explore the world and be independent is in conflict with the basic dependency on the parent. This often results in frustration and negativism. Toddlers may be difficult to examine; do not take this personally. Because they are acutely aware of being in a new environment, toddlers may be frightened and cling to the parents. Also, toddlers fear invasive procedures and dislike being restrained (Figure 9-12).

Position

- A toddler should be sitting up on the parent's lap for all of the examination. When the toddler must be supine (as in the abdominal examination), move chairs to sit knee-to-knee with the parent. Have the toddler lie in the parent's lap with the toddler's legs in your lap.
- Enlist the aid of a cooperative parent to help position the toddler during invasive procedures. The child's legs can be captured between the parent's legs. The parent can encircle the child's head with one arm, holding it against the chest, and hold the child's arms with the other arm. (See Figure 17-22.)

Preparation

- Children 1 or 2 years of age can understand symbols, and so a security object, such as a special blanket or teddy bear, is helpful.
- Begin by greeting the child and the accompanying parent by name, but with a child 1 to 6 years old, focus more on the parent. By essentially "ignoring" the child at first, you allow the child to adjust gradually and to size you up from a safe distance. Then turn your attention gradually to the child, at first to a toy or object the child is holding, or perhaps to compliment a dress, the hair, or what a big girl or boy the child is. If the child is ready, you will note these signals: eye contact with you, smiling, talking with you, or accepting a toy or a piece of equipment.
- A 2-year-old child does not like to take off his or her clothes; have the parent undress the child one part at a time.
- Children 1 or 2 years of age like to say, "No." Do not offer a choice when there really is none. Avoid saying, "May I listen to your heart now?" When the 1- or 2-year-old child says "No," and you go ahead and do it anyway, you lose trust. Instead, use clear firm instructions, in a tone that expects cooperation: "Now it is time for you to lie down so I can check your tummy."
- Also, 1- or 2-year-old children like to make choices. When possible, enhance autonomy by offering a *limited option:* "Shall I listen to your heart next, or your tummy?"
- Demonstrate the procedures on the parent (see Figure 16-11).
- Praise the child when he or she is cooperative.

Sequence

- Collect some objective data while you document the history, which is a less stressful time. While you are focusing on the parent, note the child's gross motor and fine motor skills and gait.
- Begin with "games," such as cranial nerve testing.
- Start with nonthreatening areas. Save distressing procedures—such as examination of the head, ear, nose, or throat—for last.

Preschool-Age Children

Preschool-age children display developing initiative. The preschooler takes on tasks independently, plans the tasks, and follows them through. A child of this age is often cooperative,

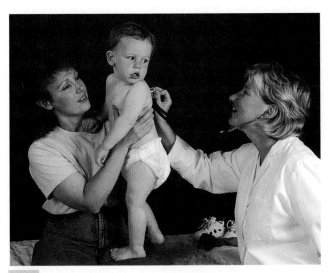

9-12

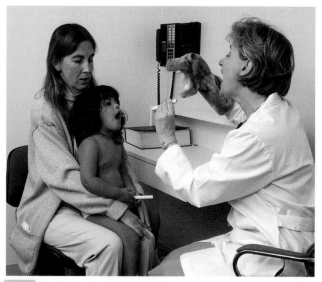

9-13

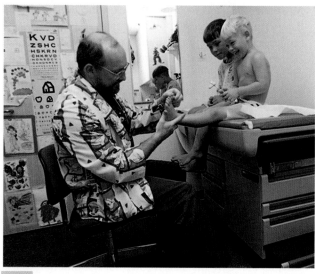

9-14

helpful, and easy to involve. However, children of this age have fantasies and may see illness as punishment for being "bad." The concept of body image is limited. The child fears any body injury or mutilation, and so he or she will recoil from invasive procedures (e.g., tongue blade, rectal temperature, injection, and venipuncture).

Position

- With a 3-year-old child, the parent should be present and may hold the child on his or her lap (Figure 9-13).
- A 4- or 5-year-old child usually feels comfortable on the "Big Girl" or "Big Boy" (examining) table, with the parent present.

Preparation

- A preschooler can talk. Verbal communication becomes helpful now, but remember that the child's understanding is still limited. Use short, simple explanations.
- The preschooler is usually willing to undress. Leave underpants on until the genital examination.
- Talk to the child and explain the steps in the examination exactly.
- Do not allow a choice when there is none.
- As with toddlers, enhance the autonomy of preschoolers by offering choice when possible.
- Allow the child to play with equipment to reduce fears (Figure 9-14).
- Preschoolers like to help; have the child hold the stethoscope for you.
- Use games. Have the child "blow out" the light on the penlight as you listen to the breath sounds or pretend to listen to the heart sounds of the child's teddy bear first. One technique that is absorbing to preschoolers is to trace their shape on the examining table paper (Perry et al., 2010). You can comment on how big the child is, then fill in the outline with a heart or stomach and listen to the

paper doll first. After the examination, the child can take the paper doll home as a souvenir.
- Use a slow, patient, deliberate approach. Do not rush.
- During the examination, give the preschooler needed feedback and reassurance: "Your tummy feels just fine."
- Compliment the child on his or her cooperation.

Sequence

- Examine the thorax, abdomen, extremities, and genitalia first. Preschoolers are usually cooperative; nevertheless, assess head, eye, ear, nose, and throat last.

School-Age Children

During the school-age period, the major task of children is developing industry. School-age children are developing basic competency in school and in social networks, and they desire the approval of parents and teachers. When successful, children have a feeling of accomplishment. During the examination, school-age children are cooperative and are interested in learning about the body. Language is more sophisticated now, but do not overestimate and treat the school-age child as a small adult. The child's level of understanding may not match that of his or her speech.

Position

- School-age children should be sitting on the examination table.
- Five-year-old children have a sense of modesty. If appropriate in the examination, let an older child (aged 11 or 12 years) decide whether parents or siblings should be present.

Preparation

- Break the ice with small talk about family, school, friends, music, or sports.

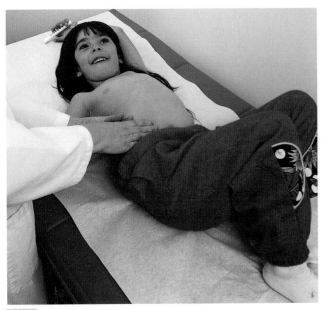

9-15

- The child should undress himself or herself, leave underpants on, and don a gown and drape.
- Demonstrate equipment; school-age children are curious about how equipment works.
- Comment on the body and how it works (Figure 9-15). An 8- or 9-year-old child has some understanding of the body and is interested to learn more. It is rewarding to see the child's eyes light up when he or she hears the heart sounds.

Sequence

- As with adults, progress from head to toes.

Adolescents

The major task in adolescence is developing a self-identity. This takes shape from various sets of values and different social roles (son or daughter, sibling, and student). In the end, each person needs to feel satisfied and comfortable with whom he or she is. In the process, the adolescent is increasingly self-conscious and introspective. Peer group values and peer acceptance are important.

Position

- An adolescent should be sitting on the examination table.
- Examine the adolescent alone, without a parent or sibling present.

Preparation

- The adolescent's body is changing rapidly. During the examination, the adolescent needs feedback that his or her own body is healthy and developing normally.
- The adolescent has a keen awareness of body image, often comparing himself or herself with peers. Apprise the adolescent of the wide variation among teenagers on the rate

of growth and development (see sexual maturity ratings, Chapters 18, 26, and 27).
- Communicate with some care. Do not treat the teenager like a child, but do not overestimate and treat him or her like an adult, either.
- Because most adolescents are idealistic, they are amenable to health teaching. Positive attitudes developed now may last throughout adult life. Focus your teaching on ways in which adolescents can achieve their own wellness.

Sequence

- As with the adult, a head-to-toe approach is appropriate. Examine genitalia last, and do so quickly.

Older Adults

During later years, the tasks are developing the meaning of life and one's own existence and adjusting to changes in physical strength and health.

Position

- An older adult should be sitting on the examination table; a frail older adult may need to be supine.
- Arrange the sequence to allow as few position changes as possible.
- Allow rest periods when needed.

Preparation

- For older adults, the pace of the examination may need to be slowed. The slower pace may dictate the ability to implement some techniques. It is better to break the complete examination into a few visits than to rush through the examination and alienate or frighten the patient.
- Use physical touch (unless there is a cultural contraindication). This is especially important with older adults because other senses, such as vision and hearing, may be diminished.
- Do not mistake diminished vision or hearing for confusion. Confusion of sudden onset may signify a disease state. It is manifested by short-term memory loss, diminished thought process, diminished attention span, and labile emotions (see Chapter 6).
- Be aware that the later years contain more of life's stress. Loss is inevitable, including changes in physical appearance of the face and body, declining energy level, loss of job through retirement, loss of financial security, loss of long-time home, and deaths of friends or spouse. How the patient adapts to these losses significantly affects health assessment.

Sequence

- Use the head-to-toe approach as in younger adults.

Ill Patients

For a patient in some distress, alter the position during the examination. For example, a patient with shortness of breath or ear pain may want to sit up, whereas a person with faintness or overwhelming fatigue may want to be supine. Initially, it may be necessary just to examine the body areas appropriate to the problem, collecting a **mini-database.** You may resume a complete assessment after the initial distress is alleviated.

REFERENCES

Berk, L. E. (2007). *Development through the lifespan* (4th ed.). Boston: Allyn & Bacon.

Perry, S., Hockenberry, M., Lowdermilk, D., & Wilson, D. (2010). *Maternal child nursing care* (4th ed.). St. Louis: Elsevier.

Public Health Agency of Canada (2007). *Infection prevention and control best practices for long term care, home and community care including health care offices and ambulatory clinics.* Retrieved from *http://www.phac-aspc.gc.ca/amr-ram/ipcbp-pepci/infection-eng.php.*

General Survey, Measurement, and Vital Signs

Written by Carolyn Jarvis, PhD, APN, CNP

Adapted by June MacDonald-Jenkins, RN, BScN, MSc

evolve WEBSITE

OUTLINE

OBJECTIVE DATA

The general survey is a study of the whole person, covering the general health state and any obvious physical characteristics. It is an introduction for the physical examination that will follow; it should give an overall impression, a "gestalt," of the patient (see Sample Charting on page 177). Objective parameters are used to form the general survey, but these apply to the whole person, not just to one body system.

Launch a general survey by observation at the moment you first encounter the patient. What leaves an immediate impression? Does the patient stand promptly as his or her name is called and walk easily to meet you? Or does the patient look sick, rising slowly or with effort, with shoulders slumped and eyes without lustre or downcast? In the hospital setting, the observation begins the moment you enter the patient's room. Is the hospitalized patient conversing with visitors, involved in reading or television, or lying still? Even as you introduce yourself and shake hands, you collect data. Does the patient fully extend the arm, shake your hand firmly, make eye contact, or smile? Are the palms dry, or are they damp and clammy? As you proceed through the health history, the measurements, and the vital signs, note the following points that will add up to the general survey. Consider these four areas: **physical appearance, body structure, mobility,** and **behaviour.**

Normal Range of Findings	Abnormal Findings

THE GENERAL SURVEY

Physical Appearance

Age. Appears his or her stated age.

Sex. Sexual development appropriate for gender and age.

Level of Consciousness. Alert and oriented, attending to your questions, and responding appropriately.

Skin Colour. Even colour tone, pigmentation varying with genetic background, and intact skin with no obvious lesions.

Facial Features. Symmetrical with movement.

No signs of acute distress.

Appears older than the stated age, as in chronic illness or chronic alcoholism.

Delayed or precocious puberty.

Confused, drowsy, or lethargic (see Table 6-1, p. 84).

Pallor, cyanosis, jaundice, erythema, or any lesions (see Chapter 13).

Immobile, masklike, asymmetrical, or drooping (see Table 14-4, p. 295).

Respiratory signs: shortness of breath, wheezing.

Pain, indicated by facial grimace and holding the affected body part.

Body Structure

Stature. Height within normal range for age and genetic heritage (see Measurement section, p. 153).

Nutrition. Weight within normal range for height and body build; even distribution of body fat.

Excessively short or tall (see Table 10-5, p. 178).

Cachectic, emaciated.

Simple obesity, with even fat distribution.

Centripetal (truncal) obesity: fat concentrated in face, neck, trunk, with thin extremities, as in Cushing's syndrome (hyperadrenalism; see Table 10-5, p. 178).

Unilateral atrophy or hypertrophy.

Symmetry. Body parts equal bilaterally and in relative proportion to each other.

Posture. Standing comfortably erect as appropriate for age; normal "plumb line" through anterior ear, shoulder, hip, patella, and ankle (exceptions: standing toddlers, who have a normally protuberant abdomen ["toddler lordosis"] and older patients, who may be stooped with kyphosis).

Asymmetrical location of a body part.

Rigid spine and neck; move as one unit (e.g., arthritis).

Patient stiff and tense, ready to spring from chair; fidgety movements.

Slumped shoulders; deflated appearance (e.g., depression).

Position. Sitting comfortably in a chair, on the bed, or on the examination table; arms relaxed at sides, head turned to examiner.

Tripod: leaning forward with arms braced on chair arms; occurs with chronic pulmonary disease.

Sitting straight up and resisting lying down (e.g., heart failure).

Curled up in fetal position (e.g., acute abdominal pain).

Body Build, Contour. Normal proportions: (a) arm span (fingertip to fingertip) equals height; (b) body length from crown to pubis approximately equal to length from pubis to sole; obvious physical deformities: note any congenital or acquired defects.

Elongated arm span, arm span greater than height (e.g., Marfan's syndrome, hypogonadism; see Table 10-5, p. 178).

Missing extremities or digits; webbed digits; shortened limb.

Mobility

Gait. Normally, base width equal to shoulder width; accurate foot placement; smooth, even, and well-balanced walk; and presence of associated movements, such as symmetrical arm swing.

Exceptionally wide base; staggering, stumbling.

Shuffling, dragging, nonfunctional leg.

Limping with injury.

Propulsion: difficulty stopping (see Table 25-5, p. 719.

Objective Data

Normal Range of Findings	Abnormal Findings

Range of Motion. Full mobility in each joint, and deliberate, accurate, smooth, and coordinated movement (see Chapter 24 for information on more detailed testing of joint range of motion).

No observation of involuntary movement.

Limited range of motion in joint.

Paralysis: absence of movement.

Jerky, uncoordinated movement.

Tics, tremors, seizures (see Table 25-4, p. 717).

Behaviour

Facial Expression. Maintaining eye contact with examiner (unless a cultural consideration exists), expressions appropriate to the situation (e.g., thoughtful, serious, or smiling; note expressions both while the face is at rest and while the patient is talking).

Flat, depressed, angry, sad, anxious (however, anxiety is common in ill people, and some people smile when they are anxious).

Mood and Affect. Comfortable and cooperative with the examiner and interacting pleasantly.

Hostile, distrustful, suspicious, crying.

Speech. Clear and understandable articulation (the ability to form words).

Dysarthria and dysphonia; speech defect, monotone, garbled speech.

Fluent stream of talking, with an even pace.

Conveying ideas clearly.

Extremes: few words or constant talking.

Word choice appropriate to culture and education.

Communicating in native language easily by himself or herself or with an interpreter.

Dress. Clothing appropriate for the climate, looks clean and fits the body, and is appropriate for the patient's culture and age group; for example, women of the Hutterite faith may wear nineteenth century–style clothing, and women of Indian descent may wear saris (culturally determined dress should not be labelled as bizarre by Western standards or by adult expectations).

Clothing too large and held up by belt: suggestive of weight loss, as does the addition of new holes in belt; belt moved to a looser fit: may indicate weight gain, obesity, or ascites.

Consistent wear of certain clothing may provide clues: long sleeves may conceal needle marks of drug abuse; broad-brimmed hats may reveal sun intolerance; Velcro fasteners instead of buttons may indicate chronic motor dysfunction.

Personal Hygiene. Appearance: clean and groomed appropriately for patient's age, occupation, and socioeconomic group (a wide variation of dress and hygiene is "normal").

Hair: groomed, brushed.

In a woman who previously was carefully groomed, unkempt hair and absence of makeup may indicate malaise or illness.

MEASUREMENT

Weight

Use a standardized *balance* or electronic standing scale. Instruct the patient to remove his or her shoes and heavy outer clothing before standing on the scale. When a sequence of repeated weights is necessary, aim for approximately the same time of day and the same type of clothing worn each time. Record the weight in kilograms and in pounds.

Show the patient how his or her own weight compares with the recommended range for height. Compare the patient's current weight with that from the previous health visit. A recent weight loss may be explained by successful dieting. A weight gain usually reflects overabundant caloric intake, unhealthy eating habits, sedentary lifestyle, or fluid accumulation.

An unexplained weight loss may be a sign of a short-term illness (e.g., fever, infection, disease of the mouth or throat) or a chronic illness (endocrine disease, malignancy, mental health dysfunction).

Obesity is weight exceeding 120% of ideal body weight and occasionally results from endocrine disorders, drug therapy (e.g., corticosteroids), or depression.

Normal Range of Findings	Abnormal Findings

Height

Use a wall-mounted device or the measuring pole on the balance scale. Align the extended headpiece with the top of the head. The patient should be shoeless, standing straight with gentle traction under the jaw, and looking straight ahead. Feet, shoulders, and buttocks should be in contact with the pole or the wall.

Body Mass Index

Body mass index (BMI) is a practical marker of optimal weight for height and an indicator of obesity or protein-calorie malnutrition. Evidence supports using BMI in obesity risk assessment because it provides a more accurate measure of total body fat, in comparison with the measure of body weight alone (Figure 10-1). BMI is calculated as follows:

$$BMI = \frac{\text{Weight (in kilograms)}}{\text{Height (in metres)}^2} \ or$$
$$\frac{\text{Weight (in pounds)}}{\text{Height (in inches)}^2} \times 703$$

For a quick determination of BMI, use a straight edge to help locate the point on the chart where height (centimetres or inches) and weight (kilograms or pounds) intersect (see Figure 10-1). Read the number on the dashed line closest to this point. For example, an individual who weighs 69 kg and is 173 cm tall has a BMI of approximately 23. Many BMI calculators are available online.

BMI interpretation for adults (World Health Organization (WHO, 2011):
  <16.0: Severe thinness
  16.0–16.99: Moderate Thinness
  17.0–18.5: Mild Thinness
  <18.5: Underweight
  18.5–24.9 Normal weight
  25.0–29.9: Overweight
  30.0–34.9: Obesity (Class 1)
  35–39.9: Obesity (Class 2)
  ≥40: Extreme obesity (Class 3)
BMI interpretation for children aged 2 to 20 years (Centers for Disease Control and Prevention, 2011): 85th to 95th percentile = risk for overweight

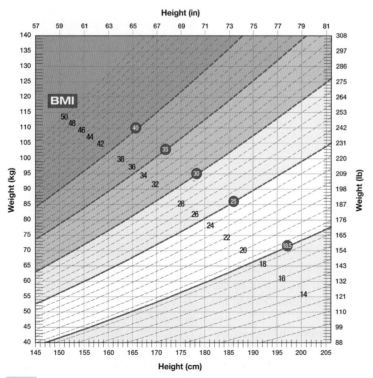

10-1 Body mass index (BMI) nomogram.

Objective Data

Normal Range of Findings	Abnormal Findings

Waist-to-Hip Ratio

The waist-to-hip ratio reflects body fat distribution as an indicator of health risk. Patients with obesity have a greater proportion of fat in the upper body, especially in the abdomen, have android obesity; obese patients with most of their fat in the hips and thighs have gynoid obesity. The equation is as follows:

$$\text{Waist-to-hip ratio} = \frac{\text{Waist circumference}}{\text{Hip circumference}}$$

where waist circumference is measured at the smallest circumference below the rib cage and above the iliac crest, and hip circumference is measured at the largest circumference of the buttocks. In addition, **waist circumference** alone can be used to predict greater health risk. Measure at the end of gentle expiration.

In the Health Canada (2003) guidelines for body weight classification in adults, BMI and waist circumference serve as as indicators of health risk. This is in keeping with internationally adopted recommendations from the WHO (2000), which are derived from population data. It is important to recognize that weight classification is only a component of a comprehensive health assessment. This classification system is not intended for use with patients younger than 18 years or with pregnant or lactating women.

> A waist-to-hip ratio of 1.0 or higher in men or of 0.8 or higher in women is indicative of android (upper body) obesity and an increased risk for obesity-related diseases and early mortality.

> A waist circumference higher than 88 cm (35 inches) in women and higher than 102 cm (40 inches) in men increases risk of cardiovascular and metabolic diseases.

VITAL SIGNS

Temperature

Cellular metabolism requires a mean stable core ("deep body") temperature of 37.2°C. The body maintains a steady temperature through a thermostat, or feedback mechanism, regulated in the hypothalamus. The thermostat balances heat production (from metabolism, exercise, food digestion, external factors) with heat loss (through radiation, evaporation of sweat, convection, conduction).

The various routes of temperature measurement reflect the body's core temperature. The normal oral temperature in a resting patient ranges from 35.8°C to 37.3°C (mean, 37°C). The rectal temperature measures 0.4°C to 0.5°C higher.

The normal temperature is influenced by

- A diurnal cycle of 1° to 1.5°C; the trough occurs in the early morning hours, and the peak occurs in late afternoon to early evening.
- The menstruation cycle in women: Progesterone secretion, occurring with ovulation at midcycle, causes a 0.5°C to 1.0°C rise in temperature that continues until menses.
- Exercise: Moderate to strenuous exercise increases body temperature.
- Age: Wider normal variations occur in infants and young children as a result of less effective heat control mechanisms. In older adults, temperature is usually lower than in other age groups, with a mean of 36.2°C.

The **oral temperature** is accurate and convenient. The oral sublingual site has a rich blood supply (from the carotid arteries) that quickly responds to changes in inner core temperature.

Shake a mercury-free glass thermometer so that the reading is down to 35.5°C, and place the thermometer at the base of the tongue in either of the posterior sublingual pockets, *not* in front of the tongue. Instruct the patient to keep his or her lips closed. Leave the thermometer in place 3 to 4 minutes if the patient is afebrile and up to 8 minutes if the patient is febrile. (Measure other vital signs during this time.) Wait 20 minutes before taking the temperature if the patient has just taken hot or iced liquids, 2 minutes if he or she has just smoked, and 5 minutes if he or she has just chewed gum.

> The thermostatic function of the hypothalamus may become disturbed during illness or central nervous system disorders.
>
> **Hyperthermia,** or fever, is caused by pyrogens secreted by toxic bacteria during infections or as a result of tissue breakdown such as that after myocardial infarction, trauma, surgery, or malignancy. Neurological disorders (e.g., a cerebral vascular accident, cerebral edema, brain trauma, tumour, or surgery) also can reset the thermostat at a higher level, resulting in heat production and conservation.
>
> **Hypothermia** is usually caused by accidental, prolonged exposure to cold. It also may be purposefully induced to lower the body's oxygen requirements during heart or peripheral vascular surgery, neurosurgery, amputation, or gastrointestinal hemorrhage.

Normal Range of Findings	Abnormal Findings

The **electronic thermometer** has the advantages of swift and accurate measurement (usually in 20 to 30 seconds) as well as safe, unbreakable, disposable probe covers. The instrument must be fully charged and correctly calibrated. Most children enjoy watching their temperature numbers advance on the box. The **axillary temperature** is safe and accurate for infants and young children when the environment is reasonably controlled (see Developmental Considerations section, p. 166).

Measure the **rectal temperature** only when the other routes are not practical—for example, in comatose or confused patients, those in shock, or those who cannot close the mouth because of breathing or oxygen tubes, wired mandible, or other facial dysfunction—or if no tympanic membrane thermometer equipment is available. Wear gloves, insert a lubricated rectal probe cover on an electronic thermometer, and insert the thermometer only 2 to 3 cm (1 in) into the adult rectum, directed toward the umbilicus. (For a glass thermometer, leave in place for 2.5 minutes.) Disadvantages to the rectal route are patient discomfort and the time-consuming and disruptive nature of the activity.

The **tympanic membrane thermometer** senses infrared emissions of the tympanic membrane (eardrum). The tympanic membrane shares the same vascular supply that perfuses the hypothalamus (the internal carotid artery).

The tympanic membrane thermometer is a noninvasive, nontraumatic device that is extremely quick and efficient. The probe tip has the shape of an otoscope, the instrument used to inspect the ear. Cover the probe tip with a tip cover, and gently place the probe tip into the patient's ear canal (see Figure 10-16 on p. 171). Do not force it in, and do not occlude the canal. Activate the device, and you can read the temperature in 2 to 3 seconds.

There is minimal chance of cross-contamination with the tympanic thermometer because the ear canal is lined with skin and not mucous membrane. However, tympanic thermometers have disposable tip covers, which are changed between patients. This thermometer is used in unconscious patients or in those who are unable or unwilling to cooperate with traditional techniques (i.e., those in critical care units, emergency departments, recovery areas, and labour and delivery units). The tympanic thermometer has the advantages of speed, convenience, safety, reduced risk of injury and infection, and noninvasiveness.

The tympanic thermometer is a commonly used temperature measurement tool in most acute care environments. However, current evidence is conflicting; some studies do not support the use of a tympanic thermometer in critically ill patients. Researchers in these studies investigated primarily normothermic patients; more research in this area is needed in the acute care setting to determine the superior method. A newer noninvasive measurement entails using infrared emissions from the *temporal artery*. This device yields measurements that agree closely with core temperature, but accuracy can be affected by diaphoresis in patients.

In Canada, Celsius is the official measurement system used for reporting body temperature. However, some older adults remain more familiar with the Fahrenheit scale.

Begin by memorizing these convenient equivalents for patients who prefer Fahrenheit measurements:

$$104°F = 40°C$$
$$98.6°F = 37°C$$
$$95°F = 35°C$$

Normal Range of Findings	Abnormal Findings

Pulse

With every beat, the heart pumps an amount of blood—the **stroke volume**—into the aorta. This is about 70 mL in adults. The force causes the arterial walls to widen and generates a pressure wave, which is felt in the periphery as the **pulse.** By palpating the peripheral pulse, you can measure the rate and rhythm of the heartbeat, as well as obtain local data on the condition of the artery. The radial pulse is usually palpated during measurement of vital signs.

Using the pads of your first three fingers, palpate the radial pulse at the flexor aspect of the wrist laterally along the radius bone (Figure 10-2). Press until you feel the strongest pulsation. If the rhythm is regular, count the number of beats in 30 seconds and multiply by 2. Although counting in 15 seconds is frequently practised, any one-beat error in counting results in a recorded error of four beats per minute. The 30-second interval is the most accurate and efficient when heart rates are normal or rapid and when rhythms are regular. However, if the rhythm is irregular, as in atrial fibrillation, always count for a full minute. It is more important to establish the rhythm so that you can accurately determine rate. Assess the pulse, including (a) rate, (b) rhythm, (c) force, and (d) equality (when comparing pulses bilaterally). All symmetrical pulses should be assessed simultaneously except for the carotid pulse.

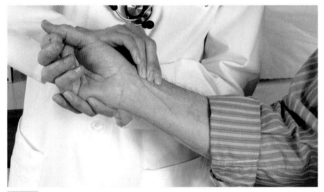

10-2

Rate

In a resting adult, the normal heart rate range is 60 to 100 beats per minute (bpm). The rate normally varies with age, being more rapid in infancy and childhood and more moderate during adult and older years. The rate also varies with gender; after puberty, girls have a slightly faster rate than do boys (Table 10-1).

In adults, a heart rate less than 60 bpm is **bradycardia.** This occurs normally in well-trained athletes, in whom the heart muscle develops along with the skeletal muscles. The stronger, more efficient heart muscle pushes out a larger stroke volume with each beat; thus fewer beats per minute are necessary to maintain a stable cardiac output. (Review the equation CO = SV × R, or Cardiac output = Stroke volume × Rate, in Chapter 20.) A heart rate faster than 100 bpm is **tachycardia.** It is normal with anxiety or with increased exercise to match the body's demand for increased metabolism.

For descriptions of abnormal rates and rhythms, see Table 21-2, p. 541.

Tachycardia occurs with fever, with sepsis, and after myocardial infarction.

Objective Data

Normal Range of Findings

Abnormal Findings

TABLE 10-1	Normal Resting Pulse Rates Across Age Groups	
Age/Condition	Average (Beats Per Minute)	Normal Limits
Newborn	120	70–190
1 yr	120	80–160
2 yr	110	80–130
4 yr	100	80–120
6 yr	100	75–115
8 yr	90	70–110
10 yr	90	70–110
12 yr		
Female	90	70–110
Male	85	65–105
14 yr		
Female	85	65–105
Male	80	60–100
16 yr		
Female	80	60–100
Male	75	55–95
18 yr		
Female	75	55–95
Male	70	50–90
Well-conditioned athlete	May be 50-60	50–100
Adult	74-76	60–100
Older adult	74-76	60–100

Rhythm

The rhythm of the pulse normally has an even tempo. However, one irregularity that is common in children and young adults is **sinus arrhythmia,** in which the heart rate varies with the respiratory cycle, speeding up at the peak of inspiration and slowing to normal with expiration. Inspiration momentarily causes a decreased stroke volume from the left side of the heart; to compensate, the heart rate increases. (See Chapter 20 for a full discussion on sinus arrhythmia.) If any other irregularities are detected, auscultate heart sounds for a more complete assessment (see Chapter 20, p. 508).

Force

The force of the pulse shows the strength of the heart's stroke volume. A "weak, thready" pulse reflects decreased stroke volume (e.g., as occurs with hemorrhagic shock). A "full, bounding" pulse denotes increased stroke volume, as occurs with anxiety, exercise, and some abnormal conditions. The pulse force is recorded on a three-point scale:

3+: Full, bounding
2+: Normal
1+: Weak, thready
0: Absent

Normal Range of Findings	Abnormal Findings

Some agencies use a four-point scale; make sure your system is consistent with that used by the rest of your staff. Either scale is somewhat subjective. Experience will improve your clinical judgement.

Respirations

Normally, a patient's breathing is relaxed, regular, automatic, and silent. Because most people are unaware of their breathing, do not mention that you will be counting the respirations; the patient's awareness that you are doing so may alter the normal pattern. Instead, maintain your position of counting the radial pulse, and unobtrusively count the respirations. Count for 30 seconds or for a full minute if you suspect an abnormality. Avoid the 15-second interval. The result can vary by a factor of ±4, which is significant with such a small number.

When you are documenting respiratory rate, ensure that you count one full cycle (inspiration and expiration) as one respiration. The first rise and fall of the chest is counted as one breath. Note that the respiratory rates presented in Table 10-2 normally are more rapid in infants and children. Also, the ratio of pulse rate to respiratory rate is fairly constant, approximately 4:1. Normally, both pulse and respiratory rates rise as a response to exercise or anxiety. Respiratory status is described in more detail in Chapter 19.

TABLE 10-2	Normal Respiratory Rates
Age	**Breaths Per Minute**
Newborn	30–40
1 yr	20–40
2 yr	25–32
4 yr	23–30
6 yr	21–26
8 yr	20–26
10 yr	20–26
12 yr	18–22
14 yr	18–22
16 yr	12–20
18 yr	16–20
Adult	10–20

Blood Pressure

Blood pressure (BP) is the force of the blood pushing against the side of the vessel wall. The strength of the push changes with the event in the cardiac cycle. The **systolic pressure** is the maximum pressure felt on the artery during left ventricular contraction, or systole. The **diastolic pressure** is the elastic recoil, or resting, pressure that the blood exerts constantly between each contraction. The **pulse pressure** is the difference between the systolic and diastolic pressures and reflects the stroke volume (Figure 10-3). The **mean arterial pressure** is the pressure forcing blood into the tissues, averaged over the cardiac cycle. This is not an arithmetic average of systolic and diastolic pressures because diastole lasts longer. Rather, it is a value closer to diastolic pressure plus one third the pulse pressure.

Objective Data

Objective Data

Normal Range of Findings	Abnormal Findings

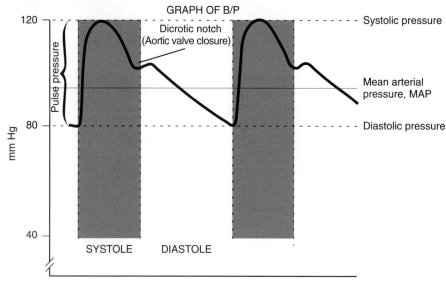

10-3 A graph of blood pressure from systole through diastole.

The average BP in the young adult is 120/80 mm Hg, although variations are normal with many factors:

- Age: Normally, BP rises gradually through childhood and into the adult years (see Figure 10-18, p. 174).
- Gender: Before puberty, no difference in BP exists between boys and girls. After puberty, girls usually have lower BP than do male counterparts. After menopause, BP is higher in women than in male counterparts.
- Ethnocultural background: In Canada, adults of African descent usually have a higher BP than do those of European descent of the same age. The incidence of hypertension is twice as high among those of African descent; reasons for the difference are not fully understood, but it appears to be a result of genetic and environmental factors.
- Diurnal rhythm: A daily cycle of a peak and a trough occurs: The BP is highest in late afternoon or early evening and then declines to an early morning low.
- Weight: BP is higher in obese patients than in patients of normal weight of the same age (including adolescents).
- Exercise: Increasing activity yields a proportionate increase in BP. Within 5 minutes of terminating the exercise, the BP normally returns to baseline.
- Emotions: The BP momentarily rises with fear, anger, and pain as a result of stimulation of the sympathetic nervous system.
- Stress: The BP is elevated in patients feeling continual tension because of lifestyle, occupational stress, or life problems.

The level of BP is determined by five factors:

1. **Cardiac output**. If the heart pumps more blood into the blood vessels, the pressure on the vessel walls increases (Figure 10-4).
2. **Peripheral vascular resistance**. Peripheral vascular resistance is the opposition to blood flow through the arteries. When the blood vessels become smaller (i.e., when constricted), greater pressure is needed to push the blood through.
3. **Volume of circulating blood**. The term *volume of circulating blood* refers to how tightly the blood is packed into the arteries. Increasing the volume of blood in the arteries increases the pressure.
4. **Viscosity**. The "thickness" of blood is determined by its formed elements, the blood cells. When the blood is thicker, the pressure increases.
5. **Elasticity of vessel walls**. When the vessel walls are stiff and rigid, more pressure is needed to push the blood through.

Normal Range of Findings			Abnormal Findings

FACTORS CONTROLLING BLOOD PRESSURE

FACTOR		CONDITION	RESULT
Cardiac output	↑	with heavy exercise to meet body demand for increased metabolism	↑ BP
	↓	with pump failure (weak pumping action after myocardial infarction, or in shock)	↓ BP
Vascular resistance	↑	resistance (vasoconstriction)	↑ BP
	↓	resistance (vasodilation)	↓ BP
Volume	↓	volume (hemorrhage)	↓ BP
	↑	volume (increased sodium and water retention, intravenous fluid overload)	↑ BP
Viscosity	↑	viscosity (increased hematocrit in polycythemia)	↑ BP
Elasticity of arterial walls	↑	rigidity, hardening as in arteriosclerosis (heart pumping against greater resistance)	↑ BP

10-4

Illustration copyright Pat Thomas, © 2006.

BP is measured with a stethoscope and an aneroid *sphygmomanometer*. The aneroid gauge is subject to drift; it must be recalibrated at least once each year, and it must rest at zero.

The cuff consists of an inflatable rubber bladder inside a cloth cover. The width of the rubber bladder should equal 40% of the circumference of the patient's arm. The length of the bladder should equal 80% of this circumference. Cuff width is 20% more than the upper arm diameter or two thirds of the length between the antecubital fossa and the axilla. When you use an automated device, ensure that you select the cuff size recommended by the manufacturer.

Cuffs are available in six sizes ranging from one that fits newborns infants to one that fits an extra-large adult, as well as tapered cuffs for the cone-shaped obese arm and thigh cuffs. Match the appropriate size cuff to the patient's arm size and shape and not to the patient's age (Figure 10-5).

The cuff size is important; using a cuff that is too narrow yields a falsely high BP because it takes extra pressure to compress the artery.

Thigh cuff or large arm cuff

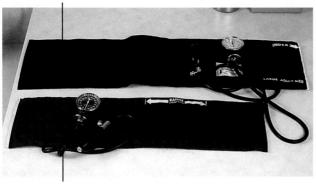

Standard adult arm cuff

10-5

Normal Range of Findings	Abnormal Findings

Arm Pressure

When a patient is comfortable and relaxed, the BP reading is valid. Many patients are anxious at the beginning of an examination; allow at least a 5-minute rest before measuring the BP. Take three BP measurements on the same arm, separating the last two by 2 minutes; discard the first reading; and average the other two. This procedure is the new recommended Canadian standard (Canadian Hypertension Education Program [CHEP], 2011).

For each patient, verify BP in both arms once, either on admission or for the first complete physical examination. It is not necessary to continue to check both arms for screening or monitoring. On occasion, a 5- to 10-mm Hg difference may occur in BP in the two arms (if values are different, record the higher value).

A difference in the two arms of more than 10 to 15 mm Hg may indicate arterial obstruction on the side with the lower reading.

The patient may be sitting or lying, with the bare arm supported at heart level. (If a mercury manometer is used, place it so that it is vertical and at your eye level.) When the patient is sitting, the feet should be flat on the floor because the BP measurement is falsely high when legs are crossed (CHEP, 2011).

Palpate the brachial artery, which is located just above the antecubital fossa, medial to the biceps tendon. Centre the deflated cuff about 2.5 cm (1 in) above the brachial artery, and wrap it evenly around the arm.

Now palpate the brachial or the radial artery (Figure 10-6). Inflate the cuff until the artery pulsation is obliterated and then 20 to 30 mm Hg beyond. This will prevent missing an **auscultatory gap,** which is a period when Korotkoff's sounds disappear during auscultation (Table 10-3).

An auscultatory gap occurs in about 5% of people, most often in those with hypertension caused by a noncompliant arterial system.

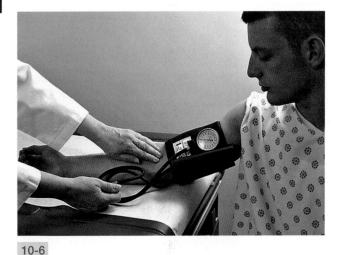

10-6

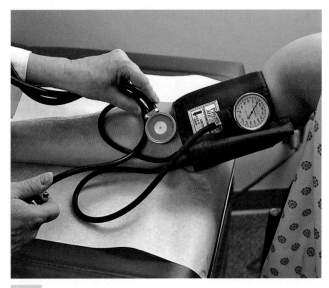

10-7

Place the bell of the stethoscope over the site of the brachial artery, making a light but airtight seal (Figure 10-7). The diaphragm endpiece is usually adequate, but the bell is designed to pick up low-pitched sounds such as the sounds of a BP reading.

Which stethoscope end chosen does not influence measurement error, but for the novice practitioner, using the bell can make the difference between hearing an accurate BP or not hearing it. Thus it is good practice to use the bell while you are acquiring skill for hearing the discrete sounds.

Normal Range of Findings	Abnormal Findings

Deflate the cuff slowly and evenly, about 2 mm Hg per heartbeat. Note the points at which you hear the first appearance of sound, the muffling of sound, and the final disappearance of sound. These are phases I, IV, and V of **Korotkoff's sounds,** which are the components of a BP reading that were first described by a Russian surgeon in 1905 (see Table 10-3).

TABLE 10-3	Korotkoff's Sounds		
Phase	Quality	Description	Rationale
Cuff correctly inflated	No sound	—	Cuff inflation compresses brachial artery. Cuff pressure exceeds heart's systolic pressure, occluding brachial artery blood flow.
I	Tapping	Soft, clear tapping, increasing in intensity	The systolic pressure: As the cuff pressure lowers to reach intraluminal systolic pressure, the artery opens, and blood first spurts into the brachial artery. Blood is at very high velocity because of small opening of artery and large pressure difference across opening. This creates turbulent flow, which is audible.
Auscultatory gap	No sound	Silence for 30–40 mm Hg during deflation: an abnormal finding	Sounds temporarily disappear during end of phase I, then reappear in phase II. This is common with hypertension. If it is undetected, systolic reading is falsely low or diastolic reading is falsely high.
II	Swooshing	Softer murmur that follows tapping	Turbulent blood flow through still partially occluded artery.
III	Knocking	Crisp, high-pitched sounds	Duration of blood flow through artery is longer. Artery closes just briefly during late diastole.
IV	Abrupt muffling	Muting of sound to a low-pitched, cushioned murmur; blowing	Artery no longer closes in any part of cardiac cycle. Change is in quality, not intensity.
V	Silence	—	Velocity of blood flow decreases. Streamlined blood flow is silent. The last audible sound (marking the disappearance of sounds) is diastolic pressure. The fifth Korotkoff sound is now used to define diastolic pressure in all age groups (Chobanian et al., 2003).
Brachial artery occluded by cuff; no blood flow		Artery intermittently compressed, blood spurts into artery	Cuff is deflated, and blood flows freely through the artery.

Brachial artery occluded by cuff, no blood flow

Artery intermittently compressed, blood spurts into artery

Cuff deflated, artery flows free

Auscultatory sound	Silence	I Clear tapping	IV Abrupt muffling	V Silence

Objective Data

Normal Range of Findings	Abnormal Findings

For all age groups, the fifth Korotkoff phase is now used to define diastolic pressure (CHEP, 2011). However, when the variance is greater than 10 to 12 mm Hg between phases IV and V, record *both* phases along with the systolic reading (e.g., 142/98/80). Seated BPs are used to determine and monitor treatment decisions. Standing BPs are used to diagnose postural hypotension. The CHEP (2011) recommended that, on initial assessment of BP, the pressure in both arms is measured. If a significant variance exists (>20 mm Hg), then measurement of bilateral pressures should be continued. Table 10-4 is a list of common errors in BP measurement.

Hypotension is abnormally low BP; **hypertension,** abnormally high BP (see parameters in Table 10-6, on p. 181).

Orthostatic (or Postural) Vital Signs

Take serial measurements of pulse and BP when you suspect volume depletion; when the patient is known to have hypertension or is taking antihypertensive medications; or when the patient reports fainting or syncope. Have the patient rest supine for 2 or 3 minutes, take baseline readings of pulse and BP, and then repeat the measurements with the patient sitting and then standing. The measurements should still be taken the recommended 2 minutes apart, to ensure that venous congestion has subsided. For a patient who is too weak or dizzy to stand, assess when the patient is first supine and then sitting with legs dangling. When the position is changed from supine to standing, a slight decrease (less than 10 mm Hg) in systolic pressure is normal. Ensure that the patient has a safe place to sit or land if he or she gets dizzy during the standing measurement.

Orthostatic hypotension—a drop in systolic pressure of more than 20 mm Hg, or an orthostatic pulse increase of 20 bpm or more—occurs with a quick change to a standing position. These changes result from abrupt peripheral vasodilatation without a compensatory increase in cardiac output. Orthostatic changes also occur with prolonged bed rest, older age, hypovolemia, and ingestion of some drugs.

Record the BP by using even numbers. Also record the patient's position, the arm used, and the cuff size, if different from the standard adult cuff. Record the pulse rate and rhythm, noting whether the pulse is regular.

Measurement of Oxygen Saturation. Use of the **pulse oximeter** is a noninvasive method to assess arterial oxygen saturation (SpO_2). A sensor attached to the patient's finger or earlobe has a diode that emits light and a detector that measures the relative amount of light absorbed by oxyhemoglobin and unoxygenated (reduced) hemoglobin. The pulse oximeter compares the ratio of light emitted to light absorbed and converts this ratio into the percentage of SpO_2. Because it measures only light absorption of pulsatile flow, the reading represents arterial SpO_2. A healthy patient with no lung disease and no anemia normally has an SpO_2 of 97% to 98%.

Select the appropriate pulse oximeter probe. The finger probe is spring-loaded and feels like a clothespin attached to the finger but does not hurt (Figure 10-8). When SpO_2 is lower, the earlobe probe is more accurate and is less affected by peripheral vasoconstriction (Grap, 2002).

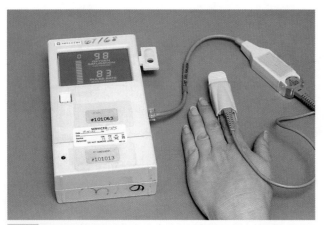

10-8

Normal Range of Findings	Abnormal Findings

TABLE 10-4	**Common Errors in Blood Pressure Measurement**	
Common Error	**Result**	**Rationale**
Taking blood pressure reading when patient is anxious or angry or has just been active	Falsely high	Sympathetic nervous system stimulation
Faulty arm position		
Above level of heart	Falsely low	Eliminates effect of hydrostatic pressure
Below level of heart	Falsely high	Additional force of gravity added to brachial artery pressure
Patient supports own arm	Falsely high diastolic	Sustained isometric muscular contraction
Faulty leg position (e.g., patient's legs are crossed)	Falsely high systolic and diastolic	Translocation of blood volume from dependent legs to thoracic area
Examiner's eyes are not level with meniscus of mercury column		
Looking up at meniscus	Falsely high	Parallax
Looking down on meniscus	Falsely low	
Inaccurate cuff size (the most common error)		
Cuff too narrow for extremity	Falsely high	Excessive pressure needed to occlude brachial artery
Cuff wrap is too loose or uneven, or bladder balloons out of wrap	Falsely high	Excessive pressure needed to occlude brachial artery
Failure to palpate radial artery while cuff is inflated	Falsely low systolic	Missing initial systolic tapping or tuning in during *auscultatory gap* (tapping sounds disappear for 10–40 mm Hg and then return; common with hypertension)
Poor inflation of the cuff		
Overinflation of the cuff	Pain	
Pushing stethoscope too hard on brachial artery	Falsely low diastolic	Distortion of artery by excessive pressure so that the sounds continue
Deflating cuff		
Too quickly	Falsely low systolic or falsely high diastolic	Insufficient time to hear tapping
Too slowly	Falsely high diastolic	Venous congestion in forearm makes sounds less audible
Halting during descent and reinflating cuff to recheck systolic	Falsely high diastolic	Venous congestion in forearm
Failure to wait 1–2 min before repeating entire reading	Falsely high diastolic	Venous congestion in forearm
Any observer error		
Examiner's haste	Any error	
Faulty technique		
Examiner's digit preference, "hears" more results that end in zero than would occur by chance alone (e.g., 130/80)		
Diminished hearing acuity		
Defective or inaccurately calibrated equipment		

Electronic Vital Signs Monitor. An automated vital signs monitor is in frequent use in hospital or clinic settings, especially when frequent monitoring is required (Figure 10-9). The artery pulsations create vibrations that are detected by the electronic sensors. The BP mode is noninvasive and fast and has automatic measurement intervals and a bright numerical display. As with manual BP machines, accuracy depends on cuff selection and placement and on calibration of the equipment.

The electronic BP monitor cannot sense vibrations of low BP or rapidly irregular pulses, as in atrial fibrillation. Do not use it if the patient's systolic BP is less than 90 mm Hg or if the patient has conditions such as shivering, tremors, or seizures. If the numerical display does not correspond to the clinical presentation of the patient, always validate your findings with a manual sphygmomanometer and your stethoscope.

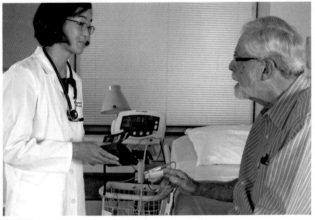

10-9

✥ DEVELOPMENTAL CONSIDERATIONS

Infants and Children

General Survey

Physical Appearance, Body Structure, Mobility. Note the same basic elements as with the adult, with consideration for age and development.

Behaviour. Note the response to stimuli and level of alertness appropriate for age.

Parental Bonding. Note the child's interactions with parents and whether parent and child show a mutual response and are warm and affectionate, appropriate to the child's condition. The parent provides appropriate physical care of child and promotes new learning (see *Promoting a Healthy Lifestyle: Health and Self-Care* box, p. 176).

Measurement

Weight. Weigh an infant on a platform-type balance scale (Figure 10-10). To check calibration, set the weight at zero and observe the beam balance. Guard the baby so that he or she does not fall. Weigh to the nearest 10 g (½ oz) for infants and 100 g (¼ lb) for toddlers.

Some signs of child abuse: the child avoids eye contact; the child exhibits no separation anxiety when you would expect it for age; the parent is disgusted by child's odour, sounds, drooling, or stools.

Deprivation of physical or emotional care (see Chapter 8).

Normal Range of Findings   **Abnormal Findings**

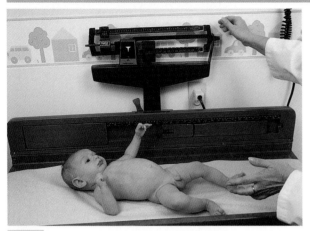

10-10

For children 2 or 3 years of age, use the upright scale. Leave underpants on the child. Some young children are fearful of the rickety standing platform and may prefer sitting on the infant scale. Use the upright scale with preschool- and school-age children, maintaining modesty with light clothing (Figure 10-11).

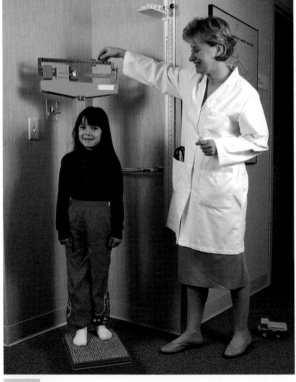

10-11

Length. For a child younger than 2 years, measure the body length when the child is supine by using a horizontal measuring board (Figure 10-12). Hold the head in the midline. Because infants normally flex their legs, extend the legs momentarily by holding the knees together and pushing them down until the legs are flat on the table. Avoid using a tape measure along the infant's length because this method yields inaccurate results. It is important to measure an infant to the nearest centimetre.

Objective Data

Normal Range of Findings	Abnormal Findings

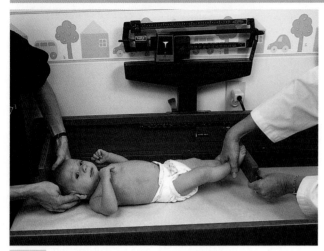

10-12

For a child 2 or 3 years of age, measure the height by standing the child against the pole on the platform scale or back against a flat ruler taped to the wall (Figure 10-13). (Sometimes a child will stand more erect against the solid wall than against the narrow measuring pole on the scale.) Encourage the child to stand straight and tall and to look straight ahead without tilting the head. The shoulders, buttocks, and heels should touch the wall. Hold a book or flat board on the child's head at a right angle to the wall. Mark just under the book, noting the measure to the nearest 1 mm (⅛ inch).

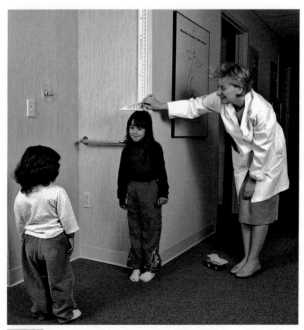

10-13

Normal Range of Findings

Physical growth is usually the best index of a child's general health. The child's height and weight are recorded at every health care visit to determine normal growth patterns. The results are plotted on growth charts based on data from the National Center for Health Statistics (NCHS). Normal limits range from the fifth to the ninety-fifth percentile on standardized charts. (See Appendix D on the Evolve Web site for samples.) In 2011, the WHO released a revised set of child growth standards that better reflect the diversity of the global population. These assessment tools—which are based on height, weight, and BMI—minimize variations noted with the NCHS tools, which are based on norms established for American children of European descent. The WHO standards are being accepted globally as a more accurate measure of growth and development. (See appendices on the Evolve Web site for growth assessment forms for boys and girls.)

Healthy childhood growth is continuous but uneven, with rapid growth spurts occurring during infancy and adolescence. Results are more reliable when numerous growth measurements over a long time are compared. These charts are also used to compare an individual child's measurements against those of the general population.

Use your judgement and consider the genetic background of the child who is small for age. Explore the growth patterns of the parents and siblings. Studies have indicated that Canadian Crees have a higher prevalence of macrosomia (birth weight >90th percentile) than their non-Aboriginal counterparts (33% versus 11%). Even after researchers controlled for gestational diabetes, which is known to contribute to higher birth weights, the rates remained significantly higher, indicating potential genetic differences in fetal growth (Rodrigues, Robinson, Kramer, & Gray-MacDonald, 2000).

Head Circumference. Measure the infant's head circumference at birth and at each well-child visit up to age 2 years and then yearly up to 6 years (Figure 10-14). Circle the tape around the head at the prominent frontal and occipital bones; the widest span is correct. Plot the measurement on standardized growth charts. Compare the infant's head size with that expected for age. A series of measurements is more valuable than a single figure to show the *rate* of head growth.

Abnormal Findings

Using NCHS Charts
Further explore any growth measurement that

- Falls below the fifth or above the ninety-fifth percentile with no genetic explanation
- Shows a wide percentile difference between height and weight; for example, a tenth-percentile height with a ninety-fifth percentile weight
- Shows that growth has suddenly stopped when it had been steady
- Fails to show normal growth spurts during infancy and adolescence

Using WHO Charts
- A child's score that is far from the median of 0, such as –3 or 3, indicates growth challenges.
- Z-score lines indicate distance from the growth average.

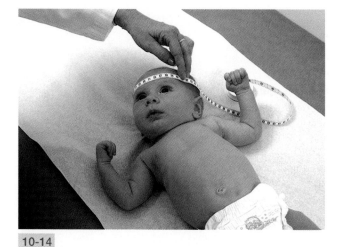

10-14

Objective Data

Normal Range of Findings	Abnormal Findings

The newborn's head measures about 32 to 38 cm (averaging around 34 cm) and is about 2 cm larger than the chest circumference. The chest grows at a faster rate than does the cranium; at some time between 6 months and 2 years, both measurements are about the same, and after 2 years, the chest circumference is greater than the head circumference.

Measurement of the chest circumference is valuable in a comparison with the head circumference, but not necessarily by itself. Encircle the tape around the chest at the nipple line. It should be snug, but not so tight that it leaves a mark (Figure 10-15).

Head circumference is enlarged with increased intracranial pressure (see Chapter 14).

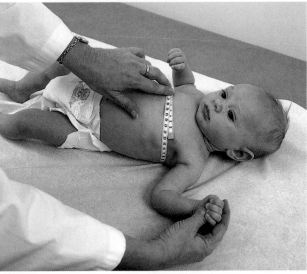

10-15

Vital Signs

Measure vital signs with the same purpose and frequency as you would in an adult. With an *infant,* reverse the order of vital sign measurement to respiration first and then pulse and temperature. Taking temperature rectally may cause the infant to cry, which will increase the respiratory and pulse rate, thus masking the normal resting values. A *preschooler's* normal fear of body mutilation is increased with any invasive procedure. If recommended, avoid the rectal route and take temperature tympanically. When this is not feasible, use the reverse order and measure the rectal temperature last. Your approach to measuring vital signs with the *adolescent* is much the same as with the adult.

Temperature

Tympanic. Tympanic temperature measurement is useful with toddlers who squirm at the restraint needed for the rectal route, and it is useful with pre-schoolers who are not yet able to cooperate for an oral temperature measurement but fear the disrobing and invasion involved with rectal measurement. The tympanic temperature measurement is so rapid that it is usually over before the child realizes it (Figure 10-16).

The data on tympanic temperature measurement with newborns and young children are conflicting. In a study of infants aged 3 to 36 months in outpatient settings, Jean-Mary, Dicanzio, Shaw, and Bernstein (2002) found the tympanic temperature measurement useful for noninvasive screening, but if the history or

Objective Data

Normal Range of Findings	Abnormal Findings

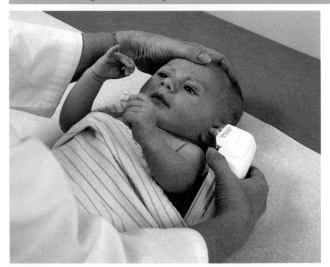

10-16

Objective Data

physical examination findings are suggestive of a febrile illness, the rectal value should be used for clinical accuracy. However, Nimah, Bshesh, Callahan, and Jacobs (2006) studied critically ill hospitalized children younger than 7 years and concluded that the tympanic temperature measurements more accurately reflected core temperatures during febrile and nonfebrile states.

Axillary. The axillary route is safer and more accessible than the rectal route; however, its accuracy and reliability have been questioned (Cusson, Madonia, & Taekman, 1997). When cold receptors are stimulated, brown fat tissue in the area releases heat through chemical energy, which artificially raises skin temperature. Studies on preterm infants show only small differences between axillary and rectal temperature measurement, which may be because brown fat is not present until 34 weeks' gestation (Bliss-Holtz, 1995). When the axillary route is used, place the tip well into the axilla, and hold the child's arm close to the body.

Oral. Use the oral route when the child is old enough to keep the mouth closed. This is usually at age 5 or 6 years, although some 4-year-old children can cooperate. Use an electronic thermometer when one is available because it is unbreakable and it registers quickly.

Rectal. The Canadian Paediatric Society's (2011) position statement on temperature measurement in infants and children articulates the advantages and disadvantages of all methods. The Society continues to recommend rectal temperature measurement as the definitive technique in infants and children 5 years of age and younger. From birth to age 2 years, rectal measurement is the definitive choice, followed by axillary for screening children at low risk for illness. For children 2 to 5 years of age, rectal measurement remains the definitive method. For children older than 5 years, oral measurement is the primary method, followed by axillary and tympanic measurement. An infant may be supine or sidelying, with the examiner's hand flexing the infant's knees up onto the abdomen. (When a baby boy is supine, cover the boy's penis with a diaper.) An infant also may lie prone across the adult's lap. Separate the buttocks with one hand, and insert the lubricated electronic rectal probe *no farther* than 2.5 cm (1 in). Insertion any deeper increases the risk of rectal perforation because the colon curves posteriorly at 3 cm (1.25 inch). (In a glass thermometer, temperature registers by 3 minutes.)

Normal Range of Findings	**Abnormal Findings**

Normally, rectal temperatures measure higher in infants and young children than in adults, with an average of 37.8°C at age 18 months. Also, the temperature normally may be elevated in the late afternoon, after vigorous playing, or after eating.

Pulse. Palpate or auscultate an apical rate with infants and toddlers. (See Chapter 20 for location of apex and technique.) In children older than 2 years, use the radial site. Count the pulse for a full minute to take into account normal irregularities, such as sinus arrhythmia. The heart rate normally fluctuates more in infants and children than in adults in response to exercise, emotion, and illness.

Respirations. Watch the infant's abdomen for movement because the infant's respirations are normally more diaphragmatic than thoracic (Figure 10-17). Count a full minute because the pattern varies significantly from rapid breaths to short periods of apnea. Note the normal rate in Table 10-2 on page 159.

Up to ages 6 to 8 years, children have higher fevers with illness than adults do. Even with minor infections, temperatures may be elevated to 40.5°C.

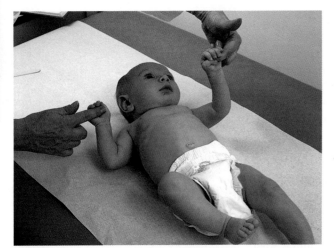

10-17

Blood Pressure. In children aged 3 years and older and in younger children at risk, take a routine BP measurement at least annually. For accurate measurement in children, make some adjustment in the choice of equipment and technique. The most common error is to use the incorrect size cuff. The cuff width must cover two thirds of the upper arm, and the cuff bladder must completely encircle it.

Use a pediatric-sized endpiece on the stethoscope to locate the sounds. If possible, allow a crying infant to become quiet for 5 to 10 minutes before measuring the BP; crying may elevate the systolic pressure by 30 to 50 mm Hg. Use the disappearance of sound (phase V Korotkoff's sound) for the diastolic reading in children, as well as in adults.

Note the new guidelines for normal BP values by age groups that are *based on the child's height* (Appendices E-1 and E-2 on the Evolve Web site). In children, height is more strongly correlated with BP than is age. For children whose BPs are at the extremes of normal, the new charts avoid misclassification as normotensive or hypertensive. Children younger than 3 years of age have such

Further explore any BP reading that is greater than the ninety-fifth percentile and refer for diagnostic evaluation. For the child whose BP falls between the ninetieth and ninety-fifth percentiles and whose high BP cannot be explained by height or weight, monitor the BP every 6 months.

Normal Range of Findings	Abnormal Findings

small arm vessels that it is difficult to hear Korotkoff's sounds with a stethoscope. Instead, use an electronic BP device that entails *oscillometry,* such as Dinamap, and gives a digital readout for systolic, diastolic, mean arterial pressure, and pulse. Or use a *Doppler* ultrasound device to amplify the sounds. This instrument is easy to use and can be used by one examiner. (Note the technique for using the Doppler device in Figure 10-19 on p. 175.)

Older Adults

General Survey

Physical Appearance. By the eighth and ninth decades, body contour is sharper, with more angular facial features, and body proportions are redistributed. (See Measurements section for weight and height, below.)

Posture. A general flexion occurs by the eighth or ninth decade.

Gait. Older adults often use a wider base to compensate for diminished balance, arms may be held out to help balance, and steps may be shorter or uneven.

Measurement

Weight. Older adults appear sharper in contour with more prominent bony landmarks than are found in younger adults. Body weight decreases during the 80s and 90s. This factor is more evident in men, perhaps because of greater muscle shrinkage. The distribution of fat also changes during the 80s and 90s. Even with good nutrition, subcutaneous fat is lost from the face and periphery (especially the forearms), whereas additional fat is deposited on the abdomen and hips.

Height. By the 80s and 90s, many people are shorter than they were in their 70s. This results from shortening in the spinal column, which is caused by thinning of the vertebral discs and shortening of the individual vertebrae, as well as slight flexion in the knees and hips and the postural changes of kyphosis. Because long bones do not shorten with age, the overall body proportion looks different: a shorter trunk with relatively long extremities.

Vital Signs

Temperature. Changes in the body's temperature regulatory mechanism leave older adults less likely to have fever but at greater risk for hypothermia. Thus the temperature is a less reliable index of the older patient's true health state. Sweat gland activity is also diminished.

Pulse. The normal range of heart rate is 60 to 100 bpm, but the rhythm may be slightly irregular. The radial artery may feel stiff, rigid, and tortuous in an older patient, although this condition does not necessarily imply vascular disease in the heart or brain. The increasingly rigid arterial wall needs a faster upstroke of blood, and so the pulse is actually easier to palpate.

Respirations. Aging causes a decrease in vital capacity and a decrease in inspiratory reserve volume. You may note a shallower inspiratory phase and an increased respiratory rate.

Blood Pressure. The aorta and major arteries tend to harden with age. As the heart pumps against a stiffer aorta, the systolic pressure increases, causing pulse pressure to increase (Figure 10-18 lists mean BP readings in apparently healthy persons from birth to older age). With many older people, both the systolic and diastolic pressures increase, which makes it difficult to distinguish normal aging values from abnormal hypertension.

Objective Data

Normal Range of Findings   **Abnormal Findings**

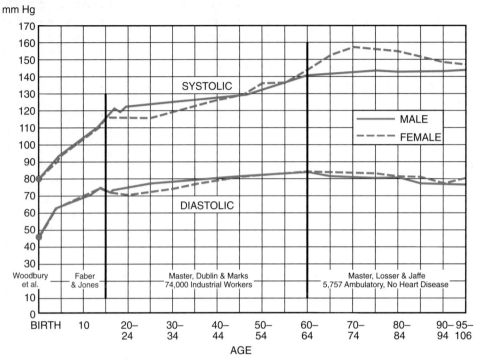

10-18   Mean blood pressure readings in apparently healthy people, birth to older age.

SPECIAL CONSIDERATIONS FOR ADVANCED PRACTICE

Normal Range of Findings   **Abnormal Findings**

Carotid Compression

Compression of both carotid arteries at the same time results in compromise of blood flow to the brain and is **never done** by any nonauthorized practitioner. It can also stimulate the cranial nerve X (vagus nerve), which causes the patient's heart rate to drop rapidly and the eventual loss of consciousness. The "carotid rub or massage" is a manoeuvre executed by cardiologists and clinicians with expertise in the area. In this manoeuvre, the practitioner rubs *only one* carotid artery at a time to slow down rapid irregular heart rates in patients with these identified cardiac considerations. Please keep in mind that this manoeuvre is *not* in the scope of practice of nurses without advanced practice credentials.

The Doppler Technique

In many situations, pulse and BP measurement are enhanced by use of an electronic device, the *Doppler ultrasonic flowmeter*. The Doppler technique works by a principle discovered in the nineteenth century by an Austrian physicist, Johannes Doppler. Sound varies in pitch in relation to the distance between the sound source and the listener; the pitch is higher when the distance is short, and the pitch lowers as the distance increases. Think of a railroad train speeding toward you: the pitch of its train whistle sounds higher the closer it gets, and the pitch of the whistle lowers as the train moves away.

Normal Range of Findings	Abnormal Findings

In this case, the sound source is the blood pumping through the artery in a rhythmic manner. A handheld transducer picks up changes in sound frequency and amplifies them as the blood flows and ebbs. The listener hears a whooshing pulsatile beat.

The Doppler technique is used to locate the peripheral pulse sites (see Chapter 21 for further discussion of this technique). For BP measurement, the Doppler technique augments Korotkoff's sounds (Figure 10-19). Through this technique, you can evaluate sounds that are hard to hear with a stethoscope, such as those in critically ill individuals with a low BP, in infants with small arms, and in obese patients in whom the sounds are muffled by layers of fat. Also, proper cuff placement is difficult on an obese patient's cone-shaped upper arm. In this situation, you can place the cuff on the more even forearm and hold the Doppler probe over the radial artery. For either location, use the following procedure:

- Apply coupling gel to the transducer probe.
- Turn the Doppler flowmeter on.
- Touch the probe to the skin, holding the probe perpendicular to the artery.
- A pulsatile whooshing sound indicates location of the artery. You may need to rotate the probe, but maintain contact with the skin. Do not push the probe too hard or you will obliterate the pulse.
- Inflate the cuff until the sounds disappear; then inflate by another 20 to 30 mm Hg beyond that point.
- Slowly deflate the cuff, noting the point at which the first whooshing sounds appear. This is the systolic pressure.
- It is difficult to hear the muffling of sounds or a reliable disappearance of sounds that indicates the diastolic pressure (phases IV and V of Korotkoff's sounds). However, the systolic pressure alone is valuable data about the level of tissue perfusion and about blood flow through patent vessels.

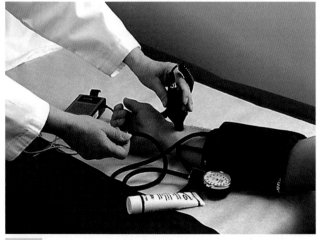

10-19

Special Considerations for Advanced Practice

Normal Range of Findings	Abnormal Findings

The Thigh Pressure

When BP measured at the arm is excessively high, particularly in adolescents and young adults, compare it with the thigh pressure to check for **coarctation** of the aorta (a congenital form of narrowing). Normally, the *thigh pressure is higher* than the pressure in the arm. If possible, turn the patient onto the prone position (on the abdomen). (If the patient must remain in the supine position, bend the knee slightly.) Wrap a large cuff, 18 to 20 cm, around the lower third of the thigh, centred over the popliteal artery on the back of the knee. Auscultate the popliteal artery for the reading (Figure 10-20). Normally, the systolic value is 10 to 40 mm Hg higher in the thigh than in the arm, and the diastolic pressures are the same.

With **coarctation of the aorta**, arm pressures are high. Thigh pressure is *lower* because the blood supply to the thigh is below the constriction.

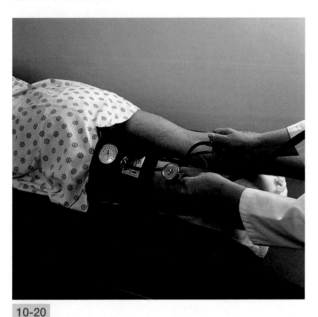

10-20

PROMOTING A HEALTHY LIFESTYLE

Health and Self-Care

As you measure height and weight and record vital signs, it is a good time to begin a teaching plan to help the patient keep these physical signs within normal limits. CHEP considers the following **health behaviours** to be the foundation of hypertension control. Even if your patient is normotensive and the body weight is within normal limits, the following recommendations help keep blood pressure (BP) under control (CHEP, 2011):

- Lose weight, if you are more than 10% above ideal weight.
- Limit alcohol intake to no more than two drinks a day: a regular-sized bottle or can of beer, 45 mL (1.5 oz) of hard liquor, or 300 mL (10.5 oz) of wine.
- Get regular aerobic exercise (e.g., a 30- to 45-minute brisk walk) most days of the week.
- Cut sodium intake from the average 3100 mg/day to less than 1500 mg/day. The recommended adequate intake for sodium is 1200 to 1500 mg for healthy adults and decreases with age.

- Include the recommended daily allowances of potassium, calcium, and magnesium in your diet.
- Stop smoking.
- Reduce dietary saturated fat and cholesterol.

Because more than 22 million visits are made to Canadian health care providers annually to manage and diagnose hypertension, CHEP recommends that the diagnosis of hypertension be expedited to ensure early intervention. See Figure 10-21 for recommendations for management. These recommendations establish a protocol for early detection; hypertension is diagnosed within one to five visits. The practice of accepting self-administered/home BP measurements has sped up the process of diagnosis significantly. Ambulatory BP monitors (ABPMs) are useful for determining readings outside the office setting for patients with suspected office-induced hypertension.

CHEP, Canadian Hypertension Education Program.

Special Considerations for Advanced Practice

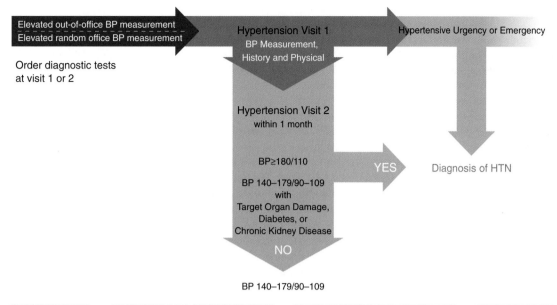

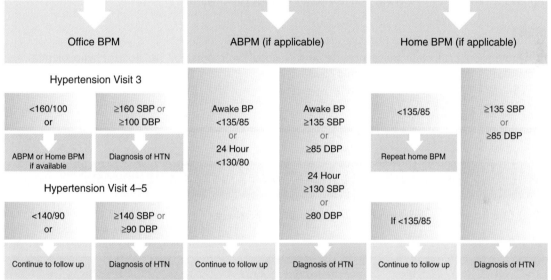

10-21   Canadian recommendations for the assessment of hypertensive patients.

Documentation &
Critical Thinking

DOCUMENTATION AND CRITICAL THINKING

Sample Charting

A. J. is a 47-year-old female African Canadian high school principal; well nourished and well developed; appears stated age. Alert, oriented, and cooperative, with no signs of acute distress. Ht, 163 cm [5 feet 4 inches]; Wt, 57 kg [126 lbs]; temp, 37°C-76-14; BP, 146/84 right arm, sitting.

Focused Assessment: Clinical Case Study*

Mrs. Grazia S. is a 76-year-old female Hispanic retired secretary, in previous good health, who is brought to the emergency department by her 83-year-old husband. Both have been ill during the night with nausea, vomiting, abdominal pain, and diarrhea, which they attribute to eating "bad food" at a buffet-style restaurant the night before. Mr. S.'s condition improved during the next day, but Mrs. S.'s is worse, with severe vomiting, diarrhea, weakness, dizziness, and abdominal pain.

*Please note that space does not allow for the inclusion of a detailed plan for each clinical case study in this text. Please consult the appropriate text for current treatment plan.

SUBJECTIVE

- Extreme fatigue. Weakness and dizziness occur whenever patient tries to sit or stand up: "Feels like I'm going to black out." Severe nausea and vomiting, thirsty but cannot keep anything down; even sips of water result in "dry heaves." Abdominal pain is moderate aching, intermittent. Diarrhea is watery brown stool, profuse during the night, somewhat diminished now.

OBJECTIVE

Helped to seated, leg-dangling position; vital signs: BP, 74/52; pulse, 138, regular rhythm; respirations, 20. Skin pale and moist (diaphoretic).

Reports being lightheaded and dizzy in seated position. Returned to supine.

Vital Signs. Temp, 37.2°C; BP (supine), 102/64; pulse (supine), 70, regular rhythm; respirations, 18.

Respiratory. Breath sounds clear in all fields; no adventitious sounds.

Cardiovascular. Regular rate (70 bpm) and rhythm when supine, S_1 and S_2 are not accentuated or diminished, no extra sounds. All pulses present, 2+ and equal bilaterally. Carotid pulses 2+ with no carotid bruit.

Abdominal. Bowel sounds hyperactive, skin pale and moist, abdomen soft and mildly tender to palpation. No enlargement of liver or spleen.

Neurological. Level of consciousness: alert and oriented; pupils equal, round, reactive to light and accommodation. Sensory status normal. Mild weakness in arms and legs. Gait and standing leg strength not tested due to inability to stand. Deep tendon reflexes 2+ and equal bilaterally. Babinski reflex → toes curl inward.

ASSESSMENT

Orthostatic hypotension, orthostatic pulse increase, and syncopal symptoms, R/T [related to] hypovolemia
Diarrhea, possibly R/T ingestion of contaminated food
Risk for hyperthermia, R/T dehydration and aging
Deficient fluid volume

ABNORMAL FINDINGS

Tables 10-5 and 10-6 list abnormalities in physique and in BP, respectively.

TABLE 10-5   Abnormalities in Body Height and Proportion

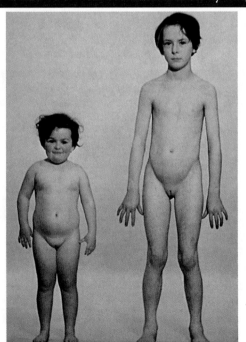

◄ **HYPOPITUITARY DWARFISM**

Deficiency in growth hormone in childhood results in retardation of growth below the third percentile, delayed puberty, hypothyroidism, and adrenal insufficiency. The 9-year-old girl at left appears much younger than her chronological age, with infantile facial features and chubbiness. The age-matched girl at right shows increased height, more mature facies, and loss of infantile fat.

TABLE 10-5   Abnormalities in Body Height and Proportion—cont'd

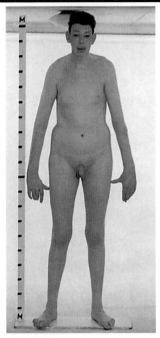

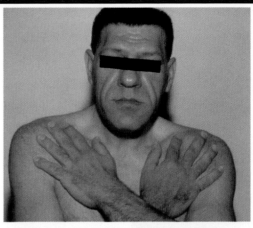

ACROMEGALY (HYPERPITUITARISM)

Excessive secretion of growth hormone in adulthood, after normal completion of body growth, causes overgrowth of bone in the face, head, hands, and feet but no change in height. Internal organs also enlarge, which may result in cardiomegaly or hepatomegaly.

GIGANTISM

Excessive secretion of growth hormone by the anterior pituitary results in overgrowth of entire body. When this occurs during childhood before closure of bone epiphyses in puberty, it causes increased height (here 2.09 m, or 6 ft 9 in) and in weight and delay in sexual development.

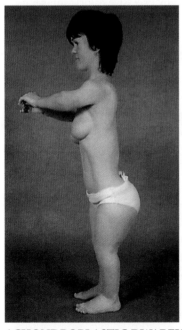

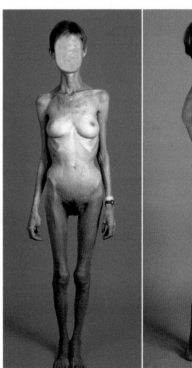

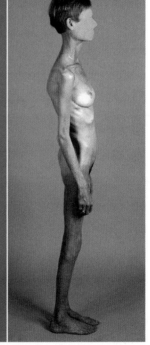

ACHONDROPLASTIC DWARFISM

Congenital skeletal malformation caused by a genetic disorder in converting cartilage to bone. Characterized by relatively large head with frontal bossing and midplace hypoplasia, short stature, and short limbs, and often thoracic kyphosis, prominent lumbar lordosis, and abdominal protrusion. The mean adult height is approximately 131.5 cm (51.8 inches) in men and approximately 125 cm (49.2 inches) in women.

ANOREXIA NERVOSA

A serious psychological disorder characterized by severe and life-threatening weight loss and amenorrhea in an otherwise healthy adolescent or young adult. Behaviour is characterized by fanatic concern about weight, aversion to food, distorted body image (perceives self as fat despite skeletal appearance), starvation diets, frenetic exercise patterns, and striving for perfection.

Continued

TABLE 10-5   Abnormalities in Body Height and Proportion—cont'd

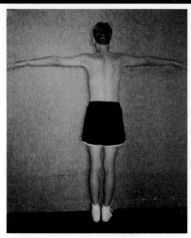

MARFAN'S SYNDROME

Michael Phelps, Niccolò Paganini, and Sergei
  Rachmaninoff are thought to have had this inherited
  connective tissue disorder, characterized by tall, thin
  stature (greater than ninety-fifth percentile),
  arachnodactyly (long, thin fingers), hyperextensible
  joints, arm span greater than height, pubis-to-sole
  measurement exceeding crown-to-pubis measurement,
  sternal deformity, high-arched narrow palate, and pes
  planus. Early morbidity and mortality occur as a result of
  cardiovascular complications such as mitral regurgitation
  and aortic dissection.

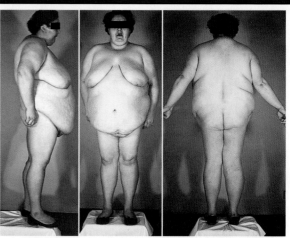

ENDOGENOUS OBESITY: CUSHING'S SYNDROME

Excessive amounts of adrenocorticotropic hormone
  (ACTH)—either administered or produced by the
  pituitary gland—stimulates the adrenal cortex to secrete
  excess cortisol. This causes Cushing's syndrome,
  characterized by weight gain and edema with central
  trunk and cervical obesity ("buffalo hump") and round
  plethoric face ("moon facies"). Excessive catabolism
  causes muscle wasting; weakness; thinness of arms and
  legs; reduced height; and thinning and fragility of skin
  with purple abdominal striae, bruising, and acne. The
  obesity in this condition is markedly different from
  exogenous obesity caused by excessive caloric intake, in
  which body fat is evenly distributed and muscle strength
  is intact.

TABLE 10-6   Abnormalities in Blood Pressure

HYPOTENSION

In normotensive adults: <95/60
In hypertensive adults: < the patient's average reading, but >95/60
In children: < expected value for age

Occurs With	Reason
Acute myocardial infarction	Decreased cardiac output
Shock	Decreased cardiac output
Hemorrhage	Decrease in total blood volume
Vasodilation	Decrease in peripheral vascular resistance
Addison's disease (hypofunction of adrenal glands)	Decrease in aldosterone production

ASSOCIATED SYMPTOMS AND SIGNS

In conditions of decreased cardiac output, low blood pressure is accompanied by faster pulse, dizziness, diaphoresis,
  confusion, and blurred vision. The skin feels cool and clammy because the superficial blood vessels constrict to shunt
  blood to the vital organs. An individual having an acute myocardial infarction may also complain of crushing substernal
  chest pain, high epigastric pain, and shoulder or jaw pain.

HYPERTENSION

Essential or Primary Hypertension

This has no known cause but is responsible for about 95% of cases of hypertension in adults.

TABLE 10-6	Abnormalities in Blood Pressure—cont'd

Cardiovascular Risk Stratification in Patients With Hypertension

Major Risk Factors	Target Organ Damage/Clinical Cardiovascular Disease
Smoking	Heart diseases
Dyslipidemia	Left ventricular atrophy
Diabetes mellitus	Angina or prior myocardial infarction
Age >60 yr	Prior coronary revascularization
Gender (men and postmenopausal women)	Heart failure
Family history of cardiovascular disease: women aged <65 yr or men aged <55 yr	Stroke or transient ischemic attack
	Nephropathy
	Peripheral arterial disease
	Retinopathy

Lifestyle Modifications for Hypertension Prevention and Management

- Lose weight if overweight
- Limit alcohol intake to no more than two drinks a day or less: a regular-sized bottle or can of beer, 45 mL (1.5 oz) of hard liquor, or 300 mL (10.5 oz) of wine
- Increase aerobic physical activity (30–45 min most days of the week)
- Reduce sodium intake to no more than 1500 mg/day
- Maintain adequate intake of dietary potassium (approximately 90 mmol/L/day)
- Maintain adequate intake of dietary calcium and magnesium for general health
- Stop smoking, and reduce intake of dietary saturated fat and cholesterol for overall cardiovascular health

Abnormal Findings

REFERENCES

Bliss-Holtz, J. (1995). Methods of newborn infant temperature monitoring: A research review. *Issues in Comprehensive Pediatric Nursing, 18,* 287–298.

Canadian Hypertension Education Program. (2011). *Canadian recommendations for the management of hypertension.* Retrieved from *http://www.hypertension.ca/images/stories/dls/2011gl/CHEPbooklet_2011.pdf.*

Canadian Paediatric Society. (2011). *CPS position statement: Temperature measurement in paediatrics.* Retrieved from *http://www.cps.ca/english/statements/cp/cp00-01.htm.*

Centers for Disease Control and Prevention. (2011). *What is a BMI percentile?* Atlanta, GA: National Center for Health Statistics in collaboration with the National Center for Chronic Disease Prevention and Health Promotion. Retrieved from *http://www.cdc.gov/healthyweight/assessing/bmi/childrens_bmi/about_childrens_bmi.html#What is BMI percentile.*

Chobanian, A. V., Bakris, G. L., Black, H. R., Cushman, W. C., Green, L. A., Izzo, J. L., Jr., ... National High Blood Pressure Education Program Coordinating Committee. (2003). The seventh report of the Joint National Committee on Prevention, Detection, Evaluation and Treatment of High Blood Pressure: The JNC 7 report. *Journal of the American Medical Association, 289,* 2560–2572.

Cusson, R. M., Madonia, J. A., & Taekmen, J. B. (1997). The effect of environment on body site temperatures in full-term neonates. *Nursing Research, 46,* 202–207.

Grap, M. J. (2002). Pulse oximetry. *Critical Care Nurse, 22*(3), 69.

Health Canada. (2003). *Canadian guidelines for body weight classifications in adults (Catalogue No. H49-179/2003E).* Ottawa: Author.

Jean-Mary, M. B., Dicanzio, J., Shaw, J., & Bernstein, H. H. (2002). Limited accuracy and reliability of infrared axillary and aural thermometers in a pediatric outpatient population. *Journal of Pediatrics, 141,* 671–676.

Nimah, M. M., Bshesh, K., Callahan, J. D., & Jacobs, B. R. (2006). Infrared tympanic thermometry in comparison with other temperature measurement techniques in febrile children. *Pediatric Critical Care Medicine, 7*(1), 48–55.

Rodrigues, S., Robinson, E. J., Kramer, M. S., & Gray-MacDonald, K. (2000). High rates of infant macrosomia: A comparison of a Canadian native and non-native population. *Journal of Nutrition, 130,* 806–812.

World Health Organization. (2000). *Obesity: Preventing and managing the global epidemic: Report of a WHO consultation on obesity.* Geneva, Switzerland: Author.

World Health Organization. (2011). BMI classification. Retrieved from *http://www.who.int/bmi/index.jsp?introPage=intro_3.html.*

CHAPTER

11

Pain Assessment

Written by Carolyn Jarvis, PhD, APN, CNP
Adapted by Lynn Haslam, RN(EC), MN, NP-Adult

evolve WEBSITE

http://evolve.elsevier.com/Canada/Jarvis/examination/

- Case Study:
  - Pain of Unknown Origin
- Examination Review Questions
- Key Points
- Quick Assessments for Common Conditions:
  - Sepsis
  - Sickle Cell Anemia

OUTLINE

STRUCTURE AND FUNCTION

NEUROANATOMICAL PATHWAY

Pain is a highly complex and subjective experience that originates from the central nervous system (CNS), the peripheral nervous system, or both. Specialized nerve endings called **nociceptors** detect painful sensations from the periphery and transmit them to the CNS. Nociceptors are located within the skin; connective tissue; muscle; and thoracic, abdominal, and pelvic viscera. These nociceptors can be stimulated directly by trauma or injury or secondarily by chemical mediators that are released from the site of tissue damage.

Nociceptors carry the pain signal to the CNS by two primary sensory (or afferent) fibres: **Aδ** and **C fibres** (Figure 11-1). Aδ fibres are myelinated and larger in diameter, and they transmit the pain signal rapidly to the CNS. Very localized, short-term, and sharp sensations result from Aδ fibre stimulation. In contrast, C fibres are unmyelinated and smaller, and they transmit the signal more slowly, which results in a diffuse and aching sensation.

Peripheral sensory Aδ and C fibres enter the spinal cord by posterior nerve roots within the dorsal horn by the tract of Lissauer. The fibres synapse with **interneurons** located

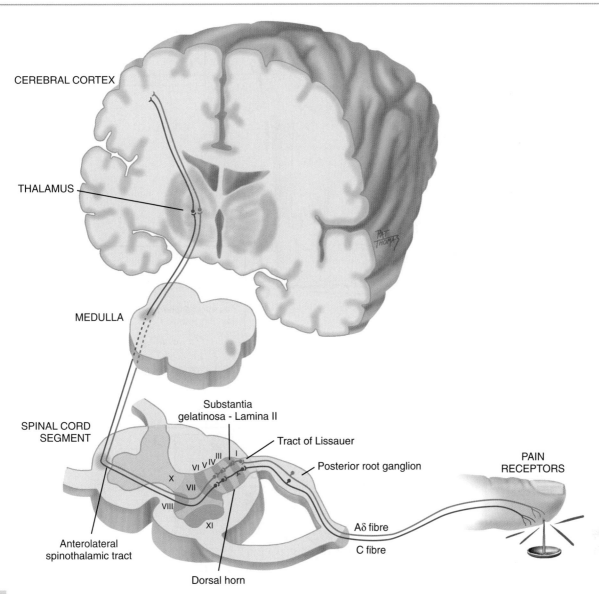

CEREBRAL CORTEX

THALAMUS

MEDULLA

SPINAL CORD
SEGMENT

Substantia
gelatinosa - Lamina II

Tract of Lissauer

Posterior root ganglion

PAIN
RECEPTORS

Aδ fibre

C fibre

Anterolateral
spinothalamic tract

Dorsal horn

11-1

within a specified area of the cord called the **substantia gelatinosa.** A cross-section shows that the grey matter of the spinal cord is divided into a series of consecutively numbered laminae (layers of nerve cells; see Figure 11-1). The substantia gelatinosa is lamina II, which receives sensory input from various areas of the body. The pain signals then cross over to the other side of the spinal cord and ascend to the brain by the **anterolateral spinothalamic tract.**

NOCICEPTION

Nociception is the term used to describe how noxious stimuli are typically perceived as pain. Nociception can be divided into four phases: (a) transduction, (b) transmission, (c) perception, and (d) modulation (Figure 11-2).

The first phase, **transduction,** occurs when a noxious stimulus in the form of traumatic or chemical injury, burn, incision, or tumour growth occurs in the periphery. These injured tissues then release a variety of chemicals (neurotransmitters), including substance P, histamine, prostaglandins, serotonin, and bradykinin. The neurotransmitters propagate a pain message, or action potential, along sensory afferent nerve fibres to the spinal cord. These nerve fibres terminate in the dorsal horn of the spinal cord. Because the initial afferent fibres stop in the dorsal horn, a second set of neurotransmitters carries the pain impulse across the synaptic cleft to the dorsal horn neurons. These neurotransmitters include substance P, glutamate, and adenosine triphosphate.

In the second phase, **transmission,** the pain impulse moves from the level of the spinal cord to the brain. Within the spinal cord, at the site of the synaptic cleft, are opioid receptors that can block this pain signalling with endogenous or exogenous opioids. However, if left uninterrupted, the pain impulse moves to the brain via various ascending fibres within the spinothalamic tract that terminate in the brain stem and thalamus. Once the pain impulse moves through the thalamus, the message is dispersed to higher cortical areas via mechanisms that are currently not clearly understood.

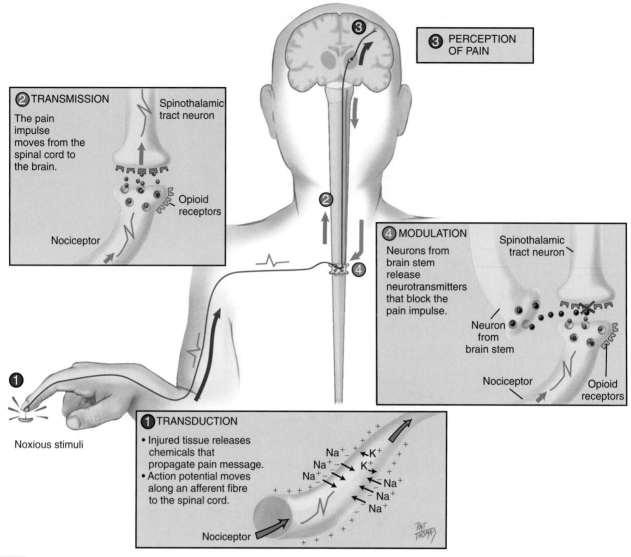

②TRANSMISSION

The pain impulse moves from the spinal cord to the brain.

Spinothalamic tract neuron

Opioid receptors

Nociceptor

③ PERCEPTION OF PAIN

④ MODULATION

Neurons from brain stem release neurotransmitters that block the pain impulse.

Spinothalamic tract neuron

Neuron from brain stem

Nociceptor

Opioid receptors

Noxious stimuli

①TRANSDUCTION

• Injured tissue releases chemicals that propagate pain message.
• Action potential moves along an afferent fibre to the spinal cord.

Na^+ K^+
Na^+ K^+
Na^+ Na^+
Na^+
Na^+

Nociceptor

11-2

The third phase, **perception,** is the conscious awareness of a painful sensation. Cortical structures such as the limbic system account for the emotional response to pain, and somatosensory areas can characterize the sensation. Only when the noxious stimuli are interpreted in these higher cortical structures can this sensation be identified as pain.

Lastly, the pain message is inhibited through the phase of **modulation.** Descending pathways from the brain stem to the spinal cord produce a third set of neurotransmitters that slow down or impede the pain impulse, producing an analgesic effect. These neurotransmitters include serotonin; norepinephrine; neurotensin; γ-aminobutyric acid (GABA); and our own endogenous opioids, β-endorphins, enkephalins, and dynorphins.

SOURCES OF PAIN

Pain is based on its origin, classified as nociceptive, neuropathic, or both. **Nociceptive pain** is caused by tissue injury. It is well-localized and often described as aching or throbbing. Nociceptive pain can be further classified as somatic or visceral. **Somatic** nociceptive pain can be superficial (superficial somatic or cutaneous pain), derived from skin surface and subcutaneous tissues, or deep (deep somatic pain), derived from joints, tendons, muscles, or bone. **Visceral** pain originates from the larger interior organs (e.g., kidney, intestine, gallbladder, and pancreas). The pain can stem from direct injury to the organ or from stretching of the organ as a result of tumour, ischemia, distension, or severe contraction. Visceral pain can be constant or intermittent, and it may be poorly localized or referred to another area of the body. Examples of conditions that cause visceral pain include ureteral colic, acute appendicitis, and pancreatitis.

Neuropathic pain is caused directly by a lesion or a disease affecting the somatosensory nervous system (Treede et al., 2008). Neuropathic pain can result from damage to the nerve pathway at any point along the nerve, from the terminals of the peripheral nociceptors to the cortical neurons in the brain. Examples of neuropathic pain may include pain caused by direct nerve trauma (spinal cord injury), infectious diseases (herpes zoster, human immunodeficiency virus infection), or metabolic problems (diabetes), or it may be drug induced (chemotherapy, antiretroviral therapy; Gold et al., 2006).

Neuropathic pain can be described as burning, shooting, or lancinating, often intensifying at night. Although affected patients may have an identical underlying cause, neuropathic pain manifestations vary between patients.

Referred pain originates in one location but is felt at another site. Both sites are innervated by the same spinal nerve, and it is difficult for the brain to differentiate the point of origin. For example, when the appendix (in the right lower quadrant of the abdomen) is inflamed, pain may be felt in the periumbilical area. It is useful to have knowledge of areas of commonly referred pain (see Table 22-2, p. 577).

TYPES OF PAIN (BY DURATION)

Acute pain is short term and self-limiting, follows a predictable trajectory, and dissipates after an injury heals. Examples of acute pain include that caused by surgery, trauma, and kidney stones. Acute pain serves a self-protective purpose: It warns of actual or potential tissue damage.

In contrast, **persistent pain** (or **chronic pain**) is defined as pain that has been present for 6 months or longer than the time of expected tissue healing (Jovey et al., 2003). Persistent pain can be categorized as malignant (cancer-related pain) or nonmalignant.

Malignant pain often parallels the pathological process created by the tumour cells. The pain is induced by tissue necrosis or stretching of an organ by the growing tumour. The severity of the pain fluctuates within the course of the disease.

Persistent nonmalignant pain is often associated with musculoskeletal conditions, such as arthritis, low back pain, and fibromyalgia. Research findings have demonstrated that unrelieved acute pain can lead to persistent pain through two processes: peripheral and central sensitization. Peripheral sensitization is the reduction of the pain threshold and an increased response of the peripheral end of the nociceptors. Central sensitization is an increase in excitability of neurons within the CNS (Kehlet, Jensen, & Woolf, 2006).

 DEVELOPMENTAL CONSIDERATIONS

Infants and Young Children

Infants have the same capacity for pain as do adults. By 20 weeks' gestation, ascending fibres, neurotransmitters, and the cerebral cortex are developed and functioning to the extent that the fetus is capable of feeling pain (Anand, 1993). Inhibitory neurotransmitters are in insufficient supply until birth at full term, which renders preterm infants more sensitive to painful stimuli.

The persistent belief that preverbal infants do not remember pain places them at higher risk for undertreatment of pain. Research indicates that repetitive and poorly controlled pain (e.g., daily heel sticks, venipunctures) can result in

lifelong adverse consequences, such as neurodevelopmental problems, poor weight gain, learning disabilities, psychiatric disorders, and alcoholism (Anand, 2000). Toddlers and children older than 2 years of age can report pain and point to its location but are unable to rate pain intensity. It is helpful to ask the parent or caregiver what words their child uses to report pain (e.g., "boo-boo," "owie"). Be aware that some children will try to act "grown up and brave" and often deny having pain in the presence of a stranger, or if they are fearful of receiving a "shot."

Older Adults

No evidence exists to suggest that older individuals perceive pain to a lesser degree or that sensitivity is diminished with age. Although pain is a common experience among older individuals, it is *not* a normal process of aging. Pain indicates disease or injury. Older adults may express fears about becoming dependent or perceive that they are taking an excessive number of medications. Active listening is the route to understanding the underlying fears that an older patient may have. You should consider the fact that older adults may need more time to respond to an assessment question. The incidence of persistent pain conditions is higher in the older adult population; such conditions include diseases such as arthritis, osteoarthritis, osteoporosis, peripheral vascular disease, peripheral neuropathies, and angina.

Gender Differences

There are gender differences in prevalence rates across painful conditions. Women are more likely to experience migraines with aura, fibromyalgia, irritable bowel syndrome, and rheumatoid arthritis. Men are more likely to experience cluster headaches, gout, coronary artery disease, and duodenal ulcers (International Association for the Study of Pain, 2007). According to findings from the Human Genome Project, genetic differences between the sexes may account for the differences in pain perception (Mogil, 2002). The pharmacological treatments for pain, and the related side effects, may not yield the same effects in both genders.

 CULTURAL AND SOCIAL CONSIDERATIONS

Ethnocultural variations are described in Chapter 3. To enhance ethnocultural sensitivity, health care providers need to work with patients and their families so that mutual goals are identified and the patients' understanding and beliefs about pain are taken into account (McCaffery & Pasero, 1999). The following are questions you can ask to assess an individual's beliefs about pain (Lasch, 2000):
- Do you have any fears about your pain or pain management options? If so, what do you fear most?
- What traditional remedies have you tried to help you with your pain?
- How do you usually behave when you are in pain? How would other people know you are in pain?
- How do you usually describe your pain?

- What does this pain mean to you? Why do you think you are having pain?
- Who, if anyone, in your family do you talk to about your pain? What is their understanding of your pain? What do you want them to know?
- Do you have family and friends who help you because of your pain? If so, who helps you?

TIMING OF THE PAIN ASSESSMENT

Nurses play a pivotal role in pain management by using current knowledge about pain assessment and relief measures. The ability to measure pain is an important component of a comprehensive or focused assessment. The assessment of pain must be timely, and you must identify variables that are creating or augmenting the pain experience. Rather than signifying a single event, pain assessment is an ongoing process. Pain is regarded as "the fifth vital sign"; thus a pain assessment should be incorporated when other vital signs are assessed. Similarly, pain should be reassessed at suitable intervals after each pharmacological or nonpharmacological intervention (e.g., 15 to 30 minutes after parenteral administration of drug therapy and 1 hour after oral administration).

The acuity of the patient's condition dictates what type of pain assessment you will conduct. For example, if you are in a health promotion type of role, or when you assess persistent pain, a comprehensive pain assessment—for example, the Brief Pain Inventory—is appropriate. In an acutely ill hospitalized patient who requires more frequent pain assessments, you would conduct a focused pain assessment with a specific tool, such as the Numerical Rating Scale or the Visual Analogue Scale. See the Critical Findings box.

CRITICAL FINDINGS

A more comprehensive assessment should be completed when the patient's pain changes notably from previous findings; sudden changes in pain may signify an underlying pathological process. Nurses at the advanced practice level (for example, Acute Pain Service nurses) often conduct comprehensive pain assessments on acutely ill patients, especially if the patient has acute or persistent pain or is undergoing multiple surgeries, to help determine the effectiveness of interventions.

SUBJECTIVE DATA

"Pain is whatever the experiencing person says it is, existing whenever he says it does" (McCaffery, 1968, p. 95). Since pain is a subjective experience, the self-report of pain is the most reliable indicator that an individual is experiencing pain. Complex physiological, genetic, and psychosocial factors contribute to the conversion of neurochemical activity to the pain experience, the individual's reaction to the painful sensation, and any related changes to an individual's mood and behaviour (Kehlet et al., 2006). Optimal use of assessment tools involves engaging the patient and the health care provider. See the box Promoting a Healthy Lifestyle: Keeping the WHO in Mind.

PROMOTING A HEALTHY LIFESTYLE: KEEPING THE WHO IN MIND

Understanding the Pain Ladder

Nurses not only play a key role in pain assessment but also devise front-line intervention plans for optimal pain management. You must understand key elements about treating pain. On the basis of the patient's report, efforts should be directed at reducing or eliminating the pain with appropriate pharmacological and non-pharmacological interventions.

Pharmacological Interventions

Nonopioid analgesics are medications such as acetaminophen and anti-inflammatory drugs.

Acetaminophen has an effect on the CNS, but the mechanism of action is not well understood. Acetaminophen is often an unrecognized player in the pain management plan. Many drugs are combined with acetaminophen to achieve a synergistic effect (Percocet, which is acetaminophen and oxycodone; Tylenol 1, 2,

and 3, which is acetaminophen with varying amounts of codeine; and Tramacet, which is paracetamol and tramadol). It is well tolerated; however, the maximum daily dose in a healthy patient should not exceed 4 g/day from all sources combined. The maximum daily dosage is best decreased for older patients and for those with impaired liver function.

A large portion of the anti-inflammatory effect is within the peripheral receptors (site of injury). Anti-inflammatory agents (ibuprofen, naproxen), which are readily available over the counter without a prescription, are generally used for muscular aches, headaches, and menstrual cramp pain. In the acute setting, they are often used to help manage postoperative pain. However, this class of drug is not free of side effects, and these drugs must be administered with caution to patients with a history of renal insufficiency, gastrointestinal bleeding, or cardiac disease and in patients about to undergo surgery because they affect clotting ability.

PROMOTING A HEALTHY LIFESTYLE: KEEPING THE WHO IN MIND—cont'd

Opioids relieve pain primarily by action in the CNS, binding to opioid receptor sites. There is no "ceiling" dose for opioids; therapy starts at a low dosage, which is titrated to effect. All opioids work similarly, but the strength may differ (for example, hydromorphone is five times stronger than morphine; therefore, the hydromorphone dose would be much lower). This concept is referred to as **equianalgesia** (a dose of one opioid whose pain-relieving effects are equivalent to a dose of another opioid). No opioids are safer than others; all opioids have similar side effects. Patients taking opioids should be assessed for respiratory rate, level of consciousness, and sedation.

Local anaesthetics (peripheral nerve blocks, epidural blocks) can help block the transmission of pain to the periphery, causing "numbness."

The World Health Organization (WHO) developed a pain management ladder for patients experiencing cancer pain; this model has also been adopted for chronic pain. When patients present with pain, management starts at the bottom of the ladder, with nonopioid analgesics (such as acetaminophen), anti-inflammatory drugs, or both. As pain progresses, so too should the treatment therapy. Most people in the hospital start on the second step, with opioids. Those on the second step should also receive adjunctive therapy with acetaminophen or anti-inflammatory drugs, or both. This method of pain management is often referred to as **multi-modal analgesia.**

Patients with chronic pain may also be taking many other adjunctive therapy medications, including, but not limited to, gabapentinoids (gabapentin, pregabalin), tricyclic antidepressants (amitriptyline, nortriptyline), and other opioids such as cannabinoid and methadone.

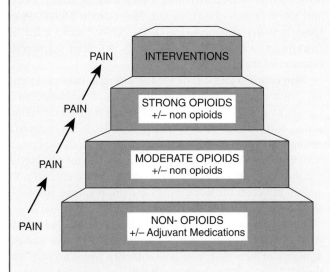

Nonpharmacological Interventions

Nurses also have a key role to play in advocating for nonpharmacological interventions in the management of pain.

Heat/Ice

The application of ice or heat to relieve pain is a simple but effective tool. Heat can help relax muscles, decrease spasm, and decrease muscle tightness.

Transcutaneous Electric Nerve Stimulation

Transcutaneous electric nerve stimulation (TENS) has been shown to be effective in the some acute pain episodes (labour and delivery, postsurgical pain). TENS has also been found to be effective in many conditions involving persistent pain, such as neuropathic pain, rheumatoid arthritis, and osteoarthritis.

Massage Therapy

Massage can be an important component in the management of persistent pain. Results of some studies have suggested that massage in the acute phase (Mitchinson, 2007) can help to decrease pain intensity and pain unpleasantness and to decrease anxiety. Massage therapy can help relieve muscle and soft tissue pain.

Physiotherapy

Many persistent pain syndromes in neurological disorders (e.g., stroke, multiple sclerosis, Parkinson's disease) may be alleviated by implementation of physiotherapy such as hydrotherapy, repositioning, active stretching, and raising limbs, as well as passive range-of-motion exercises (World Health Organization, 2006).

Pediatric Strategies

Pediatric nursing often involves potentially painful procedures. Nurses and parents can work together to optimize pain management. In addition to appropriate pharmacological interventions, physical interventions may also include the application of heat or ice, deep breathing, and distraction with activities such as bubble blowing or magic wands, musical toys, books, and video games. Ideally, the techniques should be taught and practised before the procedure, to allow the child to focus on the activity.

There are many other complementary therapies that patients with persistent pain may use. A part of the nursing assessment is to inquire about other therapies that patients may find of benefit and, when possible, to advocate for implementation of these therapies into the pain management plan.

References

Mitchinson, A., Kim, H., Rosenberg, J., Geisser, M., Kirsh, M., Cikrit, D., & Hinshaw, D. (2007). Acute postoperative pain management using massage as an adjuvant therapy: A randomized trial. Archives of Surgery, 142(12), 1158–1167.

World Health Organization (WHO). (2006). Neurological disorders: Public health challenges. In Pain associated with neurological disorders (Chapter 37). Geneva, Switzerland: Author.

Additional Resources

Adams, M., Holland, L., Bostwick, P., & King, S. (2010). Pharmacology for nurses: A pathophysiological approach (Canadian Edition). Toronto: Pearson Education Canada.

Hattan, J., King, L., & Griffiths, P. (2002). The impact of foot massage and guided relaxation following cardiac surgery. Journal of Advanced Nursing, 37(2), 199–207.

Registered Nurses Association of Ontario. (2007). Best practice guideline: Assessment and management of pain. Toronto: Author.

Rudkin, G. E., & Rudkin, A. K. (2005). Ambulatory surgery acute pain management: A review of the evidence. Acute Pain, 7, 41–49.

CNS, central nervous system.

Subjective Data

Examiner Asks	Rationale

INITIAL PAIN ASSESSMENT (PQRSTU)

1. **P: provocative or palliative**
   Does your pain increase with movement or activity?
   Are the symptoms relieved with rest?
   Were any previous treatments effective?

   To identify quality of pain and differentiate between nociceptive and neuropathic pain mechanisms; to identify alleviating and aggravating factors; and to evaluate effectiveness of current treatment

2. **Q: quality of the pain**
   What does your pain feel like?
   What words describe your pain?

   To identify mechanism of pain (terms such as "throbbing," "aching," "shooting," and "dull" may provide clues)

3. **R: region of the body/radiation**
   Where is your pain?
   Does the pain radiate, or move to other areas?

   To identify one or more areas of the body that are affected by pain, inasmuch as there may be several

4. **S: severity of pain (as appropriate)**
   How would you rate your pain on an intensity scale?

   To identify intensity (refer to various intensity scales)

   To identify degree of impairment and effect on quality of life or ability to perform activities of daily living

5. **T: timing: onset of pain**
   When did the pain start?
   Is it a constant, dull, or intermittent pain?
   Has the intensity changed over time?
   Are you pain free at night or during the day?

   To identify onset of pain (when active, or resting) or whether pain is persistent

6. **U: Understanding of pain**
   What do you believe is causing the pain?
   What is an acceptable comfort function goal?
   What medications have you been using, or what medications have worked for you in the past?

   To understand patient history of pain
   Review plan of care; set achievable pain and function goals

PAIN ASSESSMENT TOOLS

Pain is multidimensional in scope, encompassing physical, affective, and functional domains. Various tools have been developed to capture unidimensional aspects (e.g., intensity) or multidimensional components (e.g., effect on activities of daily living and quality of life). Selection of the pain assessment tool is based on its purpose, time involved in administration, and the patient's ability to comprehend and complete the tool. Specialized assessment tools should be used with very young patients, very old patients, patients with cognitive dysfunction, and patients who are unable to self-report.

Educate the patient about the pain assessment tool; this education should include instructions on how to use it, the rationale for the tool when required (e.g., help to identify the effect of pain on daily activities and quality of life), and information about when the tool is likely to be administered again.

In the **Initial Pain Assessment** (McCaffery & Pasero, 1999), the patient answers eight questions concerning location, duration, quality, and intensity of pain; aggravating/relieving factors; and effects of pain on quality of life.

On the **Brief Pain Inventory** (Daut & Cleeland, 1982), the patient rates the pain within the previous 24 hours, using graduated scales (0 to 10); indicates how much relief the patient has had; and describes how the pain interferes on areas such as general activities, mood, walking ability, work, and sleep (Figure 11-3). In the **Short-Form McGill Pain Questionnaire** (Melzack, 1987), the patient ranks a list of descriptors in terms of their intensity and rates the overall intensity of the pain.

Pain rating scales can be used to ascertain baseline intensity, track changes, and give some degree of evaluation to a treatment modality. The use of unidimensional pain rating scales, such as the **Visual Analogue Scale** or the **numeric rating scale (0-10)** (Figure 11-4), is common in clinical practice. On the Numeric Rating Scale, the patient chooses a number to rate the level of pain, wherein 0 represents no pain and 10 indicates the worst possible pain. It can be administered verbally or visually along a vertical or horizontal line.

Rating scales can be administered to patients aged 4 or 5 years. The Faces Pain Scale – Revised (FPS-R) tool has six drawings of faces that show pain intensity, from "no pain" on the left (score of 0) to "very much pain" on the right (score of 10) (Figure 11-5). The child is asked to select the face that best represents his or her pain intensity. Numbers are not shown to children, but the number scoring makes this tool compatible with the widely used 0-to-10 metric for numeric pain scales. This revised drawing has more realistic facial expressions with a furrowed brow and horizontal mouth stretch to rate pain. It avoids smiles or tears, so that children will not confuse pain intensity with happiness or sadness.

Brief Pain Inventory

Date:___/___/___   Time:_____

Name:_____
          Last   First   Middle initial

1. Throughout our lives, most of us have had pain from time to time (such as minor headaches, sprains, and tooth-aches). Have you had pain other than these everyday kinds of pain today?
   1. Yes   2. No

2. On the diagram, shade in the areas where you feel pain. Put an X on the area that hurts the most.

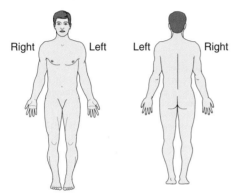

3. Please rate your pain by circling the one number that best describes your pain at its **worst** in the past 24 hours.

0	1	2	3	4	5	6	7	8	9	10

   No   Pain as bad as
   pain   you can imagine

4. Please rate your pain by circling the one number that best describes your pain at its **least** in the past 24 hours.

0	1	2	3	4	5	6	7	8	9	10

   No   Pain as bad as
   pain   you can imagine

5. Please rate your pain by circling the one number that best describes your pain on the **average**.

0	1	2	3	4	5	6	7	8	9	10

   No   Pain as bad as
   pain   you can imagine

6. Please rate your pain by circling the one number that tells how much pain you have **right now**.

0	1	2	3	4	5	6	7	8	9	10

   No   Pain as bad as
   pain   you can imagine

7. What treatments or medications are you receiving for your pain?

   _____

   _____

8. In the past 24 hours, how much **relief** have pain treatments or medications provided? Please circle the one percentage that most shows how much relief you have received.

0%	10	20	30	40	50	60	70	80	90	100%

   No   Complete
   relief   relief

9. Circle the one number that describes how, during the past 24 hours, pain has **interfered** with your:

   A: General activity

0	1	2	3	4	5	6	7	8	9	10

   Does not   Completely
   interfere   interferes

   B: Mood

0	1	2	3	4	5	6	7	8	9	10

   Does not   Completely
   interfere   interferes

   C: Walking ability

0	1	2	3	4	5	6	7	8	9	10

   Does not   Completely
   interfere   interferes

   D: Normal work (includes both work outside the home and housework)

0	1	2	3	4	5	6	7	8	9	10

   Does not   Completely
   interfere   interferes

   E: Relations with other people

0	1	2	3	4	5	6	7	8	9	10

   Does not   Completely
   interfere   interferes

   F: Sleep

0	1	2	3	4	5	6	7	8	9	10

   Does not   Completely
   interfere   interferes

   G: Enjoyment of life

0	1	2	3	4	5	6	7	8	9	10

   Does not   Completely
   interfere   interferes

Subjective Data

11-3 Brief Pain Inventory.

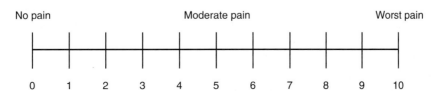

No pain   Moderate pain   Worst pain

0   1   2   3   4   5   6   7   8   9   10

11-4

Faces Pain Scale — Revised (FPS-R)

In the following instructions, say "hurt" or "pain," whichever seems right for a particular child.

"These faces show how much something can hurt. This face [point to left-most face] **shows no pain. The faces show more and more pain** [point to each from left to right] **up to this one** [point to right-most face] **— it shows very much pain. Point to the face that shows how much you hurt** [right now]."

Score the chosen face 0, 2, 4, 6, 8, or 10, counting left to right, so '0' = 'no pain' and '10' = 'very much pain.' Do not use words like 'happy' and 'sad'. This scale is intended to measure how children feel inside, not how their face looks.

Permission for use. Copyright in the FPS-R is held by the International Association for the Study of Pain (IASP) © 2001. This material may be photocopied for non-commercial clinical and research use. To request permission from IASP to reproduce the FPS-R in a publication, or for any commercial use, please e-mail **iaspdesk@iasp-pain.org**. For all other information regarding the FPS-R contact **Tiina.Jaaniste@sesiahs.health.nsw.gov.au** (Pain Medicine Unit, Sydney Children's Hospital, Randwick, NSW 2031, Austrailia).

11-5 Faces Pain Scale (Revised).

Older adults may find the numerical scale too abstract and may respond to scales in which words are used. Such an alternative scale is the simple **Descriptor Scale,** which lists words that describe different levels of pain intensity, such as *no pain, mild pain, moderate pain,* and *severe pain.*

OBJECTIVE DATA

PREPARATION

The physical examination process can help you understand the nature of the pain. Consider whether this is an acute or chronic condition.

Pain should not be discounted when objective physical evidence of it is not found. According to the American Pain Society (1992), "In cases in which the cause of acute pain is uncertain, establishing a diagnosis is a priority, but symptomatic treatment of pain should be given while the investigation is proceeding. With occasional exceptions, (e.g., the *initial* examination of the patient with an acute condition of the abdomen), it is rarely justified to defer analgesia until a diagnosis is made. In fact, a comfortable patient is better able to cooperate with diagnostic procedures" (p. 3).

EQUIPMENT NEEDED

Assessment tool that is appropriate for the patient; for example, for initial or comprehensive pain assessment, use Brief Pain Inventory; for acute/in-hospital settings, use the Numeric Rating Scale (0-10) or FACES Pain Rating Scale for children.

Normal Range of Findings	Abnormal Findings
ACUTE PAIN	
In the acute phase, patients should report their pain well controlled, with a Numeric Rating Scale intensity of 4 or higher or as "mild to moderate" in severity.	Increased heart rate or blood pressure may indicate pain.
The patient should be able to identify how much pain he or she can tolerate before it interferes with functioning or rehabilitation exercises; thus pain management goals for treatment can be set before rehabilitation interventions.	Pain may be a precursor to hypoventilation and hypoxia, inasmuch as patients may not be able to cough effectively.
Side effects such as nausea, vomiting, or pruritus should also be assessed at time of pain assessment and with pharmacological interventions.	Joint stiffness may result from limitation secondary to severe pain.
Consider preemptive analgesia for procedural pain because patients who are subjected to repetitive painful procedures (e.g., dressing changes, suctioning) may become fearful.	Nausea and vomiting may be present with severe acute pain.

Subjective Data

Objective Data

Normal Range of Findings	Abnormal Findings

NEUROPATHIC PAIN

People with neuropathic pain may have decreased or increased sensation or numbness over the affected area (e.g., as in postherpetic neuralgia).

Inspect the skin and tissues for colour, swelling, and any masses or deformity (e.g., bottoms of feet for diabetic neuropathy).

Changes in sensation may be present; patients may report an increased or decreased sensation of pinprick or cold or loss of sensation of vibration.

Neuropathic pain may increase in severity at night or at times of decreased stimulation.

Lesions, open wounds, tissue damage, change in hair distribution.

Absence of pain sensation (analgesia); increased pain sensation (hyperalgesia); or evoking of a severe pain sensation with a stimulus that does not normally induce pain (allodynia).

PERSISTENT PAIN

Pain may be present for an extended period of time after the acute phase.

Persistent pain should be manageable through timing of activities (e.g., spacing of tasks) and pain management interventions.

Physical activities should be a regular part of daily activities.

Social support systems should be in place to assist in day-to-day activities.

Financial support and psychosocial support should be in place.

Fear, anxiety, depression, isolation.
Limited mobility and function.
Family distress.
Diminished quality of life.
Possibly decreased ability to complete day-to-day activities; increasing levels of fatigue.

NONVERBAL/BEHAVIOURAL PAIN ASSESSMENT

When a patient cannot verbally communicate pain, you can assess pain by using a behavioural pain assessment tool. Behavioural pain assessment tools can help you determine the presence of pain, but they cannot help you determine the severity.

Acute Pain Behaviours

Patients may be unable to verbalize the presence of pain for a variety of reasons. However, those who are unable to report their pain are at high risk for the undertreatment of pain. Individuals who are nonverbal but are cognitively intact (e.g., intubated but alert and awake) may be able to indicate the intensity of their pain by using a numeric rating scale, by writing down a description of the quality of their pain, or by pointing to the location of their pain.

Persistent (Chronic) Pain Behaviours

Persons with persistent pain often live with the experience for months and years. A person cannot function physiologically and go on with life in a repetitive state of grimacing, diaphoresis, guarding, and so on. The person adapts over time, and clinicians must not anticipate the same behaviours as in acute pain. Patients with persistent pain may give little indication that they are in pain and therefore are at higher risk for underdetection of pain. Whenever possible, it is best to ask the patient how he or she behaves when in pain.

The Unconscious Individual

Individuals who are unconscious for physiological reasons or because they have been given sedative medications also experience pain. Assessment of pain in these individuals may be a challenge, but tools have been created to standardize key areas for assessment. Unconscious individuals experiencing moderate to intense levels of pain often exhibit grimacing, wincing, moaning, rigidity, arching, restlessness, shaking, or pushing (Puntillo et al., 2004). The Critical-Care Pain Observation Tool (Gélinas, Fillion, Puntillo, Viens, & Fortier, 2006) was developed to assess pain in patients in the critical care unit. Behaviours assessed include facial expression, body movement, muscle tension, vocalizations, and degree of compliance with ventilation (Table 11-1). The total score ranges between 0 and 8; a higher score is more indicative of pain. Physiological signs (vital signs) should not be used exclusively to rule out or confirm the presence of pain because pulse and blood pressure can also be altered by changes in fluid volume, by medications, and by blood loss.

 ## DEVELOPMENTAL CONSIDERATIONS

Neonates

Because neonates and young infants are preverbal and incapable of self-report, pain assessment is dependent on behavioural and physiological cues. Infants do feel pain; if a procedure or disease process is known to induce pain in adults (e.g., circumcision, surgery, sickle cell disease, cancer), it does induce pain in neonates and infants. Pain measures that include more than one assessment approach within a given instrument are used for measuring pain in neonates and infants. Most measures include both behavioural and physiological indicators, and some also include contextual factors, such as the gestational age or behavioural sleep/wake state of the infant. Several published measures combine behavioural and physiological indicators for assessing pain in infants with varying degrees of established reliability and

Objective Data

TABLE 11-1	The Critical-Care Pain Observation Tool		
Indicator	Description	Score	
Facial expression	No muscular tension observed	Relaxed, neutral	0
	Presence of frowning, brow lowering, orbit tightening, and levator contraction	Tense	1
	All of the above facial movements plus eyelid tightly closed	Grimacing	2
Body movements	Does not move at all (does not necessarily mean absence of pain)	Absence of movements	0
	Slow, cautious movements, touching or rubbing the pain site, seeking attention through movements	Protection	1
	Pulling tube, attempting to sit up, moving limbs/thrashing, not following commands, striking at staff, trying to climb out of bed	Restlessness	2
Muscle tension			
Evaluation by passive flexion and extension of upper extremities *and either*	No resistance to passive movements	Relaxed	0
	Resistance to passive movements	Tense, rigid	1
	Strong resistance to passive movements, inability to complete them	Very tense or rigid	2
Compliance with the ventilator (intubated patients) *or*	Alarms not activated, easy ventilation	Tolerating ventilator or movement	0
	Alarms stop spontaneously	Coughing but tolerating	1
	Asynchrony: blocking ventilation, alarms frequently activated	Fighting ventilator	2
Vocalization (extubated patients)	Talking in normal tone or no sound	Talking in normal tone or no sound	0
	Sighing, moaning	Sighing, moaning	1
	Crying out, sobbing	Crying out, sobbing	2
Total, range		0–8	

Source: From Gélinas, C., Fillion, L., Puntillo, K. A., Viens, C., & Fortier, M. (2006). Validation of the Critical-Care Observation Tool in adult patients. *American Journal of Critical Care, 15*(4), 420–427. Reprinted with permission.

validity, such as the Neonatal Pain, Agitation, and Sedation Scale and the Premature Infant Pain Profile.

The Premature Infant Pain Profile is a behavioural measure of pain for premature infants (Table 11-2). It was developed at the Universities of Toronto and McGill in Canada (Stevens, Johnston, Petryshen, & Taddio, 1996). Indicators of pain that are assessed include gestational age; behavioural state before painful stimulus; and change in heart rate, change in oxygen saturation, brow bulge, eye squeeze, and nasolabial furrow during painful stimulus.

These measures target acute pain. No biological markers have been identified for long-term persistent pain in infants or children. Therefore, evaluate the whole patient. Look for changes in temperament, expression, and activity.

Intellectual/Cognitive Disability

Although adults may have an intellectual or cognitive disability, their sensory ability to perceive pain is not diminished (Vreeling, Houx, Jolles, & Verhey, 1995). Intellectually/ cognitively impaired persons may have a limited ability to communicate information about pain, which places them at

high risk for undertreatment of pain. Patients who commonly present with a cognitive disability include those with dementia, those with Parkinson's disease, patients after a stroke, and patients with intellectual developmental disabilities. Various pain scales are available for assessment of intellectually/cognitively impaired patients; these include the PAINAD scale (Warden et al., 2003) and the Abbey scale (Abbey et al., 2004).

Discussion with the family or other health care team members can help you identify patterns that may indicate that a patient is experiencing pain. A review of medical records can also highlight potential areas for concern (e.g., diabetic neuropathy).

When you assess for behavioural cues of pain, examine facial expressions or changes in appetite, daily activities, involvement in social activities, or sleep/wake cycles. A comprehensive head-to-toe assessment should help you confirm or rule out any obvious sources of pain, such as skin tears or areas of swelling. Assess any sudden onset of acute confusion or delirium because it may indicate poor control of pain or other competing explanations such as infection or adverse reaction to medications.

TABLE 11-2	**Premature Infant Pain Profile***					
		Anchor				
Process	Indicator	0	1	2	3	Score
Chart	Gestational age	36 wk and more	32–35 wk, 6 days	28–31 wk, 6 days	<28 weeks	
Observe infant	Behavioural state	Active/awake	Quiet/awake	Active/sleep	Quiet/sleep	
15 s		Eyes open Facial movements	Eyes open No facial movements	Eyes closed Facial movements	Eyes closed No facial movements	

Observe baseline
  Heart rate
  _____
  Oxygen saturation
  _____						

Observe infant	Heart rate Max _____	0- to 4-beat/min increase	5- to 14-beat/min increase	15- to 24-beat/min increase	25-beat/min increase	
30 s	Oxygen saturation Min _____	0%–2.4% decrease	2.5%–4.9% decrease	5.0%–7.4% decrease	7.5% or more decrease	
	Brow bulge	None: 0%–9% of time	Minimum: 10%–39% of time	Moderate: 40%–69% of time	Maximum: 70% of time or more	
	Eye squeeze	None: 0%–9% of time	Minimum: 10%–39% of time	Moderate: 40%–69% of time	Maximum: 70% of time or more	
	Nasolabial furrow	None: 0%–9% of time	Minimum: 10%–39% of time	Moderate: 40%–69% of time	Maximum: 70% of time or more	
Total score						

Source: From Stevens, B., Johnston, C., Petryshen, P., and Taddio, A. (1996). Premature Infant Pain Profile: Development and initial validation. *Clinical Journal of Pain, 12*(1), 13–22.

*Scoring instructions include scoring infant's gestational age before infant is examined, scoring the behavioural state before the potentially painful event by observing the infant for 15 seconds, recording the baseline heart rate and oxygen saturation, and observing the infant for 30 seconds immediately after the painful event. Physiological and facial changes seen during this time should be scored and the scores recorded immediately. The maximum score is 21, and the higher the score, the more intense is the pain behaviour.

Objective Data

Documentation & Critical Thinking

DOCUMENTATION AND CRITICAL THINKING

Sample Charting

SUBJECTIVE

Onset within the past 2 weeks; patient states having severe epigastric pain within a half hour of eating greasy fatty foods. Pain is stabbing and squeezing in nature with radiation to right shoulder blade. Patient rates pain as a 10 on a scale of 0 to 10. Nausea accompanies pain. Patient takes antacids, with minimal relief. Pain diminishes after bringing knees to chest and "not moving" for a 1-hour period.

OBJECTIVE

Patient diaphoretic, grimacing, and having difficulty concentrating. Breathless during history. Arms guarding upper abdominal area. Abdomen distended. Severe tenderness noted on light right upper quadrant and epigastric palpation. Bowel sounds hyperactive in all four quadrants.

ASSESSMENT

Acute episodic visceral pain

Focused Assessment: Clinical Case Study 1

R. M. is a 20-year-old man with diagnosed sickle cell crisis. Admitted to the emergency department.

SUBJECTIVE

Within the past 48 hours, R. M. reports increasing pain in upper and lower extremity joints and swelling of right knee. States having "stomach flu" 1 week before with periods of vomiting and diarrhea. Pain is aching and constant in nature. Rates pain as 10+ on a scale of 0 to 10. Taking ibuprofen, one to two tablets every 4 hours, and using ice packs, with no relief.

OBJECTIVE

Requires assistance to sit on examination table. Unable to bear weight on right leg. Affect flat, clenches jaw during position changes. Tenderness localized in elbow, wrist, finger, and knee joints. Diminished range of motion in wrists and knees (right knee, 36 cm; left knee, 30 cm diameter). Right knee warm and boggy to touch.

ASSESSMENT

Acute nociceptive pain

Focused Assessment: Clinical Case Study 2

A. G. is an 85-year-old woman with a 20-year history of osteoarthritis.

SUBJECTIVE

A. G. reports increased pain and stiffness in her neck, arms, and lower back for the past month. Denies radiation of pain. Denies tingling or numbness in upper or lower extremities.

Having difficulty getting in and out of bathtub and dressing herself. Describes pain as aching, with good and bad days. Becomes frustrated when asked to rate her pain intensity; replies, "I don't know what number to give; it hurts a lot, on and off." Takes acetaminophen extra strength, two tablets, when the pain "really gets the best of me," with some degree of relief. Does not take part in "field trips" offered by assisted living facility because she "hurts too much."

OBJECTIVE

Localized tenderness noted upon palpation to C3 and C4; unable to flex neck to chest. Crepitus noted in both shoulder joints. No swelling noted. Muscle strength 1+ and equal in upper extremities. Lumbar area tender to moderate palpation. Rubs lower back frequently; limited flexion at the waist. Gait slow and unsteady. Facial expression stoic.

ASSESSMENT

Persistent (chronic) pain

SPECIAL CONSIDERATIONS FOR ADVANCED PRACTICE

SOMATOFORM DISORDERS

Medically unexplained physical symptoms occur in patients "with complaints of physical symptoms or signs for which there is inadequate objective pathophysiological evidence to explain the duress" (Neimark, Caroff, & Stinnett, 2005, p. 296).

Acute or persistent pain can be challenging, often necessitating increased pain management (e.g., involvement with Acute Pain Service nurses, as available).

Patients experiencing persistent pain may benefit from referral to chronic pain clinics and from therapies in which pain management involves integration of psychological and pharmacological support.

SICKLE CELL CRISIS

In Canada, it is hard to determine the actual incidence of sickle cell disease because no national hemoglobinopathy program exists, and no race-specific health data like that collected in the United States are available. The disease affects not only people of African descent but also people from northern and sub-Saharan Africa, as well as the Mediterranean, Caribbean, South and Central America, Arabia, and India. It is estimated that approximately 1 per 400 babies of African Canadian descent are born with sickle cell disease (Health Canada, 2000).

Sickle cell disease is characterized by an alteration of hemoglobin and by anemia and tissue injury secondary to vaso-occlusion. Any decrease in oxygenation causes alterations in the shape of the red blood cells, which causes them to stick together and ultimately block small blood vessels. The resulting vaso-occlusion (vaso-occlusive crisis) can cause severe pain, similar to that of a myocardial infarction.

Patients with sickle cell disease can experience any one of a number of pain syndromes (Tanabe & Todds, 2010):
- Acute regional pain syndrome (chest pain [acute chest syndrome], craniofacial pain, long bone and joint pain, low back pain, muscle pain)
- Persistent pain syndrome (peripheral ulcerations, avascular necrosis, osteomyelitis)
- Other pain syndromes (such as migraines, neuropathic pain, fibromyalgia, and myofascial pain)

Painful sickle cell crises can manifest early in infancy and lead to chronic pain, which can be exacerbated by acute pain in the subsequent vaso-occlusive crises. Vaso-occlusive crises can have psychological causes (e.g., stressful event) or physiological causes (such as infection, dehydration, or overexertion, and sometimes in the postoperative state). Most patients with sickle cell disease experience pain on a daily basis. Management of acute episodic pain begins with a comprehensive pain assessment and documentation of problem areas; you must recognize that many affected patients present to emergency rooms with acute pain in addition to their persistent pain. After initial assessment and intervention, these patients require frequent pain reassessments to titrate treatment dosages appropriately, and they would probably benefit from the services of advanced nursing or pain management teams to help control their pain.

Research has shown that many complementary therapies are helpful in limiting the frequency of sickle cell crises, as well as in improving patients' quality of life. Community support is beneficial for patients and their families. Many Web sites offer a source of online support for patients and health care providers; for example, the Sickle Cell Association of Ontario (see the section Web Sites of Interest) offers education and tips for families coping with the disease.

REFERENCES

Abbey, J., Piller, N., De Bellis, A., Esterman, A., Parker, D., Giles, L. & Lowcay, B. (2004). The Abbey pain scale: a 1-minute numerical indicator for people with end stage dementia. *Int J Palliat Nurs* (1), 6–13.

American Pain Society. (1992). *Principles of analgesic use in the treatment of acute and cancer pain* (3rd ed.). Glenview, IL: Author.

Anand, K. J. S. (1993). The applied physiology of pain. In K. J. S. Anand & R. J. McGrath (Eds.), *Pain in neonates*. Amsterdam: Elsevier.

Anand, K. J. S. (2000). Effects of perinatal pain and stress. *Progress in Brain Research, 122*, 117–119.

Daut, R. L., & Cleeland, C. S. (1982). The prevalence and severity of pain in cancer. *Cancer, 50*, 1913–1918.

Gélinas, C., Fillion, L., Puntillo, K.A., Viens, C., & Fortier, M. (2006). Validation of the Critical-Care Observation Tool in adult patients. *American Journal of Critical Care, 15*(4), 420–427.

Gold, M., Chessell, I., Devor, M., Dray, A., Gereau, R., et al. (2006). Peripheral nervous system targets: Rapporteur Report. In J. Campbell (Ed.), *Emerging strategies for the treatment of neuropathic pain*. Seattle: IASP Press.

Health Canada. (2000). Certain Circumstances: Issues in equity and responsiveness in access to health care in Canada. Available at *http://www.hc-sc.gc.ca/hcs-sss/alt_formats/hpb-dgps/pdf/pubs/2001-certain-equit-acces/2001-certain-equit-acces_e.pdf*.

International Association for the Study of Pain. (2007, September). *Differences in pain between women and men* [online document].

Retrieved from *www.iasp-pain.org/AM/Template.cfm?Section=Real…*

Jovey, R. D., Ennis, J., Gardner-Nix, J., Goldman, B., Hays, H., & Lynch, M. (2003). Use of opioid analgesics for the treatment of chronic non-cancer pain. A consensus statement and guidelines from the Canadian Pain Society. *Pain Research and Management, 8*(Suppl. A), 3A–14A.

Kehlet, H., Jensen, T. S., & Woolf, C. J. (2006). Persistent postsurgical pain: Risk factors and prevention. *Lancet, 367*(9522), 1618–1625.

Lasch, K. E. (2000). Culture, pain, and culturally sensitive pain care. *Pain Management Nursing, 1*(3, Suppl. 1), 16–22.

McCaffery, M. (1968). *Nursing practice theories related to cognition, bodily pain, and man-environment interactions*. Los Angeles: University of California, Los Angeles, Students' Store.

McCaffery, M., & Pasero, C. (1999). *Pain: Clinical manual* (2nd ed.). St. Louis: Mosby.

Melzack, R. (1987). The short-form McGill Pain Questionnaire. *Pain, 30*, 191–197.

Mogil, J. S. (2002). Pain genetics: Pre- and post-genomic findings. *International Association for the Study of Pain Technical Corner Newsletter, 2*, 3–6.

Neimark, G., Caroff, S., & Stinnett, J. (2005). Medically unexplained physical symptoms. *Psychiatric Annals, 35*(4), 298–306.

Puntillo, K. A., Morris, A. B., Thompson, C. L., Stanik-Hutt, J., White, C. A., & Wild, L. R. (2004). Pain behaviors observed during six common procedures: Results from Thunder Project II. *Critical Care Medicine, 32*(2), 421–427.

Stevens, B., Johnston, C., Petryshen, P., & Taddio, A. (1996). Premature Infant Pain Profile: Development and initial validation. *Clinical Journal of Pain, 12*(1), 13–22.

Tanabe, P., & Todds, K. (2010). Chapter 32: Pain in sickle cell disease. In A. Kopf & N. Patel (Eds.), *Guide to pain management in low resource settings*. Seattle: International Association for the Study of Pain.

Treede, R. D., Jensen, T. S., Campbell, J. N., Cruccu, G., Dostrovsky, J. O., Griffin, J. W., … Serra, J. (2008). Redefinition of neuropathic pain and a grading system for clinical use: Consensus statement on clinical and research diagnostic criteria. *Neurology, 70*, 1630–1635.

Vreeling, F. W., Houx, P. J., Jolles, J., & Verhey, F. R. (1995). Primitive reflexes in Alzheimer's disease and vascular dementia. *Journal of Geriatric Psychiatry and Neurology, 8*, 111–117.

Warden, V., Hurley, A. C., & Volicer, L. (1995). Development and psychometric evaluation of the pain assessment in advanced dementia (PAINAD) scale. *J Am Med Dir Assoc. 4*, 9–15.

Websites of Interest:

Canadian Pain Society: *http://www.canadianpainsociety.ca/en/*
International Association for the Study of pain (IASP): *http://www.iasp-pain.org//AM/Template.cfm?Section=Home*
Sickle Cell Association of Ontario: *http://www.sicklecellontario.org*

Nutritional Assessment and Nursing Practice

Written by Joyce K. Keithley, DNSc, RN, FAAN

Adapted by Ellen Vogel, PhD, RD, FDC; Andrea Miller, MHSc, RD; and Christina Vaillancourt, MHSc, RD, CDE

⊖volve WEBSITE

OUTLINE

STRUCTURE AND FUNCTION

Nurses, as the first point of contact for patients, collaborate with the multidisciplinary team in the development of the nutritional care plan. Nurses record the patient history, including weight history; assess vital signs; and measure current weight and height. Because nurses frequently initiate patient referrals to dietitians, it is important that they develop knowledge and skills in nutritional screening to ensure that patients' needs are met in an efficient manner. Dietitians and nurses often collaborate to facilitate optimal patient care.

Dietitians are experts in assessing the nutritional status of individuals across the life cycle and in developing nutritional care plans for wide-ranging health concerns.

Dietitians have extensive knowledge of the biochemical and nutritional components of foods and how it influences metabolic and physiologic processes. In addition, dietitians understand the feeding environment and underlying psychosocial, economic, and health determinants that influence food intake at individual/family and societal levels (Dietitians of Canada, 2011).

DEFINING NUTRITIONAL STATUS

Nutritional status is the degree of balance between nutrient intake and nutrient requirements. In addition to genetic predisposition, this balance is affected by income, education,

Structure & Function

an individual's broad physical and social environments, nutritional literacy, and access to protective foods. For example, levels of physical activity, access to healthy foods, educational attainment, and individual/family income are some of many influences that can increase or decrease the risk of overweight and obesity by shaping individual attitudes, knowledge, and behaviours about healthy lifestyles and healthy weights (Canadian Institute for Health Information, 2006).

Optimal nutritional status is achieved when nutrients are consumed in amounts that support daily requirements and any increased metabolic demands related to growth, pregnancy, or illness. Individuals who have optimal nutritional status are generally more active, have fewer physical illnesses, and live longer than those who are less well nourished.

Undernutrition occurs when nutritional reserves become depleted or when nutrient intake is inadequate to meet daily requirements or metabolic demands. Certain populations are vulnerable to undernutrition: infants, children, pregnant women, new immigrants, individuals with low incomes, hospitalized people, and older adults. Undernutrition increases the risk of impaired growth and development, lowered resistance to infection and disease, delayed wound healing, longer hospital stays, and higher health-related expenses.

Overnutrition results from the consumption of nutrients—most frequently calories, sodium, and fat—in excess of requirements. Overnutrition is a major nutritional problem, and resultant unhealthy weights can lead to chronic conditions, including heart disease, type 2 diabetes, hypertension, stroke, gallbladder disease, sleep apnea, certain cancers (e.g., breast, endometrial, colon, prostate, and kidney), and osteoarthritis (National Heart, Lung, and Blood Institute, National Institutes of Health, & U.S. Department of Health and Human Services, 2006). In 2007, the Canadian Health Measures Survey, the most comprehensive health measures survey in Canada, began collecting direct measurements of height, weight, body mass index (BMI; p. 154), skinfolds, and waist circumference from a nationally representative sample of the population. In the period 2007 to 2009, the prevalence of obesity in Canada was 24.1% (Statistics Canada, 2011a).

The proportion of overweight children and adolescents in Canada has increased significantly since the 1990s. In children, *overweight* is defined as a BMI in the 95th percentile or higher according to age- and gender-specific BMI charts. In 2004, 8% of Canadian children and adolescents were obese and 18% were overweight; in the period 1978 to 1979, in comparison, only 3% were obese and 12% were overweight. Rates of measured overweight and obesity are even higher among Aboriginal youth and young adults. In 2009, 20% of off-reserve Aboriginal youth reported being overweight and 7% obese (Statistics Canada, 2011b). A study conducted between 2008 and 2010 yielded similar results (self-reported) among on-reserve First Nation youth (aged 12 to 17 years): 30% were considered overweight and 13% obese (First Nations Information Governance Centre, 2011). Being

overweight in childhood or adolescence is associated with an increased risk of developing chronic health conditions later in life, as well as psychosocial problems, functional limitations, and impaired fertility (Public Health Agency of Canada [PHAC], 2011b).

 DEVELOPMENTAL CONSIDERATIONS

The nutrients necessary to optimize health over a lifetime are the same for all healthy individuals; however, the amount of each of those nutrients changes on the basis of stages of the life cycle. Nutrition can be viewed as a continuum over the life cycle: a continuum that changes as individuals grow, age, and respond to variations in their environment, physical activity, and health. Optimal nutrition is essential for overall health and well-being and in the prevention of chronic conditions.

Infants and Children

Early nutrition affects later development, and early feedings establish eating habits that influence nutrition throughout life. The time from birth to 4 months of age is the most rapid period of growth in the life cycle. Although infants lose weight during the first few days of life, birth weight is usually regained by the seventh to tenth day after birth. Birth weight doubles by 4 months of age and triples by the age of 1 year. An infant's length changes more slowly, increasing about 25 cm from birth to age 1 year. Growth rate then slows during the second year; an infant typically gains less than 4.5 kg and grows 12.5 cm in the second year. Brain size also increases rapidly during infancy and childhood. By 2 years of age, the brain has reached 50% of its adult size; by age 4, 75%; and by age 8, 100%.

The Canadian Paediatric Society and Health Canada recommend exclusive breastfeeding for full-term infants for the first 6 months of life, for the nutritional, physiological, social, and economic benefits it confers on the infant and mother

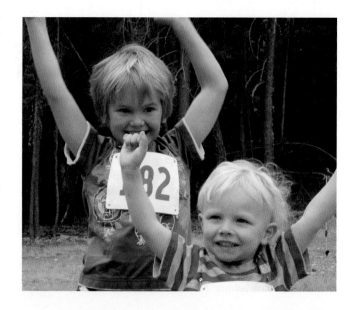

(Boland, 2005; Health Canada, 2007a). Breast milk is ideally formulated to promote normal infant growth and development and natural immunity. With the exception of vitamin D, breast milk provides all the nutrients that a healthy infant needs for the first 6 months of life. It is recommended that all breastfed and partially breastfed, full-term infants in Canada receive a daily vitamin D supplement of 10 mcg (400 IU). After 1 year, all children should have a daily vitamin D intake of 5 mcg (200 IU). Supplementation should begin at birth and continue until the infant's diet includes at least 10 mcg (400 IU) per day of vitamin D from other dietary sources, or until the breastfed infant reaches 1 year of age (Health Canada, 2007a).

Solid foods can be introduced as the infant becomes physically able to handle them. In healthy full-term infants, the introduction of iron-fortified cereal begins at 4 to 6 months of age. Whole cow's milk should *not* be offered until the end of the first year because it is associated with occult blood loss in stool, especially in the first 6 months of life (Health Canada, 2005). Lower fat milk (2% or skim) should be avoided until the age of 2 years because it has insufficient fat and calories to support optimal growth and development.

Adolescence

After a period of slower growth in late childhood, adolescence is characterized by rapid physical growth and endocrine and hormonal changes. Energy and protein requirements increase to meet these demands. In addition, because of rapid bone growth and increasing muscle mass (and, in girls, the onset of menarche), calcium and iron requirements increase during adolescence. Careful meal and snack planning is essential to meet the increased nutrient demands of adolescence.

In general, adolescent boys grow taller and accumulate less body fat than do adolescent girls. In girls, body fat increases to about 25% of total body mass; in boys, body fat decreases (replaced by muscle mass) to about 12% of total body mass. In girls, body weight doubles between the ages of 8 and 14 years; in boys, between the ages of 10 and 17 years.

Because of the societal importance placed on physical appearance, adolescent girls in particular can feel pressured to diet in order to conform to a perceived ideal body image, or they may become dissatisfied with their appearance (Sizer, Whitney, & Piche, 2009). Some adolescent girls have reported pressure to lose weight or have been exposed to body preoccupations and disordered eating at the familial level (Littleton & Ollendick, 2003). Boys increasingly tend to equate their attractiveness with increased muscle definition, mass, and body shape (Silva, 2006). Research suggests that body dissatisfaction among boys can lead to poor psychological adjustment, disordered eating behaviours (binge eating disorder, bulimia, anorexia, and dysmorphia), steroid use, and exercise dependence (Silva, 2006).

Pregnancy and Lactation

It is essential that sufficient calories, protein, vitamins, and minerals be consumed to support the synthesis of maternal and fetal tissues during pregnancy. Health Canada has adopted the 2009 U.S. Institute of Medicine's recommendations for gestational weight gain for singleton pregnancies. The Institute of Medicine's recommendations are based on observational data, which consistently show that women who gain within the recommended range experience better pregnancy outcomes (Health Canada, 2010a).

Recommended weight gain for women whose body weight is *ideal* before pregnancy is 11.5 to 16 kg (25 to 35 lb); for women who are **underweight,** recommended weight gain is 2.5 to 18 kg (28 to 40 lb); for women who begin pregnancy **overweight,** weight gain recommendations are 7 to 11 kg (15 to 24 lb). See Appendix F on the Evolve Web site for recommendations for increased nutrient requirements associated with pregnancy and lactation. Appendix G on the Evolve Web site lists recommended weight gain guidelines based on BMI and illustrates ranges of desirable weight gain during pregnancy, as recommended by the Subcommittee on Nutritional Status and Weight Gain During Pregnancy (Health Canada, 2012).

Several factors increase nutritional risk for pregnant women. These include age (adolescents are at higher risk for the development of nutrient deficiencies in pregnancy), multiple pregnancies with short (<18-month) intervals between each pregnancy, use of tobacco products, use of alcohol or illicit drugs, twin or triplet (or higher order) pregnancy, restrictive diets (including vegetarianism), and inadequate or excessive weight gain during pregnancy.

In comparison with older mothers, teenaged mothers are more likely to experience complications of pregnancy, including anemia, hypertension, preeclampsia, renal disease, and depressive disorders. Furthermore, infants born to teenaged mothers may have higher rates of perinatal mortality, higher preterm birth rates, and lower birth weights (Dryburgh, 2000).

To reduce the risk of neural tube defects in infants, women without personal health risks who are capable of becoming pregnant should take a vitamin supplement containing 400 mcg of folic acid daily. Recommendations include taking folic acid for at least 3 months before pregnancy and continuing throughout pregnancy and the postpartum period (as long as breastfeeding continues; PHAC, 2008; SickKids Motherisk, 2011).

Adulthood

Growth and nutrient requirements stabilize during adulthood. However, lifestyle factors—including use of tobacco products; stress; lack of physical activity; excessive alcohol intake; and diets high in saturated fat, cholesterol, salt, and sugar and low in fibre—contribute to the development of hypertension, obesity, atherosclerosis, some types of cancer, osteoporosis, and diabetes mellitus. The adult years provide an ideal opportunity for needs-based nutrition education, preserving health and preventing or delaying the onset of chronic disease.

Nutrition counselling is important in the prevention of overweight and obesity. Current recommendations include a diet that is rich in fruits and vegetables, low in total and saturated fat, and high in fibre. Research findings suggest that adults who consume regular meals and snacks manage their weight better than those that have more irregular or erratic eating patterns (Sizer et al., 2009).

Older Adults

With age, a number of changes take place that make individuals more prone to undernutrition or overnutrition. Poor physical or mental health, social isolation, alcoholism, limited functional ability, poverty, and polypharmacy are risk factors for undernutrition in older adults (Furman, 2006).

After the age of 50, energy requirements decrease by approximately 5% per decade. Decreasing metabolic rate, combined with an inactive lifestyle, increases the risk for chronic diseases associated with overnutrition, including obesity, type 2 diabetes, hypertension, and cardiovascular disease. Individuals older than 70 years who maintain a BMI between 25 and 32 have been observed to have the lowest mortality risk.

Normal physiological changes of aging directly affecting nutritional status in older adults include poor dentition, decreased visual acuity, decreased saliva production, slowed gastrointestinal motility, decreased gastrointestinal absorption, and diminished olfactory and taste sensitivity. Reduced socioeconomic conditions can adversely influence the nutritional status of an older adult. An overall decline in the number of extended families, in addition to the increased mobility of families, reduces available support systems. Access to facilities for meal preparation, availability of a suitable eating environment, access to grocery stores, physical limitations, limited income, and social isolation are all factors that can interfere with the acquisition and preparation of a balanced diet. Medication use must also be considered in older patients. Increasingly, older adults are prescribed multiple medications that may interact with nutrients, vitamin supplements, and other prescription drugs.

Finally, with age the synthesis of vitamin D decreases. Health Canada (2010b) recommended that, in addition to following *Eating Well With Canada's Food Guide,* all individuals older than 50 take a daily vitamin D supplement of 400 IU.

CULTURAL AND SOCIAL CONSIDERATIONS

SOCIAL DETERMINANTS OF HEALTH

At every stage of the life cycle, health is directly or indirectly influenced by key determinants of health such as education and literacy, income and social status, employment and working conditions, and social environments (PHAC, 2011a). Increasingly, evidence suggests that "the complex interaction between these determinants can influence health outcomes—both positively and negatively—and, depending on the individual, can result in the individual beginning and progressing through life stages at different times and rates" (PHAC, 2011a, p. 1).

Food Security

Food security is described as the condition in which all people, at all times, have access to nutritious, safe, personally acceptable, and culturally appropriate foods, produced in ways that are environmentally sound and socially just (Fairholm, 1999). In Canada, income-related *food insecurity* is increasingly acknowledged as a key determinant of nutritional health. Data from Health Canada (2004) indicated that in 2004, more than 2.7 million Canadians (9.2% of the population) were food insecure at some point in the previous year as a result of financial challenges. The prevalence of household food insecurity was higher in certain groups, including lone-parent families with one or more young children, those receiving social assistance, and Aboriginal people living off reserve. Isolated communities in Canada are particularly vulnerable to food insecurity as a result of decreased availability and accessibility to food. Surveys revealed a high prevalence of food insecurity (40% to 83%) in isolated Aboriginal communities (Indian Affairs and Northern Development, 2003, 2004).

Individuals and families with lower socioeconomic status are less likely to consume the nutrients needed for proper health and well-being than are those living with higher incomes (PHAC, 2011a). Studies have also linked food insecurity to the prevalence of unhealthy weights. Families with lower incomes consume more energy-dense, nutrient-poor diets, whereas families with higher incomes consume more whole grains, lean meats, low-fat dairy products, and fresh vegetables and fruit.

Because foods and eating customs are culturally distinct, each person has a unique cultural heritage that may affect nutritional status. Immigrants commonly maintain traditional eating customs long after the language and manner of dress of an adopted country become routine (especially for holidays and observance of religious customs). Occupation, socioeconomic status, religion, gender, and health awareness also have a great bearing on eating practices.

Dietary Practices and Cultural Diversity

The changing cultural profile in Canada encourages the availability of ethnically diverse foods and cuisines. This aspect of eating in Canada is reflected in updated nutrition education resources, including *Eating Well With Canada's Food Guide* (Health Canada, 2007b; Figure 12-1).

An example of a new resource designed to complement *Eating Well With Canada's Food Guide* (Health Canada, 2007b) is *Eating Well With Canada's Food Guide—First Nations, Inuit and Métis,* a food guide tailored to reflect the traditions and food choices of those population groups (Health Canada, 2007c). This guide includes listings of both traditional and store-bought foods that are generally available, affordable, and accessible to Aboriginal people across Canada. Other adaptations of *Eating Well With Canada's Food Guide* will soon be available from Health Canada, for use by specific ethnic groups.

New immigrants and refugees may be at risk for undernutrition for a variety of reasons. Some individuals come from

Structure & Function

Recommended Number of Food Guide Servings per Day

Age in Years	Children			Teens		Adults			
	2-3	4-8	9-13	14-18		19-50		51+	
Sex	Girls and Boys			Females	Males	Females	Males	Females	Males
Vegetables and Fruit	4	5	6	7	8	7-8	8-10	7	7
Grain Products	3	4	6	6	7	6-7	8	6	7
Milk and Alternatives	2	2	3-4	3-4	3-4	2	2	3	3
Meat and Alternatives	1	1	1-2	2	3	2	3	2	3

The chart above shows how many Food Guide Servings you need from each of the four food groups every day.

Having the amount and type of food recommended and following the tips in *Canada's Food Guide* will help:
- Meet your needs for vitamins, minerals and other nutrients.
- Reduce your risk of obesity, type 2 diabetes, heart disease, certain types of cancer and osteoporosis.
- Contribute to your overall health and vitality.

What is One Food Guide Serving?
Look at the examples below.

Make each Food Guide Serving count...
wherever you are – at home, at school, at work or when eating out!

▶ **Eat at least one dark green and one orange vegetable each day.**
- Go for dark green vegetables such as broccoli, romaine lettuce and spinach.
- Go for orange vegetables such as carrots, sweet potatoes and winter squash.

▶ **Choose vegetables and fruit prepared with little or no added fat, sugar or salt.**
- Enjoy vegetables steamed, baked or stir-fried instead of deep-fried.

▶ **Have vegetables and fruit more often than juice.**

▶ **Make at least half of your grain products whole grain each day.**
- Eat a variety of whole grains such as barley, brown rice, oats, quinoa and wild rice.
- Enjoy whole grain breads, oatmeal or whole wheat pasta.

▶ **Choose grain products that are lower in fat, sugar or salt.**
- Compare the Nutrition Facts table to make wiser choices.
- Enjoy the true taste of grain products. When adding sauces or spreads, use small amounts.

▶ **Drink skim, 1%, or 2% milk each day.**
- Have 500 mL (2 cups) of milk every day for adequate vitamin D.
- Drink fortified soy beverages if you do not drink milk.

▶ **Select lower fat milk alternatives.**
- Compare the Nutrition Facts table on yogurts or cheeses to make wise choices.

▶ **Have meat alternatives such as beans, lentils and tofu often.**

▶ **Eat at least two Food Guide Servings of fish each week.***
- Choose fish such as char, herring, mackerel, salmon, sardines and trout.

▶ **Select lean meat and alternatives prepared with little or no added fat or salt.**
- Trim the visible fat from meats. Remove the skin on poultry.
- Use cooking methods such as roasting, baking or poaching that require little or no added fat.
- If you eat luncheon meats, sausages or prepackaged meats, choose those lower in salt (sodium) and fat.

Oils and Fats
- Include a small amount – 30 to 45 mL (2 to 3 Tbsp) – of unsaturated fat each day. This includes oil used for cooking, salad dressings, margarine and mayonnaise.
- Use vegetable oils such as canola, olive and soybean.
- Choose soft margarines that are low in saturated and trans fats.
- Limit butter, hard margarine, lard and shortening.

Enjoy a variety of foods from the four food groups.

Satisfy your thirst with water!
Drink water regularly. It's a calorie-free way to quench your thirst. Drink more water in hot weather or when you are very active.

* Health Canada provides advice for limiting exposure to mercury from certain types of fish. Refer to www.healthcanada.gc.ca for the latest information.

12-1 Extract from *Eating Well With Canada's Food Guide.*

countries with food supplies that are limited because of poverty, poor sanitation, war, or political strife. General undernutrition, diarrhea, lactose intolerance, osteomalacia (soft bones), scurvy, and dental caries are among the more common nutrition-related problems of new immigrants from developing countries.

Upon arrival in Canada, new immigrants are faced with a new language and a new culture. They may encounter challenges related to new or unfamiliar foods, food storage requirements and facilities, food preparation difficulties, and food-buying habits. Many familiar foods are difficult or impossible to obtain. Limited income may also decrease access to familiar foods. When traditional food habits are disrupted by a new culture, borderline nutrient deficiencies may result. The best way to learn about an individual's eating pattern is to ask about his or her dietary customs. It is important to keep in mind that standard tables of weight for age, height for age, and weight for height may not be appropriate to evaluate growth and development of immigrant children. At present, no reliable standards to evaluate every immigrant group exist. Weight history in these specific population groups may be best assessed through questions related to personal and family weight history.

Lower percentages of immigrant youth and young adults were measured as overweight or obese. For example, 17% of immigrant youth were considered overweight and 5% were obese (Statistics Canada, 2007). Length of time since arrival in Canada may be a factor in immigrant overweight and obesity rates: The longer individuals reside in Canada, the higher the obesity rates are (Perez, 2002).

Important cultural factors to consider in assessing nutritional status include the cultural definition of food, frequency and number of meals eaten away from home, form and content of ceremonial meals, food preparation methods, amount and types of foods eaten, and regularity of food consumption. Because of cultural diversity, the 24-hour dietary recall or 3-day food record, traditionally used for nutritional assessment, may be insufficient for people from culturally diverse backgrounds, unless additional questions related to food type and preparation methods are included. Traditional nutrition education resources may not provide culture-specific diet information, inasmuch as nutritional content and exchange tables are generally based on Western diets.

Food itself is only one part of eating. Social interactions during meals are often as meaningful as the food itself. Understanding these social customs is an essential part of completing a nutritional assessment. Questions related to seating and serving styles, eating utensils, and the importance of how much food served is consumed may facilitate a greater understanding of the cultural diversity of food and eating.

When you work with individuals from other cultures, it is important to avoid **cultural stereotyping:** the tendency to view individuals of common cultural backgrounds similarly and according to a preconceived notion of how they "ought" to behave. Refer to topic-specific nutrition texts for detailed information about culture-specific diets and the nutritional value of ethnic foods.

Cultural food preferences are often interrelated with religious dietary beliefs and practices. Many religious customs involve foods as symbols in celebrations and rituals. Knowing how an individual's religious practices relate to food and eating may enable you to suggest modifications that do not conflict with their customs.

Other factors to consider in assessing nutritional status include fasting and other religious observations that may limit a person's food or liquid intake during specified times. This may also include customs in which specific foods are not combined at the same meal. This may be particularly important with regard to food and medication interactions during periods of fasting.

PURPOSES AND COMPONENTS OF NUTRITIONAL ASSESSMENT

Nutrition assessment is a method of collecting and evaluating data to make decisions about a nutrition-related concern or diagnosis. Best practice guidelines suggest that assessment data be compared to evidence-informed standards for evaluation. Nutrition assessment initiates the data collection process, which provides the framework for nutrition monitoring and evaluation. Nutrition assessment includes subjective data such as medical history; symptoms; dietary intake; psychosocial, behavioural, and functional factors; knowledge; readiness for potential change; and objective data, including anthropometric measurements and biochemical measurements.

Nurses, as part of the multidisciplinary health care team, often initiate the nutrition assessment on admission or with the first clinic visit. The nurse's evaluation and interpretation of the subjective and objective data collected are essential in determining next steps in the nutrition care plan. Individuals identified as being at nutritional risk can be referred to members of the health care team, including the physiotherapist, occupational therapist, speech-language pathologist, and dietitian. Each of these health care providers plays an important role in the comprehensive care of patients.

The purposes of a nutritional assessment are to (a) identify individual nutritional requirements, (b) provide information for designing a nutrition plan of care that will optimize nutrition and meet individual nutrient requirements, and (c) establish baseline data for evaluating the efficacy of nutritional care.

Nutrition screening, the first step in assessing nutritional status, can be completed in any setting (e.g., clinic, home, hospital, long-term care facilities). Based on readily obtained data, nutrition screening is an efficient way to identify individuals at nutrition risk, including those who have experienced unintentional weight loss, inadequate food intake, or recent illness. Parameters used for nutrition screening include weight and weight history, diet information, medical history, and routine laboratory data. A variety of valid tools are available for screening different populations, such as the Malnutrition Screening Tool (Anthony, 2008), which has been validated for use by nurses in hospitalized patients (Table 12-1).

TABLE 12-1	Malnutrition Screening Tool	
Have you lost weight recently without trying?		
No		0
Unsure		2
If yes, how much weight (in kilograms) have you lost?		
1–5		1
6–10		2
11–15		3
>15		4
Unsure		2
Have you been eating poorly because of decreased appetite?		
No		0
Yes		1
Total		
Score of 2 or more = patient at risk for malnutrition		

Malnutrition Screening Tool (MST). Reprinted from Ferguson, M., Capra, S., Bauer, J., & Banks, M. (1999). Development of a valid and reliable malnutrition screening tool for adult acute hospital patients. *Nutrition, 15*(6), 458-464.

The Malnutrition Screening Tool is a three-question screening tool that was developed and validated in 408 general medical/surgical adult hospital patients in Australia. It has a scoring potential of 7; a cutoff score of 2 has been determined to indicate risk of malnutrition. It is recommended that the Malnutrition Screening Tool be administered within 24 hours of the patient's hospitalization. This screen can be reliably completed by nurses and other members of the interprofessional health care team (Anthony, 2008).

Assessing Nutritional Intake

Individuals identified at nutritional risk during screening should be referred, when possible, to a dietitian to undergo a **comprehensive nutritional assessment,** which includes evaluation of dietary history and clinical information, a physical examination, and anthropometric measures.

Various methods for collecting current dietary intake information are available, including the 24-hour recall, the food frequency questionnaire, and the food diary. Documentation of nutritional intake for hospitalized patients can best be achieved through calorie counts of nutrients consumed or infused.

The 24-Hour Recall

The most common method of obtaining information about dietary intake is the **24-hour recall.** The individual or family member is asked to recall everything eaten within the past 24 hours. It is important to be aware of potential information gaps when this method is used: (a) The individual or family member may not be able to recall type or amount of food eaten; (b) intake within the past 24 hours may be atypical of usual intake; (c) the individual or family member may alter the truth for a variety of reasons; and (d) snack items and use of gravies, sauces, and condiments may be underreported.

The Food Frequency Questionnaire

To counter some of the challenges inherent in the 24-hour recall method, a **food frequency questionnaire** may also be completed. The information collected is related to how many times per day, week, or month an individual eats particular foods. The food frequency questionnaire does not quantify amount of food eaten, and, like the 24-hour recall, it relies on the individual's or family member's memory.

The Food Diary

In **food diaries,** the individual or family member writes down everything consumed for a certain period of time. Three days—two working days and one nonworking day—are customarily used. A food diary is most accurate if the individual records information immediately after eating. Potential challenges with the food diary include (a) noncompliance, (b) inaccurate recording, (c) atypical intake on the recording days, and (d) conscious alteration of diet during the recording period.

Direct Observation

Direct observation of the feeding and eating process can lead to detection of problems not readily identified through standard nutrition interviews. For example, observing the typical feeding techniques used by a parent or caregiver and the interaction between the individual and caregiver can be of value in assessing failure to thrive in children or unintentional weight loss in older adults.

Canada's Food Guide and Dietary Reference Intakes

Eating Well With Canada's Food Guide (Health Canada, 2007b) and the Dietary Reference Intakes (DRIs) are two tools commonly used to evaluate diet quality. Refer *to Canada's Food Guide* (see Figure 12-1 or online [Health Canada, 2007b]) for additional information and interactive tools ("My Food Guide") that allow you and your patients to personalize the information found in the guide.

The DRIs include four nutrient-based reference values that are used to assess and plan diets for healthy individuals (Table 12-2). The reference values include the estimated average requirement, the recommended dietary allowance, the adequate intake, and the tolerable upper intake level (Institute of Medicine, 2006). The DRIs are intended to help individuals optimize their health, prevent disease, and avoid overconsumption of any single nutrient.

The DRIs are designed for health maintenance and disease prevention in healthy individuals. They are not meant for the restoration of health or repletion of nutrients. Under the stress of an acute or chronic condition, an individual may have nutrient needs that are outside of the DRIs. Dietitians can design individualized, therapeutic diets that take into account nutrient requirements imposed by acute conditions (burns, surgery) and chronic conditions (diabetes, obesity).

There is considerable scientific and public interest in the use of vitamin supplements for the prevention and management of acute and chronic conditions. Although no nutrient

TABLE 12-2	Maintaining Healthy Eating Habits

Eating well and being active work together to promote health and well-being and provide benefits such as the following:
- Better overall health
- Lower risk of disease
- A healthy body weight
- Feeling and looking better
- More energy
- Stronger muscles and bones

Steps towards better health and a healthy body weight include the following:
- Eating the recommended amount and types of food each day
- Limiting foods and beverages high in calories, fat, sugar or salt (sodium)
- Being active every day

Following *Eating Well With Canada's Food Guide* (Health Canada, 2007b) will help people
- Meet their needs for vitamins, minerals, and other nutrients
- Reduce their risk of obesity, type 2 diabetes, heart disease, certain types of cancer, and osteoporosis
- Contribute to their overall health and vitality

Source: Adapted from Health Canada. (2007). *Maintaining healthy habits*. Retrieved from *http://www.hc-sc.gc.ca/fn-an/food-guide-aliment/maintain-adopt/index-eng.php*.

Nutrition Facts / Valeur nutritive

Per 1 25 mL (87 g) / par 1 25 mL (87 g)

Amount Teneur	% Daily Value % valeur quotidienne
Calories / Calories 80	
Fat / Lipides 0.5 g	1 %
Saturated / saturés 0 g + Trans / trans 0 g	0 %
Cholesterol / Cholestérol 0 mg	
Sodium / Sodium 0 mg	0 %
Carbohydrate / Glucides 18 g	6 %
Fibre / Fibres 2 g	8 %
Sugars / Sucres 2 g	
Protein / Protéines 3 g	
Vitamin A / Vitamine A	2 %
Vitamin C / Vitamine C	10 %
Calcium / Calcium	0 %
Iron / Fer	2 %

12-2 Nutrition Facts table.

in supplement form can replace a healthy, well-balanced diet, evidence suggests that some supplements are beneficial (e.g., vitamin D). Use caution when you recommend any vitamin or mineral supplement, to ensure that intakes do not exceed tolerable upper intake levels and that there are no nutrient–drug interactions. Referral to a dietitian may be warranted for patients using multiple nutrient supplements.

Nutrition Labelling in Canada

Nutrition labelling in Canada became mandatory for most prepackaged foods in 2007. Nutrition labelling regulations have been designed to convey information about the nutrient content of food in a standardized format, which allows for comparison among foods before purchase. The Nutrition Facts table provides information on energy (calories) and 13 nutrients, based on a stated serving size. The Nutrition Facts table must appear on the label in the prescribed manner. Clear, uniform information can support consumers in making informed food choices to achieve healthy eating goals (Canadian Food Inspection Agency, 2009).

The sample bilingual nutrition facts table shown in Figure 12-2 indicates the core information that must always be included and the order in which it must be presented. Additional nutrition information may also be required in the table or permitted either inside or outside the table, as prescribed.

The percent daily value (%DV) on a nutrition label reflects the needs of a healthy individual who consumes 2000 to 2500 calories daily. The %DV is used to express the food's content of nutrients, rather than just serving as a weight measure. The %DV can be used to make comparisons among foods. Refer to EatRight Ontario (see Links to Nutrition Information section) for additional information and interactive tools on nutrition labelling (EatRight Ontario, 2011).

SUBJECTIVE DATA

When you complete a nutrition assessment, you, as the nurse (or other health care provider), must recognize and acknowledge the patient's positive self-management behaviours, such as exercise, blood glucose monitoring, and nutrition label reading. Rapport and open communication are essential for positive outcomes.

The following represents potential areas of focus for subjective data collection in a nutrition assessment:

1. Eating patterns
2. Usual weight, recent weight changes
3. Changes in appetite, taste, smell, chewing, swallowing
4. Recent surgery, trauma, burns, infection
5. Chronic conditions
6. Nausea, vomiting, diarrhea, constipation
7. Food allergies or intolerances
8. Medications or nutritional supplements, or both

9. Self-management behaviours/access to healthy foods
10. Alcohol or illegal drug use
11. Exercise and activity patterns
12. Family history

13. Psychological symptoms
14. Physical impairments that limit ability to independently consume foods or liquids

HEALTH HISTORY QUESTIONS

Examiner Asks	Rationale/Comments
1. **Eating patterns** • Number of meals and snacks per day? • Type and amount of food eaten? • Fad, special, or alternative diets? • Where is food eaten? • Food preferences and dislikes? • Religious or cultural considerations? • Usual food preparation methods • Able to feed self?	Individuals eating fewer than three meals a day may not meet energy or nutrient requirements. Diets that restrict or eliminate entire categories of food are not recommended or supported by data. Ethnicity and religious beliefs, or feeding difficulties, may affect intake of certain foods. Include questions related to food type (e.g., light or low-fat foods); the addition of condiments, salt, or other seasonings; and an estimation of portion sizes and additional servings at meals.
2. **Usual weight.** What is your usual weight? • Recent weight change? • How much lost or gained? • Over what time period? • Reason for loss or gain?	Unintentional weight loss and obesity increase nutritional risk. Underweight individuals are vulnerable because their nutrient and energy reserves may be depleted. Obesity increases risk for chronic diseases, including hypertension, type 2 diabetes, and cancer. Protein and calorie needs should not be overlooked in acutely ill, obese individuals. Rapid weight gain over a short period of time may be an indication of a change in fluid status (e.g., edema).
3. **Changes in appetite, taste, smell, chewing, and swallowing** • Type of change? • When did change occur? • Any medical conditions and or medications associated with changes?	Poor appetite, alterations in taste and smell, and difficulties in chewing and swallowing can interfere with adequate nutrient intake and increase nutritional risk. Medication side effects can lead to changes in taste and appetite. Some medications necessitate alterations in meal timing or the avoidance of specific foods.
4. **Recent surgery, trauma, burns, and infection** • When? • Type? • How treated? • Conditions that increase nutrient loss (e.g., draining wounds, effusions, blood loss, dialysis, infection)?	With surgery, trauma, and sepsis, energy and nutrient needs may increase to two or three times greater than normal.
5. **Chronic conditions** • Type? • When diagnosed? • How managed? • Dietary modifications? • Recent cancer chemotherapy or radiation therapy?	Chronic conditions—including obesity, diabetes, metabolic syndrome, and hypertension—can increase nutrition risk as a result of the combined effects of dietary changes and medication use.

|

Subjective Data

6. **Nausea, vomiting, diarrhea, and constipation.** Do you have any of these problems?
   - Cause?
   - How long?
   - Medication use?

7. **Food allergies or intolerances**
   - Any problematic foods?
   - Type of reaction?
   - How long?
   - How treated/managed?
   - Related weight changes?
   - Medication use?

8. **Medications, nutritional supplements, and herbal supplements**
   - Prescription medications?
   - Nonprescription medications?
   - Use over a 24-hour period?

   - Type of vitamin or mineral supplement? Amount? Frequency and duration of use?
   - Herbal and botanical products? Specific type and brand and where obtained? How often used? How does it help you? Any problems?
   - Recommended by whom, and for what reason?

9. **Self-management behaviours/access to healthy foods**
   - Meal preparation facilities?
   - Transportation for travel to market?
   - Adequate income for food purchase?
   - Who prepares meals and does shopping?
   - Environment during mealtimes?
   - Current knowledge about healthy eating?

10. **Tobacco, alcohol, or illegal drug use**
    - When was last drink of alcohol?
    - Amount taken that episode?
    - Amount/type of alcohol each day? Each week?
    - Duration of use?
    - Use of other beverages with alcohol (i.e., mixed drinks)?
    - Use of tobacco products: type, how long, quantity, attempts to quit?
    - (Repeat questions for each drug used.)

11. **Exercise and activity patterns**
    - Amount?
    - Type?
    - Frequency/duration?
    - Any exercise-related injuries?

Gastrointestinal symptoms such as nausea, vomiting, diarrhea, and constipation may interfere with nutrient intake or absorption.

Many medications interfere with normal gastrointestinal function. Include a review of prescription and nonprescription medication use.

Intolerances related to the inability to digest specific foods, such as lactose in milk products, may result in gastrointestinal symptoms (i.e., gas, bloating, diarrhea) and lead to nutrient deficiencies.

Multiple food allergies or intolerances can lead to the necessary avoidance of many foods. This can result in a nutrient-deficient diet. Referral to a dietitian is warranted in cases of multiple food allergies or intolerances.

Analgesics, antacids, anticonvulsants, antibiotics, diuretics, laxatives, antineoplastic drugs, steroids, and oral contraceptives are among the drugs that can interact with nutrients, impairing their digestion, absorption, metabolism, or utilization.

Vitamin and mineral supplements may be harmful when taken in large amounts.

Use of herbal and botanical supplements is commonly underreported. Discuss use and potential adverse effects, including medication and/or nutrient interactions. Refer to the Natural Health Products Directorate (NHPD) Web site: *http://www.hc-sc.gc.ca/contact/dhp-mps/hpfb-dgpsa/nhpd-dpsn-eng.php.*

Socioeconomic factors may interfere with ingestion of adequate amounts of food and nutrients.

Distractions such as television or video games during meals may result in increased energy intake, potentially leading to weight gain.

These agents are often substituted for nutritious foods and increase requirements for some nutrients. Pregnant women who use tobacco products, drink alcohol, or use illegal drugs give birth to a disproportionate number of infants with low birth weights, failure to thrive, and other serious complications.

Energy and nutrient needs increase with greater physical activity, especially in individuals who participate in competitive sports or perform manual labour. Inactive or sedentary lifestyles often lead to excess weight gain.

Examiner Asks	Rationale/Comments

12. Family history. Family or personal history of heart disease, osteoporosis, cancer, gout, gastrointestinal disorders, obesity, or diabetes?
- Effect of each on eating patterns?
- Effect on activity patterns?

Long-term nutritional deficiencies or excesses may become apparent only when a chronic condition is diagnosed (i.e., calcium and vitamin D deficiency associated with osteoporosis). Early identification of dietary deficits allows for food and activity modifications to be implemented promptly, at a time when the body may recover more fully.

13. Psychological symptoms
- Depression or other mood-altering illness?
- Medications that affect mood?
- Psychosocial lifestyle factors?
- Disordered eating behaviours?

Psychological illness can affect the ability to access and prepare food. Mood can affect food choices and amount of food eaten. Stress, work, and home life issues may also affect eating. Distorted body image may increase the risk of eating disorders.

14. Physical impairments
- Challenges that limit the ability to independently consume foods or liquids?
- Chewing or swallowing concerns?

Conditions that affect coordination (Parkinson's disease) and chewing or swallowing (stroke, dementia) can significantly affect the ability to safely consume a healthy diet. Referral to other members of the health care team—including the speech-language pathologist, occupational therapist, and dietitian—may be warranted for such patients.

Additional History for Infants and Children

Dietary histories of infants and children are generally obtained from the child's parents or guardian. Asking caregivers to keep a thorough daily food diary and occasionally requesting 24-hour recalls during clinic visits are the most commonly employed techniques for this population group.

Nutrition assessment in infants and children include questions related to feeding (i.e., by whom), use of solid foods, and frequency and type of snacks. Inquire about beverage intake (i.e., milk vs. fruit juices) and use of sweetened vs. unsweetened foods and beverages.

Regular meal and snack times with few distractions are ideal to promote healthy eating habits and healthy weights in children.

1. Gestational nutrition
- Maternal history of alcohol or illegal drug use?
- Maternal weight gain during pregnancy?
- Any diet-related complications during gestation (i.e., hyperemesis, food avoidances, etc.)?
- Infant's birth weight?
- Any evidence of delayed physical or mental growth?

Low birth weight (<2500 g) is a risk factor in infant morbidity and mortality. Poor gestational nutrition, low maternal weight gain, and maternal alcohol and drug use—all factors in low birth weight—can lead to birth defects and delayed growth and development.

Excess weight gain in pregnancy increases risk of a high birth weight (<4500g) infant, prolonged labour, birth trauma, and caesarean birth.

2. Infant nutrition
- Type, frequency, amount, and duration of feeding?
- Any difficulties encountered?
- Timing and method of weaning?

New mothers may experience challenges with breastfeeding or bottle feeding or have questions about infant nutrition, the introduction of solid foods, and rate of infant weight gain.

Subjective Data

Examiner Asks	Rationale/Comments

3. Child nutrition
  • Any special likes or dislikes?
  • How much will child eat?
  • How do you manage non-nutritious snack foods?
  • How do you avoid food aspiration?

Use of small portions, finger foods, simple meals, and nutritious snacks are strategies to improve dietary intake. Avoid foods likely to be aspirated (e.g., hot dogs, nuts, grapes, round candies, popcorn).

Additional History for the Adolescent

1. Weight
  • What would you like to weigh?
  • How do you feel about your present weight?
  • On any special diet to lose weight?
  • Constantly think about "feeling fat"?
  • Intentionally vomit or use laxatives or diuretics after eating?

Weight gain, particularly in girls, may precipitate dieting and decreased nutrient intake. Because of adolescents' increased body awareness and self-consciousness, they are prone to eating disorders.

Eating disorders are complex psychiatric disorders strongly associated with other mental illness. Referrals to the social worker, psychologist, or psychiatrist and dietitian are warranted in suspected eating disorder cases.

2. Use of anabolic steroids or other agents to increase muscle size and physical performance?
  • When?/Why?
  • How much?
  • Prescribed by whom?

  • Use of caffeinated, energy boosting drinks? When? Type? Duration?

The use of anabolic steroids and other performance-enhancing agents now extends to junior-high, high-school, and post-secondary males and females. Adverse effects include personality disorders (aggressiveness), and liver and other organ damage.

Energy boosting drinks, such as Red Bull, contain large amounts of caffeine, other stimulants, or herbal products. Side effects include dehydration, dangerously high blood pressure and heart rate, and sleep problems.

3. What snacks or fast foods do you like to eat?
  • When?
  • How much?
4. Age first started menstruating
  • What is your menstrual flow like?

An accurate dietary history includes between-meal snacks and meals eaten away from home.

Menarche may be delayed in adolescents who are underweight, have very low body fat, or are elite athletes. Scant menstrual flow is associated with nutritional inadequacies.

Additional History for the Pregnant Woman

1. How many times have you been pregnant?
  • When?/Age at first (and subsequent) pregnancies
  • Any problems encountered during previous pregnancies?
  • Problems this pregnancy?
  • Use of vitamin/mineral/herbal supplements?
  • Use of tobacco products?
  • Caffeine intake?

A multiparous mother with pregnancies occurring less than 1 year apart has an increased risk for depleted nutritional reserves. Note previous complications of pregnancy (excessive vomiting, anemia, or gestational diabetes). Slower gastrointestinal motility and pressure from the fetus may cause constipation, hemorrhoids, and indigestion. A past history of a low-birth-weight infant suggests past nutritional problems. Giving birth to an infant weighing 4500 g (10 lb) or more may signal *latent* diabetes in the mother.

Subjective Data

Examiner Asks	Rationale/Comments
2. What foods do you prefer when pregnant? • What foods do you avoid? • Crave any particular foods?	The expectant mother is vulnerable to familial, cultural, and traditional influences for food choices. Cravings for, or aversions to, particular foods are common; evaluate for their potential contribution to, or interference with, dietary intake.
Additional History for the Older Adult 1. How does your diet differ from when you were in your 40s and 50s? • Why? • What factors affect the way you eat?	Note any physiological, psychological, or socioeconomic changes that may affect nutritional status. Use of vitamin supplements (specifically, vitamin D).

OBJECTIVE DATA

PREPARATION

An individual's general appearance—obese, cachectic (fat and muscle wasting), or edematous—can provide clues to overall nutritional status. More specific clinical signs and symptoms suggestive of nutritional deficiencies can be detected through a physical examination and laboratory testing. Laboratory tests for assessment of nutritional status are reviewed later in this chapter.

EQUIPMENT NEEDED

Measurement tape
Pen or pencil
Nutritional assessment data form

Normal Range of Findings	Abnormal Findings
ANTHROPOMORPHIC MEASURES Anthropometry is the measurement and evaluation of growth, development, and body composition. The most commonly used anthropometric measures are height, weight, waist–hip ratio, and waist circumference. Measurement of height, weight, and head circumference are described in Chapter 10.	A healthy body weight promotes general health and reduces the risk for some chronic diseases.
Derived Weight Measures Two derived weight measures are used to assess changes in body weight. The **percent usual body weight** is calculated as follows: $$\text{Percent usual body weight} = \frac{\text{Current weight}}{\text{Usual weight}} \times 100$$ **Recent weight change** is calculated with the following formula: $$\text{Weight change} = \frac{\text{Usual weight} - \text{Current weight}}{\text{Usual weight}} \times 100$$	A current weight of 85% to 95% of usual body weight indicates mild malnutrition; 75% to 84%, moderate malnutrition; and <75%, severe malnutrition. An unintentional loss of more than 5% of body weight over 1 month, more than 7.5% of body weight over 3 months, or more than 10% of body weight over 6 months is clinically significant.

Subjective Data

Objective Data

Normal Range of Findings	**Abnormal Findings**

Body Mass Index

BMI provides a practical marker of optimal weight for height and an indicator of obesity (see Figure 10-1 on p. 154). It is calculated as follows:

$$BMI = \frac{\text{Weight (in kilograms)}}{\text{Height (in metres)}^2}$$

or

$$\frac{\text{Weight (in pounds)}}{\text{Height (in inches)}^2} \times 703$$

BMI interpretation for adults (Health Canada, 2003b):

<18.5	Underweight
18.5–24.9	Normal weight
25.0–29.9	Overweight
30.0–39.9	Obesity
≥40	Extreme obesity

BMI interpretation for children aged 2 to 20 years (Centers for Disease Control and Prevention [CDC], 2000) is as follows:

85th to 95th percentiles = risk for overweight

See Appendix D on the Evolve Web site for WHO growth charts.

Waist–Hip Ratio

The waist–hip ratio reflects body fat distribution as an indicator of health risk. Obese individuals with a greater proportion of fat in the upper body, especially in the abdomen, have android obesity; obese individuals with most of their fat in the hips and thighs have gynoid obesity. Waist–hip ratio is calculated as follows:

$$\text{Waist–hip ratio} = \frac{\text{Waist circumference}}{\text{Hip circumferance}}$$

where waist circumference is measured in inches at the smallest circumference below the rib cage and above the umbilicus, and hip circumference is measured in inches at the largest circumference of the buttocks. **Waist circumference** alone can be used to predict increased health risk.

A waist–hip ratio of 1.0 or more in men or 0.8 or more in women is indicative of android (upper body obesity) and increasing risk for obesity-related diseases and early mortality.

A waist circumference exceeding 89 cm (35 in) inches in women and exceeding 102 cm (40 in) in men increases risk of cardiovascular and metabolic diseases.

 ## DEVELOPMENTAL CONSIDERATIONS

Infants, Children, and Adolescents

Weight. Because longitudinal growth is one of the best indices of nutritional status over time, height and weight should be measured at regular intervals during infancy, childhood, and adolescence. See Chapter 10 for techniques.

In 2004, approximately 18% of Canadian children and adolescents were overweight, and 8% were obese.

Pregnant Women

Weight. Measure weight monthly up to 30 weeks of pregnance and then every 2 weeks until the last month of pregnancy, at which point weight should be measured weekly. Appendix G on the Evolve Web site illustrates approximate weight gain considered normal for each week of pregnancy.

Consider the expectant mother at nutritional risk if her prepregnancy weight was 10% or more below or 20% or more above ideal weight.

Older Adults

Height. Height in men and women declines gradually from the early 30s, which results in an overall loss of height of 2.9 cm in men and 4.9 cm in women (Gabriella & Sinclair, 1997; Reuben, Greendale, & Harrison, 1995). Height measures may not be accurate in individuals confined to a bed or wheelchair or in patients with osteoporosis.

Alternative methods for height measurement can be used for patients unable to stand; these methods include knee height, forearm length, and arm span (Perry, 2009).

Objective Data

Normal Range of Findings	Abnormal Findings

LABORATORY STUDIES

Routine laboratory tests can detect preclinical nutritional deficiencies and can be used to confirm or support subjective findings. With older adults, however, use caution in interpreting test results that are outside normal ranges because they may not always indicate a nutritional problem, inasmuch as laboratory standards for older adults have not been firmly established.

Laboratory indicators of nutritional status include hemoglobin, hematocrit, cholesterol, triglycerides, total lymphocyte count, and serum albumin measurements. Glucose, low- and high-density lipoproteins, prealbumin, transferrin, and total protein levels also provide meaningful information.

Hemoglobin. Hemoglobin determination is used to detect iron deficiency anemia. Normal values are as follows:

Infants aged 1 to 3 days: 145 to 225 g/L

Infants aged 2 months: 90 to 140 g/L

Children aged 6 to 12 years: 115 to 155 g/L

Male adults: 135 to 180 g/L

Female adults: 120 to 160 g/L

Hematocrit. Hematocrit is a measure of cell volume, as well as an indicator of iron status. Normal values are as follows:

Infants aged 1 to 3 days: 0.44 to 0.72

Infants aged 2 months: 0.28 to 0.42

Children aged 6 to 12 years: 0.35 to 0.45

Male adults: 0.4 to 0.54

Female adults: 0.38 to 0.47

Cholesterol. Total cholesterol is measured to evaluate risk of cardiovascular disease. Normal cholesterol concentration is less than 5.2 mmol/L.

Triglycerides. Serum triglycerides are used to screen for hyperlipidemia and to determine the risk of coronary artery disease. Normal range is less than 1.7 mmol/L.

Blood Glucose Monitoring. Screening for type 2 diabetes with the use of fasting plasma glucose (FPG) values should be performed every 3 years in individuals older than 40 (Canadian Diabetes Association [CDA], 2008).

Glycemic targets to reduce macrovascular complications include a glycated hemoglobin (A_{1C}) value of ≤7.0% (CDA, 2008).

The CDA's *2008 Clinical Practice Guidelines* (see the section Links to Nutrition Information at the end of this chapter) contain more detailed information (CDA, 2008).

Total Lymphocyte Count. Tests of immune function include total lymphocyte count (TLC) and skin testing (also called *delayed cutaneous hypersensitivity testing*). TLC is an important indicator of visceral protein status and therefore of cellular immune function.

The TLC is derived from the white blood cell (WBC) count and the differential count:

$$TLC = WBC\ count \times \frac{Number\ of\ lymphocytes\ in\ differential}{100\ cells}$$

where TLC is calculated in cells per cubic millimetre.

Normal values for all age categories are between 1000 and 4000 cells/mm^3.

Abnormal Findings

Elevated hemoglobin levels suggest hemoconcentration as a result of polycythemia vera or dehydration.

Decreased hemoglobin levels may indicate anemia, recent hemorrhage, or hemodilution caused by fluid retention.

Decreased hematocrit indicates insufficient hemoglobin formation. Hematocrit and hemoglobin values should be interpreted together.

Risk for coronary artery disease increases with increasing serum cholesterol level.

Higher serum triglyceride levels are also associated with coronary artery disease and are categorized as *borderline* (2.26 to 4.50 mmol/L) or *high* (>4.5 mmol/L).

A 75-g oral glucose tolerance test to measure 2-hour plasma glucose should be performed in patients with a FPG of 6.1 to 6.9 mmol/L (CDA, 2008).

All patients with diabetes should be offered formal diabetes education that enhances self-management practices (CDA, 2008).

Non-nutritional factors that affect TLC include hypoalbuminemia, metabolic stress (e.g., major surgery, trauma, sepsis), infection, cancer, and chronic diseases.

Lymphopenia is a decrease in circulating lymphocytes.

Lymphocytosis is an increase in circulating lymphocytes.

Objective Data

Normal Range of Findings	Abnormal Findings

Skin Testing. Immunity can also be demonstrated by reactions to multiple skin test antigens. In these tests, a minimum of six antigens are injected intradermally in the forearm area, and the response (redness and induration) is noted at 24 and 48 hours. A response of 5 mm or larger to more than one antigen is generally considered a positive reaction (i.e., indicative of adequate immunity).

Commonly used antigens include *Candida* species, tetanus toxoid, diphtheria toxoid, *Streptococcus* species, old tuberculin, *Proteus* species, and *Trichophyton* species.

Serum Proteins. Serum albumin is a measurement of visceral protein status. Because of its relatively long half-life (17 to 20 days) and large body pool (4.0 to 5.0 g/kg), albumin is not an early indicator of protein malnutrition.

Normal serum albumin concentration in infants, in children older than 6 months, and in adults ranges from 35 to 50 g/L.

Serum transferrin, an iron-transport protein, can be measured directly or by an indirect measurement of total iron-binding capacity. Serum transferrin, which has a half-life of 8 to 10 days, may be a more sensitive indicator of visceral protein status than is albumin.

The normal values for serum transferrin are 1.90 to 3.35 g/L.

Prealbumin, or thyroxine-binding prealbumin, serves as a transport protein for thyroxine (T_4) and retinol-binding protein. Because its half-life is shorter (48 hours) than that of either albumin or transferrin, prealbumin is sensitive to acute changes in protein status and sudden demands on protein synthesis. Normal prealbumin levels range from 1.5 to 2.5 g/L.

Nitrogen Balance. Nitrogen balance is also used as an index of protein nutritional status. Nitrogen is released with the catabolism of amino acids and is excreted in the urine as urea. Nitrogen balance therefore indicates whether the person is anabolic (positive nitrogen balance) or catabolic (negative nitrogen balance).

Nitrogen balance is estimated by a formula based on urine urea nitrogen (UUN) excreted during the previous 24 hours:

$$\text{Nitrogen balance} = \text{Nitrogen intake} - \text{Nitrogen excretion}$$
$$= \text{Protein intake}/6.25 - (24 - \text{hour UUN} + 4)$$

where nitrogen balance is determined in grams; 24-hour UNN = UUN, measured in grams; and 4 = non–urea nitrogen losses via feces, skin, sweat, and lungs, measured in grams.

❖ DEVELOPMENTAL CONSIDERATIONS

In infancy and childhood, laboratory tests are performed only when undernutrition is suspected or if the child has acute or chronic conditions that affect nutritional status.

Abnormal Findings (right column):

A response smaller than 5 mm indicates anergy (immunoincompetence). Anergy occurs with malnutrition, hepatic failure, infection, and immunosuppressive drugs (e.g., chemotherapy agents, steroids).

Lymphopenia and the lack of a positive response to skin test antigens increase risk of infection and sepsis.

Serum albumin levels are low with protein-calorie malnutrition, altered hydration status, and decreased liver function.

A serum albumin level of 28 to 35 g/L represents moderate visceral protein depletion, and a level lower than 28 g/L denotes severe depletion (Chernecky & Berger, 2008).

Levels of 1.5 to 1.7 g/L suggest mild protein deficiency; 1.0 to 1.5 g/L, moderate deficiency; and levels less than 1.0 g/L, severe deficiency (Lee & Nieman, 2003). Because many clinical conditions can alter serum albumin and transferrin levels, consider the person's history in conjunction with these values for accurate interpretation.

Prealbumin levels are elevated in renal disease and reduced by surgery, trauma, burns, and infection. Prealbumin levels of 1.0 to 1.5 g/L indicate mild depletion; 0.5 to 1.0 g/L, moderate depletion; and less than 0.5 g/L, severe depletion.

In response to stress and increased protein demand, the body rapidly mobilizes its protein compartments, which results in increased production of urea and excretion of urea in the urine. With infection, an estimated loss of 9 to 11 g of UUN per day can be expected. In patients with major burns, 12 to 18 g of urea nitrogen per day may be expected in the urine (Blackburn, Bistrian, Maini, Schlamm, & Smith, 1977).

Objective Data

Normal Range of Findings	Abnormal Findings

During adolescence, unless overt disease is suspected, laboratory evaluation of hemoglobin and hematocrit levels and urinalysis for glucose and protein levels are generally considered adequate for assessment of nutritional status.

During pregnancy, hemoglobin and hematocrit values can be used to detect deficiencies of protein, folacin, vitamin B_{12}, and iron. Urine is frequently tested for glucose and protein (albumin), which can signal diabetes, preeclampsia, and renal disease.

In older adulthood, all serum and urine data must be interpreted with an understanding of declining renal efficiency and a tendency for older adults to be overhydrated or underhydrated.

SERIAL ASSESSMENT

Nutritional status in malnourished patients or individuals at risk for malnutrition is monitored through serial measurements of nutritional assessment parameters made at routine intervals. At minimum, weight and dietary intake should be evaluated weekly. Because the other nutritional assessment parameters change more slowly, data on these indicators may be collected biweekly or monthly.

Health Promotion

Essentials of a healthy diet are (a) eating a variety of foods from all food groups to ensure nutrient adequacy; (b) consuming recommended amounts of fruits and vegetables, whole grains, and fat-free or lower-fat dairy products; (c) limiting intake of foods high in saturated fats, trans fats, added sugars, starch, cholesterol, salt, and alcohol; (d) matching calorie intake with calories expended; (e) engaging in 30 to 60 minutes of moderate physical activity most days; and (f) following food safety guidelines for handling, preparing, and storing foods.

Canada's *Physical Activity Guide to Healthy Living* (*http://www.phac-aspc.gc.ca/ hp-ps/hl-mvs/pa-ap/index-eng.php*) is designed to help individuals at specific life stages (i.e., older adults, children, youth) make wise choices about physical activity. Research indicates that more than half of Canadian children and youth aged 6 to 19 are not active enough for optimal healthy growth and development (PHAC, 2011c). The majority of Canadians are unaware that insufficient physical activity is a serious risk factor for premature death, chronic disease, and disability (Health Canada, 2003a). According to Health Canada, two thirds of Canadians are currently inactive (Health Canada, 2003a).

Approaches to weight loss for people who are overweight or obese must be individualized, reflect cultural sensitivity, and account for the patient's readiness to lose weight and his or her health care and self-management behaviours. Weight loss programs involving less than 1000 to 1200 calories per day may not provide adequate nutrients. Weight loss programs that include a balance of foods from all food groups, spread over three meals and two to three snacks, will result in gradual weight loss for most people. Essential features of successful long-term weight loss plans for adults include (a) regular physical exercise; (b) eating a reduced-calorie ($\approx$1400 to 1500 kcal/day), low-fat (20% to 35% of total calories) foods; and (c) monitoring daily food intake (e.g., food diary, portion size) and body weight.

Patients should be discouraged from fad diets, diets that eliminate one or more food groups, and diets promoting weight loss in excess of 0.5 to 1.0 kg (1 to 2 lb) per week.

Patients may benefit from reminders that weight management strategies need to include a regular component of physical activity. This activity should be one that patients enjoy, can safely participate in, and fits into their daily routine on a regular basis.

Objective Data

DOCUMENTATION AND CRITICAL THINKING

Sample Charting

SUBJECTIVE

No history of diseases or surgery that would alter intake or requirements; no recent weight changes; no appetite changes. Consumes regular meals and snacks, variety of food choices.

Financial resources adequate for healthy eating. No concerns about access to healthy food. Does not use tobacco products; drink alcohol; or use illegal, prescription, or over-the-counter drugs. No vitamin/mineral or herbal supplements.

No food allergies or intolerances. Sedentary lifestyle; plays golf once per week.

OBJECTIVE

Dietary intake is adequate to meet protein and energy needs. No clinical signs of nutrient deficiencies. Height, weight, BMI, and screening laboratory test results within normal ranges.

Focused Assessment: Clinical Case Study—Type 2 Diabetes, Increased Weight, Hypertension

E.G. is 46 years old and has type 2 diabetes. She lives at home with her common-law spouse.

SUBJECTIVE

As a result of low nutrition literacy skills and depression, E.G. has been unable to keep a job. Her spouse has recently been laid off from his job. Money is very tight right now, and this has led to additional stress, which has made E.G.'s diabetes harder to manage. She has applied for Ontario Disability Support Program (Social Assistance), as well as for a Special Diet Allowance, which gives her an additional $64.00 a month because of her diabetes and hypercholesterolemia. E.G. has been trying to walk 5 to 7 days a week for 30 minutes to help manage her weight and diabetes.

OBJECTIVE

Inspection: slightly overweight female, looks older than stated age. Current weight: 71.6 kg (158 lbs). Height: 162.5 cm (5 feet 4 inches). Blood pressure: 137/88. Current medications:

- Metformin: an antidiabetic medication, used to lower blood glucose levels
- Atorvastatin: used to lower cholesterol levels
- Furosemide: used to help lower blood pressure levels
- Venlafaxine: antidepressant

Most recent laboratory values:

Test	Result	Reference Range
A_{1C}	0.071	<0.07
FBG	10.5 mmol/L	<7.0 mmol/L
LDL [low-density lipoprotein] cholesterol	3.8 mmol/L	<2.0 mmol/L
HDL [high-density lipoprotein] cholesterol	0.89 mmol/L	>1.3 mmol/L
Triglycerides	4.3 mmol/L	<1.7 mmol/L
Total cholesterol	6.6 mmol/L	<4.0 mmol/L

ASSESSMENT

Psychosocial: increased stress resulting from spouse's loss of job, limited income, recent need for social assistance; managing multiple medical concerns. Has started walking to manage weight and diabetes.

BMI = 27.1: above ideal weight

Laboratory values: elevated FBG, LDL, triglycerides. total cholesterol; low HDL level → increased risk for CVD [cardiovascular disease]

Medication review: appropriate

Diet review: challenges related to decreased income, low fruit and vegetable intake, increased intake of processed meats, few whole grains

RECOMMENDATIONS

On this visit, the nurse can discuss a number of potential behaviour changes with E.G. Each of these suggested changes should be negotiated in relation to the planning and implementation of the change. Simply telling patients what they need to do or change has been shown to be ineffective in eliciting positive behaviour change.

Short-term nutritional advice for E.G. may include the following:

- Avoiding simple sugars found in fruit juices, regular soft drinks, and other sweetened beverages.
- Following guidelines on meal planning and portion control, available from the CDA (2010, n.d.).
- Eating more fruits and vegetables daily: recommend frozen vegetables and canned (in juice) fruit because they are often more economical.
- Eating lean meats and low-fat dairy products (skim milk, low-fat cheese, and yogurt); using low-fat cooking methods (baking, broiling); and avoiding added salt.
- Continuing positive self-management behaviours (walking).

E.G. should continue being monitored for BP, blood work, and psychosocial support.

Refer to a diabetes education centre for nursing, dietitian, and social work assessment and follow-up.

ABNORMAL FINDINGS

MANAGEMENT OF CHRONIC DISEASE

Obesity

Obesity has been described as a global epidemic. It has been linked to diabetes, hypertension, cardiovascular disease, and some forms of cancer. The prevalence of obesity is 24.3% among Canadian men and 23.9% among Canadian women (Statistics Canada, 2011a).

Obese individuals more commonly suffer from chronic conditions—including hypertension, diabetes, and heart disease—than do people who are at a healthy weight. Research indicates that more than 70% of obese individuals suffer from at least one other major health problem.

Central Obesity

Even more significant than total body fat is the type and location of fat. Body fat that collects deep within the central abdominal area of the body, called *visceral fat,* is associated with increased risk for diabetes, stroke, hypertension, and cardiovascular disease. The risk of death from all causes may be higher in people with central obesity than in those whose fat accumulates elsewhere in the body.

Awareness of the social and economic factors leading to obesity is essential when you complete nutritional screening of patients. Obesity is a complex problem with genetic, environmental, and psychological components. Sensitivity to each of these factors and ensuring that all education is tailored to the individual patient may lead to more positive outcomes.

Diabetes

Diabetes, a chronic condition characterized by elevated blood glucose levels, often leads to other diseases or contributes to their development. In 2000, diabetes was diagnosed in an estimated 150 million people around the world, and that number is projected to increase to 380 million by 2025. In 2005, 5.5% of the Canadian population had diagnosed diabetes (CDA, 2008). This number is expected to grow, in view of Canada's demographic trends. An aging population, increasing immigration from high-risk populations, and growth in the Aboriginal population will increase the burden of diabetes before 2025. Of Canadians with diabetes, 11% also have three or more chronic health conditions, and in comparison with the general population, they are four times more likely to be admitted to a hospital or nursing home (CDA, 2008).

Screening for Type 2 Diabetes

Undiagnosed type 2 diabetes may be present in more than 2.8% of the general population. Tests for hyperglycemia can identify individuals who may have or be at risk for preventable diabetes complications. More frequent and earlier screening for type 2 diabetes has resulted in detecting unrecognized diabetes in individuals identified as being at risk (CDA, 2008).

Classification of Diabetes

Type 1 diabetes is the result of pancreatic β cell destruction, of which the cause is unknown. Individuals are at risk of ketoacidosis. Type 1 diabetes is often the result of an autoimmune process for which the beta cell destruction is unknown (CDA, 2008).

Type 2 diabetes has manifestations ranging from predominant insulin resistance with relative insulin deficiency to a predominant secretory defect with insulin resistance (CDA, 2008).

Gestational diabetes is glucose intolerance with onset during pregnancy (CDA, 2008).

The following parameters are diagnostic for diabetes (CDA, 2008):

- FPG level ≥7.0 mmol/L
- Casual plasma glucose level ≥11.1 mmol/L plus symptoms of diabetes
- 2-Hour plasma glucose level in a 75-g oral glucose tolerance test ≥11.1 mmol/L

Optimal glycemic control is fundamental in the management of diabetes. High plasma glucose levels, both fasting and postprandial, increase risk of diabetes-related complications. When you set management goals, it is essential to consider patients' age, prognosis, and presence of complications or comorbid conditions (CDA, 2008).

A_{1C} (previously called *hemoglobin A_{1C}*, and *HbA_{1C}*) level reflects glycemia over the 120-day life span of erythrocytes (red blood cells). This indicator of treatment effectiveness should be measured approximately every 3 months to ensure that glycemic goals are being met or maintained in individuals with diabetes (CDA, 2008).

Nutrition counselling with a dietitian is recommended for all individuals with diabetes. Nutrition therapy can reduce A_{1C} by 1.0% to 2.0% and, when used with other components of diabetes management (social work, physiotherapy), can further improve outcomes (CDA, 2008).

Metabolic Syndrome

Metabolic syndrome is a highly prevalent, multifaceted condition characterized by a distinctive collection of abnormalities, including abdominal obesity, hypertension, dyslipidemia, insulin resistance, and dysglycemia (CDA, 2008). Individuals with metabolic syndrome are at risk for developing diabetes and cardiovascular disease. Evidence supports an aggressive approach in identifying individuals with metabolic syndrome and managing the associated risk factors.

Consensus regarding operational definitions of metabolic syndrome is lacking. In 1998, the World Health Organization proposed a unifying definition that includes

TABLE 12-3	Clinical Identification of Metabolic Syndrome: ≥ 3 Measures to Make the Diagnosis
Risk Factor	**Defining Level***
Elevated FPG	≥ 5.6 mmol/L
Elevated BP	≥ 130/85 mm Hg
Elevated Triglycerides	≥ 1.7 mmol/L
Reduced HDL-C	
Men	< 1.0 mmol/L
Women	< 1.3 mmol/L
Abdominal obesity (waist circumference)	
Men	≥ 102 cm
Women	≥ 88 cm

Source: From Canadian Diabetes Association Clinical Practice Guidelines Expert Committee of the Canadian Diabetes Advisory Board (2013). Canadian Diabetes Association 2013 clinical practice guidelines for the prevention and management of diabetes in Canada. *Canadian Journal of Diabetes,* 37(Suppl. 1), S1-212. Retrieved from *http://download.journals.elsevierhealth.com/pdfs/journals/1499-2671/PIIS1499267113000129.pdf.* Reprinted with permission.
*Metabolic syndrome is diagnosed when three or more of the risk determinants are present.
BP, blood pressure; *FPG,* fasting plasma glucose; *HDL-C,* high-density lipoprotein cholesterol.

identification of the presence of insulin resistance. More recently, the Canadian Diabetes Association provided an operational definition based on three or more criteria that do not include a measure of insulin resistance (Table 12-3). Data from the Third National Health and Nutrition Survey revealed that the overall prevalence of metabolic syndrome in the United States was approximately 20% to 25%.

LINKS TO NUTRITION INFORMATION

Nurses are encouraged to further explore available resources related to nutrition. The Summary Checklist box and the following links include resources and interactive tools for the professional and the consumer. These tools may enhance understandings of the role of nutrition in health and chronic disease prevention and management.

- Canada's Nutrition and Health Atlas: *http://www.hc-sc.gc.ca/fn-an/surveill/atlas/index-eng.php*
- Canadian Diabetes Association: *http://www.diabetes.ca/for-professionals/resources/2008-cpg/*
- Dietitians of Canada: *http://www.dietitians.ca/*
- EatRight Ontario: *http://www.eatrightontario.ca/en/default.aspx*
- Health Canada, food and nutrition: *http://www.hc-sc.gc.ca/fn-an/index-eng.php*
- Public Health Agency of Canada: *http://www.phac-aspc.gc.ca/index-eng.php*
- Canadian Diabetes Association: *http://www.diabetes.ca/*

Summary Checklist: Nutritional Assessment

For a PDA-downloadable version, go to *http://evolve.elsevier.com/Canada/Jarvis/examination/*.

1. Obtain a **health history** relevant to nutritional status.
2. Elicit **dietary history**, if indicated.
3. **Inspect** skin, hair, eyes, oral cavity, nails, and musculoskeletal and neurological systems for clinical signs and symptoms suggestive of nutritional deficiencies.
4. **Measure** height, weight, and other anthropometric parameters, as indicated; calculate body mass index and waist-to-hip ratio.
5. Review relevant **laboratory tests**.
6. **Offer health promotion** teaching and referral to a dietitian or other members of the multidisciplinary health care team, as indicated.

REFERENCES

Anthony, P. S. (2008). Nutrition screening tools for hospitalized patients. *Nutrition in Clinical Practice, 23*(4), 373–382.

Blackburn, G. L., Bistrian, B. R., Maini, B. S., Schlamm, H. T., & Smith, M. F. (1977). Nutritional and metabolic assessment of the hospitalized patient. *Journal of Parenteral and Enteral Nutrition, 1*(1), 11–22.

Boland, M. (2005). Exclusive breastfeeding should continue to six months. *Pediatric Child Health, 10*(3), 148.

Canadian Diabetes Association. (2008). Canadian Diabetes Association 2008 clinical practice guidelines for the prevention and management of diabetes in Canada. *Canadian Journal of Diabetes, 32*(Suppl. 1).

Canadian Diabetes Association. (2010). *Just the basics: Tips for healthy eating, diabetes prevention and management* [Clinical Practice Guideline]. Retrieved from *http://www.diabetes.ca/files/JTB17x_11_CPGO3_1103.pdf*.

Canadian Diabetes Association. (n.d.). *Handy portion guide.* Retrieved from *http://www.diabetes.ca/Files/plan%20your%20portions.pdf*.

Canadian Food Inspection Agency. (2009). *Guide to food labelling and advertising.* Retrieved from *http://www.inspection.gc.ca/english/fssa/labeti/guide/toce.shtml*.

Canadian Institute for Health Information. (2006). *Improving the health of Canadians: Promoting healthy weights.* Ottawa: Author.

Centers for Disease Control and Prevention. (2000). *Growth charts.* Retrieved from *http://www.cdc.gov/growth_charts/clinical_charts.htm*.

Chernecky, C. C., & Berger, B. J. (2008). *Laboratory tests and diagnostic procedures* (5th ed.). St. Louis: W. B. Saunders.

Dietitians of Canada. (2011). *What we do.* Retrieved from *http://www.dietitians.ca/About-Us/What-We-Do.aspx*.

Dryburgh, H. (2000). Teenage pregnancy. *Health Reports, 12*(1), 9–19.

EatRight Ontario. (2011). *Eatright Ontario.* Retrieved from *http://www.eatrightontario.ca/en/default.aspx*.

Fairholm, J. (1999). *Urban agriculture and food security initiatives in Canada: A survey of Canadian non-governmental organizations.* Ottawa: International Development Research Centre.

First Nations Information Governance Centre. (2011). *RHS Phase 2 (2008/10) preliminary results—Adult, youth, child* (revised edition). Retrieved from *http://www.fnigc.ca/sites/default/files/First20Nations20Regional20Health20Survey20(RHS)202008-1020-20National20Report.pdf*.

Furman, E. F. (2006). Undernutrition in older adults across the continuum of care: Nutritional assessment, barriers, and interventions. *Journal of Gerontological Nursing, 32*(1), 22–27.

Gabriella, S. E., & Sinclair, A. J. (1997). Diagnosing undernutrition in elderly people. *Reviews in Clinical Gerontology, 7*, 367–371.

Health Canada. (2003a). *Canada's physical activity guide to healthy active living.* Retrieved from *http://www.phac-aspc.gc.ca/pau-uap/paguide/intro.html*.

Health Canada. (2003b). *Canadian guidelines for body weight classification in adults.* Retrieved from *http://www.hc-sc.gc.ca/fn-an/nutrition/weights-poids/guide-ld-adult/qa-qr-prof_e.html*.

Health Canada. (2004). *Canadian community health survey, Cycle 2.2, nutrition: Income-related household food security in Canada.* Retrieved from *http://www.hc-sc.gc.ca/fn-an/surveill/nutrition/commun/income_food_sec-sec_alim_e.html*.

Health Canada. (2005). *Alternate milks.* Retrieved from *http://www.healthycanadians.gc.ca/kids-enfants/infant-care-soins-bebe/nutrition-alimentation-eng.php*.

Health Canada. (2007a). *Breastfeeding.* Retrieved from *http://www.hc-sc.gc.ca/fn-an/surveill/nutrition/commun/prenatal/vit_d_sup-eng.php*.

Health Canada. (2007b). *Eating well with Canada's food guide.* Retrieved from *http://www.hc-sc.gc.ca/fn-an/food-guide-aliment/index-eng.php*.

Health Canada. (2007c). *Eating well with Canada's food guide— First Nations, Inuit and Métis.* Retrieved from *http://www.hc-sc.gc.ca/fn-an/pubs/fnim-pnim/index_e.html*.

Health Canada. (2010). *Canadian gestational weight gain recommendations.* Retrieved from *http://www.hc-sc.gc.ca/fn-an/nutrition/prenatal/qa-gest-gros-qr-eng.php*.

Health Canada. (2012). *Pregnancy weight gain calculator.* Retrieved from *http://www.hc-sc.gc.ca/fn-an/nutrition/prenatal/bmi/index-eng.php*.

Indian Affairs and Northern Development. (2003). *Nutrition and food security in Kugaaruk, Nunavut: Baseline survey for food mail pilot project.* Ottawa: Author.

Indian Affairs and Northern Development. (2004). *Nutrition and food security in Fort Severn, Ontario: Baseline survey for the food mail pilot project.* Ottawa: Author.

Institute of Medicine. (2006). *Dietary reference intakes. The essential guide to nutrient requirements.* Washington, DC: National Academies Press.

Lee, R. D., & Nieman, D. C. (2003). *Nutritional assessment* (3rd ed.). New York: McGraw-Hill.

Littleton, H. L., & Ollendick, T. (2003). Negative body image and disordered eating behavior in children and adolescents: What places youth at risk and how can these problems be prevented? *Clinical Child and Family Psychology Review, 6*(1), 51–66.

National Heart, Lung, and Blood Institute, National Institutes of Health, & U.S. Department of Health and Human Services. (2006). *Obesity education initiative.* Retrieved from *http://www.nhlbi.nih.gov/about/oei/index.htm*.

Perez, C. E. (2002). Health status and health behavior among immigrants. *Health Reports, 19*(2), 31–43.

Perry, L. (2009). Using height, weight and other body measurements in nutritional assessment. *Nursing Times.net.* Retrieved from *http://www.nursingtimes.net/using-height-weight-and-other-body-measurements-in-nutritional-assessments/1958313.article*.

Public Health Agency of Canada. (2008). *Folic acid*. Retrieved from *http://www.phac-aspc.gc.ca/fa-af/index-eng.php*.

Public Health Agency of Canada. (2011a). *The Chief Public Health Officer's report on the state of public health in Canada, 2011: Youth and young adults—Life in transition*. Ottawa: Author. Retrieved from *http://www.phac-aspc.gc.ca/cphorsphc-respcacsp/2011/index-eng.php*.

Public Health Agency of Canada. (2011b). *Curbing childhood obesity: A federal, provincial and territorial framework for action to promote healthy weights*. Ottawa: Author.

Public Health Agency of Canada. (2011c). *Physical activity*. Retrieved from *http://www.phac-aspc.gc.ca/hp-ps/hl-mvs/pa-ap/index-eng.php*.

Reuben, D. B., Greendale, G. A., & Harrison, G. G. (1995). Nutrition screening in older persons. *Journal of the American Geriatric Society, 43*, 415–425.

SickKids Motherisk. (2011). *Taking folic acid before you get pregnant*. Retrieved from *http://www.motherisk.org/women/folicAcid.jsp*.

Silva, M. A. (2006). *Body image dissatisfaction: A growing concern among men*. Milwauki: Milwaukee School of Engineering Counseling Services. Retrieved from *http://www.msoe.edu/life_at_msoe/current_student_resources/student_resources/counseling_services/newsletters_for_mental_health/body_image_dissatisfaction.shtml*.

Sizer, F. S., Whitney, E., & Piche, L. A. (2009). *Nutrition concepts and controversies* (1st Canadian edition). Toronto: Nelson.

Statistics Canada. (2007). *Canadian Health Measures Survey, 2007: Cycle 1 [Share Microdata File]*. Ottawa, Ontario: Statistics Canada as reported in Public Health Agency of Canada (2011). *The Chief Public Health Officer's report on the state of public health in Canada, 2011: Youth and young adults—Life in transition*. Ottawa: Public Health Agency of Canada. Retrieved from *http://publichealth.gc.ca/CPHOreport*.

Statistics Canada. (2011a). *Adult obesity prevalence in Canada and the United States* (Catalogue No. 82-620). Retrieved from *http://www.statcan.gc.ca/pub/82-625-x/2011001/article/11411-eng.htm*.

Statistics Canada. (2011b). *Canadian Community Health Survey, 2009: Annual [Share Microdata File]*. Ottawa, ON: Statistics Canada, as reported in Public Health Agency of Canada. (2011). *The Chief Public Health Officer's report on the state of public health in Canada, 2011: Youth and young adults—Life in transition*. Ottawa: Public Health Agency of Canada. Retrieved from *http://publichealth.gc.ca/CPHOreport*.

Skin, Hair, and Nails

Written by Carolyn Jarvis, PhD, APN, CNP
Adapted by June MacDonald-Jenkins, RN, BScN, MSc

⊖volve WEBSITE

OUTLINE

STRUCTURE AND FUNCTION

Think of the skin as the body's largest organ system. It covers 1.86 square metres of surface area in the average adult. The skin is the sentry that guards the body from environmental stresses (e.g., trauma, pathogens, dirt) and adapts it to other environmental influences (e.g., heat, cold).

SKIN

The skin has two layers: the outer highly differentiated *epidermis* and the inner supportive *dermis* (Figure 13-1). Beneath these layers is a third layer, the *subcutaneous* layer of adipose tissue.

Epidermis

The *epidermis* is thin but tough. Its cells are bound tightly together into sheets that form a rugged protective barrier. It is stratified into several zones. The inner **stratum germinativum,** or basal cell layer, forms new skin cells. Their major ingredient is the tough, fibrous protein *keratin*. The melanocytes interspersed along this layer produce the pigment *melanin*, which gives the skin and hair their brown tones. All people have the same number of melanocytes; however, the amount of melanin they produce varies with genetic, hormonal, and environmental influences.

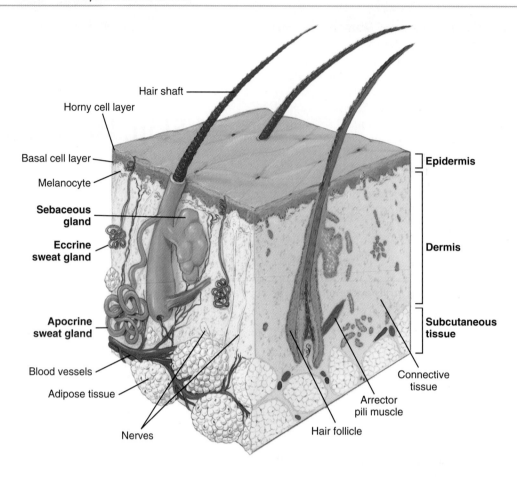

Hair shaft

Horny cell layer

Basal cell layer

Melanocyte

Sebaceous gland

Eccrine sweat gland

Apocrine sweat gland

Blood vessels

Adipose tissue

Nerves

Hair follicle

Arrector pili muscle

Connective tissue

Epidermis

Dermis

Subcutaneous tissue

13-1

From the basal layer, the new cells migrate up and flatten into the **stratum corneum.** This outer horny cell layer consists of dead keratinized cells that are interwoven and closely packed. The cells are constantly being shed, or *desquamated,* and are replaced with new cells from below. The epidermis is completely replaced every 4 weeks. In fact, each person sheds about half a kilogram of skin each year.

The epidermis is uniformly thin except on the surfaces that are exposed to friction, such as the palms and the soles. On these surfaces, skin is thicker because of work and weight bearing. The epidermis is avascular; it is nourished by blood vessels in the dermis below.

Skin colour is derived from three sources: (a) mainly from the brown pigment melanin, (b) from the yellow-orange tones of the pigment carotene, and (c) from the red-purple tones in the underlying vascular bed. All people have skin of varying shades of brown, yellow, and red; the relative proportions of these shades affect the prevailing colour. Skin colour is further modified by the thickness of the skin and by the presence of edema.

Dermis

The *dermis* is the inner supportive layer consisting mostly of connective tissue, or *collagen.* This is the tough, fibrous protein that enables the skin to resist tearing. The dermis also has resilient elastic tissue that allows the skin to stretch with body movements. The nerves, sensory receptors, blood vessels, and lymphatic vessels lie in the dermis. Also, appendages from the epidermis—such as the hair follicles, sebaceous glands, and sweat glands—are embedded in the dermis.

Subcutaneous Layer

The *subcutaneous layer* is adipose tissue, which is made up of lobules of fat cells. The subcutaneous tissue stores fat for energy, provides insulation for temperature control, and aids in protection by its soft, cushioning effect. Also, the loose subcutaneous layer gives skin its increased mobility over structures underneath.

EPIDERMAL APPENDAGES

Epidermal appendages are formed by a tubular invagination of the epidermis down into the underlying dermis.

Hair

Hair is *vestigial* for humans; it is no longer needed for protection from cold or trauma. However, hair is highly significant in most cultures for its cosmetic and psychological meaning (see the section Cultural and Social Considerations).

Hairs are threads of keratin. The hair *shaft* is the visible projecting part, and the *root* is below the surface, embedded in the follicle. At the root the *bulb matrix* is the expanded area where new cells are produced at a fast rate. Hair growth is cyclical, with active and resting phases. Each follicle functions independently so that while some hairs are resting, others are growing. Around the hair follicle are the muscular *arrector pili,* which contract and elevate the hair so that it resembles "goose flesh" during exposure to cold or in emotional states.

People have two types of hair. Fine, faint **vellus hair** covers most of the body (except the palms and soles, the dorsa of the distal parts of the fingers, the umbilicus, the glans penis, and inside the labia). The other type is **terminal hair,** the darker thicker hair that grows on the scalp and eyebrows and, after puberty, on the axillae, the pubic area, and, in men, the face and chest.

Sebaceous Glands

Sebaceous glands produce a protective lipid substance, *sebum,* which is secreted through the hair follicles. Sebum oils and lubricates the skin and hair and forms an emulsion with water that retards water loss from the skin. (Dryness of skin results from loss of water, not directly from loss of oil.) Sebaceous glands are everywhere except on the palms and soles. They are most abundant in the scalp, forehead, face, and chin.

Sweat Glands

There are two types of sweat glands. The **eccrine** glands are coiled tubules that open directly onto the skin surface and produce a dilute saline solution called *sweat.* The evaporation of sweat reduces body temperature. Eccrine glands are widely distributed through the body and are mature in 2-month-old infants.

The **apocrine** glands produce a thick, milky secretion and open into the hair follicles. They are located mainly in the axillae, anogenital area, nipples, and navel and are vestigial in humans. They become active during puberty, and secretion occurs with emotional and sexual stimulation. Bacterial flora residing on the skin surface react with apocrine sweat to produce a characteristic musky body odour. The functioning of apocrine glands decreases in older adults.

Nails

The nails are hard plates of keratin on the dorsal edges of the fingers and toes (Figure 13-2). The nail plate is clear, with fine longitudinal ridges that become prominent in aging. The pink colour of nails is derived from the underlying nail bed of highly vascular epithelial cells. The lunula is the white opaque semilunar area at the proximal end of the nail. It lies over the nail matrix, where new keratinized cells are formed. The nail folds overlap the posterior and lateral borders. The cuticle works like a gasket to cover and protect the nail matrix.

FUNCTION OF THE SKIN

The skin is a waterproof, highly resilient covering that has protective and adaptive properties:

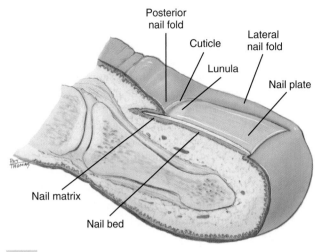

Posterior nail fold
Cuticle
Lunula
Lateral nail fold
Nail plate
Nail matrix
Nail bed

13-2

- **Protection.** Skin minimizes injury from physical, chemical, thermal, and light wave sources.
- **Prevention of penetration.** Skin is a barrier that stops invasion of microorganisms and loss of water and electrolytes from within the body.
- **Perception.** Skin is a vast sensory surface holding the neurosensory end organs for touch, pain, temperature, and pressure.
- **Temperature regulation.** Skin allows heat dissipation through sweat glands and heat storage through subcutaneous insulation.
- **Identification.** People identify one another by unique combinations of facial characteristics, hair, skin colour, and even fingerprints. Self-image is often enhanced or deterred by the way each person's perceived characteristics measure up to society's standards of beauty.
- **Communication.** Emotions are expressed in the sign language of the face and in the body posture. Vascular mechanisms such as blushing or blanching also signal emotional states.
- **Wound repair.** Skin allows cell replacement of surface wounds.
- **Absorption and excretion.** Skin allows limited excretion of some metabolic wastes, by-products of cellular decomposition such as minerals, sugars, amino acids, cholesterol, uric acid, and urea.
- **Production of vitamin D.** The skin is the surface on which ultraviolet light converts cholesterol into vitamin D.

 DEVELOPMENTAL CONSIDERATIONS

Infants and Children

The hair follicles develop in the fetus at 3 months' gestation; by midgestation, most of the skin is covered with **lanugo,** the fine downy hair of the newborn infant. In the first few months after birth, this is replaced by fine vellus hair. Terminal hair on the scalp, if present at birth, tends to be soft and to go through a period of a patchy loss, especially at the temples and occiput. Also present at birth is **vernix caseosa,** the thick, cheesy substance made up of sebum and shed epithelial cells.

A newborn's skin is similar in structure to an adult's, but many of its functions are not fully developed. A newborn's skin is thin, smooth, and elastic and is relatively more permeable than that of an adult, and so the infant is at greater risk for fluid loss. Sebum, which holds water in the skin, is present for the first few weeks of life, producing milia and cradle cap in some babies. Then sebaceous glands decrease in size and production and do not resume functioning until puberty. Temperature regulation is also ineffective. Eccrine sweat glands do not secrete in response to heat until the first few months of life and then only minimally throughout childhood. The skin cannot protect much against cold because it cannot contract and shiver and because the subcutaneous layer is inefficient. In addition, the pigment system is inefficient at birth.

As the child grows, the epidermis thickens, toughens, and darkens, and the skin becomes better lubricated. Hair growth accelerates. At puberty, secretion from apocrine sweat glands increases in response to heat and emotional stimuli, producing body odour. Sebaceous glands become more active; the skin looks oily, and acne develops. Subcutaneous fat deposits increase, especially in girls.

Secondary sex characteristics that appear during adolescence are evident in the integument (i.e., skin). In girls, the diameter of the areola enlarges and darkens, and breast tissue develops. Coarse pubic hair and then axillary hair develop in boys and girls, and then coarse facial hair develops in boys.

Pregnant Women

The change in hormone levels results in increased pigmentation in the areolae and nipples, vulva, and sometimes in the midline of the abdomen (**linea nigra**) or in the face (**chloasma**). Hyperestrogenemia probably also causes the common vascular spiders and palmar erythema. Connective tissue becomes increasingly fragile, which results in **striae gravidarum,** which may develop in the skin of the abdomen, breasts, or thighs. Metabolism is increased in pregnancy; as a way to dissipate heat, the peripheral vasculature dilates, and the sweat and sebaceous glands increase secretion. Fat deposits are laid down, particularly in the buttocks and hips, as maternal reserves for the nursing baby.

Older Adults

The skin is a mirror that reflects aging changes that proceed in *all* organ systems; it just happens to be the one organ that people can view directly. The aging process carries a slow atrophy of skin structures. The aging skin loses its elasticity; it folds and sags. By the 70s to 80s, it looks parchment thin, lax, dry, and wrinkled.

The epidermis's outer layer, the *stratum corneum,* thins and flattens. This allows chemicals easier access into the body. Wrinkling occurs because the underlying dermis also thins and flattens. Elastin, collagen, and subcutaneous fat are lost,

as is muscle tone. The loss of collagen increases the risk for shearing and tearing injuries.

Sweat glands and sebaceous glands decrease in number and function, leaving the skin dry. Decreased response of the sweat glands to thermoregulatory demand also puts older adults at greater risk for heat stroke. The vascularity of the skin diminishes while the vascular fragility increases; a minor trauma may produce dark red discoloured areas, or **senile purpura.**

Sun exposure and, to a somewhat lesser extent, cigarette smoking further accentuate aging changes in the skin. Coarse wrinkling, decreased elasticity, atrophy, speckled and uneven colouring, more pigment changes, and a yellowed, leathery texture develop. Chronic sun damage is even more prominent in pale or light-skinned persons.

An accumulation of factors increases older adults' risk for skin disease and breakdown: the thinning of the skin, the decrease in vascularity and nutrients, the loss of protective cushioning of the subcutaneous layer, a lifetime of environmental trauma to skin, the social changes of aging (e.g., less nutrition, limited financial resources), the increasingly sedentary lifestyle, and the chance of immobility. When skin breakdown does occur, subsequent cell replacement is slower, and wound healing is delayed.

In the aging hair matrix, the number of functioning melanocytes decreases, and so the hair turns grey or white and feels thin and fine. A person's genetic script determines the onset of greying and the number of grey hairs. Hair distribution changes. Men may have symmetrical W-shaped balding in the frontal areas. Some testosterone is present in both men and women; as levels of testosterone decrease with age, the amount of axillary and pubic hair decreases. As women's estrogen levels also decrease, testosterone is unopposed, and women may have some bristly facial hairs. Nails grow more slowly. Their surface is lustreless and is characterized by longitudinal ridges that result from local trauma at the nail matrix.

Because the changes of aging in the skin and hair can be viewed directly, their psychological effect is profound. For many people, self-esteem is linked to a youthful appearance. This view is compounded by media advertising in Western society. Although sagging and wrinkling skin and greying and thinning hair are normal processes of aging, they can prompt a loss of self-esteem for many adults.

CULTURAL AND SOCIAL CONSIDERATIONS

Awareness of normal biocultural differences and the ability to recognize the unique clinical manifestations of disease are especially important for people with dark pigmentation. As described earlier, melanin is responsible for the various colours and tones of skin observed among people from culturally diverse backgrounds. Melanin protects the skin against harmful ultraviolet rays, a genetic advantage that accounts for the lower incidence of skin cancer among individuals of African, Indian, or Aboriginal descent with dark skin. The incidence of melanoma is 20 times higher among individuals with lighter skin pigment.

Areas of the skin that are affected by hormones and, in some cases, differ among culturally diverse people, are the sexual skin areas, such as the nipples, areola, scrotum, and labia majora. In general, these areas are darker than other parts of the skin in both adults and children, especially among individuals of African and Asian descent.

The apocrine and eccrine sweat glands are important for fluid balance and for thermoregulation. When apocrine gland secretions are contaminated by normal skin flora, odour results. Inuit people have made an interesting environmental adaptation: In comparison with Canadians of European descent, they sweat less on their trunks and extremities but more on their faces. This adaptation allows for temperature regulation without causing perspiration and dampness of their clothes, which would decrease their ability to self-insulate against severe cold weather and would pose a serious threat to their survival.

Alcohol flush syndrome, mistakenly called "Asian flush" previously, is a condition characterized by a genetic disposition that can cause a range of symptoms such as redness and flushing of the face, heat sensation, splotchy redness of the neck, and accelerated intoxication when alcohol is ingested. It occurs in approximately 90% of individuals of Aboriginal descent and 50% of those of Asian descent. These unpleasant side effects sometimes prevent further drinking that could lead to further inebriation, but the symptoms can lead to a misassumption that the people affected are more easily inebriated than others.

Perhaps one of the most obvious and widely variable racial differences occurs with the hair. The hair of people of African descent varies widely in texture. It is very fragile and ranges from long and straight to short, spiralled, thick, and kinky. The hair and scalp have a natural tendency to be dry and require daily combing, gentle brushing, and the application of oil. Hair care products designed to specifically care for kinky hair should be available in clinical settings. In comparison, people of Asian descent generally have straight, silky hair.

Hair condition is significant in diagnosing and treating certain disease states. For example, hair texture becomes dry, brittle, and lustreless with inadequate nutrition. The hair of children of African descent with severe malnutrition (e.g., marasmus) frequently changes not only in texture but in colour. In such children, the hair often becomes less kinky and assumes a copper-red colour.

SUBJECTIVE DATA

1. Previous history of skin disease (allergies, hives, psoriasis, eczema)
2. Change in pigmentation
3. Change in mole (size or colour)
4. Excessive dryness or moisture
5. Pruritus
6. Excessive bruising
7. Rash or lesion
8. Medications
9. Hair loss
10. Change in nails
11. Environmental or occupational hazards
12. Self-care behaviours

HEALTH HISTORY QUESTIONS

Examiner Asks	Rationale
1. **Previous history of skin disease.** Any previous skin disease or problem? • How was this treated? • Any family history of allergies or allergic skin problem? • Any known allergies to drugs, plants, or animals? • Any birthmarks or tattoos?	Significant familial predisposition: allergies, hay fever, psoriasis, atopic dermatitis (eczema), acne Identification of offending allergen Risk of hepatitis C, increased with use of nonsterile equipment to apply tattoos
2. **Change in pigmentation.** Any **change in skin colour** or **pigmentation?** • Is the colour change generalized (all over), or is it localized?	Hypopigmentation: loss of pigmentation; hyperpigmentation: increase in colour Generalized change suggestive of systemic illness: pallor, jaundice, cyanosis
3. **Change in mole.** Any **change in a mole:** colour, size, shape, sudden appearance of tenderness, bleeding, or itching? • Any "sores" that do not heal?	Possible neoplasm in pigmented nevus; person may be unaware of change in nevus on back or buttocks that he or she cannot see
4. **Excessive dryness or moisture.** Any change in the feel of your skin: temperature, **moisture,** or texture? • Any excess **dryness?** Is this seasonal or constant?	Seborrhea: oily Xerosis: dry

Examiner Asks	Rationale
5. Pruritus. Any skin itching? Is this mild (prickling, tingling) or intense (intolerable)? • Does it awaken you from sleep? • Where is the itching? When did it start? • Any other skin pain or soreness? Where?	The most common of skin symptoms; occurs with dry skin, aging, drug reactions, allergy, obstructive jaundice, uremia, lice infestation Presence or absence of pruritus: possibly significant for diagnosis Excoriation of primary lesion caused by scratching
6. Excessive bruising. Any excess **bruising?** Where on the body? • How did this happen? • How long have you had it?	Multiple cuts and bruises, bruises in various stages of healing, bruises above knees and elbows, and illogical explanation: consider the possibility of abuse Frequent falls: possibly caused by dizziness of neurological or cardiovascular origin Frequent minor trauma: possibly a side effect of alcoholism or other drug abuse
7. Rash or lesion. Any skin **rash** or **lesion?** • Onset: When did you first notice it? • Location: Where did it start? • Extent: Have you noticed it spreading? If so, where? • Character or quality: Describe the colour. • Texture and odour: Is it raised or flat? Any crust, odour? Does it feel tender, warm? • Duration: How long have you had it? • Setting: Does anyone at home or work have a similar rash? Have you been camping, acquired a new pet, tried a new food, or taken a new drug? Does the rash seem to come with stress? • Alleviating and aggravating factors: What home care have you tried: bath, lotions, or heat? Do they help, or do they make it worse? • Associated symptoms: Any itching or fever? • Significance: What do you think a rash or lesion means? • Coping strategies: How has the rash or lesion affected your self-care, hygiene, and ability to function at work, at home, and socially? • Stress: Any new or increased stress in your life?	Rashes: a common reason for seeking health care A thorough history is important; it may be an accurate predictor of the type of lesion seen in the examination and its cause. Identification of the primary site; may be clue to cause Determination of migration pattern, evolution Spreading pattern: often a clue to the cause of the rash Identification of new or relevant exposure, identification of any household or social contacts with similar symptoms Myriad over-the-counter remedies are available. Many people try them and seek professional help only when they do not see improvement. Assessing person's perception of cause: fear of cancer, illnesses borne by ticks, or sexually transmitted infections Assessing effectiveness of coping strategies Chronic skin diseases may increase risk of loss of self-esteem, social isolation, and anxiety. Can exacerbate chronic skin illness
8. Medications. What **medications** do you take? • Prescription and over-the-counter? • Recent change?	Drugs that may produce allergic skin eruption: aspirin, antibiotics, barbiturates, some tonics Drugs that may increase sunlight sensitivity and produce burn response: sulphonamides, thiazide diuretics, oral hypoglycemic agents, and tetracycline Drugs that can cause hyperpigmentation: antimalarials, antineoplastic agents, hormones, metals, tetracycline

Examiner Asks	Rationale
• How long have you been taking the medication?	Sensitivity, which may develop even after a patient has taken medication for a long time
9. Hair loss. Any recent **hair loss?** • A gradual or sudden onset? Symmetrical? Associated with fever, illness, increased stress?	Alopecia is a significant loss. A full head of hair is equated with vitality in many cultures. If hair loss is treated as a trivial problem, the patient may seek alternative, unproven methods of treatment.
• Any unusual hair growth? • Any recent change in texture, appearance?	Hirsutism: shaggy or excessive hair
10. Change in nails. Any **change in nails:** shape, colour, brittleness? Do you tend to bite or chew your nails?	May indicate nutritional deficits, infections (both bacterial and viral), or trauma (see abnormal conditions of nails in Table 13-14)
11. Environmental or occupational hazards. Any **environmental** or **occupational** hazards? • Any hazard-related problems with your occupation, such as dyes, toxic chemicals, radiation? • How about hobbies? Do you perform any household or furniture repair work? • How much sun exposure do you get from outdoor work, leisure activities, sunbathing, or tanning salons? (See the Promoting Health: Tanning/Artificial Tanning and Skin Cancer Risk box.)	Majority of skin neoplasms caused by occupational or environmental agents People at risk: outdoor sports enthusiasts, farmers, sailors, outdoor workers; also creosote workers, roofers, coal workers Determining unprotected sun exposure, which accelerates aging and produces lesions; at more risk: light-skinned people, those older than 40 years, and those regularly in sun
• Have you recently been bitten by an insect: bee, tick, or mosquito? (See the Promoting Health: Lyme Disease Is on the Rise box.) • Any recent exposure to plants or animals in yard work or camping?	Identifying contactants that produce lesions or contact dermatitis To instruct people with chronic recurrent urticaria (hives) to keep diary of meals and environment to identify precipitating factors
12. Self-care behaviours. What do you do to care for your skin, hair, and nails? What cosmetics, soaps, or chemicals do you use? • Do you clip cuticles on nails or use adhesive for false fingernails?	Assessing **self-care** and influence on self-concept: may be important with society's media stress on norms of beauty Many over-the-counter remedies are costly and exacerbate skin problems.
• If you have allergies, how do you control your environment to minimize exposure? • Do you perform a skin self-examination? • Do you use sunscreen? What number sun protective factor (SPF)?	

Additional History for Infants and Children

1. Birthmarks. Does the child have any birthmarks?
2. Change in skin colour. Has there been any change in skin colour since the child's birth?
   • Any jaundice? Which day after birth?
   • Any cyanosis? What were the circumstances?
3. Rashes or sores. Have you noted any rash or sores? What seems to bring them on?
   • Have you introduced a new food or formula? When? Does your child eat chocolate, cow's milk, eggs?
4. Diaper rash. Does the child have any diaper rash? How do you care for this? How do you wash diapers? How often do you change diapers? How do you clean skin?

Generalized rash may be an allergic reaction to new food.

Irritability and general fussiness may indicate the presence of pruritus.

Rash possibly caused by occlusive diapers or infrequent changing

Possible allergy to certain detergent or to disposable wipes

Examiner Asks	Rationale
5. **Burns or bruises.** Does the child have any burns or bruises? • Where? • How did it happen?	Lesions that may indicate child abuse or neglect (versus expected childhood bumps and bruises): cigarette burns; excessive bruising, especially above knees or elbows; linear whip marks In cases of abuse, the history often does not coincide with physical appearance and location of lesion.
6. **Exposure.** Has the child had any exposure to contagious skin conditions (e.g., scabies, impetigo, lice), communicable diseases (e.g., measles, chicken pox, scarlet fever), or toxic plants (e.g., poison ivy)? • Are the child's vaccinations up to date? 7. **Self-destructive habits.** Does the child have any habits or habitual movements, such as nail-biting, twisting hair, rubbing head on mattress?	

Subjective Data (side tab)

PROMOTING HEALTH: TANNING/ARTIFICIAL TANNING AND SKIN CANCER RISK

The Dangers of Tanning Salons and the Sun

People know that prolonged sun exposure can lead to skin cancer, yet why is it that they do not realize the potential dangers of tanning booths? The skin examination is an opportunity for health care providers to educate the public about the dangers of excessive exposure to ultraviolet (UV) rays. As you examine an individual's skin, take the time to ask about the use of tanning salons. Ask about solar exposure and outdoor sun-protective precautions as well.

The popularity of indoor tanning salons appears to be growing, despite public health warnings and increasing evidence of the dangers of artificial UV radiation. The Canadian Cancer Society (2011) identified risk factors for the development of skin cancer with prolonged exposure to UV rays. Individuals most at risk are those who have a history of skin cancer, are younger than 18, are fair skinned, have freckles or moles, have a family history of skin cancer, or are using medications that increase their sensitivity to UV rays.

Many adverse effects of tanning beds have been documented, including acute sunburn, suppression of cutaneous DNA repair and immune functioning, ocular disorders, and increased risk of skin cancer, specifically squamous/basal cell carcinoma and melanoma. Health Canada (2005) stated that tanning beds and sunlamps emit light rays known to be human carcinogens. In addition, the World Health Organization has publicly recognized the dangers of tanning bed use and declared that, worldwide, no person younger than 18 years should use a tanning bed. Despite these warnings, the tanning industry appears to have convinced the public that indoor tanning is healthy, emphasizing that tanning produces a psychological sense of well-being and can even induce vitamin D production. Furthermore, they claim that getting a tan before you go out into the sun can actually prevent sunburn, a known risk factor for skin cancer. "Pretanning" before a vacation or outdoor sun exposure is a particularly dangerous practice because it not only leads to extra UV exposure but also appears to lead to decreased use of subsequent outdoor sun-protective precautions. The Canadian Skin Cancer Foundation (2011) recommended the following guidelines for safe exposure once a person heads outside:

• Stay out of the sun between 11 A.M. and 4 P.M. or any time the UV index is 3 or higher.
• Cover arms and legs with loose-fitting, tightly woven, and lightweight clothing.
• Wear a wide-brimmed hat to protect head, face, neck, and ears.
• Stay in the shade: under trees, awnings, or umbrellas.
• Wear sunglasses with UV protection.

Use sunscreen with an SPF of 30 or higher; apply it at least 20 minutes before going into the sun, and reapply every 2 or 3 hours. Although Health Canada regulates manufacturers of indoor tanning equipment and limits the amount of UV radiation that can be emitted, it does not regulate the proportion of UVB radiation emitted. Furthermore, the amount of UVA light received in a tanning salon may be two to three times more than the UVA light received from the sun and is a known risk factor for melanoma. Although one of the sources of vitamin D is exposure to UV light, an adequate level of vitamin D is typically attained through incidental exposure to the sun and normal dietary intake of vitamin D. Sources of vitamin D that do not carry an increased risk of skin cancer include vitamin D supplements or food sources supplemented with vitamin D.

Many individuals believe that tanning gives a person a "healthy glow"; on the contrary, the long-term exposure of tanning can lead to something more frightening and deadly.

Additional Resources
Canadian Cancer Society: http://www.cancer.ca/Canada-wide/ Prevention/Sun%20and%20UV/Being%20safe%20in%20 the%20sun.aspx?sc_lang=en
Canadian Skin Cancer Foundation: http://canadianskincancer foundation.com
Levine, J. A., Sorace, M., Spencer, J., & Siegel, D. M. (2005). The indoor UV tanning industry: A review of skin cancer risk, health benefit claims, and regulation, Journal of the American Academy of Dermatology, 53(6), 1038-1044.

SPF, sun-protective factor; *UVA,* ultraviolet A; *UVB,* ultraviolet B.

Examiner Asks	Rationale
8. **Sun protection.** What steps are taken to protect the child from sun exposure? What about sunscreens and sunblocks? How do you treat a sunburn?	Excessive sun exposure, especially severe or blistering sunburns in childhood, increases risk for melanoma in later life.

Additional History for the Adolescent

1. **Skin problems.** Have you noticed any skin problems such as pimples or blackheads? • How long have you had them? • How do you treat this? • How do you feel about it?	Occurs in approximately 70% of teenagers; psychological effect often more significant than physical effect; self-treatment is common Many myths surround the cause of acne. Cause is unknown; acne is not caused by poor diet, oily complexion, or contagion.

Additional History for the Older Adult

1. **Skin changes.** What changes have you noticed in your skin in the last few years?	Assessing effect of aging on self-concept; normal aging changes may cause distress Many changes attributed to aging result from chronic sun damage; most skin cancers appear in aging people, although sun damage often begins decades earlier.

PROMOTING HEALTH: LYME DISEASE IS ON THE RISE

Protection from the Ticks

In 2009, Lyme disease became a nationally reportable disease in Canada. This means that all health care providers should report cases of Lyme disease to the Public Health Agency of Canada through their provincial public health system.

Borrelia burgdorferi is the bacterium that causes Lyme disease. Small rodents are the most common reservoirs of *B. burgdorferi,* whereas larger animals serve as hosts for ticks. Ticks that transmit Lyme disease thrive in wooded areas and can lurk on the tips of grasses or shrubs, from which they can easily transfer to people or animals as they brush past. In areas where ticks are found, people should know about the risk of Lyme disease and protect themselves.

The risk for exposure to the disease is highest in regions where the ticks that transmit Lyme disease are known to be established. These regions are parts of southern and southeastern Quebec, southern and eastern Ontario, southeastern Manitoba, New Brunswick, and Nova Scotia, as well as much of southern British Columbia.

Most cases of human illness with Lyme disease occur in the late spring and summer, when the ticks are most active and human outdoor activity is greatest. The risk of contact with ticks begins in early spring when the weather warms up and lasts until permanent snow cover and subzero temperatures persist. The timing and intensity of these events vary across Canada and thus so does the risk period for exposure to ticks. Ticks may be active in the winter months in provinces with mild seasonal temperatures (4°C and above) and infrequent snow cover.

Personal Precautions to Avoid Infection
• When walking in tick-infested areas, wear long pants, with the legs tucked into boots or socks, and long-sleeved shirts that fit tightly at the wrist to keep ticks from getting to bare skin.

• Wear closed shoes, and avoid sandals.
• Wear light-coloured clothing; ticks will be seen more easily.
• Apply insect repellents containing DEET; they are safe and can effectively repel ticks. Repellents can be applied to clothing, as well as exposed skin, but should not be applied to skin underneath clothing. (*Note:* DEET may damage some materials.)
• Perform a careful self-inspection for attached ticks after being in tick-infested areas. A daily total-body inspection and prompt removal of attached ticks (within 36 hours) can reduce the transmission of *B. burgdorferi* from infected ticks. Black-legged ticks are very small, particularly during the nymph stage, so look carefully. Check children and pets as well.
• Carefully remove attached ticks by using tweezers. Grasp the tick's head and mouth parts as close to the skin as possible and pull slowly until the tick is removed. Do not twist or rotate the tick, and try not to squash or crush the tick during removal.
• After removing ticks, wash the bite site with soap and water, or disinfect it with alcohol or household antiseptic.
• Note the day of the tick bite and try to store the tick in an empty pill vial or double-zippered plastic bag.
• Contact a doctor immediately if you develop symptoms of Lyme disease, especially when you have been in an area where black-legged ticks are found. If you have stored the tick, take it with you to the doctor's office.

The black-legged ticks are primarily found in densely wooded areas and the unmaintained transitional edge habitat between woodlands and open areas. Fewer ticks are found in ornamental vegetation and lawn areas. For recommendations on reducing the risk of ticks inhabiting your surrounding property, see Public Health Agency of Canada

DEET, diethyltoluamide.

Examiner Asks	Rationale
2. **Wound healing.** Any delay in wound healing? • Any skin itching?	Pruritus: very common with aging; may be a side effect of medicine or systemic disease (e.g., liver or kidney disease, cancer, lymphoma), but senile pruritus usually results from dry skin (xerosis); exacerbated by too-frequent bathing or use of soap; excoriations produced by scratching with dirty, jagged fingernails
3. **Other skin pain.** Any other skin pain?	Some diseases, such as herpes zoster (shingles), produce more intense sensations of pain and itching in older adults. Other diseases (e.g., diabetes) may reduce pain sensation in extremities. Also, some older adults tolerate chronic pain as "part of growing old" and hesitate to "complain."
4. **Foot changes.** Any change in feet or toenails? Any bunions? Is it possible to wear shoes? 5. **Falling.** Do you experience frequent falls?	Some older adults cannot reach down to their feet to perform self-care. Assessing for multiple bruises, trauma from falls
6. **Diabetes and cardiovascular disease.** Any history of diabetes, peripheral vascular disease? 7. **Skin care.** What do you do to care for your skin?	Risk for skin lesions in feet or ankles Application of bland lotions is important to retain moisture in aging skin. Dermatitis may result from certain cosmetics, creams, ointments, and dyes applied to achieve a youthful appearance. Aging skin has a delayed inflammatory response when exposed to irritants. If the person is not alerted by warning signs (e.g., pruritus, redness), exposure may continue, and dermatitis may ensue.

OBJECTIVE DATA

PREPARATION

Try to control external variables that may influence skin colour and confuse your findings, both in light-skinned and in dark-skinned patients. Learn to consciously attend to skin characteristics. The danger is one of omission. You grow so accustomed to seeing the skin that you are likely to ignore it as you assess the organ systems underneath. However, the skin demonstrates information about the body's circulation, nutritional status, and signs of systemic diseases, as well as topical data on the integument itself.

Know the patient's normal skin colouring. Baseline knowledge is important for assessing colour or pigment changes. If this is the first time you are examining the patient, ask about his or her usual skin colour and about any self-monitoring practices.

EQUIPMENT NEEDED

Strong direct lighting (natural daylight is ideal for evaluating skin characteristics but is usually not available in the clinical area)
Small centimetre ruler
Penlight
Gloves
Needed for special procedures:
• Wood light (filtered ultraviolet light)
• Magnifying glass, for minute lesions
• Materials for laboratory tests: potassium hydroxide (KOH), glass slide

Normal Range of Findings	Abnormal Findings

The Complete Physical Examination. Although it is described alone in this chapter, skin assessment is integrated throughout the complete examination; it is not a separate step. At the beginning of the examination, assessing the patient's hands and fingernails is a nonthreatening way to accustom him or her to your touch. Many people are used to having relative strangers shake their hands or touch their arms. As you proceed through the examination, scrutinize the outer skin surface first before you concentrate on the underlying structures. Separate intertriginous areas (areas with skinfolds)—such as those under large breasts, the obese abdomen, and the groin—and inspect them thoroughly. These areas are dark, warm, and moist and provide the perfect conditions for irritation or infection. Last, always remove the patient's socks and inspect the feet, toenails, and the area between the toes.

In a hospital setting, a more formalized tool may be used to determine factors that may result in putting the patient at risk for skin tears or breakdown. One such scale that is commonly used is the Braden Risk Assessment Scale. Primarily used in the community and hospital settings, it is an efficient measurement tool for assisting in objective skin risk assessment. Table 13-1 contains the complete scale and interpretation of scores.

The Regional Examination. Some patients seek health care because of a skin change, and your assessment is focused on the skin alone. Ask the patient to remove his or her clothing. Assess the skin as one entity: Stand back at first to get an overall impression; this helps reveal distribution patterns. Then inspect lesions carefully. With a skin rash, check all areas of the body because there are some locations that the patient cannot see. You must not assume from the history alone that the rash is limited to one location. Inspect mucous membranes, too, because some disorders produce characteristic lesions in the mucosa. The skills used are inspection and palpation because some skin changes have accompanying signs that can be felt.

INSPECT AND PALPATE THE SKIN

Colour

General Pigmentation. Observe the skin tone. Normally it is consistent with genetic background and varies from pinkish tan to ruddy dark tan or from light to dark brown and may have yellow or olive overtones. Dark-skinned people normally have areas of lighter pigmentation on the palms, nail beds, and lips (Figure 13-3, *A*).

An acquired condition is **vitiligo,** the complete absence of melanin pigment in patchy areas of white or light skin on the face, neck, hands, feet, and body folds and around orifices (see Figure 13-3, *B*). Vitiligo can occur in all people, although dark-skinned people are more severely affected and the psychological effects may be more severe.

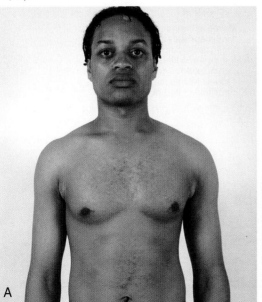

A

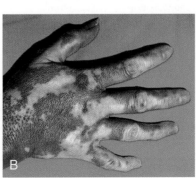

B

13-3

Objective Data

Patient's Name _____   Evaluator's Name _____

Indicate
Appropriate
Numbers
Below

Date of Assessment

Objective Data

SENSORY PERCEPTION Ability to respond meaningfully to pressure-related discomfort	**1. Completely Limited** Unresponsive (does not moan, flinch, or grasp) to painful stimuli, due to diminished level of consciousness or sedation. OR Limited ability to feel pain over most of body.	**2. Very Limited** Responds only to painful stimuli. Cannot communicate discomfort except by moaning or restlessness. OR Has a sensory impairment that limits the ability to feel pain or discomfort over ½ of body.	**3. Slightly Limited** Responds to verbal commands, but cannot always communicate discomfort or the need to be turned. OR Has some sensory impairment which limits ability to feel pain or discomfort in 1 or 2 extremities.	**4. No Impairment** Responds to verbal commands. Has no sensory deficit which would limit ability to feel or voice pain or discomfort.
MOISTURE Degree to which skin is exposed to moisture	**1. Constantly Moist** Skin is kept moist almost constantly by perspiration, urine, etc. Dampness is detected every time patient is moved or turned.	**2. Very Moist** Skin is often, but not always, moist. Linen must be changed at least once a shift.	**3. Occasionally Moist** Skin is occasionally moist, requiring an extra linen change approximately once a day.	**4. Rarely Moist** Skin is usually dry. Linen only requires changing at routine intervals.
ACTIVITY Degree of physical activity	**1. Bedfast** Confined to bed.	**2. Chairfast** Ability to walk severely limited or nonexistent. Cannot bear own weight and/or must be assisted into chair or wheelchair.	**3. Walks Occasionally** Walks occasionally during day, but for very short distances with or without assistance. Spends majority of each shift in bed or chair.	**4. Walks Frequently** Walks outside the room at least twice a day and inside room at least every 2 hours during waking hours.
MOBILITY Ability to change and control body position	**1. Completely Immobile** Does not make even slight changes in body or extremity position without assistance.	**2. Very Limited** Makes occasional slight changes in body or extremity position, but unable to make frequent or significant changes independently.	**3. Slightly Limited** Makes frequent though slight changes in body or extremity position independently.	**4. No Limitation** Makes major and frequent changes in position without assistance.
NUTRITION Usual food intake pattern	**1. Very Poor** Never eats a complete meal. Rarely eats more than ⅓ of any food offered. Eats 2 servings or less of protein (meat or dairy products) per day. Takes fluids poorly. Does not take a liquid dietary supplement. OR Is NPO and/or maintained on clear liquids or IVs for more than 5 days.	**2. Probably Inadequate** Rarely eats a complete meal and generally eats only about ½ of any food offered. Protein intake includes only 3 servings of meat or dairy products per day. Occasionally will take a dietary supplement. OR Receives less than optimum amount of liquid diet or tube feeding.	**3. Adequate** Eats over half of most meals. Eats a total of 4 servings of protein (meat or dairy products) each day. Occasionally will refuse a meal, but will usually take a supplement if offered. OR Is on tube feedings or TPN regimen, which meets most of nutritional needs.	**4. Excellent** Eats most of every meal. Never refuses a meal. Usually eats a total of 4 or more servings of meat and dairy products. Occasionally eats between meals. Does not require supplementation.
FRICTION AND SHEAR	**1. Problem** Requires moderate to maximum assistance in moving. Complete lifting without sliding against sheets is impossible. Frequently slides down in bed or chair, requiring frequent repositioning with maximum assistance. Spasticity, contractures or agitation lead to almost constant friction.	**2. Potential Problems** Moves feebly or requires minimum assistance. During a move skin probably slides to some extent against sheets, chair restraints, or other devices. Maintains relatively good position in chair or bed most of the time but occasionally slides down.	**3. No Apparent Problem** Moves in bed and chair independently and has sufficient muscle strength to lift up completely during move. Maintains good position in bed or chair.	

Total Score

NOTE:

15 to 18 = At Risk
13 to 14 = Moderate Risk
10 to 12 = High Risk
≤ 9 = Very High Risk

Assessment Schedule:

Very High to High Risk = minimum monthly
Moderate Risk = q3 months
Low/No Risk = q6 months

NOTE: Bed and chairbound individuals or those with impaired mobility to reposition should be assessed upon admission for their risk of developing pressure ulcers. Patients with established pressure ulcers should be reassessed periodically.
IVs, intravenous feedings; *NPO,* nothing by mouth; *TPN,* total parenteral nutrition.

Normal Range of Findings	Abnormal Findings

Normal Range of Findings

General pigmentation is darker in sun-exposed areas. Common (benign) pigmented areas also occur:

- **Freckles** (ephelides): small, flat macules of brown melanin pigment that occur on sun-exposed skin (Figure 13-4, *A*).
- **Mole** (nevus): a proliferation of melanocytes, tan to brown colour, flat or raised. Acquired nevi are characterized by their symmetry, small size (6 mm or less), smooth borders, and single uniform pigmentation. The **junctional nevus** (see Figure 13-4, *B*) is macular only and occurs in children and adolescents. In young adults it progresses to the **compound nevi** (see Figure 13-4, *C*) that are macular and papular. The intradermal nevus (mainly in older age) has nevus cells in only the dermis.
- **Birthmarks**: may be tan to brown in colour.

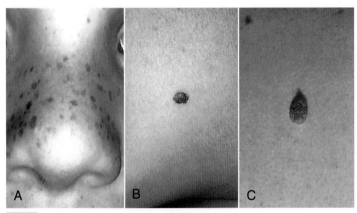

13-4   **A,** Freckles. **B,** Junctional nevus. **C,** Compound nevus.

Benign Normal	Malignant Not Normal	
Symmetrical		Asymmetrical
Borders are even		Orders are uneven
One shade		Two or more shades
Small than ¼ inch		Larger than ¼ inch

13-5   ABCDE Mole Comparison Chart.

Abnormal Findings

Danger signs: abnormal characteristics of pigmented lesions are summarized in the mnemonic **ABCDE:**

Asymmetry (*not* regularly round or oval, two halves of lesion do not look the same)

Border irregularity (notching, scalloping, ragged edges or poorly defined margins)

Colour variation (areas of brown, tan, black, blue, red, white, or combination)

Diameter greater than 6 mm (i.e., the size of a pencil eraser), although early melanomas may be diagnosed at a smaller size (Oliviero, 2002).

Elevation and enlargement

Additional symptoms: change in mole's size, a new pigmented lesion, and development of itching, burning, or bleeding in a mole. Any of these signs should raise suspicion of malignant melanoma and warrants referral.

Figure 13-5 shows a comparison of a healthy mole with one that is suspect and should be investigated further with the ABCDE assessment.

Objective Data

Normal Range of Findings	Abnormal Findings

Widespread Colour Change. Note any colour change in skin over the entire body, such as pallor (white), erythema (red), cyanosis (blue), and jaundice (yellow). Note whether the colour change is transient and expected or if it is caused by disease.

In dark-skinned people, the amount of normal pigment may mask colour changes. Lips and nail beds show some colour change, but they vary with the person's skin colour, and the colour change may not always be an accurate sign. The more reliable sites are those with the least pigmentation, such as under the tongue, the buccal mucosa, the palpebral conjunctiva, and the sclera. Table 13-2 lists specific clues to assessment.

Pallor. When the red-pink tones from the oxygenated hemoglobin in the blood are lost, the skin takes on the colour of connective tissue (collagen), which is mostly white. Pallor is common in acute high-stress states, such as anxiety or fear, because of the powerful peripheral vasoconstriction from sympathetic nervous system stimulation. The skin also looks pale with vasoconstriction from exposure to cold and cigarette smoking and in the presence of edema.

Ashen-grey colour in dark skin or marked pallor in light skin occurs with anemia, shock, and arterial insufficiency (see Table 13-2).

Look for pallor in dark-skinned people by the absence of the underlying red tones that normally give brown or black skin its lustre. Generalized pallor can be observed in the mucous membranes, lips, and nail beds. The palpebral conjunctiva and nail beds are preferred sites for assessing the pallor of anemia. When you inspect the conjunctiva, lower the eyelid sufficiently to visualize the conjunctiva near the *outer* canthus as well as the inner canthus. The coloration is often lighter near the inner canthus.

The brown-skinned individual demonstrates pallor with a more yellowish brown colour, and the black-skinned person appears ashen or grey.

The pallor of impending shock is accompanied by other subtle manifestations, such as increasing pulse rate, oliguria, apprehension, and restlessness.

Patients with anemia, particularly chronic iron-deficiency anemia, may have "spoon" nails, with a concave shape. A lemon-yellow tint of the face and a slightly yellow tint of the sclera accompany pernicious anemia, also indicated by neurological deficits and redness and pain in the tongue. Fatigue, exertional dyspnea, rapid pulse, dizziness, and impaired mental function accompany most severe anemias.

Erythema. Erythema is an intense redness of the skin from excess blood (hyperemia) in the dilated superficial capillaries. This sign is *expected* with fever, local inflammation, or with emotional reactions such as blushing in vascular flush areas (cheeks, neck, and upper chest).

When erythema is associated with fever or localized inflammation, it is characterized by increased skin temperature from the increased rate of blood flow through the blood vessels. Because you cannot see inflammation in dark-skinned persons, it is often necessary to palpate the skin for increased warmth, tautness or tightly pulled surfaces (which may be indicative of edema), and hardening of deep tissues or blood vessels.

Erythema occurs with polycythemia, venous stasis, carbon monoxide poisoning, and the extravascular presence of red blood cells (petechiae, ecchymosis, hematoma; see Table 13-2, p. 233, and Table 13-7, p. 254).

Cyanosis. This is a bluish, mottled discoloration that signifies decreased perfusion; the tissues are not adequately perfused with oxygenated blood. Be aware that cyanosis can be a nonspecific sign. A patient who is anemic could have hypoxemia without ever looking blue because not enough hemoglobin is present (either oxygenated or reduced) to colour the skin. In contrast, a patient with polycythemia (an increase in the number of red blood cells) looks ruddy blue at all times and may not necessarily be hypoxemic; this patient is just unable to fully oxygenate the massive numbers of red blood cells. Last, do not confuse cyanosis with the common and normal bluish tone on the lips of dark-skinned persons of Mediterranean origin.

Cyanosis indicates hypoxemia and occurs with shock, heart failure, chronic bronchitis, and congenital heart disease.

Normal Range of Findings		Abnormal Findings

TABLE 13-2   Detecting Colour Changes in Light and Dark Skin

	Note Appearance	
Cause	Light Skin	Dark Skin
PALLOR		
Anemia: decreased hematocrit Shock: decreased perfusion, vasoconstriction	Generalized pallor	Brown skin: appears yellow-brown, dull; black skin: appears ashen grey, dull; skin loses its healthy glow Check areas with least pigmentation, such as conjunctivae and mucous membranes.
Local arterial insufficiency	Marked localized pallor (e.g., lower extremities, especially when elevated)	Ashen grey, dull; cool to palpitation
Albinism: total absence of pigment melanin throughout the integument	Whitish pink	Tan, cream, white
Vitiligo: patchy depigmentation from destruction of melanocytes	Patchy milky white spots, often symmetrical bilaterally	Same as for light skin
CYANOSIS		
Increased amount of unoxygenated hemoglobin	Dusky blue	Dark but dull, lifeless; only severe cyanosis is apparent in skin Check conjunctivae, oral mucosa, and nail beds.
Central: chronic heart and lung disease causes arterial desaturation	Grey coloration	Dark but dull, lifeless; only severe cyanosis is apparent in skin
Peripheral: exposure to cold, anxiety	Nail beds dusky	Hard to detect
ERYTHEMA		
Hyperemia: increased blood flow through engorged arterioles, such as in inflammation, fever, alcohol intake, blushing	Red, bright pink	Purplish tinge, but difficult to see Palpate for increased warmth with inflammation, for taut skin, and for hardening of deep tissues.
Polycythemia: increased numbers of red blood cells, capillary stasis	Ruddy blue in face, oral mucosa, conjunctiva, hands, and feet	Well concealed by pigment Check for redness in lips.
Carbon monoxide poisoning	Bright cherry red in face and upper torso	Cherry-red colour in nail beds, lips, and oral mucosa
Venous stasis: decreased blood flow from area, engorged venules	Dusky rubor of dependent extremities; a prelude to necrosis with pressure sore	Easily masked Palpate for warmth or edema.
JAUNDICE		
Increased serum bilirubin (>2 to 3 mg/100 mL) as a result of liver inflammation or hemolytic disease, such as post–severe burn state and some infections	Yellow in sclera, hard palate, mucous membranes, then over skin	Check sclera for yellow near limbus; do not mistake normal yellowish fatty deposits in the periphery under the eyelids for jaundice: jaundice is best noted in junction of hard and soft palate and also palms.
Carotenemia: increased serum carotene from ingestion of large amounts of carotene-rich foods	Yellow-orange in forehead, palms and soles, and nasolabial folds, but no yellowing in sclera or mucous membranes	Yellow-orange tinge in palms and soles
Uremia: in renal failure, urochrome pigments are retained in the blood	Orange-green or grey overlying pallor of anemia; ecchymoses and purpura may also be present	Easily masked Rely on laboratory and clinical findings.
BROWN-TAN		
Addison's disease: increased melanin production stimulated by cortisol deficiency	Bronzed appearance, an "eternal tan," most apparent around nipples, perineum, genitalia, and pressure points (inner thighs, buttocks, elbow, axillae)	Easily masked Rely on laboratory and clinical findings.
Café au lait spots: caused by increased melanin pigment in basal cell layer	Tan to light brown, irregularly shaped, oval patch with well-defined borders	

Normal Range of Findings	Abnormal Findings

Cyanosis is difficult to observe in a person with dark pigmentation (see Table 13-2, p. 233). Because most conditions that cause cyanosis also cause decreased oxygenation of the brain, other clinical signs—such as changes in level of consciousness and signs of respiratory distress—will be evident.

Jaundice. Jaundice is a yellow discoloration, indicating rising amounts of bilirubin in the blood. Except for physiological jaundice in the newborn (p. 242), jaundice does not occur normally. Jaundice is *first* noted in the junction of the hard and soft palates in the mouth and in the sclera. However, do not confuse scleral jaundice with the normal yellow subconjunctival fatty deposits that are common in the outer sclera of dark-skinned persons. The scleral yellow of jaundice extends up to the edge of the iris.

As levels of serum bilirubin rise, jaundice is evident in the skin over the rest of the body. This is best assessed in direct natural daylight. Common calluses on palms and soles often look yellow; do not interpret these as jaundice.

Jaundice occurs with hepatitis, cirrhosis, sickle cell disease, transfusion reaction, and hemolytic disease of the newborn.

In both light- and dark-skinned people with jaundice, stools are often light or clay-coloured, and urine is often dark golden.

Temperature

Note the temperature of your own hands. Then use the backs (dorsa) of your hands to palpate the person and check bilaterally. The skin should be warm, and the temperature should be equal bilaterally; warmth suggests normal circulatory status. Hands and feet may be slightly cooler in a cool environment.

Hypothermia. Generalized coolness may be induced, such as in hypothermia used for surgery or high fever. Localized coolness is expected with an immobilized extremity, as when a limb is in a cast or with an intravenous infusion.

General hypothermia accompanies central circulatory problem such as shock.
Localized hypothermia occurs in peripheral arterial insufficiency and Raynaud's disease.

Hyperthermia. Generalized hyperthermia occurs with an increase in metabolic rate, as in fever or after heavy exercise. A localized area feels hyperthermic with trauma, infection, or sunburn.

Hyperthyroidism produces an increase in metabolic rate, causing warmth and moistness of skin.

Moisture

Perspiration appears normally on the face, hands, axilla, and skinfolds in response to activity, a warm environment, or anxiety. **Diaphoresis,** or profuse perspiration, accompanies an increase in metabolic rate, as occurs in strenuous activity or fever.

Look for **dehydration** in the oral mucous membranes. Normally there is none, and the mucous membranes look smooth and moist. Be aware that dark skin may normally look dry and flaky, but this does not necessarily indicate systemic dehydration.

Diaphoresis occurs with thyrotoxicosis and with stimulation of the nervous system with anxiety or pain.

With dehydration, mucous membranes look dry and the lips look parched and cracked. With extreme dryness, the skin is fissured, resembling cracks in a dry lake bed.

Texture

Normal skin feels smooth and firm, with an even surface.

Hyperthyroidism: skin feels smoother and softer, like velvet.
Hypothyroidism: skin feels rough, dry, and flaky.

Thickness

The epidermis is uniformly thin over most of the body, although thickened callus areas are normal on palms and soles. A callus is a circumscribed overgrowth of epidermis and is an adaptation to excessive pressure from the friction of work and weight bearing.

Skin is very thin and shiny (atrophic) with arterial insufficiency.

Normal Range of Findings	Abnormal Findings

Edema

Edema is fluid that accumulates in the intercellular spaces; it is not present normally. To check for edema, imprint your thumbs firmly against the ankle malleolus or the tibia. Normally, the skin surface resumes its smoothness immediately. If your pressure leaves a dent in the skin, "pitting" edema is present (Figure 13-6). Its presence is graded on a four-point scale:

1+: Mild pitting, slight indentation, no perceptible swelling of the leg

2+: Moderate pitting, indentation subsides rapidly

3+: Deep pitting, indentation remains for a short time, leg looks swollen

4+: Very deep pitting, indentation lasts a long time, leg is very swollen

This scale is somewhat subjective; ratings vary among examiners (see further content on the grading scale on p. 532 in Chapter 21).

Edema masks normal skin colour and obscures pathological conditions such as jaundice or cyanosis because the fluid lies between the surface and the pigmented and vascular layers. It makes dark skin look lighter.

Edema is most evident in dependent parts of the body (feet, ankles, and sacral areas), where the skin looks puffy and tight. Edema makes the hair follicles more prominent, so you note a pig-skin or orange-peel look (called *peau d'orange*).

Unilateral edema: Consider a local or peripheral cause.

Bilateral edema or edema that is generalized over the whole body *(anasarca)*: Consider a central problem such as heart failure or kidney failure.

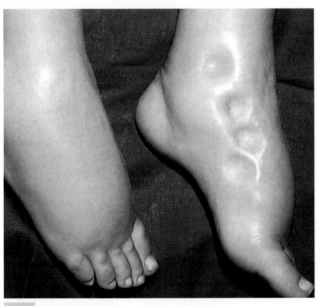

13-6   Pitting edema.

Mobility and Turgor

Pinch up a large fold of skin on the anterior aspect of the chest under the clavicle. Mobility is the skin's ease of rising, and turgor is its ability to return to place promptly when released. Together, they reflect the elasticity of the skin.

Mobility is decreased when edema is present.

Poor turgor is evident in severe dehydration or extreme weight loss; the pinched skin recedes slowly or "tents" and stands by itself.

Scleroderma, literally "hard skin," is a chronic connective tissue disorder associated with decreased mobility.

Vascularity or Bruising

Cherry (senile) angiomas are small (1–5 mm), smooth, slightly raised bright red dots that commonly appear on the trunk in all adults older than 30 years (Figure 13-7). They normally increase in size and number with aging and are not significant.

Normal Range of Findings	Abnormal Findings

Objective Data

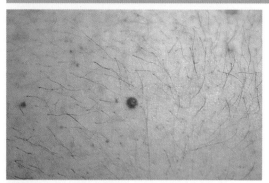

13-7 Cherry angioma.

Any bruising (ecchymosis) should be consistent with the expected trauma of life. There are normally no venous dilatations or varicosities.

Document the presence of any tattoos (a permanent skin design from indelible pigment) on the person's chart. Advise the person that the use of tattoo needles and tattoo parlour equipment of doubtful sterility increases the risk of hepatitis C.

Lesions

If any lesions are present, note these characteristics:
1. Colour.
2. Elevation: flat, raised, or pedunculated.
3. Pattern or shape: the grouping or distinctness of each lesion; for example, annular, grouped, confluent, or linear. The pattern may be characteristic of a certain disease.
4. Size, in centimetres: Use a ruler to measure. Avoid household descriptions such as "quarter size" or "pea size."
5. Location and distribution on body: Is it generalized or localized to area of a specific irritant; around jewellery, a watchband, eyes?
6. Any exudate: colour and any odour.

Palpate lesions. Wear a glove if you anticipate contact with mucosae, blood, any other body fluid, or skin lesion. Roll a nodule between the thumb and index finger to assess depth. Gently scrape a scale to see whether it comes off. Note the nature of its base or whether it bleeds when the scale comes off. Note the surrounding skin temperature. However, the erythema associated with rashes is not always accompanied by noticeable increases in skin temperature.

Does the lesion blanch with pressure or stretch? Stretching the area of skin between your thumb and index finger decreases the normal underlying red tones (blanches), thus providing more contrast and brightening the macules. Red macules from dilated blood vessels do blanch momentarily, whereas those from extravasated blood (petechiae) do not. Blanching also helps you identify a macular rash in dark-skinned patients.

Use a magnifier and light for closer inspection of the lesion (Figure 13-8). Use a Wood light (i.e., an ultraviolet light filtered through a special glass) to detect fluorescing lesions. With the room darkened, shine the Wood light on the area.

Multiple bruises at different stages of healing and excessive bruises above knees or elbows should raise concern about physical abuse (see Table 13-6, p. 253).

Needle marks or tracks from intravenous injection of street drugs may be visible on the antecubital fossae, on the forearms, or over any available vein.

Lesions are traumatic or pathological changes in previously normal structures. When a lesion develops on previously unaltered skin, it is **primary.** However, when a lesion changes over time or changes because of a factor such as scratching or infection, it is **secondary.** Table 13-3 (p. 248) lists the shapes and Tables 13-4 and 13-5 (pp. 249 and 251) list the characteristics of primary and secondary skin lesions. The terms used (e.g., *macule, papule*) are helpful for describing any lesion you note.

Note the pattern and characteristics of common skin lesions (see Table 13-10, p. 259) and malignant skin lesions (Table 13-11, p. 262), and lesions associated with acquired immune deficiency syndrome (AIDS; Table 13-12, p. 263).

Lesions with blue-green fluorescence indicate fungal infection, such as tinea capitis (scalp ringworm).

Normal Range of Findings	Abnormal Findings

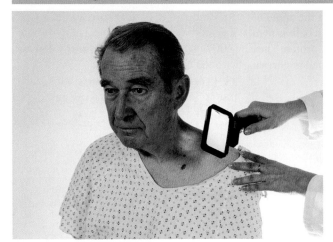

13-8

INSPECT AND PALPATE THE HAIR

Colour

Hair colour results from melanin production and may vary from pale blond to totally black. Greying normally begins as early as the third decade of life because of reduced melanin production in the follicles. Genetic factors affect the age at onset of greying.

Texture

Scalp hair may be fine or thick and may look straight, curly, or kinky. It should look shiny, although this characteristic may be lost with the use of some beauty products such as dyes, rinses, or perm materials.

Note dull, coarse, or brittle scalp hair. Grey, scaly, well-defined areas with broken hairs accompany tinea capitis, a ringworm infection found mostly in school-age children (see Table 13-13, p. 263).

Distribution

Fine vellus hair coats the body, whereas coarser terminal hairs grow at the eyebrows, eyelashes, and scalp. During puberty, distribution conforms to normal male and female patterns. At first, coarse curly hairs grow in the pubic area, then in the axillae, and last in the facial area in boys. In the genital area, the female pattern is an inverted triangle; the male pattern is an upright triangle with pubic hair extending up to the umbilicus. In individuals of Asian descent, body hair may be diminished.

Absence or with abnormal configuration of genital hair suggests endocrine abnormalities.

Hirsutism: excess body hair. In women, this is characterized by a male pattern of hair distribution on the face and chest and indicates endocrine abnormalities (see Table 13-13, p. 263).

Lesions

Separate the hair into sections and lift it, observing the scalp. When the patient has a history of itching, inspect the hair behind the ears and in the occipital area as well. All areas should be clean and free of any lesions or pest inhabitants. Many people normally have seborrhea (dandruff), which is characterized by loose white flakes.

Head or pubic lice: Distinguish dandruff from nits (eggs) of lice, which are oval, adhere to the hair shaft, and cause intense itching (see Table 13-13, p. 263).

INSPECT AND PALPATE THE NAILS

Shape and Contour

The nail surface is normally slightly curved or flat, and the posterior and lateral nail folds are smooth and rounded. When nail edges are smooth, rounded, and clean, self-care of nails is adequate.

Jagged nails, bitten to the quick, or traumatized nail folds from chronic nervous picking suggest nervous habits.

Chronically dirty nails suggest poor self-care or some occupations in which it is impossible to keep them clean.

Objective Data

Objective Data

Normal Range of Findings

The Profile Sign. View the index finger at its profile and note the angle of the nail base; it should be about 160 degrees (Figure 13-9). The nail base is firm on palpation. Curved nails are a variation of normal with a convex profile. They may look like clubbed nails, but the angle between nail base and nail is normal (i.e., 160 degrees or less).

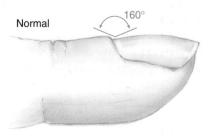 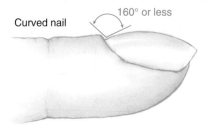 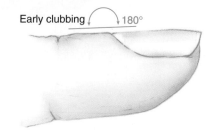

13-9

Consistency

The surface is smooth and regular, not brittle or splitting.

Nail thickness is uniform.

The nail is firmly adherent to the nail bed, and the nail base is firm on palpation.

Colour

The translucent nail plate is a window to the even, pink nail bed underneath.

Dark-skinned people may have brown-black pigmented areas or linear bands or streaks along the nail edge (Figure 13-10). All people normally may have white hairline linear markings (leukonychia strata) from trauma or picking at the cuticle (Figure 13-11). Note any abnormal marking in the nail beds.

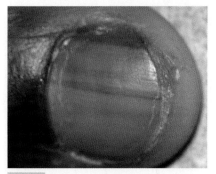

13-10   Linear pigmentation.

Abnormal Findings

Clubbing of nails occurs with congenital, chronic, and cyanotic heart disease and with emphysema and chronic bronchitis.

In early clubbing, the angle straightens out to 180 degrees, and the nail base feels spongy on palpation.

Pits, transverse grooves, or lines may indicate a nutrient deficiency or may accompany acute illness in which nail growth is disturbed (see Table 13-14, p. 264).

With arterial insufficiency, nails are thickened and ridged.

A spongy nail base accompanies clubbing.

Cyanosis or marked pallor.

Brown linear streaks (especially sudden appearance) are abnormal in light-skinned people and may indicate melanoma.

Splinter hemorrhages, transverse ridges, or Beau's lines (see Table 13-14, p. 264).

Normal Range of Findings	Abnormal Findings

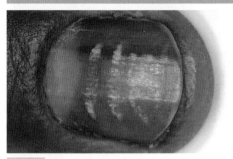

13-11   Leukonychia striata.

Capillary Refill. Depress the nail edge to cause blanching, and then release, noting the return of colour. Normally, colour returns instantly or at least within a few seconds in a cold environment. This indicates the status of the peripheral circulation. A sluggish colour return takes longer than 1 or 2 seconds.

Inspect the toenails. Separate the toes, and note the smoothness of the skin in between.

PROMOTING HEALTH AND SELF-CARE

Teach Skin Self-Examination

Teach all adults to examine their skin once a month, using the ABCDE rule (see p. 231), to detect warning signals of any suspect lesions: They should use a well-lighted room that has a full-length mirror. It helps to have a small handheld mirror. They should ask a relative to search skin areas difficult to see (e.g., behind ears, back of neck, back). They should follow the sequence outlined in Figure 13-12 and report any suspect lesions promptly to a physician or nurse.

 DEVELOPMENTAL CONSIDERATIONS

Infants

Skin Colour: General Pigmentation. Newborns of African descent initially have lighter toned skin than their parents because pigment production is not yet fully functional. Their full melanotic colour is evident in the nail beds and scrotal folds. The **mongolian spot** is a common variation of hyperpigmentation in newborns of Aboriginal, African, East Indian, or Hispanic descent (Figure 13-13). It is a blue-black to purple macular area at the sacrum or buttocks, but sometimes it occurs on the abdomen, thighs, shoulders, or arms. It results from deep dermal melanocytes. It gradually fades during the first year. By adulthood, these spots are lighter but are frequently still visible. Mongolian spots are present in 90% of individuals of African descent and 80% of individuals of Asian or Aboriginal descent. If you are unfamiliar with mongolian spots, be careful not to confuse them with bruises. Recognition of this normal variation is particularly important to avoid erroneously identifying children as victims of child abuse.

The **café au lait spot** is a large round or oval patch of light brown pigmentation (hence, the name, which means "coffee with milk"), which is usually present at birth (Figure 13-14). Most such patches are normal.

Cyanotic nail beds or sluggish colour return may be indicative of cardiovascular or respiratory dysfunction.

Bruising is a common soft tissue injury that follows a rapid, traumatic, or breech birth.

Multiple bruises in various stages of healing, or pattern injury, suggest child abuse (see Table 13-6, p. 253).

The presence of six or more café au lait macules, each more than 1.5 cm in diameter, is diagnostic of neurofibromatosis, an inherited neurocutaneous disease.

Normal Range of Findings		Abnormal Findings	
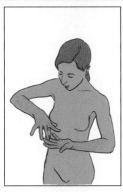	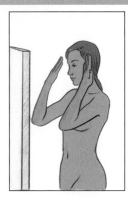	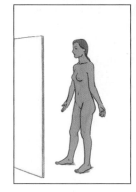	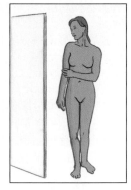
1. Undress completely. Check forearms, palms, space between fingers. Turn over hands and study the backs.	2. Face mirror; bend arms at elbow. Study arms in mirror.	3. Face mirror and study entire front of body. Start at face, neck, torso, working down to lower legs.	4. Pivot to right side facing mirror. Study sides of upper arms, working down to ankles. Repeat with left side.
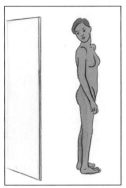	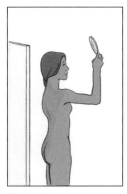	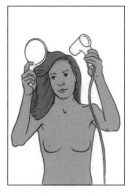	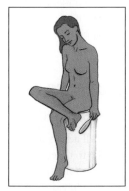
5. With back to mirror, study buttocks, thighs, lower legs.	6. Use the handheld mirror to study upper back.	7. Use the handheld mirror to study scalp, lifting the hair. A blow-dryer on a cool setting helps to lift hair.	8. Sit on chair or bed. Study insides of each leg and soles of feet. Use the small mirror to help.

13-12 Skin self-examination.

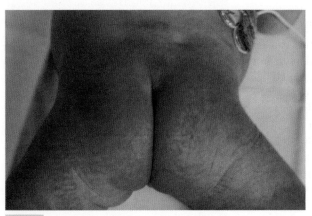

13-13 Mongolian spot.

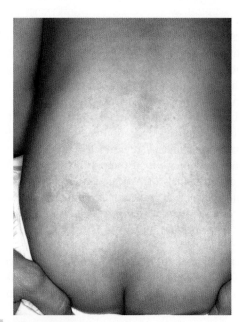

13-14 Café au lait spot.

Objective Data

Normal Range of Findings	Abnormal Findings

Skin Colour Change. Three erythematous states are common variations in the neonate:

1. The newborn's skin has a beefy-red flush for the first 24 hours because of vasomotor instability; then the colour fades to its normal shade.
2. Another finding, the **harlequin colour change,** occurs when the baby is in a side-lying position. The lower half of the body turns red, and the upper half blanches with a distinct demarcation line down the midline. The cause is unknown, and its occurrence is transient.
3. **Erythema toxicum** is a common rash that appears in the first 3 to 4 days of life. Sometimes called the "flea bite" rash or "newborn rash," it consists of tiny, punctate, red macules and papules on the cheeks, trunk, chest, back, and buttocks (Figure 13-15). The cause is unknown; no treatment is needed.

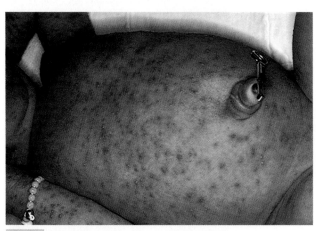

13-15   Erythema toxicum.

Two temporary cyanotic conditions may occur:

1. A newborn may have **acrocyanosis,** a bluish colour around the lips, on the hands and fingernails, and on the feet and toenails. This may last for a few hours and disappear with warming.
2. **Cutis marmorata** is a transient mottling in the trunk and extremities in response to cooler room temperatures (Figure 13-16). It is characterized by a reticulated red or blue pattern over the skin.

Persistent generalized cyanosis indicates distress, such as cyanotic congenital heart disease.

Persistent or pronounced cutis marmorata occurs with Down syndrome and prematurity.

Green-brown discoloration of the skin, nails, and umbilical cord occurs with passing of meconium in utero, which produces fetal distress.

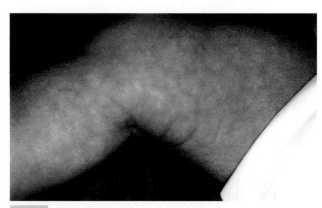

13-16   Cutis marmorata.

Objective Data

Normal Range of Findings	Abnormal Findings

Physiological jaundice is a common variation in about half of all newborns. A yellowing of the skin, sclera, and mucous membranes develops after the third or fourth day of life because of the increased numbers of red blood cells that hemolyze after birth. The hemoglobin in the red blood cells is metabolized by the liver and spleen; its pigment is converted into bilirubin.

Jaundice on the first day of life may indicate hemolytic disease. Jaundice after 2 weeks of age may indicate biliary tract obstruction.

Carotenemia also produces a yellow-orange colour in light-skinned persons but no yellowing in the sclerae or mucous membranes. It results from ingestion of large amounts of foods containing carotene, a vitamin A precursor. Carotene-rich foods are popular as prepared infant foods, and the absorption of carotene is enhanced by mashing, pureeing, and cooking. The colour is best seen on the palms and soles, the forehead, the tip of the nose and nasolabial folds, and the chin; behind the ears; and over the knuckles. It fades to normal within 2 to 6 weeks after carotene-rich foods are withdrawn from the diet.

Moisture. The vernix caseosa is the moist, white, cream cheese–like substance that covers part of the skin of all newborns. Perspiration is present after 1 month of age.

With meconium staining, vernix is green-tinged.

In children, excessive sweating may accompany hypoglycemia, heart disease, or hyperthyroidism.

Texture. A common variation occurring in infants is **milia** (Figure 13-17). Milia are tiny while papules on the cheeks, forehead, and across the nose and chin caused by sebum that occludes the opening of the follicles. Tell parents not to squeeze the lesions; milia resolve spontaneously within a few weeks.

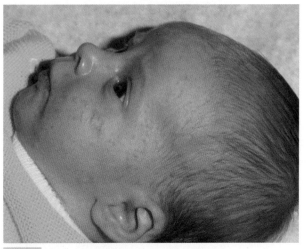

13-17   Milia.

Thickness. In neonates, the epidermis is normally thin, but you will also note well-defined areas of subcutaneous fat. The baby's skin dimples over joints, but there is no break in the skin. Check for any defect or break in the skin, especially over the length of the spine.

Subcutaneous fat may be lacking in premature and malnourished newborns.

A red sacrococcygeal dimple is present with a pilonidal cyst or sinus (see Table 25-2, p. 713).

Mobility and Turgor. Test mobility and turgor over the abdomen in an infant.

Vascularity or Bruising. Some vascular markings are common birthmarks in the newborn. A **storkbite** (salmon patch) is a flat, irregularly shaped red or pink patch found on the forehead, eyelid, or upper lip but most commonly at the back of the neck (nuchal area; Figure 13-18). It is present at birth and usually fades during the first year.

Poor turgor, or "tenting," indicates dehydration or malnutrition.

More unusual skin marks are port-wine stains, strawberry marks (immature hemangioma), and cavernous hemangiomas (see Table 13-8, p. 255).

Bruising may suggest abuse (see Table 13-7, p. 254).

Normal Range of Findings	Abnormal Findings

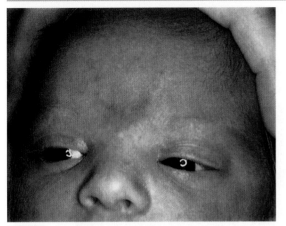

13-18   Storkbite.

Hair. A newborn's skin is covered with fine downy lanugo (Figure 13-19), especially in a preterm infant. Dark-skinned newborns have more lanugo than do light-skinned newborns. Scalp hair may be lost in the few weeks after birth, especially at the temples and occiput. It grows back slowly.

Nails. A newborn's nail beds may be blue (cyanotic) for the first few hours of life; then they turn pink.

The scalp becomes scaly and crusted with seborrheic dermatitis (cradle cap; see Table 13-13, p. 263).

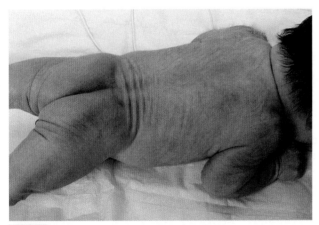

13-19   Lanugo.

Adolescents

The increase in sebaceous gland activity creates increased oiliness and **acne.** Acne is the most common skin problem of adolescence. Almost all teenagers have some acne, even if it is the milder form of open comedones (blackheads; Figure 13-20, *A*) and closed comedones (whiteheads). Severe acne includes papules, pustules, and nodules (see Figure 13-20, *B*). Acne lesions usually appear on the face and sometimes on the chest, back, and shoulders. Acne may appear in children as early as 7 to 8 years of age; then the number and severity of the lesions increase, peaking at 14 to 16 years in girls and at 16 to 19 years in boys.

Objective Data

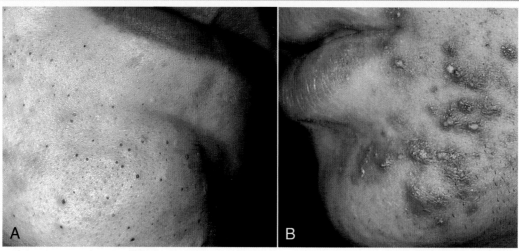

13-20   **A,** Open comedones. **B,** Severe acne.

Pregnant Women

Striae are jagged linear "stretch marks" coloured silver to pink that appear during the second trimester on the abdomen, breasts, and sometimes thighs. They occur in half of all pregnancies. They fade after delivery but do not disappear. Another skin change on the abdomen is the **linea nigra,** a brownish black line down the midline (see Figure 30-3). **Chloasma** is an irregular brown patch of hyperpigmentation on the face. It may occur with pregnancy or in women taking oral contraceptive pills. Chloasma disappears after delivery or after the woman stops taking the pills. **Vascular spiders** occur in two thirds of all pregnancies, primarily in Canadians of European descent. These lesions have tiny red centres with radiating branches and occur on the face, neck, upper chest, and arms.

Older Adults

Skin Colour and Pigmentation. Common variations of hyperpigmentation are senile lentigines and keratoses.

Senile Lentigines. Commonly called "liver spots," these are small, flat, brown macules (Figure 13-21). These circumscribed areas are clusters of melanocytes that appear after extensive sun exposure. They appear on the forearms and dorsa of the hands. They are not malignant and necessitate no treatment.

Keratoses. These lesions are raised, thickened areas of pigmentation that look crusted, scaly, and warty. One type, **seborrheic keratosis,** looks dark, greasy, and "stuck on" (Figure 13-22). They develop mostly on the trunk but also on the face and hands and on both unexposed and sun-exposed areas. It is uncommon for them to be found as cancerous.

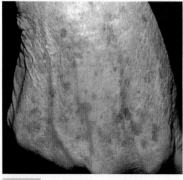

13-21   Lentigines.

Normal Range of Findings   **Abnormal Findings**

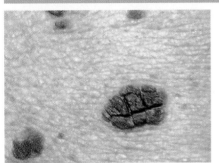

13-22   Seborrheic keratosis.

Another type, **actinic (senile** or **solar) keratosis,** is less common (Figure 13-23). These lesions are red-tan scaly plaques that enlarge over the years to become raised and roughened. A silvery white scale may adhere to the plaques. They occur on sun-exposed surfaces and are directly related to sun exposure. They are premalignant and may develop into squamous cell carcinoma.

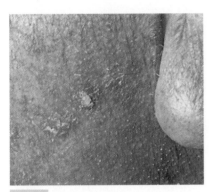

13-23   Actinic keratosis.

Moisture. Dry skin (xerosis) is common in older adults because of a decline in the size, number, and output of the sweat glands and sebaceous glands. Dry skin itches and looks flaky and loose.

Texture. Variations especially prevalent among older adults are **acrochordons,** or "skin tags," which are overgrowths of normal skin that form a stalk and are polyplike (Figure 13-24). They occur frequently on eyelids, cheeks, neck, axillae, and trunk.

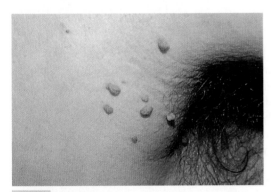

13-24   Skin tags.

Sebaceous hyperplasia appears as raised yellow papules with a central depression. They are more common in men, occurring over the forehead, nose, or cheeks. They have a pebbly look (Figure 13-25).

Normal Range of Findings	Abnormal Findings

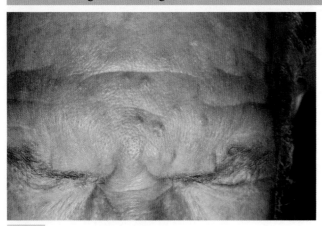

13-25   Sebaceous hyperplasia.

Thickness. With aging, the skin looks as thin as parchment, and the subcutaneous fat diminishes. Thinner skin is evident over the dorsa of the hands, forearms, lower legs, dorsa of feet, and bony prominences. The skin may feel thicker over the abdomen and chest.

Mobility and Turgor. The turgor is decreased (less elasticity), and the skin recedes slowly or "tents" and stands by itself (Figure 13-26).

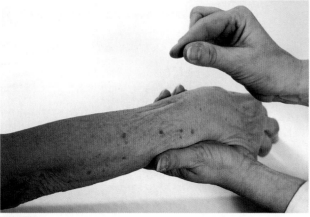

13-26

Hair. With aging, the hair growth decreases, and the amount in the axillae and pubic areas decreases. After menopause, women may develop bristly hairs on the chin or upper lip as a result of unopposed androgens. In men, coarse terminal hairs develop in the ears, nose, and eyebrows, although the beard is unchanged. Male-pattern balding, or alopecia, is a genetic trait. It is usually a gradual receding of the anterior hairline in a symmetrical W shape. In men and women, scalp hair gradually turns grey because of the decrease in melanocyte function.

Nails. With aging, the nail growth rate decreases, and local injuries in the nail matrix may produce longitudinal ridges. The surface may be brittle or peeling and sometimes yellowed. Toenails also are thickened and may grow misshapen, almost grotesque. The thickening may be a process of aging, or it may be caused by chronic peripheral vascular disease.

Fungal infections are common in aging, with thickened crumbling toenails and erythematous scaling on contiguous skin surfaces.

DOCUMENTATION AND CRITICAL THINKING

Sample Charting

SUBJECTIVE

No history of skin disease; no current change in pigmentation or in nevi; no pruritus, bruising, rash, or lesions. Taking no medications. No work-related skin hazards. Uses sunblock cream when outdoors.

OBJECTIVE

Skin: Colour tan-pink, even pigmentation, with no nevi. Warm to touch, dry, smooth, and even. Turgor good, no lesions.
Hair: Even distribution, thick texture, no lesions or pest inhabitants.
Nails: No clubbing or deformities. Nail beds pink with prompt capillary refill.

ASSESSMENT

Warm, dry, intact skin.

Focused Assessment: Clinical Case Study

Ethan E. is a 3-year-old boy presenting with his mother, who seeks health care because of Ethan's fever, fatigue, and rash of 3 days' duration.

SUBJECTIVE

- 2 weeks PTA ["prior to arrival"], Ethan was playing with a child in whom chicken pox was subsequently diagnosed.
- 3 days PTA, mother reports fever 37.7°C to 38.3°C, fatigue, and irritability. That evening noted "tiny blisters" on chest and back.
- 1 day PTA, blisters on chest changed to white with scab on top. New eruption of blisters on shoulders, thighs, face. Intense itching and scratching.

OBJECTIVE

Temperature, 38.0°C; pulse, 110; respirations, 24.
Skin: Generalized vesiculopustular rash covering face, trunk, upper arms, and thighs. Small vesicles on face, pustules and red-honey–coloured crusts on trunk. Otherwise skin is warm and dry, turgor good.
Ears: Tympanic membranes, pearl grey with landmarks intact. No discharge.
Mouth and throat: Mucosa dark pink, no lesions. Tonsils 1+, no exudate. No lymphadenopathy.
Heart: S_1, S_2 normal, not accentuated or diminished, no murmurs or extra sounds.
Lungs: Hyperresonant to percussion. Breath sounds clear, no adventitious sounds.

ASSESSMENT

Varicella
Impaired skin integrity R/T [related to] infection and scratching

ABNORMAL FINDINGS

TABLE 13-3   Common Shapes and Configurations of Lesions

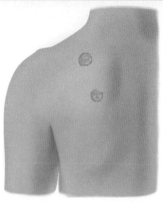

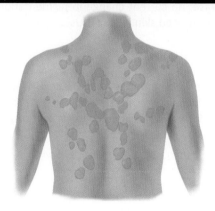

Annular
Also called *circular;* begins in centre and spreads to
 periphery
Examples: tinea corporis (ringworm), tinea versicolor,
 pityriasis rosea

Confluent
Lesions that merge together
Example: urticaria (hives)

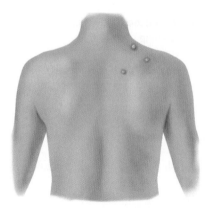

◄ ***Discrete***
    Distinct, individual lesions that remain separate

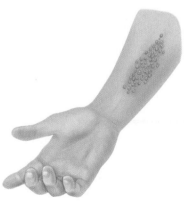

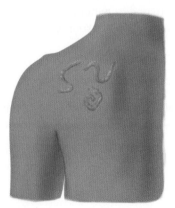

Grouped
Clusters of lesions
Example: vesicles of contact dermatitis

Gyrate
Twisted, coiled, spiral, snakelike

TABLE 13-3   Common Shapes and Configurations of Lesions—cont'd

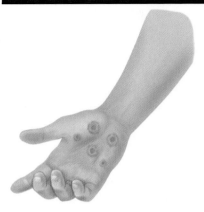

Target

Also called *iris;* resemble iris of eye, concentric rings of colour in the lesions
Example: erythema multiforme

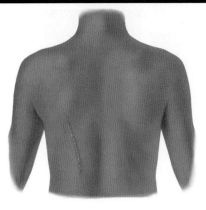

Linear

A scratch, streak, line, or stripe

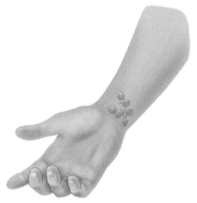

Polycyclic

Annular lesions that grow together
Examples: lichen planus, psoriasis

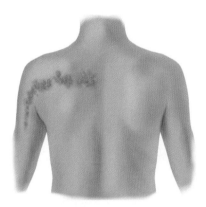

Zosteriform

Linear arrangement along a nerve route
Example: herpes zoster

TABLE 13-4   Primary Skin Lesions*

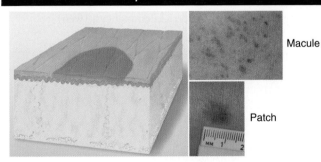

Macule

Patch

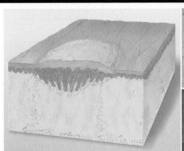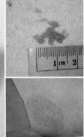

Papule

Plaque

Macule

Solely a colour change; flat and circumscribed, <1 cm diameter
Examples: freckles, flat nevi, hypopigmentation, petechiae, measles, scarlet fever

Patch

Macules >1 cm diameter
Examples: mongolian spot, vitiligo, café au lait spot, chloasma, measles rash

Papule

Palpable: solid, elevated, circumscribed, <1 cm diameter; caused by superficial thickening in the epidermis
Examples: elevated nevus (mole), lichen planus, molluscum, wart (verruca)

Plaque

Papules that coalesce to form surface elevation wider than 1 cm, a plateau-like, disc-shaped lesion
Examples: psoriasis, lichen planus

Continued

TABLE 13-4   Primary Skin Lesions—cont'd

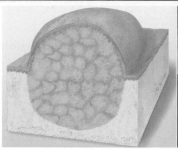
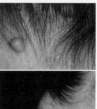
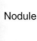

Nodule

Tumor

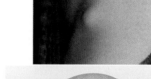

Wheal

Urticaria

Nodule
Solid, elevated, hard or soft, >1 cm diameter; may extend deeper into dermis than papule
Examples: xanthoma, fibroma, intradermal nevi

Tumour
Larger than a few centimetres in diameter, firm or soft, deeper into dermis; may be benign or malignant, although "tumour" implies "cancer" to most people
Examples: lipoma, hemangioma

Wheal
Superficial, raised, transient, and erythematous; slightly irregular shape because of edema (fluid held diffusely in the tissues)
Examples: mosquito bite, allergic reaction, dermographism

Urticaria (Hives)
Wheals that coalesce to form extensive reaction; intensely pruritic

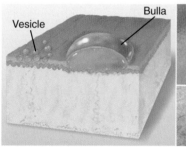
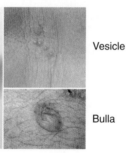

Vesicle

Bulla

Vesicle

Bulla

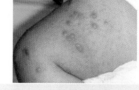

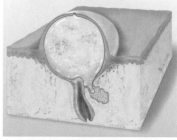

Vesicle
Also called *blister;* elevated cavity containing free fluid, up to 1 cm; clear serum flows if wall is ruptured
Examples: herpes simplex, early varicella (chicken pox), herpes zoster (shingles), contact dermatitis

Bulla
Usually single-chambered (unilocular); superficial in epidermis; >1 cm diameter; thin-walled, and so it ruptures easily
Examples: friction blister, pemphigus, burns, contact dermatitis

Cyst
Encapsulated fluid-filled cavity in dermis or subcutaneous layer, tensely elevating skin
Examples: sebaceous cyst, trichilemmal cyst (wen)

Pustule
Cavity filled with turbid fluid (pus); circumscribed and elevated
Examples: impetigo, acne

▶

*The immediate result of a specific causative factor; primary lesions develop on previously unaltered skin.

Line drawings © Pat Thomas, 2010.

TABLE 13-5   Secondary Skin Lesions*

DEBRIS ON SKIN SURFACE

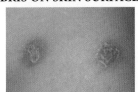

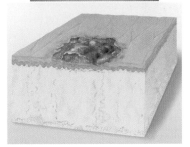

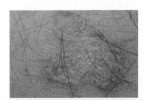

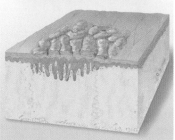

Crust

The thickened, dried-out exudate left when vesicles/
pustules burst or dry up; colour can be red-brown,
honey-like, or yellow, depending on the fluid's ingredients
(blood, serum, pus)

Examples: impetigo (dry, honey-coloured), weeping
eczematous dermatitis, scab after abrasion

Scale

Compact, desiccated flakes of skin, dry or greasy, silvery or
white, from shedding of dead excess keratin cells

Examples: lesions after scarlet fever or drug reaction
(laminated sheets), psoriasis (silver, mica-like), seborrheic
dermatitis (yellow, greasy), eczema, ichthyosis (large,
adherent, laminated), dry skin

BREAK IN CONTINUITY OF SURFACE

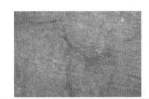

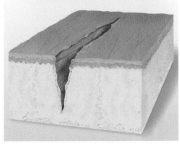

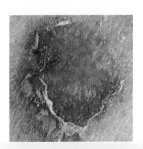

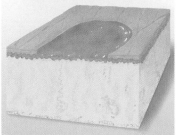

Fissure

Linear crack with abrupt edges, extending into dermis, dry
or moist

Examples: cheilosis (at corners of mouth as a result of
excess moisture); athlete's foot

Erosion

Scooped-out but shallow depression; superficial; epidermis
lost; moist but no bleeding; healing without scar because
erosion does not extend into dermis

Continued

TABLE 13-5   Secondary Skin Lesions—cont'd

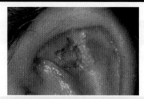

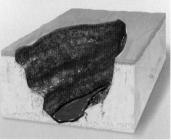

Ulcer

Deeper depression extending into dermis, irregular shape; may bleed; leaves scar when heals

Examples: stasis ulcer, pressure sore, chancre

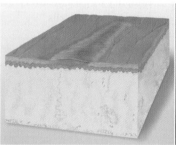

Scar

Connective tissue (collagen) that replaces normal tissue after a skin lesion is repaired; a permanent fibrotic change

Examples: healed area of surgery or injury, acne

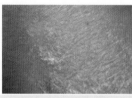

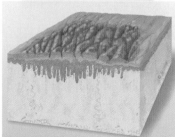

Lichenification

Thickening of skin with production of tightly packed sets of papules, caused by prolonged intense scratching; looks like surface of moss (or lichen)

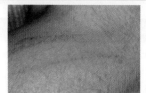

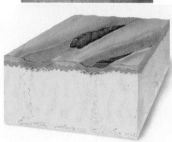

Excoriation

Self-inflicted abrasion; superficial; sometimes crusted; scratches from intense itching

Examples: lesions caused by scratching of insect bites, scabies, dermatitis, varicella

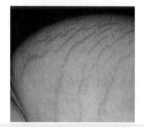

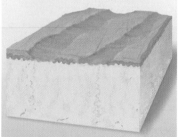

Atrophic Scar

Depression of skin level as a result of loss of tissue; a thinning of the epidermis

Example: striae

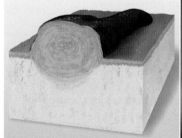

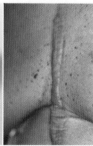

Keloid

A hypertrophic scar; elevation of the resulting skin level by excess scar tissue, which is invasive beyond the site of original injury; may increase long after healing occurs; looks smooth, rubbery, and "clawlike"; has a higher incidence among individuals of African descent

---

*Resulting from a change in a primary lesion from the passage of time; an evolutionary change.

Note: Combinations of primary and secondary lesions may coexist in the same person. Such combinations may be termed *papulosquamous, maculopapular, vesiculopustular,* or *papulovesicular.*

Line drawings © Pat Thomas, 2010.

TABLE 13-6   Pressure Ulcer (Decubitus Ulcer)

In Canada, the prevalence of pressure ulcers is estimated to be 15%–30%, with a mean occurrence at 26%. These estimates are higher than those in most other countries worldwide, perhaps because of issues regarding length of stay in hospital settings and increasing numbers of people with overall level of illness who present in acute and long-term care environments. This same study indicated that up to 53% of stage I pressure ulcers (skin breakdown on the patient's buttocks) occur in home care settings (Woodbury & Houghton, 2004).

Pressure ulcers appear on the skin over a bony prominence when circulation is impaired. This occurs when a person is confined to bed or is immobilized. Immobilization impedes delivery of blood, which carries oxygen and nutrients to the skin, and it impedes venous drainage, which carries metabolic wastes away from the skin. These impediments result in ischemia and cell death. Common sites for pressure ulcers are on the back (heel, ischium, sacrum, elbow, scapula, vertebra) and the side (ankle, knee, hip, rib, shoulder).

Risk factors for pressure ulcers include impaired mobility, thin fragile skin of aging, decreased sensory perception (which causes inability to perceive pain accompanying prolonged pressure), impaired level of consciousness (which causes inability to respond to pain), moisture from urine or stool incontinence, excessive perspiration or wound drainage, shearing injury (being pulled down or across in bed), poor nutrition, and infection. Learning about risk factors and prevention of pressure ulcers are far more easily accomplished than is treatment of existing ulcers. However, once pressure ulcers occur, they are assessed by stage depending on the pressure ulcer depth (National Pressure Ulcer Advisory Panel, 2007):

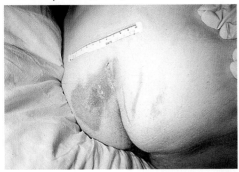

Stage I
Intact skin appears red but unbroken. Localized redness in lightly pigmented skin will blanch (turns light with pressure). Affected dark skin appears darker but does not blanch.

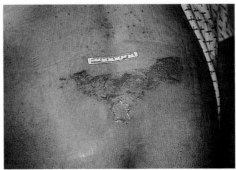

Stage II
Partial-thickness skin erosion causes loss of epidermis or also the dermis. Superficial ulcer looks shallow, like an abrasion or open blister with a red-pink wound bed.

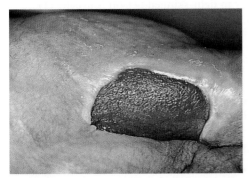

Stage III
Full-thickness pressure ulcer extends into the subcutaneous tissue and resembles a crater. Subcutaneous fat may be visible, but not muscle, bone, or tendon.

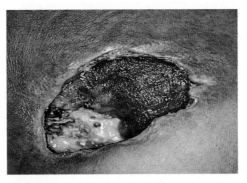

Stage IV
Full-thickness pressure ulcer involves all skin layers and extends into supporting tissue. Muscle, tendon, and bone may be exposed, and slough (stringy matter attached to wound bed) or eschar (black or brown necrotic tissue) may be present.

TABLE 13-7   Lesions Caused by Trauma or Abuse

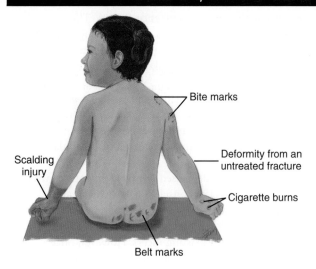

Bite marks

Deformity from an untreated fracture

Cigarette burns

Scalding injury

Belt marks

◄ Pattern Injury

Pattern injury is a bruise or wound whose shape suggests which instrument or weapon caused it (e.g., belt buckle, broomstick, burning cigarette, pinch marks, bite marks, or scalding hot liquid). Inflicted scalding-water immersion burns usually have a clear border, like a glove or sock, indicating that body part was held under water intentionally. Deformity results from an untreated fracture because the bone heals out of alignment.

In a child, these physical signs, together with a history that does not match the severity or type of injury, suggest child abuse and indicate impairment or dysfunction of the parent–child relationship. Provincial jurisdictions have legal mandates in regard to suspected/actual child abuse. What is clear nationally, however, is that members of the public, including health care providers who work with children, must promptly report to a children's aid society any suspicions that a child is or may be in need of protection.

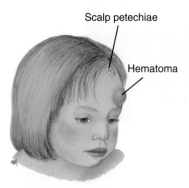

Scalp petechiae

Hematoma

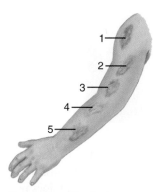

1
2
3
4
5

Hematoma

A hematoma is a bruise that you can palpate. It elevates the skin and is seen as swelling. Multiple petechiae and purpura may occur on the face when prolonged vigorous crying or coughing raises venous pressure.

Contusion (Bruise)

A contusion is a large patch of capillary bleeding into tissues. Colour in light-skinned person is usually (1) red-blue or purple immediately after or within 24 hours of trauma, which turns (2) blue to purple and then (3) blue-green, (4) yellow, and (5) brown and then disappears completely. A recent bruise in a dark-skinned person is deep, dark purple. Note that it is *not* possible to date the age of a bruise according to its colour.

Pressure on a bruise does *not* cause it to blanch. Bruises usually occurs from trauma but are also caused by bleeding disorders and liver dysfunction.

TABLE 13-8   Vascular Lesions

Hemangiomas

These are caused by a benign proliferation of blood vessels in the dermis.

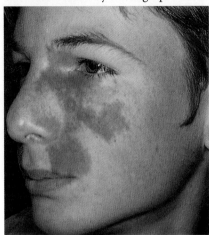

◄ *Port-Wine Stain (Nevus Flammeus)*

This is a large, flat macular patch covering the scalp or face, frequently along the distribution of cranial nerve V. The colour is dark red, bluish, or purplish and intensifies with crying, exertion, or exposure to heat or cold. The marking is formed from mature capillaries. It is present at birth and usually does not fade. The use of yellow-light lasers now makes photoablation of the lesion possible, with minimal adverse effects.

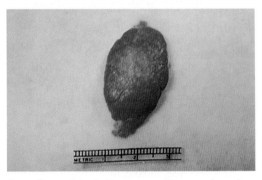

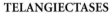

Strawberry Mark (Immature Hemangioma)

This is a raised, bright red area with well-defined borders about 2-3 cm in diameter. It does not blanch with pressure. It is formed from immature capillaries, is present at birth or develops in the first few months, and usually disappears by age 5 to 7 years. It necessitates no treatment, although parental and peer pressure may prompt treatment.

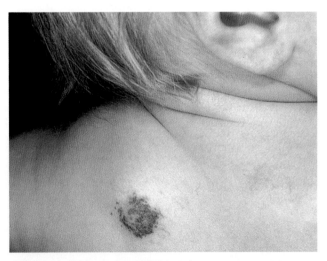

Cavernous Hemangioma (Mature)

This is a reddish blue, irregularly shaped, solid, and spongy mass of blood vessels. It may be present at birth, may enlarge during the first 10 to 15 months, and does not involve spontaneously.

TELANGIECTASES

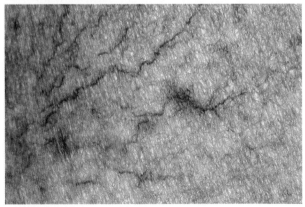

◄ *Telangiectasia*

This is the appearance of blood vessels on the skin surface. It is caused by vascular dilatation; the blood vessels are permanently enlarged and dilated.

Continued

TABLE 13-8   Vascular Lesions—cont'd

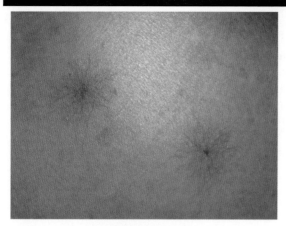

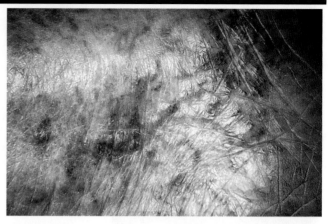

Spider or Star Angioma

This is a fiery red, star-shaped marking with a solid circular centre. Capillary radiations ("legs") extend from the central arterial body. With pressure, note a central pulsating body and blanching of extended "legs." It develops on the face, neck, or chest; may be associated with pregnancy, chronic liver disease, or estrogen therapy; or may be normal.

Venous Lake

This is a blue-purple dilatation of venules and capillaries in a star-shaped, linear, or flaring pattern. Pressure causes them to empty or disappear. They are located on the legs near varicose veins and also on the face, lips, ears, and chest.

PURPURIC LESIONS

These are caused by blood flowing out of breaks in the vessels. Red blood cells and blood pigments are deposited in the tissues (extravascularly). They are difficult to see in dark-skinned people.

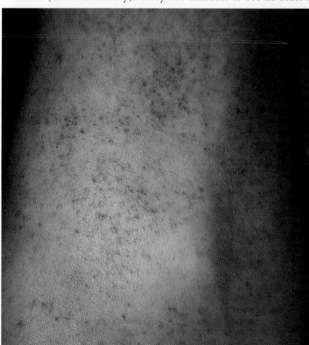

◀ *Petechiae*

These are tiny punctate hemorrhages, 1–3 mm, round and discrete, and dark red, purple, or brown. They are caused by bleeding from superficial capillaries and do not blanch. They may indicate abnormal clotting factors. In dark-skinned people, petechiae are best visualized in the areas of lighter pigmentation (e.g., the abdomen, buttocks, and volar surface of the forearm). When the skin is black or very dark brown, petechiae cannot be seen in the skin.

Most of the diseases that cause bleeding and microembolism formation—such as thrombocytopenia, subacute bacterial endocarditis, and other septicemias—are characterized by petechiae in the mucous membranes, as well as on the skin. Thus you should inspect for petechiae in the mouth, particularly the buccal mucosa, and in the conjunctivae.

TABLE 13-8   Vascular Lesions—cont'd

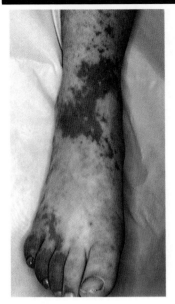

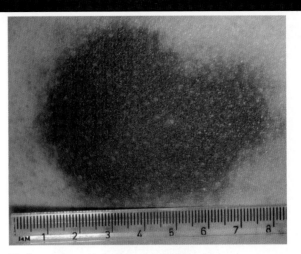

Ecchymosis

This is a purplish patch resulting from extravasation of blood into the skin, >3 mm in diameter.

Purpura

This is an extensive patch of confluent petechiae and ecchymoses, >3 mm flat, red to purple, macular hemorrhage. It occurs in generalized disorders such as thrombocytopenia and scurvy. It also occurs in old age as blood leaks from capillaries in response to minor trauma and diffuses through dermis.

TABLE 13-9   Common Skin Lesions in Children

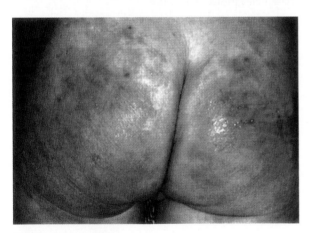

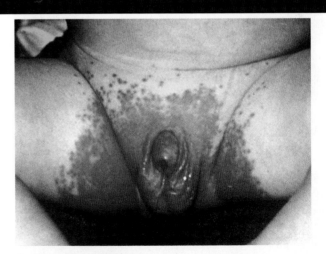

Diaper Dermatitis

Red, moist maculopapular patch with poorly defined borders in diaper area, extending along inguinal and gluteal folds. History: infrequent diaper changes or occlusive coverings. Inflammatory disease caused by skin irritation from ammonia, heat, moisture, occlusive diapers.

Intertrigo (Candidiasis)

Scalding red, moist patches with sharply demarcated borders, some loose scales. Usually in genital area, extending along inguinal and gluteal folds. Aggravated by urine, feces, heat, and moisture; *Candida* fungus infects the superficial skin layers.

Continued

TABLE 13-9 **Common Skin Lesions in Children—cont'd**

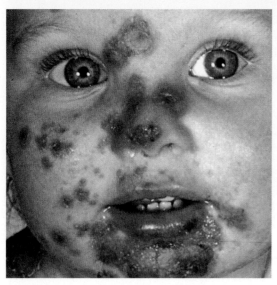

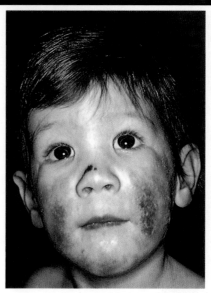

Impetigo
Moist, thin-roofed vesicles with thin, erythematous base.
Rupture is followed by formation of thick, honey-
coloured crusts. Contagious bacterial infection of skin;
most common in infants and children.

Atopic Dermatitis (Eczema)
Erythematous papules and vesicles, with weeping, oozing,
and crusting. Lesions usually on scalp, forehead, cheeks,
forearms and wrists, elbows, and backs of knees.
Paroxysmal and severe pruritus. Family history of
allergies.

Measles (Rubeola) in Dark Skin

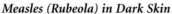

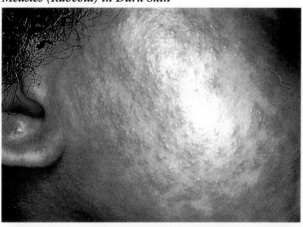

◄ Red-purple maculopapular blotchy rash in dark skin (on
top) and in light skin (on bottom) appears on third or
fourth day of illness. Rash appears first behind ears,
spreads over face, and then spreads over neck, trunk,
arms, and legs; looks "coppery" and does not blanch. Also
characterized by Koplik's spots in mouth: bluish white,
red-based elevations of 1-3 mm.

Measles (Rubeola) in Light Skin

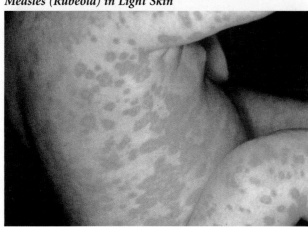

| TABLE 13-9 | **Common Skin Lesions in Children—cont'd** |

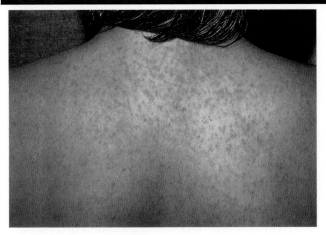

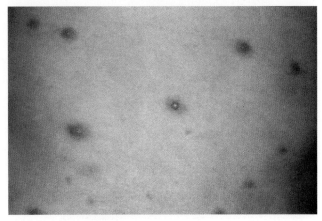

German Measles (Rubella)

Pink papular rash (similar to measles but paler) first appears on face, then spreads. Distinguished from measles by presence of neck lymphadenopathy and absence of Koplik's spots.

Chicken Pox (Varicella)

Small tight vesicles first appear on trunk and then spread to face, arms, and legs (not palms or soles). Shiny vesicles on an erythematous base are commonly described as the "dewdrop on a rose petal." Vesicles erupt in succeeding crops over several days, then become pustules, and then become crusts. Characterized by intense pruritus.

| TABLE 13-10 | **Common Skin Lesions** |

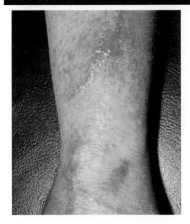

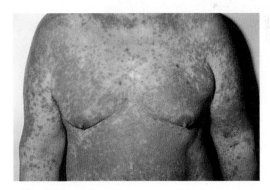

Primary Contact Dermatitis

Local inflammatory reaction to an irritant in the environment or an allergy. Characteristic location of lesions often gives clue to diagnosis. Often erythema shows first, followed by swelling, wheals (or urticaria), or maculopapular vesicles, scales. Frequently accompanied by intense pruritus. Example (in photo): poison ivy.

Allergic Drug Reaction

Erythematous and symmetrical rash, usually generalized. Some drugs produce urticarial rash or vesicles and bullae. History of drug ingestion.

Continued

TABLE 13-10   Common Skin Lesions—cont'd

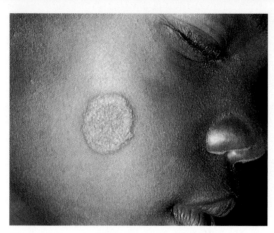

Tinea Corporis (Ringworm of the Body)

Scales: hyperpigmented in white-skinned individuals, depigmented in dark-skinned individuals. On chest, abdomen, and back of arms, forming multiple circular lesions with clear centres.

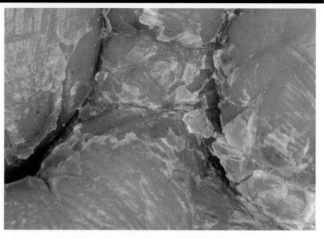

Tinea Pedis (Ringworm of the Foot)

Also known as "athlete's foot": a fungal infection, first appearing as small vesicles between toes, sides of feet, soles, and then growing scaly and hard. Found in chronically warm, moist feet: children after gymnasium activities, athletes, and older adults who cannot dry their feet well.

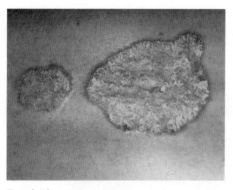

Psoriasis

Scaly erythematous patch, with silvery scales on top. Usually on scalp, outside of elbows and knees, low back, and anogenital area.

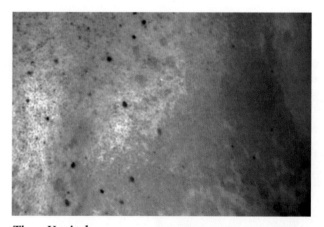

Tinea Versicolor

Fine, scaling, round patches of pink, tan, or white (hence the name) that do not tan in sunlight; caused by a superficial fungal infection. Usual distribution is on neck, trunk, and upper arms: a short-sleeved turtleneck sweater area. Most common in otherwise healthy young adults. Responds to oral antifungal medication.

TABLE 13-10   Common Skin Lesions—cont'd

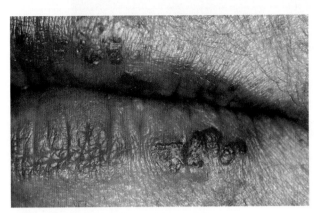

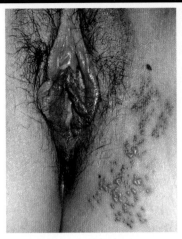

Labial Herpes Simplex (Cold Sores)

Herpes simplex virus infection has a prodrome of skin tingling sensation and sensitivity. Lesion then erupts with tight vesicles, followed by pustules, and then produces acute gingivostomatitis with many shallow, painful ulcers. Common location is upper lip; also in oral mucosa and tongue.

Herpes Zoster (Shingles)

Small grouped vesicles emerge along route of cutaneous sensory nerve, then pustules, then crusts. Caused by the varicella zoster virus, a reactivation of the dormant virus of chicken pox. Acute appearance, almost always unilateral, does not cross midline. Commonly on trunk, but can appear anywhere. If on ophthalmic branch of cranial nerve V, it poses risk to eye. Most common in adults >50 years old. Pain is often severe and long lasting in older adults, called *postherpetic neuralgia*.

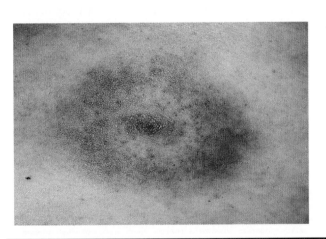

◄ ***Erythema Migrans of Lyme Disease***

The *first* sign of infection is usually a circular rash called *erythema migrans*. This rash occurs in about 70%-80% of infected people. It begins at the site of the tick bite after a delay of 3 days to 1 month and can persist for up to 8 weeks. The rash radiates from the site of the tick bite (5 cm or larger), with some central clearing, and is usually located in axilla, midriff, or inguina or behind knee, with regional lymphadenopathy. Rash fades in 4 weeks; untreated individual then may have **disseminated disease** with fatigue, anorexia, fever, chills, and joint or muscle aches. Antibiotic treatment shortens symptoms and decreases risk of progressing to disseminated disease.

TABLE 13-11   Malignant Skin Lesions

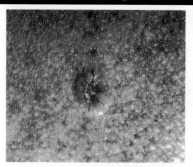

Basal Cell Carcinoma

Usually starts as a skin-coloured papule (may be deeply pigmented) with a translucent top and overlying telangiectasia. Then rounded pearly borders develop with central red ulcer, or looks like large open pore with central yellowing. One of the most common forms of skin cancer. It progresses slowly and rarely causes death.

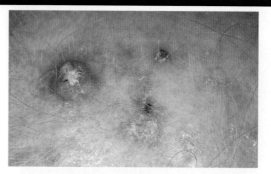

Squamous Cell Carcinoma

Erythematous scaly patch with sharp margins, ≥1 cm. Central ulcer and surrounding erythema develop. Usually on hands or head (areas exposed to solar radiation). As common as basal cell carcinoma in Canada; progresses slowly and is usually removed easily by surgery.

Malignant Melanoma

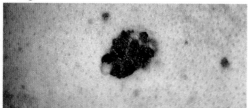

◄ Half of these lesions arise from pre-existing nevi. Usually brown; can be tan, black, pink-red, purple, or of mixed pigmentation. Often irregular or notched borders. May have scaling, flaking, oozing texture. Common locations are on the trunk and back in men and women, on the legs in women, and on the palms, soles of feet, and the nails in people of African descent. Melanoma represents only 1%-2% of all skin cancers but has the highest fatality rate; 20% of all Canadians with diagnosed melanoma die. Occurs earlier in life and progresses rapidly.

Metastatic Malignant Melanoma

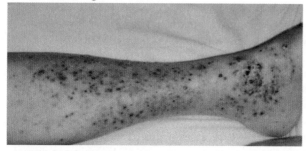

TABLE 13-12	Skin Lesions Associated With Acquired Immune Deficiency Syndrome

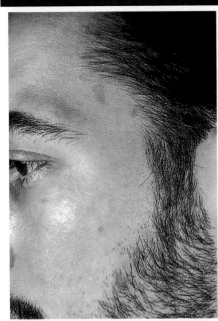

◄ *AIDS-Related Kaposi's Sarcoma: Patch Stage*
An aggressive form of Kaposi's sarcoma is one of the diseases that characterize AIDS. In the patch stage, multiple early lesions are faint pink on the temple and beard area. They could be mistaken easily for bruises or nevi and be ignored.

AIDS, acquired immune deficiency syndrome.

TABLE 13-13	Abnormal Conditions of Hair

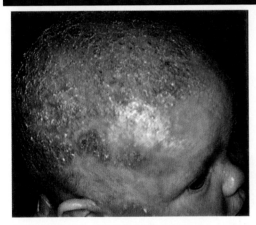

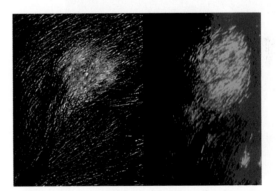

Seborrheic Dermatitis (Cradle Cap)
Thick, yellow to white, greasy, adherent scales with mild erythema on scalp and forehead; very common in early infancy. Resembles eczema lesions except cradle cap is distinguished by absence of pruritus, by "greasy" yellow-pink lesions, and by negative family history of allergy.

Tinea Capitis (Scalp Ringworm)
Rounded patchy hair loss on scalp, leaving broken-off hairs, pustules, and scales on skin. Caused by fungal infection; lesions may fluoresce blue-green under Wood light. Usually seen in children and farmers; highly contagious; routes of transmission include other people, domestic animals, and soil.

Continued

Abnormal Findings

TABLE 13-13   Abnormal Conditions of Hair—cont'd

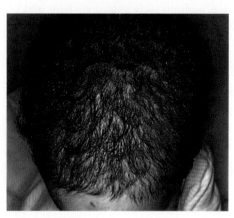

Toxic Alopecia

Patchy, asymmetrical balding that accompanies severe illness or use of chemotherapy; growing hairs are lost and resting hairs are spared. Regrowth occurs after illness ends or after discontinuation of toxin.

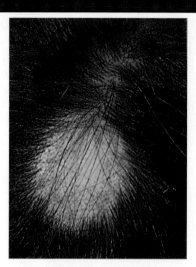

Alopecia Areata

Sudden appearance of a sharply circumscribed, round or oval balding patch, usually with smooth, soft, hairless skin underneath. Unknown cause; when limited to a few patches, person usually has complete regrowth.

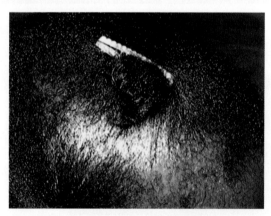

Traumatic Alopecia: Traction Alopecia

Linear or oval patch of hair loss along hairline, a part, or with scattered distribution; caused by trauma from hair rollers, tight braiding, tight ponytail, or barrettes.

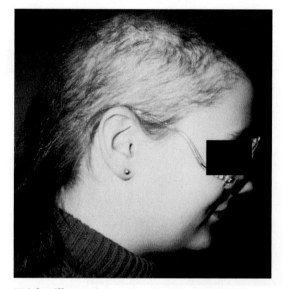

Trichotillomania

Traumatic self-induced hair loss usually the result of compulsive twisting or plucking. Forms irregularly shaped patch, with broken-off, stublike hairs of varying lengths; does not cause complete baldness. Occurs as child rubs or twists area absently while falling asleep, reading, or watching television. In adults it can be a serious problem and is usually a sign of a personality disorder.

TABLE 13-13   Abnormal Conditions of Hair—cont'd

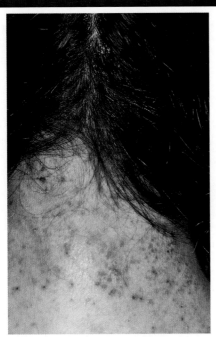

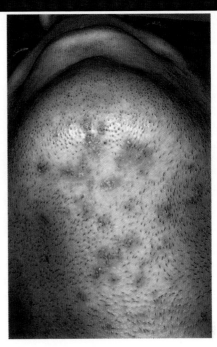

Pediculosis Capitis (Head Lice)

History includes intense itching of the scalp, especially the occiput. The nits (eggs) of lice are easier to see in the occipital area and around the ears, appearing as 2- to 3-mm oval translucent bodies, adherent to the hair shafts. Common among school-age children. Over-the-counter pediculicide shampoos are available; however, nit removal (also called *nit-picking*) by daily combing of wet hair with a fine-tooth metal comb is especially important.

Folliculitis

Superficial infection of hair follicles. Multiple pustules, "whiteheads," with hair visible at centre and erythematous base. Usually on arms, legs, face, and buttocks.

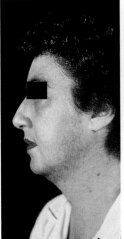
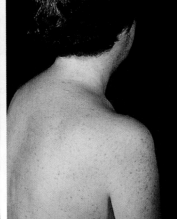

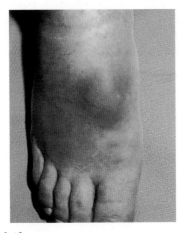

Hirsutism

Excess body hair in women that forms a male sexual pattern (upper lip, face, chest, abdomen, arms, legs); caused by endocrine or metabolic dysfunction; occasionally idiopathic.

Furuncle and Abscess

Red, swollen, hard, tender, pus-filled lesion caused by acute localized bacterial (usually staphylococcal) infection; usually on back of neck, buttocks, occasionally on wrists or ankles. Furuncles result from infection of hair follicles, whereas abscesses result from traumatic introduction of bacteria into the skin. Abscesses are usually larger and deeper than furuncles.

TABLE 13-14   Abnormal Conditions of the Nails

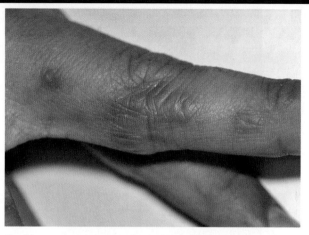

Scabies

An intensely pruritic condition caused by the scabies mite. Mites form a linear or curved elevated burrow on the fingers, web spaces of hands, and wrists. Other family members are usually infected. The patient cannot stop scratching (Habif, Campbell, Chapman, Dinulos, & Zug, 2005).

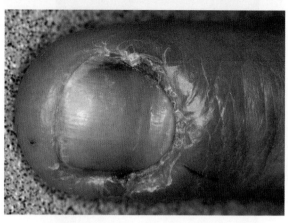

Paronychia

Red, swollen, tender inflammation of the nail folds. Acute paronychia is usually a bacterial infection; chronic paronychia is most often a fungal infection from a break in the cuticle in those who perform "wet" work.

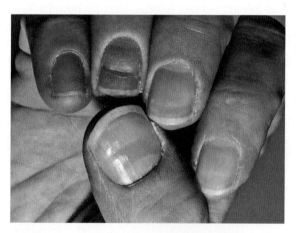

Beau's Line

Transverse furrow or groove; a depression across the nail that extends down to the nail bed. Occurs with any trauma that temporarily impairs nail formation, such as acute illness, toxic reaction, or local trauma. Dent appears first at the cuticle and moves forward as nail grows.

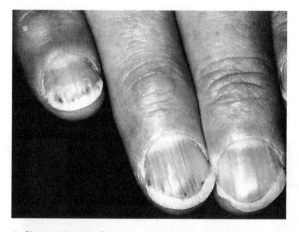

Splinter Hemorrhages

Red-brown linear streaks, embolic lesions; occur with subacute bacterial endocarditis; also may occur with minor trauma.

TABLE 13-14	Abnormal Conditions of the Nails—cont'd

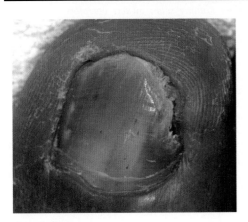

Onycholysis

This is a slow, persistent fungal infection of fingernails and, more often, toenails, common in older adults. Fungus causes change in colour (green where nail plate separates from bed), texture, and thickness, with nail crumbling or breaking and loosening of the nail plate, usually beginning at the distal edge and progressing proximally.

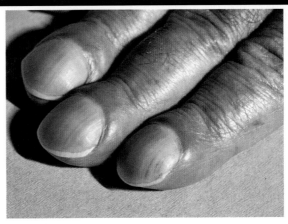

Late Clubbing*

Proximal edge of nail elevates; angle > 180 degrees. Distal phalanx looks rounder and wider. Occurs with chronic obstructive pulmonary disease and congenital heart disease with cyanosis. Occurs first in thumb and index finger.

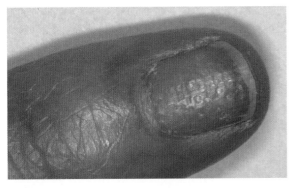

Pitting

Sharply defined pitting and crumbling of the nails with distal detachment; often occurs with psoriasis.

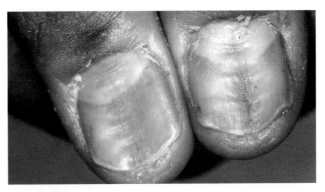

Habit-Tic Dystrophy

Depression down middle of nail or multiple horizontal ridges, caused by continuous picking of cuticle by another finger of same hand, which causes injury to nail base and matrix.

*Figure reprinted from the Clinical Slide Collection on the Rheumatic Diseases, © 1991, 1995, 1997. Used by permission of the American College of Rheumatology.

Summary Checklist: Skin, Hair, and Nails Examination

For a PDA-downloadable version, go to http://evolve.elsevier.com/Canada/Jarvis/examination/.

1. Inspect the skin:
   Colour
   General pigmentation
   Areas of hypopigmentation or hyperpigmentation
   Abnormal colour changes
2. Palpate the skin:
   Temperature
   Moisture
   Texture
   Thickness
   Edema
   Mobility and turgor
   Hygiene
   Vascularity or bruising
3. Note any lesions:
   Colour
   Shape and configuration
   Size
   Location and distribution on body
4. Inspect and palpate the hair:
   Texture
   Distribution
   Any scalp lesions
5. Inspect and palpate the nails:
   Shape and contour
   Consistency
   Colour
6. Teach skin self-examination and health promotion.

REFERENCES

Canadian Cancer Society. (2011). *Indoor tanning—Our position.* Retrieved from *http://www.cancer.ca/Canada-wide/Prevention/ Sun%20and%20UV/Indoor%20tanning/Indoor%20tanning%20 our%20position.aspx?sc_lang=en.*

Canadian Skin Cancer Foundation. (2011). Retrieved from *http:// canadianskincancerfoundation.com/.*

Habif, T. P., Campbell, J. I., Chapman, M. S., Dinulos, J. G. H., & Zug, K. A. (2005). *Skin disease: Diagnosis and treatment* (2nd ed.). St. Louis: Mosby.

Health Canada. (2005). *Guidelines for tanning salon owners, operators and users.* Retrieved from *http://www.hc-sc. gc.ca/ahc-asc/alt_formats/hecs-sesc/pdf/psp-psp/ccrpb-*
bpcrpcc/guidelines_tanning_salon_owners_operators_ users.pdf.

National Pressure Ulcer Advisory Panel. (2007). *Pressure ulcer category/Staging illustrations.* Retrieved from *http:// www.npuap.org/pr2.htm.*

Oliviero, M. C. (2002). How to diagnose malignant melanoma. *Nurse Practitioner, 27*(2), 26-37.

Public Health Agency of Canada. (2010). *Lyme disease.* Retrieved from *http://www.phac-aspc.gc.ca/id-mi/lyme-eng.php.*

Woodbury, M. G., & Houghton, P. E. (2004). Prevalence of pressure ulcers in Canadian healthcare settings. *Ostomy/Wound Management, 50*(10), 22-24, 26, 28, 30, 32, 34, 36-38.

Head, Face, and Neck, Including Regional Lymphatic System

Written by Carolyn Jarvis, PhD, APN, CNP
Adapted by June MacDonald-Jenkins, RN, BScN, MSc

℮volve WEBSITE

OUTLINE

STRUCTURE AND FUNCTION

THE HEAD

The **skull** is a rigid, bony box that protects the brain and special sense organs, and it includes the bones of the cranium and the face (Figure 14-1). Note the location of these **cranial bones:** frontal, parietal, occipital, and temporal. Use these names to describe any of your findings in the corresponding areas.

The adjacent cranial bones unite at meshed immovable joints called **sutures.** At birth, the bones are not firmly joined, which allows for the mobility and change in shape needed for the birth process. The sutures gradually ossify during early childhood. The **coronal** suture *crowns* the head from ear to ear at the union of the frontal and parietal bones. The **sagittal** suture *separates* the sides of the head lengthwise between the two parietal bones. The **lambdoid** suture separates the parietal bones crosswise from the occipital bone.

The 14 **facial bones** also articulate at sutures (note the nasal bone, zygomatic bone, and maxilla), except for the mandible (the lower jaw). It moves up, down, and sideways from the temporomandibular joints, which are anterior to the ears.

The cranium is supported by the cervical vertebra: C1, the "atlas"; C2, the "axis"; and down to C7. The C7 vertebra has a long spinous process that is palpable when the head is flexed. You can feel this useful landmark, the **vertebra prominens,** on your own neck.

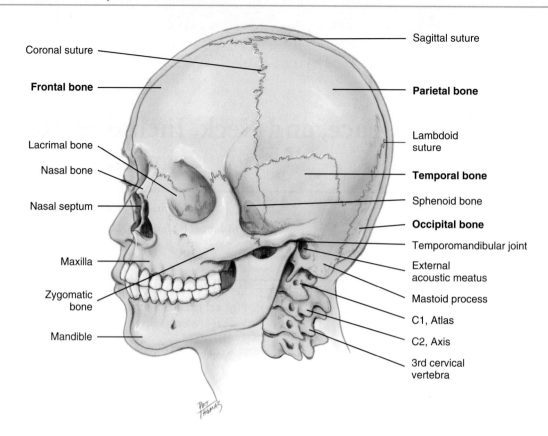

Coronal suture

Frontal bone

Lacrimal bone

Nasal bone

Nasal septum

Maxilla

Zygomatic
bone

Mandible

Sagittal suture

Parietal bone

Lambdoid
suture

Temporal bone

Sphenoid bone

Occipital bone

Temporomandibular joint

External
acoustic meatus

Mastoid process

C1, Atlas

C2, Axis

3rd cervical
vertebra

14-1

The human **face** has myriad appearances and a large array of facial expressions that reflect mood. The expressions are formed by the facial muscles (Figure 14-2), which are mediated by cranial nerve VII (the facial nerve). Facial muscle function is symmetrical bilaterally, except for an occasional quirk or wry expression.

Facial structures also are, in general, symmetrical; the eyebrows, eyes, ears, nose, and mouth appear about the same on both sides. The palpebral fissures—the openings between the eyelids—are equal bilaterally. Also, the nasolabial folds—the creases extending from the nose to each corner of the mouth—should be symmetrical. Facial sensations of pain or touch are mediated by the three sensory branches of cranial nerve V (the trigeminal nerve). (Testing for sensory function is described in Chapter 25.)

Two pairs of **salivary glands** are accessible to examination on the face (Figure 14-3). The **parotid glands** are in the cheeks over the mandible, anterior to and below the ear. They are the largest of the salivary glands but are not normally palpable. The **submandibular glands** are beneath the mandible at the angle of the jaw. A third pair, the **sublingual glands,** lie in the floor of the mouth. (Salivary gland function is described in Chapter 17.) The **temporal artery** lies superior to the temporalis muscle, and its pulsation is palpable anterior to the ear.

THE NECK

The **neck** is delimited above by the base of the skull and inferior border of the mandible and below by the manubrium sterni, the clavicle, the first rib, and the first thoracic vertebra. Think of the neck as a conduit for the passage of many structures, which are lying in close proximity: vessels, muscles, nerves, lymphatic vessels, and viscera of the respiratory and digestive systems. Blood vessels include the common and internal carotid arteries and their associated veins. The internal carotid artery branches off the common carotid artery and runs inward and upward to supply the brain; the external carotid artery supplies the face, salivary glands, and superficial temporal area. The carotid artery and internal jugular vein lie beneath the sternomastoid muscle. The external jugular vein runs diagonally across the sternomastoid muscle. (Assessment of the neck vessels is discussed in Chapter 20.)

The major **neck muscles** are the **sternomastoid** and the **trapezius** (Figure 14-4); they are innervated by cranial nerve XI (the spinal accessory nerve). The sternomastoid muscle arises from the sternum and the medial part of the clavicle and extends diagonally across the neck to the mastoid process behind the ear. It accomplishes head rotation and head flexion. The two trapezius muscles form a trapezoid shape on the upper back. Each arises from the occipital bone and the vertebrae and extends by fanning out to the scapula and clavicle. The trapezius muscles move the shoulders and extend and turn the head.

The sternomastoid muscle divides each side of the neck into two triangles. The **anterior triangle** lies in front, between the sternomastoid and the midline of the body; its base is up along the lower border of the mandible, and its apex is down at the suprasternal notch. The **posterior triangle** is behind the sternomastoid muscle, with the trapezius muscle on the

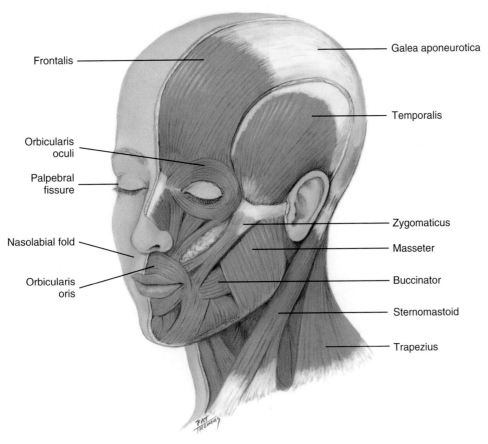

Frontalis

Galea aponeurotica

Orbicularis oculi

Palpebral fissure

Temporalis

Nasolabial fold

Orbicularis oris

Zygomaticus

Masseter

Buccinator

Sternomastoid

Trapezius

14-2   Facial muscles.

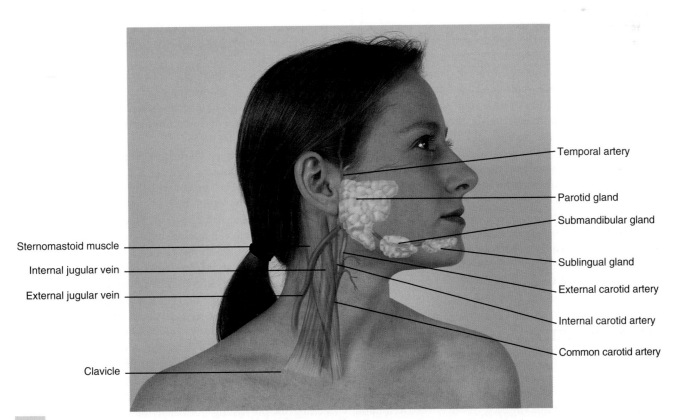

Temporal artery

Parotid gland

Submandibular gland

Sternomastoid muscle

Internal jugular vein

External jugular vein

Sublingual gland

External carotid artery

Internal carotid artery

Common carotid artery

Clavicle

14-3

Structure & Function

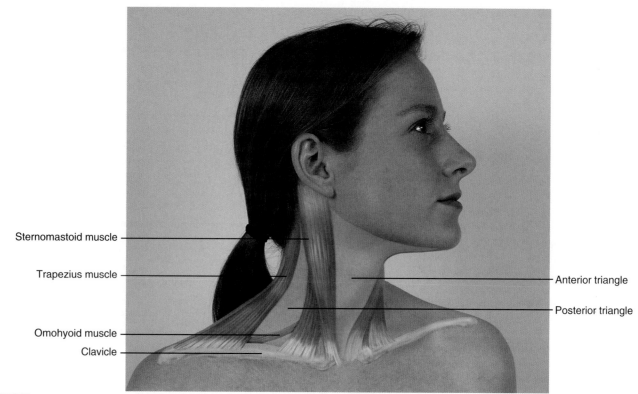

Sternomastoid muscle

Trapezius muscle

Anterior triangle

Posterior triangle

Omohyoid muscle

Clavicle

14-4

other side; its base is along the clavicle below. It contains the posterior belly of the omohyoid muscle. These triangles are helpful guidelines in describing findings in the neck.

The **thyroid gland** is an important endocrine gland with a rich blood supply. It straddles the trachea in the middle of the neck (Figure 14-5). This highly vascular endocrine gland synthesizes and secretes thyroxine (T_4) and triiodothyronine (T_3), hormones that stimulate the rate of cellular metabolism. The thyroid has two lobes, both conical in shape, each curving posteriorly between the trachea and the sternomastoid muscle. The lobes are connected in the middle by a thin isthmus lying over the second and third tracheal rings. (Sometimes a third lobe, the pyramidal lobe, is present. It too is conical, is usually on the left side, and extends up toward the hyoid bone from the isthmus or from the neighbouring lobe.)

Just above the thyroid isthmus, within about 1 cm, is the **cricoid cartilage,** or upper tracheal ring. The **thyroid cartilage** is above the cricoid cartilage, with a small palpable notch in its upper edge. This notch is the prominent "Adam's apple" in men. The highest structure in the neck is the **hyoid** bone, palpated at the level of the floor of the mouth.

LYMPHATIC SYSTEM

The lymphatic system is discussed more fully in Chapter 21. However, the head and neck have a rich supply of **lymph nodes** (Figure 14-6). Although sources differ as to their nomenclature, one commonly used system is listed as follows; note that the labels correspond to adjacent structures:

- *Preauricular:* in front of the ear
- *Posterior auricular* (mastoid): superficial to the mastoid process
- *Occipital:* at the base of the skull
- *Submental:* midline, behind the tip of the mandible
- *Submandibular:* halfway between the angle and the tip of the mandible
- *Tonsillar:* under the angle of the mandible
- *Superficial cervical:* overlying the sternomastoid muscle
- *Deep cervical:* deep under the sternomastoid muscle
- *Posterior cervical:* in the posterior triangle along the edge of the trapezius muscle
- *Supraclavicular:* just above and behind the clavicle, at the sternomastoid muscle

You also should be familiar with the direction of the drainage patterns of the lymph nodes (Figure 14-7). When nodes are abnormal, check the area in which they drain for the source of the problem. Explore the area proximal (upstream) to the location of the abnormal node.

The lymphatic system is an extensive vessel system, which is separate from the cardiovascular system and is phylogenetically older. The lymphatic vessels are a major part of the immune system, whose job is to detect and eliminate foreign substances from the body. The lymphatic vessels allow the flow of clear, watery fluid (lymph) from the tissue spaces into the circulation. Lymph nodes are small, oval clusters of lymphatic tissue that are set at intervals along the lymph vessels, like beads on a string. The nodes filter the lymph and engulf pathogens, preventing potentially harmful substances from entering the circulation. Nodes are located throughout the

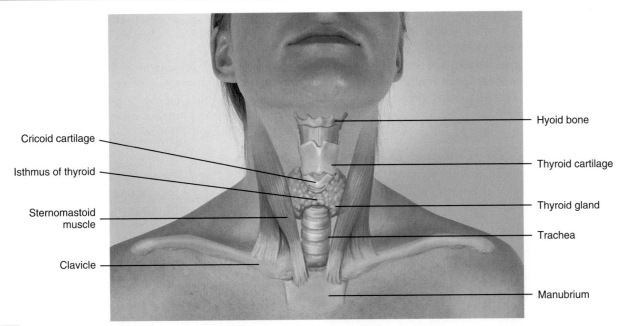

Cricoid cartilage

Isthmus of thyroid

Sternomastoid
muscle

Clavicle

Hyoid bone

Thyroid cartilage

Thyroid gland

Trachea

Manubrium

14-5

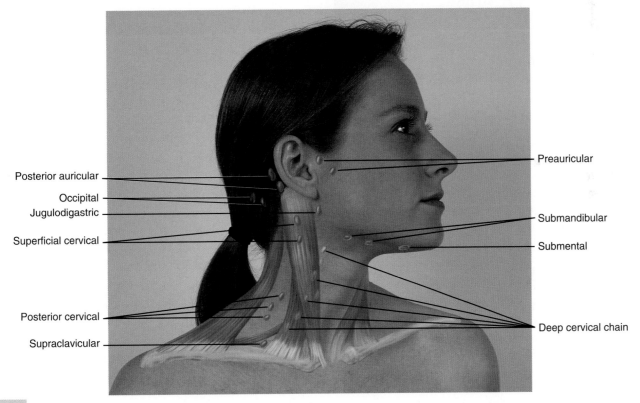

Posterior auricular

Occipital

Jugulodigastric

Superficial cervical

Posterior cervical

Supraclavicular

Preauricular

Submandibular

Submental

Deep cervical chain

14-6

body but are accessible to examination only in four areas: the head and neck, the arms, the axillae, and the inguinal region. The supply is most extensive in the head and neck.

 DEVELOPMENTAL CONSIDERATIONS

Infants and Children

The bones of the neonatal skull are separated by sutures and by **fontanelles,** the spaces where the sutures intersect (Figure 14-8). These membrane-covered "soft spots" allow for growth of the brain during the first year. They gradually ossify; the triangle-shaped posterior fontanelle is closed by age 1 to 2 months, and the diamond-shaped anterior fontanelle closes between ages 9 months and 2 years.

During the fetal period, head growth predominates. At birth, head size is greater than chest circumference. The head size grows during childhood, reaching 90% of its final size when the child is 6 years old. During infancy, however, trunk growth predominates, so that the proportion of head size to body height changes. Facial bones grow at varying rates, especially nasal and jaw bones. In the toddler, the mandible and maxilla are small and the nasal bridge is low, and so the whole face seems small in comparison with the skull.

Lymphoid tissue is well developed at birth and grows to adult size by the age of 6 years. Lymphatic tissue continues to grow rapidly until age 10 or 11 years, actually exceeding its adult size before puberty. Then the lymphatic tissue slowly atrophies.

The appearance of acne in adolescence is discussed in Chapter 13. Facial hair also appears in boys at this time: first on the upper lip, then on cheeks and lower lip, and last on the chin. The thyroid cartilage enlarges noticeably, and with enlargement, the voice deepens.

Pregnant Women

The thyroid gland enlarges slightly during pregnancy as a result of hyperplasia of the tissue and increased vascularity.

Older Adults

The facial bones and orbits appear more prominent, and the facial skin sags as a result of decreased elasticity, decreased subcutaneous fat, and decreased moisture in the skin. The lower face may look smaller if teeth have been lost.

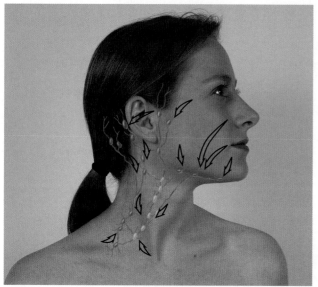

14-7

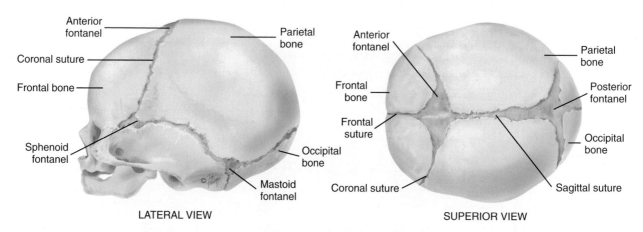

LATERAL VIEW

SUPERIOR VIEW

BONES OF THE NEONATAL SKULL

14-8

© Pat Thomas, 2006.

SUBJECTIVE DATA

Record the patient's subjective descriptions of the following abnormalities:
1. Headache
2. Head injury
3. Dizziness
4. Neck pain, limitation of motion
5. Lumps or swelling
6. History of head or neck surgery

HEALTH HISTORY QUESTIONS

Examiner Asks	Rationale
1. **Headache.** Any unusually frequent or unusually severe **headaches?** • Onset: When did this *kind* of headache start? • Gradual, over hours, or a day? • Or suddenly, over minutes, or less than 1 hour? • Ever had this *kind* of headache before? • Location: Where do you feel it: in front, on the sides, behind your eyes, like a band around the head, in the sinus area, or in the occipital area? • Is pain localized on one side, or is it all over? • Character: Throbbing (pounding, shooting) or aching (viselike, constant pressure, dull)? • Is it mild, moderate, or severe? • Course and duration: What time of day do the headaches occur: morning, evening? Do they awaken you from sleep? • How long do they last? Hours, days? • Have you noted any daily headaches, or several within a time period? • Precipitating factors: What brings it on: activity or exercise, work environment, emotional upset, anxiety, alcohol? (Examiner should also note signs of depression.) • Associated factors: Any relation to other symptoms, such as nausea and vomiting? (Examiner should note which occurred first, headache or nausea.) Any vision changes, pain with bright lights, neck pain or stiffness, fever, weakness, moodiness, stomach problems? • Do you have any other illness? • Do you take any medications? • What makes the pain worse: movement, coughing, straining, exercise? • Pattern: Any family history of headache? • What is the frequency of your headaches: once a week? Are your headaches occurring closer together? • Are they getting worse? Or are they getting better? • (For women) When do they occur in relation to your menstrual periods?	This is a more meaningful question than "Do you ever have headaches?" because most people have had at least one headache. Because headache is a symptom in many conditions, a detailed history is important. Of concern is a severe headache in an adult or child who has never had it before. Tension headaches tend to be occipital or frontal, or the sensation is of bandlike tightness; migraines (vascular) tend to be supraorbital, retro-orbital, or frontotemporal; cluster headaches (vascular) produce pain around the eye, temple, forehead, cheek. Unilateral or bilateral pain is a clue to the type of headache (e.g., with cluster headaches, pain is always unilateral and always on the same side of the head). Character is typically viselike with tension headache and throbbing with migraine or temporal arteritis. Pain is often severe with migraine and excruciating with cluster headache. On average, migraines occur at a rate of approximately two per month, each lasting 1 to 3 days; one to two cluster headaches occur per day, each lasting ½ to 2 hours for 1 or 2 months; then complete remission may last for months or years. Alcohol ingestion and daytime napping typically precipitate cluster headaches, whereas alcohol, letdown after stress, menstruation, and eating chocolate or cheese precipitate migraines. Nausea, vomiting, and visual disturbances are associated with migraines; eye reddening and tearing, eyelid drooping, rhinorrhea, and nasal congestion are associated with cluster headaches; anxiety and stress are associated with tension headaches; nuchal rigidity and fever are associated with meningitis or encephalitis. Hypertension, fever, hypothyroidism, and vasculitis can produce headaches. Oral contraceptives, bronchodilators, alcohol, nitrates, and carbon monoxide inhalation can produce headaches. Migraines are associated with family history of migraine.

Subjective Data

Examiner Asks	Rationale
• Effort to treat: What seems to help: going to sleep, medications, positions, rubbing the area?	With migraines, people lie down to feel better, whereas with cluster headaches they need to move—even to pace the floor—to feel better.
• Coping strategies: How have these headaches affected your self-care or your ability to function at work, at home, and socially?	
2. **Head injury.** Any **head injury** or blow to your head?	
• Onset: When? Please describe exactly what happened.	
• Setting: Any hazardous conditions? Were you wearing a helmet or hard hat?	
• How about yourself just before injury: Were you dizzy or lightheaded? Did you have a blackout or a seizure?	
• Did you lose consciousness and then fall? (Examiner should note which occurred first.)	Loss of consciousness *before* a fall may have a cardiovascular cause (e.g., heart block).
• Were you knocked unconscious? Or did you fall and lose consciousness a few minutes later?	
• Any history of illness (e.g., heart trouble, diabetes, epilepsy)?	
• Location: Exactly where did you hit your head?	
• Duration: How long were you unconscious?	
• Any symptoms afterward: headache, vomiting, projectile vomiting?	
• Any change in level of consciousness (dazed or sleepy) since injury?	A change in level of consciousness is of prime importance in the evaluation for a neurological deficit.
• Associated symptoms: Any pain in the head or the neck, vision change, or discharge from ear or nose (bloody or watery)? Are you able to move all extremities? Any tremors, staggered walk, numbness, or tingling?	
• Pattern: Have symptoms become worse or better, or have they remained unchanged, since injury?	
• Effort to treat: Emergency department or hospitalized? Any medications?	
3. **Dizziness.** Experienced any **dizziness?**	Dizziness is a lightheaded, swimming sensation or a feeling of falling. True *vertigo* is a sense of true rotational spinning caused by neurological disease (labyrinthine–vestibular apparatus, vestibular nuclei in brain stem).
• (Examiner should determine exactly what the person means by "dizziness.") Was it a feeling of lightheadedness or of falling? Or was it a spinning sensation?	When vertigo is *objective,* the patient's perception is that the room spins. When vertigo is *subjective,* the patient's perception is that he or she spins.
• Onset: Abrupt or gradual? After a change in position, such as sudden standing?	
• Associated factors: Any nausea and vomiting, pallor, immobility, decreased hearing acuity, or tinnitus along with the dizziness?	
4. **Neck pain, limitation of motion.** Any **neck pain?**	
• Onset: How did the pain start: injury, automobile accident, after lifting, from a fall? Or with fever? Or did it have a gradual onset?	Acute onset of stiffness with headache and fever occurs with meningeal inflammation.
• Location: Does pain radiate? If so, to the shoulders, arms?	
• Associated symptoms: Any **limitations to range of motion** (ROM)? Any numbness or tingling in shoulders, arms, or hands?	
• Precipitating factors: What movements cause pain? Do you need to lift or bend at work or home?	
• Does stress seem to trigger the pain?	
• Coping strategies: Are you able to do your work, to sleep?	Pain creates a vicious circle. Tension increases pain and disability, which produces more tension.

Examiner Asks	Rationale
5. Lumps or swelling. Any **lumps** or **swelling** in the neck?	
• Any recent infection? Any tenderness?	Tenderness is suggestive of acute infection.
• For a lump that persists, how long have you had it? Has it changed in size?	A persistent lump arouses suspicion of malignancy. For patients older than 40 years, suspect malignancy until it is proven otherwise.
• Any history of prior irradiation of head, neck, upper chest?	Such irradiation increases risk for salivary and thyroid tumours.
• Any difficulty swallowing?	**Dysphagia** is the term for this condition.
• Do you smoke? For how long? How many packs a day? Do you chew tobacco?	Smoking and chewing tobacco increase risk of oral and respiratory cancers.
• When was your last alcoholic drink? How much alcohol do you drink a day?	Smoking and large alcohol consumption together increase the risk of cancer.
• Ever had a thyroid problem? Overfunctioning or underfunctioning? How was it treated: surgery, irradiation, any medication?	
6. History of head or neck surgery. Ever had **surgery of the head or neck?**	Surgery for head and neck cancer often is disfiguring and increases risk for body image disturbance.
• For what condition? When did the surgery occur? How do you feel about results?	

Additional History for Infants and Children

1. Prenatal drug exposure. Did the mother use alcohol or street drugs during pregnancy? How often?	Alcohol increases the risk of fetal alcohol syndrome, which is characterized by distinctive facial features (see Table 14-3, p. 291). Cocaine use causes neurological, developmental, and emotional problems.
• How much was used per episode?	
2. Delivery. Was delivery vaginal or by Caesarean section? Any difficulty? Were forceps used?	Forceps may increase the risk of caput succedaneum, cephalhematoma, and Bell's palsy.
3. Growth. What were you told about the baby's growth? Was it on schedule? Did the head seem to grow and fontanelles close on schedule? At what age (in months) did the baby achieve head control?	

Additional History for Older Adults

1. Dizziness. If dizziness is a problem, how does this affect your daily activities? Are you able to drive safely, manoeuvre about the house safely?	Assess self-care. Assess potential for injury.
2. Pain. If neck pain is a problem, how does this affect your daily activities? Are you able to drive, perform at work, do housework, sleep, look down when using stairs?	

Subjective Data

Objective Data

OBJECTIVE DATA

Normal Range of Findings	Abnormal Findings
THE HEAD	
Inspect and Palpate the Skull	
Size and Shape	
Note the general size and shape. A **normocephalic** skull is round and symmetrical and is appropriately proportional to body size. Be aware that "normal" includes a wide range of sizes.	Deformities: microcephaly (abnormally small head); macrocephaly (abnormally large head), caused by hydrocephaly, acromegaly, Paget's disease (Table 14-1).

Objective Data

Normal Range of Findings	Abnormal Findings

To assess shape, place your fingers in the person's hair and palpate the scalp. The skull normally feels symmetrical and smooth. The cranial bones that have normal protrusions are the forehead, the lateral edge of each parietal bone, the occipital bone, and the mastoid process behind each ear. There is no tenderness on palpation.

Note lumps, depressions, or abnormal protrusions.

Temporal Area

Palpate the temporal artery above the zygomatic (cheek) bone between the eye and top of the ear.

With temporal arteritis, the artery looks more tortuous and feels hardened and tender.

The temporomandibular joint is just below the temporal artery and anterior to the tragus. Palpate the joint as the patient opens the mouth; normal movement is smooth, with no limitation or tenderness.

Abnormalities include crepitation, limited ROM, and tenderness.

Inspect the Face
Facial Structures

Inspect the face, noting the facial expression and its appropriateness for behaviour or reported mood. Anxiety is common in hospitalized or ill patients.

Patients may have expressions of hostility or embarrassment.
Tense, rigid muscles may indicate anxiety or pain; a flat affect may indicate depression; excessive smiling may be inappropriate.

Although the shape of facial structures may vary somewhat among races, they always should be symmetrical. Note symmetry of eyebrows, palpebral fissures, nasolabial folds, and sides of the mouth.

Marked asymmetry may occur with central brain lesion (e.g., brain attack) or with peripheral damage to cranial nerve VII (Bell's palsy; see Table 14-4, p. 293).

Note any abnormal facial structures (coarse facial features, exophthalmos, changes in skin colour or pigmentation) and any abnormal swelling. Also note any involuntary movements (tics) in the facial muscles. Normally, none occur.

Edema in the face occurs first around the eyes (periorbital) and the cheeks, where the subcutaneous tissue is relatively loose.
Note grinding of jaws, tics, fasciculations, and excessive blinking.

THE NECK

Inspect and Palpate the Neck
Symmetry

Head position is centred in the midline, and the accessory neck muscles should be symmetrical. The head should be held erect and still.

Head tilt occurs with muscle spasm. Rigidity of the head and neck occurs with arthritis.

Range of Motion

Note any limitation of movement during active motion. Ask the patient to touch the chin to the chest, turn the head to the right and left, try to touch each ear to the shoulder (without elevating shoulders), and to extend the neck backward. When the neck is supple, motion is smooth and controlled.

Note pain at any particular movement.
Note ratchety or limited movement from cervical arthritis or inflammation of neck muscles. The arthritic neck is rigid; the affected patient turns at the shoulders rather than at the neck.

Test muscle strength and the status of cranial nerve XI by trying to resist the patient's movements with your hands as the patient shrugs the shoulders and turns the head to each side.

Normal Range of Findings	Abnormal Findings

As the patient moves the head, note any enlargement of the salivary glands and lymph glands. Normally, no enlargement is present. Note a swollen parotid gland when the head is extended; look for swelling below the angle of the jaw. Also, note thyroid gland enlargement. Normally, none is present.

Also note any obvious pulsations. The carotid artery runs medial to the sternomastoid muscle, and it has a brisk localized pulsation just below the angle of the jaw. Normally, there are no other pulsations while the patient is in the sitting position (see Chapter 20).

Thyroid enlargement may be a unilateral lump, or it may be diffuse and look like a doughnut lying across the lower neck (Table 14-2).

Lymph Nodes

Using a gentle circular motion of your fingertips, palpate the lymph nodes (Figure 14-9). (Normally, the salivary glands are not palpable. When symptoms warrant, check for parotid tenderness by palpating in a line from the outer corner of the eye to the lobule of the ear.) Beginning with the preauricular lymph nodes in front of the ear, palpate the 10 groups of lymph nodes in a routine order. Many nodes are closely packed, so you must be systematic and thorough in your examination. Once you establish your sequence, do not vary, or you may miss some small nodes.

In mumps, the parotid gland is swollen (see Table 14-2, p. 290).

Parotid enlargement has been found with acquired immune deficiency syndrome (AIDS).

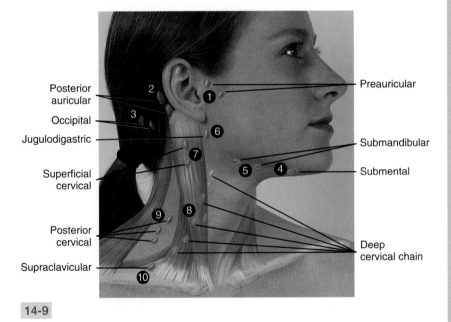

Posterior auricular
Occipital
Jugulodigastric
Superficial cervical
Posterior cervical
Supraclavicular
Preauricular
Submandibular
Submental
Deep cervical chain

14-9

Palpate gently because strong pressure could push the nodes into the neck muscles. It is usually most efficient to palpate with both hands, so that you can compare the two sides symmetrically. However, the submental gland under the tip of the chin is easier to explore with one hand. When you palpate with one hand, use your other hand to position the person's head. For the deep cervical chain, tip the person's head toward the side being examined to relax the ipsilateral muscle (Figure 14-10). Then you can press your fingers under the muscle. Search for the supraclavicular node by having the person hunch the shoulders and elbows forward (Figure 14-11); this relaxes the skin. The inferior belly of the omohyoid muscle crosses the posterior triangle here; do not mistake it for a lymph node.

Objective Data

Normal Range of Findings	**Abnormal Findings**

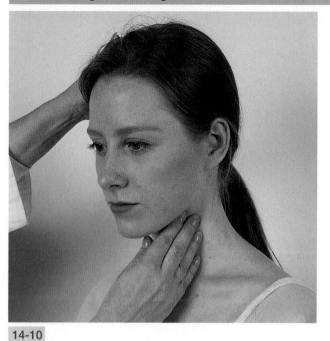

14-10

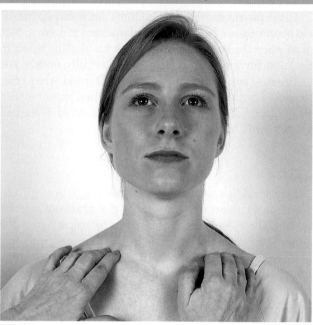

14-11

If any nodes are palpable, note their location, size, shape, delimitation (discrete or clumped together), mobility, consistency, and tenderness. Cervical nodes often are palpable in healthy persons, although this palpability decreases with age (Figure 14-12). Normal nodes feel movable, discrete, soft, and nontender.

Lymphadenopathy is enlargement of the lymph nodes (>1 cm), caused by infection, allergy, or neoplasm.

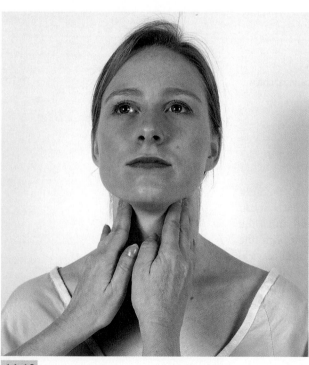

14-12

Normal Range of Findings

If nodes are enlarged or tender, check the area they drain for the source of the problem. For example, enlargement or tenderness of those in the upper cervical or submandibular area is often related to inflammation or a neoplasm in the head and neck. Follow up on your findings, or refer the patient to a specialist. An enlarged lymph node, particularly when you cannot find the source of the problem, necessitates prompt attention.

Trachea

Normally, the trachea is midline; palpate for any tracheal shift. Place your index finger on the trachea in the sternal notch, and slip it off to each side (Figure 14-13). The space should be symmetrical on both sides. Note any deviation from the midline.

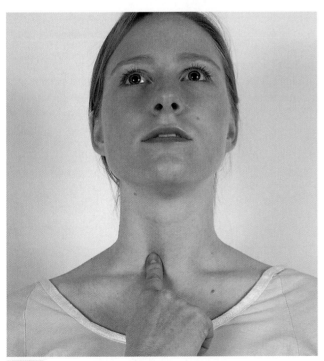

14-13

Abnormal Findings

The following criteria are common clues but are not definitive in all circumstances:

- Acute infection: Nodes are bilateral, enlarged, warm, tender, and firm but freely movable.
- Chronic inflammation: Nodes are clumped (e.g., in tuberculosis).
- Cancerous nodes: Nodes are hard, unilateral, nontender, and fixed.
- Human immunodeficiency virus (HIV) infection: Nodes are enlarged, firm, nontender, and mobile. Occipital node enlargement is common with HIV infection.
- Neoplasm in the thorax or abdomen: A single left node may be enlarged, nontender, and hard (Virchow's node).
- Hodgkin's lymphoma: Discrete nodes that are painless and rubbery gradually appear.

Conditions of tracheal shift:
- The trachea is *pushed to the unaffected* (or healthy) side with an aortic aneurysm, a tumour, unilateral thyroid lobe enlargement, and pneumothorax.
- The trachea is *pulled toward the affected* (diseased) side with large atelectasis, pleural adhesions, or fibrosis.
- Tracheal tug is a rhythmic downward pull that is synchronous with systole and that occurs with aortic arch aneurysm.

Objective Data

Normal Range of Findings	Abnormal Findings

Thyroid Gland

The thyroid gland is difficult to palpate; arrange your setting to maximize your likelihood of success. Position a standing lamp to shine tangentially across the neck to highlight any possible swelling. Supply the patient with a glass of water, and first inspect the neck as the patient takes a sip and swallows. Thyroid tissue normally moves up with a swallow.

Posterior Approach. To palpate, move behind the person (Figure 14-14, *A*). Ask the person to sit up very straight and then to bend the head slightly forward and to the right. This will relax the neck muscles. Use the fingers of your left hand to push the trachea slightly to the right.

Then curve your right fingers between the trachea and the sternomastoid muscle, retracting it slightly, and ask the patient to take a sip of water. The thyroid moves up under your fingers with the trachea and larynx as the patient swallows. Reverse the procedure for the left side.

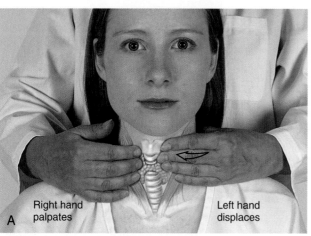

Right hand palpates   Left hand displaces

A

14-14

Usually you cannot palpate the normal adult thyroid. In some patients who have a long, thin neck, you can feel the isthmus over the tracheal rings. The lateral lobes are usually not palpable; check them for enlargement, consistency, symmetry, and the presence of nodules.

Anterior Approach. This is an alternative method of palpating the thyroid, but it is more awkward to perform, especially for a novice examiner. Stand facing the patient. Ask him or her to tip the head forward and to the right. Use your right thumb to displace the trachea slightly to the patient's right. Hook your left thumb and fingers around the sternomastoid muscle. Feel for lobe enlargement as the patient swallows (Figure 14-15).

Look for diffuse enlargement or a nodular lump.

It is important in a basic assessment to note any visible enlargement of the thyroid. Palpation of the thyroid is considered an advanced practice consideration.

Serum laboratory values related to thyroid function are as follows:
- T_4: 10 to 30 pmol/L (0.8 to 2.3 ng/dL)
- T_3 uptake: 0.25 to 0.35 (25% to 35%)
- T_3: 1.7 to 3.5 nmol/L (110 to 230 ng/dL)

Increases in T_3 level and uptake are indicative of hyperthyroidism.

Decreases in T_3 level and uptake are indicative of hypothyroidism.

Graves' disease is the most common cause of hyperthyroidism (see Table 14-4 on p. 292).

Common signs and symptoms:
- Exophthalmus (bulging eyes)
- Goitre (thickened neck)
- Fatigue, weight loss, and nervousness

Myxedema, also known as hypothyroidism, results from diminished functioning of the thyroid gland (see Table 14-4, p. 292). Common signs and symptoms are as follows:
- Periorbital edema
- Weight gain, coarsening of facial features, and dry skin
- Exhaustion, depression, or increased frequency of menses.

Abnormalities include enlarged lobes that are easily palpated before swallowing or are tender on palpation (see large goitre in Figure 14-14, *B*) and the presence of nodules or lumps (see Table 14-2, p. 290).

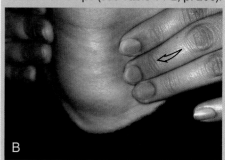

B

14-14, cont'd

Normal Range of Findings

Abnormal Findings

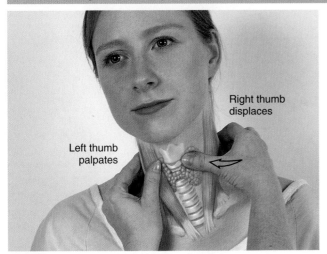

Left thumb
palpates

Right thumb
displaces

14-15

Auscultate the Thyroid

If the thyroid gland is enlarged, auscultate it for the presence of a **bruit.** This is a soft, pulsatile, whooshing, blowing sound heard best with the bell of the stethoscope. Bruits are not normally present.

A bruit occurs with accelerated or turbulent blood flow, which is indicative of hyperplasia of the thyroid (e.g., hyperthyroidism).

❖ DEVELOPMENTAL CONSIDERATIONS

Infants and Children

Skull

Measure an infant's **head size** with measuring tape at each visit up to age 2 years, then yearly up to age 6 years. (Measurement of head circumference is described in detail in Chapter 10.)

A newborn's head measures about 32 to 38 cm (average, ≈34 cm) and is 2 cm larger than chest circumference. At age 2 years, both measurements are the same. During childhood the chest circumference grows to exceed head circumference by 5 to 7 cm.

Observe the infant's head from all angles, not just the front. The contour should be symmetrical. Some racial variation in head shapes is normal; children of Nordic descent tend to have long heads, whereas those of Asian descent have broad heads.

Two common variations in the newborn cause the shape of the skull to look markedly asymmetrical: A **caput succedaneum** is edematous swelling and ecchymosis of the presenting part of the head caused by birth trauma (Figure 14-16). It feels soft, and it may extend across suture lines. It gradually resolves during the first few days of life, and no treatment is needed.

Note any abnormal increase in head size or failure to grow.

Microcephalic: Head size is below norms for age

Macrocephalic: Head is large for age or rapidly increasing in size (e.g., as in hydrocephalus [increased cerebrospinal fluid])

Frontal bulges, or "bossing," occur with prematurity or rickets.

| **Normal Range of Findings** | **Abnormal Findings** |

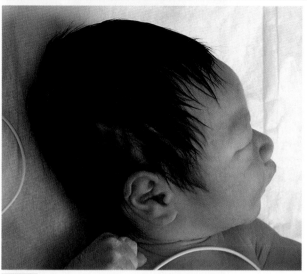

14-16   Caput succedaneum.

A **cephalhematoma,** a subperiosteal hemorrhage, is also a result of birth trauma (Figure 14-17). It is soft, fluctuant, and well defined over one cranial bone because the periosteum (i.e., the covering over each bone) holds the bleeding in place. It appears several hours after birth and gradually increases in size. No discoloration is present, but it looks bizarre, and so parents need reassurance that the fluid will be reabsorbed during the first few weeks of life without treatment. In rare cases, a large hematoma may persist as long as 3 months.

An infant with cephalhematoma is at greater risk for jaundice as the red blood cells within the hematoma are broken down and reabsorbed.

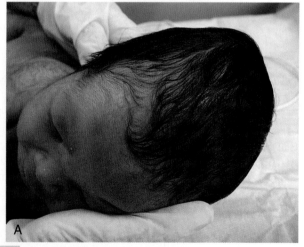

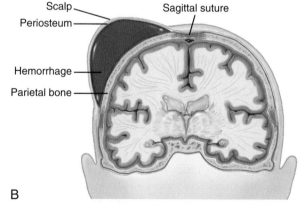

Scalp
Periosteum

Sagittal suture

Hemorrhage
Parietal bone

A

B

14-17   Cephalhematoma.

As you palpate the newborn's head, the suture lines feel like ridges. By age 5 to 6 months, they are smooth and not palpable.

A newborn's head may feel asymmetrical and the involved ridges more prominent because of *moulding* of the cranial bones during engagement and passage through the birth canal. Moulding is overriding of the cranial bones; usually, the parietal bone overrides the frontal or occipital bone. Reassure parents that this appearance lasts only a few days or a week. Babies delivered by Caesarean section usually have evenly round heads. Also, some asymmetry may occur if an infant continually sleeps in one position; this is a flattening of the dependent cranial bone, usually the occiput.

Sutures palpable when the child is older than 6 months should be investigated.

Marked asymmetry should be investigated; an example is *craniosynostosis,* a severe deformity caused by premature closure of the sutures. Premature closing of the suture results in a long, narrow head.

Flattening also occurs in children with rickets.

Normal Range of Findings	Abnormal Findings

Gently palpate the skull and fontanelles while the infant is calm and somewhat in a sitting position (crying, lying down, or vomiting may cause the anterior fontanelle to look full and bulging). The skull should feel smooth and fused except at the fontanelles. The fontanelles feel firm, slightly concave, and well defined against the edges of the cranial bones. You may see slight arterial pulsations in the anterior fontanelle.

A fontanelle may be truly tense or bulging with acute increased intracranial pressure.

Fontanelles are depressed and sunken with dehydration or malnutrition.

Pulsations may be markedly noticeable with increased intracranial pressure.

The posterior fontanelle may not be palpable at birth. If it is, it measures 1 cm and closes by 1 to 2 months. The anterior fontanelle may be small at birth and enlarges to 2.5 cm × 2.5 cm. The diameter is occasionally large (4 to 5 cm) in infants younger than 6 months. A small fontanelle usually is normal. The anterior fontanelle closes between ages 9 months and 2 years. Early closure may be insignificant if head growth proceeds normally.

Delayed closure or larger than normal fontanelle size occurs with hydrocephalus, Down's syndrome, hypothyroidism, and rickets.

A small fontanelle may be a sign of microcephaly, as is early closure.

Note the infant's **head posture** and **head control.** The infant can turn the head side to side by 2 weeks and shows the **tonic neck reflex** when supine and the head is turned to one side (extension of same arm and leg, flexion of opposite arm and leg). The tonic neck reflex disappears between ages 3 and 4 months, and then the head is maintained in the midline. Head control is achieved by age 4 months, when the baby can hold the head erect and steady when pulled to a vertical position. (See Chapters 24 and 25 for further details on the musculoskeletal and neurological systems.)

Persistence of the tonic neck reflex after age 5 months may indicate brain damage.

In children, head tilt occurs with habit spasm, poor vision, and brain tumour.

Head lag after age 4 months may indicate intellectual or motor disability.

Face

Check **facial features** for symmetry, appearance, and presence of swelling. Note symmetry of wrinkling when the infant cries or smiles (e.g., both sides of the lips rise and both sides of forehead wrinkle). Children love to comply when you ask them to "make a face." Normally, no swelling is evident. Parotid gland enlargement is most evident when the child sits and looks up at the ceiling; the swelling appears below the angle of the jaw.

Unilateral immobility indicates nerve damage (central or peripheral; e.g., note angle of mouth droop on paralyzed side).

Some facies are characteristic of congenital abnormalities or chronic allergy (Tables 14-3 and 14-4).

Neck

An infant's neck looks short; it lengthens during the first 3 to 4 years. You can see the neck better by supporting the infant's shoulders and tilting the head back a little. This positioning also facilitates palpation of the trachea, which is buried deep in the neck. Feel for the row of cartilaginous rings in the midline or just slightly to the right of the midline.

A short neck or webbing (loose, fanlike folds) may indicate a congenital abnormality (e.g., Down's or Turner's syndrome), or it may occur alone.

Assess muscle development with gentle passive ROM. Cradle an infant's head with your hands and turn it side to side, and test forward flexion, extension, and rotation. Note any resistance to movement, especially flexion. Ask an older child to actively move through the ROM, as you would an adult.

Head tilt and limited ROM occur with torticollis (wryneck) or from sternomastoid muscle injury that occurs during birth or as a congenital defect.

Resistance to flexion (nuchal rigidity) and pain on flexion indicate meningeal irritation or meningitis.

During infancy, cervical lymph nodes are normally not palpable. However, an older child's lymph nodes are; they feel more prominent than an adult's until after puberty, when lymphoid tissue begins to atrophy. Palpable nodes smaller than 3 mm are normal. They may be up to 1 cm in size in the cervical and inguinal areas but are discrete, move easily, and are nontender. Children have a higher incidence of infection, and so you should expect a higher incidence of inflammatory adenopathy among children. No other mass should occur in the neck.

Cervical nodes bigger than 1 cm are considered enlarged.

Thyroglossal duct cyst is a cystic lump high up in midline; it is freely movable and rises up during swallowing.

Supraclavicular nodes enlarge with Hodgkin's disease.

The thyroid gland is difficult to palpate in an infant because of the shortness and thickness of the neck. An older child's thyroid may be palpable normally.

Normal Range of Findings	Abnormal Findings

Special Considerations for Advanced Practice

These are procedures that would not be considered part of a basic assessment in an environment in which patients have access to diagnostic testing. In Canada, health care providers may practise in isolated health care environments in which access to computed tomography or magnetic resonance imaging is not readily available. In these environments, the health care practitioner may find the following tests a helpful addition to their toolkit.

Palpation. *Craniotabes* is a softening of the skull's outer layer. With a newborn, pressure along the suture of the parietal and occipital bones above the ear produces a snapping sensation because of the pliable skull bone. It is like indenting a Ping-Pong ball and feeling it snap back. Do not attempt this unless craniotabes is suspected on the basis of other abnormal findings, and even then avoid excessive pressure. Craniotabes may be normal, especially with premature infants.

Craniotabes may occur with rickets, hydrocephaly, or congenital syphilis.

Percussion. With an infant, you may directly percuss with your plexor finger against the head surface. This yields a resonant or "cracked pot" sound, which is normal before closure of the fontanelles.

Auscultation. Bruits are common in the skull in children younger than 4 or 5 years or in children with anemia. They are systolic or continuous and are heard over the temporal area.

The sound also occurs with hydrocephalus as a result of separation of cranial sutures (McEwen's sign).

After 5 years of age, bruits indicate increased intracranial pressure, aneurysm, or arteriovenous shunt.

Pregnant Women

During the second trimester, chloasma may show on the face. This is a blotchy, hyperpigmented area over the cheeks and forehead that fades after delivery. The thyroid gland may be palpable normally during pregnancy.

Older Adults

The temporal arteries may look twisted and prominent. In some older adults, a mild rhythmic tremor of the head may be normal. **Senile tremors** are benign and include head nodding (as if saying yes or no) and tongue protrusion. If some teeth have been lost, the lower face looks unusually small, with the mouth sunken in.

The neck may show an increased cervical concave (or inward) curve when the head and jaw are extended forward to compensate for kyphosis of the spine. During the examination, direct the older adult to perform ROM slowly; he or she may experience dizziness with side movements. An older adult may have prolapse of the submandibular glands, which could be mistaken for a tumour. Drooping submandibular glands, however, feel soft, and the drooping is bilateral.

PROMOTING HEALTH: BRAIN INJURY PREVENTION

Use Your Head. Wear a Helmet

In Canada, helmet use is legislated provincially. Safe Kids Canada currently advocates that all provinces adopt the U.S. Consumer Product Safety Commission (CPSP) recommendations in regard to helmet safety standards. Bicycle helmet laws in Canada do not specify the CPSC standard, and so cyclists may be in violation of the helmet law in their province.

When you buy a helmet in Canada, look for the Canadian Standards Association (CSA), ASTM International, or CPSC standard. The CPSC standard is comparable with the CSA standard. For guidelines and information about which helmet to choose for activities to prevent brain and head injury, go to *http://www.safekidscanada.ca* or call 1-888-SAFE-TIPS. Also ensure that you are aware of individual provincial helmet legislation, inasmuch as many provinces levy significant fines for nonuse.

In the report *Reaching for the Top: A Report by the Advisor on Healthy Children and Youth,* Leitch (2007) stated that a pan-Canadian 5-year "National Injury Prevention Strategy" would be implemented. To date, however, not all provinces in Canada have helmet legislation. Ensure that you are using the most up-to-date legislated policy to guide your decision making. For more information about CPSC standards, go to *http://www.cpsc.gov.*

In general, all helmets are designed to absorb the impact energy in a collision or fall, protecting the brain from injury and trauma. However, helmets are not created equal. Each type of helmet is specifically designed to protect the head and brain from one or more *specific* types of impact that can take place in the particular sport or activity for which it is intended.

PROMOTING HEALTH: BRAIN INJURY PREVENTION—cont'd

Wearing a properly fitted and safe bicycle helmet can reduce an individual's risk of head injury by 85% and reduce the risk of brain injury by 88%. A helmet needs to be comfortable, snug, and secured. It should not move in any direction when adjusted properly, and the chin strap needs to be securely buckled. A proper fit is as important as wearing the correct helmet. This is particularly important for children. It is important to select a helmet that fits now, not a helmet that a child will grow into.

Children and adults should wear a sport- or activity-specific helmet when participating in the following sports or recreational activities:

- Alpine skiing, snowboarding, and snowmobiling
- ATV riding and go-kart riding
- Baseball and softball
- Bicycling and electronic bicycling (E-biking)
- Football
- Horseback riding
- Ice hockey, rollerskating, and in-line skating
- Lacrosse
- Rock climbing
- Scooter and skateboard riding

Although a helmet has not yet been specifically designed for either ice-skating or sledding, wearing a bicycle, skateboard, or ski helmet may be preferable to wearing no helmet at all. Nova Scotia was the first province in Canada to pass new legislation requiring all skiers (children and adults) to wear CSA-approved helmets on the slopes.

There are also certain activities for which an individual, especially a child, should not wear a helmet: for example, playing on playgrounds or climbing. In these situations, a helmet's chin strap might get caught and pose a risk of strangulation. Furthermore, the helmet itself may also pose an entrapment hazard or risk.

For more information about CPSC standards, go to *http://www.cpsc.gov*.

Additional Resources
Leitch, K. (2007). *Reaching for the top: A report by the advisor on healthy children and youth. Ottawa: Health Canada.*
Safe Kids Canada. (2011). Safe Cycling. Retrieved from http://www.safekidscanada.ca/Professionals/Safety-Information/Wheeled-Activities/Cycling/Safe-Cycling.aspx.

PROMOTING HEALTH: PLAYING IT SAFE

Use Your Head: Understanding Postconcussion Syndrome

Sidney Crosby, Canadian National Hockey League player and Olympic gold medalist, has publicized the discussion of postconcussion syndrome. Hockey Canada (2011) has responded to this growing concern among amateur and professional athletes with an aggressive awareness program to protect young athletes. Although created by Hockey Canada, this program is an excellent resource for all sports in which a concussion could occur.

Concussions are brain injuries caused by the impact of the brain with the inside of the skull. The impact causes damage that changes how brain cells function, leading to symptoms that can be physical (headaches, dizziness), cognitive (problems remembering or concentrating), or emotional (feeling depressed). A concussion can result from a blow to the head or body in numerous activities, including sports.

Concussions are common injuries, but because they cannot be detected on radiographs or computed tomographic scans, they have been difficult to fully investigate and understand. Fortunately, many important advances in knowledge of concussions have been made, including how to identify, manage, and recover from a concussion. Although concussions are often referred to as "mild traumatic head injuries" and often resolve uneventfully, *all* concussions have the potential for serious and long-lasting symptoms, and so each must be treated carefully and in consultation with a health care practitioner. Injuries to the brain are characterized by an altered state of consciousness. The altered state of consciousness is the key finding with any head injury.

In 2012, Ontario became the first province in Canada to introduce comprehensive legislation on concussions in schools. Several national organizations are lobbying for federal legislation to protect youth. Between 2003 and 2011, emergency room visits for concussions increased by 58%.

Signs and symptoms of concussion are as follows:
- Headache
- Dizziness
- Feeling dazed
- Seeing "stars"
- Sensitivity to light
- Ringing in ears
- Tiredness
- Nausea, vomiting
- Irritability
- Confusion, disorientation

Contrary to popular belief, most concussions occur without a loss of consciousness.

It is extremely important to seek medical advice immediately upon receiving a blow to the head or body that results in signs or symptoms of a concussion. Concussions often go untreated, and symptoms may develop days or weeks after the initial injury. Ensure that patients who receive a concussion follow a recommended plan of recovery as outlined by the clinician.

Prevention is always the best approach. Ensure that patients wear a properly fitting CSA-approved helmet that is specific to the sport being played. Advise patients to report any head injuries immediately and to seek medical attention promptly.

Finally, many organizations such as the National Hockey League are mandating baseline concussion testing on all players to ensure the safety of their participants.

For more information on baseline testing or postconcussion recommendations, please visit *www.hockeycanada.ca/index.php/ci_id/60930/la_id/1.htm*.

References
Hockey Canada. (2011). *Think first: Smart hockey. Retrieved from* http://www.hockeycanada.ca.

Objective Data

DOCUMENTATION AND CRITICAL THINKING

Sample Charting

SUBJECTIVE

Denies any unusually frequent or severe headache; no history of head injury, dizziness, or syncope; no neck pain, limitation of motion, nodules, or swelling.

OBJECTIVE

Head: Normocephalic, no lumps, no lesions, no tenderness.
Face: Symmetrical, no weakness, or drooping, no involuntary movements.
Neck: Supple with full ROM, no pain. Symmetric, no lymphadenopathy or masses. Trachea midline, thyroid not palpable. No bruits.

ASSESSMENT

Normocephalic symmetrical head and neck

Focused Assessment: Clinical Case Study

Mara is a 19-year-old single female college student with a history of good health and no chronic illnesses; she enters the outpatient clinic today stating, "I think I've had a stroke!"

SUBJECTIVE

- 1 day PTA ["prior to arrival"]: first noticed at dinner at college cafeteria when joking with friends, started to stick out tongue and roll tongue and could not do it, right side of tongue was not working. Mara left room to look in mirror and became scared; when smiled, noticed right side was not working. Tried to pucker lips, could not. Could not whistle, could not raise eyebrow: "I looked like a Vulcan." No other movement disorder below neck. Mild pain behind right ear with buzzing in ear. Able to sleep last night, but roommate said Mara's right eyelid did not close completely during sleep.
- Today: still no movement on complete right side of face. Feeling self-conscious in class and during conversations with friends. Now has taste aversion; fluids with high water content taste especially bitter. No hearing loss.

OBJECTIVE

Temp, 37°C; pulse, 64; resp, 14; B/P, 108/78

Forehead appears smooth and immobile on right; patient unable to wrinkle right side. Unable to close right eye; Bell's phenomenon present with attempts to close (right eyeball rolls upward); right palpebral fissure appears wider. No corneal reflex on right. Unable to whistle or puff right cheek. Absent nasolabial fold on right. Mouth droops on right, sags on right when tries to smile. Slight drooling. Left side of face responds appropriately to all these movements. Superficial sensation intact.

Rest of musculoskeletal system intact: able to hold balance while standing, able to walk, walk heel-to-toe, do knee bend on each knee. Arm strength and ROM intact.

ASSESSMENT

Right-sided facial paralysis, consistent with Bell's palsy
Disturbed body image R/T [related to] effects of loss of facial function
Risk for deficient fluid volume R/T taste aversion and dietary alteration
Risk for sensory deficit, visual impairment, R/T effects of neurological impairment

ABNORMAL FINDINGS

TABLE 14-1 Abnormalities in Head Size and Contour

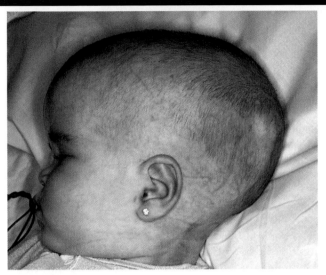

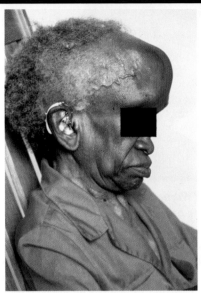

Hydrocephalus

Obstruction of drainage of cerebrospinal fluid results in excessive accumulation, increasing intracranial pressure, and enlargement of the head. The face looks small in comparison with the enlarged cranium. The increasing pressure also causes dilation of scalp veins, frontal bossing, and downcast or "setting sun" appearance of the eyes (sclera is visible above iris). The cranial bones thin, sutures separate, and percussion yields a "cracked pot" sound (MacEwen's sign).

Reprinted from the Clinical Slide Collection on the Rheumatic Diseases. ©1991, 1995, 1997. Used by permission of the American College of Rheumatology.

Paget's Disease of Bone (Osteitis Deformans)

A localized bone disease of unknown origin that softens, thickens, and deforms bone. It affects 3% of adults older than 40 years and 8%-15% older than 75 years. Symptoms occur a decade earlier in men, on average. The disease is characterized by bowed long bones, sudden fractures, frontal bossing, and enlarging skull bones that form an acorn-shaped cranium. Enlarging skull bones press on cranial nerves, causing symptoms of headache, vertigo, tinnitus, progressive deafness, and optic atrophy and compression of the spinal cord.

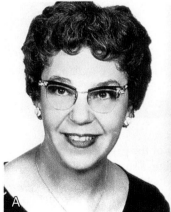
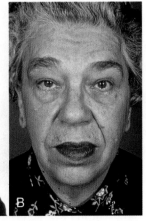

◄ Acromegaly

Excessive secretion of growth hormone from the pituitary after puberty causes enlargement of the skull and thickening of the cranial bones. In the illustration on the right, note the elongated head, massive face, prominent nose and lower jaw, heavy eyebrow ridge, and coarse facial features, especially in comparison with the same woman's face on the left, pictured several years before a pituitary tumour developed.

TABLE 14-2   Swellings on the Head or Neck

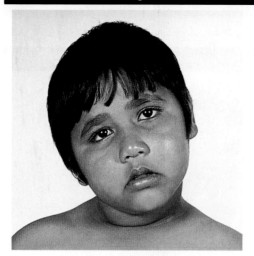

Torticollis (Wryneck)

A shortening or excessive contraction of the
sternocleidomastoid muscle in the neck; may be caused
by an idiopathic, genetic, or acquired secondary injury
that results in a lateral head tilt and chin rotation to the
opposite side. Congenital torticollis may be caused by
intrauterine malpositioning or by prenatal injury of the
muscles or blood supply in the neck. You will feel a firm,
discrete, nontender mass in the middle of the muscle on
the involved side. This necessitates treatment, or the
muscle becomes fibrotic and permanently shortened with
permanent limitation of ROM, asymmetry of head and
face, and visual problems resulting from the
nonhorizontal position of the eyes.

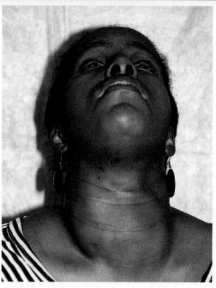

Thyroid: Multiple Nodules

Multiple nodules usually indicate inflammation or a
multinodular goitre rather than a neoplasm. However,
any rapidly enlarging or firm nodule should be further
investigated.

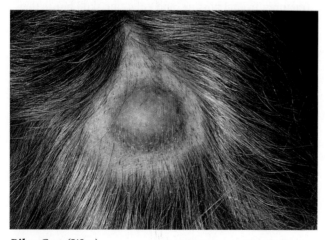

Pilar Cyst (Wen)

Smooth, firm, fluctuant swelling on the scalp. Tense
pressure of the contents causes overlying skin to be shiny
and taut. It is a benign growth.

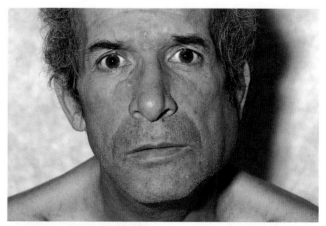

Parotid Gland Enlargement

Rapid painful inflammation of the parotid gland occurs
with mumps. Parotid swelling also occurs with blockage
of a duct, with abscess, and with tumour. Note swelling
of anterior to lower ear lobe. Stensen duct obstruction
can occur in older adults dehydrated as a result of
diuretics or anticholinergics.

ROM, range of motion.

TABLE 14-3 Pediatric Facial Abnormalities

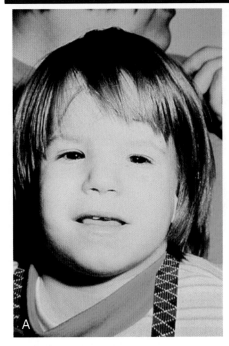

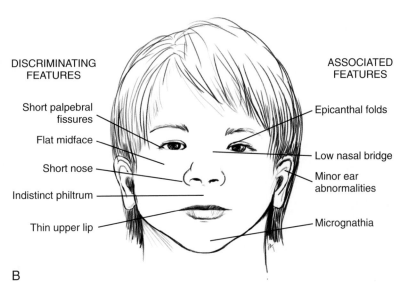

DISCRIMINATING FEATURES

Short palpebral fissures

Flat midface

Short nose

Indistinct philtrum

Thin upper lip

ASSOCIATED FEATURES

Epicanthal folds

Low nasal bridge

Minor ear abnormalities

Micrognathia

B

© Pat Thomas, 2006.

Fetal Alcohol Syndrome
A pregnant woman who abuses alcohol is at great risk of producing a baby with a wide range of growth and developmental abnormalities. Facial malformations may be recognizable at birth. Characteristic facies include narrow palpebral fissures, epicanthal folds, and midfacial hypoplasia.

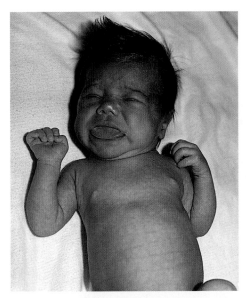

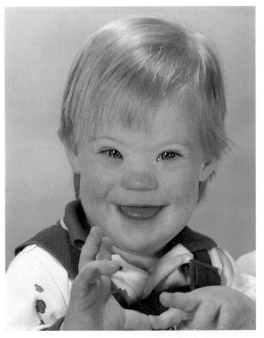

Congenital Hypothyroidism
Thyroid deficiency at an early age produces impaired growth and neurological deficit. Without neonatal screening, characteristic facies develop by 3 to 6 months of age: low hairline, hirsute forehead, swollen eyelids, narrow palpebral fissures, widely spaced eyes, depressed nasal bridge, puffy face, thick tongue protruding through an open mouth, and a dull expression. Head size is normal, but the anterior and posterior fontanelles are wide open.

Down's Syndrome
Chromosomal aberration (trisomy 21). Head and face characteristics may include upslanting eyes with inner epicanthal folds, flat nasal bridge, small broad flat nose, protruding thick tongue, ear dysplasia, short broad neck with webbing, and small hands with single palmar crease.

Continued

TABLE 14-3 Pediatric Facial Abnormalities—cont'd

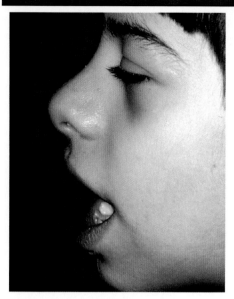

Atopic (Allergic) Facies
Children with chronic allergies such as atopic dermatitis often develop characteristic facial features. These include exhausted face, blue shadows below the eyes ("allergic shiners") from sluggish venous return, a double or single crease on the lower eyelids (Morgan's lines), central facial pallor, and open-mouth breathing (allergic gaping). The open-mouth breathing can lead to malocclusion of the teeth and malformed jaw because the child's bones are still forming.

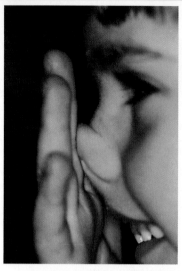

Allergic Salute and Crease
The transverse line on the nose is also a feature of chronic allergies. It is formed when the child chronically uses the hand to push the nose up and back (the "allergic salute") to relieve itching and to free swollen turbinates, which allows air passage.

TABLE 14-4 Abnormal Facial Appearances With Chronic Illnesses

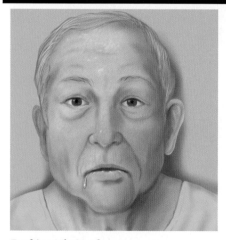

Parkinson's Syndrome
A deficiency of the neurotransmitter dopamine and degeneration of the basal ganglia in the brain. The immobility of features produces a face that is flat and expressionless, "masklike," with elevated eyebrows, staring gaze, oily skin, and drooling.

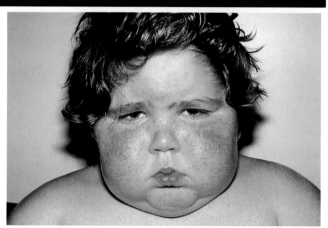

Cushing's Syndrome
With excessive secretion of adrenocorticotropic hormone (ACTH) and chronic steroid use, the person develops a plethoric, rounded, moonlike face, prominent jowls, red cheeks, hirsutism on the upper lip, lower cheeks, and chin, and acneiform rash on the chest.

TABLE 14-4   Abnormal Facial Appearances With Chronic Illnesses—cont'd

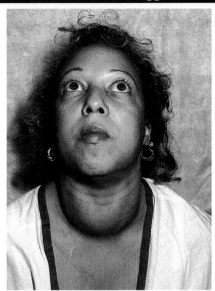

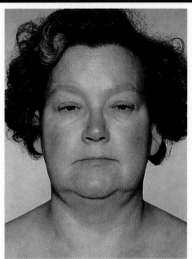

Myxedema (Hypothyroidism)
A deficiency of thyroid hormone, when severe, causes a nonpitting edema or myxedema. Note puffy edematous face, especially around eyes (periorbital edema), coarse facial features, dry skin, and dry coarse hair and eyebrows.

Hyperthyroidism
Goitre is an increase in the size of the thyroid gland and occurs with hyperthyroidism, Hashimoto's thyroiditis, and hypothyroidism. Graves' disease (shown here) is the most common cause of hyperthyroidism, manifested by goitre and exophthalmos (bulging eyeballs). Symptoms include nervousness, fatigue, weight loss, muscle cramps, and heat intolerance; signs include tachycardia, shortness of breath, excessive sweating, fine muscle tremor, thin silky hair and skin, infrequent blinking, and a staring appearance.

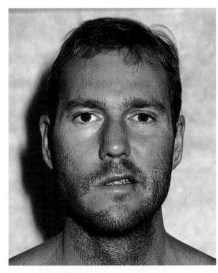

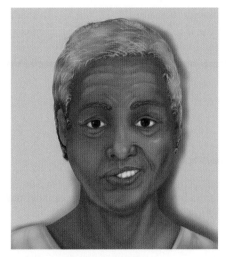

Stroke or Cerebrovascular Accident
An **upper motor neuron** lesion **(central)**. A "stroke" is an acute neurological deficit caused by an obstruction of a cerebral vessel, as in atherosclerosis, or a rupture in a cerebral vessel. Note paralysis of lower facial muscles, but also note that the upper half of face is not affected because of the intact nerve from the unaffected hemisphere. The person is still able to wrinkle the forehead and close the eyes.

Bell's Palsy (Right Side)
A **lower motor neuron** lesion **(peripheral)**, producing cranial nerve VII paralysis, which is almost always unilateral. It has a rapid onset, and the majority of cases are thought to be caused by herpes simplex virus (HSV). Note complete paralysis of one half of the face; person cannot wrinkle forehead, raise eyebrow, close eye, whistle, or show teeth on the right side. Former Canadian Prime Minister Jean Chrétien acquired Bell's palsy in his youth.

Continued

Abnormal Findings

TABLE 14-4   Abnormal Facial Appearances With Chronic Illnesses—cont'd

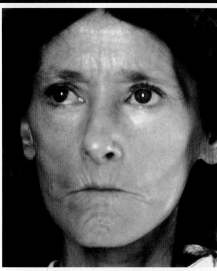

Reprinted from the Clinical Slide Collection on the Rheumatic Diseases, © 1991, 1995, 1997. Used by permission of the American College of Rheumatology.

◀ *Scleroderma*

Literally "hard skin," this rare connective tissue disease is characterized by chronic hardening and shrinking degenerative changes in the skin, blood vessels, synovium, and skeletal muscles. Changes can occur in skin, heart, esophagus, kidney, lung. Characteristic facies: hard, shiny skin on forehead and cheeks; thin, pursed lips with radial furrowing; absent skinfolds; muscle atrophy on face and neck; absence of expression.

Summary Checklist: Head, Face, and Neck, Including Examination of Regional Lymphatic System

 For a PDA-downloadable version, go to *http://evolve.elsevier.com/Canada/Jarvis/examination/*.

1. **Inspect and palpate the skull**
   General size and contour
   Any deformities, lumps, tenderness
   Palpation of temporal artery, temporomandibular joint
2. **Inspect the face**
   Facial expression

   Symmetry of movement (cranial nerve VII)
   Any involuntary movements, edema, lesions
3. **Inspect and palpate the neck**
   Active ROM

   Enlargement of salivary glands, lymph nodes, thyroid gland
   Position of the trachea
4. **Auscultate the thyroid (if enlarged) for bruit**
5. **Teaching and health promotion**

REFERENCES

Hockey Canada. (2012). *Concussion Prevention Resource Centre* Retrieved from http://www.hockeycanada.ca/index.php/ci_id/198187/la_id/1/ss_id/66201.htm

Leitch, K. (2007). *Reaching for the top: A report by the advisor on healthy children and youth.* Ottawa: Health Canada.

Safe Kids Canada. (2011). *Safe Cycling.* Retrieved from *http://www.safekidscanada.ca/Professionals/Safety-Information/Wheeled-Activities/Cycling/Safe-Cycling.aspx.*

Written by Carolyn Jarvis, PhD, APN, CNP
Adapted by Annette J. Browne, PhD, RN

⊖volve WEBSITE

http://evolve.elsevier.com/Canada/Jarvis/examination/
- Animations
- Bedside Assessment Summary Checklist
- Examination Review Questions
- Health Promotion Guide:
  - Glaucoma

- Key Points
- Physical Examination Summary Checklist
- Video—Assessment:
  - Eyes

OUTLINE

STRUCTURE AND FUNCTION

EXTERNAL ANATOMY

The eye is the sensory organ of vision. Humans are very visually oriented beings. More than half the neocortex is involved with processing visual information.

Because this sense is so important to humans, the eye is well protected by the bony orbital cavity, which is surrounded with a cushion of fat. The **eyelids** are like two movable shades that further protect the eye from injury, strong light, and dust. The upper eyelid is the larger and more mobile one. The eyelashes are short hairs in double or triple rows that curve outward from the eyelid margins, filtering out dust and dirt.

The **palpebral fissure** is the elliptical open space between the eyelids (Figure 15-1). When the eyes are closed, the eyelid margins approximate completely. When the eyes are open, the upper eyelid covers part of the iris. The lower eyelid margin is just at the **limbus,** the border between the cornea and sclera. The **canthus** is the corner of the eye, the angle where the eyelids meet. At the inner canthus, the **caruncle** is a small fleshy mass containing sebaceous glands.

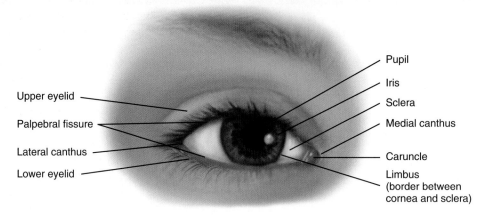

15-1

© Pat Thomas, 2006.

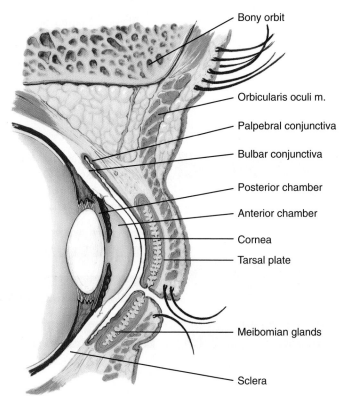

15-2

© Pat Thomas, 2006.

Within the upper eyelid, **tarsal plates** are strips of connective tissue that give it shape (Figure 15-2). The tarsal plates contain the **meibomian glands,** modified sebaceous glands that secrete an oily lubricating material onto the eyelids. This stops the tears from overflowing and helps form an airtight seal when the eyelids are closed.

The exposed part of the eye has a transparent protective covering, the **conjunctiva.** The conjunctiva is a thin mucous membrane folded like an envelope between the eyelids and the eyeball. The *palpebral* conjunctiva lines the eyelids and is clear, with many small blood vessels. It forms a deep recess and then folds back over the eye. The *bulbar* conjunctiva overlies the eyeball, with the white sclera showing through.

At the limbus, the conjunctiva merges with the cornea. The cornea covers and protects the iris and pupil.

The **lacrimal apparatus** provides constant irrigation to keep the conjunctiva and cornea moist and lubricated (Figure 15-3). The lacrimal gland, in the upper outer corner over the eye, secretes tears. The tears wash across the eye and are drawn up evenly as the eyelid blinks. The tears drain into the **puncta,** visible on the upper and lower eyelids at the inner canthus. The tears then drain into the nasolacrimal sac, through the centimetre-long nasolacrimal duct, and empty into the inferior meatus inside the nose. A tiny fold of mucous membrane prevents air from being forced up the nasolacrimal duct when the nose is blown.

Extraocular Muscles

Six muscles attach the eyeball to its orbit (Figure 15-4) and serve to direct the eye to points of the person's interest. These extraocular muscles enable both straight and rotary movements. The four straight, or *rectus,* muscles are the superior, inferior, lateral, and medial rectus muscles. The two slanting, or *oblique,* muscles are the superior and inferior oblique muscles.

Each muscle is coordinated, or yoked, with one in the other eye. This ensures that when the two eyes move, their axes always remain parallel (called *conjugate movement*). Parallel axes are important because the human brain can tolerate seeing only one image. Although some animals can perceive two different pictures through each eye, human beings have a binocular, single-image visual system. This occurs because a human's eyes move as a pair. For example, the two yoked muscles that allow looking to the far right are the right lateral rectus and the left medial rectus.

Movement of the **extraocular muscles** (see Figure 15-4) is stimulated by three **cranial nerves.** Cranial nerve VI, the abducens nerve, *innervates* (carries the nerve impulse that moves a muscle) the lateral rectus muscle (which *abducts* the eye, which means moving it laterally toward the temple); cranial nerve IV, the trochlear nerve, innervates the superior oblique muscle (downward and inward toward the nose); and cranial nerve III, the oculomotor nerve, innervates all the other nerves: the superior, inferior, and medial rectus and the

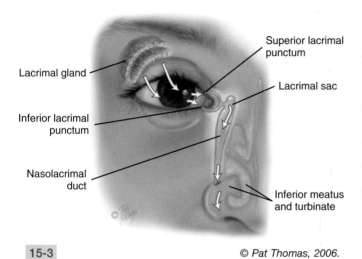

Lacrimal gland

Inferior lacrimal punctum

Nasolacrimal duct

Superior lacrimal punctum

Lacrimal sac

Inferior meatus and turbinate

15-3

© Pat Thomas, 2006.

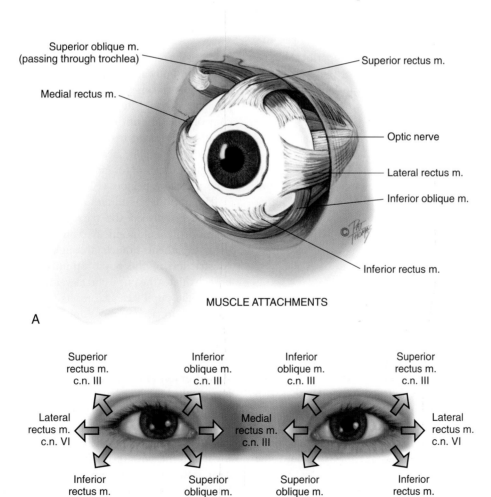

Superior oblique m. (passing through trochlea)

Medial rectus m.

Superior rectus m.

Optic nerve

Lateral rectus m.

Inferior oblique m.

Inferior rectus m.

MUSCLE ATTACHMENTS

A

| Superior rectus m. c.n. III | Inferior oblique m. c.n. III | Inferior oblique m. c.n. III | Superior rectus m. c.n. III |

Lateral rectus m. c.n. VI

Medial rectus m. c.n. III

Lateral rectus m. c.n. VI

| Inferior rectus m. c.n. III | Superior oblique m. c.n. IV | Superior oblique m. c.n. IV | Inferior rectus m. c.n. III |

B   DIRECTION OF MOVEMENT

15-4

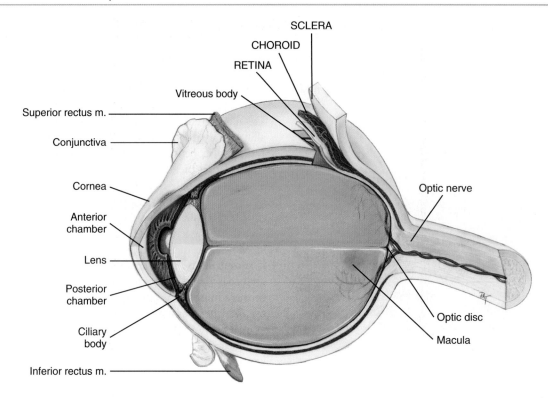

SCLERA

CHOROID

RETINA

Vitreous body

Superior rectus m.

Conjunctiva

Cornea

Anterior chamber

Lens

Posterior chamber

Ciliary body

Inferior rectus m.

Optic nerve

Optic disc

Macula

15-5

inferior oblique muscles. Note that the superior oblique muscle is located on the superior aspect of the eyeball, but when it contracts, it enables the person to look downward and inward.

INTERNAL ANATOMY

The eye is a sphere composed of three concentric coats: (a) the outer fibrous sclera, (b) the middle vascular choroid, and (c) the inner nervous retina (Figure 15-5). Inside the retina is the transparent vitreous body. The only parts accessible to examination are the sclera anteriorly and the retina through the ophthalmoscope.

The Outer Layer

The **sclera** is a tough, protective, white covering. It is continuous anteriorly with the smooth, transparent cornea, which covers the iris and pupil. The cornea is part of the refracting media of the eye, bending incoming light rays so that they are focused on the retina within.

The **cornea** is very sensitive to touch; contact with a wisp of cotton stimulates a blink in both eyes, called the *corneal reflex*. The trigeminal nerve (cranial nerve V) carries the afferent sensation into the brain, and the facial nerve (cranial nerve VII) carries the efferent message that stimulates the blink.

The Middle Layer

The **choroid** has dark pigmentation to prevent light from reflecting internally and is heavily vascularized to deliver

blood to the retina. Anteriorly, the choroid is continuous with the ciliary body and the iris. The muscles of the ciliary body control the thickness of the lens. The **iris** functions as a diaphragm, varying the opening at its centre, the pupil. This controls the amount of light admitted into the retina. The muscle fibres of the iris contract the pupil in bright light and to accommodate for near vision, and dilate the pupil when the light is dim and for far vision. The colour of the iris varies from person to person.

The **pupil** is round and regular. Its size is determined by a balance between the parasympathetic and sympathetic chains of the autonomic nervous system. Stimulation of the parasympathetic branch, through cranial nerve III, causes constriction of the pupil. Stimulation of the sympathetic branch dilates the pupil and elevates the eyelid. As mentioned earlier, the pupil size also reacts to the amount of ambient light and to accommodation (focusing an object on the retina).

The **lens** is a transparent biconvex disc located just behind the pupil. The lens serves as a refracting medium, keeping a viewed object in continual focus on the retina. Its thickness is controlled by the ciliary body; the lens bulges for focusing on near objects and flattens for far objects.

The **anterior chamber** is posterior to the cornea and anterior to the iris and lens. The **posterior chamber** lies behind the iris to the sides of the lens. These chambers contain the clear, watery aqueous humor, which is produced continually by the ciliary body. The continuous flow of this fluid serves to deliver nutrients to the surrounding tissues and to drain metabolic wastes. Intraocular pressure is determined by a balance between the amount of aqueous humor produced and resistance to its outflow at the angle of the anterior chamber.

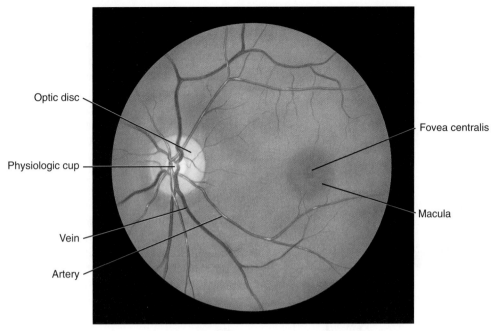

Optic disc

Physiologic cup

Vein

Artery

Fovea centralis

Macula

15-6 The retina.

The Inner Layer

The **retina** is the visual receptive layer of the eye in which light waves are changed into nerve impulses. The retina surrounds the soft gelatinous vitreous humor. The retinal structures viewed through the ophthalmoscope are the optic disc, the retinal vessels, the general background, and the macula (Figure 15-6).

The **optic disc** (or *optic papilla*) is the area in which fibres from the retina converge to form the optic nerve. Located toward the nasal side of the retina, it has these characteristics: a colour that varies from creamy yellow-orange to pink; a round or oval shape; margins that are distinct and sharply demarcated, especially on the temporal side; and a physiological cup, the smaller circular area inside the disc where the blood vessels exit and enter.

The **retinal vessels** normally include a paired artery and vein extending to each quadrant, growing progressively smaller in calibre as they reach the periphery. The arteries appear brighter red and narrower than the veins, and the arteries have a thin sliver of light (the arterial light reflex). The general background of the fundus varies in colour, depending on the person's skin colour. The **macula** is located on the temporal side of the fundus. It is a slightly darker pigmented region surrounding the **fovea centralis,** the area of sharpest and keenest vision. The macula receives and transduces light from the centre of the visual field (transduction occurs when visual pigments are broken down into neural signals that eventually travel to the visual cortex).

VISUAL PATHWAYS AND VISUAL FIELDS

Objects reflect light. The light rays are refracted through the transparent media (cornea, aqueous humor, lens, and vitreous body) and strike the retina. The retina transforms the light stimulus into nerve impulses that are conducted through the optic nerve and the optic tract to the visual cortex of the occipital lobe.

The image formed on the retina is upside down and reversed from its actual appearance in the outside world (Figure 15-7); that is, the image of an object in the upper temporal visual field of the right eye is reflected onto the lower nasal area of the retina. All retinal fibres collect to form the optic nerve, but they maintain this same spatial arrangement, with nasal fibres running medially and temporal fibres running laterally.

At the optic chiasm, nasal fibres (from both temporal visual fields) cross over. The left optic tract now has fibres only from the left half of each retina, and the right optic tract contains fibres only from the right half. Thus the right side of the brain looks at the left side of the world.

VISUAL REFLEXES

Pupillary Light Reflex

The **pupillary light reflex** is the normal constriction of the pupils when bright light shines on the retina (Figure 15-8). It is a subcortical reflex arc (i.e., a person has no conscious control over it); the afferent link is cranial nerve II, the optic nerve, and the efferent path is cranial III, the oculomotor nerve. When one eye is exposed to bright light, a *direct light reflex* occurs (constriction of that pupil), as does a *consensual light reflex* (simultaneous constriction of the other pupil). This happens because the optic nerve carries the sensory afferent message in and then synapses with both sides of the brain. For example, consider the light reflex in a person who is blind in one eye. Stimulation of the normal eye produces both a direct and a consensual light reflex. Stimulation of the blind eye causes no response because the sensory afferent in cranial nerve II is destroyed.

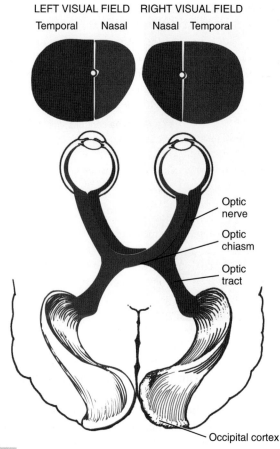

15-7 Visual pathways (viewed from above).

Fixation

This is a reflex direction of the eye toward an object attracting a person's attention. The image is fixed in the centre of the visual field, the fovea centralis. This fixing consists of very rapid ocular movements to put the target back on the fovea, and somewhat slower (smooth pursuit) movements to track the target and keep its image on the fovea. These ocular movements are impaired by drugs, alcohol, fatigue, and inattention.

Accommodation

Accommodation is adaptation of the eye for near vision. It is accomplished by increasing the curvature of the lens through movement of the ciliary muscles. Although the lens cannot be observed directly, the components of accommodation that can be observed are convergence (motion toward) of the axes of the eyeballs and pupillary constriction.

❖ DEVELOPMENTAL CONSIDERATIONS

Infants and Children

At birth, eye function is limited, but it matures fully during the early years. Peripheral vision is intact in the newborn infant. The macula, the area of keenest vision, is absent at birth but is developing by age 4 months and is mature by age 8 months. Eye movements may be poorly coordinated at birth. By 3 to 4 months of age, the infant establishes binocularity and can fixate on a single image with both eyes

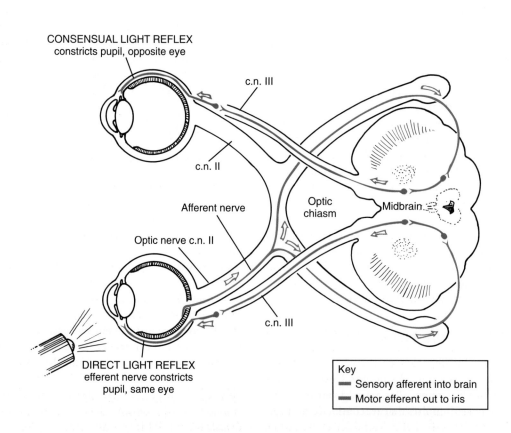

15-8

simultaneously. Most neonates (80%) are born farsighted; this gradually decreases after 7 to 8 years of age.

In structure, the eyeball reaches adult size by 8 years. At birth, the iris shows little pigmentation, and the pupils are small. The lens is nearly spherical at birth, becoming flatter throughout life. Its consistency changes from that of soft plastic at birth to that of rigid glass in old age.

Older Adults

Changes in eye structure contribute greatly to the distinct facial changes of older adults. The skin loses its elasticity, causing wrinkling and drooping; fat tissues and muscles atrophy. Lacrimal glands involute, causing decreased tear production and a feeling of dryness and burning.

On the globe itself, the cornea may show an infiltration of degenerative lipid material around the limbus (see discussion of *arcus senilis*, p. 325). Pupil size decreases. The lens loses elasticity, becoming hard and glasslike, which decreases the lens's ability to change shape to accommodate for near vision; this condition is termed **presbyopia.** The average age at onset of presbyopia is 40 years (Kaiser, Friedman, & Pineda, 2003). By 70 years of age, the normally transparent fibres of the lens begin to thicken and yellow. This is nuclear sclerosis, or the beginning of a "senile cataract."

Inside the globe, debris can accumulate in the vitreous humor (appearing in vision as "floaters") because the vitreous humor is not continuously renewed, as aqueous humor is. Visual acuity may diminish gradually after age 50 years and even more so after age 70 years. Near vision is commonly affected because of the decreased power of accommodation in the lens (presbyopia). As early as the fourth decade, a person may have blurred vision and difficulty reading. Also, older adults need more light to see because of a decreased adaptation to darkness, and this condition may affect the function of night driving.

The prevalence of age-related vision loss is increasing dramatically; one per every nine Canadians older than 65 live with significant vision loss (Canadian National Institute for the Blind [CNIB], 2004). When visual acuity declines, it is essential for nurses to assess the increased risk for falls and to support individuals and their families and friends in preventing falls. In the older adult population, the most common causes of decreased visual functioning are as follows:

1. *Macular degeneration,* or the breakdown of cells in the macula of the retina. Loss of central vision, the area of clearest vision, is the most common cause of blindness. Age-related macular degeneration (AMD) is the leading cause of blindness in Canada and remains the most common cause of legal blindness in people older than 65 (Canadian Ophthalmological Society Clinical Practice Guideline Expert Committee [COSCPGEC], 2007). It is estimated that 1 million Canadians have some form of AMD (CNIB, 2012). As the population ages, the number of people with AMD is expected to double by 2040. Studies suggest a higher incidence of AMD among women, particularly those with earlier onset of menopause, which suggests that estrogen may play a protective role in minimizing AMD risk (CNIB, 2012; Rudnicka et al., 2011).

However, part of the reason why women have a higher incidence of AMD may be the fact that women generally live longer. A person with AMD is unable to read fine print, sew, or do fine manual work and may have difficulty distinguishing faces. Depending on the extent to which the person's activities require close work, loss of central vision may cause great distress. Peripheral vision is not affected, so the person can manage self-care and does not become completely disabled.

2. *Cataract formation,* or lens opacity, which results from a clumping of proteins in the lens. Some cataract formation should be expected by age 70 years. Cataracts represent the second most common cause of correctable visual impairment after the correction of refractive error (COSCPGEC, 2007). Advancing age remains the most common risk factor; progression typically extends over a long time. Other common risk factors include diabetes mellitus, certain medications (steroids), diabetes, history of ocular trauma, and previous intraocular inflammation or surgery (CNIB, 2004). The prevalence of cataract is more than 50% among people aged 70 to 79 and almost 100% among people older than 90.

3. *Glaucoma,* or increased intraocular pressure. The age-adjusted rate among people older than 60 is 6% to 8% (Einarson et al., 2006). Chronic open-angle glaucoma is the most common type; it involves a gradual loss of peripheral vision. See the box Promoting Health: Screening for Glaucoma.

4. *Diabetic retinopathy.* This remains the leading cause of visual impairment in people younger than 65 (COSCPGEC, 2007). This risk is highest in diabetic patients with concurrent proteinuria. Patients who are diabetic should be referred regularly for screening by an ophthalmologist for diabetic retinopathy (Canadian Diabetes Association Clinical Practice Guidelines Expert Committee, 2008).*

To summarize, the number of partially sighted people is rising largely because the proportion of older adults in the population is increasing. The term *partially sighted* refers to vision that is outside normal limits (<20/60) and cannot be improved through medical or surgical means (Canadian Ophthalmological Society, 2008). In Canada, a visual acuity worse than 20/50 disqualifies people from obtaining a driver's licence or restricts their driving to daytime only, as do some visual field deficits (CNIB, 2008). Legal blindness is vision that cannot be corrected to better than 20/200 and peripheral vision that cannot be corrected to better than 20 degrees.

The Canadian Ophthalmological Society's screening recommendations for adults are listed as follows (COSCPGEC, 2007, p. 43). Screening is done for a variety of purposes: primary screening (e.g., to reduce the occurrence or incidence of disease, to encourage eye protection), secondary prevention (to reduce and control the consequences of existing disease such as diabetes mellitus [DM], glaucoma, high myopia), and tertiary prevention (e.g., to reduce the harm of a chronic disease, such as reducing intraocular pressure (IOP)

---

*New guidelines are being released in 2013, titled, *The 2013 Clinical Practice Guidelines for the Prevention and Management of Diabetes in Canada* (Canadian Diabetes Association, 2013).

in primary open-angle glaucoma, laser therapy for diabetic retinopathy (p. 40).

1. Screening intervals in asymptomic low-risk patients:
   - Age 19 to 40 years: at least every 10 years
   - Age 41 to 55 years: at least every 5 years
   - Age 56 to 65 years: at least every 3 years
   - Age older than 65 years: at least every 2 years
2. Screening in symptomatic patients:
   - Any patient noting changes in visual acuity, visual field, colour vision, or physical changes to the eye should be assessed as soon as possible.

3. Screening intervals in high-risk patients:
   - Patients at higher risk of visual impairment (e.g., those with diabetes, cataract, macular degeneration, glaucoma [verified or suspected], or a family history of these conditions) should be assessed more frequently and thoroughly (Noble & Chaudhary, 2010).
   - Age older than 40 to 50 years: at least every 3 years
   - Age older than 50 to 60 years: at least every 2 years
   - Age older than 60 years: at least annually

PROMOTING HEALTH: SCREENING FOR GLAUCOMA

Preventing Glaucoma

Glaucoma is the second leading cause of preventable blindness in Canada (Canadian Ophthalmological Society Glaucoma Clinical Practice Guideline Expert Committee ([COSGCPGEC], 2009). Glaucoma is a condition in which the optic nerve is damaged, usually as a result of increasing pressure within the eye. The risk of glaucoma increases with age, but it can occur in anyone in any age group. Glaucoma is not curable, and vision, once lost, cannot be regained. However, with medication or surgery, it is possible to prevent further loss of vision. Screening for glaucoma is the first step in early diagnosis and intervention. Primary open-angle glaucoma causes such insidious damage to the optic nerve and vision that few affected people have early awareness of the condition (COSCPGEC, 2007). As a result, it is diagnosed in time to prevent disabling vision loss in only half of affected patients in developed countries such as Canada. However, screening for this disorder is ideal because it typically progresses slowly and can be effectively managed.

The prevalence of open-angle glaucoma between the ages of 70 and 79 is 60% higher among women than among men (Canadian National Institute for the Blind [CNIB], 2004). Among people older than 80, almost 300% more women than men have open-angle glaucoma. In the United States, glaucoma-related vision compromise was reported as three times more prevalent in people of African or Hispanic descent (COSCPGEC, 2007). Increasing age and family history are major risk factors. Health care providers should encourage regular eye examinations, especially for patients with known risk factors. Risk factors for glaucoma include the following:

1. Being older than 60 years
2. Being of African descent
3. Being a woman
4. Increased intraocular pressure (IOP) (>21 mm Hg)
5. Family history of glaucoma
6. Steroid use
7. Decreased central corneal thickness (<0.5 mm)
8. Hypertension
9. Eye injury
10. Severe myopia (nearsightedness)
11. Diabetes
12. Use of certain other medications, including antihypertensives, antihistamines, anticholinergics, and antidepressants

There are two main types of glaucoma. To understand the difference, it is helpful to review the basic structure of the eye. The anterior and posterior chambers of the eye are filled with a fluid called *aqueous humor*. This fluid is produced in the posterior chamber and then passes into the anterior chamber through the pupil. The fluid moves out of the eye and into the bloodstream through a drainage area located in front of the iris. This drainage area is located in the angle formed between the iris and the point at which the iris appears to meet the inside of the cornea. If the flow of aqueous humor is blocked, IOP increases. This pressure eventually damages the optic nerve and results in a loss of vision, which is permanent because in the retina, neurons are not regenerated once they are lost.

Open-angle glaucoma is the most common type of glaucoma, accounting for more than 90% of all cases. With open-angle glaucoma, the angle between the iris and the cornea is open, but the fluid is slow to drain, which causes IOP to build. There are virtually no symptoms. Vision loss begins with the peripheral vision, which often goes unnoticed because affected individuals learn to compensate intuitively by turning their heads. As the condition progresses, the field of peripheral vision decreases until eventually affected patients may not be able to see anything on either side. This condition is referred to as *tunnel vision*.

Closed-angle glaucoma occurs when the space between the cornea and iris is narrower than normal. Anything that causes the pupil to dilate—such as dim light, eye drops, and certain medications—can block the drainage of fluid. Aging and injury also contribute to and can block the drainage of fluid. Closed-angle glaucoma causes sudden increases in IOP that result in blurred vision, sensitivity to light, nausea, and halos around lights. Affected individuals must be treated immediately.

Regular comprehensive eye examinations are extremely important because open-angle glaucoma does not produce symptoms in its early stages. These examinations should include the following:

1. Visual acuity testing
2. Visual field testing
3. Dilated eye examination
4. Tonometry to measure the IOP

The COSGCPGEC (2009) reports that Canada has not instituted a population screening program for glaucoma although it has been given serious consideration. Screening with simple IOP testing and optic nerve examination tends to yield underestimates of the prevalence of glaucoma (COSCPGEC, 2007). Although visual field testing typically reveals damage, it is usually at a more advanced stage than the very early stage ideal for diagnosis and treatment. Other testing provided by ophthalmologists include frequency-doubling perimetry to demonstrate early damage to visual function, tomography to measure IOP, and laser imaging to assess the nerve fibre layer (Einarson et al., 2006).

PROMOTING HEALTH: SCREENING FOR GLAUCOMA—cont'd

Although individuals who wear glasses appear to have more regular eye examinations, health care professionals need to remind all individuals of the risk for glaucoma and the need for regular comprehensive eye examinations.

References

Canadian National Institute for the Blind. (2004). A clear vision: Solutions to Canada's vision loss crisis. Toronto: Canterbury Communications.

Canadian Ophthalmological Society Glaucoma Clinical Practice Guideline Expert Committee (COSGCPGEC). (2009). Canadian Ophthalmological Society evidence-based clinical practice

guidelines for the management of glaucoma in the adult eye. Canadian Journal of Ophthalmology, 44:S7–93. doi:10.3129/i09.080

Canadian Ophthalmological Society Glaucoma Clinical Practice Guideline Expert Committee. (2007). Canadian Ophthalmological Society evidence-based clinical practice guidelines for the periodic eye examination in adults in Canada. Canadian Journal of Ophthalmology, 42, 39–45.

Einarson, T., Vicente, C., Machado, M., Covert, D., Trope, G., & Iskedjian, M. (2006). Screening for glaucoma in Canada: A systematic review of the literature. Canadian Journal of Ophthalmology, 41, 709–721.

 CULTURAL AND SOCIAL CONSIDERATIONS

The colour of the iris and retinal pigmentation vary greatly; darker irides have darker retinas behind them. Individuals with light retinas generally have better night vision but can have pain in an environment that has too much light.

Research from the United States shows that the rate of primary open-angle glaucoma is three to six times higher among people of African heritage than among people of European heritage, and the disease is three to six times more likely to cause blindness in people of African descent than in people of European descent (Kaiser et al., 2003). Reasons for these disparities are not known.

According to data from large-scale U.S. studies, patients with a predisposition to visual deficits include those who wear glasses or contact lenses, have diabetes, are of African

heritage, or have a strong family history of glaucoma, AMD, or retinal detachment (COSCPGEC, 2007). In Canada, outreach efforts are particularly needed among Aboriginal people, whose incidence of diabetes is three to five times higher than that of the general population (First Nations and Inuit Health, 2010). About 25% of Aboriginal people report a problem with vision, in comparison with 10% in the general population (CNIB, 2004).

Canadians between the ages of 19 and 64 must rely on private (third-party) insurance or out-of-pocket payment to see an eye specialist for routine vision screening (COSCPGEC, 2007). Nurses working in community and acute care need to consider the effect of low income on access to routine eye care and the ability to pay for corrective lenses. People who cannot afford vision testing or corrective lenses must to be referred to agencies that can provide those services free of charge or at a reduced cost.

SUBJECTIVE DATA

1. Vision difficulty (decreased acuity, blurring, blind spots)
2. Pain
3. Strabismus, diplopia
4. Redness, swelling
5. Watering, discharge
6. History of ocular problems
7. Glaucoma
8. Use of glasses or contact lenses
9. Self-care behaviours

HEALTH HISTORY QUESTIONS

Examiner Asks	Rationale
1. Vision difficulty (decreased acuity, blurring, blind spots). Any **difficulty seeing** or any blurring? Did visual difficulty or change in vision come on suddenly, or develop slowly? In one eye or both? • Is it constant, or does it come and go? • Do objects appear out of focus, or do they look clouded over? Does the problem feel like "greyness" of vision? • Do spots move in front of your eyes? One or many? In one or both eyes?	Any patient who describes a sudden change in vision is experiencing an acute ocular emergency, and should receive immediate ophthalmic evaluation. Floaters are common with myopia or after middle age as a result of condensed vitreous fibres. They are usually not significant, but acute onset of floaters ("shade" or "cobwebs") may occur with retinal detachment.

Examiner Asks	Rationale
• Any halos/rainbows around objects? Or rings around lights?	Halos around lights occur with acute narrow-angle glaucoma.
• Any blind spot? Does it move as you shift your gaze? Any loss of peripheral vision?	**Scotoma**, a blind spot in the visual field surrounded by an area of normal or decreased vision, occurs with glaucoma and with disorders of the optic nerve and visual pathway.
• Any night blindness?	Night blindness occurs with optic atrophy, glaucoma, or vitamin A deficiency.
2. **Pain.** Any **eye pain?** Please describe. • Does it come on suddenly?	*Sudden onset* of eye symptoms (pain, floaters, blind spot, loss of peripheral vision) may represent an emergency. Refer the patient immediately to the emergency department or an on-call ophthalmologist. See also Critical Findings box (p. 326).
• Quality: Is pain burning or itching? • Or is it sharp, stabbing pain or pain with bright light? • Is it a foreign body sensation? Or deep aching? Or headache in brow area?	Quality is valuable diagnostic indicator. **Photophobia** is inability to tolerate light. Note: Some common eye diseases cause no pain (e.g., refractive errors, cataract, glaucoma).
3. **Strabismus, diplopia.** Any history of crossed eyes? Now or in the past? Does this occur with eye fatigue? • Ever see double? Is this constant, or does it come and go? In one eye or both?	Strabismus is a deviation in the anteroposterior axis of the eye. **Diplopia** is the perception of two images of a single object.
4. **Redness, swelling.** Any **redness** or **swelling** in the eyes? In one eye or both? Gradual or sudden onset? • Any infections? Now or in the past? When do these symptoms occur? In a particular time of year? Are they seasonal?	
5. **Watering, discharge.** Any **watering** or excessive tearing?	Lacrimation (tearing) and epiphora (excessive tearing) are caused by irritants or obstruction in drainage of tears.
• Any **discharge?** Any matter in the eyes? Is it hard to open your eyes in the morning? What colour is the discharge? • How do you remove matter from eyes?	Purulent discharge is thick and yellow. Crusts form at night. Assess the patient's hygiene practices and knowledge of cross-contamination.
6. **History of ocular problems.** Any **history** of injury or surgery to eyes? Or any history of allergies?	Allergens (e.g., makeup, contact lens solution) may cause irritation of the conjunctiva or cornea. Research indicates that the incidence of eye injuries in Canada is extremely high, and they occur at the same rates at home and at work. Encourage the use of eye protection, both at home and at work (Gordon, 2012).
7. **Glaucoma.** Have you ever been tested for **glaucoma?** What were the results? • Any family history of glaucoma?	Glaucoma is characterized by increased intraocular pressure.
8. **Use of glasses or contact lenses.** Do you wear **glasses** or **contact lenses?** How do they work for you? • When was your prescription last checked? Was it changed? • If you wear contact lenses, are there any problems such as pain, photophobia, watering, or swelling? • How do you care for contact lenses? How long do you wear them? How do you clean them? Do you remove them for certain activities?	Assess self-care behaviours for contact lenses.

Examiner Asks	Rationale

9. **Self-care behaviours.** When was your vision last tested? Who tested it?
   • Has your colour vision ever been tested?
   • Any environmental conditions at home or at work that may affect your eyes? For example, flying sparks, metal bits, smoke, dust, chemical fumes? If so, do you wear goggles to protect your eyes?
10. **Medications.** What medications are you taking? Are they systemic or topical? Do you take any medication specifically for the eyes?
	Assess self-care behaviours for eyes and vision.
	   Eye disease can be work-related (e.g., by a foreign body from metal working or by radiation damage from welding).
	   Some medications have ocular side effects; for example, prednisone may cause cataracts or increased intraocular pressure.

11. **Coping with vision loss.** If you have experienced a vision loss, how do you cope? Do you have books with large print, books on audio tape, books printed in Braille?
   • Do you maintain your living environment the same?
   • Do you sometimes fear complete loss of vision?
	A constant spatial layout eases navigation through the home.

Additional History for Infants and Children

Examiner Asks	Rationale

1. **Delivery.** Any vaginal infections in the mother at time of delivery?
2. **Development.** Considering age of child, which developmental milestones of vision have you (parent) noted?
3. **Vision testing.** Does the child have routine vision testing at school?
4. **Safety.** Are you (parent) aware of safety measures to protect child's eyes from trauma? Do you inspect toys?
   • Have you taught the child safe care of sharp objects and how to carry and use them?
	Genital herpes and gonorrheal vaginitis have ocular sequelae for the newborn.
	   The parent is most often the one to detect vision problems.

Additional History for the Older Adult

Examiner Asks	Rationale

1. **Movement.** Have you noticed any visual difficulty with climbing stairs or driving? Any problem with night vision?
2. **Glaucoma testing.** When was the last time you were tested for glaucoma?
   • Any aching pain around eyes? Any loss of peripheral vision?
   • If you have glaucoma, how do you manage your eyedrops?
	Assess for any loss of depth perception or central vision.
	
	Compliance may be a problem if symptoms are absent. Assess the patient's ability to administer eyedrops.

3. **Cataracts.** Do you have a history of cataracts? Any loss or progressive blurring of vision? 4. **Dryness.** Do your eyes ever feel dry? Do they burn? What do you do for this? 5. **Activities.** Any decrease in usual activities, such as reading or sewing?	Tear production may be decreased with aging. Macular degeneration causes a loss in central vision acuity.

OBJECTIVE DATA

PREPARATION
Position the patient first standing for vision screening and then sitting up with the head at your eye level.

EQUIPMENT NEEDED
Snellen eye chart
Handheld visual screener
Opaque card or occluder
Penlight (some come with a pupil gauge to measure pupil size)
Applicator stick
Ophthalmoscope

Normal Range of Findings	Abnormal Findings

TEST CENTRAL VISUAL ACUITY

Snellen Eye Chart

The Snellen eye chart is the most commonly used and accurate measure of visual acuity. It has lines of letters arranged in decreasing size.

Place the Snellen eye chart in a well-lit spot at eye level. Position the patient on a mark exactly 20 feet (6.1 m) from the chart. Hand the patient an opaque card with which to shield one eye at a time during the test; inadvertent peeking may occur if the patient shields the eye with his or her own fingers (Figure 15-9). If the patient wears glasses or contact lenses, leave them on. Remove only reading glasses because they blur distance vision. Ask the patient to read through the chart to the smallest line of letters possible. Encourage the patient to try the next smallest line in addition. (Note: Use a Snellen picture chart for people who cannot read letters. See p. 320.)

Note hesitancy, squinting, leaning forward, and misreading letters.

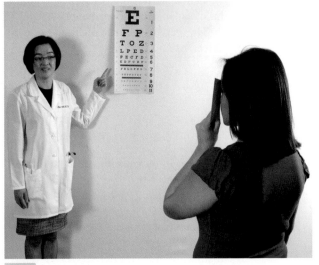

15-9

Record the result by using the numerical fraction at the end of the last line successfully read. Indicate whether the patient missed any letters (by indicating "minus 1, or minus 2")* or whether corrective lenses were worn: for example, "O.D.† 20/30-1, with glasses."

Normal visual acuity is 20/20. Contrary to some people's impression, the numerical fraction is *not* a percentage of normal vision. Instead, the top number (numerator) indicates the distance the patient is standing from the chart, and the denominator is the distance at which a normal eye could have read that particular line. Thus "20/20" means "You can read at 20 ft [6.1 m] what the normal eye could have read at 20 ft."

If the patient is unable to see even the largest letters, shorten the distance to the chart until the patient can see it, and record that distance (e.g., "10/200"). If visual acuity is even lower, assess whether the patient can count your fingers when they are spread in front of the eyes or distinguish light perception from your penlight.

The larger the denominator, the poorer the vision. If vision is poorer than 20/30, refer the patient to an ophthalmologist or optometrist. Vision may be impaired as a result of refractive error, opacity in the media (cornea, lens, vitreous), or disorder in the retina or optic pathway.

---

*Even when patients miss one or two letters on the smallest line they can read, they are still considered to have vision equal to that line. (U.S. National Library of Medicine, 2012).

†O.D., *oculus dexter,* or right eye.

Normal Range of Findings	Abnormal Findings

Near Vision

For patients older than 40 years or for those who report increasing difficulty reading, test near vision with a handheld vision screener with various sizes of print (e.g., a Jaeger card; Figure 15-10). Instruct the patient to hold the card in good light about 14 inches (35 cm) from the eye; at this distance, the print size equals that on the chart used at 20 feet (6.1 m). Test each eye separately, with glasses on. A normal result is "14/14" in each eye, reading without hesitancy and without moving the card closer or farther away. When no vision screening card is available, ask the patient to read from a magazine or newspaper.

If the patient moves the card farther away, this is a possible sign of **presbyopia**, the decrease in power of accommodation with aging.

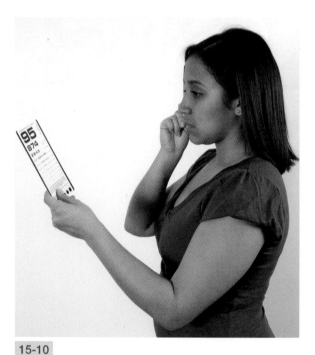

15-10

TEST VISUAL FIELDS

Confrontation Test

This is a gross measure of peripheral vision. The patient's peripheral vision is compared with your own, if yours is normal (Figure 15-11). Position yourself at eye level with the patient, about 60 cm away. Direct the patient to cover one eye with an opaque card and to look straight at you with the other eye. Cover your own eye opposite to the patient's covered one. You are testing the uncovered eye. Hold a pencil or your flicking finger as a target midline between you and the patient, at the periphery of vision, and slowly advance it inward from the periphery in several directions.

Ask the patient to say, "Now" when he or she first sees the target; this location should be the same as when you see the object also. (This works with all but the temporal visual field, with which you would need a 2-m arm to avoid being seen initially! With the temporal direction, start the object somewhat behind the patient.) Estimate the angle between the anteroposterior axis of the eye and the peripheral axis where the object is first seen. Normal results are about 50 degrees upward, 90 degrees temporal, 70 degrees down, and 60 degrees nasal (Figure 15-12).

If the patient is unable to see the object as you do, the test result suggests peripheral field loss. Refer the patient to an optometrist or ophthalmologist for more precise testing with a tangent screen (see Table 15-5 on p. 334).

Normal Range of Findings	Abnormal Findings

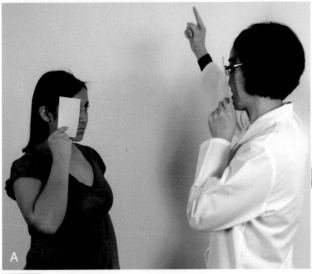

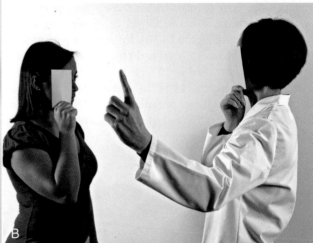

15-11

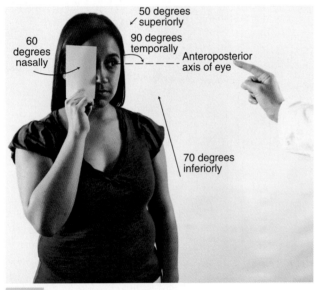

15-12   Testing range of peripheral vision.

INSPECT EXTRAOCULAR MUSCLE FUNCTION

Corneal Light Reflex (Hirschberg's Test)

Assess the parallel alignment of the eye axes by shining a light toward the patient's eyes. Direct the patient to stare straight ahead as you hold the light about 30 cm away. Note the reflection of the light on the corneas; it should be in exactly the same spot on each eye. See the bright white dots in Figure 15-30 for symmetry of the corneal light reflex.

Asymmetry of the light reflex indicates deviation in alignment as a result of eye muscle weakness or paralysis. If you see this, perform the cover-uncover test.

Cover-Uncover Test

The **cover-uncover test** detects small degrees of deviated alignment by interrupting the fusion reflex that normally keeps the two eyes parallel. Ask the patient to stare straight ahead at your nose even though the gaze may be interrupted. With an opaque card, cover one eye. As it is covered, note the uncovered eye. A normal response is a steady fixed gaze (Figure 15-13, *A*).

Meanwhile, the macular image has been suppressed on the covered eye. If muscle weakness exists, the covered eye will drift into a relaxed position.

If the eye jumps to fixate on the designated point, it was out of alignment before.

Normal Range of Findings

Now uncover the eye and observe it for movement. It should stare straight ahead (see Figure 15-13, *B*). If it jumps to reestablish fixation, eye muscle weakness exists. Repeat the test by covering the other eye.

Abnormal Findings

A **phoria** is a mild weakness noted only when fusion is blocked. **Tropia** is more severe: a constant misalignment of the eyes (see Table 15-1, p. 328).

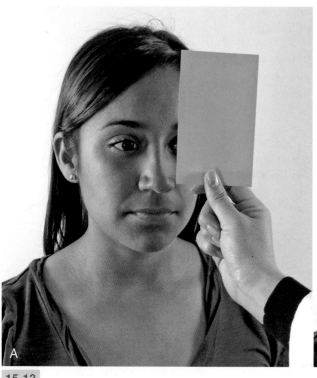
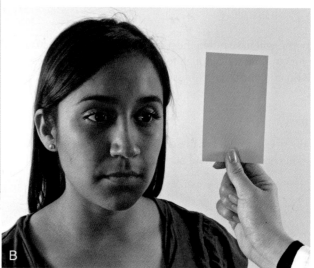

15-13

Diagnostic Positions Test

Leading the eyes through the six cardinal positions of gaze reveals any muscle weakness during movement (Figure 15-14). Ask the patient to hold the head steady and to follow the movement of your finger, pen, or penlight only with the eyes. Hold the target back about 30 cm so that the patient can focus on it comfortably, and move it to each of the six positions, hold it momentarily, then back to centre. Progress clockwise. A normal response is parallel tracking of the object with both eyes.

Eye movement that is not parallel is abnormal. Failure to follow in a certain direction indicates weakness of an extraocular muscle (EOM) or dysfunction of cranial nerve innervating it.

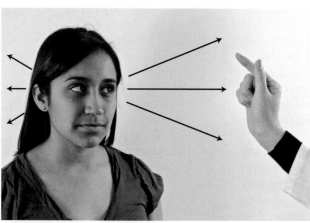

15-14   Diagnostic positions test.

Normal Range of Findings	Abnormal Findings

In addition to parallel movement, note any **nystagmus**, a fine oscillating movement best seen around the iris. Mild nystagmus at extreme lateral gaze is normal; nystagmus at any other position is not.

Finally, note that the upper eyelid continues to overlap the superior part of the iris, even during downward movement. You should not see a white rim of sclera between the eyelid and the iris. Such an appearance is termed *"lid lag."*

INSPECT EXTERNAL OCULAR STRUCTURES

Begin with the most external points, and logically work your way inward.

General

Already you will have noted the patient's ability to move around the room, with vision functioning well enough to avoid obstacles and to respond to your directions. Also note the facial expression; a relaxed expression accompanies adequate vision.

Eyebrows

Normally the eyebrows are present bilaterally, move symmetrically as the facial expression changes, and have no scaling or lesions.

Eyelids and Lashes

The upper eyelids normally overlap the superior part of the iris and approximate completely with the lower eyelids when closed. The skin is intact, without redness, swelling, discharge, or lesions.

The palpebral fissures are horizontal or slightly upward in some people of East Asian descent.

Note that the eyelashes are evenly distributed along the eyelid margins and curve outward.

Eyeballs

The eyeballs are aligned normally in their sockets with no protrusion or sunken appearance. Some people of African descent normally may have a slight protrusion of the eyeball beyond the supraorbital ridge.

Conjunctiva and Sclera

Ask the patient to look up. Using your thumbs, slide the patient's lower eyelids down along the bony orbital rim. Take care not to push against the eyeball. Inspect the exposed area (Figure 15-15). The eyeball looks moist and glossy. Numerous small blood vessels normally show through the transparent conjunctiva. Otherwise, the conjunctivae are clear and show the normal colour of the structure below: pink over the lower eyelids and white over the sclera. Note any colour change, swelling, or lesions.

The sclera is china white, although in people with dark skin, it is occasionally grey-blue or "muddy." Also in dark-skinned people, you normally may see small brown macules (like freckles) on the sclera, which should not be confused with foreign bodies or petechiae. Last, some people with dark skin may have yellowish fatty deposits beneath the eyelids away from the cornea. Do not confuse these yellow spots with the overall scleral yellowing that accompanies jaundice.

Abnormal Findings

Nystagmus occurs with disease of the semicircular canals in the ears, a paretic eye muscle, multiple sclerosis, or brain lesions.
Lid lag occurs with hyperthyroidism.

- Groping with hands
- Squinting or craning forward

Absence of lateral third of brow occurs with hypothyroidism.
Unequal or absent movement occurs with nerve damage.
Scaling occurs with seborrhea.

Lid lag occurs with hyperthyroidism.
Incomplete closure creates risk for corneal damage.
- Ptosis, drooping of upper eyelid
- Periorbital edema, lesions (see Tables 15-2 and 15-3 on pp. 330 to 331)
- Ectropion and entropion (see Table 15-2, p. 331)

Exophthalmos (protruding eyes) and enophthalmos (sunken eyes) (see Table 15-2, p. 330).

- General reddening (see Table 15-6, p. 335)
- Cyanosis of the lower eyelids
- Pallor near the outer canthus of the lower eyelid (may indicate anemia; the inner canthus normally contains less pigmentation)
- **Scleral icterus** (an even yellowing of the sclera extending up to the cornea), indicative of jaundice
- Tenderness, foreign body, discharge, or lesions

Objective Data (side tab)

Normal Range of Findings   **Abnormal Findings**

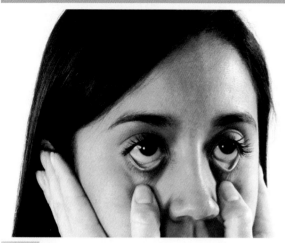

15-15

Eversion of the Upper Eyelid

This manoeuvre is not part of the normal examination, but it is useful when you must inspect the conjunctiva of the upper eyelid, as in cases of eye pain or suspicion of a foreign body. Most patients are apprehensive of any eye manipulation. Enhance their cooperation by using a calm and gentle, yet deliberate, approach.

1. Ask the patient to keep both eyes open and look down. This relaxes the eyelid, whereas closing it would tense the orbicularis muscle.
2. Slide the upper eyelid up along the bony orbit to lift up the eyelashes.
3. Grasp the lashes between your thumb and forefinger and gently pull down and outward.
4. With your other hand, place the tip of an applicator stick on the upper eyelid above the level of the internal tarsal plates (Figure 15-16, *A*).
5. Gently push down with the stick as you lift the lashes up. This uses the edge of the tarsal plate as a fulcrum and flips the eyelid inside out. Take special care not to push in on the eyeball.
6. Secure the everted position by holding the lashes against the bony orbital rim (see Figure 15-16, *B*).
7. Inspect for any colour change, swelling, lesion, or foreign body.
8. To return to normal position, gently pull the lashes outward as the patient looks up.

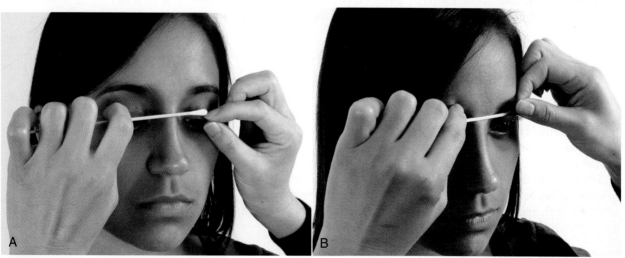

A   B

15-16

Objective Data

Normal Range of Findings	Abnormal Findings

Lacrimal Apparatus

Ask the patient to look down. With your thumbs, slide the outer part of the upper eyelid up along the bony orbit to expose under the eyelid. Inspect for any redness or swelling.

Normally, the puncta drain the tears into the lacrimal sac. Excessive tearing may indicate blockage of the nasolacrimal duct. Check this by pressing your index finger against the sac, just inside the lower orbital rim, not against the side of the nose (Figure 15-17). Pressure causes the lower eyelid to evert slightly, but no other response to pressure should occur.

Swelling of the lacrimal gland may manifest as a visible bulge in the outer part of the upper eyelid.

Puncta is red, swollen, and tender to pressure. Watch for any regurgitation of fluid out of the puncta, which confirms duct blockage.

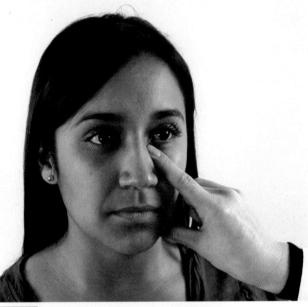

15-17

INSPECT ANTERIOR EYEBALL STRUCTURES

Cornea and Lens

Shine a light from the side across the patient's cornea, and check for smoothness and clarity. This oblique view highlights any abnormal irregularities in the corneal surface. No opacities (cloudiness) should appear in the cornea, the anterior chamber, or the lens behind the pupil. Do not confuse an *arcus senilis* with an opacity. The arcus senilis is a normal finding in older adults and is illustrated on p. 325.

A corneal abrasion causes irregular ridges in reflected light, producing a shattered appearance with light rays (see Table 15-7, p. 336).

Iris and Pupil

The iris normally appears flat, with a round regular shape and even coloration. Note the size, shape, and equality of the pupils. Normally the pupils appear round, regular, and of equal size in both eyes. In the adult, resting size is from 3 to 5 mm. A small number of people (5%) normally have pupils of two different sizes, which is termed **anisocoria**.

To test the **pupillary light reflex**, darken the room and ask the patient to gaze into the distance. (This dilates the pupils.) Advance a light in from the side* and note the response. Normally you will see (1) constriction of the same-sided pupil (a *direct light reflex*), and (2) simultaneous constriction of the other pupil (a *consensual light reflex*).

Irregular shape.

Although they may be normal, unequal-sized pupils necessitate investigation for central nervous system injury.

- Dilated pupils
- Dilated and fixed pupils
- Constricted pupils
- Sluggish pupils
- Unequal or no response to light (see Table 15-4, p. 332)

---

*Always advance the light in from the *side* to test the light reflex. If you advance from the front, the pupils constrict to accommodate for near vision; thus, you do not know what the pure response to the light would have been.

Normal Range of Findings	**Abnormal Findings**

In the acute care setting, gauge the pupil size in millimetres, both before and after the light reflex. Recording the pupil size in millimetres is more accurate when many nurses and physicians care for the same patient or when small changes may be significant signs of increasing intracranial pressure. Normally, the resting size is 3, 4, or 5 mm and decreases equally in response to light. An example of a normal response is designated by the following equation:

$$R\frac{3}{1} = \frac{3}{1}L$$

This indicates that both pupils measure 3 mm in the resting state and that both constrict to 1 mm in response to light. A graduated scale printed on a handheld vision screener or taped onto a tongue blade facilitates your measurement (see Figure 25-59 in Chapter 25).

To test for accommodation, ask the patient to focus on a distant object (Figure 15-18). This process dilates the pupils. Then have the patient shift the gaze to a near object, such as your finger held about 7 to 8 cm from the nose. A normal response includes (a) pupillary constriction and (b) convergence of the axes of the eyes.

Record the normal response to all these manoeuvres as PERRLA (**p**upils **e**qual, **r**ound, **r**eact to **l**ight, and **a**ccommodation).

- Absence of constriction or convergence
- Asymmetrical response

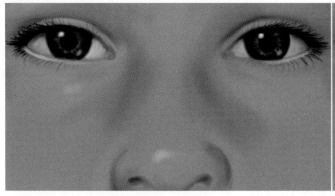 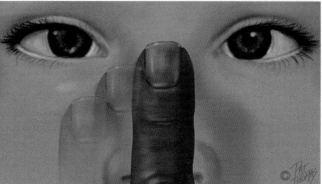

Far vision - pupils dilate   Near vision - pupils constrict

15-18   Testing accommodation. **Left,** Far vision: pupils dilate. **Right,** Near vision: pupils constrict. © *Pat Thomas, 2006.*

INSPECT THE OCULAR FUNDUS

The ophthalmoscope enlarges your view of the eye so that you can inspect the **media** (anterior chamber, lens, vitreous) and the **ocular fundus** (the internal surface of the retina). It accomplishes this by directing a beam of light through the pupil to illuminate the inner structures. Using the ophthalmoscope is thus like peering through a keyhole (the pupil) into an interesting room beyond.

The ophthalmoscope should function as an appendage of your own eye. Using it takes some practice. Practise holding the instrument and focusing at objects around the room before you use it with a real person. Hold the ophthalmoscope right up to your eye, braced firmly against the cheek and brow. Extend your index finger onto the lens selector dial so that you can refocus as necessary during the procedure without taking your head away from the ophthalmoscope to look. Now look about the room, moving your head and the instrument together as one unit. Keep both your eyes open; just view the field through the ophthalmoscope.

Recall that the ophthalmoscope contains a set of lenses that control the focus (Figure 15-19). The unit of strength of each lens is the *dioptre.* The black numbers represent positive dioptres; they focus on objects nearer in space to the ophthalmoscope. The red numbers represent negative dioptres and focus on objects farther away.

Normal Range of Findings	Abnormal Findings

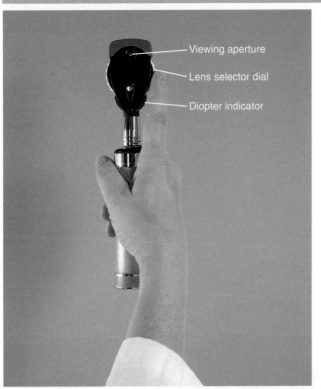

15-19

To examine a patient, darken the room to help dilate the pupils. (Dilating eye drops are not needed during a screening examination. They are used to dilate the pupils for a wider look at the fundus background and macular area. However, eye drops are used only when glaucoma can be completely ruled out because dilating the pupils in the presence of glaucoma can precipitate an acute episode.) Remove your own eyeglasses and the other patient's because they obstruct close movement; you can compensate for their correction by using the dioptre setting. Contact lenses may be left in; they pose no problem as long as they are clean.

Select the large round aperture with the white light for the routine examination. If the pupils are small, use the smaller white light. (Although the instrument has other shape and coloured apertures, as shown in Figure 15-20, these are rarely used in a screening examination.) The light must have maximum brightness; replace old or dim batteries.

◯   Large (full spot) for dilated pupils

○   Small for undilated pupils

◉   Red-free filter — a green beam, used to examine the optic disc for hemorrhage (which looks black) and melanin deposits (which look grey)

⊞   Grid — to determine fixation pattern and to assess size and location of lesions on the fundus

▯   Slit — to examine the anterior portion of the eye and to assess elevation or depression of lesions on the fundus   15-20

Instruct the patient to keep looking at a light switch (or mark) on the wall across the room, even though your head will get in the way. Staring at a distant fixed object helps dilate the pupils and hold the retinal structures still.

Match sides with the patient; that is, hold the ophthalmoscope in your *right* hand up to your *right* eye to view the patient's *right* eye. You must do this to avoid bumping noses during the procedure. Place your free hand on the patient's shoulder or forehead (Figure 15-21, *A*). This helps orient you in space, because once you have the ophthalmoscope in position, you have only a very narrow range of vision. Also, your thumb can anchor the patient's upper eyelid and help prevent blinking.

| Normal Range of Findings | Abnormal Findings |

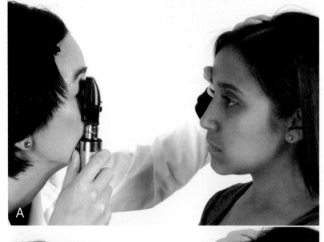

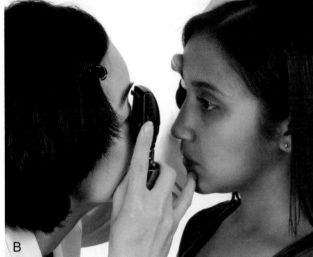

15-21

Begin about 25 cm away from the patient at an angle about 15 degrees lateral to the patient's line of vision. Note the red glow filling the patient's pupil. This is the **red reflex,** caused by the reflection of your ophthalmoscope light off the inner retina. Keep sight of the red reflex, and steadily move closer to the eye. If you lose the red reflex, the light has wandered off the pupil and onto the iris or sclera. Adjust your angle to find it again.

As you advance, adjust the lens to +6 dioptres, and note any opacities in the media. These appear as dark shadows or black dots that interrupt the red reflex. Normally, none are present.

Progress toward the patient until your foreheads almost touch (see Figure 15-21, B). Adjust the dioptre setting to bring the ocular fundus into sharp focus. If you and the patient have normal vision, this setting should be at 0. Moving the dioptres compensates for nearsightedness or farsightedness. Use the red lenses for nearsighted eyes and the black for farsighted eyes (Figure 15-22).

By moving in on the 15-degree lateral line, you should bring your view to only the optic disc. If the disc is not in sight, track a blood vessel as it grows larger, and it will lead you to the disc. Systematically inspect the structures in the ocular fundus: (a) optic disc, (b) retinal vessels, (c) general background, and (d) macula. (Figure 15-23 shows a large area of the fundus. Your actual view through the ophthalmoscope is much smaller: slightly larger than one disc diameter.)

Cataracts appear as opaque black areas against the red reflex (see Table 15-8, p. 337).

Objective Data

Normal Range of Findings	**Abnormal Findings**

NORMAL EYE

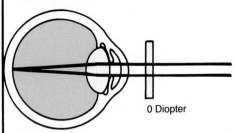

0 Diopter

The person's eye and your eye are normal. The 0 diopter (clear glass) will focus sharply on the retina.

MYOPIA (nearsighted)

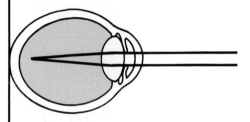

In myopia, the globe is longer than normal and light rays focus in *front* of the retina.

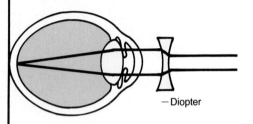

—Diopter

Compensate for myopia in yourself or the other person by using a negative diopter (red number or concave lens). This corrects the focal point onto the retina.

HYPEROPIA (farsighted)

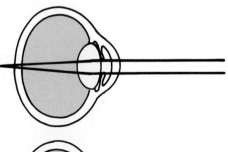

In hyperopia, the globe is shorter than normal. Light rays would focus behind the retina (if they could pass through).

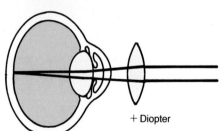

+ Diopter

Compensate for hyperopia by using a positive diopter (black number or convex lens). This bends the light rays so the focal point is on the retina.

15-22

Normal Range of Findings	Abnormal Findings

Optic Disc

The most prominent landmark is the optic disc, located on the nasal side of the retina. Explore these characteristics:

1. **Colour** — Creamy yellow-orange to pink
2. **Shape** — Round or oval
3. **Margins** — Distinct and sharply demarcated, although the nasal edge may be slightly fuzzy
4. **Cup–disc ratio** — Variable distinctness varies

When visible, the physiological cup is a brighter yellow-white than the rest of the disc. Its width is not more than half the disc diameter (Figure 15-24).

- Pallor, hyperemia
- Irregularity
- Blurred margins

- Cup extending to the disc border (see Table 15-9, p. 337)

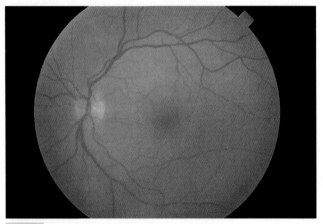

15-23 Normal ocular fundus.

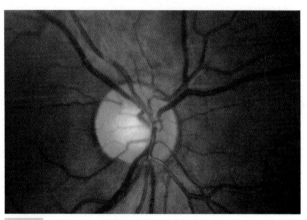

15-24 *Normal optic disc.*

Two normal variations may occur around the disc margins. A **scleral crescent** is a grey-white new moon shape. It is present when pigmentation is absent in the choroid layer, and you can see it by looking directly at the sclera. A **pigment crescent** is black; it is caused by accumulation of pigment in the choroid.

The diameter of the disc (DD) is a standard of measure for other fundus structures (Figure 15-25). To describe a finding, note its clock-face position, as well as its relationship to the disc in size and distance (e.g., "at 5:00 position, 3 DD from the disc").

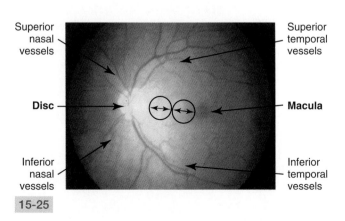

Superior nasal vessels

Superior temporal vessels

Disc

Macula

Inferior nasal vessels

Inferior temporal vessels

15-25

Objective Data

Normal Range of Findings	Abnormal Findings

Retinal Vessels

This is the only place in the body where you can view blood vessels directly. Many systemic diseases that affect the vascular system produce signs in the retinal vessels. Follow a paired artery and vein out to the periphery in the four quadrants (see Figure 15-23), noting these points:

1. **Number**   A paired artery and vein pass through each quadrant. Vessels look straighter at the nasal side.

- Absence of major vessels

2. **Colour**   Arteries are brighter red than are veins. Also, they have the arterial light reflex, with a thin stripe of light down the middle.

3. **Artery–vein ratio**   The ratio of the artery width to the vein width is 2:3 or 4:5.

- Arteries too constricted
- Veins dilated
- Focal constriction
- Neovascularization
- Crossings more than 2 DD away from disc
- Nicking or pinching of underlying vessel
- Vessel engorged peripheral to crossing (see Table 15-10, p. 338)
- Extreme tortuosity or marked asymmetry in two eyes

4. **Calibre**   Arteries and veins show a regular decrease in calibre as they extend to periphery.

5. **Arteriovenous crossing**   An artery and vein may cross paths. This is not significant if within 2 DD of disc and if no sign of interruption in blood flow is seen. There should be no indenting or displacing of vessel.

6. **Tortuosity**   Mild vessel twisting when present in both eyes is usually congenital and not significant.

7. **Pulsations**   Pulsations are visible in veins near the disc as their drainage meets the intermittent pressure of arterial systole (often hard to see).

- Absence of pulsations

General Background of the Fundus

The colour normally varies from light red to dark brown-red, generally corresponding to the patient's skin colour. Your view of the fundus should be clear; no lesions should obstruct the retinal structures.

- Abnormal lesions: hemorrhages, exudates, microaneurysms

Macula

The macula is 1 DD in size and located 2 DD temporal to the disc. Inspect this area last in the funduscopic examination. A bright light on this area of central vision causes some watering and discomfort and pupillary constriction. Note that the normal colour of the area is somewhat darker than the rest of the fundus but is even and homogeneous. Clumping of pigment may occur with aging.

Within the macula, you may note the foveal light reflex. This is a tiny white glistening dot that represents a reflection of your ophthalmoscope's light.

Clumping of pigment occurs with trauma or retinal detachment.

Hemorrhage or exudate in the macula occurs with AMD.

❖ DEVELOPMENTAL CONSIDERATIONS

Infants and Children

The eye examination is often deferred at birth because of transient edema of the eyelids from birth trauma or from the instillation of silver nitrate at birth. The eyes should be examined within a few days and at every well-child visit thereafter.

Objective Data

Normal Range of Findings	Abnormal Findings

Visual Acuity. Which screening measures to use depend on the child's age. With a newborn, test visual reflexes and attending behaviours. Test **light perception** by using the blink reflex; the neonate blinks in response to bright light (Figure 15-26). Also test for the pupillary light reflex, in which the pupils constrict in response to light. These reflexes indicate that the lower portion of the visual apparatus is intact. However, you cannot infer that the infant can *see;* that requires later observation to show that the brain has received images and can interpret them.

As you introduce an object to the infant's line of vision, note these normal attending behaviours:

Birth to 2 weeks: Refusal to reopen eyes after exposure to bright light; increasing alertness to object; possible fixation on an object

By 2 to 4 weeks: Fixating on an object

By 1 month: Fixating on and following a light or bright toy

By 3 to 4 months: Fixating on, following, and reaching for the toy

By 6 to 10 months: Fixating and following the toy in all directions

The Canadian Pediatric Society (CPS, 2009) identifies these as **clinically useful normal visual development landmarks**:

- Face follow: Birth to 4 weeks of age.
- Visual following: Three months of age.
- Visual acuity measurable with appropriate chart: 42 months of age.

The Allen chart* (picture cards) was previously often used to screen children from 30 to 35 months of age. In some cases, it may be reliable with cooperative toddlers as young as 2 years of age. The test involves seven cards depicting objects that are assumed to be familiar in most (though not all) cases (birthday cake, teddy bear, tree, house, car, telephone, and horse and rider). First, show the pictures up close to the child to make sure that the child can identify them. Then present each picture at a distance of 4.5 m. Results are normal if the child can name three of seven cards within three to five trials.

Abnormal Findings

- Absence of blinking
- Absence of pupillary light reflex, especially after 3 weeks, which indicates blindness

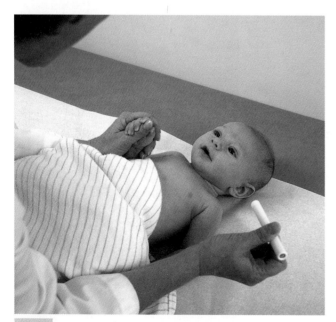

15-26

---

*The Allen chart (pictograms), previously widely used, is now thought to be too culturally specific to be helpful (CPS, 2009).

Objective Data

Normal Range of Findings

Use a picture chart or the Snellen E chart for preschoolers aged 3 to 6 years. The Snellen E chart shows the capital letter *E* in varying sizes pointing in different directions*. The child points his or her fingers in the direction the "table legs" are pointing. By 7 to 8 years of age, when the child is familiar with reading letters, begin to use the standard alphabetical Snellen eye chart. Normally, children achieve 20/20 acuity by 6 to 7 years of age (Figure 15-27).

The Canadian Paediatric Society (2009) recommends periodic screening for infants, children, and youth, outlined as follows:

Newborn to Age 3 Months
- A complete examination of the skin and external eye structures, as well as the conjunctiva, cornea, iris, and pupils, is an integral part of the physical examination of all newborns, infants, and children.
- The **red reflex** should be inspected for lenticular opacities (cataracts) and signs of posterior eye disease (retinoblastoma).
- The red reflex should be equal in brightness and colour, and should fill the pupil completely (CPS, 2009).
- Corneal light reflex should be tested to detect ocular misalignment.

Ages 6 to 12 Months
- Conduct examination as for newborns.
- Ocular alignment should again be observed to detect strabismus. The corneal light reflex should be central, and the result of the cover-uncover test normal.
- Fixation and following are observed.

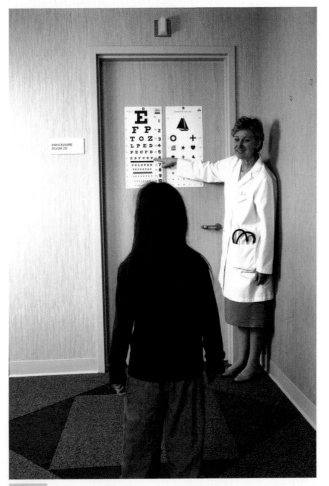

15-27

*According to the CPS (2009), most children who are four years of age can recognize Snellen letters and numbers.

Abnormal Findings

Failure of visualization or abnormalities of the red reflex are indications for immediate referral to an ophthalmologist.

The Canadian Pediatric Society (CPS, 2009, p. 3) recommends:

"School-aged children who pass visual examinations and screenings but have reading difficulties should be referred to a reading specialist educator for further assessment. Any infant or child with abnormalities on examination, or who does not pass visual screening, should be referred for further assessment. Infants and children with risk factors, such as developmental delay, should also be fully examined by a well-trained eye care professional. It is imperative that access to appropriate professional ophthalmological expertise is readily available and provided by the public health care system of Canada."

Normal Range of Findings	Abnormal Findings

Ages 3 to 5 Years
- Conduct examination as for newborns.
- Visual acuity testing with an optotype test (e.g., Snellen E acuity card or Allen test) should be completed.
- A child with visual acuity of less than 20/30 should be referred to an ophthalmologist.

Ages 6 to 18 Years
- Visual acuity should be assessed every 2 years until age 10 years and then every 3 years thereafter (e.g., with the Snellen eye chart).

Visual Fields. Assess peripheral vision with the confrontation test in children older than 3 years, when they are able to stay in position. Like adults, children should see the moving target at the same time your normal eyes do. Often a young child forgets to say "now" or "stop" as the moving object is seen. Rather, note the instant the child's eyes deviate or head shifts position to gaze at the moving object. Match this nearly automatic response with your own sighting.

Colour Vision. Colour blindness is an inherited recessive X-linked trait affecting about 8% of male Canadians of European descent. It is less common in male Canadians of African or First Nations descent, and it is rare in female Canadians. "Colour deficient" is a more accurate term because the condition is relative and not disabling. Often, it is just a social inconvenience, although it may affect the patient's ability to discern traffic lights, or it may affect school performance in which colour is a learning tool. Test only boys for colour vision, once between the ages of 4 and 8 years. Use Ishihara's test (a series of polychromatic cards). Each card has a pattern of dots of a specific colour printed against a background of dots of many other colours. Ask the child to identify each pattern. A patient with normal colour vision can see each pattern. A colour blind patient cannot see the letter against the field colour.

Extraocular Muscle Function. Testing for **strabismus** (squint, crossed eye) is an important screening measure during early childhood. Strabismus causes disconjugate vision because one eye deviates off the fixation point. To avoid diplopia or unclear images, the brain begins to suppress data from the weak eye (a suppression scotoma). Visual acuity in this otherwise normal eye then begins to deteriorate from disuse. Early recognition and treatment are essential for restoring binocular vision. When diagnosed after 6 years of age, strabismus has a poor prognosis. Test misalignment with the corneal light reflex and the cover-uncover test.

Untreated strabismus can lead to permanent visual damage. The resulting loss of vision from disuse is amblyopia ex anopsia.

When performing the **cover-uncover test**, the uncovered eye should not move. The covered eye should also not reposition when exposed. If any such movement occurs during this test, providing vision is good (fixation is well maintained), the child should be referred immediately for further assessment (CPS, 2009).

Asymmetry in the corneal light reflex after 6 months of age is abnormal and must be investigated.

Check the **corneal light reflex** by shining a light toward the child's eyes. The reflection of light should be at exactly the same spot in the two corneas (Figure 15-28). Some asymmetry (where one light falls off centre) in infants younger than 6 months is normal.

Perform the **cover-uncover test** on all children as described on p. 308. Some examiners omit the opaque card and place a hand on the child's head. The examiner's thumb extends down and blocks vision over the eye without actually touching the eye. You can use a familiar character puppet to attract the child's attention. The normal results are the same as those listed for adults.

You can assess function of the extraocular muscles during movement in the early weeks of a child's life by watching the child's gaze following a brightly coloured toy as a target. An older infant can sit on the parent's lap as you move the toy in all directions. After the child is 2 years of age, direct the child's gaze through the six cardinal positions of gaze. You may stabilize the child's chin with your hand to prevent him or her from moving the entire head.

Normal Range of Findings	Abnormal Findings

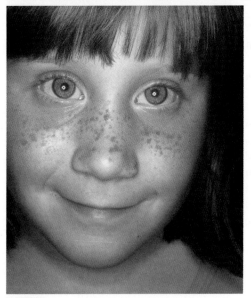

15-28

External Eye Structures. Inspect the ocular structures as described in the earlier section. A neonate usually holds the eyes tightly shut in response to a bright light. Do not attempt to pry them open; that just increases contraction of the orbicularis oculi muscle. Hold the newborn supine and gently lower the head; the eyes will open. Also, the eyes will open when you hold the infant at arm's length and slowly turn the infant in one direction (Figure 15-29). In addition to inspecting the ocular structures, this is also a test of the vestibular function reflex: The baby's eyes will look in the direction the body is being turned. When the turning stops, the eyes will shift to the opposite direction after a few quick beats of nystagmus. This reflex, also termed the *doll's-eyes reflex,* disappears by 2 months of age.

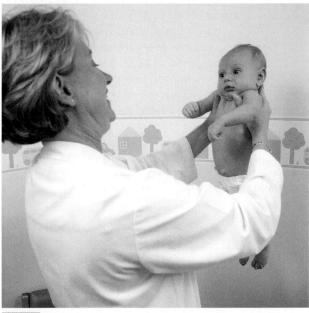

15-29

Normal Range of Findings	Abnormal Findings

Eyelids and Lashes. Normally the upper eyelids overlie the superior part of the iris. In newborns, the *setting-sun sign* is common. The eyes appear to deviate down, and you see a white rim of sclera over the iris. It may show as you rapidly change the neonate from a sitting to a supine position.

Many infants have an *epicanthal fold,* an excess skinfold extending over the inner corner of the eye, partly or totally overlapping the inner canthus. It is present in many children of Eastern Asian descent and in some people of European descent. In some children, the epicanthal folds disappear as they grow, usually by 10 years of age. While they are present, epicanthal folds give a false appearance of misalignment, termed **pseudostrabismus** (Figure 15-30). Pseudostrabismus occurs most often when a broad nasal bridge covers the nasal sclera unequally. This can be determined and distinguished from strabismus by the presence of a symmetrical corneal light reflex (CPS, 2009).

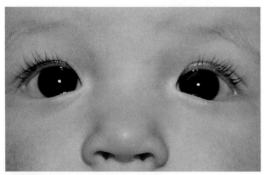

15-30   Pseudostrabismus.

Infants of Eastern Asian descent normally have an upward slant of the palpebral fissures. *Entropion,* a turning inward of the eyelid, is found normally in some children of Eastern Asian descent. If the lashes do not abrade the corneas, it is not significant.

Conjunctiva and Sclera. A newborn may have a transient chemical conjunctivitis from the instillation of silver nitrate. This appears within 1 hour and lasts not more than 24 hours after birth. The sclera should be white and clear, although it may have a blue tint as a result of thinness at birth. The lacrimal glands are not functional at birth.

Iris and Pupils. The iris normally is blue or slate grey in light-skinned newborns and brown in dark-skinned newborns. By ages 6 to 9 months, the permanent colour is established. Brushfield's spots, or white specks around the edge of the iris, are occasionally normal.

A searching nystagmus is common just after birth. The pupils are small but constrict to light.

The Ocular Fundus. The amount of data gathered during the funduscopic examination depends on the infant's ability to hold the eyes still and on your ability to glean as much data as possible in a brief time.

A complete funduscopic examination is difficult to perform on an infant, but at least check the red reflex when the infant fixates on the bright light for a few seconds. Note any interruption.

Perform a funduscopic examination on an infant between 2 and 6 months of age. Position the infant supine on the table. The fundus appears pale, and the vessels are not fully developed. The foveal light reflection is not present because the macula area is not mature until age 1 year.

Abnormal Findings (right column):

The setting-sun sign also occurs with hydrocephalus as the globes protrude.

Eyes appear blank and sunken with malnutrition, dehydration, and severe illness.

An upward lateral slope, together with epicanthal folds and hypertelorism (abnormally wide spacing between eyes), occurs with Down's syndrome.

Ophthalmia neonatorum (conjunctivitis of the newborn) is a purulent discharge caused by a chemical irritant or a bacterial or viral agent from the birth canal.

Absence of iris colour occurs with albinism.

Brushfield's spots are usually suggestive of Down's syndrome.

Constant nystagmus, prolonged setting-sun sign, marked strabismus, and slow lateral movements are suggestive of vision loss.

An interruption in the red reflex indicates an opacity in the cornea or lens. The red reflex is absent in patients with congenital cataracts or retinal disorders.

Papilledema is rare in infants because the fontanelles and open sutures absorb any increased intracranial pressure if it occurs.

Objective Data

Normal Range of Findings	Abnormal Findings

Objective Data

Inspect the fundus of young children and school-age children as described for adults. Allow a child to handle the equipment. Explain why you are darkening the room and that you will leave a small light on. Assure the child that the procedure will not hurt. Direct the young child to look at an appealing picture, or perhaps at a toy or an animal, during the examination.

Older Adults

Visual Acuity. Perform the same examination as described for adults. Central acuity may be decreased, particularly after 70 years of age. Peripheral vision may be diminished.

Ocular Structures. The eyebrows may show a loss of the outer one third to one half of hair because of a decrease in hair follicles. The remaining brow hair is coarse. As a result of atrophy of elastic tissues, the skin around the eyes may show wrinkles or crow's feet. The upper eyelid may be so elongated as to rest on the lashes, a condition called *pseudoptosis* (Figure 15-31).

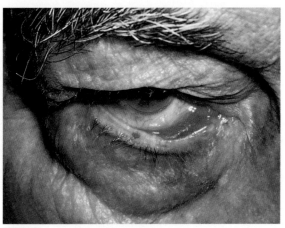

15-31 Pseudoptosis.

The eyes may appear sunken from atrophy of the orbital fat. Also, the orbital fat may herniate, causing bulging at the lower eyelids and inner third of the upper eyelids.

The lacrimal apparatus may decrease tear production, causing the eyes to look dry and lustreless and the patient to feel a burning sensation. **Pingueculae,** which commonly appear on the sclera (Figure 15-32), are yellowish elevated nodules caused by a thickening of the bulbar conjunctiva as a result of prolonged exposure to sun, wind, and dust. Pingueculae appear at the 3:00 and 9:00 positions: first on the nasal side, then on the temporal side.

- Ectropion (lower eyelid dropping away) and entropion (lower eyelid turning in; see Table 15-2, p. 331)
Distinguish pinguecula from the abnormal **pterygium,** which is also an opacity on the bulbar conjunctiva but grows over the cornea (see Table 15-7, p. 336).

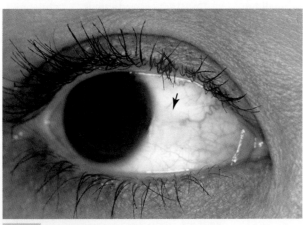

15-32 Pinguecula.

Normal Range of Findings	Abnormal Findings

Normal Range of Findings

The cornea may look cloudy with age. **Arcus senilis,** commonly seen around the cornea (Figure 15-33), is a grey-white arc or circle around the limbus; it is caused by deposition of lipid material. As more lipid accumulates, the cornea may look thickened and raised, but the arcus has no effect on vision.

Xanthelasma are soft, raised yellow plaques on the eyelids at the inner canthus (Figure 15-34). They commonly occur during the fifth decade of life and more frequently in women. They occur with both high and normal blood levels of cholesterol and have no pathological significance.

Pupils are small in old age, and the pupillary light reflex may be slowed. The lens loses transparency and looks opaque.

The Ocular Fundus. With age, retinal structures generally have less shine. The blood vessels look paler, narrower, and attenuated. Arterioles appear paler and straighter, with a narrower light reflex. More arteriovenous crossing defects occur.

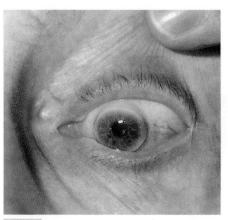

15-33   Arcus senilis.

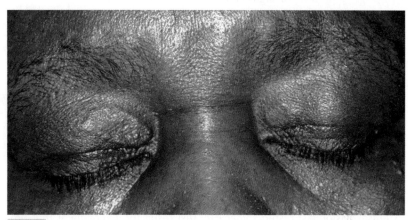

15-34   Xanthelasma.

A normal development on the retinal surface is **drusen,** or benign degenerative hyaline deposits (Figure 15-35). They are small, round, yellow dots that are scattered haphazardly on the retina. Although they do not occur in a pattern, they are usually symmetrically placed in the two eyes. They have no effect on vision.

Abnormal Findings

Drusen are easily confused with *hard exudates,* an abnormal finding that occurs with a more circular or linear pattern (see Table 15-10, p. 339). Also, drusen in the macular area occur with AMD.

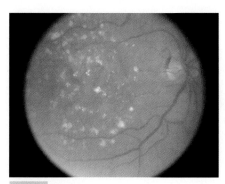

15-35   Drusen.

SPECIAL CONSIDERATIONS FOR ADVANCED PRACTICE

Assessing for AMD and other common causes of visual impairment in the adult population, including older adults, is an important aspect of advanced practice nursing. Regular examinations are important for determining whether patients may benefit from certain interventions. For example, in relation to AMD, it is recommended that patients older than 55 with no risk factors receive a comprehensive eye examination every 1 to 2 years (Noble & Chaudhary, 2010). Patients with early-stage disease or a family history of the condition need more frequent follow-up.

Advanced practice nurses frequently encounter patients with a red eye. Most patients with red eye have a benign or self-limited conditions resulting from conjunctivitis (usually viral), blepharitis, small corneal abrasions, dry eye, and subconjunctival hemorrhage (Noble & Lloyd, 2011). Ominous symptoms or signs that indicate urgent referral to an ophthalmologist are listed in the following Critical Findings box.

CRITICAL FINDINGS

Anyone who reports a sudden change in vision should be referred for urgent, immediate ophthalmic evaluation (Noble & Chaudhary, 2010, p. 1759). Ensure that such a patient is taken to the nearest emergency department; if in hospital, call for an immediate ophthalmology consultation.

For patients with red eye (see examples in Table 15-6), immediate, urgent referral to an emergency room or an on-call ophthalmologist is necessary for "a history of severe pain, visual loss, marked pain or decreased vision with the use of contact lenses, trauma, chemical injury and recent eye surgery" (Noble & Lloyd, 2011, p. 81). On examination, signs necessitating immediate, urgent referral include "decreased visual acuity, pupil irregularity, sluggish pupillary reaction to light, corneal opacification, hyphema … or hypopyon … and elevated intra-ocular pressure" (p. 81). Patients wearing contact lenses should be told to stop wearing the lenses immediately. Be especially alert when a patient has only one red eye.

DOCUMENTATION AND CRITICAL THINKING

Sample Charting

SUBJECTIVE

Vision reported good with no recent change. No eye pain, no inflammation, no discharge, no lesions. Wears no corrective lenses, vision last tested 1 year PTA, test result for glaucoma at that time was normal.

OBJECTIVE

Snellen eye chart: O.D. 20/20, O.S. [left eye] 20/20 −1. Fields normal by confrontation. Corneal light reflex symmetrical bilaterally. Diagnostic positions test shows EOMs intact. Brows and lashes present. No ptosis. Conjunctiva clear. Sclera white. No lesions. PERRLA.

Fundi: Red reflex present bilaterally. Discs flat with sharp margins. Vessels present in all quadrants without crossing defects. Retinal background has even colour with no hemorrhages or exudates. Macula has even colour.

ASSESSMENT

Healthy vision function
Healthy eye structures

Focused Assessment: Clinical Case Study 1

Emma K. is a 34-year-old married, female homemaker brought to the emergency department by police after a reported domestic quarrel.

SUBJECTIVE

- States husband struck her on the face and eyes with his fists about 1 hour PTA. "I ruined the dinner again. I can't do anything right." Pain in left cheek and both eyes felt immediately and continues. Alarmed at "bright red blood on eyeball." No bleeding from eye area or cheek. Vision intact just after trauma. Now reports difficulty opening eyelids.

OBJECTIVE

Sitting quietly and hunched over, hands over eyes. Voice tired and flat. L cheek swollen and discoloured, no laceration. Lids edematous and discoloured both eyes. No skin laceration. L lid swollen almost shut. L eye—round 1-mm bright red patch over lateral aspect of globe at 3:00 position. No active bleeding out of eye, iris intact, anterior chamber clear. R eye—conjunctiva clear, sclera white, cornea and iris intact, anterior chamber clear. PERRLA. Pupils R $\frac{4}{1} = \frac{4}{1}$ L. Vision 14/14 both eyes by Jaeger card.

ASSESSMENT

Ecchymoses L cheek and both eyes
Subconjunctival hemorrhage L eye
Pain R/T inflammation
Chronic low self-esteem R/T effects of domestic violence

Focused Assessment: Clinical Case Study 2

Sam T. is a 63-year-old married, male postal carrier admitted to the medical centre for surgery for suspected brain tumour. After postanaesthesia recovery, Sam T. is admitted to the neurology critical care unit, awake, lethargic with slowed but correct verbal responses, oriented × 3, moving all four extremities, vital signs stable. Pupils R $\frac{4}{2} = \frac{4}{2}$ L with sluggish response. Assessments are made q15 min.

SUBJECTIVE

• No response now to verbal stimuli.

OBJECTIVE

Semicomatose: no response to verbal stimuli, does withdraw R arm and leg purposefully to painful stimuli. No movement L arm or leg. Pupils R $\frac{5}{5} \neq \frac{4}{2}$ L. Vitals remain stable as noted on graphic sheet.

ASSESSMENT

Unilateral dilated and fixed R pupil
Clouding of consciousness
Focal motor deficit: no movement L side
Ineffective tissue perfusion R/T interruption of cerebral flow

Focused Assessment: Clinical Case Study 3

Trung Q. is a 4-year-old male born in Southeast Asia who arrived in this country 1 month PTA. Lives with parents, two siblings. Speaks only native language; here with uncle, who acts as interpreter.

SUBJECTIVE

• Seeks care because RN in church sponsoring family noted "crossed eyes." Uncle states vision seemed normal to parents. Plays with toys and manipulates small objects without difficulty. Identifies objects in picture books; does not read.

OBJECTIVE

With uncle interpreting directions for test to Trung, vision by Snellen E chart: O.D. 20/30, O.S. 20/50 −1. Fields seem intact by confrontation: jerks head to gaze at object entering field.
EOMs: Asymmetrical corneal light reflex with outward deviation L eye. Cover-uncover test: as R eye covered, L eye jerks to fixate, R eye steady when uncovered. As L eye covered, R eye holds steady gaze, L eye jerks to fixate as uncovered. Diagnostic positions: able to gaze in six positions, although L eye obviously misaligned at extreme medial gaze.
Eye structures: Brows and lashes present and normal bilaterally. Upward palpebral slant, epicanthal folds bilaterally: consistent with shape of eyes. Conjunctiva clear, sclera white, iris intact, PERRLA.
Fundi: Discs flat with sharp margins. Observed vessels normal. Unable to see in all four quadrants or to see macular area.

ASSESSMENT

L exotropia
Abnormal vision in L eye
Disturbed visual sensory perception R/T effects of neurological impairment

Focused Assessment: Clinical Case Study 4

Vera K. is an 87-year-old widowed, African Canadian, female homemaker living independently who is admitted to hospital for observation and adjustment of digitalis medication. Cardiac status has been stable during hospital stay.

SUBJECTIVE

- Reports desire to monitor own medication at home but fears problems because of blurred vision. First noted distant vision blurred 5 years ago but near vision seemed to improve at that time: "I started to read better without my glasses!" Since then, blurring of distant vision has increased, near vision now blurred also.
- Able to navigate home environment without difficulty. Fixes simple meals with cold foods. Receives hot meal from Meals On Wheels at lunch. Enjoys TV, although it looks somewhat blurred. Unable to write letters, sew, or read paper, which she regrets.

OBJECTIVE

Vision by Jaeger card: O.D. 20/200, O.S. 20/400 −1, with glasses on. Fields intact by confrontation. EOMs intact. Brow hair: absent lateral third. Upper lids have folds of redundant skin but lids do not droop. Lower lids and lashes intact. Xanthelasma present both inner canthi. Conjunctiva clear, sclera white, iris intact, L pupil looks cloudy, PERRLA, pupils R $\frac{3}{2} = \frac{3}{2}$ L.

Fundi: Red reflex has central dark spot, both eyes. Discs flat, with sharp margins. Observed vessels normal. Unable to see in all four quadrants or macular area because of small pupils.

ASSESSMENT

Central opacity, both eyes
Central visual acuity deficit, both eyes
Deficient diversional activity R/T poor vision

ABNORMAL FINDINGS

TABLE 15-1   Extraocular Muscle Dysfunction

Symmetrical Corneal Light Reflex   ▶
A. *Pseudostrabismus* has the appearance of strabismus because of epicanthic fold but is normal for a young child.

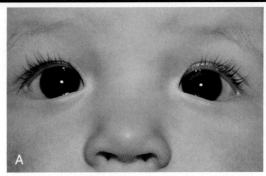

A, Pseudostrabismus.

Asymmetrical Corneal Light Reflex
Strabismus is true disparity of the eye axes. This constant misalignment is also termed *tropia* and is likely to cause amblyopia.

B. Esotropia: inward turn of the eye.   C. Exotropia: outward turning of the eyes.

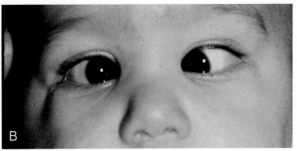

B, Left esotropia.

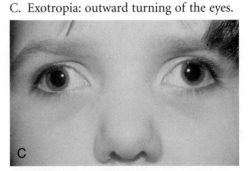

C, Exotropia.

TABLE 15-1   Extraocular Muscle Dysfunction—cont'd

Cover-Uncover Test   ▶

D. Uncovered eye: If it jumps to fixate on designated point, it was out of alignment before (i.e., when you cover the stronger eye [top], the weaker eye now tries to fixate [bottom]).

Phoria: mild weakness, apparent only with the cover test and less likely to cause amblyopia than a tropia but still possible.

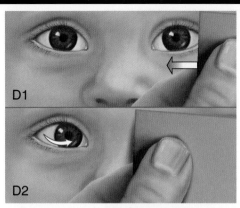

D, Right (uncovered eye) is weaker.

E. Covered eye: If this is the weaker eye, once macular ▶ image is suppressed, the eye drifts to relaxed position (top).

As eye is uncovered: If it jumps to reestablish fixation (bottom), weakness exists.

Esophoria: nasal (inward) drift.

Exophoria: temporal (outward) drift.

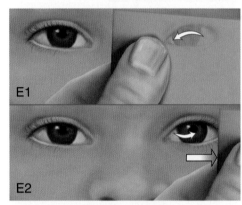

E, Left (uncovered) eye is weaker.

Diagnostic Positions Test   ▶

Paralysis is apparent during movement through six cardinal positions of gaze. This is a test of the ocular muscles: inferior oblique (IO), inferior rectus (IR), lateral rectus (LR), medial rectus (MR), superior oblique (SO), and superior rectus (SR).

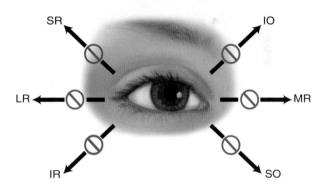

Direction That Eye Does Not Turn	Site of Paralysis	Cranial Nerve
Straight nasal	Medial rectus	III
Up and nasal	Inferior oblique	III
Up and temporal	Superior rectus	III
Straight temporal	Lateral rectus	VI
Down and temporal	Inferior rectus	III
Down and nasal	Superior oblique	IV

TABLE 15-2   Abnormalities in the Eyelids

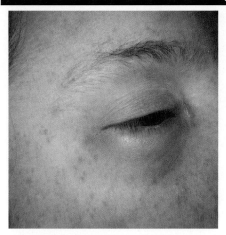

Periorbital Edema

Eyelids are swollen and puffy. Eyelid tissues are loosely connected, and so excess fluid is easily apparent. This occurs with local infections; with crying; and with systemic conditions such as heart failure, renal failure, allergy, and hypothyroidism (myxedema).

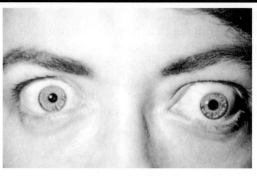

Exophthalmos (Protruding Eyes)

Eyeballs are displaced forward, and palpebral fissures are widened. Note "lid lag"; the upper eyelid rests well above the limbus, and white sclera is visible. Acquired bilateral exophthalmos is associated with thyrotoxicosis.

Enophthalmos (Sunken Eyes; Not Illustrated)

This appearance is of narrowed palpebral fissures, in which the eyeballs are recessed. Bilateral enophthalmos is caused by loss of fat in the orbits and occurs with dehydration and chronic wasting illnesses. For illustration, see "Cachectic Appearance" in Table 14-4, p. 292.

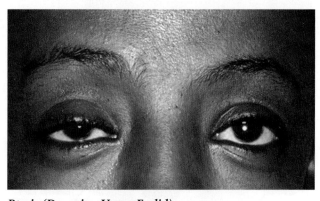

Ptosis (Drooping Upper Eyelid)

This is a positional defect that gives the patient a sleepy appearance and impairs vision. It is caused by neuromuscular weakness (e.g., myasthenia gravis with bilateral fatigue as the day progresses), oculomotor cranial nerve III damage, or sympathetic nerve damage (e.g., Horner's syndrome).

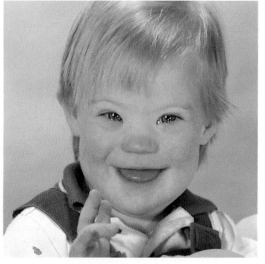

Upward Palpebral Slant

Although normal in many children, these slants—when combined with epicanthal folds, hypertelorism (wide spacing between the eyes), and Brushfield's spots (light-coloured areas in outer iris)—indicate Down's syndrome.

TABLE 15-2   Abnormalities in the Eyelids—cont'd

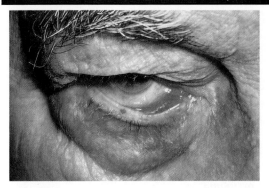

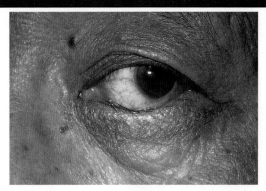

Ectropion

The lower eyelid is loose, rolls outward, and does not approximate to eyeball. Puncta cannot siphon tears effectively, and so excess tearing results. The eyes feel dry and itchy because the tears do not drain correctly over the corner and toward the medial canthus. Exposure of palpebral conjunctiva increases risk for inflammation. This occurs with aging as a result of atrophy of elastic and fibrous tissues, but it may result from trauma.

Entropion

The lower eyelid rolls inward because of spasm of eyelids or scar tissue contracting. Constant rubbing of lashes may irritate cornea. The patient feels a "foreign body" sensation.

TABLE 15-3   Lesions on the Eyelids

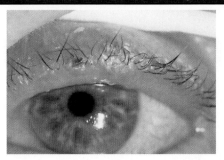

Blepharitis (Inflammation of the Eyelids)

Red, scaly, greasy flakes and thickened, crusted eyelid margins occur with staphylococcal infection or seborrheic dermatitis of the eyelid edge. Symptoms include burning sensation, itching, tearing, foreign body sensation, and some pain.

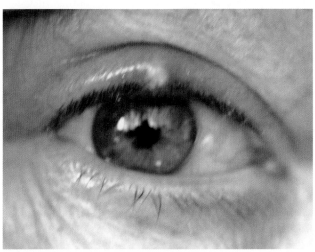

Chalazion

A beady nodule protruding on the eyelid, chalazion is an infection or retention cyst of a meibomian gland. It is a nontender, firm, discrete swelling with freely movable skin overlying the nodule. If it becomes inflamed, it points inside and not on eyelid margin (in contrast to stye).

◄ *Hordeolum (Stye)*

Hordeolum is a localized staphylococcal infection of the hair follicles at the eyelid margin. It is painful, red, and swollen: a pustule at the eyelid margin. Rubbing the eyes can cause cross-contamination and development of another stye.

Continued

TABLE 15-3   Lesions on the Eyelids—cont'd

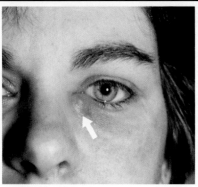

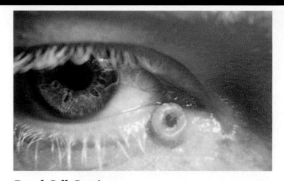

Dacryocystitis (Inflammation of the Lacrimal Sac)
Dacryocystitis is infection and blockage of sac and duct. Pain, warmth, redness, and swelling occur below the inner canthus toward the nose. Tearing is present. Pressure on sac yields purulent discharge from puncta.

Basal Cell Carcinoma
Carcinoma is rare, but it occurs most often on the lower eyelid and medial canthus. It looks like a papule with an ulcerated centre. Note the rolled-out pearly edges. It should be referred for removal, although metastasis is rare.

Dacryoadenitis (Inflammation of the Lacrimal Gland; Not Illustrated)
Dacryoadenitis is an infection of the lacrimal gland. Pain, swelling, and redness occur in the outer third of upper eyelid. It occurs with mumps, measles, and infectious mononucleosis or results from trauma.

TABLE 15-4   Abnormalities in the Pupil

Location of lesions:

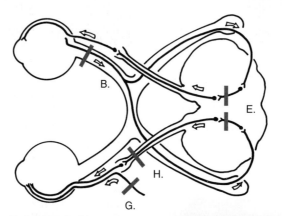

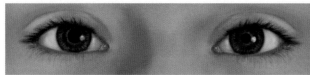

A. Unequal Pupil Size: Anisocoria
Although this exists normally in 5% of the population, consider central nervous system disease.

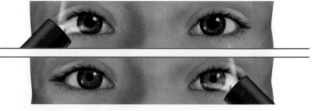

B. Monocular Blindness
When light is directed to the blind eye (in this illustration, the right eye), no response occurs in either eye. When light is directed to normal (left) eye, both pupils constrict (direct and consensual response to light) as long as the oculomotor nerve is intact.

TABLE 15-4   Abnormalities in the Pupil—cont'd

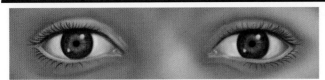

C. Constricted and Fixed Pupils: Miosis

Miosis occurs with the use of pilocarpine drops for glaucoma treatment, the use of narcotics, with iritis, and with damage of the pons in the brain.

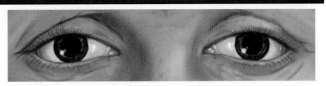

D. Dilated and Fixed Pupils: Mydriasis

Pupils become enlarged with stimulation of the sympathetic nervous system, as a reaction to sympathomimetic drugs, with use of dilating drops, and as a result of acute glaucoma and past or recent trauma. Enlarged pupils also herald central nervous system injury, circulatory arrest, or deep anaesthesia.

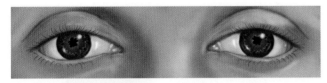

E. Argyll Robertson Pupil

Such pupils have no reaction to light but do constrict with accommodation. They are small and irregular bilaterally. Argyll Robertson pupil occurs with central nervous system syphilis, brain tumour, meningitis, and chronic alcoholism.

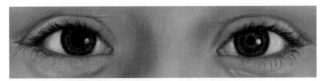

F. Tonic Pupil (Adie's Pupil)

This kind of pupil has a sluggish reaction to light and accommodation. It is usually unilateral, a large regular pupil that does react but sluggishly, after a long latent time. It has no pathological significance.

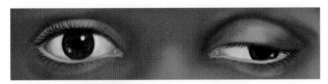

G. Cranial Nerve III Damage

Oculomotor nerve damage causes unilateral pupil dilation with no reaction to light or accommodation. Ptosis may also be present, with eye deviating downward and laterally.

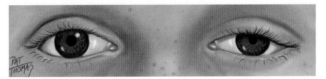

H. Horner's Syndrome

Horner's syndrome, a lesion of the sympathetic nerve, causes unilateral, small, regular pupil that does react to light and accommodation. Ptosis and absence of sweat (anhidrosis) on the same side of the face are also present.

TABLE 15-5   Visual Field Loss

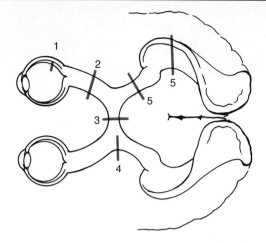

1. Retinal damage
   - Macula: central blind area (e.g., in diabetes)

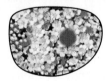 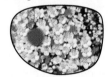

   - Localized damage: blind spot (scotoma) corresponding to particular area

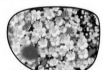 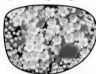

   - Increasing intraocular pressure: decrease in peripheral vision (e.g., glaucoma); starts with paracentral scotoma

 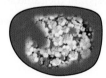

   - Retinal detachment; patient has shadow or diminished vision in one quadrant or one half of visual field

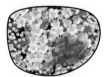 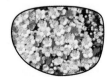

2. Lesion in globe or optic nerve; injury causes blindness in one eye, or unilateral blindness

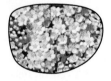 

3. Lesion at optic chiasm (e.g., pituitary tumour); injury to crossing fibres produces only a loss of nasal part of each retina and a loss of both temporal visual fields; bitemporal (heteronymous) hemianopsia

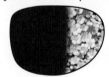 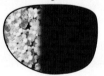

4. Lesion of outer uncrossed fibres at optic chiasm (e.g., aneurysm of left internal carotid artery exerts pressure on uncrossed fibres); injury produces left nasal hemianopsia

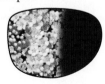 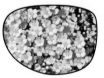

5. Lesion in right optic tract or right optic radiation; visual field loss in right nasal and left temporal fields; loss of same half visual field in both eyes is homonymous hemianopsia

 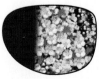

TABLE 15-6   Vascular Disorders of the External Eye

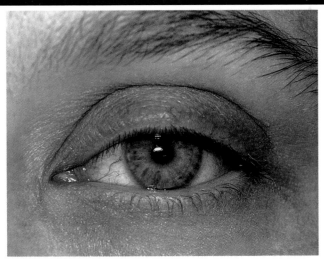

Conjunctivitis

Infection of the conjunctiva ("pink eye") causes vessels at periphery to appear red and beefy, but usually the area around the iris is clearer (although in this illustration it is severe). This is a common symptom of bacterial or viral infection, allergy, or chemical irritation. Purulent discharge accompanies bacterial infection. Preauricular lymph node is often swollen and painful, and patients have a history of upper respiratory infection. Symptoms include itching, burning sensation, foreign body sensation, and eyelids stuck together on awakening.

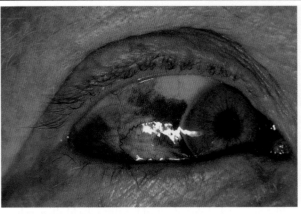

Subconjunctival Hemorrhage

A red patch on the sclera, subconjunctival hemorrhage looks alarming but is usually not serious. The red patch has clear edges, although in this illustration it is extensive. It is caused by increased intraocular pressure from coughing, sneezing, weight lifting, labour during childbirth, straining at stool, or trauma.

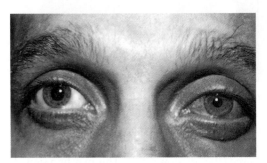

Iritis (Circumcorneal Redness)

Deep, dull red halo around the iris and cornea. Redness is around iris, in contrast to conjunctivitis, in which the redness is more prominent at the periphery. Pupil shape may be irregular from swelling of iris. Patient also has marked photophobia, constricted pupil, blurred vision, and throbbing pain. This condition warrants immediate referral.

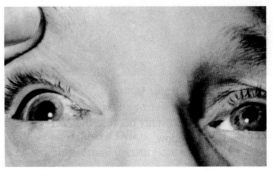

Acute Glaucoma

Acute, narrow-angle glaucoma produces a circumcorneal redness around the iris, with dilation of the pupil. Pupil is oval, dilated; cornea looks "steamy"; and anterior chamber is shallow. Acute glaucoma occurs with sudden increase in intraocular pressure caused by blockage of outflow from anterior chamber. The patient experiences a sudden clouding of vision and sudden eye pain and sees halos around lights. This necessitates emergency treatment to prevent permanent vision loss.

systematic review of the literature. *Canadian Journal of Ophthalmology, 41,* 709–721.

First Nations and Inuit Health. (2010*). Aboriginal diabetes initiative.* Retrieved from *http://recherche-search.gc.ca/s_r?t3mpl 1t34d=1&s5t34d=health&l7c1l3=eng&S_08D4T.1ct57n=searc h&S_S20RCH.p1r1m3tr5cF53lds=hcyear%2Chcsubject%2Chctyp e%2Chcsource%2Chccollection&S_S20RCH.p1r1m3tr5cS7rt=Rev erseAlphabetical&S_08D4T.s3rv5c3=basic&S_m5m3typ3. sp3c5f53r=INDEX&S_m5m3typ3.t3xt6p3r1t7r=OR&S_ m5m3typ3.v1l93=html%2Fxhtml&S_S20RCH. d7csP3rP1g3=20&S_F8LLT2XT=diabetes+initiative&submit=Sea rch&S_S20RCH.l1ng91g3=eng.*

Gordon, K. D. (2012). The incidence of eye injuries in Canada. *Canadian Journal of Ophthalmology, 47*(4), 351–353. doi:10.1016/j.jcjo.2012.03.005 or *http://www.canadianjournalofophthalmology.ca/article/S0008-4182(12)00121-4/abstract.*

Kaiser, P. K., Friedman, N. J., & Pineda, R. (2003). *The Massachusetts Eye and Ear Infirmary illustrated manual of ophthalmology* (2nd ed.). Philadelphia: W.B. Saunders.

Noble, J., & Chaudhary, V. (2010). Age-related macular degeneration. *Canadian Medical Association Journal, 182*(16), 1759. doi:10.1503/cmaj090378

Noble, J., & Lloyd, J. C. (2011). The red eye. *Canadian Medical Association Journal, 183*(1), 81. doi:10.1503/cmaj.090379

Rudnicka, A. R., Zakariya, J., Wormald, R., Cook, D. G., Fletcher, A., & Owen, C. G. (2011). Age and gender variations in age-related macular degeneration prevalence in populations of European ancestry: A meta-analysis. *Ophthalmology, 119*(3), 571–580. doi:10.1016/j.ophtha.2011.09.027

U.S. National Library of Medicine. (2012). *Visual acuity test.* Retrieved from *http://www.nlm.nih.gov/medlineplus/ency/ article/003396.htm.*

Web Sites of Interest

Canadian National Institute for the Blind: *http://www.cnib.ca/*

Canadian Ophthalmological Society: *http://www.cos-sco.ca/ clinical-practice-guidelines/*

Canadian Paediatric Society: Vision Screening in Children: *http://www.cps.ca/en/documents/position/children-vision-screening*

Written by Carolyn Jarvis, PhD, APN, CNP
Adapted by June MacDonald-Jenkins, RN, BScN, MSc

evolve WEBSITE

OUTLINE

STRUCTURE AND FUNCTION

The ear is the sensory organ for hearing and maintaining equilibrium. The ear has three parts: the external, middle, and inner ears. The external ear is called the **auricle,** or **pinna,** and consists of movable cartilage and skin (Figure 16-1). Note the landmarks of the pinna, and use these terms to describe your findings. The mastoid process—the bony prominence behind the lobule—is not part of the ear but is an important landmark.

EXTERNAL EAR

The external ear has a characteristic shape and serves to funnel sound waves into its opening, the **external auditory canal** (Figure 16-2). The canal is a cul-de-sac 2.5 to 3 cm long in adults and terminates at the eardrum, or tympanic

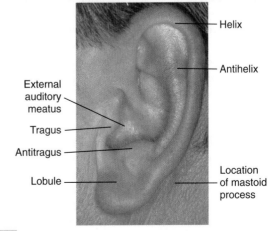

16-1 Auricle, or pinna.

Helix

Antihelix

External auditory meatus

Tragus

Antitragus

Lobule

Location of mastoid process

Structure & Function

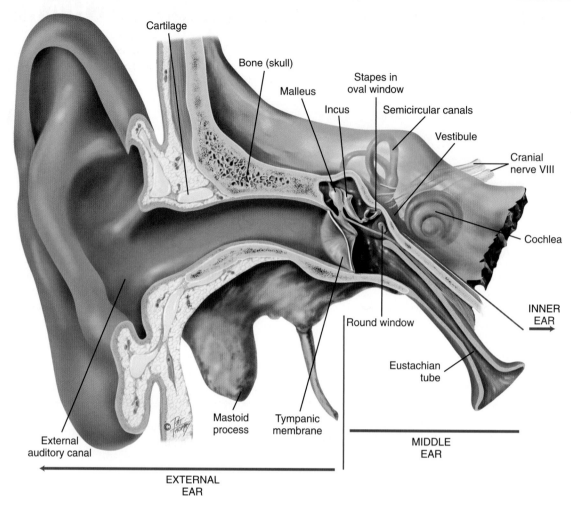

Cartilage

Bone (skull)

Malleus

Incus

Stapes in oval window

Semicircular canals

Vestibule

Cranial nerve VIII

Cochlea

INNER EAR

Round window

Eustachian tube

Mastoid process

Tympanic membrane

MIDDLE EAR

External auditory canal

EXTERNAL EAR

16-2

© Pat Thomas, 2010.

membrane. The canal is lined with glands that secrete cerumen, a yellow waxy material that lubricates and protects the ear. The wax forms a sticky barrier that helps keep foreign bodies from entering and reaching the sensitive eardrum. Cerumen migrates out to the meatus by the movements of chewing and talking.

The outer third of the canal is cartilage; the inner two thirds consists of bone covered by thin sensitive skin. The canal has a slight S-shaped curve in the adult. The outer third curves up and toward the back of the head, whereas the inner two thirds angle down and forward toward the nose.

The **tympanic membrane,** or **eardrum,** separates the external ear and middle ear and is tilted obliquely to the ear canal, facing downward and somewhat forward. It is a translucent, pearly grey membrane in which a prominent cone of light in the anteroinferior quadrant is the reflection of the otoscope light (Figure 16-3). The eardrum is oval and slightly concave, pulled in at its centre by one of the middle ear ossicles, the **malleus.** The parts of the malleus show through the translucent eardrum; these are the **umbo,** the **manubrium** (handle), and the **short process.** The small, slack, superior section of the eardrum is called the **pars flaccida.** The remainder of the eardrum, which is thicker and more taut, is the **pars tensa.** The **annulus** is the outer fibrous rim of the eardrum.

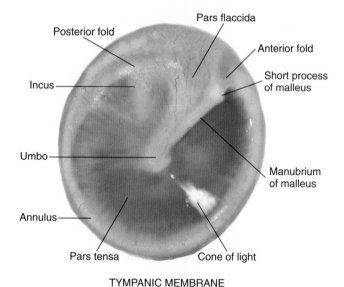

Posterior fold

Pars flaccida

Anterior fold

Short process of malleus

Incus

Umbo

Manubrium of malleus

Annulus

Pars tensa

Cone of light

TYMPANIC MEMBRANE

16-3 Tympanic membrane (eardrum).

Lymph fluid of the external ear drains into the parotid, mastoid, and superficial cervical nodes.

MIDDLE EAR

The middle ear is a tiny air-filled cavity inside the temporal bone (see Figure 16-2). It contains tiny ear bones, or auditory ossicles: the **malleus, incus,** and **stapes.** The middle ear has several openings. Its opening to the outer ear is covered by the eardrum. The openings to the inner ear are the oval window at the end of the stapes and the round window. Another opening is the **eustachian tube,** which connects the middle ear with the nasopharynx and allows passage of air. The tube is normally closed, but it opens with swallowing or yawning.

The middle ear has three functions: (a) It conducts sound vibrations from the outer ear to the central hearing apparatus in the inner ear, (b) it protects the inner ear by reducing the amplitude of loud sounds, and (c) its eustachian tube allows equalization of air pressure on each side of the eardrum so that the membrane does not rupture (e.g., during altitude changes in an airplane).

INNER EAR

The inner ear contains the **bony labyrinth,** which holds the sensory organs for equilibrium and hearing. Within the bony labyrinth, the **vestibule** and the **semicircular canals** constitute the vestibular apparatus, and the **cochlea** (Latin for "snail shell") contains the central hearing apparatus. Although the inner ear is not accessible to direct examination, its functions can be assessed.

HEARING

With regard to the function of hearing, the auditory system can be divided into three levels: peripheral, brain stem, and cerebral cortex. At the peripheral level, the ear transmits sound and converts its vibrations into electrical impulses, which can be analyzed by the brain. For example, suppose you hear an alarm bell ringing. Its sound waves travel instantly to your ears. The *amplitude* is how loud the alarm is; its *frequency* is the pitch (in this case, high), or the number of cycles per second. The sound waves produce vibrations on your eardrum. These vibrations are carried by the middle ear ossicles to the oval window. Then the sound waves travel through the cochlea, which is coiled like a snail's shell, and are dissipated against the round window. Along the way, the **basilar membrane** vibrates at a point specific to the frequency of the sound. In this case, the alarm's high frequency stimulates the basilar membrane at its base near the stapes (Figure 16-4). The numerous fibres along the basilar membrane are the receptor hair cells of the **organ of Corti,** the sensory

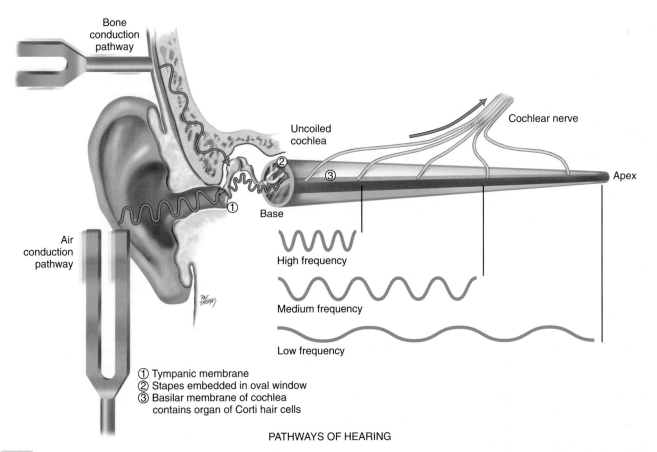

① Tympanic membrane
② Stapes embedded in oval window
③ Basilar membrane of cochlea
    contains organ of Corti hair cells

PATHWAYS OF HEARING

16-4 Pathways of hearing.

© *Pat Thomas, 2006.*

organ of hearing. As the hair cells bend, they mediate the vibrations into electric impulses. The electrical impulses are conducted by the auditory portion of cranial nerve VIII to the brain stem.

The function at the brain stem level is *binaural interaction*, which enables a person to locate the direction of a sound in space, as well as identifying the sound. How does this work? Each ear is actually one half of the total sensory organ. The ears are located on each side of a movable head. The cranial nerve VIII from each ear sends signals to both sides of the brain stem. Areas in the brain stem are sensitive to differences in intensity and timing of the messages from the two ears, depending on the way the head is turned.

The function of the cortex is to interpret the meaning of the sound and begin the appropriate response. All this happens in the split second it takes you to react to the alarm.

Pathways of Hearing

The normal pathway of hearing is air conduction, described previously; it is the most efficient. An alternative route of hearing is by bone conduction, in which the bones of the skull vibrate. These vibrations are transmitted directly to the inner ear and to cranial nerve VIII.

Hearing Loss

Anything that obstructs the transmission of sound impairs hearing. A **conductive hearing loss** involves a mechanical dysfunction of the external or middle ear. It is a partial loss because the person is able to hear if the sound amplitude is increased enough to reach normal nerve elements in the inner ear. Conductive hearing loss may be caused by impacted cerumen, foreign bodies, a perforated eardrum, pus or serum in the middle ear, or otosclerosis (a decrease in mobility of the ossicles).

Sensorineural hearing loss (or perceptive loss) signifies disease of the inner ear, cranial nerve VIII, or the auditory areas of the cerebral cortex. A simple increase in amplitude may not enable the person to understand words. Sensorineural hearing loss may be caused by *presbycusis*, a gradual nerve degeneration that occurs with aging, and by ototoxic drugs, which affect the hair cells in the cochlea.

A **mixed loss** is a combination of conductive and sensorineural types in the same ear.

Equilibrium

The labyrinth in the inner ear constantly feeds information to the brain about the body's position in space. It works like a plumb line to determine verticality or depth. The ear's plumb lines register the angle of your head in relation to gravity. If the labyrinth ever becomes inflamed, it feeds the wrong information to the brain, causing the person to have a staggering gait and a strong, spinning, whirling sensation called *vertigo*.

 DEVELOPMENTAL CONSIDERATIONS

Infants and Children

The inner ear starts to develop early in the fifth week of gestation. In early development, the ear is posteriorly rotated and low set; later it ascends to its normal placement around eye level. If maternal rubella infection occurs during the first trimester, it can damage the organ of Corti and impair hearing.

An infant's eustachian tube is relatively shorter and wider and its position is more horizontal than an adult's, and so it is easier for pathogens from the nasopharynx to migrate to the middle ear (Figure 16-5). The lumen is surrounded by lymphoid tissue, which increases during childhood; thus, the lumen is easily occluded. Because of these factors, infants are at greater risk for middle ear infections than are adults.

The external auditory canal is shorter in infants and young children than in adults, and its slope in children is opposite to that in adults (see Figure 16-5 on p. 345).

Adults

Otosclerosis is a common cause of conductive hearing loss in young adults between the ages of 20 and 40 years. It is a gradual hardening that causes the footplate of the stapes to become fixed in the oval window, which impedes the transmission of sound and causes progressive deafness.

Older Adults

In older adults, the cilia lining the ear canal become coarse and stiff. This may cause a decrease in hearing because it impedes sound waves travelling toward the eardrum. It also causes cerumen to accumulate and oxidize, which greatly reduces hearing. The cerumen itself is drier because of atrophy of the apocrine glands. Also, a life history of frequent ear infections may result in scarring on the eardrum.

Impacted cerumen is a common but reversible cause of hearing loss in older adults. After removal of cerumen, most people experience significant improvement in hearing ability. Nurses can improve the hearing health of older people by routinely performing otoscopic examinations and by performing ear canal irrigations when cerumen becomes impacted.

A person living in a noise-polluted area (e.g., near an airport or a busy highway) has a greater risk of hearing loss. However, **presbycusis** is a type of hearing loss that occurs with aging, even in people living in a quiet environment. It is a gradual sensorineural loss caused by nerve degeneration in the inner ear or auditory nerve. More than 50% of all Canadians older than 65 years have hearing loss. The affected person first notices difficulty hearing high-frequency tones; it is harder to hear consonants (high-pitched components of speech) than vowels. As a result, words sound garbled. The ability to localize sound is also impaired. This communication dysfunction is accentuated when distracting background

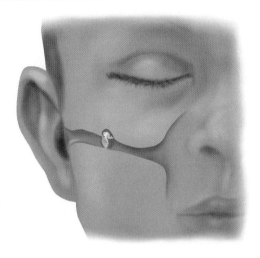
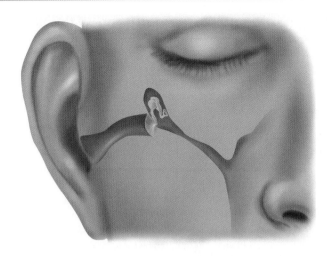

INFANT
Horizontal eustachian tube

ADULT
Sloped eustachian tube

16-5

noise is present (e.g., with music, with dishes clattering, or at a large, noisy party).

The Canadian Association of Speech-Language Pathologists and Audiologists (2011) recommends that hearing be tested every 3 years, starting at age 2, or earlier if language skills are not developing. Individuals who listen to very loud music (see the box Promoting Health: Use of Digital Music Players: Earbuds and Hearing Loss), work with high levels of industrial noise, or are older than 65 years should see an audiologist annually. There is significant evidence that neonatal hearing screening should be implemented as routine practice.

Local audiologists can test hearing and may refer patients to other health care providers on the basis of their findings. In a review of the literature, Patel and Feldman (2011) concluded that there is adequate evidence that children with an earlier diagnosis of hearing loss had improved expressive and receptive language scores. Updated evidence from multiple studies now indicate that infants who receive a diagnosis and intervention before 6 months of age score 20 to 40 percentile points higher on school-related measures (language, social adjustment, and behaviour) than do hearing-impaired children who do not receive intervention until later on (Patel & Feldman, 2011).

CULTURAL AND SOCIAL CONSIDERATIONS

Otitis media (middle ear infection) results from obstruction of the eustachian tube or of passage of nasopharyngeal secretions into the middle ear. Otitis media is one of the most common illnesses in children. The incidence and severity are especially high in children of Aboriginal descent. Rates of acute otitis media are significantly higher in Aboriginal populations than in other North American populations (Dallaire, Dewailly, Vézina, Bruneau, & Ayotte, 2006).

The incidence of otitis media is also increased among premature infants, among infants with Down's syndrome, and among infants fed by bottle in a supine position. In the supine position, the effects of gravity and sucking tend to draw the nasopharyngeal contents directly into the middle ear. Urge parents to hold the baby partly upright against the arm while feeding. Insruct parents to not prop the bottle or let the baby take a bottle to bed. Encouraging breastfeeding helps prevent this problem.

The most important side effect of acute otitis media is the persistence of fluid in the middle ear after treatment. This middle ear effusion can impair hearing, increasing the child's risk for delayed cognitive development.

Cerumen is genetically determined and comes in two major types: (a) dry cerumen, which is grey, flaky, and frequently forms a thin mass in the ear canal, and (b) wet cerumen, which is honey brown to dark brown and moist. Among individuals of Asian or Aboriginal descent, frequency of dry cerumen exceeds 80%, whereas among individuals of African or Euro-Canadian descent, the frequency of wet cerumen exceeds 97% (Overfield, 1995). The presence and composition of cerumen are not related to poor hygiene. Take caution to avoid mistaking the flaky, dry cerumen for eczematous lesions.

Almost 25% of all Canadians report some level of hearing loss, although about 10% of those identify themselves as "culturally deaf," "oral deaf," "deafened," or "hard of hearing." Hearing loss is the third most prevalent chronic condition in older adults. The Canadian Hearing Society (2011) created a series of position statements regarding the social and ethical dilemmas faced by Canadians with hearing loss. *Audism* is a form of discrimination based on a person's ability to hear or behave in the manner of people who hear. This is one of the primary issues faced by people with hearing impairments (see the Web site for the Canadian Hearing Society in the section Web Sites of Interest at the end of this chapter).

PROMOTING HEALTH: USE OF DIGITAL MUSIC PLAYERS: EARBUDS AND HEARING LOSS

Today, there is growing concern about the potential for hearing loss in young people who use digital music players and earbud headphones. Unlike earphones, which are placed over the ear, earbuds are placed directly in the ear canal, which causes the sound to be placed closer to the eardrum. Furthermore, because the sound is digital, there is virtually no distortion, no matter how loud one turns up the volume. Probably of most significance is that because digital music players can hold thousands of songs and can play for hours without recharging, users tend to listen continuously for hours at a time.

Hearing loss occurs slowly and often goes unnoticed until it is quite extensive; therefore, early prevention is the key. The risk of hearing loss increases as sound is played louder and for longer durations. For this reason, current research proposes the 60–60 rule: that individuals use their digital music players and earbuds for no more than 60 minutes a day at levels below 60% of maximum volume. Many experts are suggesting that digital music players be designed to prevent the playing of music above 90 dB, about 60% of the maximum volume (≈120 dB) of the typical digital music player today. Simply put, it means dialling down the volume to a "6" or lower and taking a break at least every hour. Other ways to avoid hearing loss include using larger headphones that rest over the ear opening and noise-cancelling headphones that eliminate background noise so that listeners do not have to increase the volume as high. It is often difficult to explain this to young people who abound with youthful optimism and tend not to worry about future damage. However, listening with earbuds boosts sound signals by as much as 6 to 9 dB, about the difference between the sound of a vacuum cleaner and a motorcycle.

The decibel scale is logarithmic; for example, 40 dB is 100 times as intense as 20 dB. Normal conversation takes place around 60 dB, whereas a chainsaw typically registers at 100 dB and a rock concert at 120 dB. Government minimum safety standards in Canada dictate that 85 dB for 8 hours daily is the limit for occupational exposure to noise. Adopted by several provinces across the country, these standards exist to protect workers from hearing loss in the workplace. As the decibel level increases, exposure time needs to be cut significantly.

Although people know not to look into the sun because its intense rays damage the eyes, people do not seem to realize that blasting their ears with intense sound is going to do damage, too. There is a certain irony in the appearance of young people donning sunglasses and earbuds.

Additional Resources

Blue, L. (2008). How bad are IPods for your hearing? Time Health & Family. Retrieved from http://www.time.com/time/health/article/0,8599,1827159,00.html.

Carter, L. (2010, May). Prevalence of hearing loss and its relationship to leisure-sound exposure: iHEAR. Paper presented at the Audiology Australia XIX National Conference, Sydney, Australia.

Gilliver, M., Carter, L., Macoun, D., Rosen, J., & Williams, W. (2012). Music to whose ears? The effect of social norms on young people's risk perceptions of hearing damage resulting from their music listening behavior. Noise and Health, 14(57), 47–51. doi:10.4103/1463-1741.95131

Health Canada. (2006). Hearing loss and leisure noise. Retrieved from http://www.hc-sc.gc.ca/iyh-vsv/environ/leisure-loisirs_e.html#is.

Selvin, J. (2005). Play it loud and you may pay for it: 4 Hearing Loss. Retrieved from http://www.4hearingloss.com/archives/2005/09/play_it_loud_an.html.

SUBJECTIVE DATA

1. Earache
2. Infections
3. Discharge
4. Hearing loss

5. Environmental noise
6. Tinnitus
7. Vertigo
8. Self-care behaviours

HEALTH HISTORY QUESTIONS

Examiner Asks	Rationale
1. Earache. Any **earache** or other pain in ears? • Location: Does it feel close to the surface or deep in the head? • Does it hurt when you push on the ear? • Character: Is it dull and aching or sharp and stabbing? Is it constant, or does it come and go? Is it affected by changing position of head? Ever had this kind of pain before? • Any accompanying cold symptoms or sore throat? Any problems with sinuses or teeth?	**Otalgia** (ear pain) may be caused directly by ear disease or may represent referred pain from a problem in the teeth or oropharynx. A virus/bacterium that causes upper respiratory tract infection may migrate up the eustachian tube to involve the middle ear.

Examiner Asks	Rationale

- Ever been hit on the ear or on the side of the head, or had any sport injury? Ever had any ear trauma from a foreign body?

Trauma may rupture the eardrum.

- What have you tried in order to relieve pain?

Assess effect of coping strategies.

2. **Infections.** Any ear **infections?** In adulthood or in childhood?

A history of chronic ear problems suggests possible sequelae.

- How frequent were they? How were they treated?
- How effective was treatment?

Repeated infections in childhood can result in progressive loss of hearing. The insertion of "tubes" (tympanoplasty) continues to be a procedure that is recommended, despite little evidence to support its benefit (reference to come).

3. **Discharge.** Any **discharge** from your ears?

Otorrhea (discharge) suggests infection of the canal or a perforated eardrum. For example:
- *External otitis:* purulent, sanguineous, or watery discharge

- Does it look like pus, or is it bloody?

- *Acute otitis media with perforation:* purulent discharge
- *Cholesteatoma:* dirty yellow or grey discharge with foul odour

- Any odour to the discharge?

With perforation: ear pain typically occurs first and stops with a popping sensation; then drainage occurs.

- Any relationship between the discharge and the ear pain?

4. **Hearing loss.** Ever had any trouble hearing?
- Onset: Did the loss come on slowly or all at once?
- Do you have a family history of otosclerosis?
- Character: Has all your hearing decreased, or just your hearing of certain sounds?

The onset of presbycusis is gradual (over years), whereas hearing loss caused by trauma is often sudden. Refer any sudden loss in one or both ears that is *not* associated with upper respiratory tract infection.

The onset of otosclerosis is generally during the second and third decades of life and is diagnosed on the basis of symptoms of conductive hearing loss. **Conductive hearing loss** is caused by fixation of the stapes (bone of the inner ear) and is present in approximately 10% of all cases. The amount of hearing loss is related directly to the degree of immobilization of the stapedial footplate (i.e., the more rigid the eardrum, the greater the hearing loss). The hearing loss may not be noticed in the early stages of otosclerosis.

- In what situations do you notice the loss: conversations, using the telephone, watching television, at a party?
- Do people seem to shout at you?

Loss is apparent when competition from background noise is present, as at a party.

Recruitment: a condition in which loss is marked when sound is initially at low intensity but actually becomes painful when repeated loudly.

- Do ordinary sounds seem hollow, as if you are hearing in a barrel or under water?
- Have you recently travelled by airplane?
- Any family history of hearing loss?
- Effort to treat: Have you tried any hearing aid or other device? Anything to help hearing?

Character of hearing loss is affected when cerumen expands and becomes impacted, as after swimming or showering.

Examiner Asks	Rationale
• Coping strategies: How does the loss affect your daily life? Any job problem? Do you feel embarrassed? Frustrated? How do your family and friends react?	Hearing loss can cause social isolation and can lessen pleasure in leisure activities.

Note to Examiner. During history documentation, note these clues from normal conversation with a patient that indicate possible hearing loss:
1. Lip reading or watching your face and lips closely rather than your eyes
2. Frowning or straining forward to hear
3. Posturing of head to catch sounds with better ear
4. Misunderstanding your questions or frequently asking you to repeat what you said
5. Acting irritable or showing startle reflex when you raise your voice (recruitment)
6. Speech sounding garbled; possible distortion of vowel sounds
7. Inappropriately loud voice
8. Flat, monotonous tone of voice

Examiner Asks	Rationale
5. **Environmental noise.** Any loud noises at home or on the job? For example, do you live in a noise-polluted area, near an airport, or near a busy traffic area? Now or in the past?	Old trauma to hearing initially goes unnoticed but results in further decibel loss in later years.
• Are you near other noises, such as heavy machinery, loud persistent music, gunshots (e.g., while hunting)?	
• Coping strategies: Have you taken any steps to protect your ears, such as using headphones or ear plugs?	
6. **Tinnitus.** Ever felt ringing, crackling, or buzzing in your ears? When did this occur?	Tinnitus originates within the person; it accompanies some hearing or ear disorders.
• Does it seem louder at night?	Tinnitus seems louder when there is no competition from environment noise.
• Are you taking any medications?	Many medications have ototoxic sequelae: aspirin, aminoglycosides (streptomycin, gentamicin, kanamycin, neomycin), ethacrynic acid, furosemide, indomethacin, naproxen, quinine, vancomycin, and local anaesthetic.
7. **Vertigo.** Ever felt **vertigo?** That is, do you feel the room spinning around or yourself spinning? (Vertigo is a true sensation of twirling.)	A true sensation of rotational spinning occurs with dysfunction of labyrinth. In **objective vertigo**, the person feels as if the room spins. In **subjective vertigo**, the person feels as if he or she spins.
• Ever felt dizzy, as if you are not quite steady, like falling or losing your balance? Giddy, lightheaded?	Distinguish true vertigo from dizziness or lightheadedness.
8. **Self-care behaviours.** How do you clean your ears?	Assess potential trauma from invasive instruments. Cotton-tipped applicators can cause impaction of cerumen, resulting in hearing loss.
• When was the last time you had your hearing checked?	Prescribe frequency of hearing assessment according to the patient's age or risk factors.
• If a hearing loss was noted, did you obtain a hearing aid? How long have you had it? Do you wear it? How does it work? Any trouble with upkeep, cleaning, or changing batteries?	

Examiner Asks	Rationale

Additional History for Infants and Children

1. **Ear Infections.** At what age was the child's first episode? How many ear infections in the last 6 months? How many total? How were these treated? How effective was the treatment?
   - Has the child had any surgery, such as insertion of ear tubes or removal of tonsils?
   - How effective was the surgical intervention?

   - Are the infections increasing in frequency, in severity, or staying the same?
   - Does anyone in the home smoke cigarettes?
   - Is there a wood-burning stove in your home?
   - Is the child breast or bottle fed? Does the child use a soother?
   - Does your child receive child care outside your home? In a day care centre or someone else's home? How many children in the group?

A first episode that occurs in the first 3 months of life increases risk of recurrent otitis media. Recurrent otitis media is three episodes in the past 3 months or four within the past year (Carlson, 2005). Children with recurrent otitis media are often prescribed low-dose long-term antibiotics for treatment, or tympanoplasty is indicated.

Removal of environmental factors is very effective in diminishing repeated infection.

The following factors are known to exacerbate infection:
- Soothers
- Bottle feeding
- Wood-burning homes
- Second-hand and gestational smoke
- Being in day care
- Exposure to cold (child should wear a hat)

2. **Hearing.** Does the child seem to be hearing well?
   - Have you noticed that the infant startles with loud noise? Did the infant start babbling at approximately 6 months of age? Does he or she talk? At what age did talking start? Was the speech intelligible?
   - Ever had the child's hearing tested? If there was a hearing loss, did it follow any diseases in the child or in the mother during pregnancy?

Children at risk for hearing deficit include those exposed to maternal rubella, syphilis, cytomegalovirus, toxoplasmosis, or maternal ototoxic drugs in utero; premature infants; infants of low birth weight; infants who suffered trauma or hypoxia at birth; and infants with congenital liver or kidney disease.

In children, an episode of meningitis, measles, mumps, otitis media, and any illness with persistent high fever may increase risk of hearing deficit.

On the basis of the available evidence, the Canadian Paediatric Society (Patel & Feldman, 2011) recommends hearing screening for all newborns.

3. **Injury.** Does the child tend to put objects in the ears? Is the older child or adolescent active in contact sports?

These children are at increased risk for trauma.

OBJECTIVE DATA

PREPARATION

An adult should be sitting up straight with his or her head at your eye level. On occasion, the ear canal is partially filled with cerumen, which obstructs your view of the eardrum. If the membrane is intact and no current infection is present, a preferred method of cleaning the adult canal is to soften the cerumen with a warmed solution of mineral oil and hydrogen peroxide. Then, with a bulb syringe or a low-pulsatile dental irrigator (Waterpik), irrigate the canal with warm water (body temperature). Direct water to the posterior wall. Leave space around the irrigator tip for water to escape. Do not irrigate if the history or the examination findings suggest perforation or infection.

EQUIPMENT NEEDED

Otoscope with bright light (fresh batteries give off white—not yellow—light)
Pneumatic bulb attachment, sometimes used with infants or young children

Normal Range of Findings	Abnormal Findings

INSPECT AND PALPATE THE EXTERNAL EAR

Size and Shape

The ears are of equal size bilaterally with no swelling or thickening. Ears of unusual size and shape may be a normal familial trait with no clinical significance.

Microtia: ears smaller than 4 cm vertically.

Macrotia: ears larger than 10 cm vertically.

Edema.

Skin Condition

The skin colour is consistent with the patient's facial skin colour. The skin is intact, with no lumps or lesions. On some people you may note **Darwin's tubercle**, a small painless nodule at the helix. This is a congenital variation and is not significant (Figure 16-6).

Reddened, excessively warm skin: indicates inflammation (see Table 16-2, p. 361).

Crusts and scaling: occur with otitis externa, eczema, contact dermatitis, seborrhea.

Enlarged, tender lymph nodes in the region: indicate inflammation of the pinna or mastoid process.

Red-blue discoloration: indicates frostbite.

Tophi, sebaceous cyst, chondrodermatitis, keloid, carcinoma (see Table 16-2, p. 361).

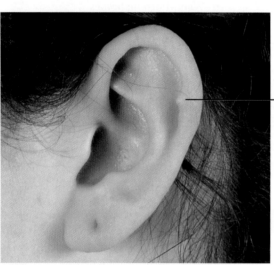
Darwin's tubercle

16-6

Tenderness

Move the pinna and push on the tragus. They should feel firm, and movement should produce no pain. Palpating the mastoid process should also produce no pain.

Pain with movement: occurs with otitis externa and furuncle.

Pain at the mastoid process: may indicate mastoiditis or lymphadenitis of the posterior auricular node.

The External Auditory Meatus

Note the size of the opening to direct your choice of speculum for the otoscope. No swelling, redness, or discharge should be present.

Atresia: absence or closure of the ear canal.

Sticky yellow discharge: accompanies otitis externa or may indicate otitis media if the eardrum has ruptured.

Impacted cerumen is a common cause of conductive hearing loss.

Some cerumen is usually present. The colour varies from grey-yellow to light brown and black, and the texture varies from moist and waxy to dry and desiccated. A large amount of cerumen obscures visualization of the canal and eardrum.

Objective Data

Normal Range of Findings

INSPECT WITH THE OTOSCOPE

As you inspect the external ear, note the size of the auditory meatus. Then choose the largest speculum that will fit comfortably in the ear canal, and attach it to the otoscope. Tilt the patient's head slightly away from you toward the opposite shoulder. This method brings the obliquely sloping eardrum into better view.

Pull the pinna up and back on adults or older children; this helps straighten the S-shaped curve of the canal (Figure 16-7). (Pull the pinna down on infants and children younger than 3 years [see Figure 16-14, p. 355]). Hold the pinna gently but firmly. Do not release traction on the ear until you have finished the examination and the otoscope is removed.

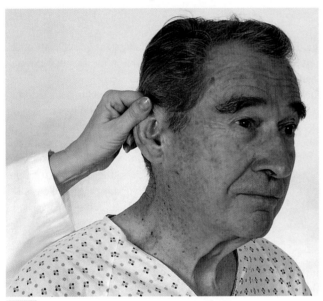

16-7

Hold the otoscope upside down along your fingers, and have the dorsa (back) of that hand along the patient's cheek braced to steady the otoscope (Figure 16-8). This position may feel awkward to you at first. It soon will feel natural, and you will find it useful in preventing forceful insertion. Also, your stabilizing hand acts as a protecting lever if the patient suddenly moves the head.

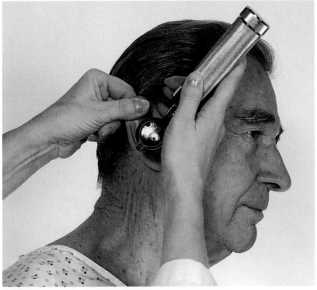

16-8

Abnormal Findings

Use caution when introducing the otoscope into an ear. Do not push the otoscope into the canal; this causes extreme pain for the patient and may result in damage to the canal. The otoscope should just "sit" in the canal. For better visualization, adjust the pinna to straighten out the canal.

Objective Data

Normal Range of Findings	Abnormal Findings

Insert the speculum slowly and carefully along the axis of the canal. Watch the insertion; then put your eye up to the otoscope. Avoid touching the inner (bony) section of the canal wall, which is covered by a thin epithelial layer and is sensitive to pain. Sometimes you cannot see anything but canal wall. If that is the case, try to reposition the patient's head, apply more traction on the pinna, and re-angle the otoscope to look forward toward the patient's nose.

Once it is in place, you may need to rotate the otoscope slightly to visualize all of the eardrum; do this gently. Perform the otoscopic examination before you test hearing; when ear canals have impacted cerumen, the hearing test will yield erroneous findings of pathological hearing loss.

The External Canal

Note any redness and swelling, lesions, foreign bodies, or discharge. If any discharge is present, note the colour and odour. (Also, clean any discharge from the speculum before examining the other ear, to avoid contamination with possibly infectious material.) For a patient with a hearing aid, note any irritation on the canal wall from poorly fitting ear moulds.

> Redness and swelling occur with otitis externa; the canal may be completely closed by swelling.
>
> Purulent otorrhea suggests otitis externa or otitis media if the eardrum has ruptured.
>
> Frank blood or clear, watery drainage (cerebrospinal fluid) after trauma suggests basal skull fracture and warrants immediate referral. Other abnormalities include foreign body, polyp, furuncle, and exostosis (see Table 16-3, pp. 362–363).

The Tympanic Membrane

Colour and Characteristics. Systematically explore the eardrum's landmarks (Figure 16-9). The normal eardrum is shiny and translucent, with pearly grey coloration. The cone-shaped light reflex is prominent in the anteroinferior quadrant (at the 5:00 position in the right eardrum and at the 7:00 position in the left eardrum). This light reflex is the reflection of your otoscope light. Sections of the malleus are visible through the translucent eardrum: the umbo, manubrium, and short process. (Infrequently, you also may see the incus behind the eardrum; it shows as a whitish haze in the upper posterior area.) At the periphery, the annulus looks whiter and denser.

> Yellow-amber eardrum discoloration: occurs with otitis media with effusion (serous).
>
> Redness: occurs with acute otitis media.
>
> Absence or distortion of landmarks.
>
> Air/fluid level or air bubbles behind eardrum: indicate otitis media with effusion (see Tables 16-4 and 16-5, p. 364 to p. 365).

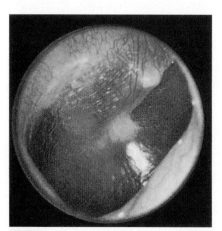

16-9   Normal tympanic membrane (right ear).

Normal Range of Findings	Abnormal Findings

Position. The eardrum is flat and slightly pulled in at the centre, and it flutters when the patient performs the Valsalva manoeuvre or holds the nose and swallows (insufflation). You may ask the patient to perform these manoeuvres so as to assess eardrum mobility. Avoid them with an older adult because they may disrupt equilibrium. In a patient with upper respiratory tract infection, also avoid middle ear insufflation because it could propel infectious matter into the middle ear.

> Retracted eardrum resulting from vacuum in middle ear with obstructed Eustachian tube.
> Bulging eardrum from increased pressure in otitis media.
> Eardrum hypomobility is an early sign of otitis media (see Table 16-5, p. 365).
> Perforation: a dark oval area or a larger opening on the eardrum (see Table 16-5, p. 365).

Integrity of Membrane. Inspect the eardrum and the entire circumference of the annulus for perforations. The normal tympanic membrane is intact. Some adults may show scarring, which is a dense white patch on the drum. This is a sequela of repeated ear infections.

TEST HEARING ACUITY

Your screening for a hearing deficit begins while you document the history; how well does the patient hear conversational speech? An audiometer gives a precise quantitative measure of hearing by assessing the patient's ability to hear sounds of varying frequency. Because this equipment is usually not available in the clinical setting, you may use alternative screening measures. These are "crude" tests, however; they are nonquantitative and do not measure the degree of loss, but they are useful for documenting the *presence* of hearing loss. Refer any abnormal findings for more accurate measures with pure tone audiometry.

Whispered Voice Test

To test one ear at a time, you must mask hearing in the other ear to prevent sound transmission around the head. To do this, place one finger on the tragus and rapidly push it in and out of the auditory meatus. Shield your lips so that the patient cannot compensate for a hearing loss (consciously or unconsciously) by lip reading or using the "good" ear. With your head 30 to 60 cm from the patient's ear, exhale and whisper slowly some two-syllable words, such as "Tuesday," "armchair," "baseball," and "fourteen." Normally, patients repeat each word correctly after you say it.

> Inability to hear whispered words (a whisper is a high-frequency sound and is used to detect high-tone loss).

Tuning Fork Tests

Tuning fork tests are used to measure hearing by air conduction or by bone conduction, in which the sound vibrates through the cranial bones to the inner ear. The air conduction route through the ear canal and middle ear is usually the more sensitive route. Traditionally, these tests have been taught for physical examination, but evidence shows that both the Weber and the Rinne tuning fork tests do not yield precise or reliable data (Bagai, Thavendiranathan, & Detsky, 2006). Thus, these tests should not be used for general screening.

THE VESTIBULAR APPARATUS

The **Romberg test** is an assessment of the ability of the vestibular apparatus in the inner ear to help maintain standing balance. Because the Romberg test is also used to assess intactness of the cerebellum and proprioception, it is discussed in Chapter 25 (see Figure 25-18, p. 675).

 ### DEVELOPMENTAL CONSIDERATIONS

Infants and Young Children

Examination of the external ear of an infant or a young child is similar to that described for an adult, with the addition of examination of position and alignment on head.

Normal Range of Findings	Abnormal Findings

Note the ear position. The top of the pinna should be horizontally aligned with the corner of the eye to the occiput. Also, the ear should be positioned within 10 degrees of vertical (Figure 16-10).

Low-set ears or deviation in alignment may indicate intellectual disability or a genitourinary malformation.

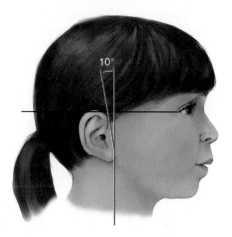

Normal alignment

16-10

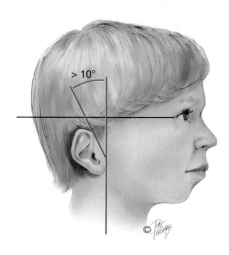

Low-set ears and deviation in alignment

© Pat Thomas, 2006.

Otoscopic Examination. In addition to its role in the complete examination, eardrum assessment is mandatory for any infant or child requiring care for illness or fever. For infants and young children, it is best to perform the otoscopic examination toward the end of the complete examination. Many young children protest vigorously during this procedure no matter how well you prepare, and it is difficult to reestablish cooperation afterward. Save the otoscopic examination until last. Then the parent can hold and comfort the child.

To help prepare the child, let the child hold your funny-looking "flashlight." You may wish to have the child look in the parent's ear as you hold the otoscope (Figure 16-11).

Ear pain and ear rubbing are associated with acute OM, as are a cloudy bulging eardrum and a distinctly red eardrum (Singh & Bond, 2006).

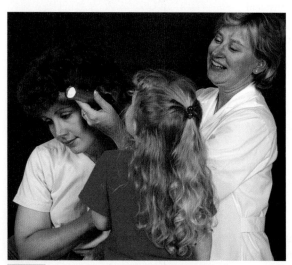

16-11

Normal Range of Findings	Abnormal Findings

Positioning of a child is important. You need a clear view of the canal. You should avoid harsh restraint, but you must protect the eardrum from injury in case of sudden head movement. Enlist the aid of a cooperative parent. Prop an infant upright against the parent's chest or shoulder, with the parent's arm around the upper part of the head (Figure 16-12). A toddler can be held in the parent's lap or may lie on the examining table with his or her arms gently secured (Figure 16-13). As you pull down on the pinna, gently push in on the child's tragus to ease insertion of the speculum tip. This sometimes helps avoid startling the child with a poke of the speculum tip.

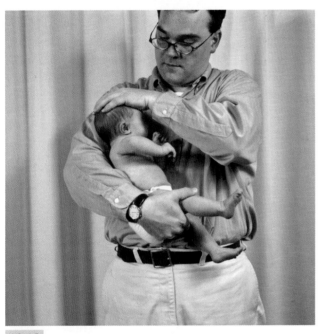

16-12

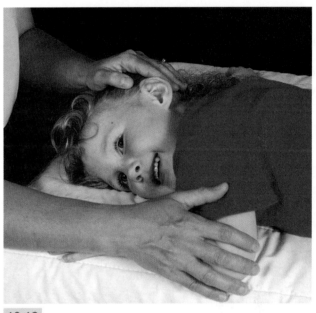

16-13

Remember to pull the pinna straight down on an infant or a child younger than 3 years. This method will help match the slope of the ear canal (Figure 16-14).

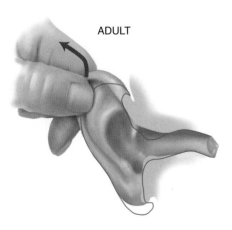

ADULT

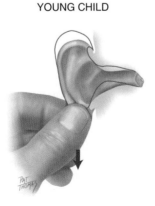

YOUNG CHILD

Adult—pull
pinna up and back

Infant/child under 3—pull
pinna straight down

16-14

Objective Data

Normal Range of Findings	**Abnormal Findings**

At birth, the patency of the ear canal is determined, but the otoscopic examination is not performed because the canal is filled with amniotic fluid and vernix caseosa. After a few days, the eardrum is examined. During the first few days, the eardrum often looks thickened and opaque. It may look infected and have a mild redness from increased vascularity. The eardrum also looks infected in infants after crying.

Atresia: absence or closure of the ear canal.

The position of the eardrum is more horizontal in the neonate, which makes it more difficult to see completely and harder to differentiate from the canal wall. By 1 month of age, the eardrum is in the oblique (more vertical) position, as in older children, and examination is a bit easier.

When you examine an infant or young child, use a pneumatic bulb attachment on the otoscope to direct a light puff of air toward the eardrum to assess its ability to vibrate (Figure 16-15). For a secure seal, choose the largest speculum that will fit in the ear canal without causing pain. A rubber tip on the end of the speculum gives a better seal. Give a small pump to the bulb (positive pressure), then release the bulb (negative pressure). Normally the eardrum moves inward with a slight puff and outward with a slight release.

Eardrums can turn pink when a child or an infant is crying. Use of the pneumatic bulb is the most reliable way to detect otitis media because with otitis media, there is little to no movement of the eardrum.

An abnormal response is no movement. Eardrum hypomobility indicates effusion or a high vacuum in the middle ear. For the newborn's first 6 weeks, eardrum immobility is the best indicator of middle ear infection.

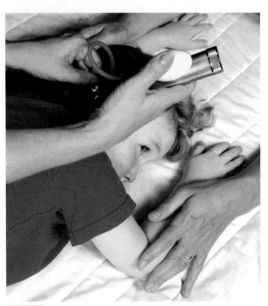

16-15

Normally the eardrum is intact. In a child being treated for chronic otitis media, you may note the presence of a tympanostomy tube in the central part of the eardrum. This is inserted surgically to equalize pressure and drain secretions. In addition, it is common, although not normal, to note a foreign body in a child's canal, such as a small stone or a bead.

Chronic otitis media relieved by tympanostomy tubes (see Table 16-3, p. 362).

Foreign body (see Table 16-3, p. 363).

Test Hearing Acuity. Use the developmental milestones mentioned in this section to assess hearing in an infant. Also, attend to the parents' concern over the infant's inability to hear; their assessment is usually well founded. The room should be silent and the baby contented. Make a loud sudden noise (hand clap or squeeze toy) out of the baby's peripheral range of vision of about 30 cm. You may need to repeat a few times, but you should note these responses:

Objective Data

Normal Range of Findings	Abnormal Findings

Normal Range of Findings

- Newborn: startle (Moro) reflex, acoustic blink reflex
- Ages 3 to 4 months: acoustic blink reflex; stopping movement and appearing to listen; halting sucking; quieting if crying, crying if quiet
- Ages 6 to 8 months: turning head to localize sound, responding to own name
- Preschool- and school-age children: must be screened with audiometry

Note that a young child may be unaware of a hearing loss because the child does not know what "ought" to be heard. Note these behavioural manifestations of hearing loss:

1. The child is inattentive in casual conversation.
2. The child reacts more to movement and facial expression than to sound.
3. The child's facial expression is strained or puzzled.
4. The child frequently asks to have statements repeated.
5. The child confuses words that sound alike.
6. The child has an accompanying speech problem: Speech is monotonous or garbled; the child mispronounces or omits sounds.
7. The child appears shy and withdrawn and "lives in a world of his or her own."
8. The child frequently complains of earaches.
9. The child hears better at times when the environment is more conducive to hearing.

Older Adults

An older adult may have pendulous earlobes with linear wrinkling because of loss of elasticity of the pinna. Coarse, wiry hairs may be present at the opening of the ear canal. During otoscopy, the eardrum normally may appear whiter, more opaque, and duller than in the younger adult. It also may look thickened.

A loss of hearing involving high-tone frequencies is apparent for those affected with presbycusis, the hearing loss that occurs with aging. This condition is manifested by difficulty hearing whispered words in the voice test and by difficulty hearing consonants during conversational speech. Many older adults believe that other people are "mumbling" and they feel isolated in family or friendship groups.

Abnormal Findings

- Absence of alerting behaviour: may indicate congenital deafness
- Failure to localize sound
- No intelligible speech by 2 years of age

DOCUMENTATION AND CRITICAL THINKING

Sample Charting

SUBJECTIVE

States hearing is good; no earaches, infections, discharge, hearing loss, tinnitus, or vertigo.

OBJECTIVE

Pinna: Skin intact with no masses, lesions, tenderness, or discharge.
Otoscope: External canals are clear with no redness, swelling, lesions, foreign body, or discharge. Both eardrums are pearly grey in colour, with light reflex and landmarks intact, no perforations.
Hearing: Responds appropriately to conversation.

ASSESSMENT

Healthy ear structures
Hearing accurate

Focused Assessment: Clinical Case Study 1

Jamal K. is a 9-month-old infant of African descent who is brought to the clinic by his mother because he "feels hot and was up crying all night."

History: Jamal is the third child of Mr. and Mrs. K. Mrs. K. received regular prenatal care. Jamal was born at 37 weeks' gestation; labour and delivery were uncomplicated. Jamal weighed 3200 g at birth, and was discharged 2 days after delivery. Jamal has been fed formula, with solids introduced at 5 months. Well-baby care has been regular; immunizations are up to date. Jamal has had two prior episodes of otitis media, no other illnesses.

Social History: Jamal lives with his family in a two-bedroom apartment over their grocery store and shares a bedroom with a 4-year-old brother and a 2-year-old brother. Mr. K. works full time in their grocery store; Mrs. K. provides child care in her own home for her children and for her sister's two young children. Both parents smoke cigarettes, one to two packs per day.

SUBJECTIVE

- 1 day PTA: Mrs. K. put Jamal down for nap with a bottle of juice, as is usual. Jamal woke up in the middle of the nap crying furiously. Quieted somewhat when held upright but still fussy. Took juice from bottle, refused solid baby food. Temperature 38°C rectally. Crying and fussy all night. Mrs. K. has given no medications to Jamal.

OBJECTIVE

Vital signs: Temp 38.4°C (tympanic), pulse 152, resp 36, Wt. 9.2 kg, Ht. 74 cm.
General: Alert, active, crying, and fussy. Developmentally appropriate for age.
Skin: Warm and dry, no rashes or lesions.
Head: Anterior fontanelle flat, 1×1.5 cm, posterior fontanelle closed.
Eyes: No exudate, conjunctivae clear, sclerae white, red reflex present bilaterally.
Ears: Both eardrums dull red and bulging, no light reflex, no mobility on pneumatic otoscopy.
Mouth/throat: Oral mucosa pink, no lesions or exudate, tonsils 1+.
Neck: Supple, no lymphadenopathy.
Heart: Regular rate and rhythm, no murmurs.
Lungs: Breath sounds clear and equal bilaterally, unlaboured.
Abdomen: Bowel sounds present, abdomen soft, nontender.

ASSESSMENT

Acute otitis media, both ears
Pain R/T inflammation in eardrums
Risk for ear infection injury R/T supine formula feeding, group child care, second-hand smoke
Deficient knowledge (parents) R/T lack of exposure to risk factors for otitis media

Focused Assessment: Clinical Case Study 2

Todd R. is a 15-year-old high school student who comes to the health centre to seek care for "cough off and on all winter and earache since last night."

SUBJECTIVE

Six weeks PTA: Nonproductive cough throughout day, no fever, no nasal congestion, no chest soreness. Todd's father gave him an over-the-counter decongestant, which helped, but cough continued off/on since. Does not smoke.

One day PTA: Intermittent cough continues, nasal congestion and thick white mucus. Also earache R ear, treated self with recommended dose of Tylenol, pain unrelieved. Pain is moderate, not deep and throbbing. Says R ear feels full, "hollow headed," voices sound muffled and far away, switches telephone to L ear to talk. No sore throat, no fever, no chest congestion or soreness.

OBJECTIVE

Vital signs: Temp 37°C oral, pulse 76, BP 106/72
Ears: L ear, canal, eardrum normal, R ear and canal normal, R eardrum retracted, with multiple air bubbles, eardrum colour is yellow/amber. No sinus tenderness.
Nose: Turbinates bright red and swollen, mucopurulent discharge.
Throat: Not reddened, tonsils 1+.
Neck: One R anterior cervical node enlarged, firm, movable, tender. All others not palpable.
Lungs: Breath sounds clear to auscultation, resonant to percussion throughout.

ASSESSMENT

Serous otitis media, R ear, with mild upper respiratory tract infection
Transient conductive hearing loss
Disturbed sensory perception (auditory) R/T excessive fluid in middle ear
Pain R/T middle ear pressure

Focused Assessment: Clinical Case Study 3

Emma S., 78 years old, has a medical diagnosis of angina pectoris, which has responded to nitroglycerin PRN [as needed] and periods of rest between activity. She has been independent in her own home, is coping well with activity restrictions through help from neighbours and family. Now hospitalized for evaluation of acute chest pain episode; MI [myocardial infarction] has been ruled out, pain diagnosed as angina, to be released to own home with a β-blocking medication and nitroglycerin PRN.

Just before this hospitalization, Mrs. S. received a hearing aid after evaluation by audiologist at senior centre. Mrs. S. was born in Germany, immigrated to Canada at age 5 years, considers English her primary language.

SUBJECTIVE

Since this hospitalization, feels "irritable and nervous." Relates this to worry about heart and also, "I get so mixed up in here, this room is so strange, and I just can't hear the nurses. They talk like cavemen, 'oo-i-ee-uou.'" Tried using her new hearing aid but no relief. "It just kept screeching in my ear, and it made the monitor beep so loud it drove me crazy." States no tinnitus, no vertigo.

OBJECTIVE

Ears: Pinna with elongated lobes but no tenderness to palpation, no discharge, no masses or lesions. Both canals clear of cerumen. Both eardrums appear grey-white, slightly opaque, and dull, although all landmarks visible. No perforation.
Hearing: Difficulty hearing room conversation. Unable to hear whispered voice bilaterally.

ASSESSMENT

Chest pain/angina pectoris
Deficient knowledge R/T lack of teaching about hearing aid
Disturbed sensory perception (auditory) R/T effects of aging
Anxiety R/T change in cardiovascular health status and inability to communicate effectively

Documentation &
Critical Thinking

ABNORMAL FINDINGS

TABLE 16-1 Abnormalities of the External Ear

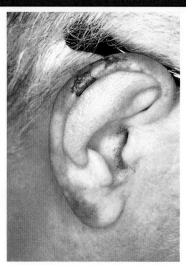

Source: From the Clinical Slide Collection on the Rheumatic Diseases, © 1991, 1995, 1997. Used by permission of the American College of Rheumatology.

Frostbite

Reddish blue discoloration and swelling of pinna after exposure to extreme cold. Vesicles or bullae may develop, the patient feels pain and tenderness, and ear necrosis may ensue.

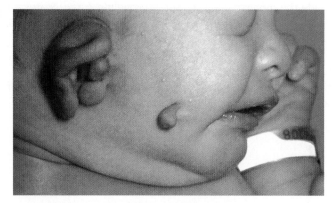

Branchial Remnant and Ear Deformity

A facial remnant or leftover of the embryological branchial arch usually appears as a skin tag; in the infant pictured, it contains cartilage. These tags occur most often in the preauricular area, in front of the tragus. When bilateral, there is increased risk of renal anomalies.

Cerebrospinal Fluid Otorrhea (not illustrated)

Skull fracture of temporal bone causes cerebrospinal fluid to leak from ear canal and pool in concha when the patient is supine. Cerebrospinal fluid feels oily and tests positive for glucose.

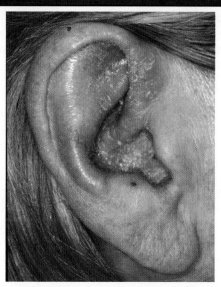

Otitis Externa (Swimmer's Ear)

An infection of the outer ear, with severe pain on movement of the pinna and tragus, redness and swelling of pinna and canal, scanty purulent discharge, scaling, itching, fever, and enlarged tender regional lymph nodes. Hearing is normal or slightly diminished. More common in hot, humid weather. Swimming causes canal to become waterlogged and swell; skinfolds are set up for infection. Prevent by using rubbing alcohol or 2% acetic acid eardrops after every swim.

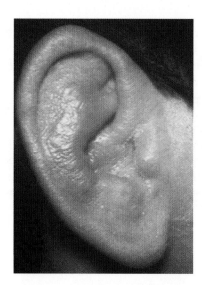

Cellulitis

Inflammation of loose, subcutaneous connective tissue. It manifests as thickening and induration of pinna with distorted contours.

TABLE 16-2   Lumps and Lesions on the External Ear

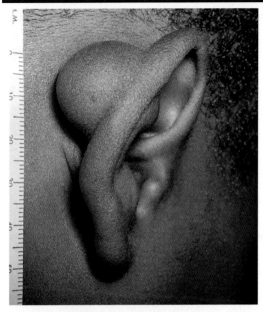

Sebaceous Cyst

Location is commonly behind lobule, in the postauricular fold. A nodule with central black punctum indicates blocked sebaceous gland. It is filled with waxy sebaceous material and is painful if it becomes infected. Often are multiple.

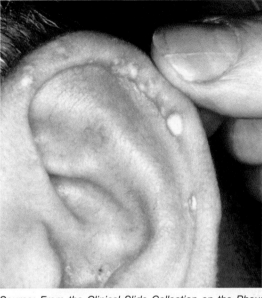

Source: From the Clinical Slide Collection on the Rheumatic Diseases, © 1991, 1995, 1997. Used by permission of the American College of Rheumatology.

Tophi

Small, whitish yellow, hard, nontender nodules in or near helix or antihelix; contain greasy, chalky material of uric acid crystals and are a sign of gout.

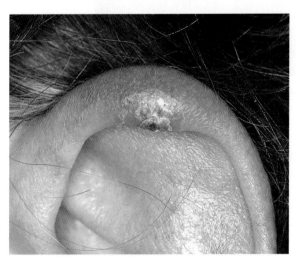

Chondrodermatitis Nodularis Helicis

Painful nodules that develop on the rim of the helix (which has no cushioning subcutaneous tissue) as a result of repetitive mechanical pressure or environmental trauma (sunlight). Small, indurated, dull red, poorly defined, and very painful.

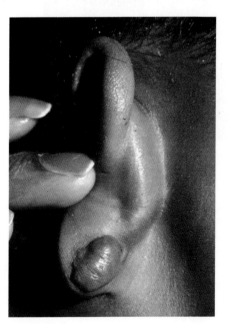

Keloid

Overgrowth of scar tissue, which invades original site of trauma. It is more common in dark-skinned people, although it also occurs in individuals with light skin. In the ear it is most common at lobule at the site of an ear piercing. Keloid shown here is unusually large.

Continued

TABLE 16-2   Lumps and Lesions on the External Ear—cont'd

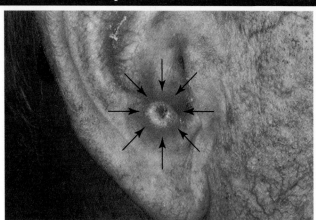

◄ *Carcinoma*
Ulcerated crusted nodule with indurated base that fails to heal. Bleeds intermittently. Must refer for biopsy. Usually occurs on the superior rim of the pinna, which has the most sun exposure. May occur also in ear canal and exude chronic discharge that is either serosanguineous or bloody.

TABLE 16-3   Abnormalities in the Ear Canal

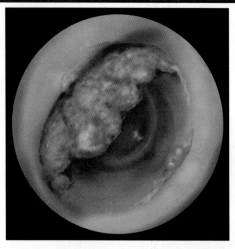

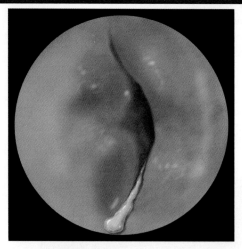

Excessive Cerumen
Excessive cerumen is produced or is impacted because canal is narrow and tortuous or as a result of poor cleaning method. May appear as round ball partially obscuring eardrum or totally occluding canal. Even when canal is 90%–95% blocked, hearing stays normal; when last 5%–10% is totally occluded (when cerumen expands after swimming or showering), patient has sensation of ear fullness and sudden hearing loss.

Otitis Externa
Severe swelling of canal, inflammation, tenderness. In this illustration, canal lumen is narrowed to one fourth of normal size. (See complete description in Table 16-2, p. 360.)

TABLE 16-3   Abnormalities in the Ear Canal—cont'd

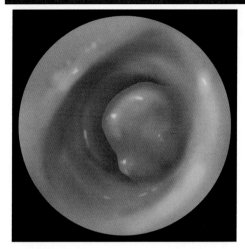

Osteoma

Single, stony hard, rounded nodule that obscures the eardrum; nontender; overlying skin appears normal. Attached to inner third (the bony part) of canal. Benign, but should be referred for removal.

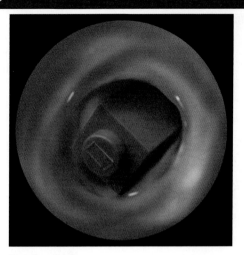

Foreign Body

Usually children are the patients who place a foreign body in the ear (here, an obstruction completely occludes the canal), which is later noted on routine examination. Common objects are beans, corn, breakfast cereals, jewellery beads, small stones, and sponge rubber. Cotton is most common in adults and becomes impacted from cotton-tipped applicators. A trapped live insect is uncommon but makes the patient especially frantic.

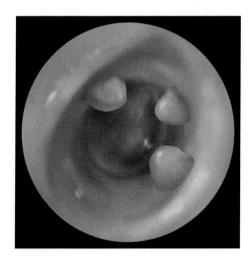

Exostosis

More common than osteoma. Small, hard, rounded nodules of hypertrophic bone, covered with normal epithelium. They arise near the eardrum but usually do not obstruct the view of the eardrum. They are usually multiple and bilateral. They may occur more frequently in cold-water swimmers. The condition needs no treatment, although it may cause accumulation of cerumen, which blocks the canal.

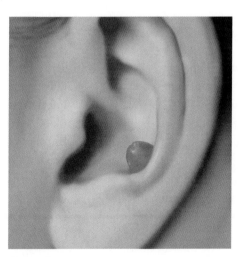

Furuncle

Exquisitely painful, reddened, infected hair follicle. In this illustration, it is on the tragus, but it also may be on cartilaginous part of ear canal. Regional lymphadenopathy often accompanies a furuncle.

Continued

TABLE 16-3   Abnormalities in the Ear Canal—cont'd

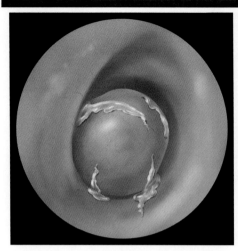

◄ *Polyp*

Arises in canal from granulomatous or mucosal tissue; redder than surrounding skin and bleeds easily; bathed in foul purulent discharge; indicates chronic ear disease. Benign, but should be referred for excision.

Images © Pat Thomas, 2010.

TABLE 16-4   Abnormal Findings Seen on Otoscopy

Appearance of Eardrum	Indicates	Suggested Condition
Yellow-amber colour	Serum or pus	Serous otitis media or chronic otitis media
Prominent landmarks	Retraction of eardrum	Negative pressure in middle ear from obstruction of eustachian tube
Air/fluid level or air bubbles	Serous fluid	Serous otitis media
Absence or distortion of light reflex	Bulging of eardrum	Acute otitis media
Bright red colour	Infection in middle ear	Acute purulent otitis media
Blue or dark red colour	Blood behind eardrum	Trauma, skull fracture
Dark oval areas	Perforation	Eardrum rupture
White, dense areas	Scarring	Sequelae of infections
Diminished or absence of landmarks	Thickened eardrum	Chronic otitis media
Black or white dots on eardrum or canal	Colony of growth	Fungal infection

Source: Adapted from Sherman, J. L., & Fields, S. K. (1988). *Guide to patient evaluation* (5th ed.). New York: Medical Examination Publishing. Reprinted by permission of Elsevier, Inc.

TABLE 16-5   Abnormal Tympanic Membranes

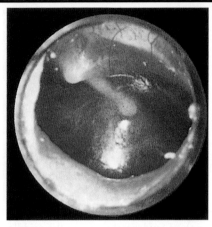

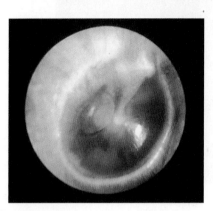

Retracted Eardrum

Landmarks look more prominent and well defined. Malleus handle looks shorter and more horizontal than normal. Short process is very prominent. Light reflex is absent or distorted. The eardrum is dull and lustreless and does not move. These signs indicate negative pressure and middle ear vacuum caused by obstruction of eustachian tube and serous otitis media.

Otitis Media With Effusion

An amber-yellow eardrum suggests serum in middle ear that transudates to relieve negative pressure from the blocked eustachian tube. Air/fluid level may be present with fine black dividing line or air bubbles visible behind eardrum. Symptoms are sensation of fullness, transient hearing loss, popping sound with swallowing. Also called *serous otitis media, glue ear.*

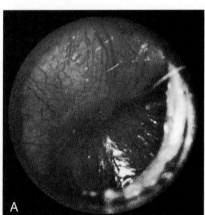

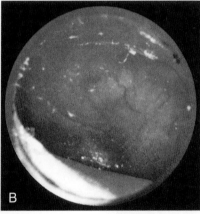

Early stage   Later stage

Acute (Purulent) Otitis Media

This results when the middle ear fluid is infected. Absence of light reflex as a result of increasing middle ear pressure is an early sign. Redness and bulging are first noted in superior part of eardrum (pars flaccida; left photo), along with earache and fever. Then fiery redness and bulging of entire eardrum (right photo), deep throbbing pain, fever, and transient hearing loss occur. Pneumatic otoscopy reveals eardrum hypomobility.

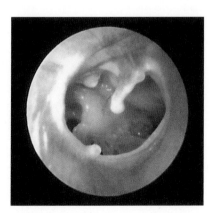

◄ Perforation

If the acute otitis media is not treated, the eardrum may rupture as a result of increased pressure. Perforations are also caused by trauma (e.g., a slap on the ear). Usually the perforation appears as a round or oval darkened area on the eardrum, but in this photo, the perforation is very large. *Central* perforations occur in the pars tensa. *Marginal* perforations occur at the annulus. When marginal perforations occur in superior part of the eardrum (the pars flaccida), they are called *attic perforations.*

Continued

TABLE 16-5   Abnormal Tympanic Membranes—cont'd

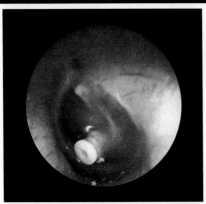

Source: From Fireman, P. (1995). Atlas of allergies (2nd ed., p. 182). St. Louis: Mosby.

Insertion of Tympanostomy Tubes

Polyethylene tubes are inserted surgically into the eardrum to relieve middle ear pressure and promote drainage of fluid from chronic or recurrent middle ear infections. Number of acute infections tends to decrease because of improved aeration. Tubes are extruded spontaneously in 12–18 months.

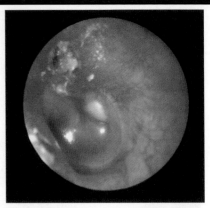

Cholesteatoma

An overgrowth of epidermal tissue in the middle ear or temporal bone may result over the years after a marginal tympanic membrane perforation. It has a pearly white, cheesy appearance. Growth of cholesteatoma can erode bone and produce hearing loss. Early signs include otorrhea, unilateral conductive hearing loss, tinnitus.

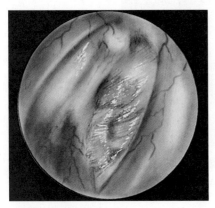

Scarred Eardrum

Dense white patches on the eardrum are sequelae of repeated ear infections. They do not necessarily affect hearing.

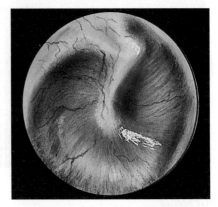

Blue Eardrum (Hemotympanum)

This indicates the presence of blood in the middle ear, as occurs when trauma results in skull fracture.

TABLE 16-5   Abnormal Tympanic Membranes—cont'd

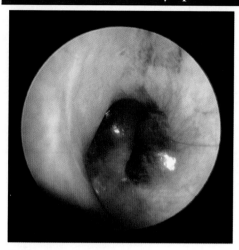

Bullous Myringitis

Small vesicles containing blood on the eardrum accompany *Mycoplasma pneumoniae* and virus infections. Affected patients may have blood-tinged discharge and severe otalgia.

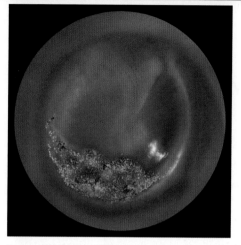

Fungal Infection (Otomycosis)

Colony of black or white dots on eardrum or canal wall suggests a yeast or fungal infection.

Summary Checklist: Ear Examination

For a PDA-downloadable version, go to *http://evolve.elsevier.com/Canada/Jarvis/examination/*.

1. Inspect external ear:
   Size and shape of pinna
   Position and alignment on head
   Skin condition: colour, lumps, lesions
   Movement of pinna and tragus (check for tenderness)
   External auditory meatus: size, swelling, redness, discharge, cerumen, lesions, foreign bodies

2. Otoscopic examination:
   External canal
   Cerumen, discharge, foreign bodies, lesions
   Redness or swelling of canal wall

3. Inspect eardrum:
   Colour and characteristics
   Position (flat, bulging, retracted)
   Integrity of membrane

4. Test hearing acuity:
   Behavioural response to conversational speech
   Voice test

5. Teaching and health promotion

Abnormal Findings

REFERENCES

Bagai, A., Thavendiranathan, P., & Detsky, A. (2006). Does this patient have hearing impairment? *Journal of the American Medical Association, 29,* 416–428.

Canadian Association of Speech-Language Pathologists and Audiologists. (2011). *CASLPA position paper on universal newborn hearing screening in Canada* (pp. 1–9). Retrieved from *http://www.caslpa.ca/PDF/position%20papers/ Universal_Newborn_Hearing_Screening_Position_ Paper_2010.pdf.*

Canadian Hearing Society. (2011). *The Canadian Hearing Society position paper on discrimination and audism.* Retrieved from *http://www.chs.ca/index.php?option=com_content&view=article &id=517%3Aposition-paper-on-discrimination-and- audism&catid=202%3Aposition-papers&Itemid=488&lang=en.*

Carlson, L. (2005). Otitis media: New information on an old disease. *Nurse Practitioner, 30,* 31–43.

Dallaire, F., Dewailly, E., Vézina, C., Bruneau S., & Ayotte, P. (2006). Portrait of outpatient visits and hospitalizations for acute infections in Nunavik preschool children. *Canadian Journal of Public Health, 97,* 362–368.

Overfield, T. (1995). *Biologic variation in health and illness: Race, age, and sex differences* (2nd ed.). New York: CRC Press.

Patel H., & Feldman, M. (2011). Universal newborn hearing screening. *Paediatrics & Child Health, 16*(5), 301–305. Retrieved from *http://www.cps.ca/english/statements/CP/ cp11-02.htm#Recommendations.*

Singh, A., & Bond, B. L. (2006). Does this child have acute otitis media? *Annals of Emergency Medicine, 47,* 113–116.

Web Sites of Interest

Canadian Hearing Society: *http://www.chs.ca*

CHAPTER

17

Nose, Mouth, and Throat

Written by Carolyn Jarvis, PhD, APN, CNP
Adapted by Barbara Wilson-Keates, RN, MS

evolve WEBSITE

http://evolve.elsevier.com/Canada/Jarvis/examination/
- Animations
- Bedside Assessment Summary Checklist
- Examination Review Questions
- Health Promotion Guide:
  - Chewing Tobacco
- Key Points
- Physical Examination Summary Checklist
- Quick Assessment for Common Conditions:
  - Rhinovirus (Common Cold)
- Video—Assessment:
  - Nose, Mouth, and Throat

OUTLINE

STRUCTURE AND FUNCTION

NOSE

The **nose** is the first segment of the respiratory system. It warms, moistens, and filters the inhaled air, and it is the sensory organ for smell. The external nose is shaped like a triangle with one side attached to the face (Figure 17-1). On its leading edge, the superior part is the *bridge,* and the free corner is the *tip.* The oval openings at the base of the triangle are the *nares;* just inside, each naris widens into the *vestibule.* The *columella* divides the two nares and is continuous inside with the nasal septum. The *ala* is the lateral outside wing of the nose on either side. The upper third of the external nose is made up of bone; the rest is cartilage.

Inside, the **nasal cavity** is much larger than the external size of the nose would indicate (Figure 17-2). It extends back over the roof of the mouth. The anterior edge of the cavity is lined with numerous coarse nasal hairs *(vibrissae).* The rest of the cavity is lined with a blanket of ciliated mucous membrane. The nasal hairs filter the coarsest matter from inhaled air, whereas the mucous blanket filters out dust and bacteria. Nasal mucosa appears redder than oral mucosa because of the rich blood supply present to warm the inhaled air.

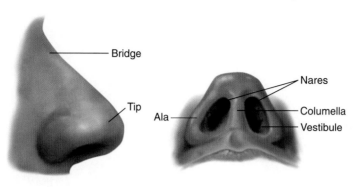

17-1 External nasal structures.

© Pat Thomas, 2006.

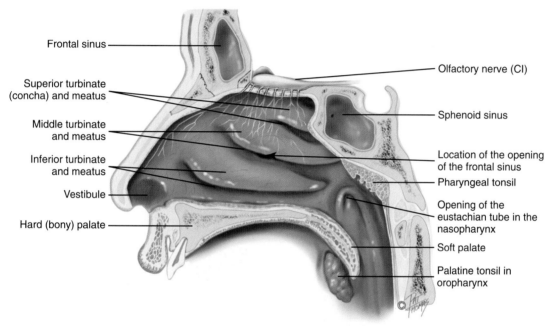

RIGHT LATERAL WALL - NASAL CAVITY

17-2

© Pat Thomas, 2006.

The nasal cavity is divided medially by the **septum** into two slitlike air passages. The anterior part of the septum holds a rich vascular network, *Kiesselbach's plexus,* the most common site of nosebleeds. In many people, the nasal septum is not absolutely straight and may deviate to one side.

The lateral walls of each nasal cavity contain three parallel bony projections: the superior, middle, and inferior **turbinates.** They increase the surface area so that more blood vessels and mucous membranes are available to warm, humidify, and filter the inhaled air. Underlying each turbinate is a cleft, the **meatus,** which is named for the turbinate above. The sinuses drain into the middle meatus, and tears from the nasolacrimal duct drain into the inferior meatus.

The olfactory receptors (hair cells) lie at the roof of the nasal cavity and in the upper one third of the septum. These receptors for smell merge into the olfactory nerve, cranial nerve I, which transmits impulses to the temporal lobe of the brain. Although it is not necessary for human survival, the sense of smell adds to nutrition by enhancing the pleasure and taste of food.

The **paranasal sinuses** are air-filled pockets within the cranium (Figure 17-3). They communicate with the nasal cavity and are lined with the same type of ciliated mucous membrane. They lighten the weight of the skull bones, serve as resonators for sound production, and provide mucus, which drains into the nasal cavity. The sinus openings are narrow and easily occluded, which may cause inflammation or sinusitis.

Two pairs of sinuses are accessible to examination: the **frontal sinuses,** in the frontal bone above and medial to the orbits, and the **maxillary sinuses,** in the maxilla (cheekbone) along the side walls of the nasal cavity. The other two sets are smaller and deeper: the **ethmoid sinuses,** between the orbits, and the **sphenoid sinuses,** deep within the skull in the sphenoid bone.

Only the maxillary and ethmoid sinuses are present at birth. The maxillary sinuses reach full size after all permanent teeth have erupted. The ethmoid sinuses grow rapidly between ages 6 and 8 years of age and after puberty. The frontal sinuses are absent at birth, are fairly well developed between 7 and 8

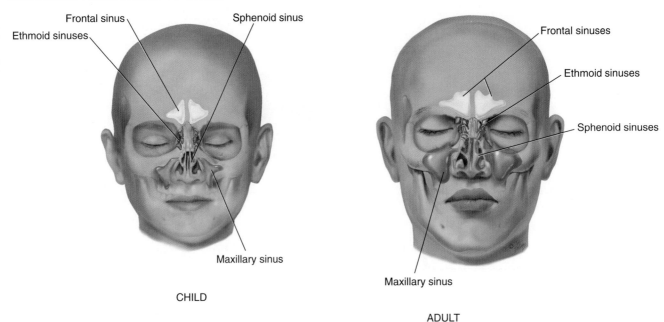

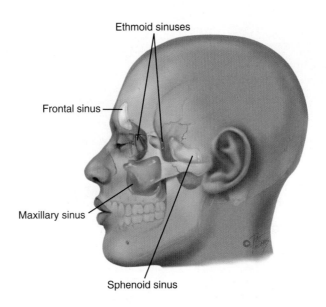

17-3 Paranasal sinuses.

© *Pat Thomas, 2006.*

years of age, and reach full size after puberty. The sphenoid sinuses are minute at birth and develop after puberty.

MOUTH

The **mouth** is the first segment of the digestive system and an airway for the respiratory system. The **oral cavity** is a short passage bordered by the lips, palate, cheeks, and tongue. It contains the teeth and gums, tongue, and salivary glands (Figure 17-4).

The **lips** are the anterior border of the oral cavity: the transition zone from the outer skin to the inner mucous membrane lining the oral cavity. The arching roof of the mouth is the palate; it is divided into two parts. The anterior **hard palate** is made up of bone and is a whitish colour. Posterior to this is the **soft palate,** an arch of muscle that is pinker

and mobile. The **uvula** is the free projection hanging down from the middle of the soft palate. The **cheeks** are the side walls of the oral cavity.

The floor of the mouth consists of the horseshoe-shaped mandible bone, the tongue, and underlying muscles. The **tongue** is a mass of striated muscle arranged in a crosswise pattern so that it can change shape and position. The **papillae** are the rough, bumpy elevations on its dorsal surface. Note the larger **vallate papillae** in an inverted V shape across the posterior base of the tongue, and do not confuse them with abnormal growths. Underneath, the ventral surface of the tongue is smooth and shiny and has prominent veins. The **frenulum** is a midline fold of tissue that connects the tongue to the floor of the mouth.

The tongue's ability to change shape and position enhances its functions in mastication, swallowing, cleansing the teeth,

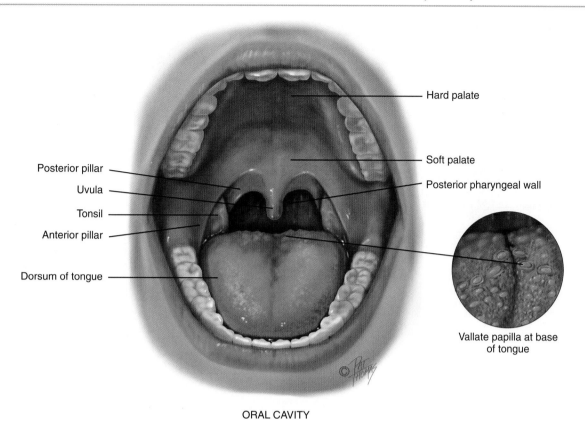

Hard palate

Soft palate

Posterior pharyngeal wall

Posterior pillar

Uvula

Tonsil

Anterior pillar

Dorsum of tongue

Vallate papilla at base
of tongue

ORAL CAVITY

17-4

© Pat Thomas, 2010.

and speech. The tongue also functions in taste sensation. Microscopic taste buds are in the papillae at the back and along the sides of the tongue and on the soft palate.

The mouth contains three pairs of **salivary glands** (Figure 17-5). The largest, the **parotid gland,** lies within the cheeks in front of the ear and extend from the zygomatic arch down to the angle of the jaw. Its duct, Stensen's duct, runs forward to open on the buccal mucosa opposite the second molar. The **submandibular gland** is the size of a walnut. It lies beneath the mandible at the angle of the jaw. Wharton's duct runs up and forward to the floor of the mouth and opens at either side of the frenulum. The smallest salivary gland, the almond-shaped **sublingual gland,** lies within the floor of the mouth under the tongue. It has many small openings along the sublingual fold under the tongue.

The glands secrete saliva, the clear fluid that moistens and lubricates the food bolus, starts digestion, and cleans and protects the mucosa.

Adults have 32 **permanent teeth,** 16 in each arch. Each tooth has three parts: the crown, the neck, and the root. The **gums** (gingivae) collar the teeth. They are thick fibrous tissues covered with mucous membrane. The gums are different from the rest of the oral mucosa because of their pale pink colour and stippled surface.

THROAT

The **throat,** or **pharynx,** is the area behind the mouth and nose. The **oropharynx** is separated from the mouth by two folds of tissue, the anterior tonsillar pillars, one on each side.

Behind the folds are the **tonsils,** each a mass of lymphoid tissue. The tonsils are the same colour as the surrounding mucous membrane, although they look more granular, and deep crypts are visible on their surface. Tonsillar tissue enlarges during childhood until puberty and then involutes. The posterior pharyngeal wall is seen behind these structures. Some small blood vessels may be visible on it.

The **nasopharynx** is continuous with the oropharynx, although it is above the oropharynx and behind the nasal cavity. The pharyngeal tonsils (adenoids) and the eustachian tube openings are located here (see Figure 17-2).

The oral cavity and throat have a rich lymphatic network. Review the lymph nodes and their drainage patterns in Chapter 14, and keep this system in mind when you evaluate the mouth.

DEVELOPMENTAL CONSIDERATIONS

Infants and Children

In infants, salivation starts at 3 months. Babies drool periodically for a few months before learning to swallow the saliva. This drooling does not herald the eruption of the first tooth, although many parents think it does.

Both sets of the teeth begin development in utero. Children have 20 temporary **deciduous teeth.** These erupt between 6 months and 24 months of age. All 20 teeth should appear by 2½ years of age. The deciduous teeth are lost beginning at age 6 years through age 12 years. They are replaced by the permanent teeth, starting with the central incisors (Figure 17-6). The permanent teeth appear earlier in girls

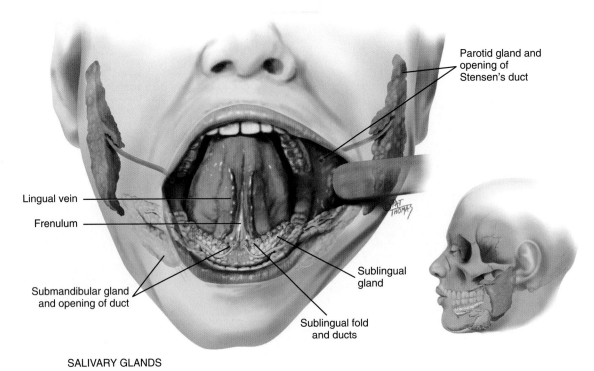

Parotid gland and
opening of
Stensen's duct

Lingual vein

Frenulum

Submandibular gland
and opening of duct

Sublingual
gland

Sublingual fold
and ducts

SALIVARY GLANDS

17-5

© Pat Thomas, 2006.

than in boys, and they erupt earlier in children of African descent than in children of European descent.

The nose develops during adolescence, along with the secondary sex characteristics. This growth starts at age 12 or 13 years, reaching full growth at age 16 years in girls and age 18 years in boys.

Pregnant Women

Nasal stuffiness and epistaxis may occur during pregnancy as a result of increased vascularity in the upper respiratory tract. Also, the gums may be hyperemic and softened and may bleed with normal toothbrushing. Contrary to superstitious folklore, no evidence shows that pregnancy causes tooth decay or loss.

Older Adults

Subcutaneous fat is gradually lost during later middle adult years, which makes the nose appear more prominent in some people. The nasal hairs grow coarser and stiffer and may not filter the air as well. The hairs protrude and may cause itching and sneezing. Many older people clip these hairs, thinking them unsightly, but this practice can cause infection. The sense of smell may diminish because of a decrease in the number of olfactory nerve fibres. The sense of smell begins decreasing after age 60 years, and it decreases progressively with age.

In the oral cavity, the soft tissues atrophy and the epithelium thins, especially in the cheek and tongue. This results in loss of taste buds, with about an 80% reduction in taste functioning. Further impairments in taste include a decrease in salivary secretion, which is needed to dissolve flavouring agents, and the presence of upper dentures, which cover secondary taste sites.

Atrophic tissues ulcerate easily, which increases older adults' risk for infections such as oral moniliasis. The risk of malignant oral lesions is also increased.

Many dental changes occur with aging. The tooth surface is abraded. The gums begin to recede, and the teeth begin to erode at the gum line. A smooth V-shaped cavity forms around the neck of the tooth, exposing the nerve and making the tooth hypersensitive. Some tooth loss may result from bone resorption (osteoporosis), which decreases the inner tooth structure and its outer support. Natural tooth loss is exacerbated by years of inadequate dental care, decay, poor oral hygiene, and tobacco use.

If tooth loss occurs, the remaining teeth drift, which causes **malocclusion.** The stress of chewing with maloccluding teeth causes further problems: (a) excessive bone resorption with further tooth loss occurs; (b) muscle imbalance results from a mandible and maxilla now out of alignment, which produces muscle spasms, tenderness of muscles of mastication, and chronic headaches; and (c) the temporomandibular joint is stressed, which leads to osteoarthritis, pain, and inability to fully open the mouth.

Diminished senses of taste and smell decrease older adults' interest in food and may contribute to malnutrition. Saliva production decreases; saliva acts as a solvent for food flavours and helps move food around the mouth. Decreased saliva also reduces the mouth's self-cleaning property. The major cause of decreased saliva flow is not the aging process itself but the use of medications that have anticholinergic effects. More than 250 medications have a side effect of dry mouth.

Because of the absence of some teeth and trouble with mastication, many older adults eat soft foods (usually high in carbohydrates) and decrease meat and fresh vegetable intake.

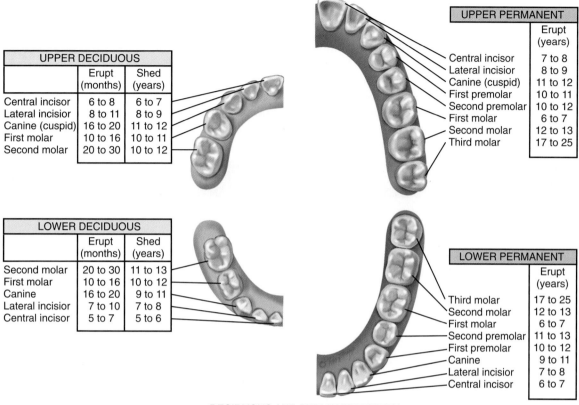

UPPER DECIDUOUS		
	Erupt (months)	Shed (years)
Central incisor	6 to 8	6 to 7
Lateral incisior	8 to 11	8 to 9
Canine (cuspid)	16 to 20	11 to 12
First molar	10 to 16	10 to 11
Second molar	20 to 30	10 to 12

UPPER PERMANENT	
	Erupt (years)
Central incisor	7 to 8
Lateral incisior	8 to 9
Canine (cuspid)	11 to 12
First premolar	10 to 11
Second premolar	10 to 12
First molar	6 to 7
Second molar	12 to 13
Third molar	17 to 25

LOWER DECIDUOUS		
	Erupt (months)	Shed (years)
Second molar	20 to 30	11 to 13
First molar	10 to 16	10 to 12
Canine	16 to 20	9 to 11
Lateral incisior	7 to 10	7 to 8
Central incisor	5 to 7	5 to 6

LOWER PERMANENT	
	Erupt (years)
Third molar	17 to 25
Second molar	12 to 13
First molar	6 to 7
Second premolar	11 to 13
First premolar	10 to 12
Canine	9 to 11
Lateral incisior	7 to 8
Central incisor	6 to 7

DECIDUOUS AND PERMANENT TEETH

17-6

This produces a risk for nutritional deficits in protein, vitamins, and minerals.

🌐 CULTURAL AND SOCIAL CONSIDERATIONS

The incidence of **cleft palate** is the same across ethnic groups, but Aboriginal populations have higher occurrence of **cleft lip** and combined cleft lip/cleft palate. Torus palatinus, a bony ridge running down the middle of the hard palate, is also more common in Aboriginal people and people of Asian descent. **Leukoedema,** a greyish-white benign lesion occurring on the buccal mucosa, may be present in people of African descent. Oral hyperpigmentation also varies according to ethnocultural groups. Usually absent at birth, hyperpigmentation increases with age. By 50 years of age, 10% of people of European descent and 50% to 90% of people of African descent show oral hyperpigmentation, a condition that is believed to be caused by a lifetime of accumulation of postinflammatory oral changes.

Although it is rare for a baby of European descent to be born with teeth (1 per 3000), the incidence is higher among Canadian Inuit infants. The size of teeth varies widely; the teeth are the smallest in people of European descent, followed by people of African descent and then people of Asian descent and Aboriginal people. Large teeth cause members of some ethnocultural groups to have prognathic, or protruding, jaws, a condition that is seen more frequently in people of African or Asian descent. The condition is normal and does not reflect an orthodontic problem.

In comparison with other Canadians, more Inuit people reported worse oral health status and greater frequency of oral pain. The increased rate of dental disease is a result of changes from traditional diets to ones higher in processed and sugary foods, lack of access to fluoridated water, and lack of access to comprehensive dental health services. Over 85% of Inuit preschoolers had dental caries, with an average of 8 affected deciduous teeth. In addition, caries remained untreated in many cases. The percentage of teeth that remained decayed for adolescents and young adults was 38% and 17% respectively, in comparison with 15% and 13% among other Canadians. Therefore, more dental disease is treated by extractions and results in a higher rate of edentulism among Inuit than among other Canadians (21% versus 6%, respectively). Furthermore, many Inuit communities lack a resident dentist. Dentists from southern Canada fly into the communities on an irregular basis to treat serious cases and dental emergencies. Consequently, restorative dental care, such as fillings and extractions, are more prevalent than dental health promotion and preventive measures.

Various socioeconomic variables are correlated with poor dental health. Individuals from lower income households have a greater prevalence of edentulism, periodontal disease, dental pain, and chewing difficulties than do people from higher income households. Consequently, Canadians from lower income groups report poorer oral health–related quality of life than do Canadians from higher income groups. Recent immigration may also potentially affect dental health. Language and cultural differences, lack of familiarity with the health care and dental care systems, and limited financial resources prevent immigrants from accessing dental care services (Dong, Levine, Loignon, & Bedos, 2011).

Access to comprehensive dental health care continues to be a major barrier to oral health promotion and maintenance for many Canadians. Aboriginal people, recent immigrants, individuals from lower socioeconomic groups, and Canadians living in rural or remote areas are less likely to have access to regular, comprehensive dental care. Thirty-two percent of Canadians lack adequate dental insurance and may not be able to pay dental care expenses. Inability to access regular and affordable dental care in their own communities results in poorer oral and overall health status for these Canadians (Quinonez & Grootendorst, 2011).

SUBJECTIVE DATA

Nose

1. Discharge
2. Frequent colds (upper respiratory infections)
3. Sinus pain
4. Trauma
5. Epistaxis (nosebleeds)
6. Allergies
7. Altered smell

3. Bleeding gums
4. Toothache
5. Hoarseness
6. Dysphagia
7. Altered taste
8. Smoking, alcohol consumption
9. Self-care behaviours
   Dental care pattern
   Dentures or appliances

Mouth and Throat

1. Sores or lesions
2. Sore throat

HEALTH HISTORY QUESTIONS

Examiner Asks	Rationale
Nose	
1. Discharge. Any **nasal discharge** or runny nose? Continuous? • Is the discharge watery, purulent, mucoid, bloody? 2. Frequent colds (upper respiratory infections). Any unusually frequent or severe colds? How often do these occur? 3. Sinus pain. Any **sinus pain** or sinusitis? How is this treated? • How would you describe your response to the treatment? • Do you have chronic postnasal drip? 4. Trauma. Ever had any **trauma** or a blow to the nose? (See Critical Findings box.) • Can you breathe through your nose? Is either side obstructed?	**Rhinorrhea** (nasal discharge) occurs with colds, allergies, sinus infection, trauma. Most people have occasional colds; thus, asking this more precise question yields more meaningful data. Trauma may cause deviated septum, which may cause nares to be obstructed.

CRITICAL FINDINGS

Trauma to the teeth, mouth, tongue, nose, and throat necessitate immediate assessment and attention. Prompt care is required for patients with slurred speech, difficulty speaking or swallowing, jaw pain, or swelling in their throats. These assessment findings suggest stroke, cardiac problems, dysphagia, or anaphylaxis. Choanal atresia in both nostrils warrants immediate insertion of an oral airway to ensure a patent airway, inasmuch as newborns are obligate nose breathers. Epistaxis that continues for more than 20 minutes necessitates urgent intervention because it may indicate life-threatening hypertension, a bleeding disorder, or a skull fracture from head trauma. Although not an emergency, unrelenting tooth pain that accompanies facial or neck swelling, redness, or bleeding necessitates prompt attention. These findings may suggest a dental abscess with systemic implications if left untreated.

Examiner Asks	Rationale

5. Epistaxis (nosebleeds). Any nosebleeds? How often?
- How much bleeding: about 5 mL or does it pour out?
- Colour of the blood: red or brown? Clots?
- From one nostril or both?
- Aggravated by nose-picking or scratching?
- How do you treat the nosebleeds? Are they difficult to stop?

Epistaxis occurs with trauma, vigorous nose blowing, or foreign body.

The patient should sit up with head tilted forward and pinch the nose between thumb and forefinger for 5 to 15 minutes.

6. Allergies. Any **allergies** or hay fever? To what are you allergic (e.g., pollen, dust, pets)?
- How was your allergy determined?
- What type of environment makes it worse? How can you avoid exposure?
- Do you use inhalers, nasal spray, nose drops? How often? Which type?
- How long have you used this?

Allergic rhinitis is "seasonal" if caused by pollen and "perennial" if the allergen is dust.

Misuse of over-the-counter nasal medications irritates the mucosa, which causes rebound swelling, a common problem.

7. Altered smell. Experienced any change in sense of smell?

Sense of smell is diminished with cigarette smoking or chronic allergies.

Mouth and Throat

1. Sores or lesions. Noticed any **sores** or **lesions** in the mouth or on the tongue or gums?
- How long have you had it? Ever had this lesion before?
- Is it single or multiple?
- Does it seem to be associated with stress, season change, food?
- How have you treated the sore? Applied any local medication?
- How would you describe your response to the treatment?

The patient's history helps determine whether oral lesions have infectious, traumatic, immunological, or malignant causes. Periodontal disease is thought to be associated with cardiovascular disease, diabetes, pulmonary infections, osteoporosis, and low birth weight.

2. Sore throat. How about **sore throats?** How frequently do you get them? Have a sore throat now? When did it start?
- Is it associated with cough, fever, fatigue, decreased appetite, headache, postnasal drip, or hoarseness?
- Is it worse when you arise? What is the humidity level in the room where you sleep? Any dust or smoke inhaled at work?
- Do you usually get a throat culture for the sore throats? Were any documented as "strep throat"?
- How have you treated this sore throat: medication, gargling? How effective are these? Have your tonsils or adenoids been taken out?

Untreated streptococcal infections may lead to the complication of rheumatic fever.

3. Bleeding gums. Any **bleeding gums?** How long have you had this?

A little bleeding is normal if a patient is just starting to floss. More frequent bleeding from brushing or flossing may indicate periodontal disease or a clotting disorder.

4. Toothache. Any **toothache?** Do your teeth seem sensitive to hot, cold? Have you lost any teeth?

5. Hoarseness. Any **hoarseness** voice change? For how long?
- Do you feel as though you have to clear your throat? Or have a "lump in your throat"?
- Do you use your voice a lot at work, recreation?
- Does the hoarseness seem associated with a cold or a sore throat?

Hoarseness is a disorder of the larynx with many causes, such as overuse of the voice, upper respiratory infection, chronic inflammation, lesions, or a neoplasm.

6. Dysphagia. Any difficulty swallowing?
- Do you feel as if food gets stopped at a certain point?
- Do you cough while drinking or eating?
- Does your voice sound "wet" or hoarse when you eat or drink?
- Any drooling or leakage of food or liquid while eating?
- Does any food get stuck in your mouth (pocketing) or in your throat?
- How long have you had the problem?
- What have you done to improve swallowing? How effective was it?
- Any pain with this?

Dysphagia may be oropharyngeal in origin, difficulty in safe transfer of liquid or food bolus from mouth to the esophagus, or esophageal dysphagia, difficulty in passing food down the esophagus to the stomach. It is present in at least half of individuals with acute stroke; other causes of dysphagia are head and neck cancer, esophageal cancer, head trauma, decreased alertness, and progressive neurological diseases.

Subjective Data

Examiner Asks	Rationale

Untreated dysphagia increases the risk of aspiration pneumonia, malnutrition, and dehydration, and it may reduce quality of life. Following training by a speech language pathologist, nursing care may include screening with a reliable and validated tool such as TOR-BSST©, which was designed specifically for stroke patients. (Figure 17-7 depicts a dysphagia screening tool.) Patients who fail dysphagia screening can be referred for a full comprehensive assessment to a speech language pathologist, who may suggest dietary modification, good oral care, resting at least 30 minutes after mealtimes in an upright position.

Odynophagia may be a burning or sharp pain, indicating mucosal inflammation, or a cramping, squeezing pain that suggests a muscular cause.

7. Altered taste. Any change in sense of taste?
8. Smoking, alcohol consumption. Do you smoke? Pipe or cigarettes? Smokeless tobacco? How many packs per day? For how many years? (See the box Promoting Health: Smokeless Tobacco and Cancer Risk.)
   - When was your last alcoholic drink? How much alcohol did you drink that time? How much alcohol do you usually drink?

Chronic tobacco use is associated with tooth loss, coronal and root caries, and periodontal disease in older adults.

Chronic tobacco use in any form and heavy alcohol consumption greatly increase risk for oral and pharyngeal cancers.

9. Self-care behaviours. Tell me about your daily dental care. How often do you use a toothbrush and floss?
   - When was your last dental examination? Do dental problems affect which foods you eat?
   - Do you have a dental appliance: braces, bridge, headgear?
   - Do you wear dentures? All the time? How long have you had this set? How do they fit?

Assess self-care behaviours for oral hygiene.

Regular dental screening, usually every 6 months, is necessary for the promotion and maintenance of oral health. Dentists may recommend more frequent checkups, depending on oral and overall health. However, dental benefit plans may provide coverage for dental screening and cleaning only every 9 months.

Lesions may be caused by ill-fitting dentures, or the presence of dentures may mask the eruption of a new lesion.

   - Any sores or irritation on the palate or gums?
   - Any problems with talking: Do the dentures whistle or drop? Can you chew all foods with them? How do you clean them?
   - Do you have dental coverage?

Nearly a third of Canadians do not have dental coverage, and this may adversely affect self-care behaviours.

Additional History for Infants and Children

1. Mouth disease. Does the child have any mouth infections or sores, such as thrush or canker sores? How frequently do these occur?
2. Throat disease. Does the child have frequent sore throat or tonsillitis? How often? How are these treated? Have they ever been documented as "strep throat" (streptococcal infections)?
3. Tooth development. Did the child's teeth erupt about on time?
   - Do the teeth seem straight to you?

Eruption is delayed with Down's syndrome, cretinism, and rickets, and this delay may impair nutrition.

Malocclusion may impair nutrition.

   - Is the child using a bottle? How often during the day? Does the child go to sleep with a bottle at night?
   - Have you noticed any thumb-sucking after the child's secondary teeth came in?

Prolonged use of a bottle increases risk for tooth decay and middle ear infections.

Prolonged thumb-sucking (after age 6 to 7 years) may affect occlusion.

TOR-BSST©
The Toronto Bedside Swallowing
Screening Test©

(addressograph)

DATE: _____ *(mm/dd/yyyy)*   TIME: _____ *(hh/mm)*

A) Before water intake: (Mark either abnormal or normal for each task.)

	Abnormal	Normal
1. Have patient say 'ah' and judge voice quality	☐	☐
2. Ask patient to stick their tongue out and then move it from side to side.	☐	☐

B) Water intake: Have the patient **sit upright** and give water. Ask patient to **say "ah"** after each intake. Mark as abnormal if you note any of the following signs: **coughing, change in voice quality** *or* **drooling.** If abnormal, stop water intake and advance to 'D'.

1) One Tsp Swallows	Cough during/after swallow	Voice change after swallow	Drooling during/after swallow	Normal
Swallow 1	☐	☐	☐	☐
Swallow 2	☐	☐	☐	☐
Swallow 3	☐	☐	☐	☐
Swallow 4	☐	☐	☐	☐
Swallow 5	☐	☐	☐	☐
Swallow 6	☐	☐	☐	☐
Swallow 7	☐	☐	☐	☐
Swallow 8	☐	☐	☐	☐
Swallow 9	☐	☐	☐	☐
Swallow 10	☐	☐	☐	☐
2) Cup drinking	☐	☐	☐	☐

C) After water intake: (Administer at least a minute after you finish Section B.)

	Abnormal	Normal
1. Have patient say 'ah' again and judge voice quality.	☐	☐

D) Results: ☐ **Passed**   ☐ **Failed** → **Initiate referral to SLP**
                    (no abnormal signs)   (1 or more abnormal signs)

TOR-BSST© Screener's Signature: _____

June 2007 version

17-7 *Toronto Bedside Swallowing Screening Test (TOR-BSST©). NOTE: Screeners may be health care professionals, such as nurses, who have received proper training using the standardized 4-hour training program. © 2003. The TOR-BSST© form is copyrighted. It may not be altered, sold, translated, or adapted without the permission of Rosemary Martino, rosemary.martino@utoronto.ca.*

Examiner Asks	Rationale
• Have you noticed the child grinding his or her teeth? Does this happen at night?	Bruxism usually occurs in sleep and results from dental problems or nervous tension.
4. **Self-care behaviours.** How are the child's dental habits? Does the child use a toothbrush regularly? How often does the child see a dentist? • Do you use fluoridated water or fluoride supplement?	Evaluate child's self-care. When baby teeth have erupted (age 2 to 3 years), begin regular 6-month dental check-ups to evaluate self-care and identify potential problems. To prevent fluorosis, adults should brush teeth of children younger than 3 years, using a smear of toothpaste. Children 3 to 6 years of age should brush with a pea-sized portion of toothpaste.
• Does the child wear a mouth protector or mouthguard when participating in sporting activities?	Mouth protectors and mouthguards help reduce risk of damage to teeth, cheeks, lips, and tongue during participation in sports or recreational activities.

Additional History for Older Adults

1. **Mouth dryness.** Any dryness in the mouth? Are you taking any medications? (Note prescribed and over-the-counter medications.)	**Xerostomia** (dry mouth) is a side effect of many drugs: antidepressants, anticholinergics, antispasmodics, antihypertensives, antipsychotics, bronchodilators.
2. **Teeth.** Have you had any loss of teeth? Can you chew all types of food?	Note a decrease in eating meat, fresh vegetables, and tooth-cleansing foods such as apples.
3. **Mouth care.** Are you able to care for your own teeth or dentures?	Self-care may be decreased by physical disability (arthritis), vision loss, confusion, or depression.
4. **Taste and smell.** Have you noticed a change in your sense of taste or smell?	Some people add extra salt and sugar to enhance food when taste begins to wane. Also, diminished smell may decrease the patient's ability to detect food spoilage, natural gas leaks, or smoke from a fire.

Subjective Data

PROMOTING HEALTH: SMOKELESS TOBACCO AND CANCER RISK

Smokeless (Tobacco) Does Not Mean Harmless!

Known as "snuff," "spit," or "chew," smokeless tobacco (SLT) carries significant health risks and is not a safe substitute for smoking. SLT, like cigarettes, contains nicotine and can lead to nicotine addiction and dependence.

Two types of SLT are commonly used in Canada. The first type, chewing tobacco, comes in loose leaf, plug, and twist forms, and, as the name implies, it is chewed or sucked. The leaves are air cured, shredded into flakes, and treated with sweet flavouring solutions. Snuff, the second type, is finely ground tobacco that is either dry or moist. Dry snuff is inhaled through the nose. Moist snuff, available in either small pouches or tins, is taken orally. It is popular because the tobacco stays in one place and generates less saliva. Most users of chewing tobacco and moist snuff place the product between their gingival and buccal mucosa, suck on the tobacco, and spit out the juices. A Scandinavian-style snuff called *snus* has been introduced into Canada. Similar to chewing tobacco and moist snuff, it is less noticeable because users do not need to spit it out.

More than 3000 chemicals, including 28 carcinogens, have been identified in SLT. Using SLT can lead to oral cancer, esophageal cancer or pancreatic cancer (Canadian Cancer Society, 2012). Holding one pinch of SLT in your mouth for 30 minutes typically delivers as much nicotine as four cigarettes. Consequently, the health consequences of nicotine from smoking are also found in SLT users. Nicotine may play a role in the pathogenesis of diseases, including coronary artery and peripheral vascular diseases, hypertension, peptic ulcer disease, and fetal mortality and morbidity.

The use of SLT has also been associated with an even greater risk of oral cancer than smoking. Early signs of oral cancer include the following:

- An ulcer or sore that does not heal
- White or red patches
- A prolonged sore throat or feeling that something is in the throat
- Difficulty chewing
- Unexplained bleeding
- Numbness or tingling
- Restricted movement of the tongue or jaw
- A small lump or thickening in the lip, tongue, floor or roof, cheeks, gums, tonsil

Pain is rarely an early symptom of oral cancer, which is why a thorough examination of the mouth is important. The risk for cancers of the pharynx, larynx, esophagus, stomach, and pancreas may also be an increased. SLT use is associated with other oral effects besides oral cancer. Because tobacco has an unpleasant taste, many brands are heavily sweetened with sugars. This concentrated sugar is then held in the mouth next to the teeth, which promotes tooth decay. Other oral health effects of SLT use include leukoplakia, periodontal disease, dental caries, and delayed wound healing. In addition, tobacco leaves contain gritty materials that wear down the surfaces of teeth, exacerbating the problem. Furthermore, the gritty materials scratch the soft tissues in the mouth, allowing the nicotine and other chemicals to enter directly into the bloodstream. The flavouring salts found in SLT also contribute to abnormal blood pressure and kidney disease.

SLT use is higher among professional athletes, men, and individuals living in rural areas. In 2009, 6% of Canadian youth aged 15 to 19 reported having tried SLT, in comparison with 11% of adults aged 25 or older. Adolescents who use SLT are more likely to become cigarette smokers. There has been a shift in distribution of SLT users from youth to older adults. From 2003 to 2009, the proportion of SLT users aged 15 to 19 years decreased from 23% to 16%, whereas that of SLT users in the 45+ age group increased from 14% to 33%. Across the nation, 13% of male Canadians, in comparison with 2% of female Canadians, reported using SLT.

SLT is not a healthy alternative to smoking, nor should it be encouraged for smokers who find themselves in smoke-free zones. The Public Health Agency of Canada (2012) offers *Enough Snuff,* a self-help program to help all SLT users quit. A nonprofit U.S. organization, Oral Health America, provides an educational program, *National Spit Tobacco Education Program (NSTEP),* to dissuade young people from using SLT and to help all SLT users quit.

Additional Resources

Canadian Cancer Society. (2012). *Any tobacco use can hurt your body.* Retrieved from http://www.cancer.ca/Canada-wide/Prevention/Smoking%20and%20tobacco/Why%20should%20I%20quit/Any%20tobacco%20use%20can%20hurt%20your%20body.aspx?sc_lang=en.

Ontario Tobacco Research Unit. (2006). What population surveys say about smokeless tobacco use. *Retrieved from* http://www.otru.org/pdf/updates/update_oct2006.pdf.

Walsh, P. M., & Epstein, J. B. (2000). The oral effects of smokeless tobacco. Journal of the Canadian Dental Association, 66, 22–25.

Subjective Data

OBJECTIVE DATA

PREPARATION

Position the patient sitting up straight with his or her head at your eye level. If the patient wears dentures, offer a paper towel and ask the patient to remove them.

EQUIPMENT NEEDED

Otoscope with short, wide-tipped nasal speculum attachment
Penlight
Two tongue blades
Cotton gauze pad (10 × 10 cm)
Gloves
Occasionally: long-stem light attachment for otoscope

Normal Range of Findings	Abnormal Findings

INSPECT AND PALPATE THE NOSE

External Nose

Normally, the nose is symmetrical, in the midline, and in proportion to other facial features (Figure 17-8). Inspect for any deformity, asymmetry, inflammation, or skin lesions. If an injury is reported or suspected, palpate gently for any pain or break in contour.

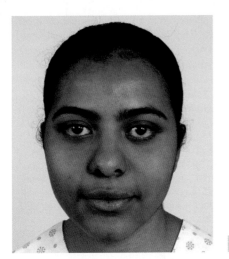

17-8

Test the patency of the nostrils by pushing one nasal wing shut with your finger while asking the patient to sniff inward through the other naris, and repeat on the other side. This reveals any obstruction, which later is explored with the use of the nasal speculum. The sense of smell, mediated by cranial nerve I, is usually not tested in a routine examination. The procedure for assessing smell is described with cranial nerve testing in Chapter 25.

Absence of sniff indicates obstruction (e.g., common cold, nasal polyps, rhinitis).

Normal Range of Findings	**Abnormal Findings**

Nasal Cavity

Attach the short wide-tipped speculum to the otoscope head and insert this combined apparatus into the nasal vestibule, avoiding pressure on the nasal septum. Gently lift up the tip of the nose with your finger before inserting.

View each nasal cavity with the patient's head erect and then with the head tilted back. Inspect the nasal mucosa, noting its normal red colour and smooth moist surface (Figure 17-9). Note any swelling, discharge, bleeding, or foreign body.

With rhinitis and an upper respiratory infection, the nasal mucosa is swollen and bright red.

Discharge is common with rhinitis and sinusitis, varying from watery and copious to thick, purulent, and green-yellow.

With chronic allergy, the mucosa looks swollen, boggy, pale, and grey.

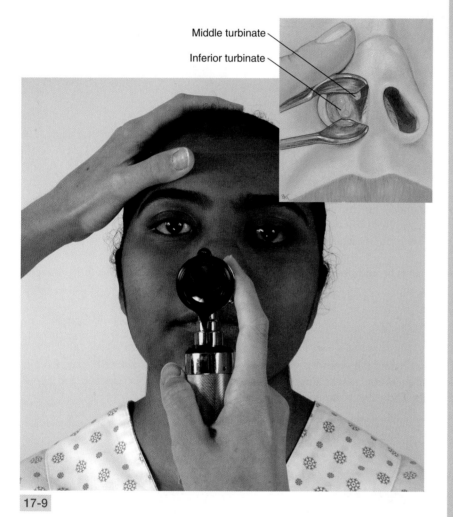

Middle turbinate
Inferior turbinate

17-9

Objective Data

Normal Range of Findings

Observe the nasal septum for deviation (Figure 17-10). A deviated septum is common and is not significant unless air flow is obstructed. (If present in a hospitalized patient, document the deviated septum in the event that the patient needs nasal suctioning or a nasogastric tube.) Also note any perforation or bleeding in the septum.

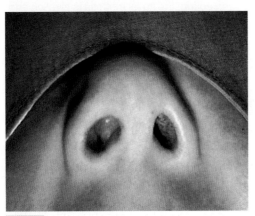

17-10 Deviated septum.

Inspect the turbinates, the bony ridges curving down from the lateral walls. The superior turbinate is not in your view, but the middle and inferior turbinates appear the same light red colour as the nasal mucosa. Note any swelling, but do not try to push the speculum past it. Turbinates are quite vascular and tender if touched.

Note any polyps, benign growths that accompany chronic allergy, and distinguish them from the normal turbinates.

PALPATE THE SINUS AREAS

Using your thumbs, press over the frontal sinuses below the eyebrows (Figure 17-11, *A*) and over the maxillary sinuses below the cheekbones (see Figure 17-11, *B*). Take care not to press directly on the eyeballs. The patient should feel firm pressure but no pain.

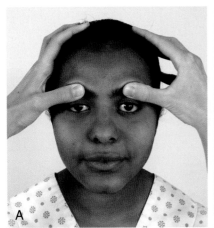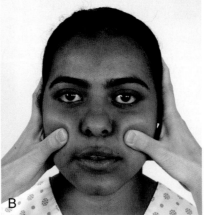

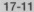
17-11

Abnormal Findings

A deviated septum looks like a hump or shelf in one nasal cavity.

Perforation is visible as a spot of light from the penlight shining in the other naris and occurs with cocaine use.

Epistaxis commonly originates from the anterior septum (see Table 17-1 on p. 396).

Polyps are smooth, pale grey, avascular, mobile, and nontender (see Table 17-1, p. 396).

Sinus areas are tender to palpation in patients with chronic allergies and acute infection (sinusitis).

Normal Range of Findings	Abnormal Findings

Transillumination

There is no evidence to support the practice of transillumination of the frontal or maxillary sinuses when you suspect sinus inflammation (Godley, 1992). The diagnosis requires distinct differences in the illumination of one of the sinus pair. Thus the technique would not help in chronic sinusitis characterized by diffuse swelling of all sinus mucosa. Although fluid collection is more extensive with acute sinusitis, the asymmetry of light illumination is nonetheless not valid because many healthy sinuses normally cannot be transilluminated.

INSPECT THE MOUTH

Begin with anterior structures, and move posteriorly. Use a tongue blade to retract structures and a bright light for optimal visualization.

Lips

Inspect the lips for colour, moisture, cracking, and lesions. Retract the lips, and note their inner surface as well (Figure 17-12). Individuals with darker complexions may normally have bluish lips and a dark line on the gingival margin.

In light-skinned people, circumoral pallor occurs with shock and anemia; cyanosis, with hypoxemia and chilling; cherry red coloration of lips, with carbon monoxide poisoning; and acidosis, with aspirin poisoning or ketoacidosis.

Cheilitis (perlèche): cracking at the corners.

Herpes simplex, other lesions (see Table 17-2, p. 396).

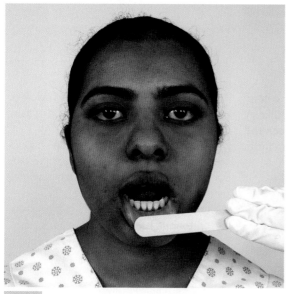

17-12

Nearly one third of Canadians do not have dental coverage, and this may adversely affect self-care behaviours.

Teeth and Gums

The condition of the teeth is an index of the patient's general health. Your examination should not replace the regular dental examination, but you should note any diseased, absent, loose, or abnormally positioned teeth. The teeth normally look white, straight, evenly spaced, and clean and free of debris or decay.

Compare the number of teeth with the number expected for the patient's age. Ask the patient to bite as if chewing something, and note alignment of upper and lower jaw. In normal occlusion in the back, the upper teeth rest directly on the lower teeth; in the front, the upper incisors slightly override the lower incisors.

Discoloured teeth appear brown with excessive fluoride use and yellow with tobacco use.

Grinding down of tooth surface.
Plaque: soft debris.
Caries: decay.
Enamel erosion: eating disorder.
Malocclusion (poor biting relationship), protrusion of upper or lower incisors (Table 17-3, p. 397).

Objective Data

Normal Range of Findings	Abnormal Findings

Normal Range of Findings

Normally, the gums look pink or coral with a stippled (dotted) surface. The gum margins at the teeth are tight and well defined (Figure 17-13). Check for swelling; retraction of gingival margins; and spongy, bleeding, or discoloured gums. Individuals with darker complexions may normally have a dark melanotic line along the gingival margin.

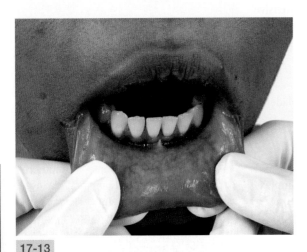

17-13

Tongue

Check the tongue for colour, surface characteristics, and moisture. The colour is pink and even. The dorsal surface is normally roughened from the papillae. A thin white coating may be present (Figure 17-14). Ask the patient to touch the tongue to the roof of the mouth. Its ventral surface looks smooth, glistening, and shows veins. Saliva is present.

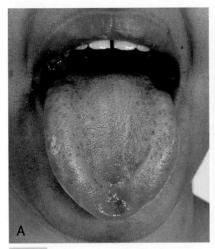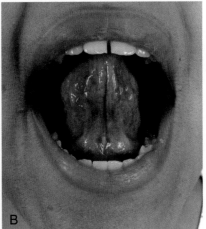

A B

17-14

With a glove*, hold the tongue with a cotton gauze pad for traction, and pull the tongue out and to each side (Figure 17-15). Inspect for any white patches or lesions: normally, none are present. If any are present, palpate these lesions for induration.

---

*Always wear gloves to examine mucous membranes. This is in accordance with routine practices to prevent the spread of possible communicable disease.

Abnormal Findings

Gingival hyperplasia (see Table 17-3, p. 398), crevices between teeth and gums, pockets of debris.

Bleeding of gums with slight pressure, indicating gingivitis.

Dark line on gingival margins: occurs with lead and bismuth poisoning.

Tongue appears beefy red and swollen; some areas may be smooth and glossy (Table 17-5, p. 400).

Enlargement of the tongue occurs with intellectual disability, hypothyroidism, acromegaly; the tongue may be small with malnutrition.

Dry mouth occurs with dehydration, fever; tongue has deep vertical fissures.

Saliva is decreased while the patient is taking anticholinergic and other medications.

Excess saliva and drooling occur with gingivostomatitis and neurological dysfunction.

Normal Range of Findings	Abnormal Findings

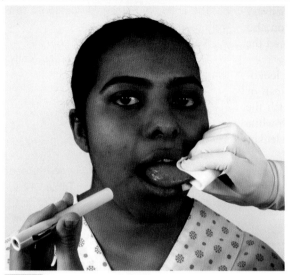

17-15

Inspect carefully the entire U-shaped area under the tongue behind the teeth. Oral malignancies are most likely to develop there. Note any white patches, nodules, or ulcerations. If lesions are present, or in any patient older than 50 years or with a positive history of smoking or alcohol use, use your gloved hand to palpate the area. Place your other hand under the jaw to stabilize the tissue and to detect any abnormality (Figure 17-16). Note any induration.

Any lesion or ulcer persisting for more than 2 weeks must be investigated.

An indurated area may be a mass or lymphadenopathy, and it must be investigated.

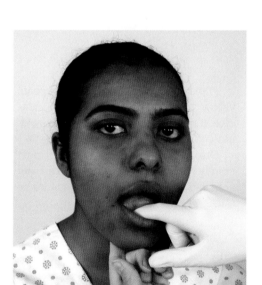

17-16

Buccal Mucosa

Hold the cheek open with a wooden tongue blade, and check the buccal mucosa for colour, nodules, and lesions. It normally looks pink, smooth, and moist, although patchy hyperpigmentation is common and normal in dark-skinned people.

Dappled brown patches are present with Addison's disease (chronic adrenal insufficiency).

Objective Data

Normal Range of Findings

An expected finding is **Stensen's duct,** the opening of the parotid salivary gland. It looks like a small dimple opposite the upper second molar. You also may see a raised occlusion line on the buccal mucosa parallel with the level the teeth meet. This is caused by the teeth closing against the cheek.

A larger patch also may be present along the buccal mucosa. This is leukoedema, a benign greyish opaque area, more common in people of African or South Asian descent. When it is mild, the patch disappears as you stretch the cheeks. The severity of the condition increases with age, looking greyish white and thickened. The cause of the condition is unknown. Do not mistake leukoedema for oral infections such as candidiasis (thrush).

Fordyce's granules are small, isolated white or yellow papules on the mucosa of the cheeks, tongue, and lips (Figure 17-17). These little sebaceous cysts are painless and not significant.

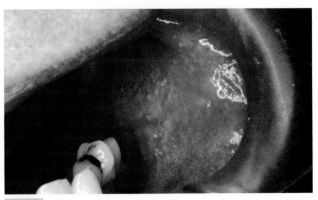

17-17   Fordyce's granules.

Palate

Shine your light up to the roof of the mouth. The more anterior hard palate is white with irregular transverse rugae. The posterior soft palate is pinker, smooth, and upwardly movable. A normal variation is a nodular bony ridge, called a **torus palatinus,** down the middle of the hard palate, which lies in the roof of the mouth (Figure 17-18). This benign growth arises after puberty and is a more common finding in Aboriginal people and people of African or Asian descent.

Abnormal Findings

The orifice of Stensen's duct looks red with mumps.

Koplik's spots (see Table 17-4, p. 399) are an early prodromal (early warning) sign of measles.

Leukoplakia, a chalky white raised patch, is abnormal (see Table 17-4, p. 399).

Candida infection will usually rub off, leaving a clear or raw denuded surface.

With jaundice, the hard palate appears yellow. In dark-skinned people with jaundice, it may look yellow, muddy yellow, or green-brown.

Oral Kaposi's sarcoma is the most common early lesion in people with acquired immune deficiency syndrome (AIDS; see Table 17-6, p. 402).

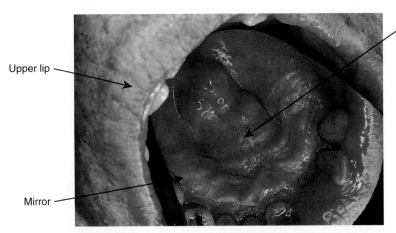

Torus in upper hard palate

Upper lip

Mirror

17-18   Torus palatinus (viewed in a mirror).

Normal Range of Findings

Observe the uvula; it normally looks like a fleshy pendant hanging in the midline (Figure 17-19). Ask the patient to say "ahhh," and note the soft palate and uvula rise in the midline. This is a test of one function of cranial nerve X, the vagus nerve.

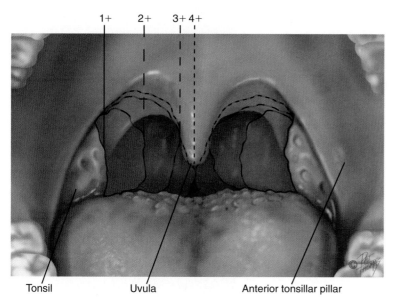

1+   2+   3+ 4+

Tonsil   Uvula   Anterior tonsillar pillar

17-19   © Pat Thomas, 2006.

During the examination, notice any breath odour (*halitosis*). This is common and usually has a local cause, such as poor oral hygiene, consumption of odoriferous foods, alcohol consumption, heavy smoking, or dental infection. On occasion, it indicates a systemic disease.

INSPECT THE THROAT

With your light, observe the oval, rough-surfaced tonsils behind the anterior tonsillar pillar (see Figure 17-19). Their colour is the same pink as the oral mucosa, and their surface is peppered with indentations, or crypts. In some people the crypts collect small plugs of whitish cellular debris. This does not indicate infection. However, there should be no exudate on the tonsils. Tonsils are graded in size as follows:

1+: Visible
2+: Halfway between tonsillar pillars and uvula
3+: Touching the uvula
4+: Touching each other

You may normally see grade 1+ or grade 2+ tonsils in healthy people, especially in children, because lymphoid tissue is proportionately enlarged until puberty.

Abnormal Findings

A **bifid uvula** looks as if it is split in two; it is more common in Aboriginal people (see Table 17-6, p. 402).

Any deviation to the side or absence of movement indicates nerve damage, which also occurs with poliomyelitis and diphtheria.

Diabetic ketoacidosis produces a sweet, fruity breath odour; this acetone smell also occurs in children with malnutrition or dehydration. Other breath odours are one of ammonia, which occurs with uremia; a musty odour, with liver disease; a foul, fetid odour, with dental or respiratory infections; alcohol odour, with ingestion of alcohol or chemicals; and a mouselike smell of the breath, with diphtheria.

With an acute infection, tonsils are bright red and swollen and may have exudates or large white spots.

A white membrane covering the tonsils may accompany infectious mononucleosis, leukemia, and diphtheria.

Tonsils are enlarged to 2+, 3+, or 4+ with an acute infection.

Normal Range of Findings	**Abnormal Findings**

Enlarge your view of the posterior pharyngeal wall by depressing the tongue with a tongue blade (Figure 17-20). Push down halfway back on the tongue; if you push on its tip, the tongue will hump up in back. Press slightly off-centre to avoid eliciting the gag reflex. You can help the patient with an easily triggered gag reflex by offering to let him or her depress the tongue with the tongue blade. (Some people can lower their own tongue so the tongue blade is not needed.) Scan the posterior wall for colour, exudate, or lesions. When you are finished, discard the tongue blade.

Although eliciting the gag reflex is usually not done in the screening examination, you can do so by touching the posterior wall with the tongue blade. This is a test of cranial nerves IX and X, the glossopharyngeal and vagus nerves.

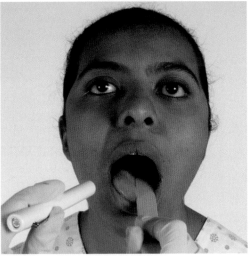

17-20

Test cranial nerve XII, the hypoglossal nerve, by asking the patient to stick out the tongue. It should protrude in the midline. Children enjoy this request! Note any tremor, loss of movement, or deviation to the side.

With cranial nerve XII damage, the tongue deviates *toward* the paralyzed side.

A fine tremor of the tongue occurs with hyperthyroidism; a coarse tremor, with cerebral palsy and alcoholism.

 DEVELOPMENTAL CONSIDERATIONS

Infants and Children

Because the oral examination is intrusive for the infant or young child, the timing is best toward the end of the complete examination, along with the ear examination. If any crying episodes occur earlier, however, seize the opportunity to examine the open mouth and oropharynx.

As with the ear examination, let the parent help position the child. Place the infant supine on the examining table, with the arms restrained (Figure 17-21).

Older infants and toddlers may be held on the parent's lap, with one of the parent's hands holding the arms down and the other hand securing the child's head against the parent's chest. Although it is not often needed, the parent's leg can be used to reach over and hold the child's legs between the parent's own (Figure 17-22).

Normal Range of Findings	Abnormal Findings

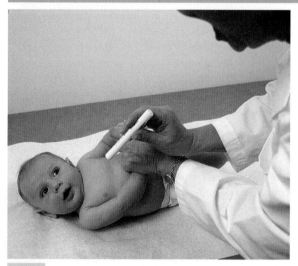

17-21

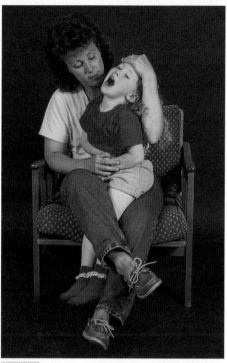

17-22

Use a game to help prepare the young child. Encourage preschool-age children to use a tongue blade to look into a puppet's mouth, or place a mirror so that they can look into the mouth while you do. School-age children are usually cooperative and love to show off missing or new teeth (Figure 17-23).

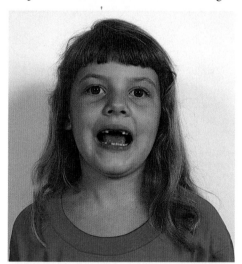

17-23

Be discriminating in your use of the tongue blade. It may be necessary for a full view of oral structures, but it produces a strong gag reflex in infants. You may avoid the tongue blade completely with cooperative preschool-age and school-age children. Try asking a young child to open the mouth "as big as a lion" and to move the tongue in different directions. To enlarge your view of the oropharynx, ask the child to stick out the tongue and "pant like a dog."

At some point, you will encounter an uncooperative young child who clenches the teeth and refuses to open the mouth. If all your other efforts have failed, slide the tongue blade along the buccal mucosa and turn it between the back teeth. Push down to depress the tongue. This stimulates the gag reflex, and the child opens the mouth wide for a few seconds. You will have a *brief* look at the throat. Make the most of it.

Objective Data

Normal Range of Findings	Abnormal Findings

Nose. The newborn may have milia across the nose. The nasal bridge may be flat in Aboriginal children and in children of Asian or African descent. There should be no nasal flaring or narrowing with breathing.

Nasal flaring in the infant indicates respiratory distress.

Many children with chronic allergy have a transverse ridge across the nose, caused by wiping the nose upward with palm (see Table 14-3 on p. 291). Nasal narrowing on inhalation is seen with chronic nasal obstruction and mouth breathing.

Inability to pass a catheter through the nasal cavity indicates choanal atresia, which necessitates immediate intervention (see Table 17-1 on p. 394).

It is essential to determine the patency of the nares in the immediate newborn period because most newborns are obligate nose breathers. Nares blocked with amniotic fluid are suctioned gently with a bulb syringe. If obstruction is suspected, a small-lumen (5- to 10-Fr) catheter is passed down each naris to confirm patency.

Avoid using the nasal speculum when you examine infants and young children. Instead, gently push up the tip of the nose with your thumb while using your other hand to shine the light into the naris. With a toddler, be alert for the possibility of a foreign body lodged in the nasal cavity (see Table 17-1).

Only in children older than 8 years do you need to palpate the child's sinus areas. In younger children, sinus areas are too small for palpation.

Mouth and Throat. A normal finding in infants is the **sucking tubercle,** a small pad in the middle of the upper lip from friction of breastfeeding or bottle-feeding. Note the number of teeth and whether this number is appropriate for the child's age. Also note pattern of eruption, position, condition, and hygiene. Use this guide for children younger than 2 years; the child's age in months minus the number 6 should equal the expected number of deciduous teeth. Normally, all 20 deciduous teeth are in by age 2½ years. Saliva is present after 3 months of age and shows in excess with teething children.

No teeth by age 1 year is abnormal.

Discoloured teeth appear yellow or yellow-brown in infants taking tetracycline or whose mothers took the drug during the last trimester; they appear green or black with excessive iron ingestion, although this reverses when the iron is stopped. White specks may indicate that a child getting too much fluoride (fluorosis). It is a cosmetic condition, not health threatening.

Malocclusion: Upper or lower dental arch is out of alignment.

Ankyloglossia, a short lingual frenulum, can limit tongue protrusion and impair speech development (see Table 17-5, p. 400).

Mobility should allow the tongue to extend at least as far as the alveolar ridge.

Trauma may indicate forced feeding of bottle or spoon, which may be child abuse.

Note any bruising or laceration on the buccal mucosa or gums of an infant or a young child.

A high-arched palate is usually normal in newborns, but a very narrow or very high arch also occurs with Turner's syndrome, Ehlers-Danlos syndrome, Marfan's syndrome, and Treacher Collins syndrome. It also develops in mouth-breathers with chronic allergies, and from thumb sucking.

On the palate, **Epstein pearls** are a normal finding in newborns and infants (Figure 17-24). They are small, whitish, glistening, pearly papules along the median raphe of the hard palate and on the gums, where they look like teeth. They are small retention cysts and disappear in the first few weeks.

Bednar aphthae are traumatic areas or ulcers on the posterior hard palate on either side of the midline. They result from abrasions during sucking.

Nursing bottle caries are brown discolourations on upper front teeth (see photo in Table 17-3).

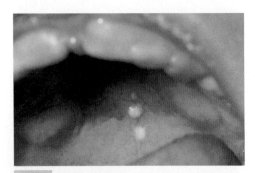

17-24 Epstein pearls.

Normal Range of Findings	Abnormal Findings

The tonsils are not visible in newborns. They gradually enlarge during childhood, remaining proportionately larger until puberty. Tonsils appear even larger in an infant who is crying or gagging. Normally, newborns can produce a strong, lusty cry.

Insert your gloved finger into the baby's mouth and palpate the hard and soft palates as the baby sucks. The sucking reflex can be elicited in infants up to 12 months old.

As teeth begin to erupt in the older infant and child, check age at eruption, sequence, and condition. Teeth should emerge straight up or down from the gums, and enamel should be clear white and smooth. Lift the upper lip to check for dental caries (tooth decay); normally there are none.

Pregnant Women

Gum hypertrophy (surface looks smooth and stippling disappears) may occur normally at puberty or during pregnancy (pregnancy gingivitis; Figure 17-25). Gums may bleed as a result of increased hormone production, which causes increased vascularity and fragility. Proper oral hygiene and healthy food choices help prevent pregnancy gingivitis.

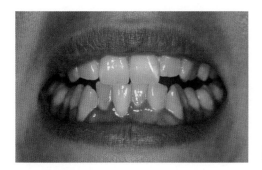

17-25 Early gingivitis.

Older Adults

The nose may appear more prominent on the face from a loss of subcutaneous fat. In edentulous patients the mouth and lips fold in, giving a "purse-string" appearance. Teeth that are present may look slightly yellowed, although the colour is uniform. Yellowing appears because the dentin is visible through worn enamel. The surface of the incisors may show vertical cracks from a lifetime of exposure to extreme temperatures. The teeth may look longer as the gum margins recede (Figure 17-26).

The tooth surfaces look worn down or abraded. Old dental work deteriorates, especially at the gum margins. The teeth loosen with bone resorption and may move with palpation.

The tongue looks smoother as a result of papillary atrophy. An older adult's buccal mucosa is thinned and may look shinier, as though it were varnished.

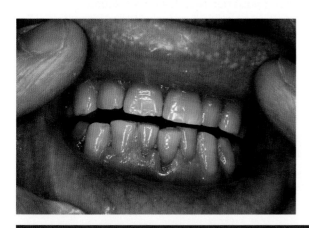

17-26 Receded gums.

Objective Data

DOCUMENTATION AND CRITICAL THINKING

Sample Charting

SUBJECTIVE

Nose: No history of discharge, sinus problems, obstruction, epistaxis, or allergy. Colds: one to two per year, mild. Nose fractured during high school sports, treated by MD.

Mouth and Throat: No pain, lesions, bleeding gums, toothache, dysphagia, or hoarseness. Occasional sore throat with colds. Tonsillectomy, age 8. Smokes cigarettes 1 PPD × 9 years. Alcohol: one to two drinks socially, about 2×/month. Visits dentist annually, dental hygienist 2×/year, flosses daily. No dental appliance.

OBJECTIVE

Nose: Symmetrical, no deformity or skin lesions. Nares patent. Mucosa pink; no discharge, lesions, or polyps; no septal deviation or perforation. Sinuses: no tenderness to palpation.

Mouth: Can clench teeth. Mucosa and gingivae pink, no masses or lesions. Teeth are all present, straight, and in good repair. Tongue smooth, pink, no lesions, protrudes in midline, no tremor.

Throat: Mucosa pink, no lesions or exudate. Uvula rises in midline on phonation. Tonsils out. Gag reflex present.

ASSESSMENT

Structures intact and appear healthy

Focused Assessment: Clinical Case Study 1

Brad D., a 34-year-old electrician, seeks care for "sore throat for 2 days."

SUBJECTIVE

- 2 days PTA experienced sudden onset of sore throat, swollen glands, fever 38.3°C, occasional shaking chills, extreme fatigue.
- Today: symptoms remain. Cough productive of yellow sputum. Treated self with aspirin with minimal relief. Unable to eat past 2 days because "throat on fire." Taking adequate fluids, on bed rest. Not aware of exposure to other sick persons. Does not smoke.

OBJECTIVE

Ears: Tympanic membranes pearl grey with landmarks intact.
Nose: No discharge. Mucosa pink, no swelling.
Mouth: Mucosa and gingivae pink, no lesions.
Throat: Tonsils 3+. Pharyngeal wall bright red with yellow-white exudate; exudate also on tonsils.
Neck: Enlarged anterior cervical nodes bilaterally, painful to palpation. No other lymph adenopathy.
Chest: Resonant to percussion throughout. Breath sounds clear anterior and posterior. No adventitious sounds.

ASSESSMENT

Pharyngitis
Pain R/T inflammation
Imbalanced nutrition: less than body requirements R/T dysphagia

Focused Assessment: Clinical Case Study 2

Calvin W., a 53-year-old man, is in the hospital awaiting coronary bypass surgery for coronary artery disease. He is allergic to dust and animal hair. As part of a preoperative teaching plan for coughing and deep breathing, a respiratory assessment is performed.

SUBJECTIVE

- States understanding of reason for admission to hospital and extent of coronary artery disease. Unaware of details of surgical procedure and postoperative care. Interested: "I do better when I know what I'm dealing with." History of exertional angina after walking one short block or climbing one flight of stairs, treats self with nitroglycerine. Does not smoke. Chronic watery nasal discharge, "comes and goes, but present most of the time."

OBJECTIVE

Nose: Only R naris patent. Mucosa grey and boggy bilaterally. L naris has mobile, grey, nontender mass, obstructing view of turbinates and rest of nasal cavity.

Mouth and Throat: Mucosa pink, no lesions. Uvula midline, rises on phonation. Tonsils absent. No lumps or lesions on palpation.

Chest: Thorax symmetrical, AP [anteroposterior] < transverse diameter, respirations 18/min, effortless. Resonant to percussion. Breath sounds are clear. No adventitious sounds.

ASSESSMENT

L nasal mass, possibly polyp
Deficient knowledge for surgery and expected postoperative course R/T lack of exposure

Focused Assessment: Clinical Case Study 3

E.V. is a 61-year-old professor who has been admitted to the hospital for chemotherapy for carcinoma of the breast. This is her fifth day in the hospital. An oral assessment is performed when she complains of "soreness and a white coating" in the mouth.

SUBJECTIVE

- Felt soreness on tongue and cheeks during night. Now pain persists, and E.V. can see a "white coating" on tongue and cheeks. "I'm worried. Is this more cancer?"

OBJECTIVE

E.V. generally appears restless and overly aware.

Oral mucosa pink. Large white, cheesy patches covering most of dorsal surface of tongue and buccal mucosa. Will scrape off with tongue blade, revealing red eroded area beneath.

Bleeds with slight contact. Posterior pharyngeal wall pink, no lesions. Patches are soft to palpation. No palpable lymph nodes.

ASSESSMENT

Oral lesion, appears as candidiasis
Impaired oral mucous membrane R/T effects of chemotherapy
Pain R/T infectious process
Anxiety R/T threat to health status

ABNORMAL FINDINGS

TABLE 17-1   Abnormalities of the Nose

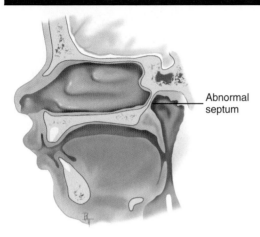

Abnormal septum

Choanal Atresia

A bony or membranous septum between the nasal cavity and the pharynx of the newborn. When the condition is bilateral, an oral airway must be established immediately to prevent asphyxia because most newborns are obligate nose breathers. When the condition is unilateral, the infant may have no symptoms until the onset of the first respiratory infection.

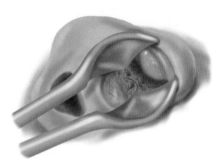

Epistaxis

The most common site of a nosebleed is Kiesselbach's plexus in the anterior septum. It may be spontaneous from a local cause or a sign of underlying illness. Causes include nose picking, forceful coughing or sneezing, fracture, foreign body, rhinitis, heavy exertion, or a coagulation disorder. Bleeding from the anterior septum is easily controlled and rarely severe. A posterior hemorrhage is less common (<10% of cases) but is more profuse, harder to manage, and more serious.

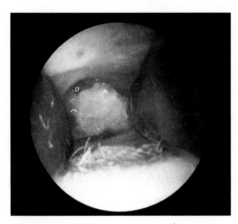

Foreign Body

Children are particularly apt to put an object up the nose (here, yellow plastic foam), which leads to unilateral mucopurulent drainage and foul odour. Because of some risk for aspiration, removal should be prompt.

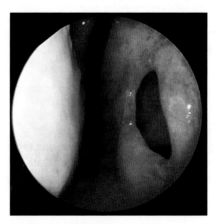

Perforated Septum

A hole in the septum, usually in the cartilaginous part, may be caused by snorting cocaine, chronic infection, trauma from continual picking of crusts, or nasal surgery. It is seen directly or as a spot of light when the penlight is directed into the other naris.

TABLE 17-1   Abnormalities of the Nose—cont'd

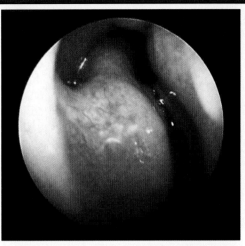

Reprinted from Fireman, P. (1995). Atlas of allergies (2nd ed.). St. Louis: Mosby, by permission of the publisher.

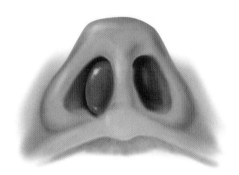

Furuncle

A small boil located in the skin or mucous membrane; appears red and swollen and is quite painful. Avoid any manipulation or trauma that may spread the infection.

Acute Rhinitis

The first sign is a clear, watery discharge, rhinorrhea, which later becomes purulent. This is accompanied by sneezing and swollen mucosa, which causes nasal obstruction. Turbinates are dark red and swollen.

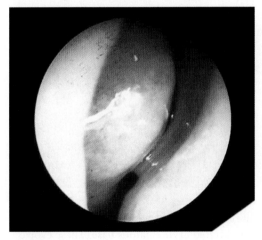

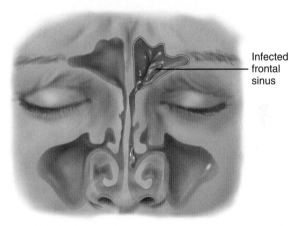

Infected frontal sinus

Allergic Rhinitis

Rhinorrhea, itching of nose and eyes, lacrimation, nasal congestion, and sneezing are present. Note serous edema and swelling of turbinates to fill the air space. Turbinates are usually pale (but may appear violet), and their surface looks smooth and glistening. May be seasonal or perennial, depending on allergen. Affected individual often has a strong family history of seasonal allergies.

Sinusitis

Facial pain, after upper respiratory infection; signs include red swollen nasal mucosa, swollen turbinates, and purulent discharge. Patient also has fever, chills, and malaise. With maxillary sinusitis, dull throbbing pain occurs in cheeks and teeth on the same side, and pain with palpation is present. With frontal sinusitis, pain is above the supraorbital ridge.

Continued

TABLE 17-1 Abnormalities of the Nose—cont'd

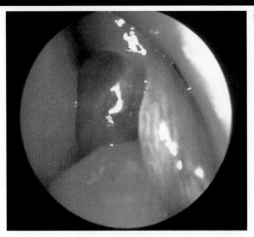

◄ *Nasal Polyps*
Smooth, pale grey nodules, which are overgrowths of mucosa, most commonly caused by chronic allergic rhinitis. May be stalked. A common site is protrusion from the middle meatus. Often multiple, they are mobile and nontender in contrast to turbinates. They may obstruct air passageways as they get larger. Symptoms include the absence of a sense of smell and a "valve that moves" in the nose as the patient breathes.

TABLE 17-2 Abnormalities of the Lips

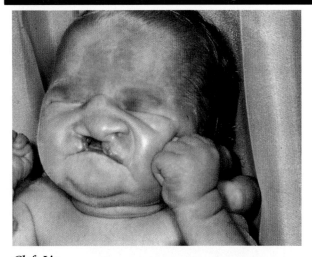

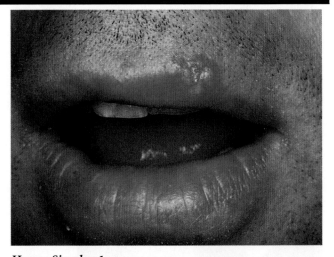

Cleft Lip
Maxillofacial clefts are the most common congenital deformities of the head and neck. The incidence varies widely among ethnocultural groups, with a higher frequency among Aboriginal people than among people of European descent. Although a reliable birth registry is not present in all countries, birth records do show a relatively high incidence in Scandinavia and middle European countries (e.g., 1 per 550 in Denmark and Finland, 1 per 575 in Poland and the former Czechoslovakia [Bluestone, Stool, & Kenna, 1996]). Early treatment preserves the functions of speech and language formation and deglutition (swallowing).

Herpes Simplex 1
"Cold sores" are groups of clear vesicles with a surrounding indurated erythematous base. These evolve into pustules, which rupture, weep, crust, and heal in 4–10 days. The most likely site is the lip–skin junction; infection often recurs in same site. Caused by the herpes simplex virus (HSV-1), the lesion is highly contagious and is spread by direct contact. Recurrent herpes infections may be precipitated by sunlight, fever, colds, and allergy. It is a very common lesion, affecting 50% of adults.

TABLE 17-2 Abnormalities of the Lips—cont'd

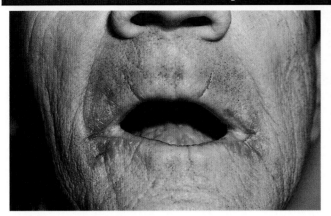

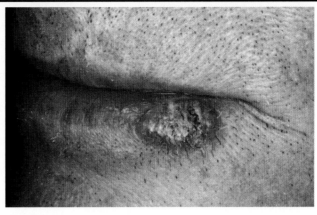

Angular Cheilitis (Stomatitis, Perlèche)
Erythema, scaling, and shallow, and painful fissures at the corners of the mouth occur with excess salivation and *Candida* infection. Cheilitis is often seen in edentulous patients and in those with poorly fitting dentures that cause the corners of the mouth to fold in, creating a warm, moist environment favourable for the growth of yeast.

Carcinoma
The initial lesion is round and indurated, and then it becomes crusted and ulcerated with an elevated border. The majority occur between the outer and middle thirds of the lip. Any lesion that is still unhealed after 2 weeks should be investigated.

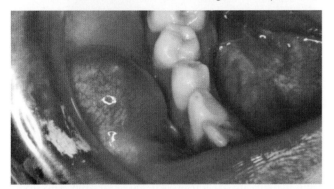

◄ **Retention "Cyst" (Mucocele)**
A round, well-defined translucent nodule that may be very small or up to 2 cm in diameter. It is a pocket of mucus that forms when a duct of a minor salivary gland ruptures. The benign lesion also may occur on the buccal mucosa, on the floor of the mouth, or under the tip of the tongue.

TABLE 17-3 Abnormalities of the Teeth and Gums

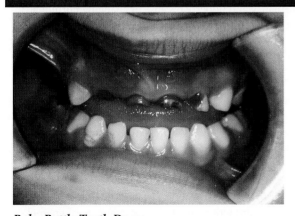

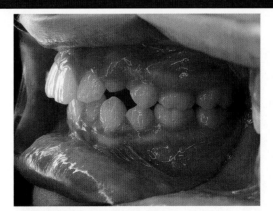

Baby Bottle Tooth Decay
Destruction of numerous deciduous teeth may occur in older infants and toddlers who take a bottle of milk, juice, or sweetened drink to bed and prolong bottle-feeding past the age of 1 year. Liquid pools around the upper front teeth. Mouth bacteria act on carbohydrates in the liquid, especially sucrose, forming metabolic acids. Acids break down tooth enamel and destroy its protein.

Malocclusion
Upper or lower dental arches are not in alignment, and incisors protrude as a result of a developmental problem of the mandible or maxilla or because of incompatibility between jaw size and tooth size. The condition increases risk of facial deformity, negative body image, chewing problems, and speech dysfluency.

Continued

TABLE 17-3   Abnormalities of the Teeth and Gums—cont'd

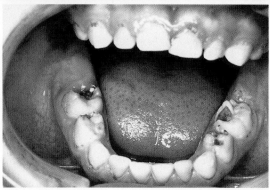

Dental Caries

Progressive destruction of tooth. Decay initially looks chalky white. Later, it turns brown or black and forms a cavity. Early decay is apparent only on radiographs. Susceptible sites are tooth surfaces where food debris, bacterial plaque, and saliva collect.

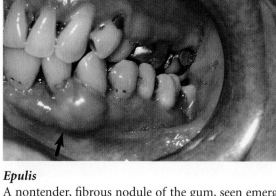

Epulis

A nontender, fibrous nodule of the gum, seen emerging between the teeth *(arrow)*; an inflammatory response to injury or hemorrhage.

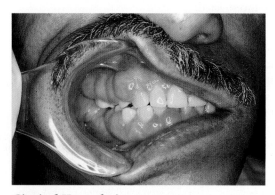

Gingival Hyperplasia

Painless enlargement of the gums, sometimes overreaching the teeth. This occurs with puberty, pregnancy, leukemia, and long-term therapeutic use of phenytoin (Dilantin).

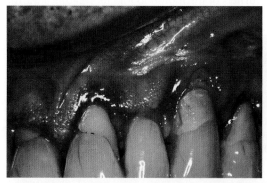

Gingivitis

Gum margins are red and swollen and bleed easily. This case is severe; gingival tissue has desquamated, exposing roots of teeth. Inflammation is usually a result of poor dental hygiene or vitamin C deficiency. The condition may occur in pregnancy and puberty because of changing hormonal balance.

◄ Meth Mouth

Illicit methamphetamine abuse ("crystal meth," "meth ice") leads to extensive dental caries, gingivitis, tooth cracking, and tooth loss. Methamphetamine causes vasoconstriction and a decrease in saliva, and its use increases the urge to consume sugars and starches and to neglect oral hygiene. Absence of the buffering saliva leads to increased acidity in the mouth, and the increased plaque encourages bacterial growth. These conditions and the presence of carbohydrates set up an oral environment prone to caries, cracking of enamel, and the damage seen here.

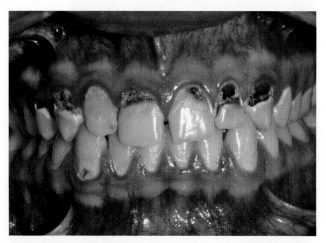

From Neville, B. W., Damm, D. D., Allen, C. M., & Bouquot, J. E. (2009). Oral and maxillofacial pathology (3rd ed.). St. Louis: W. B. Saunders.

TABLE 17-4	Abnormalities of the Buccal Mucosa

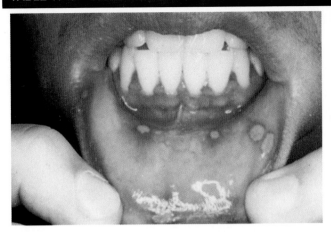

Aphthous Ulcers

Also called *canker sore;* are vesicles at first and then become small, round, "punched-out" ulcers with a white base surrounded by a red halo. They are quite painful and last for 1 to 2 weeks. The cause is unknown, although they are associated with stress, fatigue, and food allergy. They are common, affecting 20%–60% of the population.

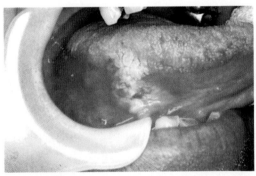

Leukoplakia

Chalky white, thick, raised patch with well-defined borders. The lesion is firmly attached and cannot be scraped off. It may occur on the lateral edges of tongue. It is caused by chronic irritation and occurs more frequently with heavy smoking and heavy alcohol use. Lesions are precancerous, and the patient should be referred. Here, the lesion is associated with squamous carcinoma.

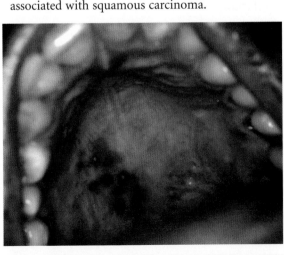

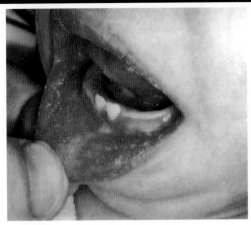

Koplik's Spots

Small blue-white spots with irregular red halo that are scattered over mucosa opposite the molars. They are an early sign, and pathognomonic, of measles.

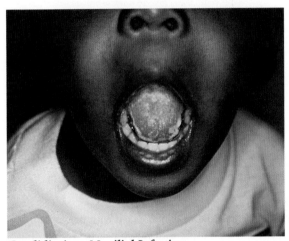

Candidiasis or Monilial Infection

A white, cheesy, curdlike patch on the buccal mucosa and tongue. It scrapes off, leaving a raw, red surface that bleeds easily. Termed *thrush* in newborns. It is an opportunistic infection that occurs after the use of antibiotics or corticosteroids and in immunosuppressed patients.

◄ **Herpes Simplex 1**

Herpes infection on the hard palate (see discussion in Table 17-2).

TABLE 17-5	Abnormalities of the Tongue

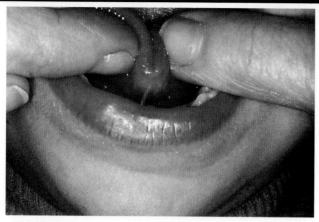

Ankyloglossia

Also known as *tongue-tie*. A short lingual frenulum, here fixing the tongue tip to the floor of the mouth and gums. This limits mobility and will affect speech (pronunciation of *a, d, n*) if the tongue tip cannot be elevated to the alveolar ridge. A congenital defect.

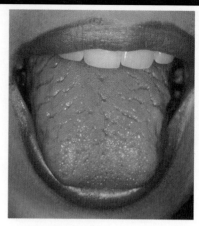

Fissured or Scrotal Tongue

Deep furrows divide the papillae into small irregular rows. The condition occurs in 5% of the general population and in Down's syndrome. The incidence increases with age. (Vertical, or longitudinal, fissures also occur with dehydration because of reduced volume of the tongue.)

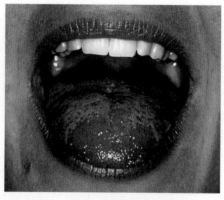

Geographic Tongue (Migratory Glossitis)

Pattern of normal coating interspersed with bright red, shiny, circular bald areas with raised pearly borders. The pattern resembles a map that changes as lesions heal in one area and migrate to a different area of the tongue. Not significant, and its cause is not known.

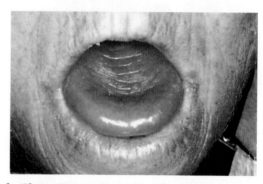

Smooth, Glossy Tongue (Atrophic Glossitis)

The surface is slick and shiny; the mucosa thins and looks red as a result of decreased papillae. Accompanied by dryness of tongue and burning sensation. Occurs with vitamin B_{12} deficiency (pernicious anemia), folic acid deficiency, and iron-deficiency anemia. Here, also note angular cheilitis.

TABLE 17-5   Abnormalities of the Tongue—cont'd

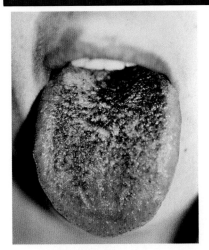

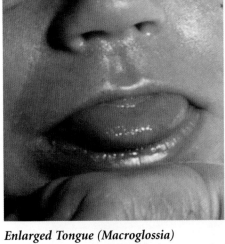

Black Hairy Tongue

The black appearance is not really hair but the elongation of filiform papillae and painless overgrowth of mycelial threads of fungus infection on the tongue. Colour varies from black-brown to yellow. It occurs after use of antibiotics, which inhibit normal bacteria and allow proliferation of fungus.

Enlarged Tongue (Macroglossia)

The tongue is enlarged and may protrude from the mouth. The condition is not painful but may impair speech development. Here, it occurs with Down's syndrome; it also occurs with cretinism, myxedema, and acromegaly. Also a transient swelling can occur with local infections.

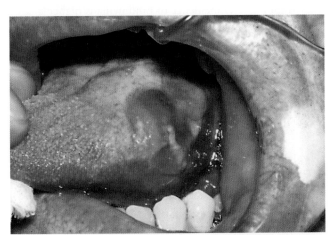

◄ Carcinoma

An ulcer with rolled edges; indurated. Occurs particularly at sides, base, and under the tongue. When it is in the floor of the mouth, it may cause movement of the tongue to be painful or limited. Risk of early metastasis is high because of rich lymphatic drainage. Heavy smoking and heavy alcohol use increase the risk.

TABLE 17-6   Abnormalities of the Oropharynx

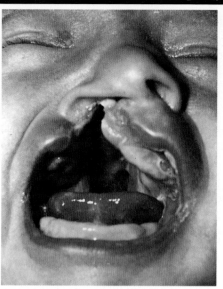

Cleft Palate

A congenital defect involving the failure of fusion of the maxillary processes. Wide variation occurs in the extent of cleft formation: from upper lip only, palate only, or uvula only to clefts of the nostril and the hard and soft palates.

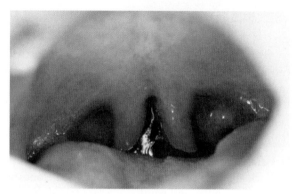

Bifid Uvula

The uvula looks partly severed. May indicate a submucous cleft palate, which feels like a notch at the junction of the hard and soft palates. The submucous cleft palate may affect speech development because it prevents necessary air trapping. The incidence of bifid uvula is higher among Aboriginal people.

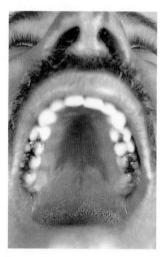

Oral Kaposi's Sarcoma

Bruiselike, dark red or violet, confluent macule, usually on the hard palate, may be on soft palate or gingival margin. Oral lesions may be among the earliest lesions to develop with AIDS.

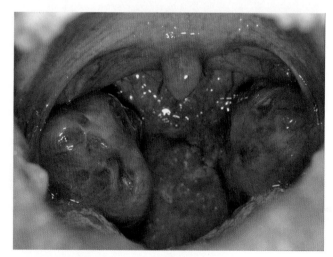

Acute Tonsillitis and Pharyngitis

Bright red throat; swollen tonsils; white or yellow exudate on tonsils and pharynx; swollen uvula; and enlarged, tender anterior cervical and tonsillar nodes. Accompanied by severe sore throat, painful swallowing, and fever (temperature >38.3°C) of sudden onset.

Caution: Bacterial infection cannot be distinguished from viral infection on the basis of clinical data alone; all patients with sore throats need a throat culture. Bacterial pharyngitis caused by group A β-hemolytic *Streptococcus* species, if untreated, may lead to the complication of rheumatic fever. This is a serious, complex illness characterized by fever, malaise, swollen joints, rash, and scarring on the heart valves.

AIDS, acquired immune deficiency syndrome.

Summary Checklist: Nose, Mouth, and Throat Examination

For a PDA-downloadable version, go to *http://evolve.elsevier.com/Canada/Jarvis/examination/*.

Nose

1. Inspect nose for symmetry, any deformity, or lesions
2. Palpation: test patency of each nostril
3. Inspect with nasal speculum:
   Nasal mucosa: note colour and integrity
   Septum: note any deviation, perforation, or bleeding
   Turbinates: note colour, exudates, swelling, or polyps
4. Palpate the sinus areas: note any tenderness

Mouth and Throat

1. Inspect with penlight:
   Lips, teeth and gums, tongue, buccal mucosa: note colour; whether structures are intact; any lesions
   Palate and uvula: note integrity and mobility as patient phonates
   Grade tonsils
   Pharyngeal wall: note colour, any exudates, or lesions
2. Palpation:
   When indicated in adults, palpate mouth bimanually
   With the neonate, palpate for integrity of the palate and to assess sucking reflex

REFERENCES

Bluestone, C. D., Stool, S. E., & Kenna, M. A. (1996). *Pediatric otolaryngology* (3rd ed.). Philadelphia: W. B. Saunders.

Dong, M., Levine, A., Loignon, C., & Bedos, C. (2011). Chinese immigrants' dental care pathways in Montreal, Canada. *Journal of the Canadian Dental Association, 77,* b131.

Godley, F. A. (1992). Chronic sinusitis: An update. *American Family Physician, 45*(5), 2190–2199.

Public Health Agency of Canada. (2012). Enough snuff. Retrieved from *http://66.240.150.14/intervention/225/view-eng.html.*

Quinonez, C., & Grootendorst, P. (2011). Equity in dental care among Canadian households. *International Journal for Equity in Health, 10*(4), 14. doi:10.1186/1475-9276-10-14

CHAPTER

18

Breasts and Regional Lymphatic System

Written by Carolyn Jarvis, PhD, APN, CNP
Adapted by Denise S. Tarlier, PhD, MSN, NP(F), NCMP

evolve WEBSITE

OUTLINE

The assessment of breast health is always performed in the context of health promotion; it offers a prime opportunity for teaching about health promotion and preventive health care practices related to women's health in general, as well as breast health more specifically. Most women and some men are well aware of the prevalence of breast cancer and are motivated to have regular breast examinations and to follow their health practitioner's health promotion and disease prevention recommendations.

STRUCTURE AND FUNCTION

The breasts, or mammary glands, are present in both women and men, although in men they are rudimentary throughout life. The female breasts are accessory reproductive organs whose function is to produce milk for nourishing the newborn.

404

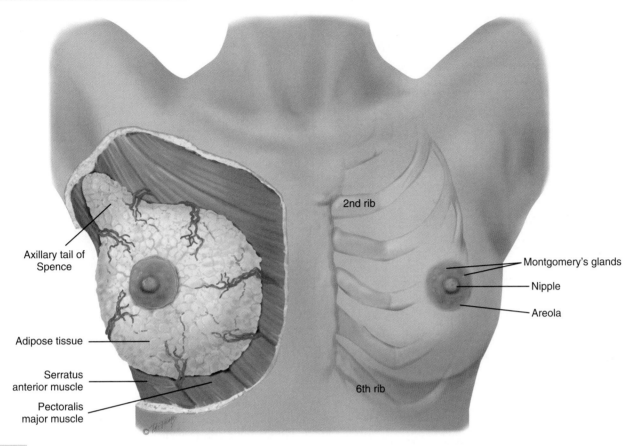

© Pat Thomas, 2010.

18-1

SURFACE ANATOMY

The **breasts** lie anterior to the pectoralis major and serratus anterior muscles (Figure 18-1). The breasts are located between the second and sixth ribs, extending from the side of the sternum to the midaxillary line. The superior lateral corner of breast tissue, called the axillary **tail of Spence,** projects up and laterally into the axilla.

The **nipple** is just below the centre of the breast. It is rough, round, and usually protuberant; its surface looks wrinkled and is indented with tiny milk duct openings. The **areola** surrounds the nipple for a 1- to 2-cm radius. In the areola are small elevated sebaceous glands, called *Montgomery's glands.* These glands secrete a protective lipid material during lactation. The areola also has smooth muscle fibres that cause nipple erection when stimulated. Both the nipple and areola are more darkly pigmented than the rest of the breast surface; the colour varies from pink to brown, depending on the person's skin colour and parity.

INTERNAL ANATOMY

The breast is composed of (a) glandular tissue; (b) fibrous tissue, including the suspensory ligaments; and (c) adipose tissue (Figure 18-2). The **glandular tissue** contains 15 to 20 lobes radiating from the nipple, and these are composed of lobules. Within each lobule are clusters of **alveoli** that produce milk. Each lobe empties into a **lactiferous** duct. The 15 to 20 lactiferous ducts

form a collecting duct system that converges at the nipple. There, the ducts form ampullae, or lactiferous sinuses, behind the nipple, which are reservoirs for storing milk.

The suspensory ligaments, or **Cooper's ligaments,** are fibrous bands extending vertically from the surface to attach on chest wall muscles. These support the breast tissue. They become contracted in cancer of the breast, which produces pits or dimples in the overlying skin.

The lobes are embedded in **adipose tissue.** These layers of subcutaneous and retromammary fat actually provide most of the bulk of the breast. The relative proportions of glandular, fibrous, and fatty tissue vary, depending on age, cycle, pregnancy, lactation, and general nutritional state.

The breast may be viewed as four quadrants, with imaginary horizontal and vertical lines intersecting at the nipple (Figure 18-3). This mapping is convenient for describing clinical findings. The upper outer quadrant includes the axillary tail of Spence, the cone-shaped breast tissue that projects up into the axilla, close to the pectoral group of axillary lymph nodes. The upper outer quadrant is the site of most breast tumours.

LYMPHATIC SYSTEM

The breast has extensive lymphatic drainage. Most of the lymph, more than 75%, drains into the ipsilateral (same side) axillary nodes. Four groups of axillary nodes are present (Figure 18-4):

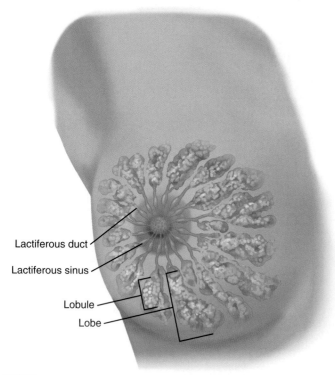

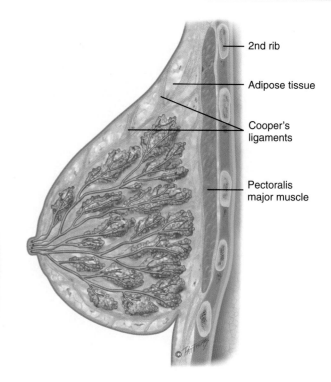

18-2

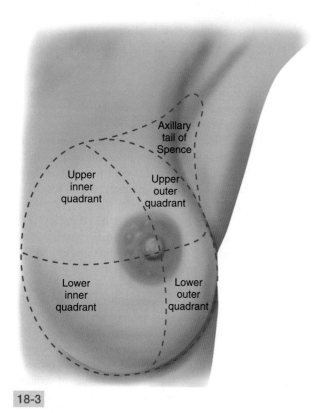

18-3

1. **Central axillary nodes:** high up in the middle of the axilla, over the ribs and serratus anterior muscle. These receive lymph from the other three groups of nodes.
2. **Pectoral** (anterior): along the lateral edge of the pectoralis major muscle, just inside the anterior axillary fold.

3. **Subscapular** (posterior): along the lateral edge of the scapula, deep in the posterior axillary fold.
4. **Lateral:** along the humerus, inside the upper arm.

From the central axillary nodes, lymph flows up to the infraclavicular and supraclavicular nodes.

A smaller amount of lymph does not drain through these channels but flows directly up to the infraclavicular group, deep into the chest, or into the abdomen, or directly across to the opposite breast.

❖ DEVELOPMENTAL CONSIDERATIONS

During embryonic life, ventral epidermal ridges, or "milk lines," are present; these curve down from the axilla to the groin bilaterally (Figure 18-5). The breast develops along the ridge over the thorax, and the rest of the ridge usually atrophies. On occasion, a **supernumerary nipple** (i.e., an extra nipple) persists and is visible somewhere along the track of the mammary ridge (see Figure 18-8 on p. 416).

At birth, the only breast structures present are the lactiferous ducts within the nipple. No alveoli have developed. Little change occurs until puberty.

Adolescents

At puberty the estrogen hormones stimulate breast changes. The breasts enlarge, mostly as a result of extensive fat deposition. The duct system also grows and branches, and masses of small, solid cells develop at the duct endings. These are potential alveoli.

On occasion, one breast grows faster than the other, which results in a temporary asymmetry. This may cause some

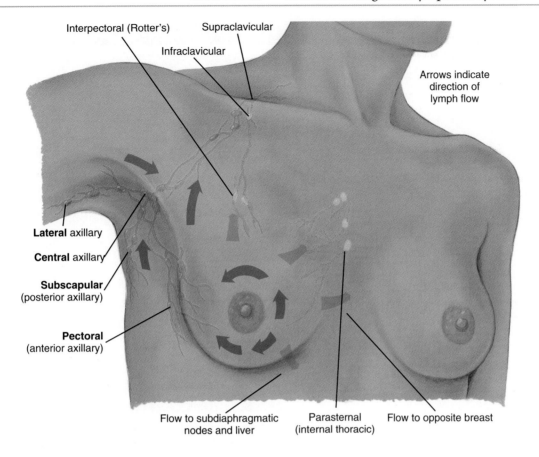

Interpectoral (Rotter's)
Supraclavicular
Infraclavicular
Arrows indicate direction of lymph flow

Lateral axillary
Central axillary
Subscapular (posterior axillary)
Pectoral (anterior axillary)

Flow to subdiaphragmatic nodes and liver
Parasternal (internal thoracic)
Flow to opposite breast

18-4

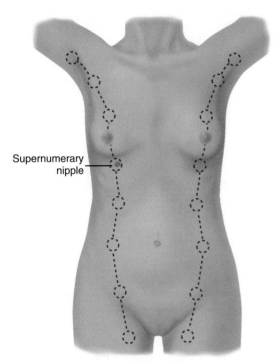

Supernumerary nipple

18-5

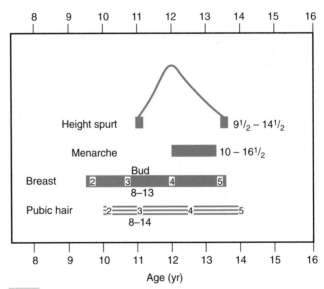

18-6 Relationship of puberty events in girls.

distress; reassurance is necessary. Tenderness in the developing breasts is also common. Although the age at onset varies widely, the breasts develop in five stages according to the classic description of sexual maturity rating, or **Tanner staging** (Table 18-1).

Full development from stage 2 to stage 5 takes an average of 3 years, although the range is 1.5 to 6 years. During this time, pubic hair appears, and axillary hair appears 2 years after the appearance of pubic hair. **Thelarche,** the beginning of breast development, precedes **menarche** (beginning of menstruation) by about 2 years. Menarche occurs during breast development stage 3 or 4, usually just after the peak of the adolescent growth spurt, at approximately age 12 years. Note the relationship of these events (Figure 18-6). This aids

Structure & Function

TABLE 18-1	Sexual Maturity Rating in Girls

Stage 1 (preadolescent): Only a small elevated nipple is present.

Stage 2 (breast bud stage): A small mound of breast and nipple develops; the areola widens.

Stage 3: The breast and areola enlarge; the nipple is flush with the breast surface.

Stage 4: The areola and nipple form a secondary mound over the breast.

Stage 5 (mature breast): Only the nipple protrudes; the areola is flush with the breast contour (the areola may continue as a secondary mound in some normal women).

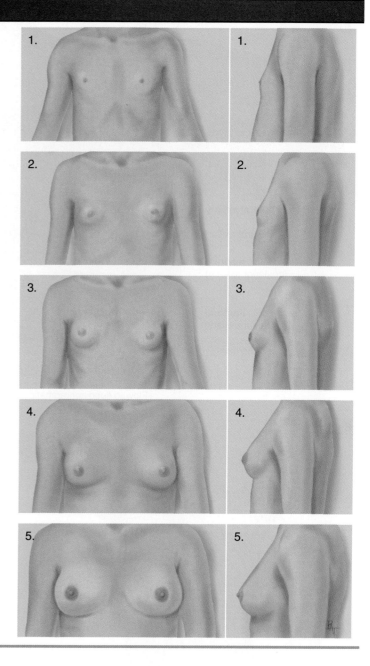

in assessing the development of adolescent girls and increases their knowledge about their own development.

Breasts of nonpregnant women change with the ebb and flow of hormones during the monthly menstrual cycle. Nodularity increases from midcycle up to menstruation. During the 3 to 4 days before menstruation, the breasts feel full, tight, heavy, and occasionally sore. The breast volume is smallest on days 4 to 7 of the menstrual cycle.

Pregnant Women

During pregnancy, breast changes start during the second month and are an early sign of pregnancy for most women. Pregnancy stimulates the expansion of the ductal system and supporting fatty tissue, as well as development of the true secretory alveoli. Thus the breasts enlarge and feel more nodular. The nipples are larger, darker, and more erectile, and the areolae become larger and darken as pregnancy progresses. (The colour fades after lactation, but the areolae never return to the original colour.) The tubercles become more prominent. A venous pattern is prominent over the skin surface (see Figure 30-4 on p. 827).

After the fourth month, **colostrum** may be expressed. This thick yellow fluid is the precursor of milk, containing the same amount of protein and lactose but practically no fat. The breasts produce colostrum for the first few days after delivery. It is rich with antibodies that protect the newborn against infection, and so breastfeeding is important. Milk production (lactation) begins 1 to 3 days post partum. The whitish colour is caused by the presence of emulsified fat and calcium caseinate.

Older Women

After menopause, ovarian secretion of estrogen and progesterone decreases, which causes the breast glandular tissue to atrophy. This is replaced with fibrous connective tissue. The fat envelope also atrophies, beginning in the middle years and becoming marked in the eighth and ninth decades. These changes decrease breast size and elasticity, so that the breasts droop and sag, looking flattened and flabby. Drooping is accentuated by the kyphosis in some older women.

As a result of decreased breast size, the inner structures become more prominent. A breast lump that may have been present for years but not detected becomes palpable. Around the nipple, the lactiferous ducts are more palpable and feel firm and stringy because of fibrosis and calcification. The axillary hair decreases.

THE MALE BREAST

The male breast is a rudimentary structure consisting of a thin disk of undeveloped tissue underlying the nipple. The areola is well developed, although the nipple is relatively very small. During adolescence, it is common for the breast tissue to temporarily enlarge; such enlargement represents **gynecomastia** (see Figure 18-21). This condition is usually unilateral and temporary. Reassurance is necessary for adolescent boys, to whom body image is extremely important. Gynecomastia may reappear in older men and may be a result of testosterone deficiency.

CULTURAL AND SOCIAL CONSIDERATIONS

Few health initiatives across Canada have been taken up by the public in the way that women's breast screening has. Long-term, proactive public awareness initiatives and access to screening measures such as mammography are paying off in declining rates of mortality from breast cancer (Canadian Cancer Society [CCS] Steering Committee on Cancer Statistics, 2011). Breast cancer is being diagnosed at earlier stages of cancer development, and patients are receiving treatment sooner and surviving longer. Despite these successes, breast cancer remains the most common cancer among women in Canada and is the second most common cause of cancer-related death in women (CCS Steering Committee on Cancer Statistics, 2011).

The lifetime risk for breast cancer in Canada is approximately 1 per 9, and 1 per 29 women may be expected to die from breast cancer (CCS Steering Committee on Cancer Statistics, 2011). Incidence and mortality rates for breast cancer, and related risk factors, are heavily influenced by socioeconomic level, ethnocultural background, rural locations, and inequities in access to health services. For example, women of higher socioeconomic status have a slightly increased risk for breast cancer; researchers speculate that this may be related to an average older age at childbearing, having fewer children, or a greater likelihood of receiving postmenopausal hormone replacement therapy (CCS, 2012). However, researchers and health care providers are focusing increasingly on how social determinants of health, such as low socioeconomic level, education, living in a rural or remote area, and ethnocultural background, along with an identified lack of culturally safe health service options, present barriers to women's access to and use of health care resources. For example, Ahmad, Cameron, and Stewart (2005) found that offering "socioculturally tailored and language specific health education materials" (p. 575) to South Asian immigrant women residing in Toronto not only increased the women's knowledge about breast cancer but also improved their self-efficacy and practice of clinical breast examination (CBE). Similarly, research findings show that Canadian Aboriginal women are more likely to access and understand breast cancer education when it is culturally relevant, presented respectfully, and offered in easily understood language (Friedman & Hoffman-Goetz, 2007).

The growing obesity "epidemic" in Canada has important implications for breast cancer risk: obesity is an identified risk factor for breast cancer (Table 18-2). Some studies have also

TABLE 18-2	**Risk Factors for Breast Cancer**	
Unmodifiable Risk Factors	**Modifiable Risk Factors**	**Possible Risk Factors***
Female sex, age between 50 and 69 years	Nulliparity or first child after age 30 years	Physical inactivity
Personal history of breast cancer	Hormonal contraceptive use	Adult weight gain
Family history of breast cancer	Hormone replacement therapy	Smoking and second-hand smoke exposure
Dense breasts	Alcohol intake of ≥1 drink daily	High birth weight
BRCA gene mutation	Obesity	Night shift work
Ashkenazi Jewish ancestry	High socioeconomic status	Certain benign breast conditions
Specific rare genetic conditions		
Early menarche (before age 11 years) or late menopause (age 55 or older)		
Exposure to ionizing radiation		
Atypical hyperplasia		
Tall adult height		

*Although possible risk factors have some association with breast cancer, evidence at the time of publication is insufficient to identify these as known risk factors.
Data adapted from Canadian Cancer Society. Retrieved from *http://www.cancer.ca/Canada-wide/About%20cancer/Types%20of%20cancer/Causes%20of%20breast%20cancer.aspx?sc_lang=en.*

revealed that a diet rich in certain fats strongly promotes development of breast cancer and that breast cancer is less common in countries where the diet is low in total fat, low in polyunsaturated fat, and low in saturated fat (Buzdar, 2006). Although obesity is an identified breast cancer risk factor, the relationship of breast cancer to dietary fat is not yet clear. It is clear, however, that the relationship between obesity, high-fat diets, and breast cancer has implications for Canadians who consume a "typical" high-fat North American–style diet and, in particular, for those who lack the socioeconomic resources to eat more nutritious foods. For example, Aboriginal people living in Canada's far northern and remote communities may not be able to make more nutritious food choices because of both the high cost and the lack of availability of such foods in their communities.

SUBJECTIVE DATA

Breast

1. Pain
2. Lump
3. Discharge
4. Rash
5. Swelling
6. Trauma
7. History of breast disease
8. Surgery
9. Self-care behaviours
   Perform breast self-examination
   Last mammogram

Axilla

1. Tenderness, lump, or swelling
2. Rash

In Western culture the female breasts signify more than their primary purpose of lactation. Women are surrounded by messages that feminine norms of beauty and desirability are enhanced by and dependent on the size of the breasts and their appearance. Women leaders have tried to refocus this attitude, stressing women's self-worth as individual human beings, not as stereotyped sexual objects. The intense cultural emphasis is gradually changing, but the breasts still are crucial to many women's self-concept and their perception of their femininity. Matters pertaining to the breast affect a woman's body image and generate deep emotional responses.

This emotionality may take strong forms that you observe as you discuss the woman's history. One woman may be acutely embarrassed talking about her breasts, as evidenced by lack of eye contact, minimal response, nervous gestures, or inappropriate humour. Another woman may talk wryly and disparagingly about the size or development of her breasts. A young adolescent is acutely aware of her own development in relation to her peers. A woman who has found a breast lump may exhibit fear, high anxiety, and even panic. Although many breast lumps are benign, women initially assume the worst possible outcome: cancer, disfigurement, and death. While you are collecting the subjective data, tune in to cues for these behaviours, which necessitate a straightforward and reasoned attitude on your part.

HEALTH HISTORY QUESTIONS

Examiner Asks	Rationale
Breast	
1. Pain. Any **pain** or tenderness in the breasts? When did you first notice it? • Where is the pain? Localized or all over? • Is the painful spot sore to touch? Do you feel a burning or pulling sensation?	**Mastalgia** occurs with trauma, inflammation, infection, and benign breast disease.
• Is the pain cyclical? Any relation to your menstrual period?	Cyclical pain is common with normal breasts, oral contraceptives, and benign breast disease.
• Is the pain brought on by strenuous activity, especially involving one arm; a change in activity; manipulation during sex; part of an underwire bra; or exercise?	Determine whether pain is related to specific cause.

|

2. **Lump.** Ever noticed a **lump** or **thickening** in the breast? Where?
   - When did you first notice it? Has it changed at all since then?
   - Does the lump have any relation to your menstrual period?
   - Have you noticed any change in the overlying skin: redness, warmth, dimpling, swelling?

3. **Discharge.** Any **discharge** from the nipple?
   - When did you first notice this?
   - What colour is the discharge?
   - Consistency: Is it thick or runny?
   - Does it have an odour?

Carefully explore the presence of any lump. A lump present for many years and exhibiting no change may not be serious but still should be investigated. Approach any recent change or new lump with suspicion.

Galactorrhea refers to the secretion of milky-white discharge from one or both breasts in a man, or in a woman who is neither pregnant nor breastfeeding.

Note medications that may cause clear nipple discharge: oral contraceptives, phenothiazines, diuretics, digitalis, steroids, methyldopa, calcium channel blockers.

Bloody or blood-tinged discharge should always be investigated. Any discharge with a lump should be investigated.

Paget's disease starts with a small crust on the nipple apex and then spreads to the areola (see Table 18-6, Abnormal Nipple Discharge, p. 429).

4. **Rash.** Any **rash** on the breast?
   - When did you first notice this?
   - Where did it start? On the nipple, areola, or surrounding skin?

Eczema or other dermatitis rarely starts at nipple unless it is caused by breastfeeding. It usually starts on the areola or surrounding skin and then spreads to the nipple.

5. **Swelling.** Any **swelling** in the breasts? In one spot or all over?
   - Related to your menstrual period, pregnancy, or breastfeeding?
   - Any change in bra size?

6. **Trauma.** Any **trauma** or injury to the breasts?
   - Did it result in any swelling, lump, or break in skin?

A lump from an injury is caused by local hematoma or edema and should resolve shortly. Trauma may also cause a woman to feel the breast and find a lump that really was there before.

7. **History of breast disease and breast cancer risk factors.** Do you have any personal history of breast disease?
   - What type? How was this diagnosed? For example, has a health care provider ever told you that you have "dense" breasts or "atypical hyperplasia" of your breasts?
   - When did this occur?
   - How is it being treated?
   - Any breast cancer in your family? In whom: sister, mother, maternal grandmother, maternal aunts, daughter?
   - At what age did this relative have breast cancer?
   - At what age did your menses start?
   - (If postmenopausal) What was your age at menopause?
   - Have you experienced any changes in your weight?
   - Have you had any exposure to ionizing radiation (e.g., chest radiographs, computed tomography [CT])? What is your alcohol intake? Do you have Ashkenazi Jewish ancestry or any genetic conditions?
   - Reproductive history: How many times have you been pregnant? How old were you when your first child was born? Have you used hormonal contraceptives or (if perimenopausal) hormone replacement therapy?

Past breast cancer increases the risk of recurrent cancer (see Table 18-2, p. 409).

The presence of benign breast disease makes the breasts more difficult to examine; the general lumpiness conceals a new lump.

Women who have a first-degree relative with breast cancer have approximately double the lifetime risk of developing breast cancer (CCS, 2012). Genetic factors are also implicated as risk factors but to a lesser extent: only 5%-10% of cancers are characterized by an identifiable breast cancer gene (*BRCA1* or *BRCA2*; see Table 18-2, Risk Factors for Breast Cancer, p. 409).

8. **Surgery.** Have you ever had **surgery** on your breasts? Was this a biopsy?
   - What were the biopsy results?
   - Did you undergo mastectomy? Have you undergone mammoplasty (augmentation or reduction)?

Subjective Data

Examiner Asks	Rationale

9. Current breast health behaviours
- Have you ever discussed your breast cancer risk and screening recommendations with a health care provider?
- Have you ever had mammography, a screening x-ray examination of the breasts? (If yes) How often?
- Do you have your breasts examined by a trained health care provider as part of your routine health checkup?
- Do you ever examine your own breasts? Have you ever been taught breast self-examination (BSE)?
  - (If yes) I would like you to show me your technique after I complete your examination.
  - (If no) If you decide you would like to practise BSE after a discussion of the benefits and risks, I will teach you the technique.

Axilla

1. **Tenderness, lump, or swelling.** Any **tenderness** or **lump** in the underarm area?
   - Where? When did you first notice this?
2. **Rash.** Any axillary **rash?** Please describe it.
   - Does it seem to be a reaction to deodorant?

Breast tissue extends up into the axilla. Also, the axilla contains many lymph nodes.

Additional History for Preadolescents

1. **Female breast changes.** Have you noticed your breasts changing?
   - How long has this been happening?
2. **Other pubertal changes.** Many girls notice other changes in their bodies, too, that come with growing up. What have you noticed?
   - What do you think about all this?

Developing breasts are the most obvious sign of puberty and the focus of attention for most girls, especially in comparison with peers. Assess each girl's perception of her own development, and provide teaching and reassurance as indicated.

Additional History for Pregnant Women

1. **Breast changes.** Have you noticed any enlargement or fullness in the breasts?
   - Is there any tenderness or tingling?

   - Do you have a history of **inverted** nipples?

2. **Breastfeeding.** Are you planning to breastfeed your baby?

Breast changes are expected and normal during pregnancy. Assess the woman's knowledge, and provide reassurance.

Inverted nipples (i.e., that are depressed or invaginated) may need special care in preparation for breastfeeding.

Breastfeeding provides the perfect food and antibodies for the baby, decreases risk of ear infections, promotes bonding, and provides relaxation.

Additional History for Menopausal Women

1. **Breast changes.** Have you noticed any change in the breast contour, size, or firmness? (Note: Change may not be as apparent to obese women or to the woman whose earlier pregnancies already have produced breast changes.)

Decreased estrogen level causes decreased firmness. Rapid decrease in estrogen level causes actual shrinkage.

SPECIAL CONSIDERATIONS FOR ADVANCED PRACTICE

The breast health history offers an ideal opportunity to provide information about risk assessment and counselling related to hormone therapy in perimenopausal women. Many women are afraid to broach the question of hormone therapy with health practitioners because of concerns about its safety. Reassure women that risk assessment and counselling about using hormone therapy is an individual matter; with adequate risk analysis and by following evidence-informed guidelines, many women may safely use hormone therapy for the relief of uncomfortable perimenopausal symptoms, such as hot flashes (North American Menopause Society, 2012). See the box Promoting Health: Breast Cancer.

PROMOTING HEALTH: BREAST CANCER

Best Practice for Breast Cancer Risk Assessment and Screening Recommendations

Breast cancer is the second major cause of death from cancer in women. However, early detection and improved treatment have increased survival rates. The 5-year relative survival ratio (RSR) for breast cancer across Canada is 88% (CCS Steering Committee on Cancer Statistics, 2011). The RSR is defined as the "observed survival of a group of persons diagnosed with a cancer [in comparison with that of] the survival of people in the same general population" (CCS Steering Committee on Cancer Statistics, 2011, p. 60). For example, a RSR of 88% means women with breast cancer have an 88% likelihood of living for 5 or more years after diagnosis, in comparison with women in the general population without breast cancer, who are presumed to have a 100% likelihood of living 5 or more years.

Health assessment offers an opportunity to review the patient's knowledge about breast cancer risk and screening. It is also an opportunity to assess the patient's breast cancer risk, offer education and counselling about current breast cancer screening recommendations, and, in collaboration with the patient, develop a breast cancer screening plan customized to the patient's level of risk and her individual preferences about screening methods (North American Menopause Society, 2012).

The best way to detect a patient's risk for breast cancer is by asking the correct history questions. Table 18-2 highlights risk factors for breast cancer, and from these you can fashion your questions. Be aware that most breast cancers occur in women with no identifiable risk factors, other than gender and age. Just because a woman does not report the cited risk factors does not mean that you or she should fail to consider breast cancer seriously.

According to the recommendations by the Canadian Task Force on Preventive Health Care and colleagues (2011) for breast cancer screening (see Box 18-1), neither BSE nor CBE is now routinely recommended to Canadian women who have an average or low risk for breast cancer. Current evidence suggests that these procedures lack specificity and result in excessive benign or false-positive results of biopsies, lead to overdiagnosis and overtreatment, and create anxiety. In other words, the harms outweigh the benefits. However, of importance is that these guidelines are directed only to women between the ages of 40 and 74 years and of average risk. *Average risk* is defined by the guideline as having (a) no previous history of breast cancer, (b) no history of breast cancer in a first-degree relative, (c) no known *BRCA/BRCA2* gene mutations, and (d) no previous exposure of the chest wall to radiation. Also of importance is that the recommendations are considered *weak,* being informed by moderate- or low-quality evidence. Thus your assessment of individual risk directs how you implement the guideline in clinical practice with any individual patient.

The value of early detection of breast cancer is clear. Although screening mammography is available for many groups of women in developed countries, BSE is available to virtually all women. BSE is valuable to women who are younger or older than the ages recommended for screening mammography or who have barriers to access mammography. BSE has no cost, is noninvasive, can be accomplished without visits to expert professionals, and enhances self-care action.

The CCS (2012) continues to recommend that it is important for all women to be familiar with their own breasts, regardless of their risk of breast cancer or what screening protocol is followed. The seeming discrepancy between the evidence-informed guideline of the Canadian Task Force on Preventive Health Care and colleagues (2011) and the CCS's (2012) recommendation underscores what is *most important* about counselling and teaching women about BSE: the decision to do BSE is an *individual* informed decision made by each woman based on her *individual* breast cancer risk assessment, and a comprehensive discussion with her health care provider about the risks and benefits to her as an *individual* of breast cancer screening, including BSE and CBE.

BSE, breast self-examination; *CBE,* clinical breast examination.

SPECIAL CONSIDERATIONS FOR ADVANCED PRACTICE

BREAST CANCER SCREENING TOOLS

The use of breast cancer risk assessment tools in the clinical setting (Box 18-1) supports more effective early detection programs for individuals at high risk for breast cancer. The Gail Model, a breast cancer risk assessment tool, is widely used for calculating individual risk estimates for breast cancer. This model takes into account identified risk factors, including current age, age at menarche, age at first live birth, and family history of breast cancer in first-degree relatives. It also calculates 5-year and lifetime cumulative absolute risk estimates for the individual. It is easy to complete, and many computer-based data programs are available to clinicians (for an example, see the Halls MD Health Calculators and Charts,

listed in the section Other Web Sites of Interest at the end of this chapter). The U.S. National Cancer Institute also provides an interactive online tool that is based on the Gail Model to assist health care providers in estimating a woman's risk for developing breast cancer (see the section Other Web Sites of Interest).

However, the Gail Model may underestimate the breast cancer risk in the subgroup of women with family cancer histories suggestive of hereditary breast cancer syndromes, such as those caused by the oncogenes *BRCA1* and *BRCA2.*

The Pedigree Assessment Tool (PAT) was developed to identify this subgroup of women and can be used along with the Gail Model to screen for breast cancer risk. The PAT score is calculated by adding the points assigned to

---

BOX 18-1 SUMMARY OF BREAST CANCER SCREENING RECOMMENDATIONS FOR CLINICIANS AND POLICYMAKERS

Recommendations are presented for the use of mammography, magnetic resonance imaging (MRI), breast self-examination, and clinical breast examination to screen for breast cancer. These recommendations apply only to women at average risk of breast cancer aged 40–74 years. They do not apply to women at higher risk because of personal history of breast cancer, history of breast cancer in first-degree relatives, known mutations of the *BRCA1/BRCA2* genes, or previous exposure of the chest wall to radiation. No recommendations are made for women aged 75 years and older, given the lack of data available for this group.

Mammography
- For women aged 40–49 years, we recommend not routinely screening with mammography. (Weak recommendation; moderate-quality evidence.)
- For women aged 50–69 years, we recommend routinely screening with mammography every two to three years. (Weak recommendation; moderate-quality evidence.)

- For women aged 70–74 years, we recommend routinely screening with mammography every two to three years. (Weak recommendation; low-quality evidence.)

Magnetic Resonance Imaging
- We recommend not routinely screening with MRI scans. (Weak recommendation; no evidence.)

Clinical Breast Examination
- We recommend not routinely performing clinical breast examinations alone or in conjunction with mammography to screen for breast cancer. (Weak recommendation; low-quality evidence.)

Breast Self-Examination
- We recommend not advising women to routinely practise breast self-examination. (Weak recommendation; moderate-quality evidence.)

Source: From Canadian Task Force on Preventive Health Care, Tonelli, M., Connor Gorber, S., Joffres, M., Dickinson, J., Singh, H., … Liu, Y. Y. (2011). Recommendations on screening for breast cancer in average-risk women aged 40–74 years. *Canadian Medical Association Journal, 183*(17), 1991–2001 (p. 1995). doi:10.1503/cmaj.110334

every family member, including second- and third-degree relatives, with a breast or ovarian cancer diagnosis. Additional points for each individual are calculated for bilateral disease, the occurrence of both breast and ovarian cancers, and for the age at diagnosis. A separate score is calculated for the individual's maternal and paternal family histories. The higher of the two scores is used. The specific inclusion of both sides of a woman's family is important because many women often disregard or overlook paternal lineage altogether when thinking about or reporting family history of breast cancer. For more information about the Gail Model

and PAT risk assessment tools, as well as instructions on calculating a PAT score, please see the section Web Sites of Interest.

Although breast cancer screening tools such as the Gail Model and PAT provide useful information to health practitioners, it is important to remember the limitations of each tool, as described previously. Screening tools provide additional valuable assessment data that must be considered critically and within the context of the whole assessment, in order to best counsel a woman about her individual breast cancer risk.

OBJECTIVE DATA

PREPARATION
The woman is sitting up and facing the examiner. An alternative draping method is to use a short gown, open at the back, and lift it up to the woman's shoulders during inspection. During palpation, when the woman is supine, cover one breast with the gown while examining the other. Be aware that many women are embarrassed to have their breasts examined; use a sensitive but matter-of-fact approach.

EQUIPMENT NEEDED
Small pillow
Ruler marked in centimetres

Normal Range of Findings	Abnormal Findings

INSPECT THE BREASTS

General Appearance

Note symmetry of size and shape (Figure 18-7). It is common to have a slight asymmetry in size; often the left breast is slightly larger than the right.

A sudden increase in the size of one breast signifies inflammation or new growth.

Normal Range of Findings	Abnormal Findings

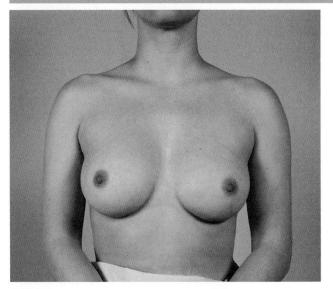

18-7

Skin

The skin is normally smooth and of even colour. Note any localized areas of redness, bulging, or dimpling. Also, note any skin lesions or focal vascular pattern. A fine blue vascular network is normally visible during pregnancy. Pale linear **striae**, or stretch marks, often follow pregnancy.

Normally, no edema is present. Edema exaggerates the hair follicles, giving a "pig-skin" or "orange-peel" look (also called ***peau d'orange***).

Hyperpigmentation.
Redness and heat with inflammation.
Unilateral dilated superficial veins in a nonpregnant woman.
Edema (see Table 18-3, p. 426).

Lymphatic Drainage Areas

Observe the axillary and supraclavicular regions. Note any bulging, discoloration, or edema.

Nipple

The nipples should be symmetrical, on the same plane on the two breasts. Nipples usually protrude, although some are flat and some are inverted. They tend to stay in their original condition. Distinguish a recently retracted nipple from one that has been inverted for many years or since puberty. Normal nipple inversion may be unilateral or bilateral, and usually the nipple can be pulled out (i.e., it is not fixed).

Note any dry scaling, any fissure or ulceration, and bleeding or other discharge.

Deviation in nipple pointing (see Table 18-3, p. 426).
Recent nipple retraction: signifies acquired disease (see Table 18-3, p. 426).

Explore any discharge, especially in the presence of a breast mass. (See the Critical Findings box.)

CRITICAL FINDINGS

Unexplained discharge or bleeding from nipples, open or ulcerating nontraumatic lesions, or a breast mass in a patient with previously diagnosed cancer indicate further investigation on an urgent basis. Patients with these conditions may require referral to a practitioner who can requisition the appropriate diagnostic tests (such as a nurse practitioner, physician, or surgeon). Tests may include diagnostic mammography, ultrasonography, biopsy, or magnetic resonance imaging (MRI), depending on the specific findings and the patient's history (see Table 18-6, Abnormal Nipple Discharge, p. 428).

Objective Data

Normal Range of Findings	Abnormal Findings

A supernumerary nipple is a normal and common variation (Figure 18-8). An extra nipple along the embryonic "milk line" on the thorax or abdomen (see Figure 18-5) is a congenital occurrence. Usually, it is 5 to 6 cm below the breast near the midline and has no associated glandular tissue. It looks like a mole, although a close look reveals a tiny nipple and areola. It is not significant; merely distinguish it from a mole.

In rare cases, additional glandular tissue, called a *supernumerary breast,* is present.

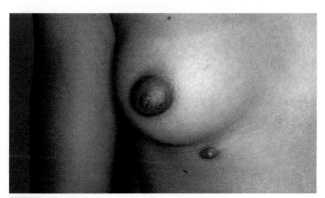

18-8   Supernumerary nipple and areolar complex.

Manoeuvres to Screen for Retraction

Direct the woman to change position while you check the breasts for skin retraction signs. First, ask her to lift the arms slowly over the head. Both breasts should move up symmetrically (Figure 18-9).

Retraction signs result from fibrosis in the breast tissue, usually caused by growing neoplasms. The fibrosis shortens with time, causing signs that are in contrast to the normally loose breast tissue.

Note a lag in movement of one breast.

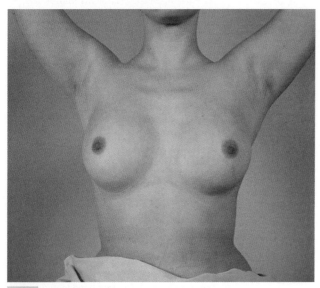

18-9   Retraction manoeuvre.

Next, ask her to push her hands onto her hips (Figure 18-10) and then to push her two palms together (Figure 18-11). These manoeuvres contract the pectoralis major muscle. Both breasts are lifted slightly.

Note a dimpling or a pucker, which indicates skin retraction (see Table 18-3, p. 426).

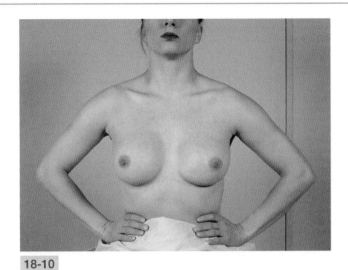

18-10

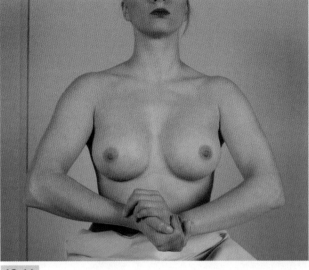

18-11

Normal Range of Findings	Abnormal Findings
Ask a woman with large, pendulous breasts to lean forward while you support her forearms. Note the symmetrical free-forward movement of both breasts (Figure 18-12).	Note fixation to chest wall or skin retraction (see Table 18-3, p. 426).

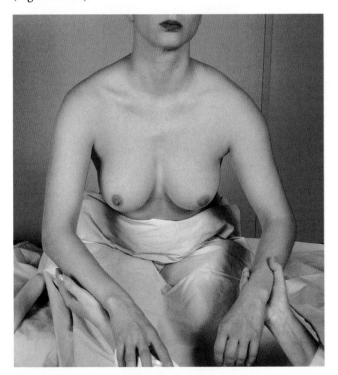

18-12

INSPECT AND PALPATE THE AXILLAE

Examine the axillae while the woman is sitting. Inspect the skin, noting any rash or infection. Lift the woman's arm and support it yourself, so that her muscles are loose and relaxed. Use your right hand to palpate the left axilla for tenderness or palpable lymph nodes (Figure 18-13). Reach your fingers high into the axilla. Move them firmly down in four directions: (a) down the chest wall in a line from the middle of the axilla, (b) along the anterior border of the axilla, (c) along the posterior border, and (d) along the inner aspect of the upper arm. Move the woman's arm through the range of motion to increase the surface area you can reach.

Normal Range of Findings	Abnormal Findings

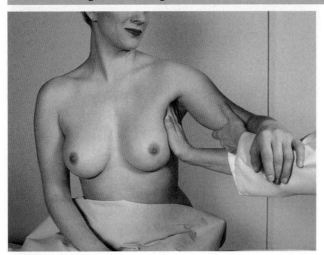

18-13

Usually nodes are not palpable, although you may feel a small, soft, nontender node in the central group. Expect some tenderness when palpating high in the axilla. Note any enlarged and tender lymph nodes.

Nodes enlarge with any local infection of the breast, arm, or hand, and with breast cancer metastases.

PALPATE THE BREASTS

Help the woman to a supine position. Tuck a small pad under the side to be palpated and raise her arm over her head. These manoeuvres will flatten the breast tissue and displace it medially. Any significant lumps will then feel more distinct (Figure 18-14).

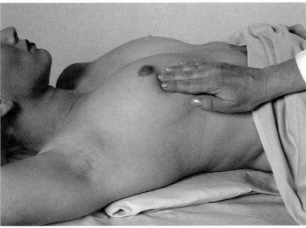

18-14

Use the pads of your first three fingers, and make a gentle rotary motion on the breast. Vary your pressure so you are palpating light, medium, and deep tissues in each location. The vertical strip pattern (Figure 18-15, *A*) currently is recommended as the best to detect a breast mass, but two other patterns are in common use: from the nipple palpating out to the periphery, as if following spokes on a wheel, and in concentric circles out to the periphery (see Figure 18-15, *B* and *C*).

Objective Data

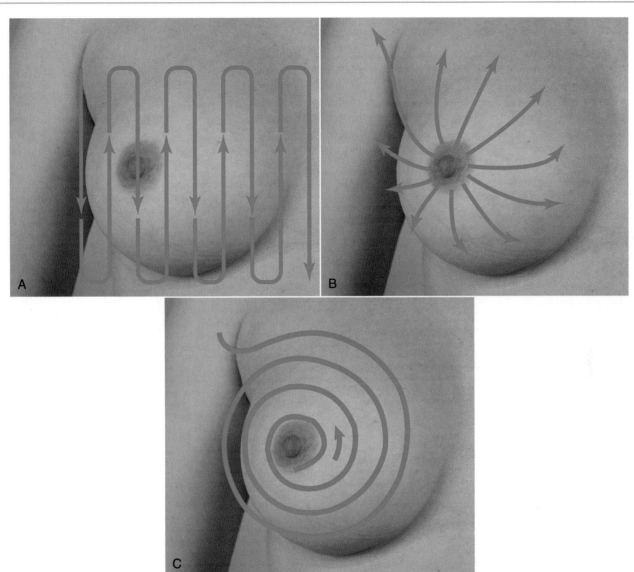

18-15   Patterns of breast palpation. **A,** Vertical strip pattern. **B,** Spokes-on-a-wheel pattern. **C,** Concentric circles pattern.

Normal Range of Findings	Abnormal Findings
For the vertical strip pattern, start high in the axilla and palpate down just lateral to the breast. Proceed in overlapping vertical lines, ending at the sternal edge. In every pattern, take care to palpate every square centimetre of the breast and to examine the tail of Spence high into the axilla. Be consistent and thorough in your approach to each woman.	
In nulliparous women, normal breast tissue feels firm, smooth, and elastic. After pregnancy, the tissue feels softer and looser. Premenstrual engorgement from increasing progesterone is normal. This consists of a slight enlargement, tenderness to palpation, and a generalized nodularity; the lobes feel prominent and their margins more distinct.	In women who are not lactating and not post partum, heat, redness, and swelling in the breasts indicate inflammation.
Also, normally you may feel a firm transverse ridge of compressed tissue in the lower quadrants. This is the **inframammary ridge,** and it is especially noticeable in large breasts. Do not confuse it with an abnormal lump.	

Objective Data

Normal Range of Findings	**Abnormal Findings**

After palpating over the four breast quadrants, palpate the nipple (Figure 18-16). Note any induration or subareolar mass. With your thumb and forefinger, gently depress the nipple tissue into the well behind the areola. The tissue should move inward easily. If the woman reports spontaneous nipple discharge, press the areola inward with your index finger; repeat from a few different directions. If any discharge appears, note its colour and consistency.

Except during pregnancy and lactation, discharge is abnormal (see Table 18-6, p. 428). Note the number of discharge droplets and the quadrant or quadrants producing them. Blot the discharge on a white gauze pad to ascertain its colour. Test any abnormal discharge for the presence of blood.

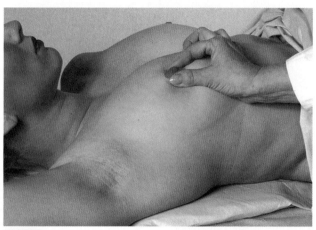

18-16

For the woman with large, pendulous breasts, you may palpate by using a bimanual technique (Figure 18-17). The woman should sit up and lean forward. Support the inferior part of the breast with one hand. Use your other hand to palpate the breast tissue against your supporting hand.

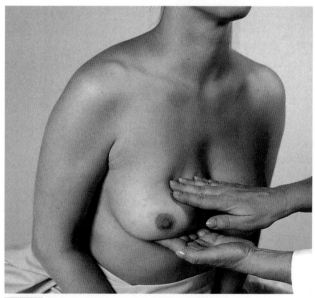

18-17

If the woman mentions a breast lump that she has discovered herself, examine the unaffected breast first to learn a baseline of normal consistency for this woman. If you do feel a lump or mass, note these characteristics (Figure 18-18):

Normal Range of Findings	Abnormal Findings

Normal Range of Findings

1. Location: Using the breast as a clock face, describe the distance in centimetres from the nipple (e.g., "7:00 position, 2 cm from the nipple"). Or diagram the breast in the woman's record and mark in the location of the lump.
2. Size: Judge in centimetres in three dimensions: width × length × thickness.
3. Shape: State whether the lump is oval, round, lobulated, or indistinct.
4. Consistency: State whether the lump is soft, firm, or hard.
5. Movable: Note whether the lump is freely movable or is fixed when you try to slide it over the chest wall.
6. Distinctness: Note whether the lump is solitary or multiple.
7. Nipple: Determine whether the lump is displaced or retracted.
8. Note the skin over the lump: erythematous, dimpled, or retracted.
9. Tenderness: Note whether the lump is tender to palpation.
10. Lymphadenopathy: Determine whether any regional lymph nodes are palpable.

Abnormal Findings

See Tables 18-4 and 18-5 (pp. 427 and 428) for descriptions of common breast lumps with these characteristics.

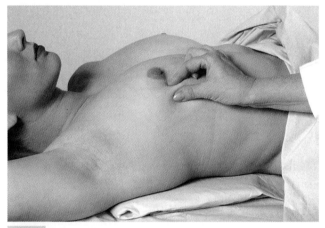

18-18

TEACH BREAST SELF-EXAMINATION

On its Web site, the CCS (2012) states, "There really isn't a right or wrong way for women to examine their breasts, as long as they get to know the whole area of their breast tissue—up to the collarbone, under the armpits and including the nipples—well enough to notice changes." Reinforce to patients that self-examination will familiarize them with their own breasts and their normal variation. Emphasize the absence of lumps (not the presence of them). However, do encourage women to report any unusual finding promptly.

While teaching women about the importance of being familiar with their own breasts, focus on the positive aspects of breast self-examination. Avoid citing frightening mortality statistics about breast cancer. This may generate excessive fear and denial that actually obstructs a woman's self-care action. Rather, be selective in your choice of factual material:

- The majority of women never get breast cancer.
- The great majority of breast lumps are benign.
- Early detection of breast cancer is important; if the cancer is not invasive, the survival rate is close to 100%.

Emphasize self-care through knowledge of risk factors and early referral for any suspect findings.

Objective Data

Normal Range of Findings	Abnormal Findings

Keep your teaching simple! The simpler the plan, the more likely the patient is to comply. Suggest that women inspect their breasts in front of a mirror while disrobed to the waist. Encourage women to learn how their breasts feel while in the shower, where soap and water assist palpation, and while lying supine so that breast tissue is flattened. Encourage each woman to palpate her own breasts while you are there to monitor her technique. Many examiners use a breast model (Figure 18-19) so that the woman can palpate a simulated "lump." Pamphlets are also helpful reinforcers. Use the return demonstration to assess the patient's technique and understanding of the procedure.

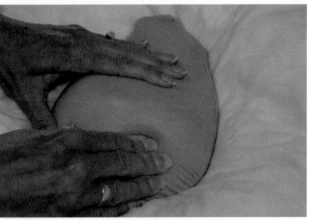

18-19

THE BREAST EXAMINATION IN MEN

Your examination of the male breast can be much more abbreviated, but do not omit it. Combine the breast examination with that of the anterior thorax. Inspect the chest wall, noting the skin surface and any lumps or swelling. Palpate the nipple area for any lump or tissue enlargement (Figure 18-20). It should feel even, with no nodules. Palpate the axillary lymph nodes.

The incidence of breast cancer in men is 1%, or fewer than 200 cases per year in Canada (CCS Steering Committee on Cancer Statistics, 2011).

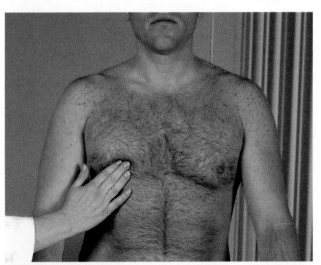

18-20

Normal Range of Findings	Abnormal Findings

The normal male breast has a flat disc of undeveloped breast tissue beneath the nipple. Gynecomastia is an enlargement of this breast tissue, which makes it clinically distinguishable from the other tissues in the chest wall (Figure 18-21). It feels like a smooth, firm, movable disc. This occurs normally during puberty. It usually affects only one breast and is temporary. Male adolescents are acutely aware of body image. Reassure them that this change is normal, common, and temporary. In contrast, an obese adolescent boy has an increase of fatty, not glandular, tissue.

Gynecomastia also occurs with use of anabolic steroids, some medications, and some disease states. See Table 18-8, p. 430.

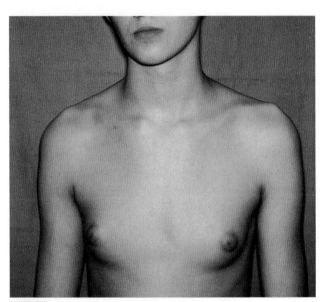

18-21   Adolescent gynecomastia.

DEVELOPMENTAL CONSIDERATIONS

Infants and Children

In neonates, the breasts may be enlarged and visible as a result of maternal estrogen crossing the placenta. They may secrete a clear or white fluid, called "witch's milk." These signs are not significant and are resolved within a few days to a few weeks.

Note the position of the nipples on the prepubertal child. They should be symmetrical, just lateral to the midclavicular line, between the fourth and fifth ribs. The nipple is flat, and the pigmentation of the areola is darker than that of the surrounding skin.

Premature thelarche is early breast development with no other hormone dependent signs (pubic hair, menses).

Adolescents

Adolescent breast development begins, on average, between 8 and 10 years of age. Expect some asymmetry during growth. (Distinguish breast development from extra adipose tissue present in obese children.) Record the stage of development by using Tanner (1962) staging, described on p. 408. Use the chart to teach the adolescent normal developmental stages and to assure her of her own normal progress.

Note precocious development, which occurs before age 8 years. It is usually normal but also occurs with thyroid dysfunction, stilbestrol ingestion, or ovarian or adrenal tumour.

Note delayed development, which occurs with hormonal failure, anorexia nervosa beginning before puberty, or severe malnutrition.

With maturing adolescents, palpate the breasts as you would with the adult. The breasts normally feel firm and uniform. Note any mass.

At this age, a mass is almost always a benign **fibroadenoma** or a cyst (see Table 18-4, p. 427).

Objective Data

Normal Range of Findings	Abnormal Findings

Pregnant Women

A delicate blue vascular pattern is visible over the breasts. The breasts increase in size, as do the nipples. Jagged linear stretch marks, or striae, may develop if breast size increases significantly. The nipples also become darker and more erectile. The areolae widen; grow darker; and contain the small, scattered, elevated Montgomery's glands. On palpation, the breasts feel more nodular, and thick yellow colostrum can be expressed after the first trimester.

Lactating Women

Colostrum changes to milk production around the third postpartum day. At this time, the breasts may become engorged, appearing enlarged, reddened, and shiny and feeling warm and hard. Frequent nursing helps drain the ducts and sinuses and stimulate milk production. Nipple soreness is normal, appearing around the twentieth nursing, lasting 24 to 48 hours, then disappearing rapidly. The nipples may look red and irritated. They may even crack but will heal rapidly if kept dry and exposed to air. Frequent nursing is also the best treatment for nipple soreness.

If one section of the breast surface appears red and tender, a duct is plugged (see Table 18-7, p. 428).

Older Women

On inspection, the breasts look pendulous, flattened, and sagging. Nipples may be retracted but can be pulled outward. On palpation, the breasts feel more granular, and the terminal ducts around the nipple feel more prominent and stringy. Thickening of the inframammary ridge at the lower breast is normal, and it feels more prominent with age.

Reinforce the value of routine breast health behaviours. Women older than 50 years have an increased risk of breast cancer. Older women may have problems with arthritis, limited range of motion, or decreased vision that may inhibit self-care. Suggest aids to the self-examination; for example, talcum powder helps fingers glide over skin.

Because atrophy causes shrinkage of normal glandular tissue, cancer detection is somewhat easier in older women. Any palpable lump that cannot be positively identified as a normal structure should be investigated.

DOCUMENTATION AND CRITICAL THINKING

Sample Charting: Female

SUBJECTIVE

52-y.o. woman. States no breast pain, lump, discharge, rash, swelling, or trauma. No history of breast disease herself; mother does have benign breast disease. No history of breast surgery. Never been pregnant. Hormonal contraceptive use aged 20 through 40 yrs. Perimenopausal but no hormone replacement. Last CBE, 1 yr ago. Mammogram q 2 years, due next month.

OBJECTIVE

Inspection: Breasts symmetrical. Skin smooth with even colour and no rash or lesions. Arm movement shows no dimpling or retractions. No nipple discharge, no lesions.
Palpation: Breast contour and consistency firm and homogeneous. No masses or tenderness. No lymphadenopathy.

ASSESSMENT

Healthy breast structure
Knowledgeable regarding breast screening recommendations

Sample Charting: Male

SUBJECTIVE

No pain, lump, rash, or swelling.

OBJECTIVE

No masses or tenderness. No lymphadenopathy.

Focused Assessment: Clinical Case Study 1

J.G. is a 32-year-old female high school teacher, married, with no children. She reports good health until finding "lump in my right breast 2 weeks ago."

SUBJECTIVE

- 2 weeks PTA: noticed lump in R breast while showering. Lump firm, nonmovable area "the size of a quarter," in upper outer quadrant of breast, tender on touch only. No skin changes, no nipple discharge, on no medications. No history of breast disease in self or family. Gravida 0. No known genetic risk factors. CXR [chest radiograph] age 15 (chest infection). Menarche age 13. Hormonal contraceptive use, ages 21–30 yr. Moderate alcohol use, 2 glasses of wine a week.
- 2 days PTA: saw MD, who confirmed presence of lump and recommended biopsy as outpatient. Last menstrual period 1/25 (2½ weeks PTA). States that the last 2 days she has been so nervous that she has been unable to sleep well or to concentrate at work: "I just know it's cancer."

OBJECTIVE

Voice trembling and breathless during history. Sitting posture stiff and rigid. B/P 148/78. Temp 37°C, pulse 92, resp 16.

Inspection: Breasts symmetrical, nipples everted. No skin lesions, no dimpling, no retraction, no fixation.

Palpation: Left breast firm, no mass, no tenderness, no discharge. Right breast firm, with 2 cm × 2 cm × 1 cm mass at 10:00 position, 5 cm from the nipple. Lump is firm, oval, with smooth discrete borders, nonmovable, tender to palpation. No other mass. No discharge. No lymphadenopathy.

ASSESSMENT

Lump in R breast
Anxiety

Focused Assessment: Clinical Case Study 2

D.B. is a 62-year-old female bank comptroller, married, with no children. History of hypertension, managed by diuretic medication and diet. No other health problems until yearly company physical examination 3 days PTA, when NP [nurse practitioner] "found a lump in my right breast."

SUBJECTIVE

- 3 days PTA: NP noted lump in R breast during yearly physical examination. NP did not describe lump but told D.B. it was "serious" and needed immediate biopsy. D.B. has not felt it herself. States has noted no skin changes, no nipple discharge. No previous history of breast disease. Mother died aged 54 years of breast cancer; no other relative with breast disease. *BRCA/BRCA2* status unknown. D.B. has had no term pregnancies; two spontaneous abortions, ages 28 and 31 years. Menarche age 11, menopause completed at age 52 years. No hormone replacement. No hormonal contraceptive use. No alcohol use. No history of chest wall irradiation.
- Married 43 years. States husband supportive but "I just can't talk to him about this. I can't even go near him now."

OBJECTIVE

Inspection: Breasts symmetrical when sitting, arms down. Nipples flat. No lesions, no discharge. As lifts arms, left breast elevates, right breast stays fixed. Dimple in right breast, 9:00 position, apparent at rest and with muscle contraction. Leaning forward reveals left breast falls free, right breast flattens.

Palpation: Left breast feels soft and granular throughout, no mass. Right breast soft and granular, with large, stony hard mass in upper outer quadrant. Lump is 5 cm × 4 cm × 2 cm, at 9:00 position, 3 cm from nipple. Borders irregular, mass fixed to tissues, no pain with palpation.

One firm, palpable lymph node in centre of right axilla. No palpable nodes on the left.

ASSESSMENT

Lump in R breast
Situational stress R/T breast lump

ABNORMAL FINDINGS

TABLE 18-3	Signs of Retraction and Inflammation in the Breast

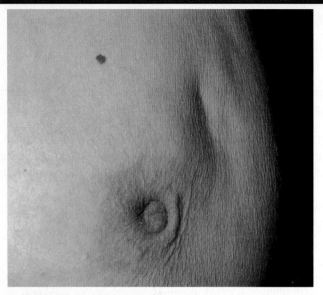

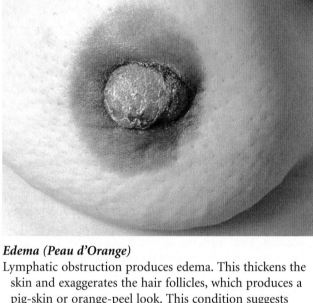

Dimpling

The shallow dimple (also called a *skin tether*) shown in this photo is a sign of skin retraction. Cancer causes fibrosis, which contracts the suspensory ligaments. The dimple may be apparent at rest, with compression, or with lifting of the arms. Also note the distortion of the areola in this photo as the fibrosis pulls the nipple toward it.

Nipple Retraction

The retracted nipple looks flatter and broader, like an underlying crater. A recent retraction suggests cancer, which causes fibrosis of the whole duct system and pulls in the nipple. It also may occur with benign lesions such as ectasia of the ducts. Do not confuse retraction with the normal longstanding type of nipple inversion, which has no broadening and is not fixed.

Edema (Peau d'Orange)

Lymphatic obstruction produces edema. This thickens the skin and exaggerates the hair follicles, which produces a pig-skin or orange-peel look. This condition suggests cancer. Edema usually begins in the skin around and beneath the areola, the most dependent area of the breast. Also note nipple infiltration in this photo.

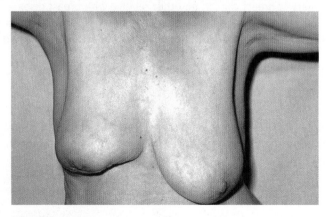

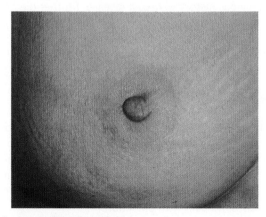

Fixation

Asymmetry, distortion, or decreased mobility with the elevated arm manoeuvre. As cancer becomes invasive, the fibrosis fixes the breast to the underlying pectoral muscles. In this photo, note that the right breast is held against the chest wall.

Deviation in Nipple Pointing

An underlying cancer causes fibrosis in the mammary ducts, which pulls the nipple angle toward it. In this photo, note the swelling behind the right nipple and that the nipple tilts laterally.

TABLE 18-4   Breast Lump

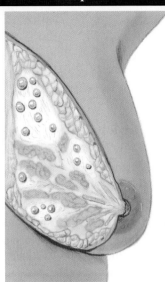

◄ *Benign Breast Disease*
Multiple tender masses. Formerly called *fibrocystic breast disease*; this is a meaningless term because it covers too many entities. Actually, six diagnostic categories exist, based on symptoms and physical findings (Love & Lindsey, 2005):
- Swelling and tenderness (cyclical discomfort)
- Mastalgia (severe pain, both cyclical and noncyclical)
- Nodularity (significant lumpiness, both cyclical and noncyclical)
- Dominant lumps (including cysts and fibroadenomas)
- Nipple discharge (including intraductal papilloma and duct ectasia)
- Infections and inflammations (including subareolar abscess, lactational mastitis, breast abscess, and Mondor's disease)

About 50% of all women have some form of benign breast disease. Nodularity occurs bilaterally; regular, firm nodules that are mobile, well demarcated, and feel rubbery, like small water balloons. Pain may be dull, heavy, and cyclical or just before menses as nodules enlarge. Some women have nodularity but no pain, and some vice versa. Cysts are discrete, fluid-filled sacs. Dominant lumps and nipple discharge must be investigated carefully, and biopsy may be needed to rule out cancer. Nodularity itself is not premalignant but may cause difficulty in detecting truly cancerous lumps.

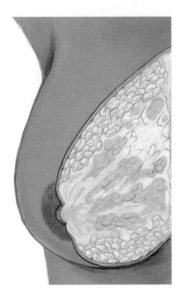

Cancer
Solitary unilateral nontender mass. Single focus in one area, although it may be interspersed with other nodules. Solid, hard, dense, and fixed to underlying tissues or skin as cancer becomes invasive. Borders are irregular and poorly delineated. Grows constantly. Often painless, but may cause pain. Most common in upper outer quadrant. Usually found in women 30–80 years of age; risk increases at ages 50–69 years. As cancer advances, signs include firm or hard irregular axillary nodes; skin dimpling; and nipple retraction, elevation, and discharge.

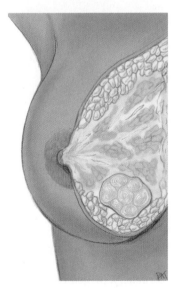

Fibroadenoma
Solitary nontender benign mass. Most common between 15 and 30 years of age but can occur up to age 55 years; is most commonly self-detected in late adolescence. Solid, firm, rubbery, and elastic. Round, oval, or lobulated; 1–5 cm. Freely movable, slippery; fingers slide it easily through tissue. Usually no axillary lymphadenopathy. Grows quickly and constantly. Diagnosis is based on history, physical examination, ultrasonography; suspect tumours (i.e., large, rapidly growing, or other suspect findings) may necessitate biopsy, surgical excision, or both (Jayasinghe & Simmons, 2009).

TABLE 18-5	Differentiating Breast Lumps		
Characteristic	Fibroadenoma	Benign Breast Disease	Cancer
Likely age	15-30 years; can occur up to 55 years	30-55 years; conditions tend to decrease after menopause	30-80 years; risk increases after 50 years
Shape	Round, lobular	Round, lobular	Irregular, star-shaped
Consistency	Usually firm, rubbery	Firm to soft, rubbery	Firm to stony hard
Demarcation	Well demarcated, clear margins	Well demarcated	Poorly defined
Number	Usually single	Usually multiple, may be single	Single
Mobility	Very mobile, slippery	Mobile	Fixed
Tenderness	Usually none	Present, usually increases before menses, may be noncyclical	Usually none but may be present
Skin retraction	None	None	Usually
Pattern of growth	Grows quickly and constantly	Size may increase or decrease rapidly	Grows constantly
Risk to health	None; they are benign and must be diagnosed through biopsy	Benign, although general lumpiness may mask other cancerous lump	Serious, necessitates early treatment

TABLE 18-6	Abnormal Nipple Discharge

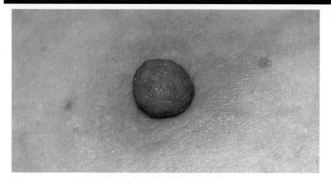

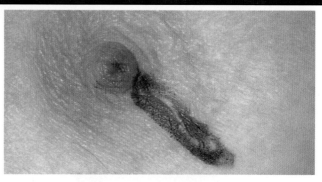

Mammary Duct Ectasia

Pastelike matter in subareolar ducts produces sticky, purulent discharge that may be white, grey, brown, green, or bloody. A light green, single duct discharge is shown in this photo. Caused by stagnation of cellular debris and secretions in the ducts, leading to obstruction, inflammation, and infection. Occurs in women who have lactated; usually occurs in perimenopausal period.

Itching, burning sensation, or pulling pain occurs around nipple. May have subareolar redness and swelling. Ducts are palpable as rubbery, twisted tubules under areola. May have palpable mass, soft or firm, poorly delineated. Not malignant, but biopsy is needed to rule out cancer.

Intraductal Papilloma

Serous or serosanguineous discharge, which is spontaneous, unilateral, or from a single duct. Lesion consists of tiny tumours, 2 to 3 mm in diameter. Often there is a palpable nodule in the underlying duct (highlighted by black marker in this photo). Papillomas affect women 40–60 years of age; most are benign. Refer any patient with bloody discharge for careful evaluation, including biopsy, to rule out cancer.

TABLE 18-6	**Abnormal Nipple Discharge—cont'd**

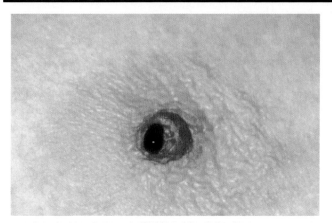

Carcinoma

Bloody nipple discharge that is unilateral and from a single duct necessitates further investigation. Although there was no palpable lump associated with the discharge shown in this photo, mammography revealed a 1-cm, centrally located, ill-defined mass.

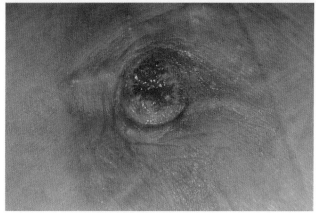

Paget's Disease (Intraductal Carcinoma)

Early lesion has unilateral, clear, yellow discharge and dry, scaling crusts, friable at nipple apex. Spreads outward to areola with erythematous halo on areola and crusted, eczematous, retracted nipple. In later stages of lesion, nipple is reddened, excoriated, and ulcerated, with bloody discharge when surface is eroded, and an erythematous plaque surrounds the nipple. Symptoms include tingling sensation, burning sensation, itching.

Except for the redness and occasional cracking from initial breastfeeding, any dermatitis of the nipple area must be carefully explored and investigated immediately.

TABLE 18-7	**Disorders Occurring During Lactation**

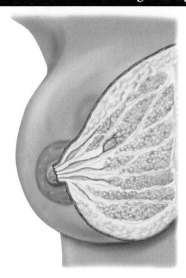

Plugged Duct

A fairly common and not serious condition. One milk duct is clogged. One section of the breast is tender and may be reddened. No infection. It is important to keep breast as empty as possible and milk flowing. The woman should nurse frequently, on affected side first to ensure complete emptying, and manually express any remaining milk. A plugged duct usually resolves in less than 1 day.

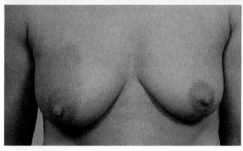

Mastitis

This is uncommon; an inflammatory mass before abscess formation. Usually occurs in single quadrant. Area is red, swollen, tender, very hot, and hard; in this photo, redness is forming outward from areola upper edge, in right breast. The woman in this photo also has a headache, malaise, fever, chills and sweating, increased pulse, and flulike symptoms. Mastititis may occur during first 4 months of lactation from infection or from stasis from plugged duct. Treat with rest, local heat to area, antibiotics, and frequent nursing to keep breast as empty as possible. Weaning must not be undertaken now, or the breast will become engorged and the pain will increase. Antibiotic administered to mother is not harmful to infant. Condition usually resolves in 2–3 days.

Continued

TABLE 18-7   Disorders Occurring During Lactation—cont'd

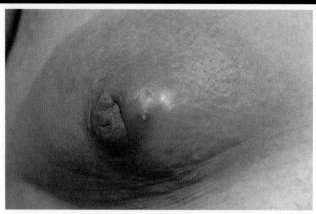

◀ *Breast Abscess*

A rare complication of generalized infection (e.g., mastitis) if untreated. A pocket of pus accumulates in one local area. This photo shows extensive nipple edema, and abscess is "pointing" at the 3:00 position on the areolar margin. Nursing on affected breast must be discontinued temporarily; manually express milk and discard. Continue to nurse on unaffected side. Treat with antibiotics, and refer patient for surgical incision and drainage.

TABLE 18-8   Abnormalities in the Male Breast

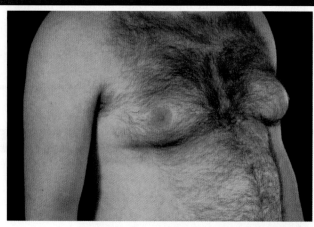

◀ *Gynecomastia*

Noninflammatory enlargement of male breast tissue. This is physiological at puberty, unilateral, usually mild and transient. Gynecomastia occurs commonly in older men because of changing hormone levels. It is bilateral and may be tender. It also occurs bilaterally as a result of hormone stimulation (e.g., estrogen for cancer of prostate); Cushing's syndrome; cirrhosis of liver, because the patient is unable to metabolize estrogen completely; leukemia occasionally; sometimes drugs (digitalis, isoniazid, spironolactone, phenothiazines, and marijuana); testicular tumour or lung cancer; adrenal disease; and thyrotoxicosis.

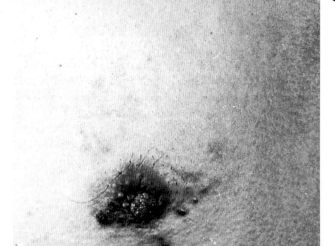

◀ *Breast Carcinoma in Men*

Fewer than 1% (about 200 cases) of all breast cancers occur in men per year in Canada (CCS Steering Committee on Cancer Statistics, 2011). Breast cancer may be diagnosed in men of any age but is most commonly diagnosed in men older than 60 years. The lesion is a hard, irregular, nontender mass, most often directly under the areola, fixed to the area, and the nipple may be retracted. Mass is noticeable early because of minimal breast tissue; however, nipple discharge with or without a palpable mass is a significant warning of early breast cancer (Morrogh & King, 2009). Spread to axillary lymph nodes occurs early because breast tissue is minimal. The ulcerating mass shown in this photo had been present for 3½ years and is advanced carcinoma.

Summary Checklist: Breasts and Regional Lymphatic Examination

For a PDA-downloadable version, go to *http://evolve.elsevier.com/Canada/Jarvis/examination/*.

1. Inspect breasts as the woman sits, raises arms overhead, pushes hands on hips, and leans forward.
2. Inspect the supraclavicular and infraclavicular areas.
3. Palpate the axillae and regional lymph nodes.
4. With woman supine, palpate the breast tissue, including tail of Spence, the nipples, and areolae.
5. Perform teaching and health promotion.

REFERENCES

Ahmad, F., Cameron, J. I., & Stewart, D. E. (2005). A tailored intervention to promote breast cancer screening among South Asian immigrant women. *Social Science & Medicine, 60,* 575–586.

Buzdar, A. (2006). Dietary modification and risk of breast cancer. *Journal of the American Medical Association, 295,* 691–692. doi:10.1001/jama.295.6.691

Canadian Cancer Society Steering Committee on Cancer Statistics. (2011). *Canadian cancer statistics 2011.* Toronto: Canadian Cancer Society. Retrieved from *http://www.cancer.ca/Canada-wide/About%20cancer/Cancer%20statistics/Past%20statistics.aspx?sc_lang=en.*

Canadian Cancer Society. (2012). *Screening for breast cancer.* Retrieved from *http://info.cancer.ca/cce-ecc/default.aspx?Lang=E&toc=10&cceid=194#Knowing_your_breasts.*

Canadian Task Force on Preventive Health Care, Tonelli, M., Connor Gorber, S., Joffres, M., Dickinson, J., Singh, H., … Liu, Y. Y. (2011). Recommendations on screening for breast cancer in average-risk women aged 40–74 years. *Canadian Medical Association Journal, 183*(17), 1991–2001. doi:10.1503/cmaj.110334

Friedman, D. B., & Hoffman-Goetz, L. (2007). Assessing cultural sensitivity of breast cancer information for older Aboriginal women. *Journal of Cancer Education: The Official Journal of the American Association for Cancer Education, 22*(2), 112–118. doi:10.1080/08858190701372927

Jayasinghe, Y., & Simmons, P. S. (2009). Fibroadenomas in adolescence. *Current Opinion in Obstetrics & Gynecology, 21*(5), 402–406. doi:10.1097/GCO.0b013e32832fa06b

Love, S., & Lindsey, K. (2005). *Dr. Susan Love's breast book* (4th ed.). Cambridge, MA: Da Capo Lifelong Books.

Morrogh, M., & King, T. A. (2009). The significance of nipple discharge of the male breast. *Breast Journal, 15*(6), 632–638. doi:10.1111/j.1524-4741.2009.00818.x

North American Menopause Society. (2012). Position statement. The 2012 hormone therapy position statement of the North American Menopause Society. *Menopause: The Journal of The North American Menopause Society, 19*(3), 257–271. doi:10.1097/gme.0b013e31824b970a

Tanner, J. M. (1962). *Growth at adolescence* (2nd ed.). Oxford, UK: Blackwell Scientific.

Web Sites of Interest

Breast Cancer.ca: *http://www.breast-cancer.ca/*
Breast Cancer Society of Canada: *http://www.bcsc.ca/*
Canadian Breast Cancer Foundation: *http://www.cbcf.org/Pages/default.aspx*
Canadian Cancer Society, About Breast Cancer: *http://www.cancer.ca/Canada-wide/About%20cancer/Types%20of%20cancer/Causes%20of%20breast%20cancer.aspx?sc_lang=en*
Canadian Task Force on Preventive Health Care, Screening for Breast Cancer: *http://www.canadiantaskforce.ca/recommendations/2011_01_eng.html*
Halls MD Health Calculators and Charts: *http://www.halls.md/*
OSF HealthCare: *https://myosfhealth.osfhealthcare.org/sites/OSF/BCRA/Web_Pages/ABOUT%20THE%20BCRA%20TOOL.htm*
North American Menopause Society: *http://www.menopause.org/*
U.S. National Institutes of Health, National Cancer Institute, Breast Cancer Risk Assessment Tool: *http://www.cancer.gov/bcrisktool/*

CHAPTER

19

Thorax and Lungs

Written by Carolyn Jarvis, PhD, APN, CNP

Adapted by June MacDonald-Jenkins, RN, BScN, MSc

evolve WEBSITE

http://evolve.elsevier.com/Canada/Jarvis/examination/

- Animations
- Audio—Lung Sounds
- Bedside Assessment Summary Checklist
- Case Study:
  - Exacerbation of COPD
  - Persistent Cough
  - Respiratory Assessment
  - Respiratory Problems
- Examination Review Questions
- Health Promotion Guide:
  - Smoking Cessation
- Key Points
- Physical Examination Summary Checklist
- Quick Assessment for Common Conditions:
  - Asthma
  - Pneumonia
- Video—Assessment
  - Anterior Chest and Upper Extremities
  - Posterior and Lateral Chest

OUTLINE

STRUCTURE AND FUNCTION

POSITION AND SURFACE LANDMARKS

The **thoracic cage** is a bony structure with a conical shape, which is narrower at the top (Figure 19-1). It is defined by the sternum, 12 pairs of **ribs,** and 12 thoracic **vertebrae.** Its "bottom" is the **diaphragm,** a musculotendinous septum that separates the thoracic cavity from the abdomen. The anterior aspects of the first seven ribs attach directly to the sternum via their costal cartilages; those of ribs 8, 9, and 10 attach to the costal cartilage above; and those of ribs 11 and 12 are

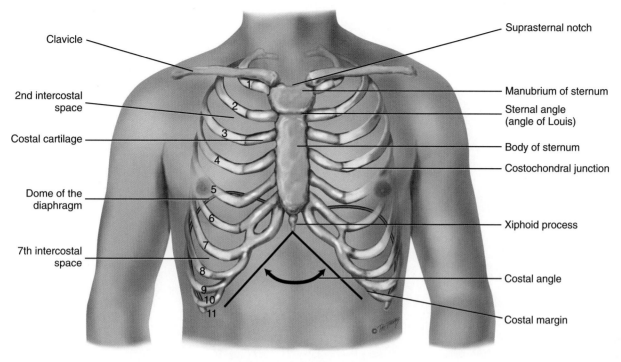

ANTERIOR THORACIC CAGE

19-1 Anterior thoracic cage. © *Pat Thomas, 2010.*

"floating," with free palpable tips. The **costochondral junctions** are the points at which the ribs join their cartilages. They are not palpable.

Anterior Thoracic Landmarks

Surface landmarks on the thorax are signposts for underlying respiratory structures. Knowledge of landmarks will help you localize a finding and will facilitate communication of your findings to other professionals.

Suprasternal Notch. Feel this hollow U-shaped depression just above the sternum, in between the clavicles.

Sternum. The **sternum,** or "breastbone," has three parts: the manubrium, the body, and the xiphoid process. Walk your fingers down the manubrium a few centimetres until you feel a distinct bony ridge, the manubriosternal angle.

Sternal Angle. The sternal angle, often called the *angle of Louis,* is the articulation of the manubrium and body of the sternum, and it is continuous with the second rib. The angle of Louis is a useful place to start counting ribs, which helps localize a respiratory finding horizontally. Identify the angle of Louis, palpate lightly to the second rib, and slide down to the second intercostal space. Each intercostal space is numbered by the rib above it. Continue counting down the ribs in the middle of the hemithorax, not close to the sternum, where the costal cartilages lie too close together to count. You can palpate easily down to the tenth rib.

The angle of Louis also marks the site of tracheal bifurcation into the right and left main bronchi; it corresponds with the upper border of the atria of the heart, and it lies above the fourth thoracic vertebra on the back.

Costal Angle. The right and left costal margins form an angle where they meet at the xiphoid process. Usually 90 degrees or less, this angle increases when the rib cage is chronically overinflated, as in emphysema.

Posterior Thoracic Landmarks

Counting ribs and intercostal spaces on the back is a bit harder because of the muscles and soft tissue surrounding the ribs and spinal column (Figure 19-2).

Vertebra Prominens. Start at the base of your neck. Flex your head and feel for the most prominent bony protrusion there. This is the spinous process of C7. If two bumps seem equally prominent, the upper one is C7 and the lower one is T1.

Spinous Processes. Count down the vertebrae, which stack together to form the spinal column. Note that the spinous processes align with their same-numbered ribs only down to T4. After T4, the spinous processes angle downward from their vertebral bodies, and each overlies the vertebral body and rib below.

Inferior Border of the Scapula. The scapulae are located symmetrically in each hemithorax. The lower tip is usually at the level of the seventh or eighth rib.

Twelfth Rib. Palpate midway between the spine and the patient's side to identify the free tip of the twelfth rib.

Reference Lines

Use the reference lines to pinpoint a finding vertically on the chest. On the chest, note the **midsternal line** and the

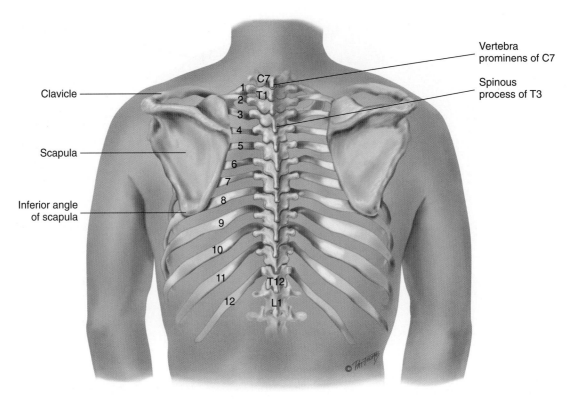

Clavicle

Scapula

Inferior angle of scapula

C7
T1
1
2
3
4
5
6
7
8
9
10
11
12
T12
L1

Vertebra prominens of C7

Spinous process of T3

POSTERIOR THORACIC CAGE

19-2 Posterior thoracic cage.

© Pat Thomas, 2010.

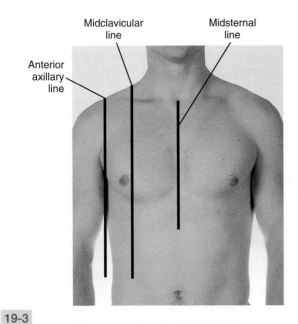

Anterior axillary line

Midclavicular line

Midsternal line

19-3

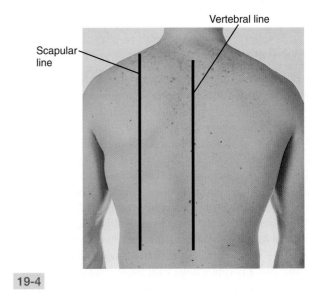

Scapular line

Vertebral line

19-4

midclavicular line. The midclavicular line bisects the centre of each clavicle at a point halfway between the palpated sternoclavicular and acromioclavicular joints (Figure 19-3).

The posterior chest wall can be demarcated by the **vertebral line** (or *midspinal line*) and the **scapular line,** which extends through the inferior angle of the scapula when the arms are at the sides of the body (Figure 19-4).

Lift up one of the patient's arms 90 degrees, and observe the lateral chest. It can be demarcated by three lines: The **anterior axillary line** extends down from the anterior axillary fold, where the pectoralis major muscle inserts; the **posterior axillary line** continues down from the posterior axillary fold, where the latissimus dorsi muscle inserts; and the **midaxillary line** runs down from the apex of the axilla and lies between and parallel to the other two (Figure 19-5).

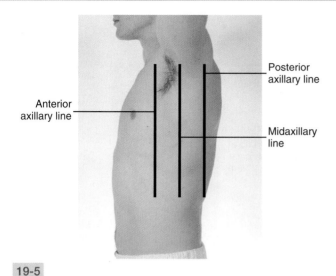

Anterior
axillary line

Posterior
axillary line

Midaxillary
line

19-5

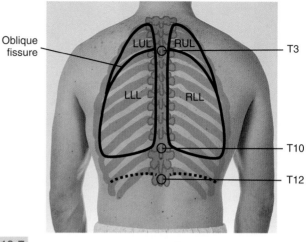

Oblique
fissure

LUL   RUL   T3

LLL   RLL

T10

T12

19-7

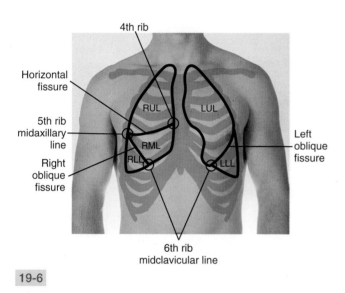

4th rib

Horizontal
fissure

RUL   LUL

5th rib
midaxillary
line

RML

Right
oblique
fissure

RLL   LLL

Left
oblique
fissure

6th rib
midclavicular line

19-6

THE THORACIC CAVITY

The **mediastinum** is the middle section of the thoracic cavity, and it contains the esophagus, trachea, heart, and great vessels. The right and left **pleural cavities,** on either side of the mediastinum, contain the lungs.

Lung Borders. In the anterior chest, the **apex,** or highest point, of lung tissue is 3 or 4 cm above the inner third of the clavicles. The **base,** or lower border, rests on the diaphragm at about the sixth rib in the midclavicular line. Laterally, lung tissue extends from the apex of the axilla down to the seventh or eighth rib. Posteriorly, the location of C7 marks the apex of lung tissue, and T10 usually corresponds to the base. Deep inspiration expands the lungs, and their lower border drops to the level of T12.

Lobes of the Lungs

The lungs are paired but not precisely symmetrical structures (Figure 19-6). The right lung is shorter than the left lung

because of the underlying liver. The left lung is narrower than the right lung because the heart bulges to the left. The right lung has three lobes, and the left lung has two lobes. These lobes are not arranged in horizontal bands like dessert layers in a parfait glass; rather, they stack in diagonal sloping segments and are separated by **fissures** that run obliquely through the chest.

Anterior. On the anterior chest, the **oblique fissure** (the major or diagonal fissure) crosses the fifth rib in the midaxillary line and terminates at the sixth rib in the midclavicular line. The right lung also contains the **horizontal fissure** (minor fissure), which divides the right upper and middle lobes. This fissure extends from the fifth rib in the right midaxillary line to the third intercostal space or fourth rib at the right sternal border. The anterior chest contains primarily upper and middle lobes.

Posterior. The most remarkable point about the posterior chest is that its contents consist almost entirely of lower lobe (Figure 19-7). The upper lobes occupy a smaller band of tissue from their apices at T1 down to T3 or T4. At this level, the lower lobes begin, and their inferior border reaches down to the level of T10 on expiration and to T12 on inspiration. Note that the right middle lobe does not project onto the posterior chest at all. If the patient abducts the arms and places the hands on the back of the head, the division between upper and lower lobes corresponds to the medial border of the scapulae.

Lateral. Laterally, lung tissue extends from the apex of the axilla down to the seventh or eighth rib. The right upper lobe extends from the level of the apex of the axilla down to the level of the horizontal fissure at the fifth rib (Figure 19-8). The right middle lobe extends from the level of the horizontal fissure down and forward to the level of the sixth rib at the midclavicular line. The right lower lobe continues from the level of the fifth rib to that of the eighth rib in the midaxillary line.

The left lung contains only two lobes, upper and lower (Figure 19-9). These appear laterally as two triangular areas separated by the oblique fissure. The left upper lobe extends from the level of the apex of the axilla down to the

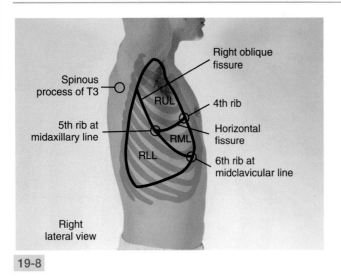

19-8

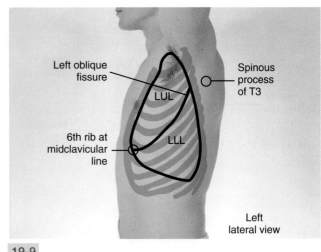

19-9

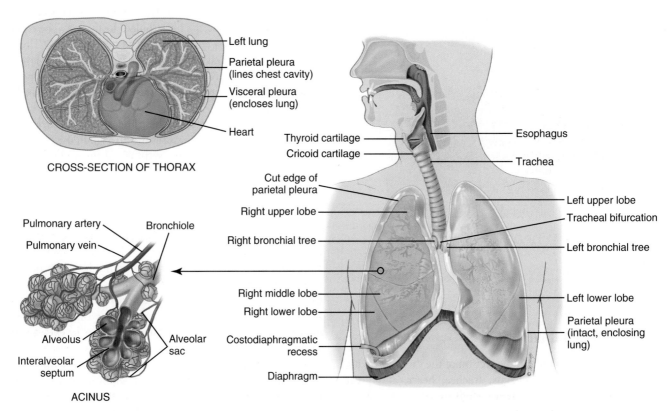

19-10 Pleurae and tracheobronchial tree.

© Pat Thomas, 2006.

level of the fifth rib at the midaxillary line. The left lower lobe continues down to the level of the eighth rib in the midaxillary line.

Using these landmarks, try determining the outline of each lobe on a willing partner. Take special note of the three points that commonly confuse beginning examiners:

1. The left lung has no middle lobe.
2. The anterior chest contains mostly upper and middle lobe with very little lower lobe.
3. The posterior chest contains almost all lower lobe.

Pleurae

The thin, slippery **pleurae** form an envelope between the lungs and the chest wall (Figure 19-10). The **visceral pleura** lines the outside of the lungs, dipping down into the fissures. It is continuous with the **parietal pleura,** which lines the inside of the chest wall and diaphragm.

The inside of the envelope, the pleural cavity, is a potential space filled only with a few millilitres of lubricating fluid. It normally has a vacuum, or negative pressure, which holds the lungs tightly against the chest wall. The lungs slide smoothly and noiselessly up and down during respiration, lubricated by a few millilitres of fluid. Think of this as similar to two glass slides with a drop of water between them; although it is difficult to separate the slides, they slide smoothly back and forth. The pleurae extend about 3 cm below the level of the lungs, forming the **costodiaphragmatic recess.** This is a potential space; when it abnormally fills with air or fluid, it compromises lung expansion.

Trachea and Bronchial Tree

The **trachea** lies anterior to the esophagus and is 10 to 11 cm long in the adult. It begins at the level of the cricoid cartilage in the neck and bifurcates just below the sternal angle into the right and left main bronchi. Posteriorly, tracheal bifurcation is at the level of T4 or T5. The right main bronchus is shorter, wider, and more vertical than the left main bronchus.

The trachea and bronchi transport gases between the environment and the lung parenchyma. They constitute the *dead space,* or space that is filled with air but is not available for gaseous exchange. In adults, its capacity is approximately 150 mL. The bronchial tree also protects alveoli from small particulate matter in the inhaled air. The bronchi are lined with goblet cells, which secrete mucus that entraps the particles, and with cilia, which sweep the particles upward where they can be swallowed or expelled.

An **acinus** is a functional respiratory unit that consists of the bronchioles, alveolar ducts, alveolar sacs, and the alveoli. Gaseous exchange occurs across the respiratory membrane in the alveolar duct and in the millions of alveoli. The alveoli are clustered like grapes around each alveolar duct. As a result, there are millions of interalveolar septa (walls) that tremendously increase the working space available for gas exchange. This bunched arrangement creates a surface area for gas exchange that is as large as a tennis court.

MECHANICS OF RESPIRATION

The respiratory system has four major functions: (a) supplying oxygen to the body for energy production, (b) removing carbon dioxide as a waste product of energy reactions, (c) maintaining homeostasis (acid–base balance) of arterial blood, and (d) maintaining heat exchange (less important in humans).

By supplying oxygen to the blood and eliminating excess carbon dioxide, respiration maintains the pH, or the acid–base balance, of the blood. The body tissues are bathed by blood, whose normal acceptable pH has a narrow range. Although a number of compensatory mechanisms regulate the pH, the lungs help maintain the balance by adjusting the level of carbon dioxide through respiration; that is, hypoventilation (slow, shallow breathing) causes carbon dioxide to build up in the blood, and hyperventilation (rapid, deep breathing) causes carbon dioxide to be blown off.

Control of Respirations

Normally, a person's breathing pattern changes, without the person's awareness, in response to cellular demands. This involuntary control of respiration is mediated by the respiratory centre in the brainstem (pons and medulla). The major feedback loop is humoral regulation, or the change in carbon dioxide and oxygen levels in the blood and, of less importance, the hydrogen ion level. The *normal stimulus to breathe* for most people is an increase of carbon dioxide in the blood, or **hypercapnia.** A decrease of oxygen in the blood (**hypoxemia**) also increases respirations but is less effective than hypercapnia.

Changing Chest Size

Respiration is the physical act of breathing; air rushes into the lungs as the chest size increases (inspiration) and is expelled from the lungs as the chest recoils (expiration). The mechanical expansion and contraction of the chest cavity alters the size of the thoracic container in two dimensions: (a) The vertical diameter lengthens or shortens, which is accomplished by downward or upward movement of the diaphragm, and (b) the anteroposterior diameter increases or decreases, which is accomplished by elevation or depression of the ribs (Figure 19-11).

In inspiration, increasing the size of the thoracic container creates a slightly negative pressure in relation to the atmosphere, and so air rushes in to fill the partial vacuum. The major muscle responsible for this increase is the diaphragm. During inspiration, contraction of the bell-shaped diaphragm causes it to descend and flatten. This lengthens the vertical diameter. Intercostal muscles lift the sternum and elevate the ribs, making them more horizontal. This increases the anteroposterior diameter.

Expiration is primarily passive. As the diaphragm relaxes, elastic forces within the lung, thoracic cage, and abdomen cause it to expand upward and form a dome. All this squeezing creates a relatively positive pressure within the alveoli, and the air flows out.

In forced inspiration, such as that after heavy exercise or occurring pathologically with respiratory distress, the accessory neck muscles are used to heave up the sternum and rib cage. These neck muscles are the sternomastoid, scalene, and the trapezius muscles. In forced expiration, the abdominal muscles contract powerfully to push the abdominal viscera forcefully in and up against the diaphragm, causing it to expand upward as a dome and squeeze against the lungs.

 DEVELOPMENTAL CONSIDERATIONS

Infants and Children

During the first 5 weeks of fetal life, the primitive lung bud emerges; by 16 weeks, the conducting airways reach the same number as in the adult; at 32 weeks, **surfactant,** the complex lipid substance needed for sustained inflation of the air sacs, is present in adequate amounts; and by birth, the lungs have

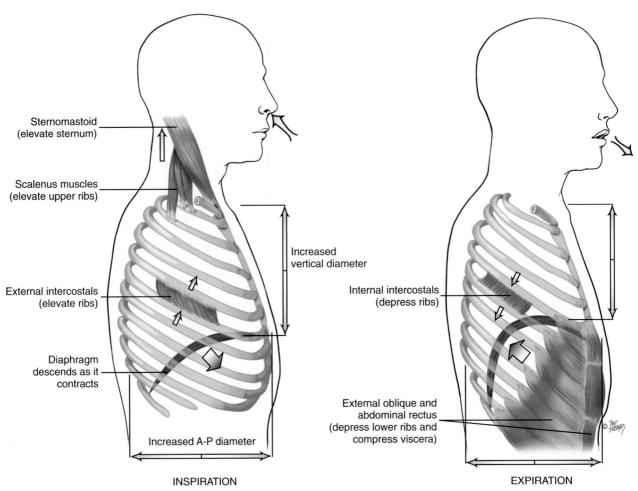

Sternomastoid (elevate sternum)

Scalenus muscles (elevate upper ribs)

External intercostals (elevate ribs)

Diaphragm descends as it contracts

Increased vertical diameter

Increased A-P diameter

INSPIRATION

Internal intercostals (depress ribs)

External oblique and abdominal rectus (depress lower ribs and compress viscera)

EXPIRATION

19-11

© *Pat Thomas, 2010.*

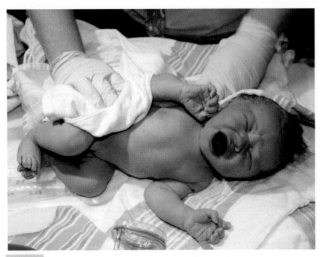

19-12

70 million primitive alveoli ready to start the job of respiration.

Breath is life. When the newborn inhales the first breath, the lusty cry that follows reassures anxious parents that their baby is all right (Figure 19-12). The baby's body systems all develop in utero, but the respiratory system alone

does not function until birth. Birth necessitates its instant performance.

When the umbilical cord is cut, blood is cut off from the placenta, and it gushes into the pulmonary circulation. Relatively less resistance exists in the pulmonary arteries than in the aorta, and so the foramen ovale in the heart closes just after birth. (See the discussion of fetal circulation in Chapter 20 on p. 484.) The ductus arteriosus (linking the pulmonary artery and the aorta) contracts and closes several hours later, and pulmonary and systemic circulation become functional.

Respiratory development continues throughout childhood, with increases in the diameter and length of airways and in the size and number of alveoli, reaching the adult range of 300 million by adolescence.

The relatively smaller size and immaturity of children's pulmonary systems and the presence of people who smoke result in enormous vulnerability and increased risks to child health. Prenatal exposure results in chronic hypoxia and low birth weight. Also, it sensitizes the fetal brain to nicotine, which increases risk for addiction when the child is exposed to nicotine at a later age. Postnatal exposure to environmental tobacco smoke is linked to increased rates of otitis media, sudden infant death syndrome, lower respiratory tract infections, and childhood asthma (Best, 2009; Håberg et al., 2010).

(See the box Promoting Health: Environmental Tobacco Smoke.)

Pregnant Women

The enlarging uterus elevates the diaphragm 4 cm during pregnancy. This decreases the vertical diameter of the thoracic cage, but this decrease is compensated for by an increase in the horizontal diameter. The increase in estrogen level relaxes the thoracic cage ligaments. This allows an increase in the transverse diameter of the thoracic cage by 2 cm, and the costal angle widens. The total circumference of the thoracic cage increases by 6 cm. Although the diaphragm is elevated, it is not fixed. It moves with breathing even more

---

PROMOTING HEALTH: ENVIRONMENTAL TOBACCO SMOKE

Second-Hand/Third-Hand Smoke: There Is No Risk-Free Level of Exposure!

Second-hand smoke, also referred to as environmental tobacco smoke, is a mixture of *sidestream smoke* (the smoke from the burning end of a cigarette, pipe, or cigar) and *mainstream smoke* (the smoke exhaled from the lungs of the smoker). Health Canada (2006) determined that there is *no safe level* of exposure to the carcinogens in cigarette smoke. Exposure to second-hand smoke, which is primarily involuntary, increases risk for adverse health effects. Furthermore, the exposure to second-hand smoke, for the general public, both smokers and others, is much higher than most people realize.

Second-hand smoke is especially harmful to young children, increasing rates of respiratory infections and inner ear infections and aggravating asthma. In 2010, 17% of Canadian households reported at least one person who smoked inside the home every day or almost every day. Of households without someone who regularly smoked inside the home, 86% did not allow smoking inside their homes.

Since 2001, provincial legislation in Canada has been implemented to restrict smoking in the workplace. In addition to the increase in the prevalence of smoke-free and smoke-restricted workplaces, many provincial and territorial governments have enacted legislation requiring public places to be smoke free: Northwest Territories, Prince Edward Island, Nunavut, New Brunswick, and Manitoba in 2004; Saskatchewan, Newfoundland, and Labrador in 2005; Ontario, Quebec, and Nova Scotia in 2006; and Alberta and British Columbia in 2007. Not all provinces have enacted 100% smoke-free legislation, but many provinces such as Alberta and British Columbia have implemented some of the most aggressive nonsmoking laws in the country.

Second-hand smoke contains hundreds of chemicals known to be toxic or carcinogenic, including formaldehyde, benzene, vinyl chloride, arsenic, and cyanide. It can linger in the air for hours long after the cigarette, cigar, or pipe has been extinguished and is involuntarily inhaled by nonsmokers. *Third-hand smoke* is a new name for an old problem: the toxic chemicals in smoke that linger in the air, even after the smoker has put out the cigarette, cigar, or pipe. Third-hand smoke gets trapped in hair, skin, fabric, carpet, furniture, and toys, and it builds up over time.

Exposure to second-hand smoke places nonsmokers at risk for the same diseases that active smoking does. Nonsmokers exposed to second-hand smoke are 25% more likely to have heart disease and 20% more likely to have lung cancer than are nonsmokers not exposed to smoke. Separating smokers from nonsmokers, cleaning the air indoors, and ventilating buildings do not eliminate the exposure risk to nonsmokers. However, eliminating smoking in indoor spaces does fully protect the nonsmoker.

With eliminating smoking in mind in January of 2010, the federal government announced a reinvestment into "Extending Tobacco Treatment Excellence: A National Dissemination of Systems." The goal of this project was to implement a smoking cessation program in 21 outpatient clinics that would provide advice to 15,000 smokers and facilitate best practices and knowledge sharing. The project also provided training to 2000 health care providers on tobacco addiction treatment, including the development of policies and training tools. Partners include the Vancouver Coastal Authority, Regional Health Authority B (New Brunswick), the Heart and Stroke Foundation of Ontario, and Atlantic Canada. In the same year, the government launched an aggressive national labelling campaign to require all tobacco products to visually depict the harmful of effects of tobacco on humans; this campaign has placed Canada at the forefront of addressing this international issue.

Where do you start? First, do not smoke or allow smoking in your home. Tell smokers that you do mind if they smoke indoors, and ask them to go outside while they smoke. It is important to protect children from the harmful effects of second-hand smoke, inasmuch as research has demonstrated that children have an especially high risk of health problems from exposure. Children breathe in more air than do adults in relation to their body weight—which means they absorb more tobacco smoke—and their immune systems are less developed; moreoever, they have less power and ability to complain about being around second-hand smoke. The Canadian Lung Association in 2008 launched a national strategy to ban smoking in vehicles with children. Smoking when anyone younger than 16 is present in a vehicle is currently banned in the provinces of British Columbia, Newfoundland and Labrador, Manitoba, Ontario, New Brunswick, Prince Edward Island, Saskatchewan, and Yukon Territory. In Nova Scotia, smoking is banned in vehicles when persons younger than 19 are present.

For more information about smoking cessation programs, visit the following Web sites:

- Canadian Lung Association: *http://www.lung.ca/home-accueil_e.php*
- Ministry of Health, B.C. Smoking Cessation Program: *http://www.health.gov.bc.ca/pharmacare/stop-smoking/*
- Health Canada, Tobacco Product Labelling Information (Cigarettes and Little Cigars): *http://www.hc-sc.gc.ca/hc-ps/tobac-tabac/legislation/reg/label-etiquette/index-eng.php*

References

Health Canada. (2006). Second-hand smoke. *Retrieved from* http://www.hc-sc.gc.ca/hl-vs/tobac-tabac/second/index_e.html.

Health Canada. (2006). Smoke-free public places: You can get there. Ottawa: Author.

Sources: American Lung Association. (2006). *Secondhand smoke facts sheet.* Retrieved from *http://www.lung.org/stop-smoking/about-smoking/health-effects/secondhand-smoke.html;* Canadian Lung Association. (2008). *Lung Association to launch Clean Air for Kids Campaign on January 23.* Ottawa: Author; Health Canada. (2006). *Second-hand smoke.* Retrieved from *http://www.hc-sc.gc.ca/hl-vs/tobac-tabac/second/index_e.html;* and Health Canada. (2006). *Smoke-free public places: You can get there.* Ottawa: Author.

during pregnancy, which results in an increase in tidal volume (Cunningham et al., 2005).

The growing fetus increases the oxygen demand on the mother's body. This is met easily by the increasing tidal volume (deeper breathing). Little change occurs in the respiratory rate. An increased awareness of the need to breathe develops, even early in pregnancy, and some pregnant women may interpret this as dyspnea, although structurally nothing is wrong.

Older Adults

In older adults, the costal cartilages become calcified, which reduces mobility of the thorax. Respiratory muscle strength declines after age 50 years and continues to decrease into the 70s. A more significant change is the decrease in elastic properties within the lungs, which makes them less distensible and lessens their tendency to contract and recoil. In summary, the aging lung is a more rigid structure that is harder to inflate.

These changes result in an increase in small airway closure, and that causes a decrease in *vital capacity* (the maximum amount of air that a person can expel from the lungs after first filling the lungs to maximum) and an increase in *residual volume* (the amount of air remaining in the lungs even after the most forceful expiration). From an assessment point of view, this means a decrease in the ability to take a deep breath and exhale it.

With aging, histological changes (i.e., a gradual loss of intra-alveolar septa and a decrease in the number of alveoli) also occur, so that less surface area is available for gas exchange. Also, the lung bases become less ventilated as a result of the closing off of a number of airways. This increases the risk for shortness of breath with exertion beyond an older person's usual workload.

The histological changes also increase older persons' risk for postoperative pulmonary complications. That is, older persons have a greater risk for postoperative atelectasis and infection as a result of a decreased ability to cough, a loss of protective airway reflexes, and increased secretions.

CULTURAL AND SOCIAL CONSIDERATIONS

In 2010, 1577 new active and re-emergent cases of tuberculosis were reported to the Canadian Tuberculosis Reporting System, with a corresponding incidence rate of 4.6 per 100,000 population. This represents an unprecedented national low since collection of tuberculosis data began in Canada in 1924. However, reported tuberculosis incidence rates varied by jurisdiction, and a disproportionately high number of cases were reported in Nunavut in particular. In 2010, 66% of all reported tuberculosis cases were among foreign-born individuals, 21% among Canadian-born Aboriginal people and 12% of cases were among Canadian-born non-Aboriginal people.

Since 2005, the total number of reported cases of active **tuberculosis** disease has remained relatively stable. The three most populous provinces (British Columbia, Ontario, and Quebec) accounted for 66% of the total number of reported cases.

Mycobacterium tuberculosis, which causes this disease, is an airborne pathogen. Therefore, isolation of infected individuals and early diagnosis are essential for minimizing spread of the disease (Public Health Agency of Canada, 2010b).

In 2010, 2.4 million Canadians were identified as having active cases of **asthma;** this number was down from 2.7 million in 2005. The two most important preventable risk factors for respiratory disease are tobacco smoke (both personal and second-hand) and poor air quality (indoor and outdoor). Asthma was a contributing factor in approximately 10% of the hospital admissions of children younger than 5 years and in 8% of those aged 5 to 14 years (Public Health Agency of Canada, 2010a).

Respiratory diseases, including lung cancer, are a major cause of death in Canada. In 2013 an estimated 25,600 Canadians will receive a diagnosis of lung cancer, and 20,100 are estimated to die of it. Lung cancer remains the leading cause of cancer death in both men and women. One per 11 men is expected to develop lung cancer during his lifetime, and 1 per 13 will die of it. One per 15 women is expected to develop lung cancer during her lifetime, and 1 per 17 is expected to die of it. The incidence rate among women, although still elevated, appears to be stabilizing. In men, the incidence has been decreasing (Canadian Lung Association, 2013).

Women and Chronic Obstructive Pulmonary Disease

With regard to chronic obstructive pulmonary disease (COPD), a national report (Lung Association, 2006) called for increased awareness, screening, and advocacy. Spirometry in women should be as routine as mammography for breast screening. Women seem to incur greater lung damage from exposure to environmental tobacco than do men. This devastating breathing disease has been diagnosed in more than 425,000 women in Canada, and more than 4300 die of it every year, according to the most recent statistics in the report. Moreover, the report indicates that the percentage of women who undergo appropriate screening for the disease is unacceptably low (Canadian Lung Association, 2013).

SUBJECTIVE DATA

1. Cough
2. Shortness of breath
3. Chest pain with breathing
4. History of respiratory infections
5. Smoking history
6. Environmental exposure
7. Self-care behaviours

HEALTH HISTORY QUESTIONS

Examiner Asks	Rationale

1. **Cough.** Do you have a cough? When did it start? Gradual or sudden?
  • How long have you had it?
  • How often do you cough? At any special time of day or just on arising? Does the cough wake you up at night?
	Acute cough lasts less than 2 or 3 weeks; chronic cough lasts more than 2 months.
	  In some conditions, the timing of a cough is characteristic:
	• Continuous throughout day: acute illness (e.g., respiratory infection)
	• Afternoon/evening: may reflect exposure to irritants at work
	• Night: postnasal drip, sinusitis
	• Early morning: chronic bronchial inflammation of smokers

• Do you cough up any phlegm or sputum? How much? What colour is it?	Chronic bronchitis is characterized by a history of productive cough for 3 months of the year for 2 years in a row.
	  Green phlegm is indicative of a viral or bacterial infection.
	  In some conditions, sputum production is characteristic:

• Cough up any blood **(hemoptysis)?** Does this look like streaks or frank blood? Does the sputum have a foul odour?	• White or clear mucoid: colds, bronchitis, viral infections • Yellow or green: bacterial infections • Rust coloured: tuberculosis, pneumococcal pneumonia • Pink, frothy: pulmonary edema, some sympathomimetic medications (side effect of pink-tinged mucus)
• How would you describe your cough: hacking, dry, barking, hoarse, congested, bubbling?	Some conditions are accompanied by a characteristic cough: • *Mycoplasma* pneumonia: hacking • Early heart failure: dry • Croup: barking • Colds, bronchitis, pneumonia: congested

• Does cough seem to come with anything: activity, position (lying), fever, congestion, talking, anxiety?
  • Does activity make it better or worse?
  • What treatment have you tried: prescription or over-the-counter medications, vaporizer, rest, position change?
  • Does the cough bring on anything: chest pain, ear pain? Is it tiring? Are you concerned about it?
	Assess effectiveness of coping strategies.
	
	Note severity.

2. **Shortness of breath.** Ever had any **shortness of breath** or a hard-breathing spell? What brings it on? How severe is it? How long does it last?	Determine how much activity precipitates the shortness of breath; state specific number of blocks walked, number of stairs.

Examiner Asks	Rationale

- Is it affected by position, such as lying down?

Orthopnea is difficulty breathing in the supine position. State number of pillows needed to achieve comfort (e.g., "two-pillow orthopnea").

- Does it occur at any specific time of day or night?

Paroxysmal nocturnal dyspnea is awakening from sleep with shortness of breath and needing to be upright to achieve comfort.
This condition is diaphoresis.
The bluish colour is cyanosis.

- Are the episodes associated with night sweats?
- Are they associated with cough, chest pain, or bluish colour around lips or nails? Wheezing sound?
- Do episodes seem to be related to food, pollen, dust, animals, season, or emotion?
- What do you do in a hard-breathing attack: take a special position, or use pursed-lip breathing? Use any oxygen, inhalers, or medications?
- How does the shortness of breath affect your work or home activities? Is it getting better or worse, or is it staying about the same?

Asthma attacks may be associated with a specific allergen, extreme cold, or anxiety.
Assess effect of coping strategies and the need for more teaching.
Assess effect on activities of daily living.

3. Chest pain with breathing. Any **chest pain with breathing**? Please point to the exact location.
   - When did it start? Is it constant, or does it come and go?
   - Describe the pain: burning, stabbing?
   - Is it brought on by respiratory infection, coughing, or trauma? Is it associated with fever, deep breathing, or unequal rising and falling of the chest?
   - What have you done to treat it? Medication or heat application?

Chest pain of thoracic origin occurs with muscle soreness from coughing or from inflammation of pleura overlying pneumonia. Distinguish this from chest pain of cardiac origin (see Chapter 20) or from heartburn of stomach acid.

4. History of respiratory infections. Any past history of breathing trouble or lung diseases such as bronchitis, emphysema, asthma, pneumonia?
   - Have you had unusually frequent or unusually severe colds?

Consider sequelae after these conditions.
Because most people have had some colds, it is more meaningful to ask about excess number or severity.
Assess possible risk factors.

   - Any family history of allergies, tuberculosis, or asthma?
5. Smoking history. Do you **smoke** cigarettes or cigars? At what age did you start? How many packs per day do you smoke now? For how long?
   - Have you ever tried to quit? What helped? Why do you think it did not work? What activities do you associate with smoking?
   - Do you live with someone who smokes?

State number of packs per day and the number of years smoked.
Most people who smoke already know they should quit smoking. Instead of admonishing, assess smoking behaviour and ways to modify daily smoking activities, identify triggers, and to manage withdrawal.

6. Environmental exposure. Are there any **environmental conditions** that may affect your breathing? Where do you work: at a factory, chemical plant, coal mine, farm, outdoors in a heavy traffic area?

Pollution exposure.
Farmers may be at risk for grain inhalation and pesticide inhalation. "Farmer's lung" (**extrinsic allergic alveolitis**) occurs in about 2% to 10% of farm workers, depending on the region. The disease is most common in Canada in regions with wet weather at harvest time. Coal miners have a risk of pneumoconiosis. Stone cutters, miners, and potters are at risk for silicosis. Other irritants include asbestos and radon.
Assess **self-care** measures.

- Do you do anything to protect your lungs, such as wear a mask or have the ventilatory system checked at work? Do you do anything to monitor your exposure? Do you have periodic examinations, pulmonary function tests, radiographic examination?

Examiner Asks	Rationale
• Do you know what specific symptoms to note that may signal breathing problems?	General symptoms: cough, shortness of breath. Some gases produce specific symptoms: • Carbon monoxide: dizziness, headache, fatigue • Sulphur dioxide: cough, congestion
7. **Self-care behaviours.** When was your most recent tuberculosis skin test, chest radiographic study, pneumonia immunization, or influenza immunization?	"Flu" vaccine is modified yearly; it is recommended for adults with chronic medical conditions, for residents of nursing homes, for health care workers, and for people who are immunosuppressed.

Additional History for Infants and Children

Examiner Asks	Rationale
1. **Illness.** Has the child had any frequent or very severe colds?	No more than four to six uncomplicated upper respiratory infections per year are expected in early childhood.
2. **Allergy.** Is there any history of allergy in the family? • For a child younger than 2 years: At what age were new foods introduced? Was the child breastfed or formula-fed?	Consider new foods or formula as possible allergens.
3. **Chronic respiratory illness.** Does the child have a cough? Seem congested? Have noisy breathing or wheezing? (Further questions similar to those listed in the section on adults.)	Document onset, and follow course of childhood chronic respiratory problems: asthma, bronchitis.
4. **Safety.** What measures have you taken to childproof your home and yard? Is there any risk that the child could inhale or swallow toxic substances? • Has anyone taught you emergency care measures in case of accidental choking or a hard-breathing spell?	Young children are at risk for accidental aspiration, poisoning, and injury. Assess knowledge level of parents and caregivers.
5. **Environmental smoke.** Any smokers in the home or in the car with the child?	Environmental smoke increases the risk for acute and chronic ear and respiratory infections in children (DiFranza, Aligne, & Weitzman, 2004).

Additional History for Older Adults

Examiner Asks	Rationale
1. **Activity intolerance.** Have you noticed any shortness of breath or fatigue with your daily activities?	In older adults, the respiratory system is less efficient (decreased vital capacity, less surface area for gas exchange), and so they have less tolerance for activity.
2. **Level of activity.** Tell me about your usual amount of physical activity.	Older patients may have reduced capacity to perform exercise because of pulmonary function deficits of aging. Sedentary or bedridden people are at risk for respiratory dysfunction. Assess coping strategies.
3. **Lung disease.** For patients with a history of COPD, lung cancer, or tuberculosis: How are you getting along each day? Any weight change in the last 3 months? How much? • How about energy level? Do you tire more easily? How does your illness affect you at home? At work?	Activities may decrease because of increasing shortness of breath or pain.
4. **Pain.** Do you have any chest pain with breathing? • Any chest pain after a bout of coughing? After a fall?	Some older adults feel pleuritic pain less intensely than do younger adults. When pain is precisely localized and sharp (patient points to it with one finger): consider fractured rib or muscle injury.

OBJECTIVE DATA

PREPARATION

Ask the patient to sit upright and to leave the gown on and open at the back. When you examine the anterior chest, lift up the gown and drape it on the patient's shoulders, rather than removing it completely. This promotes comfort by giving the patient the feeling of being somewhat clothed. To ensure further comfort, use a warm room and a warm diaphragm endpiece, and provide private examination time with no interruptions.

Perform the inspection, palpation, percussion, and auscultation on the posterior and lateral thorax. Then move to face the patient, and repeat these four manoeuvres on the anterior chest. This avoids repetitiously moving front to back around the patient.

Finally, clean your stethoscope endpiece with an alcohol wipe. Because your stethoscope touches many people, it could be a possible vector for both aerobic and anaerobic bacteria. Cleaning with an alcohol wipe is very effective.

EQUIPMENT NEEDED
Stethoscope
Small ruler, marked in centimetres
Marking pen
Alcohol wipe

Normal Range of Findings	Abnormal Findings

INSPECT THE POSTERIOR CHEST

Thoracic Cage

Note the *shape and configuration* of the chest wall. The spinous processes should appear in a straight line. The thorax is symmetrical, in an elliptical shape, with downward sloping ribs, angled at approximately 45 degrees in relation to the spine. The scapulae are symmetrically placed in each hemithorax.

The anteroposterior diameter should be less than the transverse diameter. The normal ratio of anteroposterior diameter to transverse diameter is approximately 1:2.

The neck muscles and trapezius muscles should have developed normally for age and occupation.

Note the **position** the patient takes to breathe. This includes a relaxed posture and the ability to support his or her own weight with arms comfortably at the sides or in the lap.

Assess the *skin colour and condition*. Colour should be consistent with the patient's genetic background, with allowance for sun-exposed areas on the chest and the back. No cyanosis or pallor should be present. Note any lesions. Inquire as to any change in a nevus in a place where the patient may have difficulty monitoring, such as on the back (see Chapter 13).

> Skeletal deformities may limit thoracic cage excursion: scoliosis, kyphosis (see Table 19-4, p. 463).
>
> Anteroposterior diameter equals transverse diameter ("barrel chest"). Ribs are horizontal, chest appears as if held in continuous inspiration. This occurs in chronic emphysema as a result of hyperinflation of the lungs (see Table 19-4, p. 462).
>
> Neck muscles are hypertrophied in COPD as a result of aiding in forced respirations.
>
> Patients with COPD often sit in a tripod position, leaning forward with arms braced against their knees, chair, or bed. This gives them leverage so that their rectus abdominis, intercostal, and accessory neck muscles all can aid in expiration.
>
> Cyanosis occurs with tissue hypoxia.

PALPATE THE POSTERIOR CHEST

Symmetrical Expansion

Confirm *symmetrical chest expansion* by placing your warmed hands on the patient's posterolateral chest wall, with your thumbs at the level of T9 or T10. Slide your hands medially to pinch up a small fold of skin between your thumbs (Figure 19-13).

Normal Range of Findings

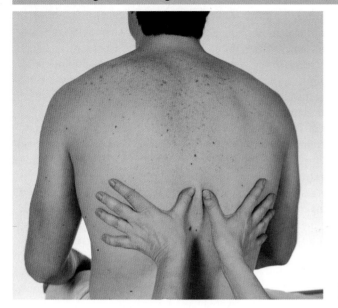

19-13

Ask the patient to take a deep breath. Your hands serve as mechanical amplifiers; as the patient inhales deeply, your thumbs should move apart symmetrically. Note any lag in expansion.

Tactile Fremitus

Assess **tactile** (or **vocal**) **fremitus.** Fremitus is a palpable vibration. Sounds generated from the larynx are transmitted through patent bronchi and through the lung parenchyma to the chest wall, where you feel them as vibrations.

Use either the palmar base (the ball) of the fingers or the ulnar edge of one of your hands, and touch the patient's chest while he or she repeats the words "ninety-nine" or "blue moon." These are resonant phrases that generate strong vibrations. Start over the lung apices, and palpate from one side to another (Figure 19-14).

Fremitus intensity varies among persons, but symmetry is most important; the vibrations should feel the same in the corresponding area on each side. However, just between the scapulae, fremitus may feel stronger on the right side than on the left side because the right side is closer to the bronchial bifurcation. Avoid palpating over the scapulae because bone damps sound transmission.

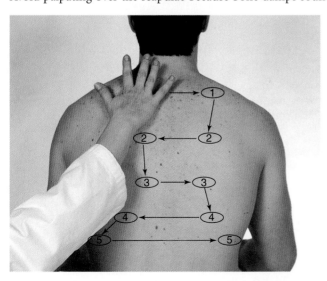

19-14

Abnormal Findings

Chest expansion is unequal with marked atelectasis or pneumonia; with thoracic trauma such as fractured ribs; and with pneumothorax.

Pain accompanies deep breathing when the pleurae are inflamed.

Objective Data

Normal Range of Findings	Abnormal Findings

The following factors affect the normal intensity of tactile fremitus:

- Location of bronchi in relation to the chest wall: Normally, fremitus is most prominent between the scapulae and around the sternum, sites where the major bronchi are closest to the chest wall. Fremitus normally decreases lower down because more and more tissue impedes sound transmission.
- Thickness of the chest wall: Fremitus feels greater over a thin chest wall than over an obese or heavily muscular one, in which thick tissue damps the vibration.
- Pitch and intensity: A loud, low-pitched voice generates more fremitus than does a soft, high-pitched one.

Note any areas of abnormal fremitus. Sound is conducted better through a uniformly dense structure than through a porous one, which changes in shape and solidity (as does the lung tissue during normal respiration). Thus conditions that increase the density of lung tissue make a better conducting medium for sound vibrations and increase tactile fremitus.

Using the fingers, gently palpate the entire chest wall. This enables you to note any areas of tenderness, to note skin temperature and moisture, to detect any superficial lumps or masses, and to explore any skin lesions noted on inspection.

Decreased fremitus occurs when anything obstructs transmission of vibrations (e.g., obstructed bronchus, pleural effusion or thickening, pneumothorax, or emphysema). Any barrier between the sound and your palpating hand decreases fremitus.

Increased fremitus occurs with compression or consolidation of lung tissue (e.g., lobar pneumonia). This occurs only when the bronchus is patent and when the consolidation extends to the lung surface. Note that only gross changes increase fremitus. Small areas of early pneumonia do not significantly affect fremitus.

Rhonchal fremitus is palpable with thick bronchial secretions.

Pleural friction fremitus is palpable with inflammation of the pleura (see Table 19-6, p. 465).

Crepitus is a coarse crackling sensation palpable over the skin surface. It occurs in subcutaneous emphysema when air escapes from the lung and enters the subcutaneous tissue, as after open thoracic injury or surgery.

PERCUSS THE POSTERIOR CHEST

Lung Fields

Determine the **predominant note over the lung fields.** Start at the apices and percuss the band of normally resonant tissue across the tops of both shoulders (Figure 19-15). Then, percussing in the interspaces, make a side-to-side comparison all the way down the lung region. Percuss at 5-cm intervals. Avoid the damping effect of the scapulae and ribs.

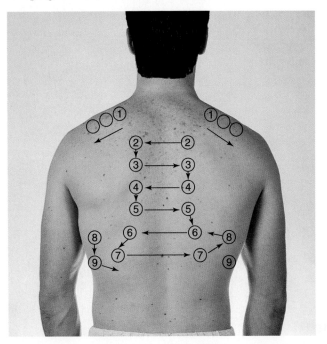

19-15

Normal Range of Findings	Abnormal Findings

Resonance is the low-pitched, clear, hollow sound that predominates in healthy lung tissue in adults (Figure 19-16). However, *resonance* is a relative term and has no constant standard. The resonant note may be modified somewhat in an athlete with a heavily muscular chest wall and in an obese adult, in whom subcutaneous fat produces scattered dullness.

The depth of penetration of percussion has limits. Percussion sets into motion only the outer 5 to 7 cm of tissue. It does not penetrate to reveal any change in density deeper than that. Also, any abnormal tissue must be 2 to 3 cm wide to yield an abnormal percussion note. Lesions smaller than that are not detectable by percussion.

Hyperresonance is a lower-pitched, booming sound found when too much air is present, as in emphysema or pneumothorax.

A **dull note** (soft, muffled thud) signals abnormal density in the lungs, as with pneumonia, pleural effusion, atelectasis, or tumour.

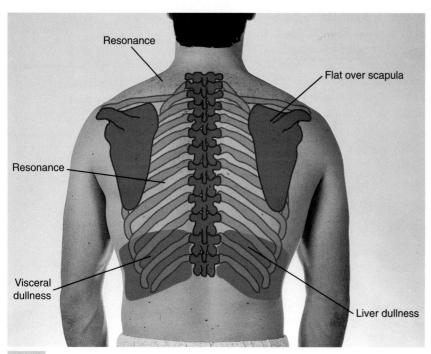

Resonance
Flat over scapula
Resonance
Visceral dullness
Liver dullness

19-16   Expected percussion notes.

AUSCULTATE THE POSTERIOR CHEST

The passage of air through the tracheobronchial tree creates a characteristic set of noises that are audible through the chest wall. These noises also may be modified by obstruction within the respiratory passageways or by changes in the lung parenchyma, the pleura, or the chest wall.

Breath Sounds

Evaluate the presence and quality of **normal breath sounds.** The patient should be sitting, leaning forward slightly, with arms resting comfortably across the lap. Instruct the patient to breathe through the mouth, a little bit deeper than usual, but to stop if he or she begins to feel dizzy. Be careful to monitor the breathing throughout the examination and allow times for the patient to rest and breathe normally. Many patients are willing to comply with your instructions in an effort to please you and to be a "good patient." Watch that the patient does not hyperventilate to the point of fainting.

Clean the flat diaphragm endpiece of the stethoscope and hold it firmly on the patient's chest wall. Listen to at least one full respiration in each location. Side-to-side comparison is most important.

Crackles are abnormal lung sounds (see Table 19-7, Adventitious Lung Sounds, p. 465).

Objective Data

Normal Range of Findings	Abnormal Findings

Do not confuse background noise with lung sounds. Become familiar with these extraneous noises that may be confused with lung pathology if not recognized:
1. Examiner's breathing on stethoscope tubing
2. Stethoscope tubing bumping together
3. Patient shivering
4. Patient's hairy chest: Movement of hairs under stethoscope sounds like crackles (rales) (see p. 450); minimize this movement by pressing harder or by wetting the hair with a damp cloth
5. Rustling of paper gown or paper drapes

While standing behind the patient, listen to the following lung areas: posterior from the apices at C7 to the bases (around T10) and laterally from the axilla down to the seventh or eighth rib. Use the sequence illustrated in Figure 19-17.

Continue to visualize approximate locations of the lobes of each lung so that you correlate your findings to anatomical areas. As you listen, think about (a) what you are hearing over this spot and (b) what you should expect to be hearing. You should expect to hear three types of normal breath sounds in adults and older children: **bronchial** (sometimes called *tracheal* or *tubular*), **bronchovesicular**, and **vesicular.** Study the characteristics of these normal breath sounds presented in Table 19-1.

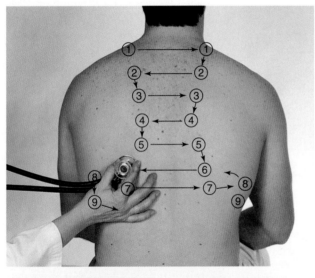

19-17 Sequence for auscultation.

TABLE 19-1	Characteristics of Normal Breath Sounds				
Type of Breath Sound	Pitch	Amplitude	Duration	Quality	Normal Location
BRONCHIAL (TRACHEAL)	High	Loud	Inspiration < expiration	Harsh, hollow, tubular	Trachea and larynx
BRONCHOVESICULAR	Moderate	Moderate	Inspiration = expiration	Mixed	Over major bronchi, where fewer alveoli are located: posterior, between scapulae especially on right; anterior, around upper sternum in first and second intercostal space
VESICULAR	Low	Soft	Inspiration > expiration	Rustling, like the sound of the wind in the trees	Over peripheral lung fields, where air flows through smaller bronchioles and alveoli

Objective Data

Normal Range of Findings

Note the normal location of the three types of breath sounds on the chest wall of adults and older children (Figures 19-18 and 19-19).

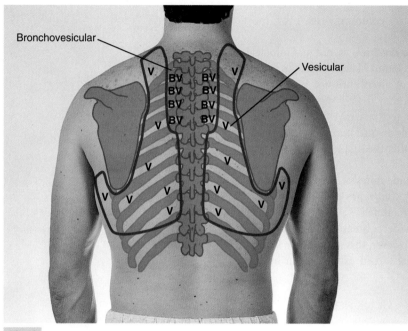

Bronchovesicular

Vesicular

19-18

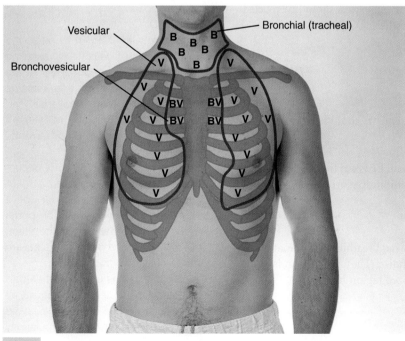

Vesicular

Bronchial (tracheal)

Bronchovesicular

19-19

Abnormal Findings

Decreased or **absent breath sounds** are indications of the following situations:
1. Obstruction of the bronchial tree at some point by secretions, mucus plug, or a foreign body
2. Emphysema, as a result of loss of elasticity in the lung fibres and decreased force of inspired air; also, because the lungs are already hyperinflated, the inhaled air does not make as much noise
3. Obstruction of the transmission of sound between the lung and your stethoscope, as in pleurisy or pleural thickening or by air (pneumothorax) or fluid (pleural effusion) in the pleural space

A silent chest means no air is moving in or out, which is an ominous sign.

Increased breath sounds mean that sounds are louder than they should be (e.g., bronchial sounds heard over an abnormal location, the peripheral lung fields, are abnormal). They have a high-pitched, tubular quality, with a prolonged expiratory phase and a distinct pause between inspiration and expiration. They sound very close to your stethoscope, as if they were right *in* the tubing close to your ear. They occur when consolidation (e.g., pneumonia) or compression (e.g., fluid in the intrapleural space) increases the density in a lung area, which enhances the transmission of sound from the bronchi. When the inspired air reaches the alveoli, it hits solid lung tissue that conducts sound more efficiently to the surface.

Normal Range of Findings	Abnormal Findings

Adventitious Sounds

Note the presence of any **adventitious sounds.** These are additional sounds that are *not* normally heard in the lungs. If present, they are heard as being superimposed on the breath sounds. They are caused by the collision of moving air with secretions in the tracheobronchial passageways or by the popping open of previously deflated airways. Sources differ as to the classification and nomenclature of these sounds (see Table 19-7, p. 466), but **crackles** (or rales) and **wheeze** (or rhonchi) are terms commonly used by most examiners.

One type of adventitious sound, **atelectatic crackles,** is not pathological. These are short, popping, crackling sounds that sound like fine crackles but do not last beyond a few breaths. When sections of alveoli are not fully aerated (as in people who are asleep or in older adults), they deflate slightly and accumulate secretions. Crackles are heard when these sections are expanded by a few deep breaths. Atelectatic crackles are heard only in the periphery, usually in dependent portions of the lungs, and disappear after the first few breaths or after a cough.

Charting of normal breath sound would include notes of both air entry and adventitia. Thus when breath sounds are normal, your notes will read as follows: "Good bilateral A/E [air entry] with no adventitia noted."

In the past, patients were asked to "take a deep breath and blow it out hard" to screen for the presence of wheezing. However, this manoeuvre is futile because slight wheezing may occur on maximal forced exhalation in healthy people.

Study Table 19-7, pp. 465–467, for a complete description of these abnormal adventitious breath sounds.

During normal tidal flow, high-pitched wheeze occurs with asthma.

INSPECT THE ANTERIOR CHEST

Note the *shape and configuration* of the chest wall. The ribs are sloping downward with symmetrical interspaces. The costal angle is within 90 degrees. Development of abdominal muscles is as expected for the patient's age, weight, and athletic condition.

Note the patient's **facial expression.** The facial expression should be relaxed and benign, indicating unconscious effort of breathing.

Assess the **level of consciousness.** The patient should be alert and cooperative.

Note skin *colour and condition.* The lips and nail beds are free of cyanosis or unusual pallor. The nails are of normal configuration. Explore any skin lesions.

Assess the quality of **respirations.** Normal relaxed breathing is automatic and effortless, regular and even, and produces no noise. The chest expands symmetrically with each inspiration. Note any localized lag on inspiration.

Barrel chest is characterized by horizontal ribs and a costal angle exceeding 90 degrees.

Hypertrophy of abdominal muscles occurs in chronic emphysema.

Facies appear tense, strained, and tired in COPD.

The patient with COPD may purse the lips in a whistling position. By exhaling slowly and against a narrow opening, the pressure in the bronchial tree remains positive, and fewer airways collapse.

Cerebral hypoxia may be manifested by excessive drowsiness or by anxiety, restlessness, and irritability.

Clubbing of the distal phalanx occurs with chronic respiratory disease.

Cutaneous angiomas (spider nevi) associated with liver disease or portal hypertension may be evident on the chest.

Breathing may be noisy with severe asthma or chronic bronchitis.

Chest expansion is unequal when part of the lung is obstructed or collapsed, as with pneumonia, or in guarding to avoid postoperative incisional pain or pleurisy pain.

Normal Range of Findings	Abnormal Findings

No retraction or bulging of the interspaces should occur on inspiration.

Retraction suggests obstruction of the respiratory tract or that increased inspiratory effort is needed, as in atelectasis. Bulging indicates trapped air, as in forced expiration associated with emphysema or asthma.

Normally, accessory muscles are not used to augment respiratory effort. However, with very heavy exercise, the accessory neck muscles (scalene, sternomastoid, trapezius) are used momentarily to enhance inspiration.

Accessory muscles are used in acute airway obstruction and massive atelectasis.

In COPD, the rectus abdominis and internal intercostal muscles are used to force expiration.

The respiratory rate is within normal limits for the patient's age (see Table 10-3, p. 163), and the pattern of breathing is regular. Occasional sighs normally punctuate breathing.

Tachypnea and hyperventilation, bradypnea and hypoventilation, and periodic breathing are abnormal (see Table 19-5, p. 463).

PALPATE THE ANTERIOR CHEST

Palpate for *symmetrical chest expansion.* Place your hands on the anterolateral wall with the thumbs along the costal margins and pointing toward the xiphoid process (Figure 19-20).

With emphysema, the costal angle is abnormally wide, and little inspiratory variation occurs.

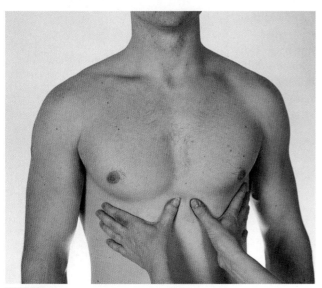

19-20

Ask the patient to take a deep breath. Watch your thumbs move apart symmetrically, and note smooth chest expansion with your fingers. Any limitation in thoracic expansion is easier to detect on the anterior chest because the range of motion is greater with breathing.

A lag in expansion occurs with atelectasis, pneumonia, and postoperative guarding.

A palpable grating sensation with breathing indicates pleural friction fremitus (see Table 19-6, p. 465).

Assess tactile (vocal) fremitus. Begin palpating over the lung apices in the supraclavicular areas (Figure 19-21). Compare vibrations from one side to the other as the patient says, "ninety-nine." Avoid palpating over female breast tissue because breast tissue normally damps sounds.

Palpate the anterior chest wall to note any tenderness (normally none is present) and to detect any superficial lumps or masses (again, normally none is present). Note skin mobility and turgor, and note skin temperature and moisture.

If any lumps are found in male breast tissue, refer the man to a specialist.

Normal Range of Findings	Abnormal Findings

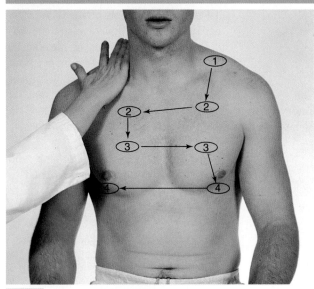

19-21   Assess tactile fremitus.

PERCUSS THE ANTERIOR CHEST

Begin percussing the apices in the supraclavicular areas. Then, percussing the interspaces and comparing one side with the other, move down the anterior chest.

Interspaces are easier to palpate on the anterior chest than on the back. Do not percuss directly over female breast tissue because this would produce a dull note. Shift the breast tissue over slightly with the edge of your stationary hand. In women with large breasts, percussion may yield little useful data. With all people, use the sequence illustrated in Figure 19-22.

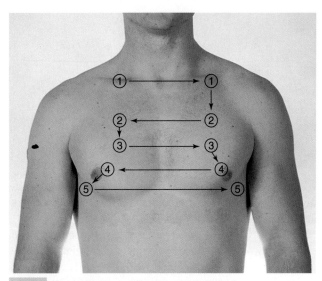

19-22   Sequence for percussion and auscultation.

Note the borders of cardiac dullness normally found on the anterior chest, and do not confuse these with suspected lung disease (Figure 19-23). In the right hemithorax, the upper border of liver dullness is located in the fifth intercostal space in the right midclavicular line. On the left, tympany is evident over the gastric space.

Lungs are hyperinflated with chronic emphysema; therefore, you would hear hyperresonance where you would expect cardiac dullness.

Normal Range of Findings	Abnormal Findings

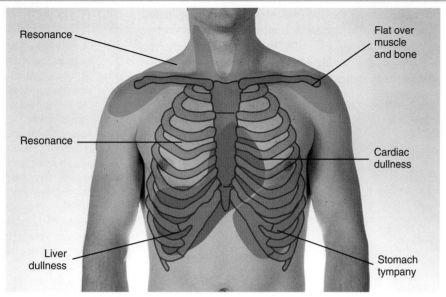

Resonance

Flat over muscle and bone

Resonance

Cardiac dullness

Liver dullness

Stomach tympany

19-23 Expected percussion notes.

AUSCULTATE THE ANTERIOR CHEST

Breath Sounds

Auscultate the lung fields over the anterior chest from the apices in the supra-clavicular areas down to the sixth rib. Progress from side to side as you move downward, and listen to one full respiration in each location. Use the sequence indicated for percussion. Do not place your stethoscope directly over the female breast. Displace the breast and listen directly over the chest wall.

Evaluate normal breath sounds, noting any abnormal breath sounds and any adventitious sounds. If the situation warrants, assess the voice sounds on the anterior chest.

Study Table 19-8, pp. 467–473, for a complete description of abnormal respiratory conditions.

THE LATERAL CHEST

Often forgotten—but equally important in the inspection, palpation, percussion, and auscultation of the thorax—is including the lateral chest wall. It is an extension of the vesicular lung field that wraps around the sides of the patient. The only way to ensure that you are aware what is happening in the right middle lobe is to extend your assessment into the lateral chest area.

Women, in particular, are prone to accumulating excretions into the right middle lobe secondary to postural drainage and the size of their breast tissue, which can impede movement of the chest wall. It is a common site of pneumonia and often the forgotten lobe, because it is the small third lobe of the right lung.

Right middle lobe syndrome generally refers to atelectasis in the right middle lobe of the lung. This condition is most common in children with a history of asthma. Although the mechanism by which asthma leads to lobar atelectasis is unknown, associated inflammation, bronchospasm, and secretions that cause mucus plugging are probably major contributors, as is the structural location of the lobe itself. (See the Critical Findings box.)

Objective Data

Normal Range of Findings	Abnormal Findings

The **pulse oximeter** is a noninvasive method of assessing arterial oxygen saturation (SpO_2) and is described in Chapter 10. A healthy person with no lung disease and no anemia normally has an SpO_2 of 97% to 98%. However, every SpO_2 value must be evaluated in the context of the patient's hemoglobin level, acid–base balance, and ventilatory status.

CRITICAL FINDINGS

- O_2 saturation of less than 93% on room air must be attended to immediately: Sit the patient up and have him or her take a few deep breaths to see whether this brings the O_2 saturation back to a normal range.
- Apply O_2 as indicated in standing orders or clinician orders for the acute area in which you are working.
- Ensure that your patient is not a CO_2 retainer (such patients may have COPD or other obstructive or restrictive disorder). Normal O_2 levels for such patients range from 88% to 92%, and many are receiving low-flow O_2 (1–2 L/min).
- If you are unsure, *go and find help* from a health care provider who is capable of determining the best course of action.

The **6-minute distance walk** is a safer, simple, inexpensive, clinical measure of functional status in aging adults (Enright, 2003). The 6-minute distance walk is used as an outcome measure for patients in pulmonary rehabilitation because it mirrors conditions that are used in everyday life. Locate a flat-surfaced corridor that has little foot traffic, is wide enough to enable comfortable turns, and has a controlled environment. Ensure that the patient is wearing comfortable shoes, and equip him or her with a pulse oximeter to monitor oxygen saturation. Ask the patient to set his or her own pace to cover as much ground as possible in 6 minutes, and assure the patient that it is all right to slow down or to stop to rest at any time. Use a stopwatch to time the walk. A patient who walks more than 300 m in 6 minutes is more likely to engage in activities of daily living.

Ask the patient to stop the walk if the SpO_2 is below 85% to 88% or if extreme breathlessness occurs.

✥ DEVELOPMENTAL CONSIDERATIONS

Infants and Children

To prepare, let the parent hold an infant supported against the chest or shoulder. Do not let the usual sequence of the physical examination restrain you; seize the opportunity with a sleeping infant to inspect and then to listen to lung sounds. This way you can concentrate on the breath sounds before the baby wakes up and possibly cries. The crying does not have to be a problem for you, however, because it actually enhances palpation of tactile fremitus and auscultation of breath sounds.

An older child may sit upright on the parent's lap. Offer the stethoscope and let the child handle it. This reduces any fear of the equipment. Promote the child's participation; school-age children usually are delighted to hear their own breath sounds when you place the stethoscope properly. While you listen to breath sounds, ask the young child to take a deep breath and "blow out" your penlight while you hold the stethoscope with your other hand. Time your letting go of the penlight button so the light goes off after the child blows. Or ask the child to "pant like a dog" while you auscultate.

Normal Range of Findings

Inspection. In infants, the thorax is rounded, and the anteroposterior-to-transverse ratio is 1 (Figure 19-24). By age 6 years, the thorax reaches the adult ratio of 1:2. The newborn's chest circumference is 30 to 36 cm and is 2 cm smaller than the head circumference until 2 years of age. The chest wall is thin, with little musculature. The ribs and the xiphoid process are prominent; you can both see and feel the sharp tip of the xiphoid process. The thoracic cage is soft and flexible.

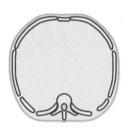 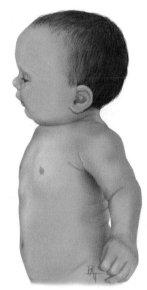

19-24   Round thorax in an infant.

In male and female newborns, the breasts may look enlarged by the second or third day as a result of maternal estrogen. On occasion, a white fluid, sometimes referred to as "witch's milk," can be expressed. This resolves within a week.

Some children have a horizontal groove in the rib cage at the level of the insertion of the diaphragm, extending from the sternum to the midaxillary line. This is called Harrison's groove, and it is normal.

The newborn's first respiratory assessment is part of the **Apgar scoring system** to measure the success of transition to extrauterine life (Table 19-2). The five standard parameters are scored at 1 minute and at 5 minutes after birth. A 1-minute total Apgar score of 7 to 10 indicates that the newborn is in good condition, needing only suctioning of the nose and mouth and otherwise routine care.

Newborns breathe through the nose rather than the mouth and are obligate nose breathers until age 3 months. Slight flaring of the lower costal margins may occur with respirations, but normally no flaring of the nostrils and no sterna retractions or intercostal retractions occur. The diaphragm is the newborn's major respiratory muscle. Intercostal muscles are not well developed. Thus you observe the abdomen bulge with each inspiration but see little thoracic expansion.

Abnormal Findings

A barrel shape that persists after age 6 years may develop with chronic asthma or cystic fibrosis.

Harrison's groove also occurs in rickets as a result of the pull of the diaphragm on weakened ribs.

In the immediate neonatal period, respirations may be depressed as a result of maternal drugs, interruption of the uterine blood supply, or obstruction of the tracheobronchial tree by mucus or fluid.

A 1-minute total Apgar score of 3 to 6 indicates that the newborn's status is moderately depressed and that more resuscitation and subsequent close observation are needed. A score of 0 to 2 indicates severe depression and necessitates full resuscitation, ventilatory assistance, and subsequent intensive care.

Marked retractions of sternum and intercostal muscles indicate increased inspiratory effort, as in atelectasis, pneumonia, asthma, and acute airway obstruction.

Normal Range of Findings				Abnormal Findings

TABLE 19-2	Apgar Scoring System			
Characteristic	2	1	0	Score
Heart rate	Over 100	Slow (below 100)	Absent	_____
Respiratory effort	Good, sustained cry; regular respiration	Slow, irregular, shallow	Absent	_____
Muscle tone	Active motion, spontaneous flexion	Some flexion of extremities; some resistance to extension	Limp, flaccid	_____
Reflex irritability (response to catheter nares)	Sneeze, cough, cry	Grimace, frown	No response	_____
Colour	Completely pink	Body pink, extremities pale	Cyanotic, pale	_____
				Total score _____

Count the respiratory rate for 1 full minute. Normal rates for the newborn are 30 to 40 breaths per minute but may spike up to 60 per minute. The respiratory rate is counted most accurately when the infant is asleep; when awake, infants reach rapid rates with very little excitation. The respiratory pattern may be irregular with extremes in room temperature or during feeding or sleeping. Brief periods of apnea lasting less than 10 or 15 seconds are common. This periodic breathing is more common in premature infants.

Palpation. Palpate symmetrical chest expansion by encircling the infant's thorax with both hands. Further palpation should reveal no lumps, masses, or crepitus, although you may feel the costochondral junctions in some normal infants.

Percussion. Percussion is of limited usefulness in newborns and especially in premature newborns because your adult fingers are too large in relation to the infant's tiny chest. The percussion note of hyperresonance occurs normally in infants and young children because the chest wall is relatively thin. Anything less than hyperresonance would have the same clinical significance as dullness in an adult. Diaphragmatic excursion measures about one to two rib interspaces in children.

Auscultation. Auscultation normally reveals bronchovesicular breath sounds in the peripheral lung fields of infants and young children up to ages 5 to 6 years. Their relatively thin chest walls with underdeveloped musculature do not damp the sound as do the thicker walls of adults; thus breath sounds are louder and harsher.

Fine crackles are the adventitious sounds commonly heard in the immediate neonatal period as a result of the opening of the airways and clearing of fluid. Because the newborn's chest wall is so thin, transmission of sounds is enhanced, and sound is heard easily all over the chest; thus localization of breath sounds is difficult. Even bowel sounds are easily heard in the chest. Try using the smaller pediatric diaphragm endpiece of a stethoscope, or place the bell of the stethoscope over the infant's interspaces and not over the ribs. Use the pediatric diaphragm on an older infant or toddler (Figure 19-25).

Respiratory rates are rapid pneumonia, fever, pain, heart disease, and anemia.

In an infant, tachypnea (rate of 50 to 100 per minute) during sleep may be an early sign of heart failure.

Asymmetrical expansion occurs with diaphragmatic hernia or pneumothorax.

Crepitus is palpable around a fractured clavicle, which may occur with difficult forceps delivery.

Breath sounds are diminished with pneumonia, atelectasis, pleural effusion, and pneumothorax.

Persistent fine crackles that are scattered over the chest occur with pneumonia, bronchiolitis, or atelectasis.

Crackles only in upper lung fields occur with cystic fibrosis; crackles only in lower lung fields occur with heart failure.

Expiratory wheezing occurs with lower airway obstruction (e.g., asthma or bronchiolitis). When unilateral, it may be caused by foreign body aspiration.

Persistent peristaltic sounds with diminished breath sounds on the same side may indicate diaphragmatic hernia.

Stridor is a high-pitched inspiratory crowing sound heard without the stethoscope, occurring with upper airway obstruction (e.g., croup, foreign body aspiration, or acute epiglottitis).

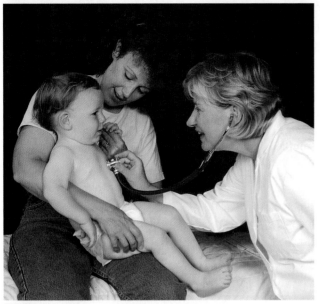

19-25

Pregnant Women

The thoracic cage may appear wider, and the costal angle may feel wider than in the nonpregnant state. Respirations may be deeper, although this can be quantified only with pulmonary function tests.

Older Adults

The thoracic cage commonly has an increased anteroposterior diameter, which produces a round barrel shape, and **kyphosis,** an outward curvature of the thoracic spine (see Table 19-4, p. 463). The patient compensates by holding the head extended and tilted back. You may palpate marked bony prominences because of decreased subcutaneous fat. Chest expansion may be somewhat decreased in an older patient, although it still should be symmetrical. The costal cartilages become calcified with aging, resulting in less mobility of the thorax.

Older patients may fatigue easily, especially during auscultation when deep mouth breathing is required. Take care that such patients do not hyperventilate and become dizzy. Allow brief rest periods or quiet breathing. If a patient does feel faint, instruct him or her to hold the breath for a few seconds; this will restore equilibrium.

Acutely Ill Patients

Ask a second examiner to hold the patient's arms and to support him or her in the upright position. If a second examiner is not available, you need to roll the patient from side to side, examining the uppermost half of the thorax. This obviously prevents you from comparing findings from one side to another. Also, side flexion of the trunk alters percussion findings because the ribs of the upward side may flex closer together.

SPECIAL CONSIDERATIONS FOR ADVANCED PRACTICE

Normal Range of Findings	Abnormal Findings

SPECIAL CONSIDERATIONS FOR ADVANCED PRACTICE

Voice Sounds

Determine the quality of **voice sounds** or **vocal resonance.** The spoken voice can be auscultated over the chest wall just as it can be felt in tactile fremitus described earlier. Ask the patient to repeat a phrase such as "ninety-nine" while you listen over the chest wall. Normal voice transmission is soft, muffled, and indistinct; you can hear sounds through the stethoscope but cannot distinguish exactly what is being said. Disease that increases lung density enhances transmission of voice sounds.

Voice sounds are usually *not* elicited in routine examination. Rather, this testing consists of supplemental manoeuvres that are performed if you suspect lung disease on the basis of earlier data. When they are performed, you are testing for possible presence of **bronchophony, egophony,** and **whispered pectoriloquy** (see Table 19-3, p. 461).

If Not Now, When?

The voice test is not considered part of a basic health assessment; however, it can be used to further investigate abnormal findings noted in the traditional auscultation, as a method of confirming your findings.

TABLE 19-3	Voice Sounds		
Technique	**Normal Finding**	**Abnormal Finding**	
Bronchophony Ask the patient to repeat "ninety-nine" while you listen with the stethoscope over the chest wall; listen especially if you suspect disease.	Normal voice transmission is soft, muffled, and indistinct; you can hear sound through the stethoscope but cannot distinguish exactly what is being said.	Disease that increases lung density enhances transmission of voice sounds; when auscultating, you clearly hear the words "ninety-nine." The words are more distinct than normal and sound close to your ear.	

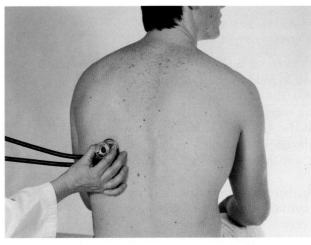

Egophony* Auscultate the chest while the patient phonates a long "eeeeeeee" sound.	Normally, you should hear "eeeeeeee" through your stethoscope.	Over area of consolidation or compression, the spoken "eeeeeeee" sounds like a bleating, long "aaaaa."
Whispered Pectoriloquy Ask the patient to whisper a phrase such as "one-two-three" as you auscultate.	Normal voice transmission is faint, muffled, and almost inaudible.	With only small amounts of consolidation, the whispered voice is transmitted very clearly and distinctly, although it is still somewhat faint; it sounds as if the patient is whispering, "one-two-three" right into your stethoscope.

*From Greek, referring to the voice of a goat.

Normal Range of Findings	Abnormal Findings

Voice sounds are assessed primarily in advance practice settings. One caution in using the voice test: if the patient has sustained a facial injury or has a chronic upper respiratory issue with the nasal cavity, all voice sounds coming through the oropharyngeal area are distorted because the test sounds, such as "ninety-nine," are nasally generated.

It may be more beneficial in this case to use egophony or whispered pectoriloquy.

Consolidation or compression of lung tissue will enhance the voice sounds, making the words more distinct.

Diaphragmatic Excursion

Determine **diaphragmatic excursion,** a measurement of distance between the base of the lungs on inspiration and expiration as the diaphragm recoils (Figure 19-26, A). Percuss to map out the lower lung border, both in expiration and in inspiration. First, ask the patient to "exhale and hold it" briefly while you percuss down the scapular line until the sound changes from resonant to dull on each side (see Figure 19-26, B). This helps you estimate the level of the diaphragm where the lungs are separated from the abdominal viscera. It may be somewhat higher on the right side (about 1 to 2 cm) because of the presence of the liver. Mark the spot.

Now ask the person to "take a deep breath and hold it." Continue percussing down from your first mark, and mark the level where the sound changes to dull on this deep inspiration. Measure the difference. This diaphragmatic excursion should be equal bilaterally and measure about 3 to 5 cm in adults, although it may be up to 7 to 8 cm in well-conditioned patients (Figure 19-26, B).

Often the beginning examiner becomes so involved in the subtle differences of percussion notes that he or she extends the patient's limits of breath-holding. Always hold your own breath when you ask your patient to. When you run out of air, the other person surely has too, especially if that person has a respiratory problem.

If Not Now, When?

Not traditionally considered part of a basic assessment for beginning practitioners. The procedure is then done in advanced practice settings when access to diagnostic imaging tools is not readily available. However, it is an excellent tool when the stethoscope is not an option for the practitioner, such as transporting a patient in a helicopter.

Note any abnormally high level of dullness and absence of diaphragmatic excursion. These characterize pleural effusion (fluid in the space between the visceral and parietal pleura) and atelectasis of the lower lobes.

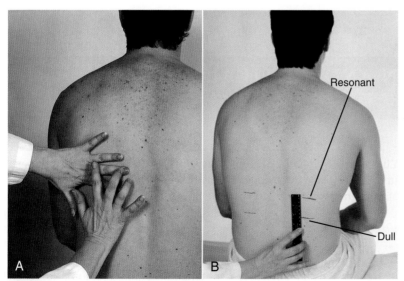

Resonant

Dull

A   B

19-26

Normal Range of Findings	Abnormal Findings

Measurement of Pulmonary Function Status

The **forced expiratory time** is the number of seconds it takes for the patient to exhale from total lung capacity to residual volume. It is a screening measure of airflow obstruction. Although the test usually is *not* performed in the respiratory assessment, it is useful when you wish to screen for pulmonary function.

Ask the patient to inhale the deepest breath possible and then to blow it all out hard, as quickly as possible, with the mouth open. Listen with your stethoscope over the sternum. The normal time for full expiration is 4 seconds or less.

In the ambulatory care setting, a handheld **spirometer** is used to measure lung health in chronic conditions, such as asthma. Ask the patient to inhale deeply and then exhale into the spirometer as fast as possible, until the most air is exhaled. The **forced vital capacity** (FVC) is the total volume exhaled. The **forced expiratory volume in 1 second** (FEV_1) is the volume exhaled in the first measured second. A normal finding is a FEV_1/FVC ratio of 75% to 80%, or greater, meaning that no significant obstruction of airflow is present.

If Not Now, When?

Measuring forced expiratory time is not a part of the basic assessment for beginning practitioners. However, an understanding of pulmonary function is helpful in certain situations:

- As a means of identifying early pulmonary disease
- As a means of testing FVC before discharge from hospital
- As a means of monitoring ongoing chronic respiratory disease in the community setting

With obstructive lung disease, forced expiration takes 6 seconds or more. In such cases, refer patients for more precise pulmonary function studies.

The ratio of FEV_1 to FVC is an indication of the severity of airflow obstruction:

- Mild obstruction of airflow: FEV_1/FVC = 60% to 70%
- Moderate obstruction of airflow: FEV_1/FVC = 50% to 60%
- Severe obstruction of airflow: FEV_1/FVC < 50%

DOCUMENTATION AND CRITICAL THINKING

Sample Charting

SUBJECTIVE

No cough, shortness of breath, or chest pain with breathing. No history of respiratory diseases. Has "one or no" colds per year. Has never smoked. Works in well-ventilated office; smoking by coworkers is restricted to lounge. Last TB [tuberculin] skin test: 4 years PTA, negative. Never had chest radiography.

OBJECTIVE

Inspection: AP [anteroposterior] < transverse diameter. Respirations: 16/min, relaxed and even.
Palpation: Chest expansion: symmetrical. Tactile fremitus: equal bilaterally. No tenderness to palpation. No lumps or lesions.

Special Considerations for Advanced Practice

Documentation & Critical Thinking

Percussion: Resonant to percussion over lung fields. Diaphragmatic excursion: 5 cm bilaterally.
Auscultation: Vesicular breath sounds: clear over lung fields. No adventitious sounds.

ASSESSMENT

Intact thoracic structures
Lung sounds clear

Focused Assessment: Clinical Case Study

Thomas G. is a 58-year-old, thin, male traffic patrolman who appears older than stated age. Face is anxious and tense, although in no acute distress at this time. Seeks care for "increasing shortness of breath and fatigue in last couple months."

SUBJECTIVE

- 1 year PTA: noticed more "winded" than usual when walking >3–4 blocks. Early morning cough present daily × 10 years, but now increased sputum production to 2 T per morning, frothy white.
- 6 mo. PTA: had a "cold" with severe harsh coughing, productive of "½ cup" thick white sputum per day. Noted midsternal chest pain (mild) with cough. Lasted 2 weeks. Treated self with humidifier and OTC [over-the-counter] cough syrup—minimal relief.
- 3 mo. PTA: noticed increasing SOB [shortness of breath] with less activity. Fatigue and SOB when working outside during traffic rush hours. Unable to take evening walks (usually 2–3 blocks) because of SOB and fatigue. Has two-pillow orthopnea. Wakes 3–4 times during night.
- Now: feels he is "worse and needs some help." Continues with two-pillow orthopnea. Unable to walk >2 blocks or climb >1 flight stairs without resting. Unable to blow out birthday candles on cake last week. Morning cough productive of "¼ cup" thin white sputum, cough continues sporadically during day.
- No chest pain, hemoptysis, night sweats, or paroxysmal nocturnal dyspnea. No history of allergies, hospitalizations, or injuries to chest. No family history of TB [tuberculosis], allergies, asthma, or cancer. Smokes cigarettes 2 packs per day × 30 years. Alcohol: <1 six-pack beer/week, summer months only.

OBJECTIVE

Inspection: Sitting on side of bed with arms propped on bedside table. Resp. resting: 24/min, regular, shallow with prolonged expiration; resp. ambulating: 34/min. Increased use of accessory muscles, AP = transverse diameter (barrel chest) with widening of costal angle, slightly flushed face, tense expression.
Palpation: Minimal but symmetrical chest expansion. Tactile fremitus = bilaterally. No lumps, masses, or tenderness to palpation.
Percussion: Diaphragmatic excursion is 1 cm and = bilaterally. Hyperresonance over lung fields.
Auscultation: Breath sounds diminished. Expiratory wheeze throughout posterior chest, R > L. No crackles.

ASSESSMENT

Chronic and increasing SOB
Ineffective airway clearance R/T bronchial secretions and obstruction
Activity intolerance R/T imbalance between oxygen supply and demand
Insomnia R/T dyspnea and decreased mobility
Anxiety R/T change in health status

Documentation & Critical Thinking

ABNORMAL FINDINGS

TABLE 19-4   Configurations of the Thorax

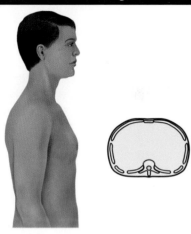

Normal Adult (for comparison)

The thorax has an elliptical shape with an anteroposterior-to-transverse ratio of 1:2 to 5:7.

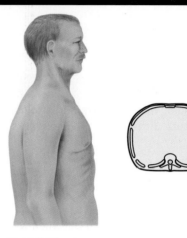

Barrel Chest

Note equal anteroposterior-to-transverse ratio and that ribs are horizontal instead of the normal downward slope. This is associated with normal aging and also with chronic emphysema and asthma as a result of hyperinflation of lungs.

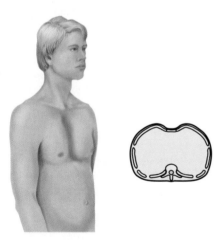

Pectus Excavatum

A markedly sunken sternum and adjacent cartilages (also called *funnel breast*). Depression begins at second intercostal space, becoming depressed most at junction of xiphoid process with body of sternum. More noticeable on inspiration. Congenital, usually not symptomatic. When severe, sternal depression may cause embarrassment and a negative self-concept. Surgery may be indicated.

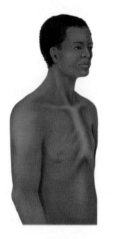

Pectus Carinatum

A forward protrusion of the sternum, with ribs sloping back at either side, and vertical depressions along costochondral junctions (pigeon breast). Less common than pectus excavatum, this minor deformity necessitates no treatment. If severe, surgery may be indicated.

TABLE 19-4   Configurations of the Thorax—cont'd

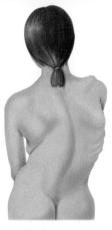 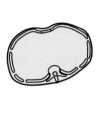

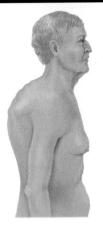 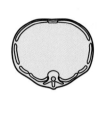

Scoliosis

A lateral S-shaped curvature of the thoracic and lumbar spine, usually with involved vertebrae rotation. Note unequal shoulder and scapular heights, unequal hip levels, and rib interspaces flared on convex side. Onset is more prevalent in adolescent age groups, especially girls. Mild deformities are asymptomatic. If deviation is severe (>45 degrees), scoliosis may reduce lung volume; then the patient is at risk for impaired cardiopulmonary function. Primary impairment is cosmetic deformity, negatively affecting self-image. Refer early for treatment, often surgery.

Kyphosis

An exaggerated posterior curvature of the thoracic spine (humpback) that causes significant back pain and limited mobility. Severe deformities impair cardiopulmonary function. If the neck muscles are strong, patient compensates by hyperextension of head to maintain level of vision.

Kyphosis has been associated with aging, especially in cases of "dowager's hump" in postmenopausal women with osteoporosis. However, it is common well before menopause. It is related to physical fitness; women with adequate exercise habits are less likely to have kyphosis.

TABLE 19-5   Respiration Patterns*

Inspiration   Expiration

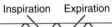

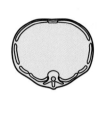

Normal Adult (for Comparison)

Rate: 10-20 breaths per minute.

Depth: 500 mL to 800 mL.

Pattern: even.

Depth: air moving in and out with each respiration.

The ratio of pulse to respirations is fairly constant, about 4 : 1. Both values increase as a normal response to exercise, fear, or fever.

Sigh

Occasional sighs punctuate the normal breathing pattern and help expand alveoli. Frequent sighs may indicate emotional dysfunction. Frequent sighs also may lead to hyperventilation and dizziness.

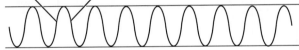

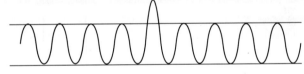

Tachypnea

Rapid, shallow breathing. Increased rate is more than 24 per minute. This is a normal response to fever, fear, or exercise. Rate also increases with respiratory insufficiency, pneumonia, alkalosis, pleurisy, and lesions in the pons.

Hyperventilation

Increase in both rate and depth. Normally occurs with extreme exertion, fear, or anxiety. Also occurs with diabetic ketoacidosis (Kussmaul's respirations), hepatic coma, salicylate overdose (hyperventilation produces a respiratory alkalosis to compensate for the metabolic acidosis), lesions of the midbrain, and alteration in blood gas concentration (either an increase in carbon dioxide or decrease in oxygen). Hyperventilation causes the level of carbon dioxide in the blood to decrease (alkalosis).

*Assess (a) rate, (b) depth (tidal volume), and (c) pattern.

Continued

TABLE 19-5   Respiration Patterns—cont'd

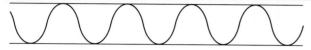

Bradypnea

Slow breathing. A decreased but regular rate (<10 per minute), as in drug-induced depression of the respiratory centre in the medulla, increased intracranial pressure, and diabetic coma.

Hypoventilation

An irregular, shallow pattern caused by an overdose of narcotics or anaesthetics. May also occur with prolonged bed rest or conscious splinting of the chest to avoid respiratory pain.

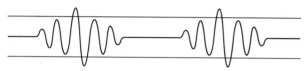

Cheyne-Stokes Respiration

A cycle in which respirations gradually wax and wane in a regular pattern, increasing in rate and depth and then decreasing. The breathing periods last 30 to 45 seconds, with periods of apnea (20 seconds) alternating the cycle. The most common cause is severe heart failure; other causes are renal failure, meningitis, drug overdose, and increased intracranial pressure. Occurs normally in infants and older adults during sleep.

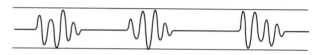

Biot's Respiration

Similar to Cheyne-Stokes respiration, except that the pattern is irregular. A series of normal respirations (three to four) is followed by a period of apnea. The cycle length is variable, lasting anywhere from 10 seconds to 1 minute. Occurs with head trauma, brain abscess, heat stroke, spinal meningitis, and encephalitis.

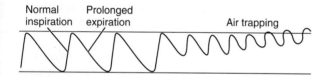

Normal inspiration   Prolonged expiration   Air trapping

◀ Chronic Obstructive Breathing

Normal inspiration and prolonged expiration to overcome increased airway resistance. In a patient with chronic obstructive lung disease, any situation calling for increased heart rate (exercise) may lead to dyspneic episode (air trapping) because then the patient does not have enough time for full expiration.

TABLE 19-6   Abnormal Tactile Fremitus

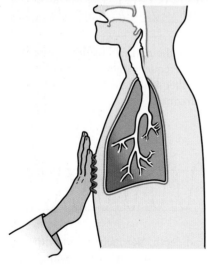

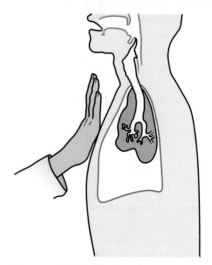

Increased Tactile Fremitus

Occurs with conditions that increase the density of lung tissue, thereby making a better conducting medium for vibrations (e.g., compression or consolidation [pneumonia]). For increased fremitus to be apparent, at least one bronchus must be patent, and consolidation must extend to lung surface.

Decreased Tactile Fremitus

Occurs when anything obstructs transmission of vibrations (e.g., an obstruction in bronchus, pleural effusion or thickening, pneumothorax, and emphysema).

TABLE 19-6   Abnormal Tactile Fremitus—cont'd

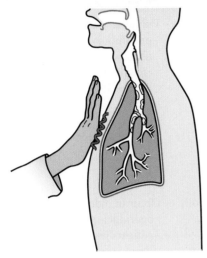

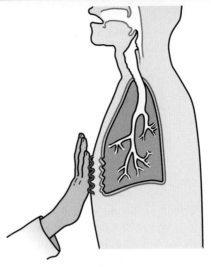

Rhonchal Fremitus
Vibration felt when inhaled air passes through thick secretions in the larger bronchi. This may decrease somewhat after coughing.

Pleural Friction Fremitus
Produced when inflammation of the parietal or visceral pleura causes a decrease in the normal lubricating fluid. Then the opposing surfaces make a coarse grating sound when rubbed together during breathing. Although this sound is best detected by auscultation, it may sometimes be palpable and feels like two pieces of leather grating together. It is synchronous with respiratory excursion. Also called a *palpable friction rub*.

TABLE 19-7   Adventitious Lung Sounds

Sound	Description	Mechanism	Clinical Example
Discontinuous Sounds These are discrete, crackling sounds. *Crackles:* fine (formerly called rales) Inspiration — Expiration	Discontinuous, high-pitched, short crackling, popping sounds heard during inspiration that are not cleared by coughing; you can simulate this sound by rolling a strand of hair between your fingers near your ear, or by moistening your thumb and index finger and separating them near your ear	Inhaled air collides with previously deflated airways; airways suddenly pop open, creating crackling sound as gas pressures between the two compartments equalize (Forgacs, 1978).	*Late inspiratory crackles* occur with restrictive disease: pneumonia, heart failure, and interstitial fibrosis. *Early inspiratory crackles* occur with obstructive disease: chronic bronchitis, asthma, and emphysema. *Posturally induced crackles* (PICs) are fine crackles that appear with a change from sitting to the supine position or with a change from supine to supine with legs elevated. PICs that appear after acute myocardial infarction have been associated with increased mortality (Deguchi, Hirakawa, Gotoh, Yagi, & Ohshima, 1993).

Continued

TABLE 19-7	Adventitious Lung Sounds—cont'd		
Sound	**Description**	**Mechanism**	**Clinical Example**
Crackles: (coarse)	Loud, low-pitched, bubbling and gurgling sounds that start in early inspiration and may be present in expiration; may decrease somewhat after suctioning or coughing but will reappear shortly: sounds like opening a Velcro fastener.	Inhaled air collides with secretions in the trachea and large bronchi.	Pulmonary edema, pneumonia, pulmonary fibrosis, and a depressed cough reflex in terminally ill patients.
Atelectatic crackles (atelectatic rales)	Sound like fine crackles but do not last and are not indications of disease; disappear after the first few breaths; heard in axillae and bases (usually dependent) of lungs.	When sections of alveoli are not fully aerated, they deflate and accumulate secretions. Crackles are heard when these sections re-expand with a few deep breaths.	Occur in older adults, bedridden patients, and in patients just aroused from sleep.
Pleural friction rub	A very superficial sound that is coarse and low-pitched; it has a grating quality as if two pieces of leather are being rubbed together; sounds just like crackles, but *close* to the ear; sounds louder if you push the stethoscope harder onto the chest wall; sound is inspiratory and expiratory.	Caused when pleurae become inflamed and lose their normal lubricating fluid; their opposing roughened pleural surfaces rub together during respiration; heard best in anterolateral wall, where lung mobility is greatest.	Pleuritis, accompanied by pain with breathing (rub disappears after a few days if pleural fluid accumulates and separates pleurae).

Continuous Sounds

These are connected, musical sounds.

Wheeze: high-pitched (sibilant)	High-pitched, musical squeaking sounds that sound polyphonic (multiple notes as in a musical chord); predominate in expiration but may occur in both expiration and inspiration.	Air squeezed or compressed through passageways narrowed almost to closure by collapsing, swelling, secretions, or tumours; the passageway walls oscillate in apposition between the closed and barely open positions; the resulting sound is similar to that from a vibrating reed (Forgacs, 1978).	Diffuse airway obstruction from acute asthma or chronic emphysema.

TABLE 19-7   Adventitious Lung Sounds—cont'd

Sound	Description	Mechanism	Clinical Example
Wheeze: low-pitched (sonorous rhonchi)	Low-pitched; monophonic single note, musical snoring, moaning sounds; they are heard throughout the cycle, although they are more prominent on expiration; may clear somewhat after coughing.	Airflow obstruction as described by the vibrating reed mechanism for high-pitched wheeze; the pitch of the wheeze cannot be correlated with the size of the passageway that generates it.	Bronchitis, single bronchus obstruction from airway tumour.
Stridor	High-pitched, monophonic, inspiratory, crowing sound, louder in neck than over chest wall.	Originating in larynx or trachea; upper airway obstruction from swollen, inflamed tissues or lodged foreign body.	Croup and acute epiglottitis in children, foreign body inhalation, and obstructed airway (all may be life-threatening).

TABLE 19-8   Assessment of Common Respiratory Conditions

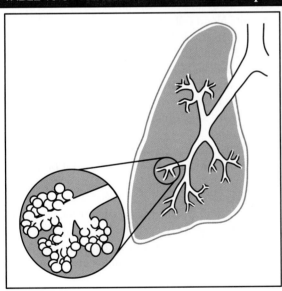

◄ *Normal Lung (for Comparison)*

Inspection: Anteroposterior < transverse diameter, relaxed posture, normal musculature; rate 10-18 breaths per minute, regular, no cyanosis or pallor.

Palpation: Symmetrical chest expansion. Tactile fremitus present and equal bilaterally, diminishing toward periphery. No lumps, masses, or tenderness.

Percussion: Resonant. Diaphragmatic excursion 3 to 5 cm and equal bilaterally.

Auscultation: Vesicular over peripheral fields. Bronchovesicular parasternally (anterior) and between scapulae (posterior). Infants and young children: bronchovesicular throughout.

Adventitious sounds: None.

Continued

TABLE 19-8   Assessment of Common Respiratory Conditions—cont'd

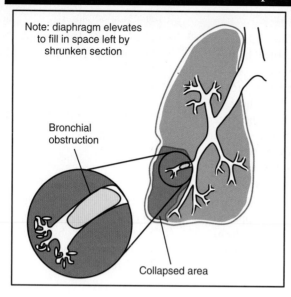

Note: diaphragm elevates to fill in space left by shrunken section

Bronchial obstruction

Collapsed area

◄ *Atelectasis (Collapse)*

Condition: Collapsed shrunken section of alveoli, or an entire lung, as a result of (a) airway obstruction (e.g., the bronchus is completely blocked by thick exudate, aspirated foreign body, or tumour), the alveolar air beyond it is gradually absorbed by the pulmonary capillaries, and the alveolar walls cave in; (b) compression on the lung; and (c) lack of surfactant (hyaline membrane disease).

Inspection: Cough. Lag on expansion on affected side. Increased respiratory rate and pulse. Possible cyanosis.

Palpation: Chest expansion decreased on affected side. Tactile fremitus decreased or absent over area. With large collapse, tracheal shift toward affected side.

Percussion: Dull over area (remainder of thorax sometimes has hyperresonant note).

Auscultation: Vesicular decreased or absent over area. Voice sounds variable, usually decreased or absent over affected area.

Adventitious sounds: None if bronchus is obstructed. Occasional fine crackles if bronchus is patent.

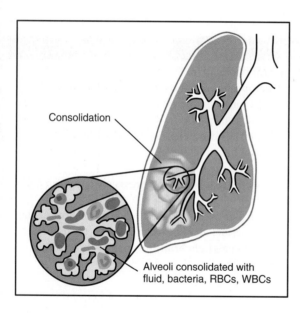

Consolidation

Alveoli consolidated with fluid, bacteria, RBCs, WBCs

◄ *Lobar Pneumonia*

Condition: Infection in lung parenchyma leaves alveolar membrane edematous and porous, and so red blood cells (RBCs) and white blood cells (WBCs) pass from blood to alveoli. Alveoli progressively fill up (become consolidated) with bacteria, solid cellular debris, fluid, and blood cells, all of which replace alveolar air. This results in decreased surface area of the respiratory membrane, which causes hypoxemia.

Inspection: Increased respiratory rate. Guarding and lag on expansion on affected side. Children: sternal retraction, nasal flaring.

Palpation: Chest expansion decreased on affected side. Tactile fremitus increased if bronchus patent, decreased if bronchus obstructed.

Percussion: Dull over lobe.

Auscultation: Breath sounds louder with patent bronchus, as if coming directly from larynx. Voice sounds have increased clarity, bronchophony, egophony, whispered pectoriloquy present. Children: diminished breath sounds may occur early in pneumonia.

Adventitious sounds: Crackles, fine to medium.

TABLE 19-8   Assessment of Common Respiratory Conditions—cont'd

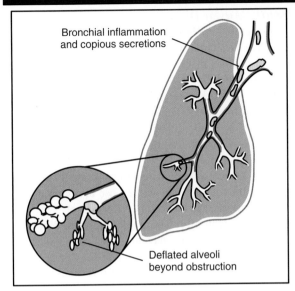

Bronchial inflammation and copious secretions

Deflated alveoli beyond obstruction

◀ *Bronchitis*

Condition: Proliferation of mucous glands in the passageways, resulting in excessive mucus secretion. Inflammation of bronchi with partial obstruction of bronchi by secretions or constrictions. Sections of lung distal to obstruction may be deflated. Bronchitis may be acute or chronic with recurrent productive cough. Chronic bronchitis is usually caused by cigarette smoking.

Inspection: Hacking, rasping cough productive of thick mucoid sputum. Chronic: dyspnea, fatigue, cyanosis, possible clubbing of fingers.

Palpation: Tactile fremitus normal.

Percussion: Resonant.

Auscultation: Normal vesicular. Voice sounds normal. Chronic: prolonged expiration.

Adventitious sounds: Crackles over deflated areas. Wheeze may be present.

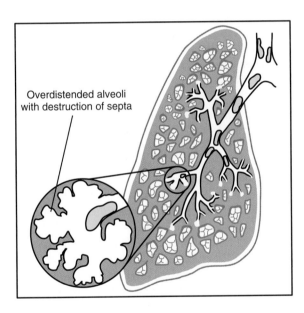

Overdistended alveoli with destruction of septa

◀ *Emphysema*

Condition: Caused by destruction of pulmonary connective tissue (elastin, collagen); characterized by permanent enlargement of air sacs distal to terminal bronchioles and rupture of interalveolar walls. Airway resistance is increased, especially on expiration, which causes hyperinflation of the lung and an increase in lung volume. Cigarette smoking accounts for 80%-90% of cases of emphysema.

Inspection: Increased anteroposterior diameter. Barrel chest. Use of accessory muscles to aid respiration. Tripod position. Shortness of breath, especially on exertion. Respiratory distress. Tachypnea.

Palpation: Decreased tactile fremitus and chest expansion.

Percussion: Hyperresonant. Decreased diaphragmatic excursion.

Auscultation: Decreased breath sounds. Expiration may be prolonged. Muffling of heart sounds as a result of overdistension of lungs.

Adventitious sounds: Usually none; occasionally, wheeze.

Continued

TABLE 19-8   Assessment of Common Respiratory Conditions—cont'd

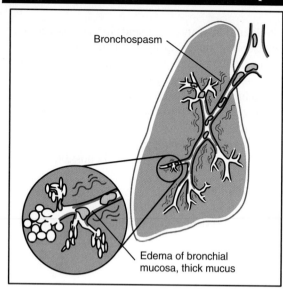

Bronchospasm

Edema of bronchial mucosa, thick mucus

◄ *Asthma (Reactive Airway Disease)*

Condition: An allergic hypersensitivity to certain inhaled allergens (pollen), irritants (tobacco, ozone), microorganisms, stress, or exercise that produces a complex response characterized by bronchospasm, and inflammation, edema in walls of bronchioles, and secretion of highly viscous mucus into airways. These factors greatly increase airway resistance, especially during expiration, and produce the symptoms of wheezing, dyspnea, and sensation of tightness in the chest.

Inspection: During severe attack: increased respiratory rate, shortness of breath with audible wheeze, use of accessory neck muscles, cyanosis, apprehension, retraction of intercostals spaces. Expiration laboured, prolonged. When asthma is chronic, barrel chest may develop.

Palpation: Tactile fremitus decreased; tachycardia.

Percussion: Resonant. May be hyperresonant if asthma is chronic.

Auscultation: Diminished air movement. Breath sounds decreased, with prolonged expiration. Voice sounds decreased.

Adventitious sounds: Bilateral wheezing on expiration; sometimes inspiratory and expiratory wheezing.

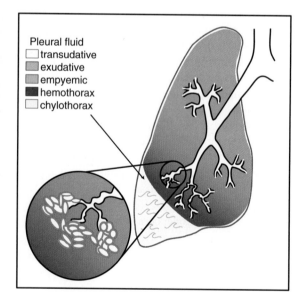

Pleural fluid
☐ transudative
☐ exudative
☐ empyemic
■ hemothorax
☐ chylothorax

◄ *Pleural Effusion (Fluid) or Thickening*

Condition: Collection of excess fluid in the intrapleural space, with compression of overlying lung tissue. Effusion may contain watery capillary fluid (transudative), protein (exudative), purulent matter (empyemic), blood (hemothorax), or milky lymphatic fluid (chylothorax). Gravity settles fluid in dependent areas of thorax. Presence of fluid subdues all lung sounds.

Inspection: Increased respirations, dyspnea; patient may have dry cough, tachycardia, cyanosis, abdominal distension.

Palpation: Tactile fremitus decreased or absent. Tracheal shift away from affected side. Chest expansion decreased on affected side.

Percussion: Dull to flat. No diaphragmatic excursion on affected side.

Auscultation: Breath sounds decreased or absent. Voice sounds decreased or absent. When remainder of lung is compressed near the effusion, bronchial breath sounds may be heard over the compression along with bronchophony, egophony, whispered pectoriloquy.

Adventitious sounds: None.

TABLE 19-8   Assessment of Common Respiratory Conditions—cont'd

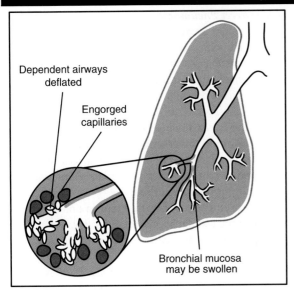

◄ *Heart Failure*

Condition: Pump failure with increasing pressure of cardiac overload causes pulmonary congestion or an increased amount of blood present in pulmonary capillaries. Dependent air sacs are deflated. Pulmonary capillaries engorged. Bronchial mucosa may be swollen.

Inspection: Increased respiratory rate, shortness of breath on exertion, orthopnea, paroxysmal nocturnal dyspnea, nocturia, ankle edema, pallor in light-skinned people.

Palpation: Skin moist, clammy. Tactile fremitus normal.

Percussion: Resonant.

Auscultation: Normal vesicular. Heart sounds include S_3 gallop.

Adventitious sounds: Crackles at lung bases.

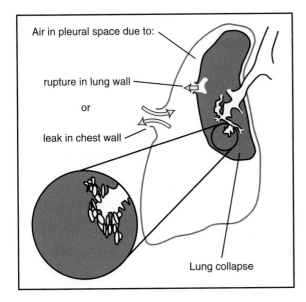

◄ *Pneumothorax*

Condition: Free air in pleural space causes partial or complete lung collapse. Air in pleural space neutralizes the usual negative pressure present; thus lung collapses. Usually unilateral. Pneumothorax can be (a) *spontaneous* (air enters pleural space through rupture in lung wall), (b) *traumatic* (air enters through opening or injury in chest wall), or (c) *tension* (trapped air in pleural space increases, compressing lung and shifting mediastinum to the unaffected side).

Inspection: Unequal chest expansion. If pneumothorax is large, patient may have tachypnea, cyanosis, apprehension, bulging in interspaces.

Palpation: Tactile fremitus decreased or absent. Tracheal shift to opposite side (unaffected side). Chest expansion decreased on affected side. Tachycardia, decreased blood pressure.

Percussion: Hyperresonant. Decreased diaphragmatic excursion.

Auscultation: Breath sounds decreased or absent. Voice sounds decreased or absent.

Adventitious sounds: None.

Continued

TABLE 19-8   Assessment of Common Respiratory Conditions—cont'd

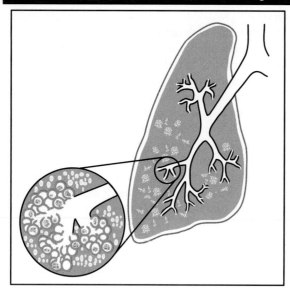

◀ *Pneumocystis jiroveci Pneumonia*

Condition: This virulent form of pneumonia is a protozoal infection associated with AIDS. The parasite *P. jiroveci* (formerly known as *Pneumocystis carinii*) is common in Canada and harmless to most people except in immunocompromised patients, in whom a diffuse interstitial pneumonitis ensues. More than 75% of children are seropositive by the age of 4, which suggests a high rate of background exposure to the organism. Cysts containing the organism and macrophages form in alveolar spaces, alveolar walls thicken, and the disease spreads to bilateral interstitial infiltrates of foamy, protein-rich fluid.

Inspection: Anxiety, shortness of breath, dyspnea on exertion, malaise are common; also tachypnea; fever; a dry, nonproductive cough; intercostal retractions in children; cyanosis.

Palpation: Decreased chest expansion.

Percussion: Dull over areas of diffuse infiltrate.

Auscultation: Breath sounds may be diminished.

Adventitious sounds: Crackles may be present but often are absent.

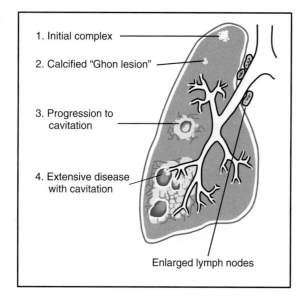

1. Initial complex
2. Calcified "Ghon lesion"
3. Progression to cavitation
4. Extensive disease with cavitation

Enlarged lymph nodes

◀ *Tuberculosis*

Condition: Inhalation of tubercle bacilli into the alveolar wall starts course of disease: (a) Initial complex is acute inflammatory response; macrophages engulf bacilli but do not kill them. Tubercle forms around bacilli. (b) Scar tissue forms, and lesion calcifies and is visible on radiograph. (c) Previously healed lesion is reactivated. Dormant bacilli now multiply, producing necrosis, cavitation, and caseous lung tissue (cheeselike appearance). (d) Extensive destruction occurs as lesion erodes into bronchus, forming air-filled cavity. Apex usually has the most damage.

Subjective data: Initially no symptoms, manifests as positive result of skin test or on radiograph. Progressive tuberculosis involves weight loss, anorexia, easy fatigability, low-grade afternoon fevers, night sweats. Patient may have pleural effusion, recurrent lower respiratory infections.

Inspection: Cough initially nonproductive, later productive of purulent, yellow-green sputum, may be blood-tinged. Dyspnea, orthopnea, fatigue, weakness.

Palpation: Skin moist at night from night sweats.

Percussion: Resonant initially. Dull over any effusion.

Auscultation: Normal or decreased vesicular breath sounds.

Adventitious sounds: Crackles over upper lobes common, persist after full expiration and cough.

TABLE 19-8   Assessment of Common Respiratory Conditions—cont'd

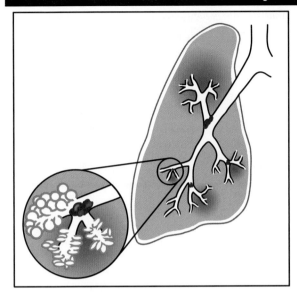

◄ Pulmonary Embolism

Condition: Undissolved materials (e.g., thrombus, or air bubbles, fat globules) originating in legs or pelvis, detach and travel through venous system returning blood to right heart and lodge to occlude pulmonary vessels. More than 95% arise from deep vein thrombi in lower legs as a result of stasis of blood, vessel injury, or hypercoagulability. Pulmonary occlusion results in ischemia of downstream lung tissue, increased pulmonary artery pressure, decreased cardiac output, and hypoxia. In rare cases, a saddle embolus in bifurcation of pulmonary arteries leads to sudden death from hypoxia. More often, small to medium pulmonary branches occlude, leading to dyspnea. These may resolve by fibrolytic activity.

Subjective data: Chest pain, worse on deep inspiration, dyspnea.

Inspection: Apprehensiveness, restlessness, anxiety, mental status changes, cyanosis, tachypnea, cough, hemoptysis, PaO_2 < 80 on pulse oximetry. Arterial blood gases show respiratory alkalosis.

Palpation: Diaphoresis, hypotension.

Auscultation: Tachycardia, accentuated pulmonic component of S_2 heart sound.

Adventitious sounds: Crackles, wheezes.

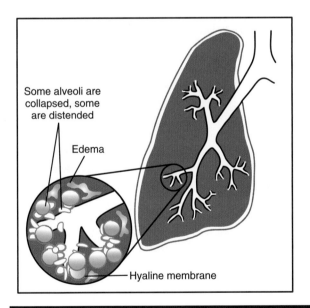

Some alveoli are collapsed, some are distended

Edema

Hyaline membrane

◄ Acute Respiratory Distress Syndrome (ARDS)

Condition: An acute pulmonary insult (trauma, gastric acid aspiration, shock, sepsis) damages alveolar capillary membrane, leading to increased permeability of pulmonary capillaries and alveolar epithelium, and to pulmonary edema. Gross examination (autopsy) would show dark red, firm, airless tissue, with some alveoli collapsed, and hyaline membranes lining the distended alveoli.

Subjective: Acute onset of dyspnea, apprehension.

Inspection: Restlessness; disorientation; rapid, shallow breathing; productive cough; thin, frothy sputum; retractions of intercostal spaces and sternum. Decreased PaO_2, blood gases show respiratory alkalosis, radiographs show diffuse pulmonary infiltrates, a late sign is cyanosis.

Palpation: Hypotension.

Auscultation: Tachycardia.

Adventitious sounds: Crackles, rhonchi.

AIDS, acquired immune deficiency syndrome; *PaO₂,* arterial partial pressure of oxygen.

Summary Checklist: Thorax and Lung Examination

For a PDA-downloadable version, go to *http://evolve.elsevier.com/Canada/Jarvis/examination/*.

1. Inspection
   Assess thoracic cage.
   Measure respirations.
   Assess skin colour and condition.
   Evaluate patient's position.
   Observe patient's facial expression.
   Assess level of consciousness.
2. Palpation
   Confirm symmetrical expansion.

   Assess tactile fremitus.
   Detect any lumps, masses, tenderness.
3. Percussion
   Percuss over lung fields.
   Estimate diaphragmatic excursion.
4. Auscultation
   Assess normal breath sounds.
   Note any abnormal breath sounds.

   If breath sounds are abnormal, perform bronchophony, whispered pectoriloquy, and egophony.
   Note any adventitious sounds.
5. Teaching and health promotion

REFERENCES

Best, D. (2009). Technical report: Secondhand smoke and prenatal tobacco exposure. *Pediatrics, 124*(5), e1017–e1044.

Canadian Lung Association. (2008). *Lung Association to launch Clean Air for Kids Campaign on January 23*. Ottawa: Author. Retrieved from *http://www.lung.ca/media-medias/news-nouvelles_e.php?id=100*.

Canadian Lung Association. (2013). Statistics: Lung Cancer. Retrieved from *http://www.lung.ca/lung101-renseignez/statistics-statistiques/lungdiseases-maladiespoumon/index_e.php#lungcancer*.

Cunningham, F. G., Leveno, K. J., Bloom, S. L., Hauth, J. C., Gilstrap, L. C., & Wenstrom, K. D. (2005). *Williams' obstetrics* (22nd ed.). New York: McGraw-Hill Professional.

Deguchi, F., Hirakawa, S., Gotoh, K., Yagi, Y., & Ohshima, S. (1993). Prognostic significance of posturally induced crackles: Long term follow-up of patients after recovery from acute myocardial infarction. *Chest, 103*, 1457–1462.

DiFranza, J. R., Aligne, A., & Weitzman, M. (2004). Prenatal and postnatal environmental tobacco smoke exposure and children's health. *Pediatrics, 113*, 1007–1015.

Enright, P. L. (2003). The six-minute walk test. *Respiratory Care, 48*, 783–785.

Forgacs, P. (1978). The functional basis of pulmonary sounds. *Chest, 73*, 399–405.

Håberg, S. E., Bentdal, Y. E., London, S. J., Kvaerner, K. J., Nystad, W., & Nafstad, P. (2010). Prenatal and postnatal parental smoking and acute otitis media in early childhood. *Acta Paediatrica, 99*(1), 99–105.

Lung Association. (2006). *Women & COPD: A national report*. Ottawa: Author. Retrieved from *http://www.lung.ca/_resources/Women_COPD_Report_2006.pdf*.

Public Health Agency of Canada. (2010a). Asthma, by age group and sex. Ottawa: Minister of Health.

Public Health Agency of Canada. (2010b). *Tuberculosis in Canada 2010*. Ottawa: Minister of Health.

Heart and Neck Vessels

Written by Carolyn Jarvis, PhD, APN, CNP

Adapted by June MacDonald-Jenkins, RN, BScN, MSc

⊖volve WEBSITE

- Animations
- Audio—Heart Sounds
- Bedside Assessment Summary Checklist
- Case Study:
  - Chest Pain
  - Shortness of Breath
- Examination Review Questions
- Health Promotion Guide:
  - Heart Disease

- Key Points
- Physical Examination Summary Checklist
- Quick Assessment for Common Conditions:
  - Congestive Heart Failure (CHF)
  - Hyperlipidemia
  - Myocardial Infarction
- Video—Assessment:
  - Neck Vessels and Heart

OUTLINE

STRUCTURE AND FUNCTION

The cardiovascular system consists of the **heart,** a muscular pump, and the **blood vessels.** The blood vessels are arranged in two continuous loops: the *pulmonary circulation* and the *systemic circulation* (Figure 20-1). When the heart contracts, it pumps blood simultaneously into both loops.

POSITION AND SURFACE LANDMARKS

The **precordium** is the area on the anterior chest overlying the heart and great vessels (Figure 20-2). The great vessels are the major arteries and veins connected to the heart. The heart and the great vessels are located between the lungs in the middle third of the thoracic cage; this area is called the **mediastinum.** The heart extends from the levels of the second to the fifth intercostal spaces and from the right border of the sternum to the left midclavicular line.

Think of the heart as an upside-down triangle in the chest. The "top" of the heart is the broader *base,* and the "bottom" is the *apex,* which points down and to the left (Figure 20-3). During contraction, the apex beats against the chest wall, producing an apical impulse. This is palpable in most people, normally at the fifth intercostal space, 7 to 9 cm from the midsternal line.

Inside the body, the heart is positioned so that its right side is anterior and its left side is mostly posterior. Of the heart's four chambers, the right ventricle forms the greatest area of anterior cardiac surface. The left ventricle lies behind the right ventricle and forms the apex and slender area of the left border. The right atrium lies to the right and above the right ventricle and forms the right border. The left atrium is located posteriorly, and only a small portion, the left atrial appendage, is visible anteriorly when the chest is open.

The **great vessels** lie bunched above the base of the heart. The **superior** and **inferior venae cavae** return unoxygenated venous blood to the right side of the heart. The **pulmonary artery** leaves the right ventricle, bifurcates, and carries the venous blood to the lungs. The **pulmonary veins** return the freshly oxygenated blood to the left side of the heart, and the **aorta** carries it out to the body. The aorta ascends from the left ventricle, arches back at the level of the sternal angle, and descends behind the heart.

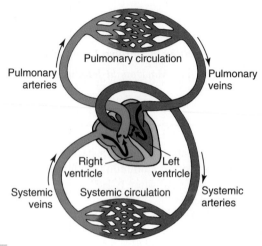

20-1 Two loops—separate but interdependent.

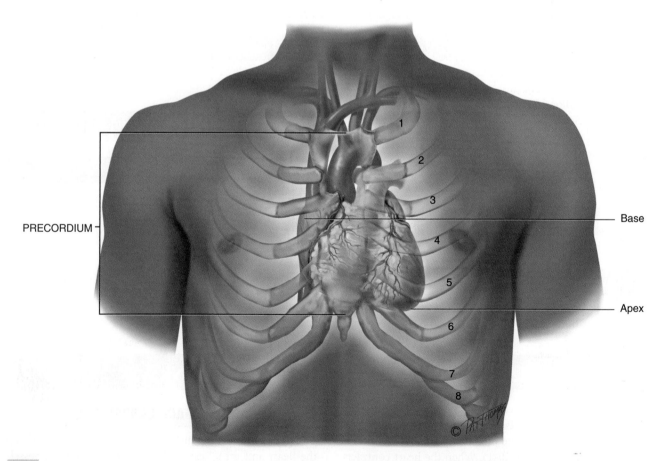

20-2

HEART WALL, CHAMBERS, AND VALVES

The **heart wall** has numerous layers. The **pericardium** is a tough, fibrous, double-walled sac that surrounds and protects the heart (Figure 20-4). It has two layers that contain a few millilitres of serous *pericardial fluid.* This ensures smooth, friction-free movement of the heart muscle. The pericardium is adherent to the great vessels, esophagus, sternum, and pleurae and is anchored to the diaphragm. The **myocardium** is the muscular wall of the heart; it does the pumping. The **endocardium** is the thin layer of endothelial tissue that lines the inner surface of the heart chambers and valves.

The common metaphor is to think of the heart as a pump. However, the heart is actually *two* pumps: The right side of the heart pumps blood into the lungs, and the left side of the heart simultaneously pumps blood into the body. The two pumps are separated by an impermeable wall, the septum. Each side has an atrium and a ventricle. The **atrium** (Latin for "anteroom") is a thin-walled reservoir for holding blood, and the thick-walled **ventricle** is the muscular pumping chamber.

The four **chambers** are separated by swinging-door–like structures, called *valves,* whose main purpose is to prevent backflow of blood. The valves are unidirectional; they can open only one way. The valves open and close *passively* in response to pressure gradients in the moving blood.

There are four **valves** in the heart (see Figure 20-4). The two **atrioventricular (AV) valves** separate the atria and the ventricles. The right AV valve is the **tricuspid valve,** and the left AV valve is the bicuspid or **mitral valve.** The valves' thin leaflets are anchored by collagenous fibres (**chordae tendineae**) to papillary muscles embedded in the ventricle

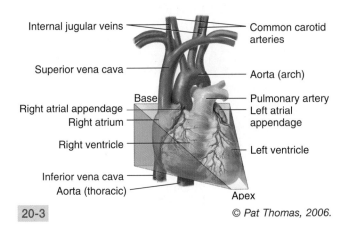

Internal jugular veins
Common carotid arteries
Superior vena cava
Aorta (arch)
Base
Pulmonary artery
Right atrial appendage
Left atrial appendage
Right atrium
Right ventricle
Left ventricle
Inferior vena cava
Aorta (thoracic)
Apex

20-3

© Pat Thomas, 2006.

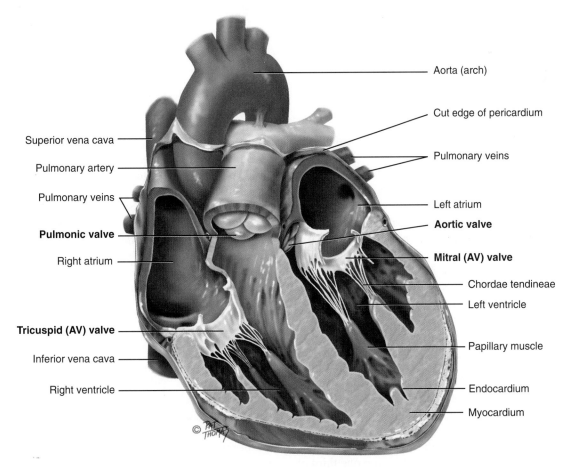

Aorta (arch)
Cut edge of pericardium
Superior vena cava
Pulmonary veins
Pulmonary artery
Pulmonary veins
Left atrium
Aortic valve
Pulmonic valve
Mitral (AV) valve
Right atrium
Chordae tendineae
Left ventricle
Tricuspid (AV) valve
Inferior vena cava
Papillary muscle
Right ventricle
Endocardium
Myocardium

floor. The AV valves open during the heart's filling phase (diastole) to allow the ventricles to fill with blood. During the pumping phase (systole), the AV valves close to prevent regurgitation of blood back up into the atria. The papillary muscles contract at this time, so that the valve leaflets meet and unite to form a perfect seal without turning themselves inside out.

The **semilunar valves** are located between the ventricles and the pulmonary arteries. Each semilunar valve has three cusps that look like half moons. The semilunar valves are the **pulmonic valve** in the right side of the heart and the **aortic valve** in the left side of the heart. They open during pumping, or systole, to allow blood to be ejected from the heart.

Note that there are no valves between the venae cavae and the right atrium, nor between the pulmonary veins and the left atrium. For this reason, abnormally high pressure in the left side of the heart produces symptoms of pulmonary congestion, or heart failure, and abnormally high pressure in the right side of the heart manifests as bulging neck veins and abdominal distension.

DIRECTION OF BLOOD FLOW

Think of an unoxygenated red blood cell being drained downstream into the venae cavae. It is swept along with the flow of venous blood and follows the route illustrated in Figure 20-5:

1. Blood flows from liver to right atrium through inferior vena cava.
   Superior vena cava drains venous blood from the head and upper extremities.
   From right atrium, venous blood travels through tricuspid valve to right ventricle.
2. From right ventricle, venous blood flows through pulmonic valve to pulmonary artery.
   Pulmonary artery delivers unoxygenated blood to lungs.
3. Lungs oxygenate blood.
   Pulmonary veins return fresh blood to left atrium.
4. From left atrium, arterial blood travels through mitral valve to left ventricle.
   Left ventricle ejects blood through aortic valve into aorta.
5. Aorta delivers oxygenated blood to body.
   Remember that the circulation is a continuous loop. The blood is kept moving along by continually shifting pressure gradients. The blood flows from an area of higher pressure to one of lower pressure.

CARDIAC CYCLE

The rhythmic movement of blood through the heart is the **cardiac cycle.** It has two phases, diastole and systole. In **diastole,** the ventricles relax and fill with blood. This takes up two thirds of the cardiac cycle. During **systole,** the heart's contraction, blood is pumped from the ventricles and fills the pulmonary and systemic arteries. This takes up one third of the cardiac cycle.

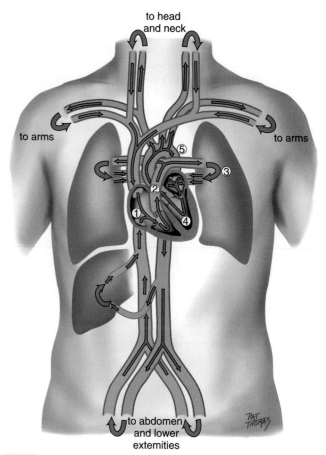

to head and neck
to arms
to arms
⑤
③
②
①
④
to abdomen and lower extemities

20-5

Diastole

In diastole, the ventricles are relaxed, and the AV valves (i.e., the tricuspid and mitral valves) are open (Figure 20-6). (Opening of the normal valve is acoustically silent.) The pressure in the atria is higher than that in the ventricles, and so blood pours rapidly into the ventricles. This first passive filling phase is called **early** or **protodiastolic filling.**

Toward the end of diastole, the atria contract and push the last amount of blood (about 25% of stroke volume) into the ventricles. This active filling phase is called **presystole,** or **atrial systole,** sometimes referred to as the *atrial kick.* It causes a small rise in left ventricular pressure. (Note that atrial systole occurs during ventricular diastole, a confusing but important point.)

Systole

At this point, a large volume of blood has been pumped into the ventricles. This volume raises ventricular pressure so that it is finally higher than that in the atria, and the mitral and tricuspid valves swing shut. The closure of the AV valves contributes to the first heart sound (S_1) and signals the beginning of systole. The AV valves close to prevent any regurgitation of blood back up into the atria during contraction.

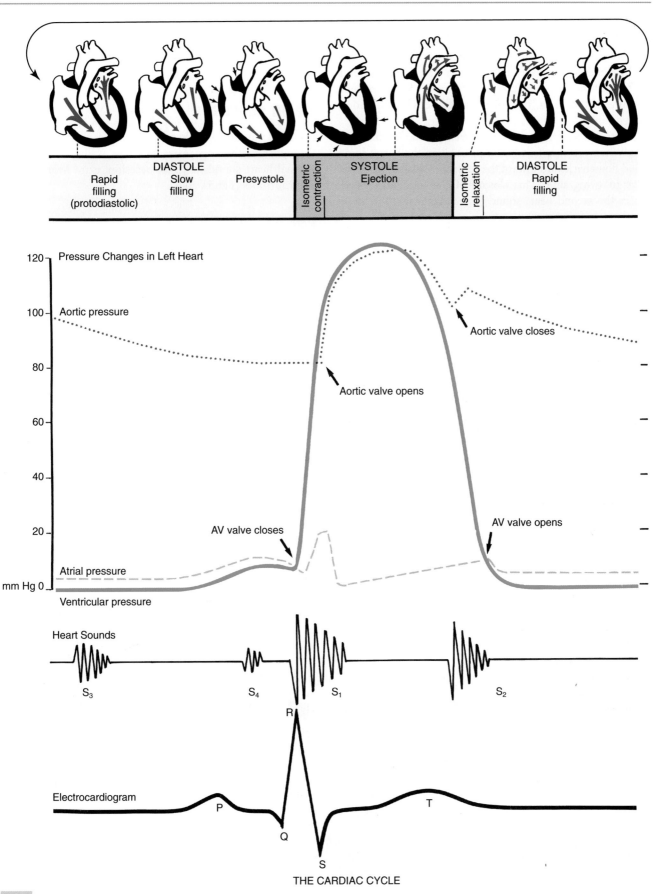

DIASTOLE

Rapid filling (protodiastolic) | Slow filling | Presystole

Isometric contraction

SYSTOLE
Ejection

Isometric relaxation

DIASTOLE
Rapid filling

Pressure Changes in Left Heart

Aortic pressure

Aortic valve closes

Aortic valve opens

AV valve opens

AV valve closes

Atrial pressure

mm Hg 0

Ventricular pressure

Heart Sounds

S_3 S_4 S_1 S_2

R

Electrocardiogram

P

Q

S

T

THE CARDIAC CYCLE

20-6

For a very brief time, all four valves are closed. The ventricular walls contract. This contraction against a closed system works to build pressure inside the ventricles to a high level (**isometric contraction**). Consider first the left side of the heart. When the pressure in the ventricle finally exceeds pressure in the aorta, the aortic valve opens and blood is ejected rapidly.

After the ventricle's contents are ejected, its pressure falls. When pressure falls below pressure in the aorta, some blood flows backward toward the ventricle, causing the aortic valve to swing shut. This closure of the semilunar valves causes the second heart sound (S_2) and signals the end of systole.

Diastole Again

At this point in the cardiac cycle, all four valves are closed and the ventricles relax (called **isometric** or **isovolumic relaxation**). Meanwhile, the atria have been filling with blood delivered from the lungs. Atrial pressure is now higher than the relaxed ventricular pressure. The mitral valve drifts open, and diastolic filling begins again.

Events in the Right and Left Chambers

The same events are happening in the right side of the heart, but pressures in the right chambers of the heart are much lower than those of the left chambers because less energy is needed to pump blood to its destination, the pulmonary circulation. Also, events occur just slightly later in the right side of the heart because of the route of myocardial depolarization. As a result, each of the heart sounds has two distinct components, and sometimes you can hear them separately.

In the first heart sound, closure of the mitral valve (M_1) can be heard just before tricuspid valve closure (T_1). In S_2, aortic valve closure (A_2) occurs slightly before pulmonic valve closure (P_2).

HEART SOUNDS

Events in the cardiac cycle generate sounds that can be heard through a stethoscope over the chest wall. These include normal heart sounds and, on occasion, extra heart sounds and murmurs (Figure 20-7).

Normal Heart Sounds

The **first heart sound** (S_1) occurs with closure of the AV valves and thus signals the beginning of systole. The mitral component of the first sound (M_1) slightly precedes the tricuspid component (T_1), but you usually hear these two components fused as one sound. You can hear S_1 over all the precordium, but it is usually loudest at the apex.

The **second heart sound** (S_2) occurs with closure of the semilunar valves and signals the end of systole. The aortic component of the second sound (A_2) slightly precedes the pulmonic component (P_2). Although it is heard over all the precordium, S_2 is loudest at the base.

Effect of Respiration

The volumes of right and left ventricular systole are just about equal, but this balance can be affected by respiration. To learn this, consider the following mnemonic:

> *MoRe to the Right,*
> *Less to the Left*

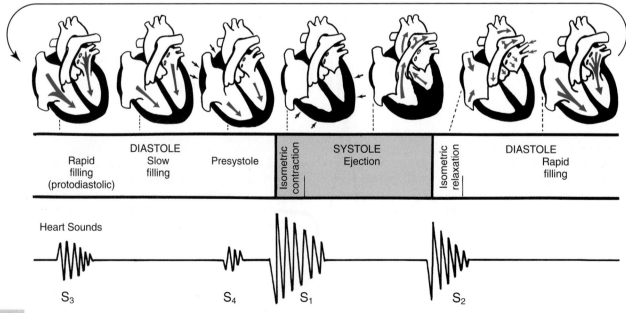

	DIASTOLE		Isometric contraction	SYSTOLE	Isometric relaxation	DIASTOLE
Rapid filling (protodiastolic)	Slow filling	Presystole		Ejection		Rapid filling

Heart Sounds

S_3 S_4 S_1 S_2

20-7

That means that during inspiration, intrathoracic pressure is decreased. This pushes more blood into the venae cavae, increasing venous return to the right side of the heart, which increases right ventricular stroke volume. The increased volume prolongs right ventricular systole and delays pulmonic valve closure.

Meanwhile on the left side, a greater amount of blood is sequestered in the lungs during inspiration. This momentarily decreases the amount returned to the left side of the heart, decreasing left ventricular stroke volume. The decreased volume shortens left ventricular systole and allows the aortic valve to close a bit earlier. When the aortic valve closes significantly earlier than the pulmonic valve, you can hear the two components separately. This is a *split S₂*.

Extra Heart Sounds

Third Heart Sound (S₃)

Normally diastole is a silent event. However, in some conditions, ventricular filling creates vibrations that can be heard over the chest. These vibrations constitute the S_3. The S_3 is heard when the ventricles are resistant to filling during the early rapid filling phase (protodiastole). This occurs immediately after S_2, when the AV valves open and atrial blood first pours into the ventricles. (See a complete discussion of S_3 in Table 20-7 on p. 510.)

Fourth Heart Sound (S₄)

The S_4 occurs at the end of diastole, at presystole, when the ventricle is resistant to filling. The atria contract and push blood into a noncompliant ventricle. This creates vibrations that are heard as S_4. The S_4 occurs just before S_1.

Murmurs

Blood circulating through normal cardiac chambers and valves usually makes no noise. However, some conditions create turbulence in blood flow and collision currents. These result in a murmur, much like the sound of noisy water flow created by a pile of stones or a sharp turn in a stream. A murmur is a gentle, blowing, swooshing sound that can be heard on the chest wall.

The following conditions result in a murmur:
1. Increases in velocity of blood flow (flow murmur; e.g., in exercise, thyrotoxicosis)
2. Decreases in viscosity of blood (e.g., in anemia)
3. Structural defects in the valves (narrowed valve, incompetent valve) or unusual openings in the chambers (dilated chamber, wall defect)

Characteristics of Sound

All heart sounds are described by four characteristics:
1. Frequency (pitch): heart sounds are described as high-pitched or low-pitched, although these terms are relative because all are low-frequency sounds, and you need a high-quality stethoscope to hear them
2. Intensity (loudness): loud or soft
3. Duration: very short for heart sounds; silent periods are longer
4. Timing: systole or diastole

CONDUCTION

Of all organs, the heart has a unique ability: automaticity. The heart can contract by itself, independently of any signals or stimulation from the body. The heart contracts in response to an electrical current conveyed by a conduction system (Figure 20-8). Specialized cells in the sinoatrial node near the superior vena cava initiate an electrical impulse. (Because the sinoatrial node has an intrinsic rhythm, it is the "pacemaker.") The current flows in an orderly sequence, first across the atria to the AV node low in the atrial septum. At the AV node, it is delayed slightly so that the atria have time to contract before the ventricles are stimulated. Then the impulse travels to the Bundle of His, a collection of heart muscle cells specialized for electrical conduction that transmits the electrical impulses to the point of the apex of the fascicular branches, called the right and left bundle branches, and then through the ventricles.

The electrical impulse stimulates the heart to do its work, which is to contract. A small amount of electricity spreads to the body surface, where it can be measured and recorded on the electrocardiogram (ECG). The electrocardiographic waves are arbitrarily labelled *PQRST*, which stand for the following elements:

P wave: depolarization of the atria
P–R interval: the interval from the beginning of the P wave to the beginning of the QRS complex (the time necessary for atrial depolarization plus time for the impulse to travel through the AV node to the ventricles)
QRS complex: depolarization of the ventricles
T wave: repolarization of the ventricles

Electrical events slightly *precede* the mechanical events in the heart. The phases of the cardiac cycle are labelled on an illustration of the ECG in Figure 20-8.

PUMPING ABILITY

In the resting adult, the heart normally pumps between 4 and 6 L of blood per minute throughout the body. This **cardiac output** (CO) equals the volume of blood in each systole (called the *stroke volume* [SV]) times the number of beats per minute (*rate* [R]); that is,

$$CO = SV \times R$$

The heart can alter its cardiac output to adapt to the metabolic needs of the body. Preload and afterload affect the heart's ability to increase cardiac output.

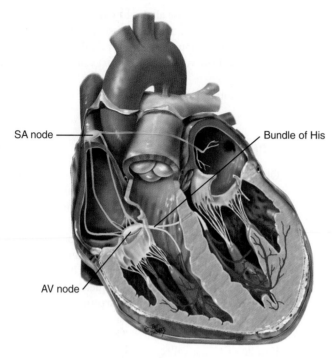

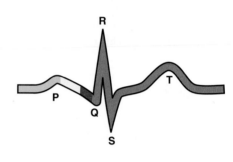

CONDUCTION SYSTEM

ELECTROCARDIOGRAPH
(ECG) WAVE

20-8

© Pat Thomas, 2006.

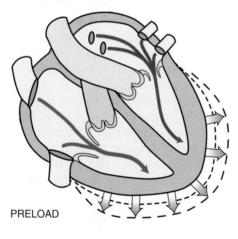

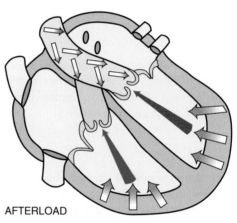

PRELOAD

AFTERLOAD

20-9

© Pat Thomas, 2006.

Preload is the venous return that builds during diastole. It is the length to which the ventricular muscle is stretched at the end of diastole just before contraction (Figure 20-9).

When the volume of blood returned to the ventricles is increased (as when exercise stimulates skeletal muscles to contract and force more blood back to the heart), the muscle bundles are stretched beyond their normal resting state to accommodate it. The force of this switch is the preload. According to the Frank-Starling law, the greater the stretch, the stronger is the heart's contraction. This increased contractility results in an increase in the volume of blood ejected (increased stroke volume).

Afterload is the opposing pressure that the ventricle must generate to open the aortic valve against the higher aortic

pressure. It is the resistance against which the ventricle must pump its blood. Once the ventricle is filled with blood, the ventricular end-diastolic pressure is 5 to 10 mm Hg, whereas that in the aorta is 70 to 80 mm Hg. To overcome this difference, the ventricular muscle *tenses* (isovolumic contraction). After the aortic valve opens, rapid ejection occurs.

THE NECK VESSELS

Cardiovascular assessment includes the survey of vascular structures in the neck: the carotid artery and the jugular veins (Figure 20-10). These vessels reflect the efficiency of cardiac function.

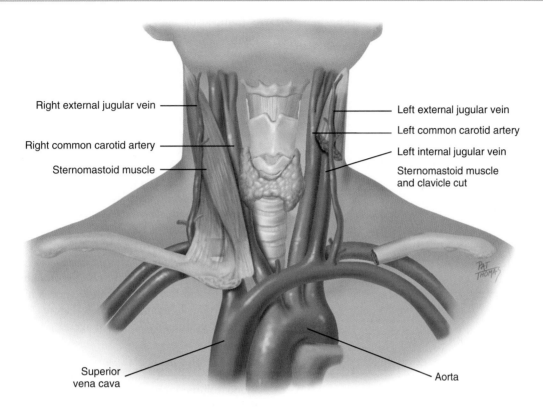

Right external jugular vein

Right common carotid artery

Sternomastoid muscle

Left external jugular vein

Left common carotid artery

Left internal jugular vein

Sternomastoid muscle and clavicle cut

Superior vena cava

Aorta

NECK VESSELS

20-10

Carotid Artery Pulse

Chapter 10 describes the pulse as a pressure wave generated by each systole as blood is pumped into the aorta. The carotid artery is a central artery; that is, it is close to the heart. The timing of the carotid artery pulse closely coincides with ventricular systole. (Assessment of the peripheral pulses is described in Chapter 21, and blood pressure assessment is described in Chapter 10.)

The **carotid artery** is located in the groove between the trachea and the sternomastoid muscle, medial to and alongside that muscle. Note the characteristics of its waveform (Figure 20-11): a smooth rapid upstroke, a summit that is rounded and smooth, and a downstroke that is more gradual and that has a dicrotic notch caused by closure of the aortic valve (marked *D* in the figure).

Jugular Venous Pulse and Pressure

The **jugular veins** empty unoxygenated blood directly into the superior vena cava. Because no cardiac valve exists to separate the superior vena cava from the right atrium, the jugular veins give information about activity on the right side of the heart. Specifically, they reflect filling pressure and volume changes. When the right side of the heart fails to pump efficiently, the volume and pressure increase, as exposed by the jugular veins.

Two jugular veins are present in each side of the neck (see Figure 20-10). The larger **internal jugular vein** lies deep and

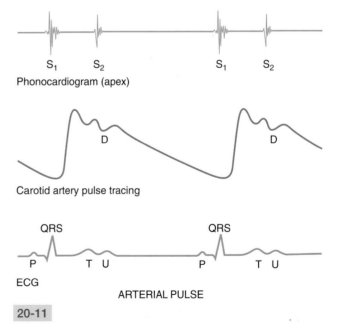

S_1 S_2 S_1 S_2

Phonocardiogram (apex)

D   D

Carotid artery pulse tracing

QRS   QRS

P   T U   P   T U

ECG

ARTERIAL PULSE

20-11

medial to the sternomastoid muscle. It is usually not visible, although its diffuse pulsations may be seen in the sternal notch when the person is supine. The **external jugular vein** is more superficial; it lies lateral to the sternomastoid muscle, above the clavicle.

Although an arterial pulse is caused by a forward propulsion of blood, the jugular vein pulse is different. The jugular

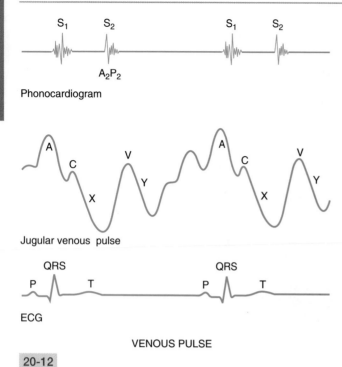

S_1 S_2 S_1 S_2

A_2P_2

Phonocardiogram

A
C
V
Y
X
A
C
V
Y
X

Jugular venous pulse

QRS   QRS
P   T   P   T

ECG

VENOUS PULSE

20-12

vein pulse results from movement of a waveform backward as a result of events upstream. The jugular vein pulse has five components, as shown in Figure 20-12.

The five components of the jugular vein pulse occur because of events in the right side of the heart. The A wave reflects atrial contraction because some blood flows backward to the vena cava during right atrial contraction. The C wave, or ventricular contraction, is backflow from the bulging upward of the tricuspid valve when it closes at the beginning of ventricular systole (not from the neighbouring carotid artery pulsation). Next, the X descent shows atrial relaxation when the right ventricle contracts during systole and pulls the bottom of the atria downward. The V wave occurs with passive atrial filling because of the increasing volume in the right atria and increased pressure. The Y descent reflects passive ventricular filling when the tricuspid valve opens and blood flows from the right atrium to the right ventricle.

✦ DEVELOPMENTAL CONSIDERATIONS

Infants and Children

The fetal heart functions early; it begins to beat at the end of 3 weeks' gestation. The lungs are nonfunctional, but the fetal circulation compensates for this (Figure 20-13). Oxygenation takes place at the placenta, and the arterial blood is returned to the right side of the heart. There is no point in pumping all this freshly oxygenated blood through the lungs; it is therefore rerouted in two ways. First, about two thirds of it is shunted through an opening in the atrial septum, the **foramen ovale,** into the left side of the heart, where it is pumped out through the aorta. Second, the rest of the oxygenated blood

is pumped by the right side of the heart out through the pulmonary artery, but it is detoured through the **ductus arteriosus** to the aorta. Because they are both pumping into the systemic circulation, the right and left ventricles are equal in weight and muscle wall thickness.

Inflation and aeration of the lungs at birth produces circulatory changes. The blood is oxygenated through the lungs rather than through the placenta. The foramen ovale closes within the first hour after birth because of the new lower pressure in the right side of the heart than in the left side. The ductus arteriosus closes later, usually within 10 to 15 hours of birth. The left ventricle has the greater workload of pumping into the systemic circulation, so that when the baby has reached 1 year of age, the left ventricle's mass increases to reach the adult proportion; the ratio of the left ventricle to the right ventricle is 2:1.

The heart's position in the chest is more horizontal in the infant than in the adult; thus the apex is higher, located at the fourth left intercostal space (Figure 20-14). It reaches the adult position by 7 years of age.

Pregnant Women

Blood volume increases by 30% to 40% during pregnancy; the expansion is most rapid during the second trimester. This expansion causes an increase in stroke volume and cardiac output and an increase in pulse rate by 10 to 15 beats per minute. Despite the increase in cardiac output, arterial blood pressure decreases in pregnancy as a result of peripheral vasodilation. The blood pressure drops to its lowest point during the second trimester and then rises. The blood pressure varies with the person's position.

Older Adults

It is difficult to isolate the "aging process" of the cardiovascular system per se because it is so closely interrelated with lifestyle, habits, and diseases. Lifestyle is known to be a modifying factor in the development of cardiovascular disease (CVD); smoking, diet, alcohol use, exercise patterns, and stress have an influence on the development of coronary artery disease (CAD). Lifestyle also affects the aging process; cardiac changes once thought to be caused by aging result partially from the increasingly sedentary lifestyle accompanying aging (Figure 20-15). What is left to be attributed to the aging process alone?

Hemodynamic Changes With Aging

- With aging, systolic blood pressure increases as a result of stiffening of the large arteries, which, in turn, is caused by calcification of vessel walls (arteriosclerosis). This stiffening creates an increase in pulse wave velocity because the less compliant arteries cannot store the volume ejected.
- The overall size of the heart does not increase with age, but left ventricular wall thickness increases. This is an adaptive mechanism to accommodate the vascular stiffening mentioned earlier that creates an increased workload on the heart.

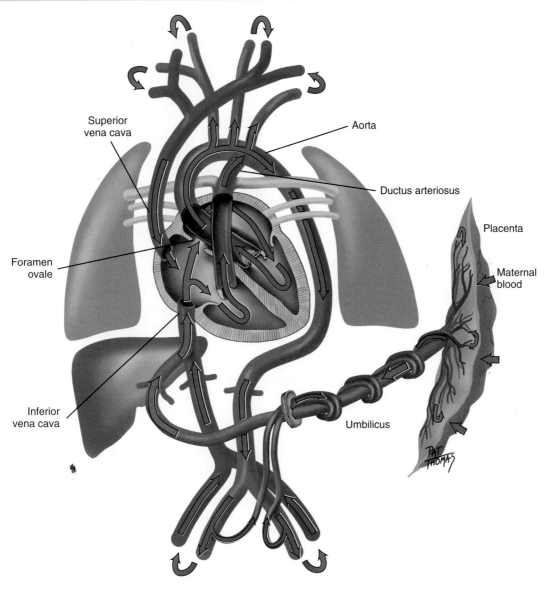

Superior
vena cava

Aorta

Ductus arteriosus

Placenta

Foramen
ovale

Maternal
blood

Inferior
vena cava

Umbilicus

FETAL CIRCULATION

20-13

- No significant change in diastolic pressure occurs with age. A rising systolic pressure with a relatively constant diastolic pressure increases the pulse pressure (the difference between the two).
- No change in resting heart rate occurs with aging.
- Cardiac output at rest is not changed with aging.
- The ability of the heart to augment cardiac output with exercise is decreased. This is shown by a decrease in maximum heart rate with exercise and a diminishing of sympathetic response.

Noncardiac factors also cause a decrease in maximum work performance with aging: decrease in skeletal muscle performance, increase in muscle fatigue, increased sense of dyspnea. Persistent exercise conditioning modifies many of the aging changes in cardiovascular function (Zipes, Libby, Bonow, & Braunwald, 2005).

Arrhythmias. The presence of supraventricular and ventricular arrhythmias increases with age. Ectopic beats are common in older adults; although these are usually asymptomatic in healthy older people, they may compromise cardiac output and blood pressure when disease is present.

Tachyarrhythmias may not be tolerated as well by older people. The myocardium is thicker and less compliant, and early diastolic filling is impaired at rest. Thus a tachycardia is not tolerated as well because of shortened diastole. Also, tachyarrhythmias may further compromise a vital organ whose function has already been affected by aging or disease. For example, a ventricular tachycardia produces a 40% to 70% decrease in cerebral blood flow. Although a younger person may tolerate this, an older person with cerebrovascular disease may experience syncope (Libby, Bonow, Mann, & Zipes, 2008).

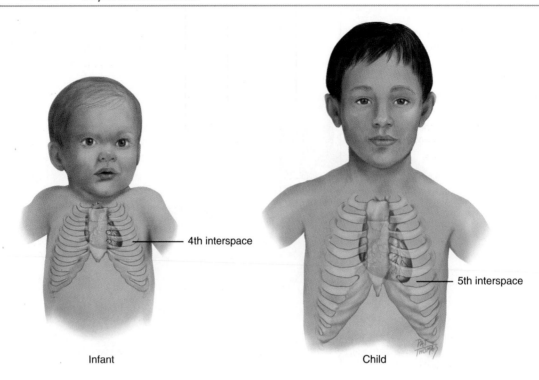

4th interspace

5th interspace

Infant

Child

HEART'S POSITION IN THE CHEST

20-14

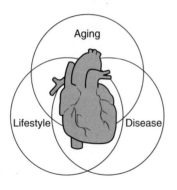

Aging

Lifestyle

Disease

20-15

Electrocardiography. Age-related changes in the ECG occur as a result of histological changes in the conduction system:

- Prolonged P–R interval (first-degree AV block) and prolonged Q–T interval, but no change in the QRS complex
- Left axis deviation from mild age-related hypertrophy of the left ventricle and fibrosis in the left bundle branch
- Increased incidence of bundle branch block

Although the hemodynamic changes associated with aging alone do not seem severe or portentous, the fact remains that the incidence of CVD increases with age. The incidence of CAD increases sharply with advancing age, and this disease accounts for about half the deaths of older people. The incidence of hypertension (systolic, >140 mm Hg; diastolic, >90 mm Hg) and heart failure also increases, with age.

Lifestyle habits (smoking, chronic alcohol use, lack of exercise, poor diet) certainly play a significant role in the acquisition of heart disease. Also, increasing the physical activity of older adults—even at a moderate level—is associated with a reduction in risk of death from CVD and respiratory illnesses. Both points underscore the need for health education as an important treatment parameter.

CULTURAL AND SOCIAL CONSIDERATIONS

In Canada the prevalence of death from CVD is sharply decreasing on an annual basis, and yet the incidence of CVD itself continues to increase. Better medications, early intervention, and public health awareness are some of the factors contributing to the reduction in deaths. According to Statistics Canada (2010), men and women in Canada have almost equal rates of death from CVD, a trend noted since 2000. Interestingly, as CVD death rates have diminished (29%), rates of death from cancer have increased (29.6%), and so cancer is the number one killer of Canadians in all provinces for the first time. Of interest, however, is that CVD remains the primary killer of Canadian women. The prevalence of heart disease and stroke is higher among adults of African descent than in any other ethnic group. These differences in prevalence show the crucial need to improve early detection, screening, and treatment.

Socioeconomic factors also influence the incidence of CVD in Canadians. Concerns about food security continue to be in the forefront of arguments for action to diminish heart disease. *Food security* is defined as economic and physical access by all people to sufficient, safe, and nutritious food necessary to meet both their dietary needs and their food preferences to lead an active, healthy life (this was discussed in Chapter 12). A lack of food security as a result of economic or geographic barriers, as in most northern communities, is a significant determinant of health and an important heart health issue for many Canadians (Heart and Stroke Foundation, 2009). Income and employment, access to resources, and extended health care plans also influence the ability to support a heart-healthy lifestyle. The major risk factors for heart disease and stroke are high blood pressure, smoking, high cholesterol levels, obesity, physical inactivity, and diabetes. In addition, for some women, the use of oral contraceptives and the presence of postmenopausal hormones are risk factors.

High Blood Pressure. In 2010, nearly 5 million Canadians (17.1%) aged 20 years and older had received a diagnosis of **hypertension.** These rates are lower than the self-reported numbers noted in 2010 by the Canadian Health Survey (19.4%). This discrepancy could reflect the number of Canadians self-managing their hypertension without pharmaceutical intervention. Age-specific prevalence rates are similar between men and women younger than 50, although the prevalence increases among women after the age of 55. The Atlantic provinces have the highest prevalence of hypertension in the nation; the western and the northern provinces (Yukon, British Columbia, and Northwest Territories) have the lowest rates (Statistics Canada, 2011).

Smoking. The Canadian Tobacco Use Monitoring Survey revealed an 8% decline in the overall prevalence of smoking in Canada from 1999 to 2010 (Health Canada, 2011). An estimated 4.7 million Canadians, or 17% of the population aged 15 and older, reported smoking daily or occasionally in 2010. The national smoking cessation strategy discussed in Chapter 19 highlights the country's desire to manage this contributing factor. Smoking cessations programs are available at public health units.

Serum Cholesterol. During childhood (ages 4 to 19), children and adolescents of African descent have higher levels of total cholesterol, low-density lipoprotein cholesterol (the "bad" cholesterol), and high-density lipoprotein cholesterol (the "good" cholesterol) than do children and adolescents of Euro-Canadian descent. These differences reverse during adulthood, so that individuals of African descent have lower serum cholesterol levels than do those of Euro-Canadian descent.

Obesity. *Overweight* is defined by a body mass index (BMI) of 25 to 29.9 kg/m² and *obesity* by a BMI of 30 kg/m²

or higher. These problems have reached epidemic proportions in Canada. Among Canadian men, the prevalence of obesity, at 24.3%, is only slightly higher than that among women, at 23.9%. Since 2000, the percentage of obesity rates has increased by 10% in Canada. Overweight and obesity among children are of national concern; 25% of girls and 29% of boys between the ages of 2 and 17 years weigh in above the national average BMI. There is significant evidence that obesity is at least partly genetic. Certain ethnic groups are more vulnerable to obesity and obesity-related disorders. Genome-wide association studies show that some genes are associated with a higher BMI. However, genes are not the whole story: The significant change in obesity rates since the 1990s is evidence against genetic drift and in favour of strong environmental influences interacting with existing genes.

Children are particularly vulnerable to their environment because they have less ability to shape it. Children's eating habits and physical activity patterns tend to be similar to those of their parents, which is one environmental reason why obesity and obesity-related disorders often run in families. There is growing evidence that the environment in the womb helps to "program" a child's metabolism. Exposure to gestational diabetes or maternal obesity, high birth weight, and intrauterine growth retardation with rapid catch-up growth are all associated with obesity later on. In contrast, breastfeeding in infancy may reduce the risk of obesity, as may other health practices, such as getting enough sleep, and eating only in response to appetite cues.

Diabetes. More than 9 million Canadians live with diabetes or are prediabetic. It is estimated that the prevalence will increase significantly by 2025, in part because the population is aging, obesity rates are rising, Canadian lifestyles are increasingly sedentary, and nearly 80% of all new Canadians belong to Hispanic, Asian, South Asian, and African populations, which are at increased risk of developing type 2 diabetes. The personal cost of diabetes may include a reduced quality of life and an increased likelihood of complications, such as heart disease, stroke, kidney disease, blindness, need for amputation, and erectile dysfunction. Approximately 80% of people with diabetes die as a result of heart disease or stroke. Medical costs for individuals with diabetes are two to three times higher than those for individuals without the disease. By 2020, it is estimated that diabetes will cost the Canadian health care system $16.9 billion (Canadian Diabetes Association, 2011).

SUBJECTIVE DATA

1. Chest pain
2. Dyspnea
3. Orthopnea
4. Cough
5. Fatigue
6. Cyanosis or pallor
7. Edema
8. Nocturia
9. Past cardiac history
10. Family cardiac history
11. Personal habits (cardiac risk factors)

HEALTH HISTORY QUESTIONS

Examiner Asks	Rationale
1. Chest pain. Any *chest pain* or tightness?	Angina, an important cardiac symptom, occurs when heart's vascular supply cannot keep up with metabolic demand. Chest pain also may be of pulmonary, musculoskeletal, or gastrointestinal origin; it is important to differentiate.
• Onset: When did it start? How long have you had it *this* time? Have you had this type of pain before? How often?	
• Location: Where did the pain start? Does the pain radiate to any other spot?	
• Character: How would you describe it: crushing, stabbing, burning, vise-like? (Allow the patient to offer adjectives before you suggest them. Note whether the patient uses a clenched fist to describe pain.)	A squeezing "clenched fist" sign is characteristic of angina, but the symptoms listed as follows may be anginal equivalents in the absence of chest pain.
• Is the pain brought on by activity (what type), rest, emotional upset, eating, sexual intercourse, or cold weather?	
• Do you have any associated symptoms: sweating, ashen grey or pale skin, heart skipping a beat, shortness of breath, nausea or vomiting, heart racing?	Diaphoresis, cold sweats, pallor, greyness Palpitations, dyspnea, nausea, tachycardia, fatigue
• Is the pain made worse by moving the arms or neck, by breathing, or by lying flat?	Try to differentiate pain of cardiac versus noncardiac origin.
• Is the pain relieved by rest or nitroglycerine? How many sprays?	
2. Dyspnea. Any shortness of breath?	**Dyspnea** on exertion (DOE): quantify exactly (e.g., DOE after walking two level blocks)
• What type of activity, and how much, brings on shortness of breath? How much activity brought it on 6 months ago?	
• Onset: Does the shortness of breath come on unexpectedly?	Paroxysmal dyspnea
• Duration: constant or does it come and go?	Constant or intermittent dyspnea
• Seem to be affected by position: lying down?	Recumbent dyspnea
• Awaken you from sleep at night?	Paroxysmal nocturnal dyspnea occurs with heart failure. Lying down increases volume of intrathoracic blood, and the weakened heart cannot accommodate the increased load. Affected patients classically awaken after 2 hours of sleep with the perception of needing fresh air.
• Does the shortness of breath interfere with activities of daily living?	
3. Orthopnea. How many pillows do you use when sleeping or lying down?	*Orthopnea* is the need to assume a more upright position to breathe. Note the exact number of pillows used.
4. Cough. Do you have a **cough?**	
• Duration: How long have you had it?	Sputum production, mucoid or purulent
• Frequency: Is it related to time of day?	
• Type: Is it dry, hacking, barky, hoarse, or productive?	
• Do you cough up mucus? What colour is it? Any odour? Blood-tinged (hemoptysis)?	Hemoptysis is often a pulmonary disorder but also occurs with mitral stenosis.
• Is the cough associated with activity, position (lying down), anxiety, talking?	
• Does activity make it better or worse (sit, walk, exercise)?	
• Is it relieved by rest or medication?	
5. Fatigue. Do you seem to tire easily? Are you able to keep up with your family and coworkers?	
• Onset: When did fatigue start? Was it sudden or gradual? Has any *recent* change occurred in energy level?	Fatigue from decreased cardiac output is worse in the evening, whereas fatigue from anxiety or depression is present all day or is worse in the morning.
• Is fatigue related to time of day: all day, morning, evening?	

Subjective Data

Examiner Asks	Rationale
6. Cyanosis or pallor. Ever noted your facial skin turn blue or ashen?	**Cyanosis** or **pallor** occurs with myocardial infarction or low cardiac output states as a result of decreased tissue perfusion.
7. Edema. Any swelling of your feet and legs? • Onset: When did you first notice this? • Any recent change? • What time of day does the swelling occur? Do your shoes feel tight at the end of day? • How much swelling would you say there is? Are both legs equally swollen? • Does the swelling go away with rest, with elevation, or after a night's sleep? • Do you have any associated symptoms, such as shortness of breath? If so, does the shortness of breath occur before leg swelling or after?	**Edema** is dependent when caused by heart failure. Cardiac edema is worse at evening and better in morning after legs are elevated all night. Cardiac edema is bilateral; unilateral swelling has a local vein cause.
8. Nocturia. Do you awaken at night with an urgent need to urinate? How long has this been occurring? Any recent change?	Recumbency at night promotes fluid reabsorption and excretion; **nocturia** occurs with heart failure in patients who are ambulatory during the day.
9. Cardiac history. Do you have any history of hypertension, elevated cholesterol or triglyceride levels, heart murmur, congenital heart disease, rheumatic fever or unexplained joint pains in childhood or youth, recurrent tonsillitis, anemia, or diabetes? • Ever had heart disease? When was this? Was it treated by medication or heart surgery? • Have you ever had a heart attack? If so, when, and what treatment or intervention did you receive? (See the box Promoting Health: Women and Heart Attack.) • When was your most recent ECG, stress ECG, serum cholesterol measurement, or other heart tests?	
10. Family cardiac history. Any family history of hypertension, obesity, diabetes, CAD, sudden death at a young age?	
11. Personal habits (cardiac risk factors) • Nutrition: Please describe your usual daily diet. (Note whether this diet is representative of the basic food groups, and note the amount of calories, cholesterol, and any additives such as salt.) What is your usual weight? Has your weight changed recently? • Smoking: Do you smoke cigarettes or other tobacco? At what age did you start? How many packs per day? For how many years have you smoked this amount? Have you ever tried to quit? If so, how did this go? • Alcohol: How much alcohol do you usually drink each week or each day? When was your most recent drink? What was the number of drinks that episode? Have you ever been told you had a drinking problem? • Exercise: What is your usual amount of exercise each day or week? How many minutes per day do you exercise? What type of exercise (state type or sport)? If a sport, what is your usual amount (light, moderate, heavy)? • Drugs: Do you take any antihypertensives, β-blockers, calcium channel blockers, digoxin, diuretics, aspirin and anticoagulants, over-the-counter drugs, or street drugs? • Do you take any nutritional supplements? • Do you use any street drugs? Marijuana? • Stress: Tell me about stress in your life. What are the main causes? How do you manage it? How does it affect you?	**Risk factors for CAD:** Collect data regarding elevated cholesterol level, elevated blood pressure, random plasma glucose level value in excess of 11.1 mmol/L or known diabetes mellitus, obesity, cigarette smoking, low activity level, and, for postmenopausal women, length of any hormone replacement therapy.

Subjective Data

Subjective Data

PROMOTING HEALTH: WOMEN AND HEART ATTACK

The Heart Truth: Women and Heart Attacks

When someone complains of chest pain or pain radiating down the left arm, the person almost always thinks "heart attack." After all, these are the typical symptoms, correct? Well, yes and no. In the past it was believed that women experienced different warning signs than men. The Heart and Stroke Foundation (2009) notes that this may not actually be the case. Both women and men may experience typical or atypical symptoms, such as nausea; sweating; pain in the arm, throat, or jaw; or pain that is unusual. However, women may describe their pain differently than men. Nevertheless, the most common symptom in women is still chest pain.

Many of the symptoms that women experience are easily attributable to something else, other than the heart, and are therefore often ignored. According to the Women's Heart Foundation (2013) almost one third of affected women experience little to no chest pain at all when having a heart attack. In fact, 71% reported flu-like symptoms, including extreme fatigue, for up to a month before the attack. Women are more likely to feel hot or cold burning sensations or a tenderness to touch on their back, shoulder, arms, or jaw—not sharp pain. Other symptoms include nausea, vomiting, indigestion, and shortness of breath, which are easily attributed to other conditions. Scientific evidence now shows that women tend to minimize the significance of the symptoms of cardiac disease. However, the reason for this may be a lack of awareness.

Heart disease is the leading cause of death in women older than 55 years. Women tend to be safeguarded from heart disease before menopause because of the protective effect of naturally occurring estrogen, but not always. For example, in premenopausal women with diabetes, the risk is similar to that of men of the same age because diabetes cancels out the protective effect that estrogen provides to premenopausal women.

Some factors directly influence a woman's risk of cardiovascular disease. During a woman's reproductive life cycle, from approximately ages 12 to 50, the naturally occurring estrogen provides a protective effect on women's cardiovascular health. However, estrogen's protective effect can change, depending on a variety of factors and conditions.

Oral contraceptives are much safer now than the forms used in the past. In women younger than 35 who do not smoke, contraceptive use generally does not increase the risk of stroke. However, in a small proportion of women, oral contraceptives increase the risk of high blood pressure and blood clots. The risk increases if the woman smokes or already has high blood pressure or other risk factors for heart disease or stroke.

During the menopausal transition, which occurs around age 51, a woman's risk for heart disease and stroke increases. During this period, the ovaries slowly decrease the production of the hormone estrogen, which, as previously mentioned, has a protective effect on the heart. A menopausal woman may experience an increase in LDL ("bad") cholesterol and triglyceride levels and a decrease in HDL ("good") cholesterol. She may also develop a tendency toward higher blood pressure. Reduced estrogen levels may also increase body fat above the waist, have harmful effects on the way blood clots, and affect the way the body metabolizes sugar, a precursor condition to diabetes.

Until the 2000s, it was thought that hormone replacement therapy (HRT) could help reduce the risk of cardiac disease in menopausal women. However, studies have shown that taking certain types of hormones (estrogen with progestin) can actually increase the risk of heart attack, stroke, blood clots, and breast cancer for some women. As a result of these studies, HRT is no longer recommended for the prevention of heart disease, although it may be helpful for some women in treating other symptoms of menopause, such as hot flashes. Women should always consult their physician for recommendations regarding HRT.

Naturally occurring estrogen also helps to keep cholesterol levels in a healthy range. Overall, however, 40% of Canadian women between the ages of 18 and 74 have cholesterol levels that are too high. After menopause, as estrogen levels drop, the incidence of high cholesterol increases. A health care provider should be consulted about how often cholesterol levels should be checked.

Exercise and weight control are paramount for mitigating the risk of heart disease. Inactive women have twice the risk of developing heart disease than do active women. Thirty minutes of physical activity, four to six times a week, helps to keep the heart strong and prevent heart disease. Even losing a small amount of extra weight can also help reduce the risk.

The Heart Truth is a national public health education campaign to raise awareness that heart disease and stroke is the most common killer of women in Canada. The Heart and Stroke Foundation of Canada adopted this U.S.-based initiative in 2008 because of its overwhelming success. The Heart Truth campaign introduced the *Red Dress* as the national symbol for women and heart disease awareness. Since its introduction, many women have taken ownership of the symbol. Each year, the Red Dress is featured on runways as top Canadian fashion designers create original red dress creations, modelled by some of Canada's most celebrated women.

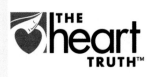 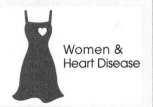

For more information about women and heart disease, consult the following Web sites:

- Women with Heart Disease: Living a Good Life. *http://www.phac-aspc.gc.ca/cd-mc/cvd-mcv/women-femmes_04-eng.php*
- Heart and Stroke Foundation of Canada: *http://www.heartandstroke.ca*
- Women's Heart Foundation. (2013). Women and Heart Disease Facts. Retrieved from *http://www.womensheart.org/content/HeartDisease/heart_disease_facts.asp*

HDL, high-density lipoprotein; *LDL,* low-density lipoprotein.

Examiner Asks	Rationale

Additional History for Infants

1. **Maternal health.** How was the mother's health during pregnancy: any unexplained fever, rubella during first trimester, other infection, hypertension, drugs taken?

2. **Feeding.** Have you noted any cyanosis while the baby is nursing or crying? Is the baby able to eat, nurse, or finish bottle without tiring?

To screen for heart disease in an infant, note fatigue during feeding. Infants with heart failure take fewer ounces each feeding; become dyspneic with sucking; may be diaphoretic and then fall into exhausted sleep; and awaken after a short time hungry again.

3. **Growth.** Has the baby grown as expected by growth charts and about the same as siblings or peers?

Poor weight gain

4. **Activity.** Were the baby's motor milestones achieved as expected? Is the baby able to play without tiring? How many naps does the baby take each day? How long does a nap last?

Additional History for Children

1. **Growth.** Has the child grown as expected by growth charts?

Poor weight gain

2. **Activity.** Is the child able to keep up with siblings or age mates? Is the child willing or reluctant to go out to play? Is the child able to climb stairs, ride a bike, walk a few blocks? Does the child squat to rest during play or to watch television, or assume a knee-chest position while sleeping? Have you noted "blue spells" during exercise?

Fatigue: Record specific limitations.
Cyanosis

3. **Joint pain and fever.** Has the child had any unexplained joint pains or unexplained fever?

4. **Headache and nosebleed.** Does the child have frequent headaches or nosebleeds?

5. **Respiratory disease.** Does the child have frequent respiratory infections? How many per year? How are they treated? Have any of these proved to be streptococcal infections?

6. **Family history.** Does the child have a sibling with heart defect? Is anyone in the child's family known to have chromosomal abnormalities, such as Down's syndrome?

Additional History for Pregnant Women

1. **Hypertension.** Have you had any high blood pressure during this or earlier pregnancies?
   - What was your usual blood pressure level before pregnancy? How has your blood pressure been monitored during the pregnancy?
   - If you have high blood pressure, what treatment has been started?
   - Any associated symptoms: weight gain; protein in urine; swelling in feet, legs, or face?

2. **Hypotension.** Have you had any faintness or dizziness with this pregnancy?

Additional History for Older Adults

1. **Disease.** Do you have any known heart or lung disease: hypertension, CAD, chronic emphysema, or bronchitis?
   - What efforts to treat this have been started?
   - Have your usual symptoms changed recently? Does your illness interfere with activities of daily living?

2. **Medication.** Do you take any medications for your heart, such as water pills, blood pressure pills, or heart pills? Are you aware of side effects? Have you recently stopped taking your medication? Why?

Noncompliance with a treatment regimen may be related to side effects or lack of finances.

3. **Environment.** Does your home have any stairs? How often do you need to climb them? Does this have any effect on activities of daily living?

OBJECTIVE DATA

PREPARATION

To evaluate the carotid arteries, the patient can be sitting up. To assess the jugular veins and the precordium, the patient should be supine with the head and chest slightly elevated.

Stand on the patient's right side; this will facilitate your hand placement and auscultation of the precordium.

The room must be warm; chilling makes the patient uncomfortable, and shivering interferes with heart sounds. Take scrupulous care to ensure *quiet*; heart sounds are very soft, and any ambient room noise masks them.

Ensure privacy by keeping the chest draped. A woman's left breast overrides part of the area you need to examine. Gently displace the breast upward, or ask the woman to hold it out of the way.

Perform a regional cardiovascular assessment in this order:
1. Pulse and blood pressure (see Chapter 10)
2. Extremities (see Chapter 21)
3. Neck vessels
4. Precordium

The logic of this order is that you will begin observations peripherally and move in toward the heart. For choreography of these steps in the complete physical examination, see Chapter 28.

EQUIPMENT NEEDED
Marking pen
Small centimetre ruler
Stethoscope with diaphragm and bell end pieces
Alcohol wipe (to clean end piece)

Normal Range of Findings	Abnormal Findings

THE NECK VESSELS

Auscultate the Carotid Artery

For middle-aged or older patients or patient who show symptoms or signs of CVD, auscultate each carotid artery for the presence of a **bruit** (pronounced *bru'-ee;* Figure 20-16). This is a blowing, swishing sound indicating blood flow turbulence; normally none is present.

Keep the neck in a neutral position. Lightly apply the bell of the stethoscope over the carotid artery at three levels: (1) the angle of the jaw, (2) the midcervical area, and (3) the base of the neck (see Figure 20-16). Avoid compressing the artery because this could create an artificial bruit, and it could compromise circulation if the carotid artery is already narrowed by atherosclerosis. Ask the patient to take a breath, exhale, and hold still briefly without breathing while you listen so that tracheal breath sounds do not mask or mimic a carotid artery bruit. (Holding the breath on inhalation will also tense the levator scapulae muscles, which makes it hard to hear the carotid arteries.) Sometimes you can hear normal heart sounds transmitted to the neck; do not confuse these with a bruit.

A bruit indicates turbulence with a local vascular cause, such as atherosclerotic narrowing.

A carotid bruit is audible when the lumen is half to two-thirds occluded. Bruit loudness increases as the atherosclerosis worsens until the lumen is two-thirds occluded. After that, bruit loudness decreases. When the lumen is completely occluded, the bruit disappears. Thus absence of a bruit does not ensure absence of a carotid lesion.

A murmur sounds much the same but is caused by a cardiac disorder. Some aortic valve murmurs (aortic stenosis) radiate to the neck and must be distinguished from a local bruit.

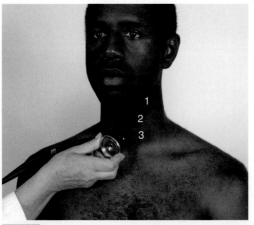

20-16

Normal Range of Findings	Abnormal Findings

Palpate the Carotid Artery

Located central to the heart, the carotid artery yields important information about cardiac function.

Palpate each carotid artery medial to the sternomastoid muscle in the neck (Figure 20-17). Avoid excessive pressure on the carotid sinus area higher in the neck; excessive vagal stimulation here could slow down the heart rate, especially in older adults. Take care to palpate gently. To avoid compromising arterial blood flow to the brain, palpate only one carotid artery at a time.

Carotid sinus hypersensitivity is the condition in which pressure over the carotid sinus leads to a decrease in heart rate, a decrease in blood pressure, and cerebral ischemia with syncope. This may occur in older adults with hypertension or occlusion of the carotid artery

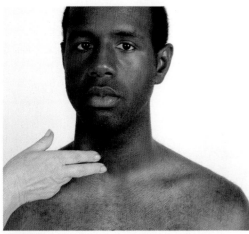

20-17

Feel the contour and amplitude of the pulse. Normally the contour is smooth with a rapid upstroke and slower downstroke, and the normal strength is 2+ or moderate (see Chapter 21). The findings should be the same bilaterally.

Diminished pulse feels small and weak (decreased stroke volume).

Increased pulse feels full and strong (hyperkinetic states; see Table 21-2, p. 541).

Estimate the Jugular Venous Pressure

Think of the jugular veins as a **central venous pressure** (CVP) manometer attached directly to the right atrium. You can "read" the CVP at the highest level of pulsations (Figure 20-18). Use the angle of Louis (sternal angle) as an arbitrary reference point, and compare it with the highest level of venous pulsation.

Hold a vertical ruler on the sternal angle. Align a straight edge on the ruler like a T-square, and adjust the level of the horizontal straight edge to the level of pulsation. Read the level of intersection on the vertical ruler; normal jugular venous pulsation is 2 cm or less above the sternal angle. Also state the patient's position: for example, "internal jugular vein pulsations 3 cm above sternal angle when elevated 30 degrees."

Elevated pressure is a level of pulsation that is more than 3 cm above the sternal angle while at 45 degrees. This occurs with heart failure.

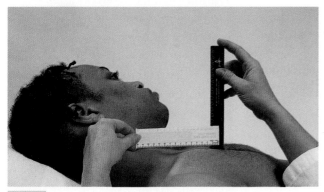

20-18

Normal Range of Findings	Abnormal Findings

If you cannot find the internal jugular veins, use the external jugular veins and note the point where they look collapsed. Be aware that the technique of estimating venous pressure is difficult and is not always a reliable predictor of CVP. Consistency in grading among examiners is difficult to achieve.

If venous pressure is elevated, or if you suspect heart failure, perform **hepatojugular reflux** (Figure 20-19). Position the patient comfortably supine and instruct him or her to breathe quietly through an open mouth. Hold your right hand on the right upper quadrant of the patient's abdomen just below the rib cage. Watch the level of jugular pulsation as you push in with your hand. Exert firm sustained pressure for 30 seconds. This empties venous blood out of the liver sinusoids and adds its volume to the venous system. If the heart is able to pump this additional volume (i.e., if CVP is not elevated), the jugular veins will rise for a few seconds and then recede back to the previous level.

If heart failure is present, the jugular veins will stay elevated as long as you push.

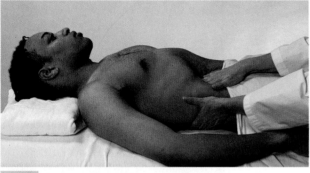

20-19   Hepatojugular reflux.

THE PRECORDIUM

Inspect the Anterior Chest

Arrange tangential lighting to accentuate any flicker of movement.

Pulsations. You may or may not see the **apical impulse,** the pulsation created as the left ventricle rotates against the chest wall during systole. When visible, it appears at the level of the fourth or fifth intercostal space, at or inside the midclavicular line. It is easier to see in children and in patients with thin chest walls.

A **heave** or **lift** is a sustained forceful thrusting of the ventricle during systole. It occurs with ventricular hypertrophy as a result of increased workload. A right ventricular heave is seen at the sternal border; a left ventricular heave is seen at the apex (see Table 20-8, p. 512).

Palpate the Apical Impulse

(This used to be called the *point of maximal impulse.* Because some abnormal conditions may cause a maximal impulse to be felt elsewhere on the chest, use the term *apical impulse* specifically for the apex beat.)

Localize the apical impulse precisely by using one finger pad (Figure 20-20, *A*). Asking the patient to "exhale and then hold it" aids the examiner in locating the pulsation. You may need to roll the patient midway to the left to find it; note that this also displaces the apical impulse farther to the left (see Figure 20-20, *B*).

Objective Data

Normal Range of Findings	**Abnormal Findings**

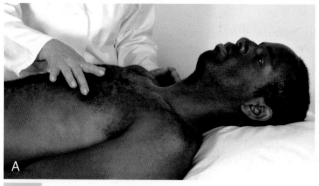
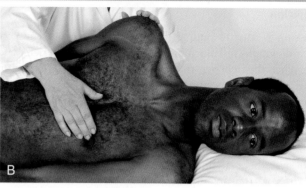

20-20   Checking the apical impulse. **A,** With the patient supine. **B,** With the patient rolled laterally.

Note the following characteristics:
- Location: The apical impulse should occupy only one interspace, the fourth or fifth, and be at or medial to the midclavicular line
- Size: Normally 1 × 2 cm
- Amplitude: Normally a short, gentle tap
- Duration: Short; normally occupies only first half of systole

The apical impulse is palpable in about half of adults. It is not palpable in obese patients or in patients with thick chest walls. In states of high cardiac output (anxiety, fever, hyperthyroidism, anemia), the apical impulse increases in amplitude and duration.

Palpate Across the Precordium

Using the palmar aspects of your four fingers, gently palpate over the apex, the left sternal border, and the base, searching for any other pulsations (Figure 20-21). Normally none are felt. If any are felt, note the timing. Use the carotid artery pulsation as a guide, or auscultate as you palpate.

Cardiac enlargement is characterized as follows:
- Left ventricular dilatation (volume overload) displaces impulse down and to left and increases size more than one space.
- Increased force and duration but no change in location occurs with left ventricular hypertrophy and no dilatation (pressure overload; see Table 20-8, p. 513).

Cardiac enlargement is not palpable with pulmonary emphysema because of the overriding lungs.

A **thrill** is a palpable vibration. It feels like the throat of a purring cat. The thrill signifies turbulent blood flow and accompanies loud murmurs. Absence of a thrill, however, does not necessarily rule out the presence of a murmur.

Accentuated first and second heart sounds and extra heart sounds also may cause abnormal pulsations.

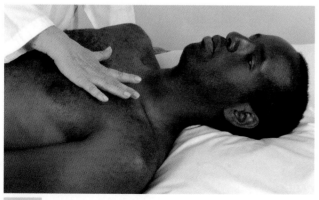

20-21

Objective Data

Normal Range of Findings	**Abnormal Findings**

Percussion

Percussion is used to outline the heart's borders, but chest radiography and echocardiography are much more accurate methods of detecting heart enlargement. When the right ventricle enlarges, it does so in the anteroposterior diameter, which is better seen on radiographs. Evidence from numerous comparison studies shows the cardiac border defined by percussion is correlated "only moderately" with the true cardiac border (McGee, 2007). Also, percussion is of limited usefulness with the female breast tissue, in an obese patient, and in a patient with a muscular chest wall.

However, there are times when your percussing hands are the only tools you have with you, as in an outpatient setting, an extended-care facility, or a patient's home. When you need to search for cardiac enlargement, place your stationary finger over the patient's fifth intercostal space on the left side of the chest near the anterior axillary line. Slide your stationary hand toward yourself, percussing as you go, and note the change of sound from resonance (over the lung) to dull (over the heart). Normally, the left border of cardiac dullness is at the midclavicular line in the fifth interspace and slopes in toward the sternum as you progress upward, so that by the second interspace the border of dullness coincides with the left sternal border. The right border of dullness normally matches the sternal border.

Auscultation

Identify the auscultatory areas where you will listen. These include the four traditional valve "areas" (Figure 20-22). The valve areas are not over the actual anatomical locations of the valves but are the sites on the chest wall where sounds produced by the valves are best heard. The sound radiates with the direction of blood flow. The valve areas are as follows:

- Second right interspace: aortic valve area
- Second left interspace: pulmonic valve area
- Fifth intercostal space at left lower sternal border: tricuspid valve area
- Fifth interspace at approximately left midclavicular line: mitral valve area

Abnormal Findings

Cardiac enlargement is caused by increased ventricular volume or wall thickness; it occurs with hypertension, CAD, heart failure, and cardiomyopathy.

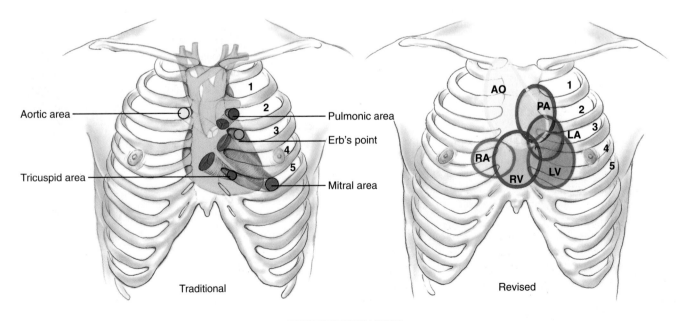

Aortic area — Pulmonic area — Erb's point — Tricuspid area — Mitral area

Traditional

AO — PA — LA — RA — RV — LV

Revised

AUSCULTATORY AREAS

20-22   Auscultatory areas.

Normal Range of Findings	**Abnormal Findings**

Do not limit your auscultation to only four locations. Sounds produced by the valves may be heard all over the precordium. (For this reason, many experts even discourage the naming of the valve areas.) Thus learn to inch your stethoscope in a rough Z pattern, from the base of the heart across and down, then over to the apex. Or start at the apex and work your way up. Include the sites shown in Figure 20-22.

Recall the characteristics of a high-quality stethoscope (see Chapter 9). Clean the earpiece and endpiece with an alcohol wipe; you will use both. Although all heart sounds are low frequency, the diaphragm is for relatively higher pitched sounds, and the bell is for relatively lower pitched ones.

Before you begin, alert the patient: "I always listen to the heart in a number of places on the chest. Just because I am listening a long time, it does not necessarily mean that something is wrong."

After you place the stethoscope, try closing your eyes briefly to tune out any distractions. Concentrate, and listen selectively to *one* sound at a time. Consider that at least two, and perhaps three or four, sounds may be happening in less than 1 second. You cannot process everything at once. Begin with the diaphragm endpiece and use the following routine: (a) Note the rate and rhythm, (b) identify S_1 and S_2, (c) assess S_1 and S_2 separately, (d) listen for extra heart sounds, and (e) listen for murmurs.

Note the Rate and Rhythm. The rate ranges normally from 60 to 100 beats per minute. (Review the full discussion of the pulse in Chapter 10 and the normal rates across age groups.) The rhythm should be regular, although **sinus arrhythmia** occurs normally in young adults and children. With sinus arrhythmia, the rhythm varies with the patient's breathing, increasing at the peak of inspiration and slowing with expiration. Note any other irregular rhythm. If one occurs, check whether it has any pattern or if it is totally irregular.

When you notice any irregularity, check for a pulse deficit by auscultating the apical beat while simultaneously palpating the radial pulse. Count a serial measurement (one after the other) of apical beat and radial pulse. Normally, with every beat you hear at the apex, the pulse should perfuse to the periphery and be palpable. The two counts should be identical. When they are different, subtract the radial rate from the apical rate, and record the remainder as the pulse deficit.

Identify S_1 and S_2. This is important because S_1 is the start of systole and thus serves as the reference point for the timing of all other cardiac sounds. Usually, you can identify S_1 instantly because you hear a pair of sounds close together ("lub-dup"), and S_1 is the first of the pair. This guideline works except in the cases of the tachyarrhythmias (rates >100 per minute). In those cases, the diastolic filling time is shortened, and the beats are too close together to distinguish. Other guidelines to distinguish S_1 from S_2 are as follows:

- S_1 is louder than S_2 at the apex; S_2 is louder than S_1 at the base.
- S_1 coincides with the carotid artery pulse. Feel the carotid pulse gently as you auscultate at the apex; the sound you hear as you feel each pulse is S_1 (Figure 20-23).
- If the patient is on an electrocardiographic monitor, the monitor will show S_1 coinciding with the R wave (the upstroke of the QRS complex).

Listen to S_1 and S_2 Separately. Note whether each heart sound is normal, accentuated, diminished, or split. Inch your diaphragm across the chest as you do this.

Abnormal Findings:

Premature beat: An isolated beat is early, or a pattern occurs in which every third or fourth beat sounds early.

Irregularly irregular: Sounds have no pattern; beats come rapidly and at random intervals.

A **pulse deficit** signals a weak contraction of the ventricles; it occurs with atrial fibrillation, premature beats, and heart failure.

Objective Data

Normal Range of Findings	Abnormal Findings

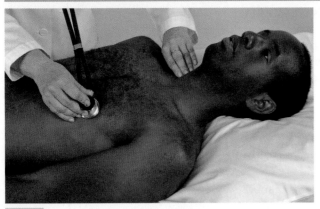

20-23

First Heart Sound (S₁). Caused by closure of the AV valves, S_1 signals the beginning of systole. You can hear it over the entire precordium, although it is loudest at the apex (Figure 20-24). (Sometimes the two sounds are equally loud at the apex because S_1 is lower pitched than S_2.)

You can hear S_1 with the diaphragm of the stethoscope when the patient is in any position and equally well during inspiration and expiration. A split S_1 is normal, but it is rare. A split S_1 means you are hearing the mitral and tricuspid components separately. It is audible in the tricuspid valve area (the left lower sternal border). The split is very rapid, with the two components only 0.03 second apart.

Causes of accentuated or diminished S_1 are listed in Table 20-3 (p. 508).

Both heart sounds are diminished with conditions in which the amount of tissue between the heart and your stethoscope is increased: emphysema (hyperinflated lungs), obesity, pericardial fluid.

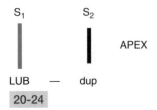

20-24

Second Heart Sound (S₂). The S_2 is associated with closure of the semilunar valves. You can hear it with the diaphragm over the entire precordium, although S_2 is loudest at the base (Figure 20-25).

Accentuated or diminished S_2 is described in Table 20-4 ("Variations in S_2," on p. 508).

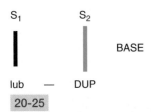

20-25

Splitting of S₂. A split S_2 is a normal phenomenon that occurs toward the end of inspiration in some people. Recall that closure of the aortic and pulmonic valves is nearly synchronous. Because of the effects of respiration on the heart described earlier, inspiration separates the timing of closure of the two valves, and the aortic valve closes 0.06 seconds before the pulmonic valve. Instead of one "DUP," you hear a split sound: "T-DUP" (Figure 20-26). During expiration, synchrony returns, and the aortic and pulmonic components fuse together. A split S_2 is heard only in the pulmonic valve area (the second left interspace).

Normal Range of Findings	Abnormal Findings

SPLITTING OF THE SECOND HEART SOUND

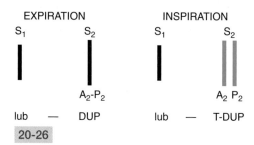

20-26

Listen for Murmurs. A murmur is a blowing, swooshing sound that occurs with turbulent blood flow in the heart or great vessels. Except for the innocent murmurs described in the "Posture" section, murmurs are abnormal. If you hear a murmur, describe it by indicating the following characteristics.

Timing. It is crucial to define the murmur by its occurrence in systole or diastole. You must be able to identify S_1 and S_2 accurately to do this. Try to further describe the murmur as being in early, middle, or late systole or diastole; throughout the cardiac event (termed *pansystolic, holosystolic/pandiastolic,* or *holodiastolic*); and whether it obscures or muffles the heart sounds.

Loudness. Describe the intensity in terms of six "grades." For example, record a grade II murmur as "II/VI."
Grade I: barely audible, heard only in a quiet room and then with difficulty
Grade II: clearly audible, but faint
Grade III: moderately loud, easy to hear
Grade IV: loud, associated with a thrill palpable on the chest wall
Grade V: very loud, heard with one corner of the stethoscope lifted off the chest wall
Grade VI: loudest, still heard with entire stethoscope lifted just off the chest wall

Pitch. Describe the pitch as high, medium, or low. The pitch depends on the pressure and the rate of blood flow producing the murmur.

Pattern. The intensity may follow a pattern during the cardiac phase, growing louder (crescendo), tapering off (decrescendo), or increasing to a peak and then decreasing (crescendo–decrescendo, or diamond-shaped). Because the whole murmur is just milliseconds long, it takes practice to diagnose any pattern.

Quality. Describe the quality as musical, blowing, harsh, or rumbling.

Location. Describe the area of maximum intensity of the murmur (where it is best heard) by noting the valve area or intercostal spaces.

Radiation. The murmur may be transmitted downstream in the direction of blood flow and may be heard in another place on the precordium, on the neck, on the back, or on the axilla.

Posture. Some murmurs disappear or are enhanced by a change in position. Some murmurs are common in healthy children or adolescents and are termed *innocent* or *functional*. **Innocent murmurs** have no valvular or other pathological cause; **functional murmurs** are caused by increased blood flow in the heart (e.g., in anemia, fever, pregnancy, hyperthyroidism). The contractile force of the heart is greater in children. This increases blood flow velocity. Because of the increased velocity and a smaller chest measurement, a murmur is audible.

Although it is important to distinguish innocent murmurs from pathological ones, it is best to suspect all murmurs as pathological until they are proved otherwise. Diagnostic tests such as electrocardiography, phonocardiography, and echocardiography are needed to establish an accurate diagnosis.

Abnormal Findings

Murmurs may be caused by congenital defects and acquired valvular defects. Study Tables 20-9 and 20-10, pp. 513 and 515, for a complete description.

A systolic murmur may occur with a normal heart or with heart disease; a diastolic murmur always indicates heart disease.

The murmur of mitral stenosis is rumbling, whereas that of aortic stenosis is harsh (see Table 20-10, p. 516).

The innocent murmur is generally soft (grade II), midsystolic, short, crescendo–decrescendo, and with a vibratory or musical quality (like fiddle strings). Also, the innocent murmur is heard at the second or third left intercostal space and disappears with sitting, and the young person has no associated signs of cardiac dysfunction.

Objective Data

Normal Range of Findings	Abnormal Findings

Change Position. After auscultating in the supine position, roll the patient toward his or her left side. Listen with the bell at the apex for the presence of any diastolic filling sounds (i.e., the S_3 or S_4; Figure 20-27).

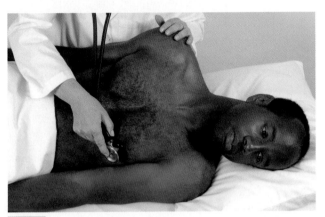

20-27

Ask the patient to sit up, lean forward slightly, and exhale. Listen with the diaphragm firmly pressed at the base, right, and left sides. Check for the soft, high-pitched, early diastolic murmur of aortic or pulmonic regurgitation (Figure 20-28).

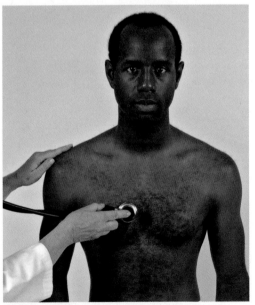

20-28

 DEVELOPMENTAL CONSIDERATIONS

Infants

The transition from fetal to pulmonic circulation occurs in the immediate neonatal period. Fetal shunts normally close within 10 to 15 hours after birth but may take up to 48 hours. Thus you should assess the cardiovascular system during the first 24 hours and again in 2 to 3 days.

S_3 and S_4, and the murmur of mitral stenosis are sometimes heard only when on the left side.

Murmur of aortic regurgitation sometimes may be heard only when the patient is leaning forward in the sitting position.

Failure of shunts to close (e.g., patent ductus arteriosus, atrial septal defect); see Table 20-9, p. 513.

Normal Range of Findings	Abnormal Findings

Note any extracardiac signs that may reflect heart status (particularly in the skin), liver size, and respiratory status. The skin colour should be pink to pinkish brown, depending on the infant's genetic heritage. If cyanosis is present, determine its first appearance: at or shortly after birth versus after the neonatal period. Normally, the liver is not enlarged, and the respirations are not laboured. Also, note the expected parameters of weight gain throughout infancy.

Cyanosis at or just after birth signals oxygen desaturation of congenital heart disease (Table 20-9, p. 514).

The most important signs of heart failure in an infant are persistent tachycardia, tachypnea, and liver enlargement. Engorged veins, gallop rhythm, and pulsus alternans are additional signs. Respiratory crackles (rales) is an important sign in adults but not in infants.

Failure to thrive occurs with cardiac disease.

Palpate the apical impulse to determine the size and position of the heart. Because the infant's heart has a more horizontal placement, expect to palpate the apical impulse at the fourth intercostal space just lateral to the midclavicular line. It may or may not be visible.

The apex is displaced in certain conditions:
- Cardiac enlargement: shifts to the left
- Pneumothorax: shifts away from affected side
- Diaphragmatic hernia: shifts usually to right because this hernia occurs more often on the left
- Dextrocardia: a rare anomaly in which the heart is located on right side of chest

The heart rate is best auscultated because radial pulses are hard to count accurately. Use the small (pediatric size) diaphragm and bell (Figure 20-29). The heart rate may range from 100 to 180 per minute immediately after birth and then stabilize to an average of 120 to 140 per minute. Infants normally have wide fluctuations with activity, from 170 per minute or more during crying or other activity to 70 to 90 per minute during sleep. Variations are greatest at birth and are even more so with premature babies.

Persistent tachycardia is a heart rate of more than 200 per minute in newborns and more than 150 per minute in older infants.

Bradycardia is a heart rate of less than 90 per minute in newborns and less than 60 in older infants or children. This causes a serious drop in cardiac output because the small muscle mass of their hearts cannot increase stroke volume significantly.

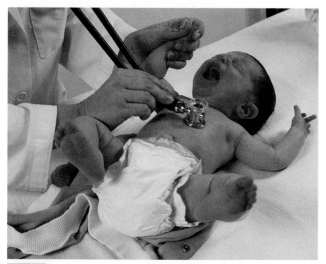

20-29

Expect the heart rhythm to have sinus arrhythmia, the phasic speeding up or slowing down with the respiratory cycle.

Investigate any irregularity except sinus arrhythmia.

Normal Range of Findings	Abnormal Findings
Rapid rates make it more challenging to evaluate heart sounds. Expect heart sounds to be louder in infants than in adults because of the infant's thinner chest wall. Also, S_2 has a higher pitch and is sharper than S_1. Splitting of S_2 just after the height of inspiration is common, not at birth, but beginning a few hours after birth.	Fixed split S_2 indicates atrial septal defect (see Table 20-5, p. 509).
Murmurs in the immediate neonatal period do not necessarily indicate congenital heart disease. Murmurs are relatively common in the first 2 to 3 days because of fetal shunt closure. These murmurs are usually grade I or II, are systolic, accompany no other signs of cardiac disease, and disappear in 2 to 3 days. The murmur of patent ductus arteriosus is a continuous machinery-like murmur, which disappears by 2 to 3 days. On the other hand, absence of a murmur in the immediate neonatal period does not ensure that the heart is perfect; congenital defects can be present but not signalled by an early murmur. It is best to listen frequently and to note and describe any murmur according to the characteristics listed on p. 499.	Persistent murmur after 2 to 3 days, holosystolic murmurs or those that last into diastole, and those that are loud all warrant further evaluation.
To help facilitate the assessment of an infant, you should listen to the heart sounds while the infant is quiet. This may mean that you need to alter the traditional sequence of assessment.	

Children

Note any extracardiac or cardiac signs that may indicate heart disease: poor weight gain, developmental delay, persistent tachycardia, tachypnea, DOE, cyanosis, and clubbing. Note that clubbing of fingers and toes usually does not appear until late in the first year, even with severe cyanotic defects.	
The apical impulse is sometimes visible in children with thin chest walls. Note any obvious bulge or any heave; these are not normal.	A precordial bulge to the left of the sternum with a hyperdynamic precordium signals cardiac enlargement. The bulge occurs because the cartilaginous rib cage is more compliant.
	A substernal heave occurs with right ventricular enlargement, and an apical heave occurs with left ventricular hypertrophy.
Palpate the apical impulse: in the fourth intercostal space to the left of the midclavicular line until age 4 years; at the fourth interspace at the midclavicular line from ages 4 to 6 years; and in the fifth interspace to the right of the midclavicular line at age 7 years (Figure 20-30).	The apical impulse moves laterally with cardiac enlargement.
The average heart rate slows as the child grows older, although it still varies with rest and activity (see Table 10-2, p. 159).	Thrill (palpable vibration) is abnormal.

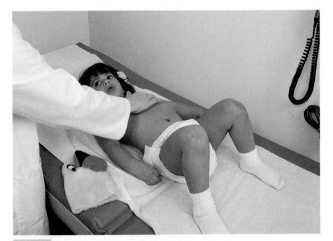

20-30

Normal Range of Findings	Abnormal Findings

The heart rhythm remains characterized by sinus arrhythmia. Physiological S_3 is common in children (see Table 20-7, p. 511). It occurs in early diastole, just after S_2, and is a dull, soft sound that is best heard at the apex.

A **venous hum**—which represents turbulence of blood flow in the jugular venous system—is common in healthy children and has no pathological significance. It is a continuous, low-pitched, soft hum that is heard throughout the cycle, although it is loudest in diastole. Listen with the bell over the supraclavicular fossa at the medial third of the clavicle, especially on the right or over the upper anterior thorax.

The venous hum is usually not affected by respiration, may sound louder when the child stands, and is easily obliterated by occluding the jugular veins in the neck with your fingers.

> This latter manoeuvre helps differentiate the venous hum from other cardiac murmurs (e.g., that of patent ductus arteriosus).
>
> Distinguish innocent murmurs from pathological ones. This may involve referral to another examiner or the performance of diagnostic tests such as electrocardiography or ultrasonography.

Heart murmurs that are innocent (or functional) in origin are very common throughout childhood. Results of some studies indicate that they have a 30% occurrence, and others indicate that nearly all children may demonstrate a murmur at some time. Most innocent murmurs have these characteristics: soft, relatively short systolic ejection murmur; medium pitch; vibratory; and best heard at the left lower sternal or midsternal border, with no radiation to the apex, base, or back.

For a child whose murmur has been shown to be innocent, it is very important that the parents understand this completely. They need to believe that this murmur is just a "noise" and has no pathological significance. Otherwise, the parents may become overprotective and limit activity for the child, which may cause the child to develop a negative self-concept.

Pregnant Women

The vital signs usually reveal that the resting pulse rate is increased by 10 to 15 beats per minute and that blood pressure is lower than the normal prepregnancy level. The blood pressure decreases to its lowest point during the second trimester and then slowly rises during the third trimester. The blood pressure varies with position. It is usually lowest in left lateral recumbent position, a bit higher in the supine position, and highest in the sitting position (Cunningham et al., 2005).

> Suspect pregnancy-induced hypertension with a sustained rise of 30 mm Hg systolic or 15 mm Hg diastolic under basal conditions.

Inspection of the skin often reveals a mild hyperemia in light-skinned women because the increased cutaneous blood flow is an attempt to eliminate the excess heat generated by the increased metabolism. Palpation of the apical impulse is higher and lateral than when the heart is in the normal position, as the enlarging uterus elevates the diaphragm and displaces the heart up and to the left and rotates it on its long axis.

Auscultation of the heart sounds reveals changes caused by the increased blood volume and workload:
- Heart sounds
  Exaggerated splitting of S_1 and increased loudness of S_1
  A loud, easily heard S_3
- Heart murmurs
  A systolic murmur in 90%, which disappears soon after delivery
  A soft, diastolic murmur heard transiently in 19%
  A continuous murmur from breast vasculature in 10% (Cunningham et al., 2005)

The last-mentioned murmur is termed a **mammary souffle** (pronounced *soof'fl*), which occurs near term or when the mother is lactating; it is caused by increased blood flow through the internal mammary artery. The murmur is heard in the second, third, or fourth intercostal space; it is continuous, although it is accented in systole. You can obliterate it by pressure with the stethoscope or one finger lateral to the murmur.

> Murmurs of aortic valve disease cannot be obliterated.

Normal Range of Findings	Abnormal Findings

The ECG shows no changes except for a slight left axis deviation as a result of the change in the heart's position.

Older Adults

A gradual rise in systolic blood pressure is common in older patients; the diastolic blood pressure stays fairly constant, with a resulting widening of pulse pressure. Some older adults experience **orthostatic hypotension,** a sudden drop in blood pressure when rising to sit or stand.

Use caution in palpating and auscultating the carotid artery. Avoid pressure in the carotid sinus area, which could cause a reflex slowing of the heart rate. Also, pressure on the carotid artery could compromise circulation if the artery is already narrowed by atherosclerosis.

When measuring jugular venous pressure, view the right internal jugular vein. The aorta stiffens, dilates, and elongates with aging, which may compress the left neck veins and obscure pulsations on the left side (Fleg, 1990).

The chest often increases in anteroposterior diameter in older patients. This makes it more difficult to palpate the apical impulse and to hear the splitting of S_2. The S_4 often occurs in older people with no known cardiac disease. Systolic murmurs are common, occurring in more than 50% of older people (Fleg, 1990).

Occasional premature ectopic beats are common and do not necessarily indicate underlying heart disease. When in doubt, obtain an ECG. However, consider that the ECG is a recording of only 1 isolated minute in time and may need to be supplemented by a test of 24-hour ambulatory heart monitoring.

The S_3 is associated with heart failure and is always abnormal when present after 40 years of age (see Table 20-7, p. 511).

SPECIAL CONSIDERATIONS FOR ADVANCED PRACTICE

Normal Range of Findings	Abnormal Findings

INSPECT THE JUGULAR VENOUS PULSE

From the jugular veins you can assess the CVP and thus judge the heart's efficiency as a pump. Although the external jugular vein is easier to see, the internal (especially the right) jugular vein is attached more directly to the superior vena cava and thus is more reliable for assessment. You cannot see the internal jugular vein itself, but you can see its pulsation.

Position the patient supine at a 30- to a 45-degree angle, wherever you can best see the pulsations. In general, the higher the venous pressure is, the higher the position you need. Remove the pillow to avoid flexing the neck; the head should be in the same plane as the trunk. Turn the patient's head slightly away from the examined side, and direct a strong light tangentially onto the neck to highlight pulsations and shadows.

Note the external jugular veins overlying the sternomastoid muscle. In some patients, the veins are not visible at all, whereas in others they are full in the supine position. As the patient is raised to a sitting position, these external jugular veins flatten and disappear, usually at 45 degrees.

Now look for pulsations of the internal jugular veins in the area of the suprasternal notch or around the origin of the sternomastoid muscle around the clavicle. You must be able to distinguish pulsation of the internal jugular vein from that of the carotid artery. It is easy to confuse them because they lie close together. Use the guidelines shown in Table 20-1.

This inspection is considered by many authorities to be an advanced skill for practitioners in the cardiopulmonary environments in particular. It is not considered part of the basic cardiac assessment when no other abnormal cardiac findings are evident.

Unilateral distension of external jugular veins has a local cause (kinking or aneurysm).

Full distended external jugular veins above 45 degrees signify increased CVP, as with heart failure.

Normal Range of Findings		Abnormal Findings

TABLE 20-1	Characteristics of Jugular Versus Carotid Pulsations	
Characteristic	Internal Jugular Pulse	Carotid Pulse
Location	Lower, more lateral, under or behind the sternomastoid muscle	Higher and medial to this muscle
Quality	Undulant and diffuse; two visible waves per cycle	Brisk and localized; one wave per cycle
Respiration	Varies with respiration; its level descends during inspiration when intrathoracic pressure is decreased	Does not vary
Palpability	None	Yes
Pressure	Light pressure at the base of the neck easily obliterates	No change
Position of patient	Level of pulse drops and disappears as the patient is brought to a sitting position	Unaffected

SPLITTING OF S₂

When you first hear the split S_2, do *not* be tempted to ask the patient to hold his or her breath so that you can concentrate on the sounds. Breath-holding will only equalize ejection times in the right and left sides of the heart and cause the split to go away. Instead, concentrate on the split as you watch the patient's chest rise up and down with breathing. The split S_2 occurs about every fourth heartbeat, fading in with inhalation and fading out with exhalation.

A **fixed split** is unaffected by respiration; the split is always there.

A **paradoxical split** is the opposite of what you would expect; the sounds fuse on inspiration and split on expiration (see Table 20-5, p. 509).

Focus on Systole, Then on Diastole, and Listen for Any Extra Heart Sounds

Listen with the diaphragm, and then switch to the bell, covering all auscultatory areas (Figure 20-31). Usually, these are silent periods. When you do detect an extra heart sound, listen carefully to note its timing and characteristics. During systole, the **midsystolic click** (which is associated with mitral valve prolapse) is the most common extra sound (see Table 20-6, p. 510). The third and fourth heart sounds occur in diastole; either may be normal or abnormal (see Table 20-7, pp. 511–512).

A pathological S_3 (ventricular gallop) occurs with heart failure and volume overload; a pathological S_4 (atrial gallop) occurs with CAD (see Table 20-7, p. 510, for a full description).

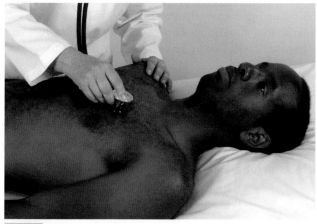

20-31

Special Considerations for Advanced Practice

DOCUMENTATION AND CRITICAL THINKING

Sample Charting

SUBJECTIVE

No chest pain, dyspnea, orthopnea, cough, fatigue, or edema. No personal history of hypertension, abnormal blood tests, heart murmur, or rheumatic fever. Last ECG 2 yr PTA, result normal. No stress ECG or other heart tests.

Family history: father with obesity, smoking, and hypertension, treated with diuretic medication. No other family history significant for CVD.

Personal habits: diet balanced in 4 food groups, 2 to 3 regular coffee/day; no smoking; alcohol, 1 to 2 beers occasionally on weekend; exercise, runs 5 km, 3 to 4 ×/week; no prescription or OTC medications or street drugs.

OBJECTIVE

Neck: Carotids 2+ and = bilaterally. Internal jugular vein pulsations present when supine, and disappear when elevated to a 45-degree position.

Precordium: Inspection. No visible pulsations, no heave or lift.

Palpation: Apical impulse in fifth ICS [intercostal space] at left midclavicular line, no thrill.

Auscultation: Rate 68 beats per minute, rhythm regular, S_1–S_2 are normal, not diminished or accentuated, no S_3, no S_4 or other extra sounds, no murmurs.

ASSESSMENT

Neck vessels healthy by inspection and auscultation
Heart sounds normal

Focused Assessment: Clinical Case Study

Mr. N. V. is a 53-year-old Euro-Canadian male woodcutter admitted to the critical care unit at Toronto General Hospital (TGH) with chest pain.

SUBJECTIVE

- 1 year PTA: N. V. admitted to TGH with crushing substernal chest pain, radiating to L shoulder, accompanied by nausea, vomiting, diaphoresis.
- Diagnosis, MI [myocardial infarction]; hospitalized 7 days, discharged with nitroglycerine prn [as needed] for anginal pain.
- Did not return to work. Activity included walking 2 km/day, hunting. Had occasional episodes of chest pain with exercise, relieved by rest.
- 1 day PTA: had increasing frequency of chest pain, about every 2 hours, lasting few minutes, saw pain as warning to go to doctor.
- Day of admission: severe substernal chest pain ("like someone sitting on my chest") unrelieved by rest. Saw personal doctor; while in office had episode of chest pain same as last year's, accompanied by diaphoresis, no N & V [nausea and vomiting] or shortness of breath, relieved by 1 nitroglycerine. Transferred to TGH by paramedics. No further pain since admission 2 hours ago.
- Family hx: mother died of MI at age 57.
- Personal habits: smokes 1½ pack cigarettes daily × 34 years, no alcohol; diet; trying to limit fat and fried food, still high in added salt.

OBJECTIVE

Extremities: Skin pink, no cyanosis. Upper extrem.: capillary refill sluggish, no clubbing. Lower extrem.: no edema, no hair growth 10 cm below knee bilaterally.

Pulses:
  Carotid: 2+
  Brachial: 2+
  Radial: 2+
  Femoral: 2+
  Popliteal: 0
  P.T. [posterior tibial]: 0

D.P. [dorsalis pedis]: 1+

B/P [blood pressure] R arm, 104/66

Neck: External jugular veins flat. Internal jugular pulsations present when supine and absent when elevated to 45 degrees.

Precordium: Inspection. Apical impulse visible fifth ICS, 7 cm left of midsternal line, no heave.

Palpation: Apical impulse palpable in fifth and sixth ICSs. No thrill.

Auscultation: Apical rate, 92 regular; S_1–S_2 are normal, not diminished or accentuated; no S_3 or S_4; grade III/VI systolic murmur present at left lower sternal border.

ASSESSMENT

Substernal chest pain

Systolic murmur

Ineffective tissue perfusion R/T interruption in flow

Decreased cardiac output R/T reduction in stroke volume

ABNORMAL FINDINGS

TABLE 20-2   Clinical Portrait of Heart Failure

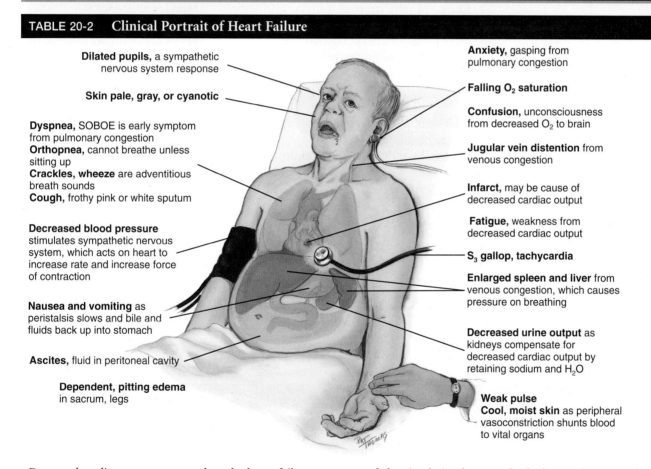

Dilated pupils, a sympathetic nervous system response

Skin pale, gray, or cyanotic

Dyspnea, SOBOE is early symptom from pulmonary congestion
Orthopnea, cannot breathe unless sitting up
Crackles, wheeze are adventitious breath sounds
Cough, frothy pink or white sputum

Decreased blood pressure stimulates sympathetic nervous system, which acts on heart to increase rate and increase force of contraction

Nausea and vomiting as peristalsis slows and bile and fluids back up into stomach

Ascites, fluid in peritoneal cavity

Dependent, pitting edema in sacrum, legs

Anxiety, gasping from pulmonary congestion

Falling O$_2$ saturation

Confusion, unconsciousness from decreased O$_2$ to brain

Jugular vein distention from venous congestion

Infarct, may be cause of decreased cardiac output

Fatigue, weakness from decreased cardiac output

S$_3$ gallop, tachycardia

Enlarged spleen and liver from venous congestion, which causes pressure on breathing

Decreased urine output as kidneys compensate for decreased cardiac output by retaining sodium and H$_2$O

Weak pulse
Cool, moist skin as peripheral vasoconstriction shunts blood to vital organs

Decreased cardiac output occurs when the heart fails as a pump and the circulation becomes backed up and congested.

Signs and symptoms of heart failure come from two basic mechanisms: (a) the heart's inability to pump enough blood to meet the metabolic demands of the body and (b) the kidney's compensatory mechanisms of abnormal retention of sodium and water to compensate for the decreased cardiac output. This increases blood volume and venous return, which causes further congestion.

Onset of heart failure may be (a) *acute,* as after a myocardial infarction, when direct damage to the heart's contracting ability has occurred, or (2b) *chronic,* as with hypertension, when the ventricles must pump against chronically increased pressure.

In illustration: *CO,* cardiac output; *SOBOE,* shortness of breath on exertion.

TABLE 20-3   **Variations in S_1**

The intensity of S_1 depends on three factors: (a) position of AV valve at the start of systole, (b) structure of the valve leaflets, and (c) how quickly pressure rises in the ventricle.

Variation	Factor	Examples
Loud (Accentuated) S_1	1. Position of AV valve at start of systole: wide open and no time for leaflets to drift together.	Hyperkinetic states in which blood velocity is increased: exercise, fever, anemia, hyperthyroidism
	2. Change in valve structure: calcification of valve, increasing ventricular pressure needed to close the valve against increased atrial pressure.	Mitral stenosis with leaflets still mobile
Faint (Diminished) S_1	1. Position of AV valve: delayed conduction from atria to ventricles. Mitral valve drifts shut before ventricular contraction closes it.	First-degree heart block (prolonged PR interval)
	2. Change in valve structure: extreme calcification, which limits mobility.	Mitral insufficiency
	3. More forceful atrial contraction into noncompliant ventricle; delays or diminishes ventricular contraction.	Severe hypertension: systemic or pulmonary
Varying Intensity of S_1	1. Position of AV valve varies before closing from beat to beat.	Atrial fibrillation: irregularly irregular rhythm
	2. Atria and ventricles beat independently.	Complete heart block with changing PR interval
Split S_1	Mitral and tricuspid components are heard separately.	Normal but uncommon

AV, atrioventricular.

TABLE 20-4   **Variations in S_2**

	Condition	Example
Accentuated S_2	1. Higher closing pressure	Systemic hypertension, ringing or booming S_2
	2. Increased pressure in aorta	Exercise and excitement
	3. Pulmonary hypertension	Mitral stenosis, heart failure
	4. Semilunar valves calcified but still mobile	Aortic or pulmonic stenosis
Diminished S_2	1. Decrease in valve strength, caused by a fall in systemic blood pressure	Shock
	2. Semilunar valves thickened and calcified, with decreased mobility	Aortic or pulmonic stenosis

TABLE 20-5   Variations in Split S₂

Variation	Condition	Example
Normal Splitting		
Fixed Split	A fixed split is unaffected by respiration; the split is always there.	Atrial septal defect Right ventricular failure
Paradoxical Split	Conditions that delay aortic valve closure cause the opposite of a normal split. In inspiration, P₂ is normally delayed so with a paradoxical split, the sounds fuse. In expiration you hear the split, in the order of P₂A₂.	Aortic stenosis Left bundle branch block Patent ductus arteriosus
Wide Split	When the right ventricle has delayed electrical activation, the split is very wide on inspiration and is still there on expiration.	Right bundle branch block (which delays P₂)

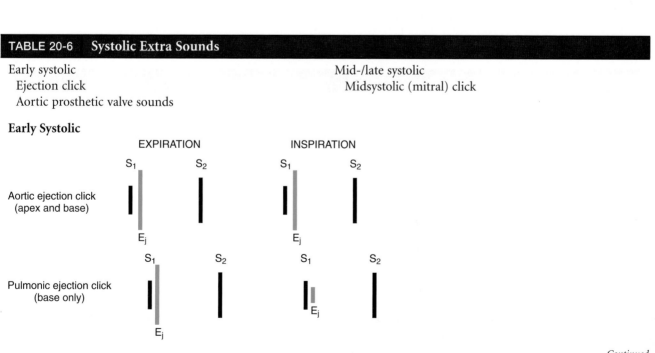

TABLE 20-6   Systolic Extra Sounds

Early systolic
  Ejection click
  Aortic prosthetic valve sounds

Mid-/late systolic
  Midsystolic (mitral) click

Early Systolic

Aortic ejection click (apex and base)

Pulmonic ejection click (base only)

Continued

TABLE 20-6 Systolic Extra Sounds—cont'd

Ejection Click

The ejection click occurs early in systole at the start of ejection because it results from opening of the semilunar valves. Normally, the semilunar valves open silently, but in the presence of stenosis (e.g., aortic stenosis, pulmonic stenosis), their opening makes a sound. It is short and high pitched, with a click quality, and is heard better with the diaphragm of the stethoscope.

The aortic ejection click is heard at the second right interspace and apex and may be loudest at the apex. Its intensity does not change with respiration. The pulmonic ejection click is best heard in the second left interspace and often grows softer with inspiration.

"Ball-in-cage"
AO = aortic opens
AC = aortic closes

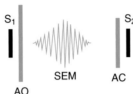

Aortic Prosthetic Valve Sounds*

As a sequela of modern technological intervention for heart problems, some people now have *iatrogenically* induced heart sounds. The opening of an aortic ball-in-cage prosthesis (e.g., Starr-Edwards prosthesis) produces an early systolic sound. This sound is less intense with a tilting disc prosthesis (e.g., Bjork-Shiley prosthesis) and is absent with a tissue prosthesis (e.g., porcine).

Mid-/Late Systolic

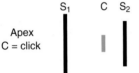

Apex
C = click

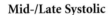

Midsystolic (Mitral) Click

Although it is systolic, this is not an ejection click. It is associated with *mitral valve prolapse,* in which the mitral valve leaflets not only close with contraction but balloon back up into the left atrium. During ballooning, the sudden tensing of the valve leaflets and the chordae tendineae creates the click.

The sound occurs in mid- to late systole and is short and high pitched, with a click quality. It is best heard with the diaphragm of the stethoscope at the apex, but it also may be heard at the left lower sternal border. The click usually is followed by a systolic murmur. The click and murmur move with postural change; when the patient assumes a squatting position, the click may sound sooner after S_2, and the murmur may sound louder and delayed. The Valsalva manoeuvre also moves the click sooner after S_2.

*In illustration: *SEM,* soft ejection murmur.

TABLE 20-7 Diastolic Extra Sounds

Early diastole	Mid-diastole	Late diastole
Opening snap	Third heart sound	Fourth heart sound
Mitral prosthetic valve sound	Summation sound ($S_3 + S_4$)	Pacemaker-induced sound

Early Diastole

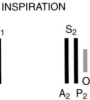

Opening Snap

Normally the opening of the AV valves is silent. In the presence of stenosis, increasingly higher atrial pressure is needed to open the valve. The deformed valve opens with a noise: the opening snap. It is sharp and high pitched, with a snapping quality. It sounds after S_2 and is best heard with the diaphragm of the stethoscope at the third or fourth left interspace at the sternal border, less well heard at the apex.

TABLE 20-7 Diastolic Extra Sounds—cont'd

The opening snap (*OS* in the illustration) usually is not an isolated sound. As a sign of mitral stenosis, the opening snap usually ushers in the low-pitched diastolic rumbling murmur of that condition.

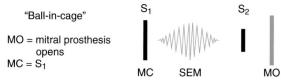

Mitral Prosthetic Valve Sound*

An iatrogenic sound, the opening of a ball-in-cage mitral prosthesis produces an early diastolic sound: an opening click just after S_2. It is loud, is heard over the whole precordium, and is loudest at the apex and left lower sternal border.

Mid-Diastole

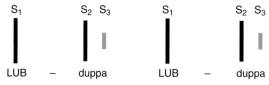

Third Heart Sound

The S_3 is a ventricular filling sound. It occurs in early diastole during the rapid filling phase. Your hearing quickly accommodates to the S_3, so it is best heard when you listen initially. It sounds after S_2 but later than an opening snap would be. It is a dull, soft sound, and it is low pitched, like "distant thunder." It is heard best in a quiet room, at the apex, with the bell of the stethoscope held lightly (just enough to form a seal), and with the patient in the left lateral position.

The S_3 can be confused with a split S_2. Use these guidelines to distinguish the S_3:

- *Location*: The S_3 is heard at the apex or left lower sternal border; the split S_2 is heard at the base.
- *Respiratory variation*: The S_3 does not vary in timing with respirations; the split S_2 does.
- *Pitch*: The S_3 is lower pitched; the pitch of the split S_2 stays the same.

The S_3 may be normal (physiological) or abnormal (pathological). The *physiological* S_3 is heard frequently in children and young adults; it occasionally persists after age 40 years, especially in women. The normal S_3 usually disappears when the patient sits up.

In adults, the S_3 is usually abnormal. The *pathological* S_3 is also called a *ventricular gallop* or an S_3 *gallop,* and it persists when the patient is sitting up. The S_3 indicates decreased compliance of the ventricles, as in heart failure. The S_3 may be the earliest sign of heart failure. The S_3 may originate from either the left or the right ventricle; a left-sided S_3 is heard at the apex in the left lateral position, and a right-sided S_3 is heard at the left lower sternal border with the patient supine and is louder on inspiration.

The S_3 occurs also with conditions of volume overload, such as mitral regurgitation and aortic or tricuspid regurgitation. The S_3 is also found in states of high cardiac output in the absence of heart disease, such as hyperthyroidism, anemia, and pregnancy. When the primary condition is corrected, the gallop disappears.

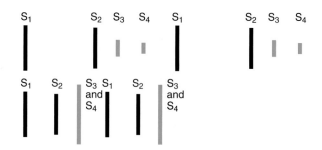

Summation Sound

When both the pathological S_3 and S_4 are present, a quadruple rhythm is heard. Often, in cases of cardiac stress, one response is tachycardia. During rapid rates, the diastolic filling time shortens, and the S_3 and S_4 move closer together. They sound superimposed in mid-diastole, and you hear one loud, prolonged, summated sound, often louder than either S_1 or S_2.

Continued

TABLE 20-7   Diastolic Extra Sounds—cont'd

Late Diastole

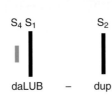

S₄ S₁	S₂	S₄ S₁	S₂
daLUB	– dup	daLUB	– dup

Fourth Heart Sound

The S_4 is a ventricular filling sound. It occurs when the atria contract late in diastole. It is heard immediately before S_1. This is a very soft sound, of very low pitch. You need a good bell, and you must listen for it. It is heard best at the apex, with the patient in left lateral position.

A *physiological S_4* may occur in adults older than 40 or 50 years with no evidence of cardiovascular disease, especially after exercise.

A *pathological S_4* is termed an *atrial gallop* or an *S_4 gallop.* It occurs with decreased compliance of the ventricle (e.g., coronary artery disease, cardiomyopathy) and with systolic overload (afterload), including outflow obstruction to the ventricle (aortic stenosis) and systemic hypertension. A left-sided S_4 occurs with these conditions. It is heard best at the apex, in the left lateral position.

A right-sided S_4 is less common. It is heard at the left lower sternal border and may increase with inspiration. It occurs with pulmonary stenosis or pulmonary hypertension.

Extracardiac Sounds

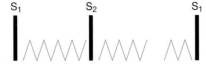

S₁	S₂	S₁

Pericardial Friction Rub

Inflammation of the precordium gives rise to a friction rub. The sound is high pitched and scratchy, like sandpaper being rubbed. It is best heard with the diaphragm of the stethoscope, with the patient sitting up and leaning forward, and with the breath held in expiration.

A friction rub can be heard any place on the precordium but usually is best heard at the apex and left lower sternal border, places where the pericardium comes in close contact with the chest wall. Timing may be systolic and diastolic. The friction rub of pericarditis is common during the first week after a myocardial infarction and may last only a few hours.

*In illustration: *SEM,* soft ejection murmur.
AV, atrioventricular.

TABLE 20-8   Abnormal Pulsations on the Precordium

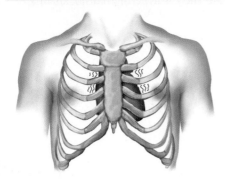

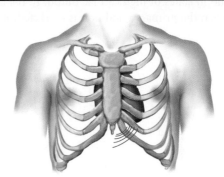

Base

A *thrill* in the second and third right interspaces occurs with severe aortic stenosis and systemic hypertension.

A thrill in the second and third left interspaces occurs with pulmonic stenosis and pulmonic hypertension.

Left Sternal Border

A *lift (heave)* occurs with right ventricular hypertrophy, as found in pulmonic valve disease, pulmonic hypertension, and chronic lung disease. You feel a diffuse lifting impulse during systole at the left lower sternal border. It may be associated with retraction at the apex because the left ventricle is rotated posteriorly by the enlarged right ventricle.

TABLE 20-8	Abnormal Pulsations on the Precordium—cont'd

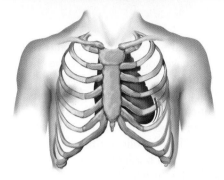

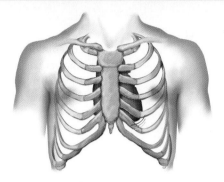

Apex

Cardiac enlargement displaces the apical impulse laterally and over a wider area when left ventricular hypertrophy and dilatation are present. This is *volume overload,* which occurs in mitral regurgitation, aortic regurgitation, and left-to-right shunts.

Apex

The apical impulse is increased in force and duration but is not necessarily displaced to the left when left ventricular hypertrophy occurs alone without dilatation. This is *pressure overload,* which occurs in aortic stenosis or systemic hypertension.

Images © Pat Thomas, 2006.

TABLE 20-9	Congenital Heart Defects

Condition	Description	Clinical Data
Patent Ductus Arteriosus (PDA) 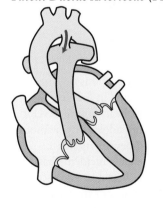	Persistence of the channel joining left pulmonary artery to aorta. This is normal in the fetus and usually closes spontaneously within hours of birth.	S: Usually no symptoms in early childhood; growth and development are normal. O: Blood pressure has wide pulse pressure and bounding peripheral pulses from rapid runoff of blood into low-resistance pulmonary bed during diastole. Thrill often palpable at left upper sternal border. The continuous murmur heard in systole and diastole is called a *machinery murmur.*
Atrial Septal Defect (ASD) 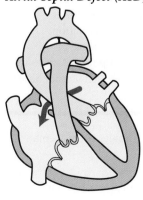	Abnormal opening in the atrial septum, resulting usually in left-to-right shunting of blood and causing large increase in pulmonary blood flow.	S: Defect is remarkably well tolerated. Symptoms in infants are rare; growth and development are normal. Affected children and young adults have mild fatigue and DOE. O: Sternal lift often present. S_2 has fixed split, with P_2 often louder than A_2. Murmur is systolic ejection, medium pitch, best heard at base in second left interspace. Murmur caused not by shunting itself but by increased blood flow through pulmonic valve.

Continued

TABLE 20-9	Congenital Heart Defects—cont'd	
Condition	Description	Clinical Data

Ventricular Septal Defect (VSD)

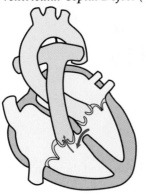

Abnormal opening in septum between the ventricles, usually subaortic area. The size and exact position vary considerably.

S: Small defects are asymptomatic. Infants with large defects have poor growth, slow weight gain; later look pale, thin, and delicate. Affected infants may have feeding problems; DOE; frequent respiratory infections; and, when the condition is severe, heart failure.

O: Loud, harsh holosystolic murmur, best heard at left lower sternal border, may be accompanied by thrill. Large defects also produce soft diastolic murmur at apex (mitral flow murmur) as a result of increased blood flow through mitral valve.

Tetralogy of Fallot

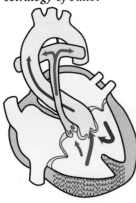

Four components: (a) right ventricular outflow stenosis, (b) VSD, (c) right ventricular hypertrophy, and (d) overriding aorta. *Result:* Large amount of venous blood is shunted directly into aorta away from pulmonary system, so that blood is never oxygenated.

S: Severe cyanosis, not in first months of life but developing as infant grows and RV outflow (i.e., pulmonic) stenosis gets worse. Cyanosis initially with crying and exertion, then at rest. Affected child uses squatting posture after starts walking. DOE common. Growth and development are slowed.

O: Thrill is palpable at left lower sternal border. S_1 is normal; in S_2, A_2 is loud and P_2 is diminished or absent. Murmur is systolic, loud, crescendo–decrescendo.

Coarctation of the Aorta

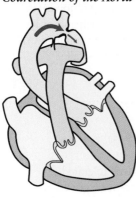

Severe narrowing of descending aorta, usually at the junction of the ductus arteriosus and the aortic arch, just distal to the origin of the left subclavian artery. Results in increased workload on left ventricle. Associated with defects of aortic valve in most cases, as well as associated patent ductus arteriosus and associated VSD.

S: In infants with associated lesions or symptoms, diagnosis occurs in first few months as symptoms of heart failure develop. For affected children and adolescents without symptoms, growth and development are normal. Diagnosis is usually incidental, as a result of blood pressure findings. Adolescents may complain of vague lower extremity cramping that is worse with exercise.

O: Upper extremity hypertension, with readings 20 mm Hg higher than those of lower extremity, is a hallmark of coarctation. Another important sign is absence of or greatly diminished femoral pulses. A systolic murmur is heard best at the left sternal border, radiating to the back.

DOE, dyspnea on exertion; *O,* objective data; *RV,* right ventricular; *S,* subjective data.

Images © Pat Thomas, 2006.

TABLE 20-10	**Murmurs Caused by Valvular Defects**	
Type of Defect	Description	Clinical Data

Midsystolic Ejection Murmurs
Caused by forward flow through semilunar valves

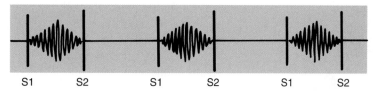

Aortic Stenosis

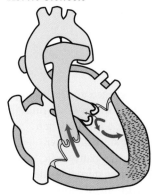

Calcification of aortic valve cusps restricts forward flow of blood during systole; hypertrophy of LV develops.

S: Fatigue, DOE, palpitation, dizziness, fainting, and anginal pain are present.
O: Pallor, slow diminished radial pulse, low blood pressure, and auscultatory gap are common. Apical impulse is sustained and displaced to left. Thrill occurs in systole over second and third right interspaces and right side of neck. S_1 is normal; ejection click is often present, paradoxical split S_2 is often present, and S_4 is present with hypertrophy of LV.
Murmur is loud, harsh, midsystolic, crescendo–decrescendo, and loudest at second right interspace; it radiates widely to side of neck, down left sternal border, or to apex.

Pulmonic Stenosis

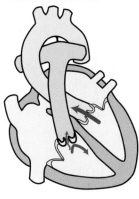

Calcification of pulmonic valve restricts forward flow of blood.

O: Thrill occurs in systole at second and third left interspace, ejection click is often present after S_1, S_2 is diminished and usually with wide split, and S_4 is common with hypertrophy of RV.
Murmur is systolic, medium pitch, coarse, crescendo–decrescendo (diamond shape), and best heard at second left interspace, and it radiates to left and neck.

Pansystolic Regurgitant Murmurs
Caused by backward flow from area of higher pressure to one of lower pressure

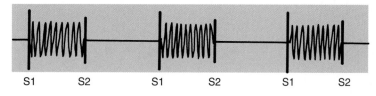

Continued

TABLE 20-10	Murmurs Caused by Valvular Defects—cont'd	
Type of Defect	Description	Clinical Data

Mitral Regurgitation

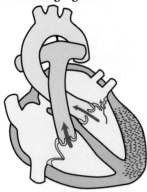

Stream of blood regurgitates back into LA during systole through incompetent mitral valve. In diastole, blood passes back into LV again along with new flow; results in dilatation and hypertrophy of LV.

S: Fatigue, palpitation, orthopnea, and PND are common.

O: Thrill occurs in systole at apex. Lift occurs at apex. Apical impulse is displaced down and to left. S_1 is diminished, S_2 is accentuated, S_3 at apex is often present.

Murmur is pansystolic, often loud, blowing, and best heard at apex, and it radiates well to left axilla.

Tricuspid Regurgitation

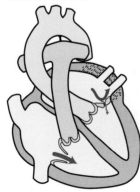

Backflow of blood through incompetent tricuspid valve into RA.

O: Neck veins are engorged and pulsating; liver is enlarged. Lift occurs at sternum if RV is hypertrophied; a thrill is often present at left lower sternal border.

Murmur is soft, blowing, pansystolic, and best heard at left lower sternal border, and it increases with inspiration.

Diastolic Rumbles of AV Valves

Filling murmurs at low pressures, best heard with bell of stethoscope lightly touching skin

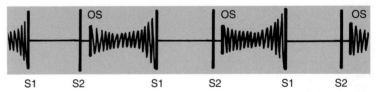

Mitral Stenosis

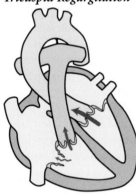

Calcified mitral valve does not open properly, impedes forward flow of blood into LV during diastole. Results in enlargement of LA and increasing pressure in LA.

S: Fatigue, palpitations, DOE, orthopnea are common; PND or pulmonary edema occasionally occur.

O: Arterial pulse is diminished and often irregular. Lift occurs at apex; diastolic thrill is common at apex. S_1 is accentuated; opening snap after S_2 is heard over wide area of precordium, followed by murmur.

Murmur is a low-pitched diastolic rumble, best heard at apex with patient in left lateral position; it does not radiate.

TABLE 20-10	Murmurs Caused by Valvular Defects—cont'd	
Type of Defect	Description	Clinical Data

Tricuspid Stenosis

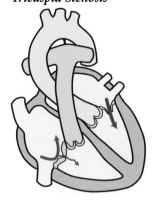

Calcification of tricuspid valve impedes forward flow into RV during diastole.

O: Arterial pulse is diminished; jugular venous pulse is prominent.

Murmur is a diastolic rumble; it is best heard at left lower sternal border and is louder in inspiration.

Early Diastolic Murmurs
Due to semilunar valve incompetence

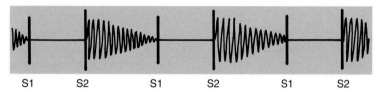

Aortic Regurgitation

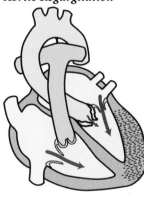

Stream of blood regurgitates back through incompetent aortic valve into LV during diastole. Dilatation and hypertrophy of LV are caused by increased stroke volume of LV. Large stroke volume is ejected rapidly into poorly filled aorta; then rapid runoff occurs in diastole as part of blood is pushed back into LV.

S: Affected patients have only minor symptoms for many years and then rapid deterioration: DOE, PND, angina, dizziness.

O: Bounding "water-hammer" pulse is present in carotid, brachial, and femoral arteries. Blood pressure has wide pulse pressure. Pulsations are palpable in cervical and suprasternal areas; apical impulse is displaced to left and down and feels brief.

Murmur starts almost simultaneously with S_2: It is soft, high-pitched, blowing diastolic, and decrescendo, best heard at third left interspace at base; as patient sits up and leans forward, murmur radiates down.

Pulmonic Regurgitation

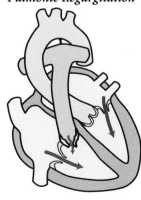

Blood flows backward through incompetent pulmonic valve, from pulmonary artery to RV.

Murmur has same timing and characteristics as that of aortic regurgitation, and the two are hard to distinguish on physical examination.

AV, atrioventricular; *DOE,* dyspnea on exertion; *LA,* left atrium; *LV,* left ventricle; *O,* objective data; *PND,* paroxysmal nocturnal dyspnea; *RA,* right atrium; *RV,* right ventricle; *S,* subjective data.

Summary Checklist: Heart and Neck Vessels Examination

For a PDA-downloadable version, go to *http://evolve.elsevier.com/Canada/Jarvis/examination/*.

Neck
1. Carotid pulse: observe and palpate
2. Jugular venous pulse: observe
3. Jugular venous pressure: estimate

Precordium
1. Inspection and palpation
   Describe location of apical impulse.
   Note any heave (lift) or thrill.
2. Auscultation
   Identify anatomical areas where you listen.

Note rate and rhythm of heartbeat.
Identify S_1 and S_2, and note any variation.
Listen in systole and diastole for any extra heart sounds.
Listen in systole and diastole for any murmurs.
Repeat sequence with bell of stethoscope.
Listen at apex with patient in left lateral position.

Listen at base with patient in sitting position.
3. Health Promotion and Teaching

REFERENCES

Canadian Diabetes Association. (2011). *The prevalence and costs of diabetes.* Retrieved from *http://www.diabetes.ca/diabetes-and-you/what/prevalence.*

Cunningham, F. G., Leveno, K. J., Bloom, S. L., Hauth, J. C., Gilstrap, L. C., & Wenstrom, K. D. (2005). *Williams' obstetrics* (22nd ed.). New York: McGraw-Hill Professional.

Fleg, J. L. (1990). Diagnostic evaluations. In W. B. Abrams & R. Berkow (Eds.), *The Merck manual of geriatrics.* Rahway, NJ: Merck, Sharp, & Dohme.

Health Canada. (2011). *Canadian tobacco use monitoring survey 2010.* Ottawa: Author.

Heart and Stroke Foundation. (2009). *Position statement: Access to affordable, healthy and nutritious foods.* Toronto: Author.

Libby, P., Bonow, R. O., Mann, D. L., & Zipes, D. P. (2008). *Braunwald's heart disease: A textbook of cardiovascular medicine* (8th ed.). Philadelphia: W. B. Saunders.

McGee, S. (2007). *Evidence based physical diagnosis* (2nd ed.). Philadelphia: W. B. Saunders.

Statistics Canada. (2010a). *Canadian community survey, 2010.* Ottawa: Author.

Statistics Canada. (2010b). *Canadian health measures survey: Adult obesity prevalence in Canada and the United States.* Ottawa: Author.

Statistics Canada. (2011). *High blood pressure, by age group and sex.* Ottawa: Author.

Zipes, D., Libby, P., Bonow, R., & Braunwald, E. (2005). *Braunwald's heart disease: A textbook of cardiovascular medicine* (7th ed.). Philadelphia: W. B. Saunders.

Peripheral Vascular System and Lymphatic System

Written by Carolyn Jarvis, PhD, APN, CNP
Adapted by June MacDonald-Jenkins, RN, BScN, MSc

⊝volve WEBSITE

http://evolve.elsevier.com/Canada/Jarvis/examination/

OUTLINE

STRUCTURE AND FUNCTION

The vascular system consists of the vessels of the body. Vessels are tubes for transporting fluid, such as the blood or lymph. Any disease in the vascular system creates problems with delivery of oxygen and nutrients to the tissues or with elimination of waste products from cellular metabolism.

ARTERIES

The heart pumps freshly oxygenated blood through the arteries to all body tissues. The pumping of the heart makes this a high-pressure system. The artery walls are strong, tough,

and tense in order to withstand pressure demands. Arteries contain elastic fibres, which allow their walls to stretch with systole and recoil with diastole. Arteries also contain muscle fibres (vascular smooth muscle), which control the amount of blood delivered to the tissues. The vascular smooth muscle contracts and dilates, which changes the diameter of the arteries to control the rate of blood flow.

Each heartbeat creates a pressure wave, which makes the arteries expand and then recoil. It is the recoil that propels blood through like a wave. All arteries have this pressure wave, or **pulse,** throughout their length, but you can feel it only at

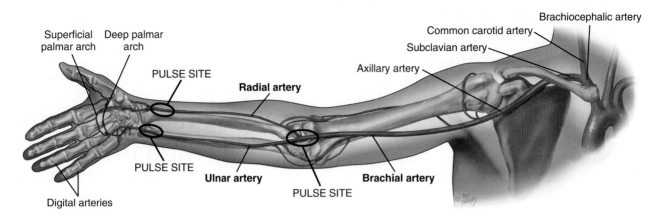

21-1

© Pat Thomas, 2010.

body sites where the artery lies close to the skin and over a bone. The arteries described in the following sections are accessible to examination.

Temporal Artery

The temporal artery is palpated in front of the ear, as discussed in Chapter 14.

Carotid Artery

The carotid artery is palpated in the groove between the sternomastoid muscle and the trachea and is discussed in Chapter 20 in the section on great vessels.

Arteries in the Arm

The major artery supplying the arm is the **brachial artery,** which runs in the biceps–triceps furrow of the upper arm and surfaces at the antecubital fossa in the elbow medial to the biceps tendon (Figure 21-1). Immediately below the elbow, the brachial artery bifurcates into the **ulnar** and **radial arteries.** These run distally and form two arches supplying the hand; these are called the *superficial* and *deep palmar arches.* The radial pulse can be palpated just medial to the radius at the wrist; the ulnar artery is located in the same relation to the ulna, but it is deeper and often difficult to palpate.

Arteries in the Leg

The major artery in the leg is the **femoral artery,** which passes under the inguinal ligament (Figure 21-2). The femoral artery travels down the thigh. At the lower thigh, it courses posteriorly; from that point, it is termed the **popliteal artery.** Below the knee, the popliteal artery divides. The anterior tibial artery travels down the front of the leg on to the dorsum of the foot, where it becomes the **dorsalis pedis artery.** In back of the leg, the **posterior tibial artery** travels down behind the medial malleolus and in the foot divides into the **plantar arteries.**

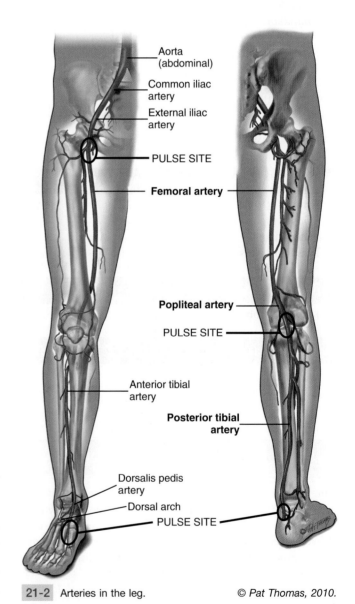

21-2 Arteries in the leg. © Pat Thomas, 2010.

The function of the arteries is to supply oxygen and essential nutrients to the tissues. **Ischemia** is a deficiency in the supply of oxygenated arterial blood to a tissue, caused by obstruction of a blood vessel. A complete blockage leads to death of the distal tissue. A partial blockage causes the supply to be insufficient, and the ischemia may be apparent only during exercise, when oxygen needs increase.

VEINS

The course of veins parallels that of arteries, but the body has more veins, and they lie closer to the skin surface. The following veins are accessible to examination.

Jugular Veins

Assessment of the jugular veins is described in Chapter 20.

Veins in the Arm

Each arm has two sets of veins: superficial and deep. The superficial veins are in the subcutaneous tissue and are responsible for most of the venous return.

Veins in the Leg

The legs have three types of veins (Figure 21-3):
1. The **deep veins** run alongside the deep arteries and conduct most of the venous return from the legs. These are the **femoral** and **popliteal veins.** As long as these veins remain intact, the superficial veins can be excised without harming the circulation.
2. The **superficial veins** are the **great** and **small saphenous veins.** The great saphenous vein, inside the leg, starts at the medial side of the dorsum of the foot. You can see it ascend in front of the medial malleolus; then it crosses the tibia obliquely and ascends along the medial side of the thigh. The small saphenous vein, in the outer portion of the leg, starts on the lateral side of the dorsum of the foot and ascends behind the lateral malleolus and up the back of the leg, where it joins the popliteal vein.
3. **Perforators** (not illustrated in Figure 21-3) are connecting veins that join the two sets. They also have one-way valves that route blood from the superficial veins into the deep veins.

VENOUS FLOW

Veins drain the deoxygenated blood and its waste products from the tissues and return it to the heart. Unlike the arteries, veins are a low-pressure system. Because veins do not have a pump to generate their blood flow, the veins need a mechanism to keep blood moving (Figure 21-4). This movement is accomplished by (a) the contracting skeletal muscles that milk the blood proximally, back toward the heart; (b) the pressure gradient caused by breathing, in which inspiration makes the thoracic pressure decrease and the abdominal pressure increase; and (c) the intraluminal valves, which ensure

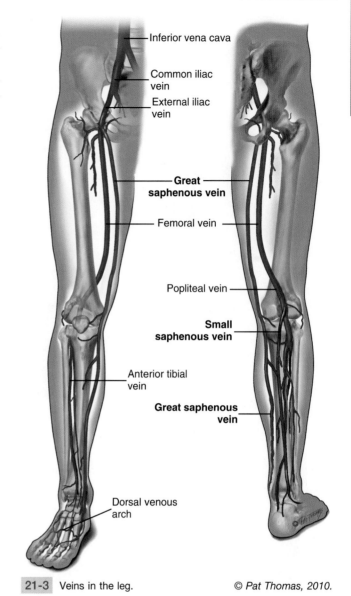

Inferior vena cava

Common iliac vein

External iliac vein

Great saphenous vein

Femoral vein

Popliteal vein

Small saphenous vein

Anterior tibial vein

Great saphenous vein

Dorsal venous arch

21-3 Veins in the leg.   © Pat Thomas, 2010.

unidirectional flow. Each valve is a paired semilunar pocket that opens toward the heart and closes tightly when filled to prevent backflow of blood.

In the legs, this mechanism is called the *calf pump,* or "peripheral heart." During walking, the calf muscles alternately contract (systole) and relax (diastole). In the contraction phase, the gastrocnemius and soleus muscles squeeze the veins and direct the blood flow proximally. Because of the valves, venous blood flows just one way: toward the heart.

Besides the presence of intraluminal valves, venous structure differs from arterial structure. Because venous pressure is lower, walls of the veins are thinner than those of the arteries. Veins have a larger diameter and are more distensible; they can expand and hold more blood when blood volume increases. This is a compensatory mechanism to reduce stress on the heart. Because of this ability to stretch, veins are called **capacitance vessels.**

Efficient venous return is dependent on contracting skeletal muscles, competent valves in the veins, and a patent

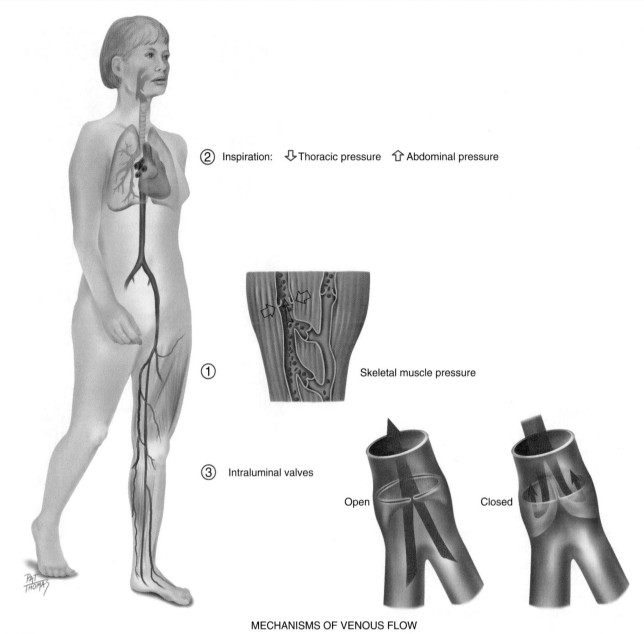

② Inspiration: ⬇Thoracic pressure   ⬆ Abdominal pressure

① Skeletal muscle pressure

③ Intraluminal valves

Open   Closed

MECHANISMS OF VENOUS FLOW

21-4

© *Pat Thomas, 2006.*

lumen. Problems with any of these three elements lead to venous stasis. The risk for venous disease is increased by prolonged standing, sitting, or bed rest because of the absence of the milking action that walking accomplishes. Hypercoagulable states and vein wall trauma are other factors that increase risk for venous disease. Also, dilated and tortuous (varicose) veins have **incompetent valves,** wherein the lumen is so wide the valve cusps cannot approximate. This condition increases venous pressure, which further dilates the vein. Some people have a genetic predisposition to varicose veins, but obesity and pregnancy are risk factors.

LYMPHATIC VESSELS

The lymphatic vessels form a completely separate vessel system, which retrieves excess fluid from the tissue spaces

and returns it to the bloodstream (Figure 21-5). During circulation of the blood, somewhat more fluid leaves the capillaries than the veins can absorb. Without lymphatic drainage, fluid would build up in the interstitial spaces and produce edema.

The lymphatic vessels converge and drain into two main trunks, which empty into the venous system at the subclavian veins (see Figure 21-5):

1. The **right lymphatic duct** empties into the right subclavian vein. It drains the right side of the head and neck, right arm, right side of thorax, right lung and pleura, right side of the heart, and right upper section of the liver.
2. The **thoracic duct** drains the rest of the body. It empties into the left subclavian vein.

The functions of the lymphatic system are (a) to conserve fluid and plasma proteins that leak out of the capillaries, (b)

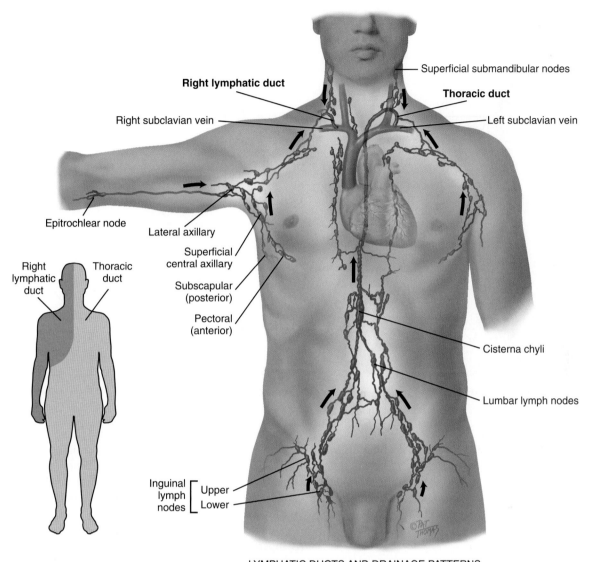

Right lymphatic duct

Thoracic duct

Superficial submandibular nodes

Right subclavian vein

Left subclavian vein

Epitrochlear node

Lateral axillary

Superficial central axillary

Subscapular (posterior)

Pectoral (anterior)

Right lymphatic duct

Thoracic duct

Cisterna chyli

Lumbar lymph nodes

Inguinal lymph nodes { Upper / Lower

LYMPHATIC DUCTS AND DRAINAGE PATTERNS

21-5

© Pat Thomas, 2010.

to form a major part of the immune system that defends the body against disease, and (c) to absorb lipids from the intestinal tract.

The immune system is a complicated network of organs and cells that work together to protect the body. The immune system detects and eliminates foreign pathogens, both those that come in from the environment and those arising from inside (abnormal or mutant cells). It accomplishes this (a) by phagocytosis (digestion) of the substances by neutrophils and by monocytes or macrophages and (b) by production of specific antibodies or specific immune responses by the lymphocytes.

The lymphatic vessels have a unique structure. Lymphatic capillaries start as microscopic open-ended tubes, which siphon interstitial fluid. The capillaries converge to form small vessels. The small vessels, like veins, drain into larger ones. The vessels have valves, and so flow is in one direction from the tissue spaces into the bloodstream. The many valves make the vessels look beaded. The flow of lymph is slower than that of the blood. Lymph flow is propelled by contracting skeletal muscles, by pressure changes secondary to breathing, and by contraction of the vessel walls themselves.

Lymph nodes are small oval clumps of lymphatic tissue located at intervals along the vessels. Most nodes are arranged in groups, both deep and superficial, in the body. Nodes filter the fluid before it is returned to the bloodstream and filter out microorganisms that could be harmful to the body. The pathogens are exposed to lymphocytes in the lymph nodes. The lymphocytes mount an antigen-specific response to eliminate the pathogens. When local inflammation occurs, the nodes in that area become swollen and tender.

The superficial groups of nodes are accessible to inspection and palpation and give clues to the status of the lymphatic system:

- **Cervical nodes** drain the head and neck. They are described in Chapter 14.
- **Axillary nodes** drain the breast and upper arm. They are described in Chapter 18.

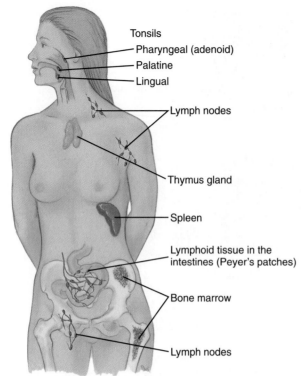

Tonsils
— Pharyngeal (adenoid)
— Palatine
— Lingual

Lymph nodes

Thymus gland

Spleen

Lymphoid tissue in the
intestines (Peyer's patches)

Bone marrow

Lymph nodes

RELATED ORGANS IN IMMUNE SYSTEM

21-6   © *Pat Thomas, 2006.*

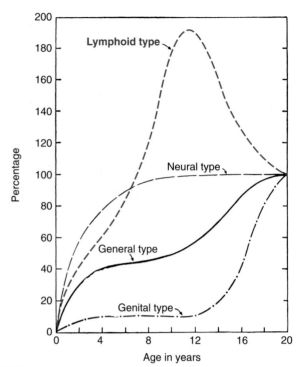

21-7 Comparison of growth rates of three types of tissues in the body.

- The **epitrochlear node** is in the antecubital fossa and drains the hand and lower arm.
- The **inguinal nodes** in the groin drain most of the lymph of the lower extremity, the external genitalia, and the anterior abdominal wall.

Related Organs

The spleen, tonsils, and thymus gland aid the lymphatic system (Figure 21-6). The **spleen** is located in the left upper quadrant of the abdomen. It has four functions: (a) to destroy old red blood cells, (b) to produce antibodies, (c) to store red blood cells, and (d) to filter microorganisms from the blood.

The **tonsils** (palatine, pharyngeal, and lingual) are located at the entrance to the respiratory and gastrointestinal tracts and respond to local inflammation.

The **thymus gland** is flat, pink-grey, and located in the superior mediastinum behind the sternum and in front of the aorta. It is relatively large in the fetus and young child and atrophies after puberty. It is important in developing the T lymphocytes of the immune system in children, but it serves no function in adults. The T and B lymphocytes originate in the bone marrow and mature in the lymphoid tissue.

DEVELOPMENTAL CONSIDERATIONS

Infants and Children

The lymphatic system has the same function in children as in adults. Lymphoid tissue has a unique growth pattern in

comparison with other body systems (Figure 21-7): It is well developed at birth and grows rapidly until age 10 or 11 years. By age 6 years, the lymphoid tissue reaches adult size; it surpasses adult size by puberty, and then it slowly atrophies. It is possible that the excessive antigen stimulation in children causes the early rapid growth.

Lymph nodes are relatively large in children, and the superficial ones are often palpable even in healthy children. With infection, excessive swelling and hyperplasia occur. Enlargement of the tonsils is a familiar sign in respiratory infections. The excessive lymphoid response also may account for the common childhood symptom of abdominal pain with seemingly unrelated problems such as upper respiratory infections. Possibly, the inflammation of mesenteric lymph nodes produces the abdominal pain.

Pregnant Women

Hormonal changes cause vasodilatation and the resulting drop in blood pressure in the first and second trimesters of the pregnancy, as described in Chapter 20. The growing uterus obstructs drainage of the iliac veins and the inferior vena cava. This condition lowers blood flow and increases venous pressure. These developments, in turn, cause dependent edema, varicosities in the legs and vulva, and hemorrhoids.

Older Adults

Peripheral blood vessels grow more rigid with age, which results in **arteriosclerosis** (once called *hardening of the arteries*). This condition produces the rise in systolic blood pressure discussed in Chapter 10. Do not confuse this process with another one, **atherosclerosis,** which is the deposition of fatty plaques on the intima of the arteries.

With aging, the intramuscular calf veins progressively enlarge. Prolonged bed rest, prolonged sitting, and heart failure increase the risk of deep venous thrombosis (DVT) and subsequent pulmonary embolism. These conditions are common in aging and also occur after myocardial infarction. However, care for myocardial infarction now includes early mobilization and low-dose anticoagulant medication, which reduce the risk of pulmonary embolism.

As a result of the loss of lymphatic tissue, fewer numbers of lymph nodes are present in older people, and the size of remaining nodes decreases.

SUBJECTIVE DATA

1. Leg pain or cramps
2. Skin changes on arms or legs
3. Swelling in the arms or legs
4. Lymph node enlargement
5. Medications

HEALTH HISTORY QUESTIONS

Examiner Asks	Rationale
1. **Leg pain or cramps.** Any leg pain (cramps)? Where? • Describe the type of pain: Is it burning, aching, cramping, stabbing? Did this come on gradually or suddenly? • Is it aggravated by activity, walking? • How many blocks (stairs) does it take to produce this pain?	Such pain and cramps are signs of peripheral vascular disease; see Table 21-4, p. 543. **Claudication distance** is the number of blocks walked or stairs climbed that produces pain.
• Has this amount changed recently? • Is the pain worse with elevation? Worse with cool temperatures? • Does the pain wake you up at night?	Note sudden decrease in claudication distance or pain not relieved by rest. Night leg pain is common in older adults. It may indicate the ischemic rest pain of peripheral vascular disease, severe night muscle cramping (usually the calf), or restless leg syndrome.
• Tell me about your exercise pattern: Any recent change in exercise, a new exercise, increasing exercise? • Do you have a foot care routine? • Tell me about your job: Are you on your feet during the day or sitting at a desk?	Determine whether pain is of musculoskeletal origin rather than vascular. Chronic venous insufficiency, musculoskeletal pain of the lower back and feet, preterm birth, and spontaneous abortions are health risks associated with working conditions that required prolonged standing.
• What relieves this pain: dangling, walking, rubbing? Is the leg pain associated with any skin changes? • Is it associated with any change in sexual function (in men)?	Aortoiliac occlusion is associated with impotence (Leriche's syndrome).
• Any history of vascular problems, heart problems, diabetes, obesity, pregnancy, smoking, trauma, prolonged standing, or prolonged bed rest?	
2. **Skin changes on arms or legs.** Any **skin changes** in arms or legs? What colour: redness, pallor, blueness, brown discolorations? • Any change in temperature: excess warmth or coolness?	Coolness is associated with arterial disease.
• Do your leg veins look enlarged or crooked? Are these areas painful? • How have you treated these? Do you use support hose?	**Varicose veins** are swollen, twisted, and sometimes painful veins that have filled with an abnormal collection of blood.

Examiner Asks	Rationale
• Any leg sores or ulcers? Where on the leg? Any pain with the leg ulcer?	Leg ulcers occur with chronic arterial and chronic venous disease (see Table 21-1, p. 534).

3. Swelling in the arms or legs. Do you have swelling in one or both legs? When did this swelling start?
  • What time of day is the swelling at its worst: morning, or after you have been up most of day?
  • Does the swelling come and go, or is it constant?
  • What seems to trigger it: trauma, standing all day, sitting?
  • What relieves swelling: elevation, support hose?
  • Is swelling associated with pain, heat, redness, ulceration, hardened skin?
	Edema is bilateral when caused by a systemic problem such as heart failure or unilateral when it is the result of a local obstruction or inflammation.

4. Lymph node enlargement. Any "swollen glands" (lumps, kernels)? Where in body? How long have you had them?
  • Any recent change?
  • How do they feel to you: hard, soft?
  • Are the swollen glands associated with pain, or local infection?
	Lymph nodes enlarge with infection, malignancies, and immunological diseases.

5. Medications. What medications are you taking (e.g., oral contraceptives, hormone replacement, aspirin)?	

OBJECTIVE DATA

PREPARATION

During a complete physical examination, examine the arms at the very beginning when you are checking the vital signs and the patient is sitting. Examine the legs directly after the abdominal examination while the patient is still supine. Then have the patient stand up to evaluate the leg veins.

Examination of the arms and legs includes peripheral vascular characteristics (described in this chapter), the skin (see Chapter 13), musculoskeletal findings (see Chapter 24), and neurological findings (see Chapter 25). A method of integrating these steps is discussed in Chapter 28.

Room temperature should be approximately 22°C (72°F) and draft free to prevent vasodilatation or vasoconstriction.

Use inspection and palpation. Compare your findings in one extremity with those in the opposite extremity.

EQUIPMENT NEEDED

Occasionally needed:
Paper tape measure
Tourniquet or blood pressure cuff
Stethoscope
Doppler ultrasonic stethoscope

Normal Range of Findings	Abnormal Findings
INSPECT AND PALPATE THE ARMS	
Lift both the patient's hands in your hands. Inspect, then turn the patient's hands over, noting colour of skin and nail beds; temperature, texture, and turgor of skin; and the presence of any lesions, edema, or clubbing. Use the **profile sign** (viewing the finger from the side) to detect early clubbing. The normal nail bed angle is 160 degrees. (See Chapter 13 for a full discussion of skin colour, lesions, and clubbing.)	Flattening of nail bed angle and clubbing (diffuse enlargement of terminal phalanges) occur with congenital cyanotic heart disease and cor pulmonale.
With the patient's hands near the level of his or her heart, check **capillary refill.** This is an index of peripheral perfusion and cardiac output. Depress and blanch the nail beds; release and note how long it takes for colour to return. Usually, the vessels refill within a fraction of a second. Consider it normal if the colour returns in less than 1 or 2 seconds. Note conditions that can skew your findings: a cool room, decreased body temperature, cigarette smoking, peripheral edema, and anemia.	Refill time of more than 1 or 2 seconds signifies vasoconstriction or decreased cardiac output (hypovolemia, heart failure, shock). The hands are cold, clammy, and pale.

Normal Range of Findings

The two arms should be symmetrical in size.

Note the presence of any scars on hands and arms. Many occur normally with usual childhood abrasions or with occupations involving hand tools.

Palpate radial pulses bilaterally, noting rate, rhythm, elasticity of vessel wall, and equal force (Figure 21-8). Grade the force (amplitude) on a four-point scale:
- 3+: increased, full, bounding
- 2+: normal
- 1+: weak
- 0: absent

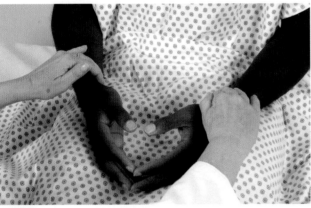

21-8

It usually is not necessary to palpate the ulnar pulses. If doing so is indicated, palpate along the medial side of the inner forearm (Figure 21-9), although the ulnar pulses often are not palpable in normal people.

Palpate the brachial pulses; their force should be equal bilaterally (Figure 21-10).

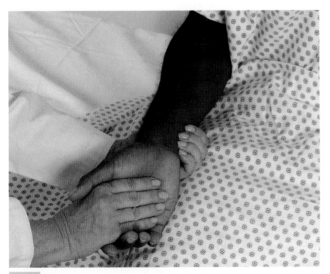

21-9

Abnormal Findings

Edema of upper extremities occurs when lymphatic drainage is obstructed, which may occur after breast surgery (see Table 21-3, p. 542).

Needle tracks in antecubital fossae occur with intravenous drug use; linear scars in wrists may signify past self-inflicted injury.

The pulse is full and bounding (3+) in hyperkinetic states (exercise, anxiety, fever), anemia, and hyperthyroidism.

The pulse is weak and "thready" in shock and peripheral arterial disease. See Table 21-2 on p. 541 for illustrations of these and irregular pulse rhythms.

Objective Data

Normal Range of Findings	Abnormal Findings

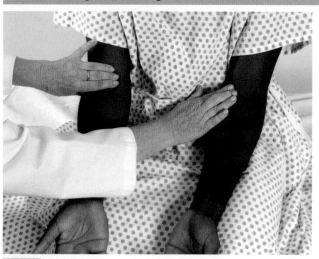

21-10

Check the epitrochlear lymph node in the depression above and behind the medial condyle of the humerus. Do this by "shaking hands" with the patient and reaching your other hand under the patient's elbow to the groove between the biceps and triceps muscles, above the medial epicondyle (Figure 21-11). This node is normally not palpable.

The epitrochlear node becomes enlarged in infection of the hand or forearm.

Epitrochlear nodes are palpable in conditions of generalized lymphadenopathy: lymphoma, chronic lymphocytic leukemia, sarcoidosis, infections, mononucleosis.

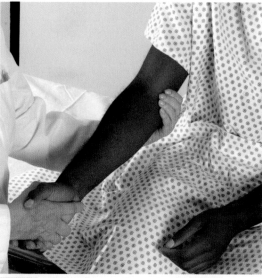

21-11

INSPECT AND PALPATE THE LEGS

Uncover the patient's legs while keeping the genitalia draped. Inspect both legs together, noting skin colour, hair distribution, venous pattern, size (swelling or atrophy), and any skin lesions or ulcers.

Normally, hair covers the legs. Even if leg hair is shaved, you will still note hair on the dorsa of the toes.

The venous pattern normally is flat and barely visible. Note obvious varicosities, although these are best assessed while the patient is standing.

Abnormalities include pallor with vasoconstriction, erythema with vasodilatation, and cyanosis.

In malnutrition, skin is thin, shiny, and atrophic; nails have thick ridges; hair loss occurs; and ulcers and gangrene may be present. Malnutrition, pallor, and coolness occur with arterial insufficiency.

Normal Range of Findings

Both legs should be symmetrical in size without any swelling or atrophy. If the lower legs look asymmetrical or if DVT is suspected, measure the calf circumference with a nonstretchable tape measure (Figure 21-12). Measure at the widest point, taking care to measure the other leg in exactly the same place: the same number of centimetres down from the patella or other landmark. If lymphedema is suspected, measure also at the ankle, distal calf, knee, and thigh. Record your findings in centimetres.

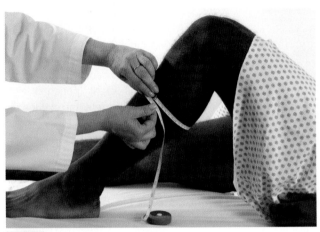

21-12

In the presence of skin discoloration, skin ulcers, or gangrene, note the size and the exact location.

Palpate for temperature (using the dorsa of your hand) along the patient's legs down to the feet, comparing symmetrical spots (Figure 21-13). The skin should be warm and of equal warmth bilaterally. Both feet may be cool because of environmental factors such as cool room temperature, apprehension, and cigarette smoking. If temperature is increased higher up the leg, note whether this increase is gradual or abrupt.

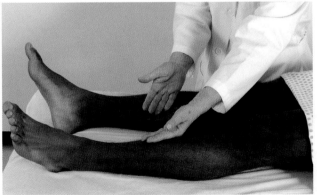

21-13

Abnormal Findings

Diffuse bilateral edema occurs with systemic illnesses.

Acute, unilateral, painful swelling and asymmetry of calves of 1 cm or more is abnormal; refer the patient to determine whether DVT is present.

Asymmetry of 1 to 3 cm occurs with mild lymphedema; 3 to 5 cm, with moderate lymphedema; and more than 5 cm, with severe lymphedema (see Table 21-3, p. 542).

Brown discoloration occurs with chronic venous stasis as a result of hemosiderin deposits from red blood cell degradation.

Venous ulcers occur usually at the medial malleolus because of bacterial invasion of poorly drained tissues (see Table 21-1 on p. 534).

With arterial deficit, ulcers occur on tips of toes, metatarsal heads, and lateral malleoli.

With arterial deficit, one foot or leg may be cool or the temperature may drop suddenly as you move down the leg.

Normal Range of Findings	Abnormal Findings

Flex the patient's knee, then gently compress the gastrocnemius (calf) muscle anteriorly against the tibia; no tenderness should be present. Or you may sharply dorsiflex the foot toward the tibia. Flexing the knee first exerts pressure on the posterior tibial vein. Normally, this does not cause pain.

Calf pain with these manoeuvres is a positive **Homan's sign,** which occurs in approximately 20% of cases of DVT. This test was once considered important but has lost its significance because of its **low sensitivity** in predicting the actual presence of a clot. A positive Homan's sign is also present in a variety of other conditions such as muscle injury, Achilles tendonitis, and plantar muscle injury. Venous ultrasonography is considered the **highly sensitive** diagnostic test to determine the presence or absence of a clot. Approximately half of all patients with DVT have no clinically detectable signs or symptoms.

Palpate the inguinal lymph nodes. It is not unusual to find palpable nodes that are small (1 cm or less), movable, and nontender.

Nodes are not normally enlarged, tender, or fixed in area.

Palpate the femoral, popliteal, dorsalis pedis, and posterior tibial arteries in both legs. Grade the force on the four-point scale. Locate the femoral arteries just below the inguinal ligament, halfway between the pubis and anterior superior iliac spines (Figure 21-14). To help expose the femoral area, particularly in obese patients, ask the patient to bend his or her knees to the side in a froglike position. Press firmly and then slowly release, noting the pulse tap under your fingertips. Should this pulse be weak or diminished, auscultate the site for a bruit.

A bruit occurs with turbulent blood flow, indicating partial occlusion (see Table 21-5, p. 544).

The **popliteal pulse** is a more diffuse pulse and can be difficult to localize. With the leg extended but relaxed, anchor your thumbs on the knee, and curl your fingers around into the popliteal fossa (Figure 21-15). Press your fingers forward hard to compress the artery against the bone (the lower edge of the femur or the upper edge of the tibia). Often the pulse is just lateral to the medial tendon.

If you have difficulty with this manoeuvre, turn the patient prone and lift up the lower leg (Figure 21-16). Let the leg relax against your arm, and press in deeply with your two thumbs. Often a normal popliteal pulse is impossible to palpate.

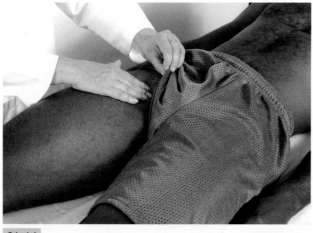

21-14

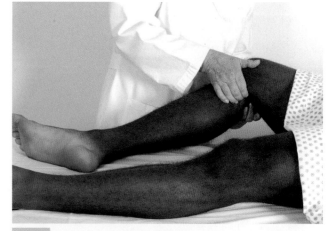

21-15

Normal Range of Findings	Abnormal Findings

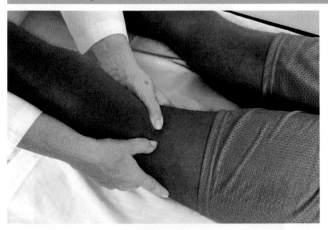

21-16

For the **posterior tibial pulse,** curve your fingers around the medial malleolus (Figure 21-17). You will feel the tapping right behind it in the groove between the malleolus and the Achilles tendon. If you cannot feel it, try passive dorsiflexion of the foot to make the pulse more accessible.

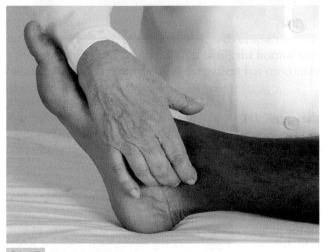

21-17   Posterior tibial pulse.

Palpating the **dorsalis pedis pulse** requires a very light touch. Normally the pulse is just lateral to and parallel with the extensor tendon of the big toe (Figure 21-18). Do not mistake the pulse in your own fingertips for that of the patient.

In adults older than 45 years, occasionally either the dorsalis pedis or the posterior tibial pulse may be hard to find, but not both on the same foot.

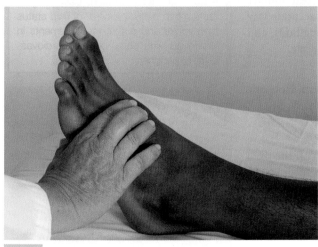

21-18   Dorsalis pedis pulse.

Objective Data

CHAPTER

22

The Abdomen

Written by Carolyn Jarvis, PhD, APN, CNP
Adapted by Marian Luctkar-Flude, RN, MScN

⊘volve WEBSITE

http://evolve.elsevier.com/Canada/Jarvis/examination/
- Animations
- Audio—Abdomen Sounds
- Bedside Assessment Summary Checklist
- Examination Review Questions
- Key Points

- Physical Examination Summary Checklist
- Quick Assessment for Common Conditions:
  - Peptic Ulcer Disease
- Video—Assessment:
  - Abdomen and Inguinal Hernia

OUTLINE

STRUCTURE AND FUNCTION

SURFACE LANDMARKS

The **abdomen** is a large oval cavity extending from the diaphragm down to the top of the pelvis. It is bordered in back by the vertebral column and paravertebral muscles and at the sides and front by the lower rib cage and abdominal muscles (Figure 22-1). Four layers of large, flat muscles form the ventral abdominal wall. These are joined at the midline by a tendinous seam, the **linea alba.** One muscle, the **rectus abdominis,** forms a strip extending the length of the midline, and its edge is often palpable. The muscles protect and hold the organs in place, and they flex the vertebral column.

INTERNAL ANATOMY

Inside the abdominal cavity, all the internal organs are called the **viscera.** It is important that you know the location of these organs so well that you could draw a map of them on the skin (Figure 22-2). You must be able to visualize each organ that you listen to or palpate through the abdominal wall.

The **solid viscera** are those that maintain a characteristic shape (liver, pancreas, spleen, adrenal glands, kidneys, ovaries, and uterus). The **liver** fills most of the right upper quadrant (RUQ) and extends over to the left midclavicular line. The lower edge of the liver and the right kidney may normally be

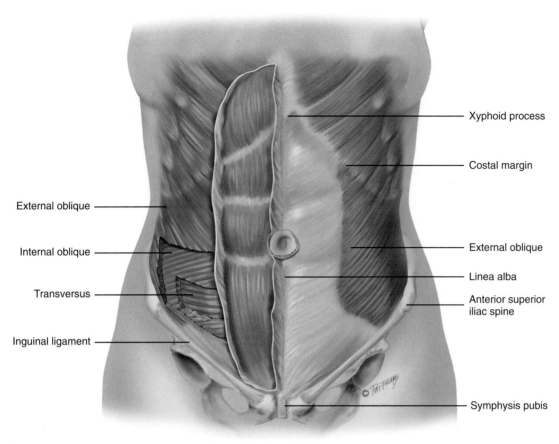

External oblique

Internal oblique

Transversus

Inguinal ligament

Xyphoid process

Costal margin

External oblique

Linea alba

Anterior superior
iliac spine

Symphysis pubis

22-1

© Pat Thomas, 2006.

palpable. The ovaries normally are palpable only on bimanual assessment during the pelvic examination.

The shape of the **hollow viscera** (stomach, gallbladder, small intestine, colon, and bladder) depends on the contents. They are usually not palpable, although you may feel a colon distended with feces or a bladder distended with urine. The stomach is just below the diaphragm, between the liver and spleen. The gallbladder rests under the posterior surface of the liver, just lateral to the right midclavicular line. Note that the small intestine is located in all four quadrants. It extends from the stomach's pyloric valve to the ileocecal valve in the right lower quadrant (RLQ), where it joins the colon.

The **spleen** is a soft mass of lymphatic tissue on the posterolateral wall of the abdominal cavity, immediately under the diaphragm (Figure 22-3). It lies obliquely with its long axis behind and parallel to the tenth rib, lateral to the midaxillary line. Its width extends from the ninth to the eleventh ribs, approximately 7 cm. It is normally not palpable. If it becomes enlarged, its lower edge moves downward and toward the midline.

The **aorta** is just to the left of midline in the upper part of the abdomen (Figure 22-4). It descends behind the peritoneum, and at 2 cm below the umbilicus, it bifurcates into the right and left common iliac arteries opposite the fourth lumbar vertebra. You can palpate the aortic pulsations easily in the upper anterior abdominal wall. The right and left iliac arteries become the femoral arteries in the groin area. Their pulsations are easily palpated as well, at a point halfway between the anterior superior iliac spine and the symphysis pubis.

The **pancreas** is a soft, lobulated gland located behind the stomach. It stretches obliquely across the posterior abdominal wall to the left upper quadrant (LUQ).

The bean-shaped **kidneys** are retroperitoneal, or posterior to the abdominal contents (Figure 22-5). They are well protected by the posterior ribs and musculature. The twelfth rib forms an angle, the **costovertebral angle,** with the vertebral column. The left kidney lies at that point, at the eleventh and twelfth ribs. Because of the placement of the liver, the right kidney rests 1 to 2 cm lower than the left kidney and is sometimes palpable.

For convenience in description, the abdominal wall is divided into **four quadrants** by a vertical and a horizontal line bisecting the umbilicus (Figure 22-6). (According to an older, more complicated scheme, the abdomen was divided into nine regions. Although the old system is generally not used, some regional names persist, such as **epigastric** for the area between the costal margins, **umbilical** for the area around the umbilicus, and **hypogastric** or **suprapubic** for the area above the pubic bone.)

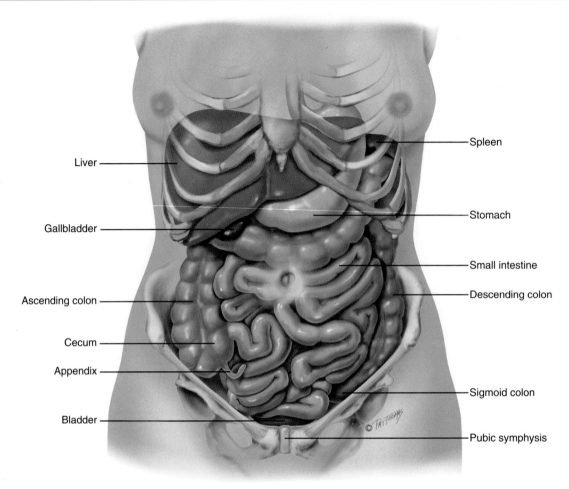

Liver

Gallbladder

Ascending colon

Cecum

Appendix

Bladder

Spleen

Stomach

Small intestine

Descending colon

Sigmoid colon

Pubic symphysis

22-2

© Pat Thomas, 2006.

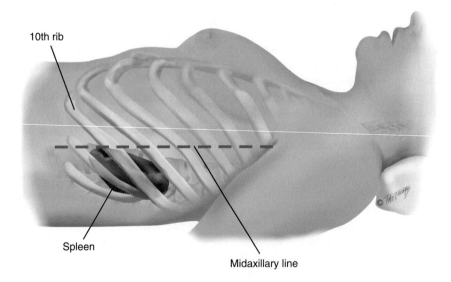

10th rib

Spleen

Midaxillary line

22-3

© Pat Thomas, 2006.

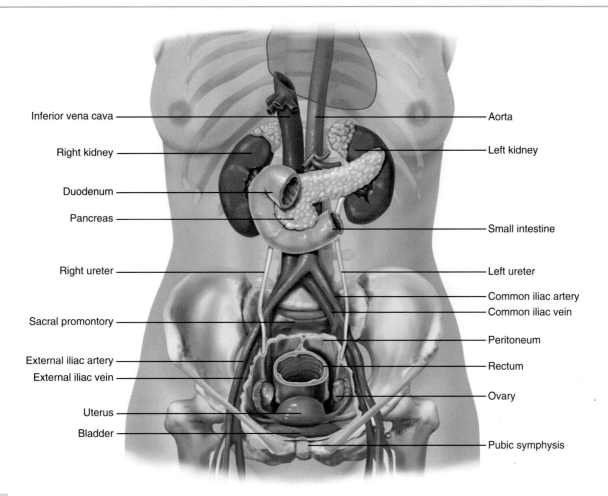

Inferior vena cava

Right kidney

Duodenum

Pancreas

Right ureter

Sacral promontory

External iliac artery

External iliac vein

Uterus

Bladder

Aorta

Left kidney

Small intestine

Left ureter

Common iliac artery

Common iliac vein

Peritoneum

Rectum

Ovary

Pubic symphysis

22-4

© Pat Thomas, 2006.

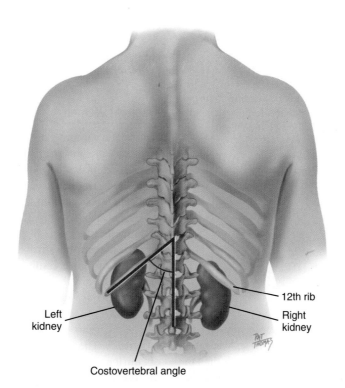

Left
kidney

12th rib

Right
kidney

Costovertebral angle

22-5

© Pat Thomas, 2006.

Structure & Function

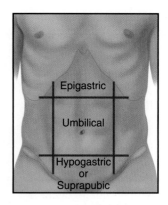

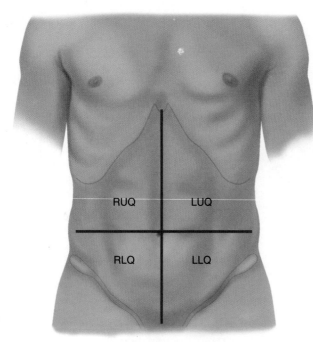

Four quadrants

22-6

The anatomical location of each organ by quadrants is listed as follows:

RIGHT UPPER QUADRANT (RUQ)

Liver
Gallbladder
Duodenum
Head of pancreas
Right kidney and adrenal
   gland
Hepatic flexure of colon
Parts of ascending and
   transverse colon

RIGHT LOWER QUADRANT (RLQ)

Cecum
Appendix
Right ovary and fallopian tube
Right ureter
Right spermatic cord

MIDLINE

Aorta
Uterus (if enlarged)
Bladder (if distended)

LEFT UPPER QUADRANT (LUQ)

Stomach
Spleen
Left lobe of liver
Body of pancreas
Left kidney and adrenal
   gland
Splenic flexure of colon
Parts of transverse and
   descending colon

LEFT LOWER QUADRANT (LLQ)

Part of descending colon
Sigmoid colon
Left ovary and fallopian
   tube
Left ureter
Left spermatic cord

❖ DEVELOPMENTAL CONSIDERATIONS

Infants and Children

In newborns, the umbilical cord shows prominently on the abdomen. It contains two arteries and one vein. The liver takes up proportionately more space in the abdomen at birth than in later life. In healthy full-term newborns, the lower edge may be palpated 0.5 to 2.5 cm below the right costal margin. Age-related values of expected liver size are listed in the Objective Data

section. The urinary bladder is located higher in the abdomen in newborns than in adults. It lies between the symphysis and the umbilicus. Also, during early childhood, the abdominal wall is less muscular, and so the organs may be easier to palpate.

Children younger than 10 years are at highest risk for acute gastrointestinal illness involving vomiting or diarrhea (Majowicz, Horrocks, & Bocking, 2007). Children with gastroenteritis, particularly those younger than 1 year, are at increased risk for dehydration because of their relatively small body weights and high turnover of water and electrolytes. Signs of clinical dehydration that indicate increased risk of progression to shock include altered responsiveness (irritability, lethargy), sunken eyes, tachycardia, tachypnea, and reduced skin turgor (Khanna, Lakhanpaul, Burman-Roy, & Murphy, 2009).

Pregnant Women

Nausea and vomiting, or "morning sickness," is an early sign of pregnancy in many pregnant women, starting between the first and second missed periods. The cause is unknown but may be related to hormone changes, such as the production of human chorionic gonadotropin. Another symptom is "acid indigestion," or heartburn, caused by esophageal reflux. Elevated levels of progesterone relax all smooth muscle, which leads to a decrease in gastrointestinal motility and prolongation of gastric emptying time. As a result of decreased motility, more water is reabsorbed from the colon, which leads to constipation. The constipation, as well as increased venous pressure in the lower pelvis, may lead to the formation of hemorrhoids.

The enlarging uterus displaces the intestines upward and posteriorly. The gradual upward displacement of the appendix during pregnancy was confirmed by two studies through the use of magnetic resonance imaging (Oto et al., 2006; Pates, Avendanio, Zaretsky, McIntire, & Twickler, 2009); however, appendicitis-related pain during pregnancy may still be felt in the RLQ (Mourad, Elliott, Erickson, & Lisboa, 2000). Bowel sounds are diminished. Skin changes on the abdomen, such as striae and linea nigra, are discussed later in this chapter and in Chapter 13.

Older Adults

Aging alters the appearance of the abdominal wall. During and after middle age, some fat accumulates in the suprapubic area in women as a result of decreased estrogen levels. Men also show some fat deposits in the abdominal area, which results in the "big belly." This development is accentuated in adults with a sedentary lifestyle. With further aging, adipose tissue is redistributed away from the face and extremities and to the abdomen and hips, and the abdominal musculature relaxes. Changes of aging occur in the gastrointestinal system but do not significantly affect function as long as no disease is present.

- Salivation decreases, causing dryness of the mouth and a decrease in the sense of taste. Further changes are discussed in Chapter 17.
- Esophageal emptying is delayed. Feeding an older adult in the supine position increases risk of aspiration.
- Gastric acid secretion decreases with aging. As a result, the absorption of orally administered drugs may be impaired or delayed. This may cause pernicious anemia (as a result of impaired vitamin B_{12} absorption), iron deficiency anemia, and malabsorption of calcium.
- Older adults are more susceptible to dehydration because the ability to conserve water is reduced, as are the ability to respond to changes in temperature and the acuteness of thirst.
- Liver size decreases with age, particularly after 80 years, although most liver function remains normal. Drug metabolism may be impaired in older adults as a result of decreased blood flow to the liver and decreased oxidative processes (Howland, 2009). In addition, renal function decreases with age, which contributes to the increased risk for adverse or toxic effects, inasmuch as most drugs are eventually cleared through the kidneys after metabolism in the liver. Older adults who drink alcohol and take medications are at even greater risk for adverse medication reactions, including exacerbation of therapeutic and adverse effects and interference with effectiveness of medications (Moore, Whiteman, & Ward, 2007).
- The incidence of gallstones increases with age, occurring in up to 20% of Canadian women and 10% of Canadian men by age 60 (Canadian Liver Foundation, 2011).
- Age-related changes alone do not account for the frequent reports of constipation by older adults. Common risk factors in older adults include functional impairments such as decreased mobility, pathological conditions such as hypothyroidism, adverse medication effects, and poor dietary habits, including inadequate intake of fluids and fibre (Miller, 2012). Additional lifestyle factors that contribute to constipation include prolonged use and overuse of laxatives; ignoring the defecation urge; sedentary lifestyle; and polypharmacy (Registered Nurses Association of Ontario, 2005). Medications associated with constipation

PROMOTING HEALTH: HEPATITIS RISK

How's Your Liver Doing?

The liver is the largest organ in the body. It has an immense capacity to heal and regenerate, but that capacity is not infinite. Unfortunately, signs of severe liver damage or disease usually do not become apparent until the liver has been significantly harmed. The best protection for the liver is to prevent damage *before* it occurs!

Many self-management measures can be taken to protect the liver:

- *Practise safe sex.* Do not have unprotected sex with a man or woman.
- *Do not share items that may have bodily fluids on them.* This means needles, razors, nail clippers, cuticle scissors, and toothbrushes. If you are getting a tattoo, make sure that a new bottle of ink is opened and used only for you. Access clean needle exchange programs if you use injected drugs.
- *Be aware of your environment.* Be careful with aerosol cleaners. Make sure rooms are well ventilated. Wear a mask, a hat, or protective clothing when you use insecticides, fungicides, paint, or other toxic chemicals. The liver can be damaged by what you breathe or absorb through your skin.
- *Monitor your diet and weight.* Obesity can cause a condition called *nonalcoholic fatty liver disease,* which may include cirrhosis.
- *Travel wisely.* Visit a travel medicine clinic before travelling. If you travel to an area with an increased rate of hepatitis A, such as Mexico, Central America, and the Caribbean, get vaccinated; avoid eating uncooked food, including raw vegetables; avoid drinking unboiled or unbottled water (including ice cubes); and brush your teeth with boiled or bottled water.

- *Use medications wisely.* Use prescription and over-the-counter medications only when needed. Be sure to take only the recommended doses.
- *Do not mix medications without consulting a health care provider.* Mixing certain medications can cause the formation of toxic compounds that can cause liver damage. Be certain that all medications, including over-the-counter and herbal preparations, are approved by a health care provider.
- *Drink alcohol in moderation.* More than one drink a day for women or two drinks a day for men over many years may be enough to lead to cirrhosis. A cirrhotic liver shrinks to a fraction of its former size and ability.
- *Do not mix medications and alcohol.* Acetaminophen can be toxic to the liver even if a person drinks alcohol in moderation.
- *Do not use illegal drugs.* Cocaine is one of many illegal drugs known to cause liver damage.
- *Get vaccinated.* A vaccine is available for both hepatitis A and hepatitis B. Universal immunization of children and adolescents against hepatitis B is now part of the publicly funded vaccine programs offered in all Canadian provinces and territories.
- *Be aware of your risk for hepatitis.* Six hepatitis viruses have been identified, but three—hepatitis A (HAV), hepatitis B (HBV), and hepatitis C (HCV)—cause approximately 90% of acute hepatitis cases in Canada. The annual incidence of HAV illness has been estimated at 2.9 cases per 100,000 persons in Canada; the annual incidence of HBV illness is higher, at approximately 4.9 cases per 100,000 persons; and the annual

Continued

PROMOTING HEALTH: HEPATITIS RISK—cont'd

incidence of HCV illness is highest, at between 10 and 20 cases per 100,000 persons.

HAV is spread primarily through food or water contaminated by feces from an infected patient. Risk factors for HAV infection include the following:

- Eating food that has been prepared by someone who has HAV infection and poor hygiene
- Eating raw or undercooked shellfish (such as oysters or clams)
- Eating uncooked food, including unpeeled fruits and vegetables
- Travelling to HAV-endemic areas
- Having homosexual relations
- Sharing a household with an HAV-infected patient

HBV is spread primarily through contact with infected blood or bodily fluids. Risk factors for HBV infection include the following:

- Having unprotected sex, especially with someone with HBV infection or whose sexual history is unknown
- Sharing needles or other drug use equipment, including spoons, water, and cotton, to inject illegal drugs

- Handling blood or bodily fluids as a routine part of your job (such jobs include those of nurses and other health care providers, as well as morticians and embalmers)
- Getting body piercings or tattoos from a site in which infection control practices are poor
- Travelling to HBV-endemic areas
- Sharing a household with an HBV-infected patient
- Receiving dialysis treatment

HCV is spread primarily through contact with infected blood. Risk factors for HCV infection include the following:

- Having received a transfusion before 1992 or clotting factors before 1987
- Using illegal intravenous drugs or intranasal cocaine
- Handling blood or bodily fluids as a routine part of a job
- Receiving dialysis treatment
- Getting body piercings or tattoos from a site in which infection control practices are poor
- Sharing a household with an HCV-infected patient

Sources: Data from Canadian Liver Foundation. (2012). *Viral hepatitis A, B, C.* Retrieved from *http://www.liver.ca/liver-disease/types/viral-hepatitis-a-b-c.aspx*; from Health Canada. (2008). *Hepatitis.* Retrieved from *http://www.hc-sc.gc.ca/hc-ps/dc-ma/hep-eng.php;* and from Public Health Agency of Canada. (2006). *Canadian immunization guide* (Evergreen ed.). Retrieved from *http://www.phac-aspc.gc.ca/publicat/cig-gci/index-eng.php.*

include nonsteroidal anti-inflammatory drugs (NSAIDs), diuretics, calcium channel blockers, opioids, antiparkinsonian agents, antacids, and calcium or iron supplements (Mauk, 2005).

- The risk for colorectal cancer increases with age. See Chapter 23 for screening recommendations.

 ### CULTURAL AND SOCIAL CONSIDERATIONS

Lactase is the digestive enzyme necessary for absorption of the carbohydrate lactose (milk sugar). In some individuals, lactase activity is high at birth but declines to low levels by adulthood. These people are **lactose intolerant** and have abdominal pain, bloating, and flatulence when they consume milk products. Lactose intolerance affects as much as 70% of the world's population. The prevalence of lactose intolerance is higher among Aboriginal Canadians and Canadians of African, Asian, Middle Eastern, or South American descent, and it is rarer in Canadians of European descent.

Rates of celiac disease have nearly doubled since the 1980s in Western countries; it has been diagnosed in more than 330,000 Canadians, including more than 73,000 children (Canadian Digestive Health Foundation, 2012). Celiac disease is an inherited autoimmune condition in which intestinal tissue is damaged in response to eating gluten, which creates a risk for malabsorption of nutrients, which in turn may result in conditions such as iron-deficiency anemia and osteoporosis (American Celiac Disease Alliance, 2013).

Between 10% and 20% of the Canadian population experience the troublesome symptoms of heartburn and regurgitation associated with gastroesophageal reflux disease (GERD; Fedorak, van Zanten, & Bridges, 2010). Modifiable risk factors for GERD include obesity, smoking, and a high-cholesterol diet. Older adults and patients with cystic fibrosis are also at higher risk for developing GERD.

Canada has the highest incidence of gastrointestinal ulcers in the world. Peptic ulcer disease occurs with frequent use of NSAIDS, alcohol, smoking, and infection with *Helicobacter pylori.* Eight to 10 million Canadians have *H. pylori* infection; approximately 75% of First Nations people are infected (Canadian Digestive Health Foundation, 2012).

Canada also has one of the highest incidences of inflammatory bowel disease (IBD) in the world. More than 200,000 Canadians live with IBD: 112,000 with Crohn's disease and 88,500 with ulcerative colitis (Crohn's and Colitis Foundation of Canada, 2008). IBD can be diagnosed at any age, but usual onset is in the 20s for Chrohn's disease and throughout adulthood for ulcerative colitis; incidence for both diseases peaks by age 30 and does not decline until age 80. A diagnosis of IBD is associated with a higher risk for colorectal cancer.

Infectious diseases such as hepatitis A and gastrointestinal illnesses are often related to socioeconomic factors such as inadequate housing, sewage, and water-treatment facilities (see the box Promoting Health: Hepatitis Risk). These conditions are often present in Aboriginal communities (Noël & Larocque, 2009).

SUBJECTIVE DATA

1. Appetite
2. Dysphagia

3. Food intolerance
4. Abdominal pain

5. Nausea/vomiting
6. Bowel habits
7. Past abdominal history

8. Medications
9. Alcohol and tobacco
10. Nutritional assessment

HEALTH HISTORY QUESTIONS

Examiner Asks	Rationale
1. **Appetite.** Any change in **appetite?** Is this change a loss of appetite? • Any change in weight? How much weight gained or lost? Over what time period? Is the weight loss due to diet?	**Anorexia** is a loss of appetite that occurs with gastrointestinal disease, is a side effect of some medications, occurs with pregnancy, or occurs with psychological disorders. Loss of appetite and unexplained weight loss may be a sign of gastrointestinal cancers such as stomach, esophageal, and pancreatic cancer.
2. **Dysphagia.** Any difficulty swallowing? When did you first notice this?	**Dysphagia** occurs with disorders of the throat or esophagus, such as the later stages of esophageal cancer.
3. **Food intolerance.** Are there any foods you cannot eat? • What happens if you do eat them: allergic reaction, heartburn, belching, bloating, indigestion? • Do you use antacids? How often?	Examples of food intolerance are lactase deficiency (resulting in bloating or excessive gas after ingesting milk products) and wheat allergy or gluten intolerance (resulting in abdominal pain, distension, or diarrhea). **Pyrosis** (heartburn) is a burning sensation in esophagus and stomach, caused by reflux of gastric acid. Excessive eructation (belching) may occur with food intolerance.
4. **Abdominal pain.** Do you have any **abdominal pain?** Please point to it. • Is the pain in one spot, or does it move around? • How did it start? How long have you had it? • Is the pain constant, or does it come and go? Does it occur before or after meals? Does it peak? When? • How would you describe the character: cramping (colic type), burning in pit of stomach, dull, stabbing, aching? • Is the pain relieved by food, or is it worse after eating? • Is the pain associated with the menstrual period or menstrual irregularities, stress, dietary indiscretion, fatigue, nausea and vomiting, gas, fever, rectal bleeding, frequent urination, vaginal or penile discharge?	Abdominal pain may be *visceral,* from an internal organ (dull, general, poorly localized); *parietal,* from inflammation of overlying peritoneum (sharp, precisely localized, aggravated by movement); or *referred,* from a disorder in another site (see Table 22-2 on p. 577). Acute pain that necessitates urgent diagnosis occurs with appendicitis, cholecystitis, bowel obstruction, or perforation of an organ. Pain in the upper abdomen is a symptom that may occur in the later stages of gastrointestinal neoplasms, such as liver or pancreatic cancer. Chronic pain of gastric ulcers usually occurs on an empty stomach; pain of duodenal ulcers occurs 2 to 3 hours after a meal and is relieved by more food.
• What makes the pain worse: food, position, stress, medication, activity? • What have you tried in order to relieve pain: rest, heating pad, change in position, medication?	
5. **Nausea/vomiting.** Any **nausea** or **vomiting?** • How often? How much comes up? What is the colour? Does it have an odour? • Is it bloody? • Are the nausea and vomiting associated with colicky pain, diarrhea, fever, chills?	Nausea/vomiting is a common side effect of many medications, with gastrointestinal disease, and in early pregnancy. Nausea/vomiting may occur in later stages of gastrointestinal neoplasms, such as stomach, liver, or pancreatic cancer. **Hematemesis** occurs with stomach or duodenal ulcers and esophageal varices.

Examiner Asks	Rationale

- What foods did you eat in the past 24 hours? Where: at home, school, a restaurant? Has anyone else in the family had the same symptoms in the past 24 hours?

Consider food poisoning.

6. Bowel habits. How often do you have a **bowel movement?**
   - What is the colour? Consistency?
   - Any diarrhea or constipation? How long?
   - Any recent change in bowel habits?
   - Do you use laxatives? Which ones? How often do you use them?

Assess usual **bowel habits.**

Stools may be black and tarry because of occult blood (melena) from gastrointestinal bleeding, or they may be black but nontarry because of iron medications. Grey stools occur with hepatitis.

Red blood in stools occurs with gastrointestinal bleeding or localized bleeding around the anus. A change in bowel habits, stools that are narrower than usual, blood in the stool, diarrhea, and constipation are possible symptoms of colorectal cancer and necessitate further investigations.

7. Past abdominal history. Any **history** of gastrointestinal problems: ulcer, gallbladder disease, hepatitis/jaundice, appendicitis, colitis, hernia?
   - Any **family history** of irritable bowel disease (IBD), colorectal cancer, or familial adenomatous polyposis (FAP)?
   - Ever had any operations in the abdomen? Please describe.
   - Any problems after surgery?
   - Any abdominal X-ray studies? How were the results?

FAP is caused by a genetic mutation that can be inherited. In individuals with FAP, the risk for colon cancer is 87% by age 45.

8. Medications. What **medications** are you currently taking?
   - Do you take over-the-counter remedies?
   - Do you take natural or herbal supplements?

Many prescription and over-the-counter medications, such as acetaminophen and salicylates, can have toxic effects on the liver. Peptic ulcer disease occurs with frequent use of NSAIDs, alcohol, smoking, and *H. pylori* infection.

Herbal supplements such as ginkgo biloba may cause gastrointestinal upset, nausea and vomiting, or prolonged bleeding.

9. Alcohol and tobacco. How much alcohol would you say you drink each day? Each week? When was your most recent alcoholic drink?
   - Do you smoke? How many packs per day? How long have you smoked?

Heavy alcohol drinking is a risk factor for esophageal cancer, liver cancer, and cirrhosis of the liver. Alcohol can also increase the toxic effects of medications such as acetaminophen on the liver.

Smoking is a risk factor for esophageal, stomach, and pancreatic cancers.

10. Nutritional assessment. Now I would like to ask you about your diet. Please tell me all the food you ate yesterday, starting with breakfast.
    - Does the diet follow Canada's Food Guide?

Nutritional assessment is based on a 24-hour recall (see Chapter 12 for a complete discussion).

Additional History for Infants Children

1. Feeding infants. Are you breastfeeding the baby, or are you feeding the baby formula? If formula-feeding, how does the baby tolerate the formula?
2. Table foods. What table foods have you introduced? How does the infant tolerate the food?

Consider a new food as a possible allergen. Adding only one new food at a time to the infant's diet helps identify allergies.

3. Eating patterns. How often does your toddler/child eat? Does he or she eat regular meals?
   - Does the child's diet follow *Canada's Food Guide*?
   - How do you feel about your child's eating problems?
   - Please describe all that your child had to eat yesterday, starting with breakfast. What foods does the child eat for snacks?

Irregular eating patterns are common among children and a source of parental anxiety. As long as a child shows normal growth and development and only nutritious foods are offered, parents may be reassured. Refer to *Canada's Food Guide* in Chapter 12.

Examiner Asks	Rationale
• Does the toddler or child ever eat nonfoods (grass, dirt, paint chips)?	Although a toddler may attempt to eat nonfoods (**pica**) at some time, he or she should recognize which materials are edible by age 2 years.
4. **Constipation.** Does your child have constipation: How long? • What are the number of stools per day? Stools per week? • How much water or juice is in the diet? • Does the constipation seem to be associated with toilet training? • What have you tried in order to treat the constipation?	
5. **Abdominal pain.** Does the child have abdominal pain? Please describe what you have noticed and when it started.	This symptom is hard to assess with young children. Many conditions of unrelated organ systems (e.g., otitis media) are associated with vague abdominal pain. The children cannot articulate specific symptoms and often focus on "the tummy." Abdominal pain accompanies inflammation of the bowel, constipation, urinary tract infection, and anxiety.
6. **Overweight children.** How long has weight been a problem? • At what age did the child first seem overweight? Did any change in diet pattern occur then? Is the *Canada Food Guide* being followed? • Describe the diet pattern now. • Do any other family members have a similar problem? • How does child feel about his or her own weight?	Reduced physical activity and poor food marketing practices contribute to the current obesity epidemic (Keith, Redden, & Katzmarzyk, 2006). Assess for family history of obesity. Assess body image.

Additional History for Adolescents

Examiner Asks	Rationale
1. **Schedule and content.** What do you eat at regular meals? Do you eat breakfast? What do you eat for snacks?	Adolescents take control of eating and may reject family values (e.g., skipping breakfast, consuming junk foods, soft drinks). The only control parents have is over what food is in the home.
• How many calories do you figure you consume?	You probably cannot change an adolescent's eating pattern, but you can supply nutritional facts.
2. **Exercise.** What is your exercise pattern?	Boys need, on average, 4000 calories/day to maintain weight and more calories if they participate in sports. Girls need 20% fewer calories and the same nutrients as boys. Fast food is high in fat, calories, and salt, and it has no fibre.
3. **Underweight.** If weight is less than body requirements: How much have you lost? By diet, exercise, or how?	Screen any extremely thin adolescent for **anorexia nervosa,** a serious psychosocial disorder that includes loss of appetite, voluntary starvation, and grave weight loss. Such patients may augment weight loss by purging (self-induced vomiting) and using laxatives.
• How do you feel? Tired, hungry? How do you think your body looks?	Denial of hunger and tiredness is common in anorexia. Although thin, such patients insist that they look fat and "disgusting." Body image is distorted.
• What is your activity pattern?	Patients with anorexia may have healthy activity and exercise, but many are hyperactive.
• Is the weight loss associated with any other body change, such as menstrual irregularity?	Amenorrhea is common with anorexia nervosa.

Subjective Data

Examiner Asks	Rationale
• What do your parents say about your eating? Your friends?	This is a family problem involving control issues. Anyone at risk requires immediate referral to a physician or psychologist.

Additional History for Older Adults

1. Food access. How do you acquire your groceries and prepare your meals?

Assess risk for nutritional deficit: limited access to grocery store, limited income, or limited cooking facilities; physical disability (impaired vision, decreased mobility, decreased strength, neurological deficit).

2. Emotional characteristics. Do you eat alone or share meals with others?

Assess risk for nutritional deficit if the patient is living alone; he or she may not bother to prepare all meals. Assess for social isolation and depression.

3. Recall. Please tell me all that you had to eat yesterday, starting with breakfast.

Note: 24-hour recall may not be sufficient because daily pattern may vary. The patient should attempt a week-long diary of intake. Food pattern may be different during a month if monthly income (e.g., Old Age Security pension cheque) runs out.

• Do you have any trouble swallowing these foods?
• What do you do right after eating: walk, take a nap?

4. Bowel movements. How often do your bowels move?

   • If the patient reports constipation: What do you mean by "constipation"? How much liquid is in your diet? How much bulk or fibre?

To prevent constipation, fluid intake should be between 1500 and 2000 mL/day; dietary fibre intake should be from 25 to 30 g/day (Registered Nurses Association of Ontario, 2005).

   • Do you take anything for constipation, such as laxatives? Which ones? How often?
   • What medications do you take?

Consider gastrointestinal side effects (e.g., nausea, upset stomach, anorexia, dry mouth).

OBJECTIVE DATA

PREPARATION

The lighting should include a strong overhead light and a secondary stand light. Expose the patient's abdomen so that it is fully visible. Drape the genitalia and female breasts.

The following measures will enhance abdominal wall relaxation:

- Instruct the patient to empty the bladder, saving a urine specimen if needed.
- Keep the room warm to avoid chilling and tensing of muscles.
- Position the patient supine, with the head on a pillow, the knees bent or on pillow, and the arms at the sides or across the chest. (Note: Discourage the patient from placing his or her arms over the head, because this tenses abdominal musculature.)
- To avoid abdominal tensing, warm the stethoscope endpiece and your hands, and keep your fingernails very short.
- Inquire about any painful areas. Examine such an area last to avoid any muscle guarding.
- Finally, learn to use distraction: enhance muscle relaxation through breathing exercises and/or emotive imagery; keep your voice low and soothing; and encourage the patient to relate his or her abdominal history while you palpate.

EQUIPMENT NEEDED

Stethoscope
Small centimetre ruler
Skin-marking pen
Alcohol wipe (to clean endpiece)

Subjective Data

Objective Data

Normal Range of Findings	Abnormal Findings

INSPECT THE ABDOMEN

Contour

Stand on the patient's right side and look down on the abdomen. Then stoop or sit to gaze across the abdomen. Your head should be slightly higher than the abdomen (Figure 22-7). Determine the profile from the rib margin to the pubic bone. The contour describes the nutritional state and normally ranges from flat to rounded (Figure 22-8).

A scaphoid abdomen caves in. Protuberant abdomen and abdominal distension (see Table 22-1, p. 575) are abnormal.

Flat

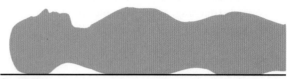

Scaphoid

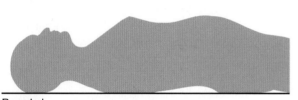

Rounded

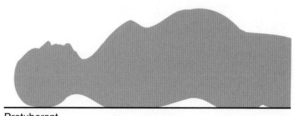

Protuberant

22-7

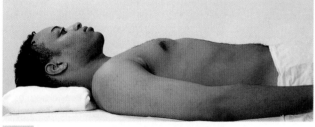

22-8

Symmetry

Shine a light across the abdomen toward you, or shine it lengthwise across the patient. The abdomen should be symmetrical bilaterally. Note any localized bulging, visible mass, or asymmetrical shape. Even small bulges are highlighted by shadow. Step to the foot of the examination table to recheck symmetry.

Ask the patient to take a deep breath to further highlight any change. The abdomen should stay smooth and symmetrical. You can also ask the patient to perform a sit-up without pushing up with his or her hands.

Bulges, masses.
Hernia: protrusion of abdominal viscera through abnormal opening in muscle wall (see Table 22-3, p. 578).
Note any localized bulging.
Hernia, enlarged liver, or spleen may show.

Umbilicus

Normally the umbilicus is midline and inverted, with no sign of discoloration, inflammation, or hernia. It becomes everted and pushed upward during pregnancy.

The umbilicus is a common site for piercings in young women. The site should not be red or crusted.

Everted: with ascites or underlying mass (see Table 22-1, p. 576).
Deeply sunken: with obesity.
Enlarged and everted: with umbilical hernia.
Bluish periumbilical colour: with intra-abdominal bleeding (Cullen's sign), although rare.

Normal Range of Findings	Abnormal Findings

Skin

The surface is smooth and even, with homogeneous colour. This area is helpful for judging pigment because it is often protected from sun.

Redness: with localized inflammation.

Jaundice (shows best in natural daylight).

Glistening and tautness of skin: with ascites.

One common pigment change is **striae** (lineae albicantes), which are silvery white, linear, jagged marks approximately 1 to 6 cm long (Figure 22-9). They occur when elastic fibres in the reticular layer of the skin are broken after rapid or prolonged stretching, as in pregnancy or excessive weight gain. Recent striae are pink or blue; then they turn silvery white.

Striae also occur with ascites.

Striae look purple-blue in patients with Cushing's syndrome (because excess adrenocortical hormone causes the skin to be fragile and easily broken from normal stretching).

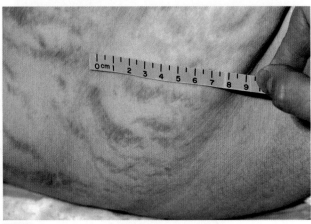

22-9 Striae.

Pigmented nevi (moles), which are circumscribed brown macular or papular areas, are common on the abdomen.

Normally, no lesions are present, although you may note well-healed surgical scars. If a scar is present, draw its location in the patient's record, indicating the length in centimetres (Figure 22-10). (Note: Sometimes patients forget a past operation while providing the history. If you note a scar, ask about it.) A surgical scar alerts you to the possible presence of underlying adhesions and excess fibrous tissue.

Unusual colour or change in shape of mole (see Chapter 13).

Petechiae.

Cutaneous angiomas (spider nevi) occur with portal hypertension or liver disease.

Lesions and rashes warrant investigation (see Chapter 13).

Underlying adhesions are inflammatory bands that connect opposite sides of serous surfaces after trauma or surgery.

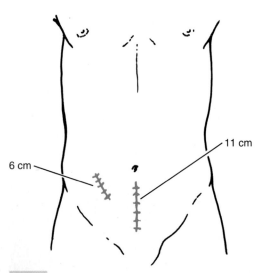

22-10

Normal Range of Findings	Abnormal Findings

Veins usually are not seen, but a fine venous network may be visible in thin patients.

Veins may become prominent and dilated with portal hypertension, cirrhosis, ascites, or vena caval obstruction. Veins are more visible with malnutrition as a result of thinned adipose tissue.

Good skin turgor reflects healthy nutrition. Gently pinch up a fold of skin; then release to note the skin's immediate return to original position.

Turgor is poor with dehydration, which often accompanies gastrointestinal disease.

Pulsation or Movement

Normally, you may see the pulsations from the aorta beneath the skin in the epigastric area, particularly in thin patients with good muscle wall relaxation. Respiratory movement also shows in the abdomen, particularly in men. Waves of peristalsis are sometimes visible in very thin patients. They ripple slowly and obliquely across the abdomen.

Pulsation of the aorta is marked with widened pulse pressure (e.g., hypertension, aortic insufficiency, thyrotoxicosis) and with aortic aneurysm.

Markedly visible peristalsis, together with abdominal distension, indicates intestinal obstruction.

Hair Distribution

The pattern of pubic hair growth normally has a diamond shape in men and an inverted triangle shape in women (see Chapters 26 and 27).

Patterns alter with endocrine or hormone abnormalities and with chronic liver disease.

Demeanour

A comfortable patient is relaxed quietly on the examining table, has a benign facial expression, and has slow, even respirations.

Restlessness and constant turning to find comfort occur with the colicky pain of gastroenteritis or bowel obstruction.

Absolute stillness, resisting any movement, occurs with the pain of peritonitis.

Upward flexing of the knees, facial grimacing, and rapid, uneven respirations also indicate pain.

AUSCULTATE BOWEL SOUNDS AND VASCULAR SOUNDS

Depart from the usual examination sequence and auscultate the abdomen next. Auscultation is done first because percussion and palpation can increase peristalsis, which would give a false interpretation of bowel sounds. Also, if you hear a bruit during auscultation, you should avoid percussion and palpation. Use the diaphragm endpiece because bowel sounds are relatively high pitched. Hold the stethoscope lightly against the skin; pushing too hard may stimulate more bowel sounds (Figure 22-11). Listen in all four quadrants, beginning in the RLQ at the ileocecal valve area because bowel sounds are normally always present here.

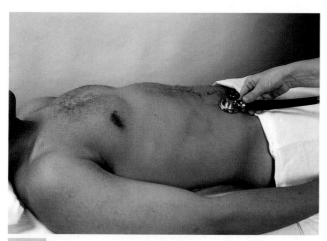

22-11

Objective Data

Normal Range of Findings	Abnormal Findings

Bowel Sounds

Note the character and frequency of bowel sounds. Bowel sounds originate from the movement of air and fluid through the small intestine. Depending on the time elapsed since eating, normal sounds range widely. Bowel sounds are high-pitched, gurgling, cascading sounds, occurring irregularly anywhere from 5 to 30 times per minute. Do not bother to count them. Judge whether they are normal, hypoactive, or hyperactive.

One type of hyperactive bowel sounds is fairly common. This is the hyper-peristalsis when you feel your "stomach growling," termed **borborygmus.** A perfectly "silent abdomen" is uncommon; you must listen for 5 minutes by your watch before deciding that bowel sounds are completely absent.

Abnormal bowel sounds have two distinct patterns:
1. **Hyperactive sounds** are loud, high-pitched, rushing, tinkling sounds that signal increased motility and may indicate bowel obstruction.
2. Sounds may be **hypoactive** or **absent** after abdominal surgery or with inflammation of the peritoneum (see Table 22-4, p. 579).

Vascular Sounds

Using firmer pressure, listen with the bell of the stethoscope to check over the aorta and the renal arteries, iliac, and femoral arteries, especially in patients with hypertension (Figure 22-12). Note the presence of any vascular sounds or **bruits.** Usually, no such sound is present.

Note location, pitch, and timing of a vascular sound.

A systolic bruit is a pulsatile blowing sound and occurs with stenosis or occlusion of an artery.

Venous hum and peritoneal friction rub are rare (see Table 22-5, p. 580 and the Critical Findings box below).

CRITICAL FINDINGS

If a bruit is heard over the aorta, you should *not* palpate the area, to avoid rupturing a possible aortic aneurysm. Report findings immediately.

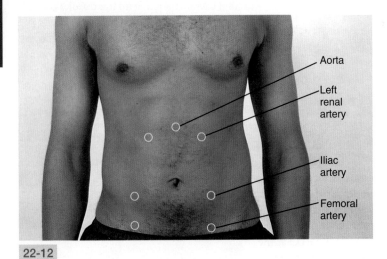

Aorta

Left renal artery

Iliac artery

Femoral artery

22-12

PERCUSS GENERAL TYMPANY, LIVER SPAN, AND SPLENIC DULLNESS

Percuss to assess the relative density of abdominal contents, to locate organs, and to screen for abnormal fluid or masses.

General Tympany

First, percuss lightly in all four quadrants to determine the prevailing amount of tympany and dullness (Figure 22-13). Move clockwise. Tympany should predominate because air in the intestines rises to the surface when the patient is supine.

Dullness is heard over a distended bladder, adipose tissue, fluid, or a mass.

Hyperresonance is heard with gaseous distension.

Normal Range of Findings	Abnormal Findings

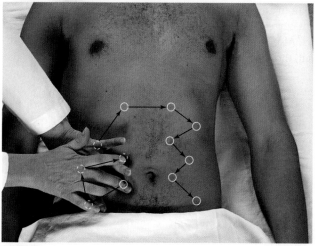

22-13

SPECIAL CONSIDERATIONS FOR ADVANCED PRACTICE

Liver Span

Next, percuss to map out the boundaries of certain organs. Measure the height of the liver in the right midclavicular line. (For a consistent placement of the midclavicular line landmark, remember to palpate the acromioclavicular and the sternoclavicular joints, and judge the line at a point midway between the two.)

Begin in the area of lung resonance, and percuss down the intercostal spaces until the sound changes to a dull quality (Figure 22-14). Mark the spot on the patient's body, usually in the fifth intercostal space. Then find abdominal tympany and percuss up in the midclavicular line. Mark the spot on the patient's body where the sound changes from tympany to a dull sound, normally at the right costal margin.

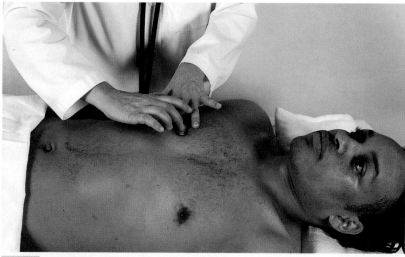

22-14

Objective Data

Normal Range of Findings

Measure the distance between the two marks; the normal liver span in adults ranges from 6 to 12 cm (Figure 22-15). The height of the liver span is correlated with with the height of the patient; taller people have longer livers. Also, men have a longer liver span than do women of the same height. Overall, the mean liver span is 10.5 cm in men and 7 cm in women.

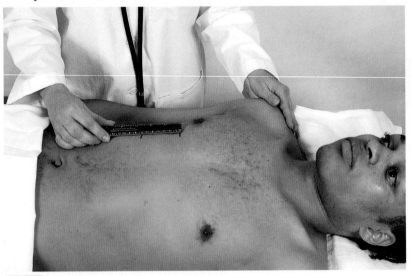

22-15

One variation occurs in people with chronic emphysema, in which the liver is displaced downward by the hyperinflated lungs. Although you hear a dull percussion note well below the right costal margin, the overall span is still within normal limits.

Clinical estimation of liver span is important in screening for hepatomegaly and in monitoring changes in liver size. However, this measurement is a gross estimate; the liver span may be underestimated because of inaccurate detection of the upper border.

Scratch Test. Another assessment technique is the *scratch test,* which may help define the liver border when the abdomen is distended or the abdominal muscles are tense. Place your stethoscope over the liver. With one fingernail, scratch short strokes over the abdomen, starting in the RLQ and moving progressively up toward the liver (Figure 22-16). When the scratching sound in your stethoscope becomes magnified, you will have crossed the border from over a hollow organ to over a solid one.

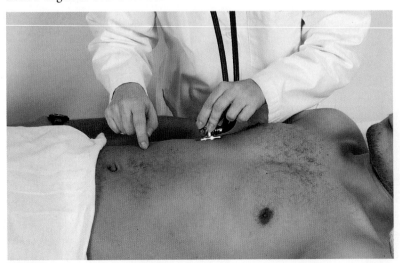

22-16

Abnormal Findings

Elongation of the liver span indicates liver enlargement **(hepatomegaly).**

Detection of liver borders is rendered inaccurate by dullness above the fifth intercostal space, which occurs with lung disease (e.g., pleural effusion or consolidation). Detection at the lower border is rendered inaccurate when dullness is pushed up with ascites or pregnancy or with gas distension in colon, which obscures the lower border.

Normal Range of Findings	Abnormal Findings

Splenic Dullness

Often the spleen is obscured by stomach contents, but you may locate it by percussing for a dull note from the ninth to eleventh intercostal spaces just behind the left midaxillary line (Figure 22-17). The area of splenic dullness normally is not wider than 7 cm in the adult and should not encroach on the normal tympany over the gastric air bubble.

A dull note forward of the midaxillary line indicates enlargement of the spleen, as occurs with mononucleosis, trauma, and infection.

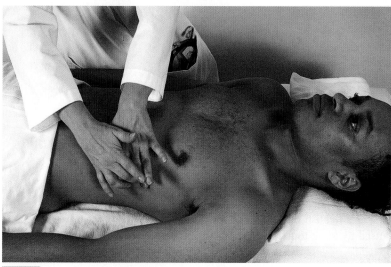

22-17

Now percuss in the lowest intercostal space in the left *anterior* axillary line. You should hear tympany. Ask the patient to take a deep breath. Normally, tympany remains through full inspiration.

In the anterior axillary line, a change in percussion from tympany to a dull sound with full inspiration is a **positive spleen percussion sign,** indicating splenomegaly. This method helps detect mild to moderate splenomegaly before the spleen becomes palpable, as in mononucleosis, malaria, or hepatic cirrhosis.

Costovertebral Angle Tenderness

Indirect fist percussion causes the tissues to vibrate instead of producing a sound. To assess the kidney, place one hand over the twelfth rib at the costovertebral angle on the back (Figure 22-18). Thump that hand with the ulnar edge of your other fist. The patient normally feels a thud but no pain. Perform the assessment bilaterally. (Although this step is explained here with percussion techniques, its usual sequence in a complete examination is with thoracic assessment, when the patient is sitting up and you are standing behind him or her.)

Sharp pain occurs with inflammation of the kidney or paranephric area.

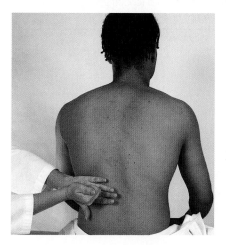

22-18

Normal Range of Findings	Abnormal Findings

PALPATE SURFACE AND DEEP AREAS

Perform palpation to judge the size, location, and consistency of certain organs and to screen for an abnormal mass or tenderness. Review comfort measures on p. 559. Because most people are naturally inclined to protect their abdomen, you need to use additional measures to enhance complete muscle relaxation:

1. Bend the patient's knees.
2. Keep your palpating hand low and parallel to the abdomen. Holding the hand high and pointing down would make anyone tense up.
3. Teach the patient to breathe slowly (in through the nose, and out through the mouth).
4. Keep your own voice low and soothing. Conversation may relax the patient.
5. Try "emotive imagery." For example, you might say, "Now I want you to imagine you are dozing on the beach, with the sun warming your muscles and the sound of the waves lulling you to sleep. Let yourself relax."
6. With a very ticklish patient, keep the patient's hand under your own with your fingers curled over his or her fingers. Move both hands around as you palpate; people are not ticklish to themselves.
7. Alternatively, perform palpation just after auscultation. Keep the stethoscope in place and curl your fingers around it, palpating as you pretend to auscultate. People generally do not perceive a stethoscope as a ticklish object. You can slide the stethoscope out when the patient is used to being touched.

Light Palpation

Begin with **light palpation.** With the first four fingers close together, depress the skin approximately 1 cm (Figure 22-19). Make a gentle rotary motion, sliding the fingers and skin together. Then lift the fingers (do not drag them) and move clockwise to the next location around the abdomen. The objective here is not to search for organs but to form an overall impression of the skin surface and superficial musculature. Save the examination of any identified tender areas until last. In this way, you avoid causing pain and the resulting muscle rigidity that would obscure deep palpation later in the examination.

Muscle guarding.
Rigidity.
Large masses.
Tenderness (see the Critical Findings box below).

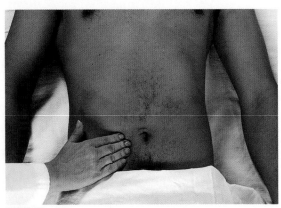

22-19

As you circle the abdomen, discriminate between voluntary muscle guarding and involuntary rigidity. **Voluntary guarding** occurs when the patient is cold, tense, or ticklish. It is bilateral, and you will feel the muscles relax slightly during exhalation. Use the relaxation measures described previously to try to eliminate this type of guarding, or it will interfere with deep palpation. If the rigidity persists, it is probably involuntary.

CRITICAL FINDINGS

RLQ tenderness on palpation in a patient with acute abdominal pain migrating from the umbilicus to the RLQ is indicative of **appendicitis,** the most common abdominal surgical emergency (Flaser & Goldberg, 2006).

Immediate referral to a surgeon is required. Associated symptoms include nausea, vomiting, fever, and loss of appetite. Additional signs include guarding, rigidity, rebound tenderness, and iliopsoas (see pp. 564–569).

RLQ, right lower quadrant.

Involuntary rigidity is a constant boardlike hardness of the muscles. It is a protective mechanism accompanying **peritonitis,** an acute inflammation of the peritoneum. It may be unilateral, and the same area usually becomes painful when the patient increases intra-abdominal pressure by attempting a sit-up.

Normal Range of Findings	Abnormal Findings

SPECIAL CONSIDERATIONS FOR ADVANCED PRACTICE

Deep Palpation

If appropriate, perform **deep palpation** by using the same technique described earlier, but push down approximately 5 to 8 cm (Figure 22-20). Moving clockwise, palpate the entire abdomen.

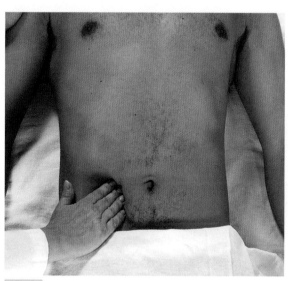

22-20

To overcome the resistance of a very large or obese abdomen, use a bimanual technique. Place your two hands on top of each other (Figure 22-21). The top hand does the pushing; the bottom hand is relaxed and can concentrate on the sense of palpation. With either technique, note the location, size, consistency, and mobility of any palpable organs and the presence of any abnormal enlargement, tenderness, or masses.

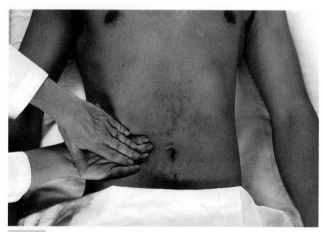

22-21

Making sense of what you are palpating is more difficult than it seems. Inexperienced examiners complain that the abdomen "all feels the same," as if they are pushing their hand into a soft sofa cushion. It helps to memorize the anatomy and visualize what is under each quadrant as you palpate. Also remember that some structures are normally palpable, as illustrated in Figure 22-22.

Objective Data

Normal Range of Findings	Abnormal Findings

Objective Data

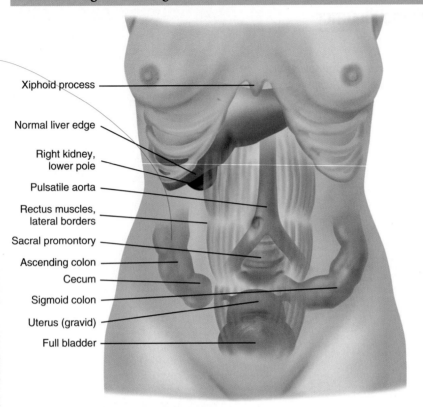

Xiphoid process

Normal liver edge

Right kidney, lower pole

Pulsatile aorta

Rectus muscles, lateral borders

Sacral promontory

Ascending colon

Cecum

Sigmoid colon

Uterus (gravid)

Full bladder

NORMALLY PALPABLE STRUCTURES

22-22

Mild tenderness normally is present when the sigmoid colon is palpated. Any other tenderness should be investigated.

If you identify a mass, first distinguish it from a normally palpable structure or an enlarged organ. Then note the following:

1. Location
2. Size
3. Shape
4. Consistency (soft, firm, hard)
5. Surface (smooth, nodular)
6. Mobility (including movement with respirations)
7. Pulsatility
8. Tenderness

Liver

Next, palpate for specific organs, beginning with the liver in the RUQ (Figure 22-23). Place your left hand under the patient's back, parallel to the eleventh and twelfth ribs, and lift up to support the abdominal contents. Place your right hand on the RUQ, with fingers parallel to the midline. Push deeply down and under the right costal margin. Ask the patient to take a deep breath. It is normal to feel the edge of the liver bump your fingertips as the diaphragm pushes it down during inhalation. It feels like a firm, regular ridge. However, the liver is often not palpable, and you feel nothing firm.

Hooking Technique. An alternative method of palpating the liver is to stand up at the patient's right shoulder and swivel your body to the right so that you face the patient's feet (Figure 22-24). Hook your fingers over the costal margin from above. Ask the patient to take a deep breath. Try to feel the liver edge bump your fingertips.

Tenderness occurs with local inflammation, with inflammation of the peritoneum or underlying organ, and with an enlarged organ whose capsule is stretched.

Except with a depressed diaphragm, a liver palpated more than 1 to 2 cm below the right costal margin is enlarged. Record the number of centimetres it descends, and note its consistency (hard, nodular) and tenderness (see Table 22-6, p. 580).

Normal Range of Findings	**Abnormal Findings**

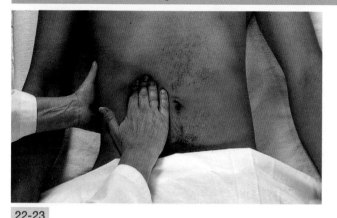

22-23

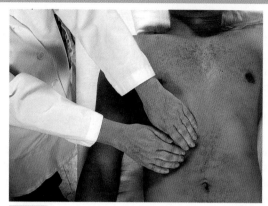

22-24

Spleen

Normally, the spleen is not palpable and must be enlarged to three times its normal size to be felt. To search for it, reach over the abdomen with your left hand and behind the left side at the eleventh and twelfth ribs (Figure 22-25, *A*). Lift up for support. Place your right hand obliquely on the LUQ with the fingers pointing toward the left axilla and just inferior to the rib margin. Push your hand deeply down and under the left costal margin, and ask the patient to take a deep breath. You should feel nothing firm.

When enlarged, the spleen slides out and bumps your fingertips (see the Critical Findings box to the right). It can grow so large that it extends into the lower quadrants. When this condition is suspected, start low on the abdomen so that you will not miss it. An alternative position is to roll the patient onto his or her right side to displace the spleen more forward and downward (see Figure 22-25, *B*). Then palpate as described earlier.

> ### CRITICAL FINDINGS
>
> The spleen becomes enlarged with mononucleosis and trauma (see Table 22-6, p. 581). If you feel enlargement of the spleen, refer the patient, but do *not* continue to palpate it. An enlarged spleen is friable and can rupture easily with overpalpation.
>
> Describe the number of centimetres that the spleen extends below the left costal margin.

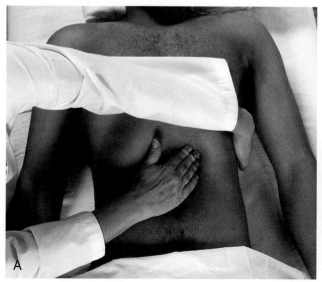

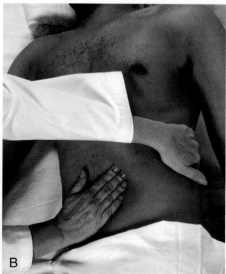

22-25

Normal Range of Findings	Abnormal Findings

(sidebar, rotated) Objective Data

Kidneys

Search for the right kidney by placing your hands together in a "duck bill" position at the patient's right flank (Figure 22-26, *A*). Press your two hands together firmly (you need deeper palpation than that used with the liver or spleen), and ask the patient to take a deep breath. In most people, you will feel no change. On occasion, you may feel the lower pole of the right kidney as a round, smooth mass slide between your fingers. Either condition is normal.

The left kidney sits 1 cm higher than the right kidney and is normally not palpable. Search for it by reaching your left hand across the abdomen and behind the left flank for support (see Figure 22-26, *B*). Push your right hand deep into the abdomen, and ask the patient to breathe deeply. You should feel no change with the inhalation.

Enlarged kidney.
Kidney mass.

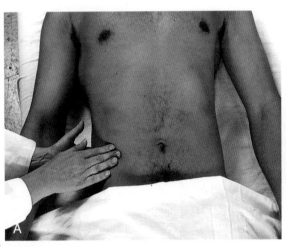 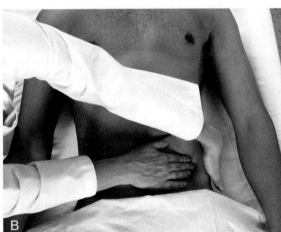

22-26

Aorta

Using your opposing thumb and fingers, palpate the aortic pulsation in the upper abdomen slightly to the left of midline (Figure 22-27). In adults, it is normally 2.5 to 4 cm wide and pulsates in an anterior direction.

Widened pulsation with aneurysm (see Tables 22-5 and 22-6, pp. 580–581).

Prominent lateral pulsation with aortic aneurysm (see the Critical Findings box below).

CRITICAL FINDINGS

If a bruit was heard on auscultation, you should *not* palpate the area, to avoid rupturing an aortic aneurysm. Report findings immediately.

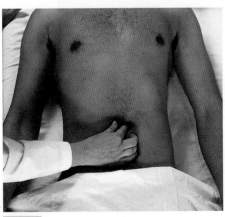

22-27

Normal Range of Findings	Abnormal Findings

Rebound Tenderness (Blumberg's Sign). Assess rebound tenderness when the patient reports abdominal pain or when you elicit tenderness during palpation. Choose a site away from the painful area. Hold your hand 90 degrees, or perpendicular, to the abdomen. Push down slowly and deeply (Figure 22-28, *A*); then lift up *quickly* (see Figure 22-28, *B*). This makes structures that are indented by palpation rebound suddenly. A normal, or negative, response is no pain on release of pressure. Perform this test at the end of the examination, because it can cause severe pain and muscle rigidity.

Pain on release of pressure confirms rebound tenderness, which is a reliable sign of peritoneal inflammation. Peritoneal inflammation accompanies appendicitis.

Cough tenderness that is localized to a specific spot also signals peritoneal irritation. Refer the patient with suspected appendicitis for computed tomographic scanning.

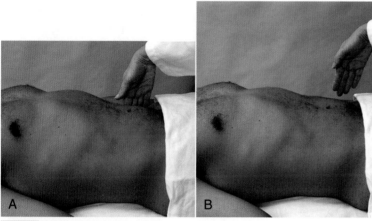

22-28   Rebound tenderness.

Inspiratory Arrest (Murphy's Sign). Normally, palpating the liver causes no pain. In a patient with inflammation of the gallbladder, or cholecystitis, pain occurs. Hold your fingers under the liver border. Ask the patient to take a deep breath. A normal response is to complete the deep breath without pain. (Note: This sign is less accurate in patients older than 60 years: Evidence shows that 25% of older patients do not have any abdominal tenderness; McGee, 2007.)

Iliopsoas Muscle Test. Perform the iliopsoas muscle test when the acute abdominal pain is suspect for appendicitis. With the patient supine, lift the right leg straight up, flexing at the hip (Figure 22-29); then push down over the lower part of the right thigh as the patient tries to hold the leg up. When the test result is negative, the patient feels no change.

(Note: Evidence shows that the obturator test, another technique that stretches the obturator muscle, does not work to diagnose appendicitis; Berry & Malt, 1984; McGee, 2012, p. 446.)

When the test result is positive, as the descending liver pushes the inflamed gallbladder onto the examining hand, the patient feels sharp pain and abruptly stops inspiration midway.

When the iliopsoas muscle is inflamed (which occurs with an inflamed or perforated appendix), pain is felt in the RLQ.

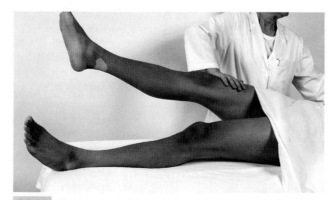

22-29   Iliopsoas muscle test.

Normal Range of Findings	Abnormal Findings

Ascites

At times, you may suspect that a patient has ascites (free fluid in the peritoneal cavity) because the abdomen is distended, the flanks are bulging, and the umbilicus is protruding and displaced downward. You can differentiate ascites from gaseous distension by performing the following two percussion tests.

Fluid Wave. First, test for a **fluid wave** by standing on the patient's right side. Place the ulnar edge of another examiner's hand or the patient's own hand firmly on the abdomen in the midline (Figure 22-30). (This will stop transmission across the skin of the upcoming tap.) Place your left hand on the patient's right flank. With your right hand, reach across the abdomen and give the left flank a firm strike.

Ascites occurs with heart failure, portal hypertension, cirrhosis, hepatitis, pancreatitis, and cancer.

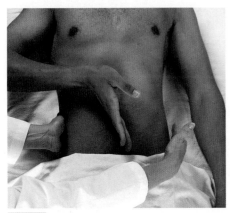

22-30   Fluid wave.

If ascites is present, the blow will generate a fluid wave through the abdomen, and you will feel a distinct tap on your left hand. If the abdomen is distended from gas or adipose tissue, you will feel no change.

Shifting Dullness. The second test for ascites is percussing for **shifting dullness.** In a supine patient, ascitic fluid settles by gravity into the flanks, displacing the air-filled bowel upward. You will hear a tympanitic note as you percuss over the top of the abdomen because gas-filled intestines float over the fluid (Figure 22-31). Then percuss down the side of the abdomen. If fluid is present, the note will change from tympany to dull as you reach its level. Mark this spot on the patient's body.

A fluid wave occurs with large amounts of ascitic fluid.

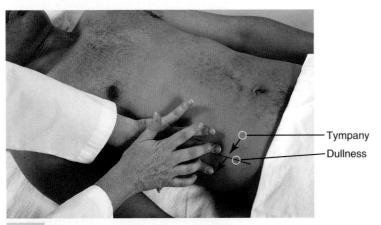

— Tympany
— Dullness

22-31

Normal Range of Findings	Abnormal Findings

Now turn the patient onto the right side (roll the patient toward you; Figure 22-32). The fluid will gravitate to the dependent (in this case, right) side, displacing the lighter bowel upward. Begin percussing the upper side of the abdomen and move downward. The sound changes from tympany to a dull sound as you reach the fluid level, but this time the level of dullness is higher, upward toward the umbilicus. This **shifting level of dullness** indicates the presence of fluid.

Shifting dullness is present with a large volume of ascitic fluid; it cannot be detected when the amount of fluid is less than 500 mL.

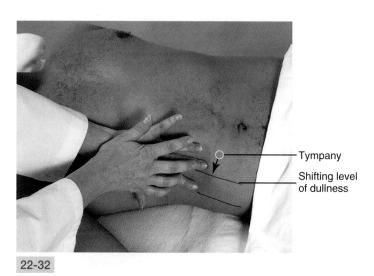

- Tympany

Shifting level of dullness

22-32

Both the fluid wave and shifting dullness tests are not completely reliable. Ultrasonography study is the definitive tool for detecting ascites.

DEVELOPMENTAL CONSIDERATIONS

Infants

Inspection. The contour of the abdomen is protuberant because of the immature abdominal musculature. The skin exhibits a fine, superficial venous pattern. This may be visible in lightly pigmented children until puberty.

Inspect the umbilical cord throughout the neonatal period. At birth, it is white and contains two umbilical arteries and one vein surrounded by mucoid connective tissue, called *Wharton's jelly*. The umbilical stump dries within a week, hardens, and falls off by 10 to 14 days after birth. Skin covers the area by 3 to 4 weeks.

The abdomen should be symmetrical, although two bulges are common. You may note an **umbilical hernia.** It appears 2 to 3 weeks after birth and is especially prominent when the infant cries. The hernia reaches maximum size at 1 month (up to 2.5 cm) and usually disappears by the age of 1 year. Another common variation is **diastasis recti,** a separation of the rectus muscles with a visible bulge along the midline. The condition is more common in infants of African descent, and it usually disappears by early childhood.

The abdomen shows respiratory movement. The only other abdominal movement you should note is occasional peristalsis, which may be visible because of the thin musculature.

Auscultation. Auscultation yields only bowel sounds, the metallic tinkling of peristalsis. No vascular sounds should be heard.

Scaphoid shape: occurs with dehydration.

Dilated veins.

The presence of only one artery signals the possibility of congenital defects.

Inflammation should be investigated.

Drainage after cord stump falls off is abnormal and should be investigated.

Refer for investigation any umbilical hernia that is larger than 2.5 cm (see Table 22-3, p. 578); that is continuing to grow after 1 month; or that lasts for more than 2 years in a child of European descent or for more than 7 years in a child of African descent.

Refer for investigation diastasis recti that lasts more than 6 years.

Marked peristalsis with pyloric stenosis (see Table 22-4, p. 579).

Bruit.
Venous hum.

Normal Range of Findings	Abnormal Findings

Objective Data

Percussion. Percussion reveals tympany over the stomach (the infant swallows some air with feeding) and dullness over the liver. The spleen is not percussed in infants. The abdomen sounds tympanitic, although it is normal to percuss dullness over the bladder. This dullness may extend up to the umbilicus.

Palpation. Aid palpation by flexing the baby's knees with one hand while palpating with the other (Figure 22-33). Alternatively, you may hold the upper back and flex the neck slightly with one hand. Offer a pacifier to a crying baby. The liver fills the RUQ. It is normal to feel the liver edge at the right costal margin or 1 to 2 cm below. Normally, you may palpate the spleen tip, both kidneys, and the bladder. Also easily palpated are the cecum in the RLQ and the sigmoid colon, which feels like a sausage in the left inguinal area.

Make note of the newborn's first stool, a sticky, greenish black meconium stool within 24 hours of birth. By the fourth day, stools of breastfed babies are golden yellow and pasty and smell like sour milk, whereas those of formula-fed babies are brown-yellow, firmer, and more fecal smelling.

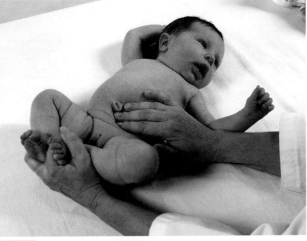

22-33

Children

At ages younger than 4 years, the abdomen looks protuberant when the child is both supine and standing. After age 4 years, the potbelly remains when the child stands because of lumbar lordosis, but the abdomen looks flat when the child is supine. Normal movement on the abdomen includes respirations, which remain abdominal until 7 years of age.

To palpate the abdomen, position a young child on the parent's lap as you sit knee to knee with the parent (Figure 22-34). Flex the child's knees up, and elevate the head slightly. You can ask the child to "pant like a dog" to further relax abdominal muscles. Hold your entire palm flat on the abdominal surface for a moment before starting palpation. This accustoms the child to being touched. If the child is very ticklish, hold his or her hand under your own as you palpate, or apply the stethoscope and palpate around it.

The liver remains easily palpable 1 to 2 cm below the right costal margin. The edge is soft and sharp and moves easily. On the left, the spleen also is easily palpable as a soft, sharp, movable edge. Usually you can feel 1 to 2 cm of the right kidney and the tip of the left kidney. Percussion of the liver span reveals measurements of approximately 3.5 cm at age 2 years, 5 cm at age 6 years, and 6 to 7 cm during adolescence.

A scaphoid abdomen is associated with dehydration or malnutrition.

Before age 7 years of age, abdominal respirations are absent with inflammation of the peritoneum.

Normal Range of Findings	Abnormal Findings

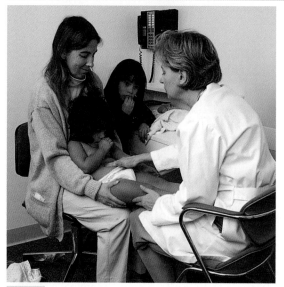

22-34

When asking young children about abdominal tenderness, remember that they often answer this question affirmatively no matter how the abdomen actually feels. Use objective signs to aid assessment, such as a cry changing in pitch as you palpate, facial grimacing, movement away from you, and guarding.

The school-age child has a slim abdominal shape as he or she loses the potbelly. This slimming trend continues into adolescence. Many adolescents are easily embarrassed by exposure of the abdomen, and adequate draping is necessary. The physical findings are the same as those listed for adults.

Older Adults

On inspection, you may note increased deposits of subcutaneous fat on the abdomen and hips because it is redistributed away from the extremities. The abdominal musculature is thinner and has less tone than that of younger adults; therefore, in the absence of obesity, you may note peristalsis.

Because the abdominal wall is thinner and softer, the organs may be easier to palpate (in the absence of obesity). The liver is easier to palpate. Normally, you can feel the liver edge at or just below the costal margin. When the lungs are distended and the diaphragm is depressed, the liver is palpated lower, descending 1 to 2 cm below the costal margin with inhalation. The kidneys are easier to palpate.

Abdominal rigidity with acute abdominal conditions is less common in older adults.

Older adults with conditions that cause severe abdominal pain ("acute abdomen") often complain of less pain than do younger patients.

Objective Data

Documentation & Critical Thinking

DOCUMENTATION AND CRITICAL THINKING

Sample Charting

SUBJECTIVE

States appetite is good with no recent change, no dysphagia, no food intolerance, no pain, no nausea/vomiting. Has one formed BM [bowel movement]/day. Takes vitamins, no other prescribed or over-the-counter medication. No history of abdominal disease, injury, or surgery. Diet recall of past 24 hours listed at end of history.

OBJECTIVE

Inspection: Abdomen flat, symmetrical, with no apparent masses. Skin smooth with no striae, scars, or lesions.
Auscultation: Bowel sounds present, no bruits.

Percussion: Tympany predominates in all four quadrants; liver span is 8 cm in right midclavicular line. Splenic dullness located at tenth intercostal space in left midaxillary line.

Palpation: Abdomen soft; no organomegaly, no masses, no tenderness.

ASSESSMENT

Healthy abdomen, bowel sounds present

Focused Assessment: Clinical Case Study 1

George E. is a 58-year-old unemployed, divorced man with chronic alcoholism who enters the chemical dependency treatment centre.

SUBJECTIVE

States past 6 months has been drinking 500 mL whisky/day. Last alcohol use 1 week PTA, with "5 or 6" drinks that episode. Estranged from family, lives alone. Makes a few meals on hot plate. States never has appetite. Has fatigue and weakness.

OBJECTIVE

Inspection: Appears older than stated age. Oriented, although verbal response time slowed. Weight loss of 5.5 kg in last 3 months. Abdomen protuberant, symmetrical, no visible masses. Poor skin turgor. Dilated venous pattern over abdominal wall. Hair sparse in axillary, pubic areas.

Auscultation: Bowel sounds present. No vascular sounds.

Percussion: Tympany predominates over abdomen. Liver span is 16 cm in right midclavicular line. No fluid wave. No shifting dullness.

Palpation: Soft. Liver palpable 10 cm below right costal margin, smooth and nontender. No other organomegaly or masses.

ASSESSMENT

Alcohol dependence, severe, with physiological dependence
Imbalanced nutrition: less than body requirements R/T impaired absorption
Ineffective coping R/T effects of chronic alcoholism
Social isolation

Focused Assessment: Clinical Case Study 2

Edith J. is a 63-year-old, retired homemaker who has a history of lung cancer with metastasis to the liver.

SUBJECTIVE

Feeling "puffy and bloated" for the past week. States unable to get comfortable. Also short of breath "all the time now." Difficulty sleeping. "I feel like crying all the time now."

OBJECTIVE

Inspection: Weight increase of 3.7 kg in 1 week. Abdomen is distended with everted umbilicus and bulging flanks. Girth at umbilicus is 85 cm. Prominent dilated venous pattern present over abdomen.

Auscultation: Bowel sounds present, no vascular sounds.

Percussion: When supine, tympany present at dome of abdomen, dullness over flanks. Shifting dullness present. Positive fluid wave present. Liver span is 12 cm in right midclavicular line.

Palpation: Abdominal wall firm, able to feel liver with deep palpation at 6 cm below right costal margin. Liver feels firm, nodular, nontender. 4+ pitting edema in both ankles.

ASSESSMENT

Ascites
Grieving
Ineffective breathing pattern R/T increased intra-abdominal pressure
Pain R/T distended abdomen
Risk for impaired skin integrity: R/T ascites, edema, and faulty metabolism
Insomnia

Focused Assessment: Clinical Case Study 3

Dan G. is a 17-year-old male high school student who enters the emergency department with abdominal pain of 2 days' duration.

SUBJECTIVE

2 days PTA: Dan noted general abdominal pain in umbilical region. Now pain is sharp and severe, and Dan points to location in RLQ. No BM for 2 days. Nausea and vomiting off and on 1 day.

OBJECTIVE

Inspection: BP 112/70, temp 38°C, pulse 116, resp 18.

Lying on side with knees drawn up under chin. Resists any movement. Face tight and occasionally grimacing. Cries out with any sudden movement.

Auscultation: No bowel sounds present. No vascular sounds.

Percussion: Tympany. Percussion over RLQ leads to tenderness.

Palpation: Abdominal wall is rigid and boardlike. Extreme tenderness to palpation in RLQ. Rebound tenderness is present in RLQ. Positive iliopsoas muscle test.

ASSESSMENT

Acute abdominal pain in RLQ
Nausea

ABNORMAL FINDINGS

TABLE 22-1   Abdominal Distension*

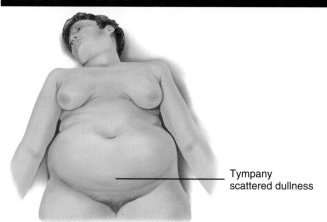

Tympany
scattered dullness

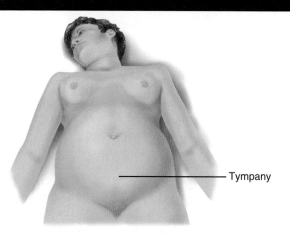

Tympany

Obesity

Inspection: Uniformly rounded; umbilicus sunken (it adheres to peritoneum, and layers of fat are superficial to it)

Auscultation: Normal bowel sounds

Percussion: Tympany; scattered dullness over adipose tissue

Palpation: Normal; may be hard to feel through thick abdominal wall

Air or Gas

Inspection: Single round curve

Auscultation: Depends on cause of gas (e.g., decreased or absent bowel sounds with ileus); hyperactive with early intestinal obstruction)

Percussion: Tympany over large area

Palpation: May have muscle spasm of abdominal wall

Continued

TABLE 22-1   Abdominal Distension—cont'd

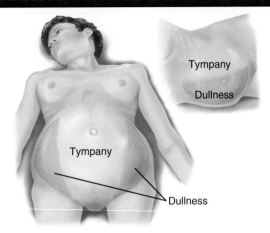

Ascites

Inspection: Single curve; everted umbilicus; bulging flanks in supine position; taut, glistening skin; recent weight gain; increase in abdominal girth

Auscultation: Normal bowel sounds over intestines; diminished over ascitic fluid

Percussion: Tympany at top where intestines float; dull over fluid; produces fluid wave and shifting dullness

Palpation: Limited by taut skin and increased intra-abdominal pressure

Ovarian Cyst (Large)

Inspection: Curve in lower half of abdomen, midline; everted umbilicus

Auscultation: Normal bowel sounds over upper abdomen where intestines are pushed superiorly

Percussion: Top dull over fluid; intestines pushed superiorly; large cyst produces fluid wave and shifting dullness

Palpation: Aortic pulsation present (in ascites, it is not)

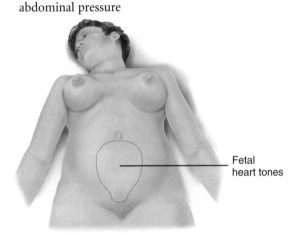

Pregnancy†

Inspection: Single curve; umbilicus protruding; breasts engorged

Auscultation: Fetal heart tones; diminished bowel sounds

Percussion: Tympany over intestines; dull over enlarging uterus

Palpation: Fetal parts; fetal movements

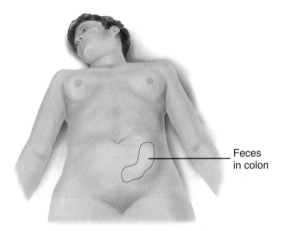

Feces

Inspection: Localized distension

Auscultation: Normal bowel sounds

Percussion: Tympany predominates; scattered dullness over fecal mass

Palpation: Plastic-like or ropelike mass with feces in intestines

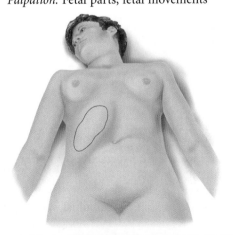

◄ Tumour

Inspection: Localized distension

Auscultation: Normal bowel sounds

Percussion: Dull over mass if mass reaches up to skin surface

Palpation: Used to define borders and distinguish from enlarged organ or normally palpable structure

*A mnemonic device to recall the common causes of abdominal distension is the seven *F*s: fat, flatus, fluid, fetus, feces, fetal growth, and fibroid.

†Obviously a normal finding, pregnancy is included for comparison of conditions causing abdominal distension.

TABLE 22-2   Common Sites of Referred Abdominal Pain

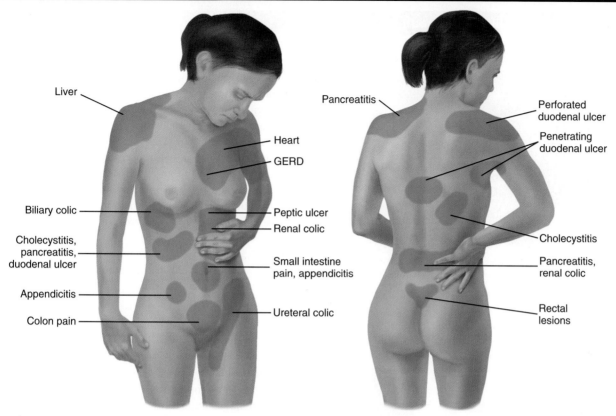

When a patient gives a history of abdominal pain, the location of the pain may not necessarily be directly over the involved organ. That is because the human brain has no felt image for internal organs. Rather, pain is referred to a site where the organ was located in fetal development. Although the organ migrates during fetal development, its nerves persist in referring sensations from the former location. The following are examples, not a complete list.

Liver

Hepatitis may produce mild to moderate, dull pain in RUQ or epigastrium, along with anorexia, nausea, malaise, and low-grade fever.

Esophagus

Gastroesophageal reflux disease (GERD) is a complex of symptoms of esophagitis, including burning pain in midepigastrium or behind lower sternum that radiates upward, or "heartburn." The pain occurs 30–60 minutes after eating; it is aggravated by lying down or bending over.

Gallbladder

Cholecystitis is biliary colic, sudden pain in right upper quadrant that may radiate to the right or left scapula and that builds over time, lasting 2 to 4 hours, after ingestion of fatty foods, alcohol, or caffeine. It is associated with nausea and vomiting and a positive Murphy sign (sudden stop in inspiration with RUQ palpation).

Pancreas

Pancreatitis produces acute, boring midepigastric pain radiating to the back and sometimes to the left scapula or flank, severe nausea, and vomiting.

Duodenum

Duodenal ulcer typically produces dull, aching, gnawing pain; it does not radiate, may be relieved by food, and may awaken the patient from sleep.

Stomach

Gastric ulcer pain is dull, aching, gnawing epigastric pain, usually brought on by eating; it radiates to the back or substernal area. Perforated ulcer produces burning epigastric pain of sudden onset that is referred to one or both shoulders.

Appendix

Appendicitis typically starts as dull, diffuse pain in periumbilical region that later shifts to severe, sharp, persistent pain and tenderness localized in RLQ (McBurney's point). Pain is aggravated by movement, coughing, and deep breathing; it is associated first with anorexia, then with nausea and vomiting, and later with fever.

Kidney

Kidney stones prompt a sudden onset of severe, colicky flank or lower abdominal pain.

Small Intestine

Gastroenteritis produces diffuse, generalized abdominal pain, with nausea and diarrhea.

Colon

Large bowel obstruction produces moderate, colicky pain of gradual onset in lower abdomen, with bloating. Irritable bowel syndrome (IBS) is accompanied by sharp or burning, cramping pain over a wide area; the pain, which does not radiate, is triggered by meals and relieved by bowel movement.

RLQ, right lower quadrant; *RUQ,* right upper quadrant.

Image © Pat Thomas, 2006.

Abnormal Findings

TABLE 22-3   Abnormalities on Inspection

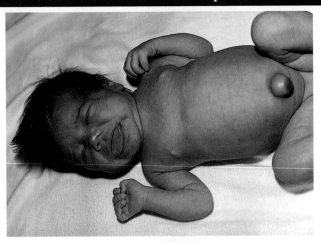

◄ *Umbilical Hernia*

Umbilical hernia is a soft, skin-covered mass, which is the protrusion of the omentum or intestine through a weakness or incomplete closure in the umbilical ring. It is accentuated by increased intra-abdominal pressure, which occurs with crying, coughing, vomiting, or straining, but the bowel rarely becomes incarcerated or strangulated. It is more common in infants of African or Asian descent and in premature infants. Most umbilical hernias resolve spontaneously by age 1 year; parents should avoid affixing a belt or coin at the hernia because this will not speed closure and may cause contact dermatitis.

In an adult, it occurs with pregnancy and chronic ascites, or it may result from chronic intrathoracic pressure (e.g., asthma, chronic bronchitis).

Epigastric Hernia (Not Illustrated)

Epigastric hernia is a small, fatty nodule at the epigastrium in the midline, through the linea alba. Usually it can be palpated rather than observed. It may be palpable only when the patient is standing.

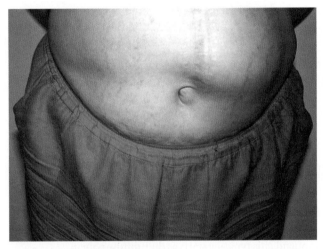

◄ *Incisional Hernia*

A bulge near an old operative scar that may not show when patient is supine but is apparent when the patient increases intra-abdominal pressure by a sit-up, by standing, or by performing the Valsalva manoeuvre.

Diastasis Recti (Not Illustrated)

Diastasis recti, a midline longitudinal ridge, is a separation of the abdominal rectus muscles. The ridge is revealed when intra-abdominal pressure is increased by raising the head while in the supine position. It occurs congenitally and as a result of pregnancy or marked obesity in which distension is prolonged or muscle tone has decreased. It is not clinically significant.

TABLE 22-4	**Abnormal Bowel Sounds**

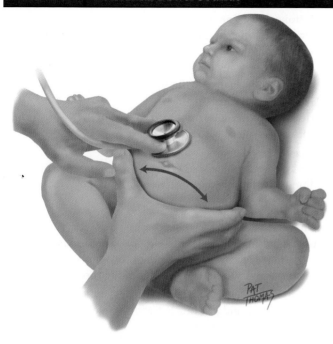

◄ *Succussion Splash*

Unrelated to peristalsis, this is a very loud splash auscultated over the upper abdomen when the infant is rocked side to side. It indicates increased air and fluid in the stomach, as occurs with pyloric obstruction or large hiatus hernia.

Marked peristalsis, together with projectile vomiting in the newborn, is suggestive of **pyloric stenosis**, an obstruction of the stomach's pyloric valve. Pyloric stenosis is a congenital defect and appears in the second or third week after birth. After feeding, pronounced peristaltic waves cross from left to right, leading to projectile vomiting. Then the examiner can palpate an olive-sized mass in the RUQ midway between the right costal margin and umbilicus. Affected infants must be referred promptly because of the risk of weight loss.

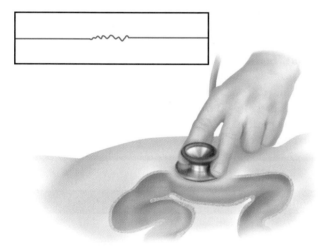

Hypoactive Bowel Sounds

Diminished or absence of bowel sounds signal decreased motility that results from inflammation, as with peritonitis; from paralytic ileus, as after abdominal surgery; or from late bowel obstruction. It also occurs with pneumonia.

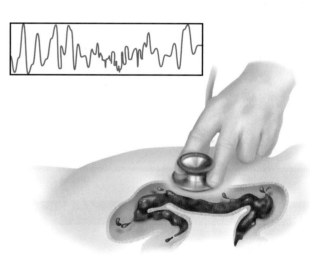

Hyperactive Bowel Sounds

Loud, gurgling sounds (borborygmi) signal increased motility. They occur with early mechanical bowel obstruction (high-pitched), gastroenteritis, brisk diarrhea, laxative use, and subsiding paralytic ileus.

RUQ, right upper quadrant.

TABLE 22-5   Abdominal Friction Rubs and Vascular Sounds

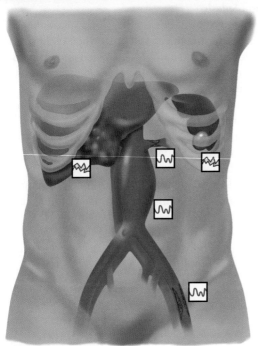

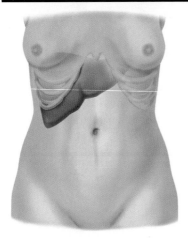 Peritoneal friction rub

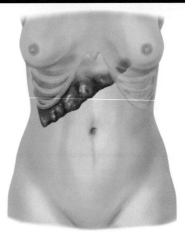 Vascular sounds

◀ **Peritoneal Friction Rub**
A rough, grating sound, like two pieces of leather rubbed together, indicates peritoneal inflammation. Occurs rarely. Usually occurs over organs with a large surface area in contact with the peritoneum.

Liver
Friction rub over lower right rib cage, caused by abscess or metastatic tumour.

Spleen
Friction rub over lower left rib cage in left anterior axillary line, caused by abscess, infection, or tumour.

Vascular Sounds
Arterial
A *bruit* indicates turbulent blood flow, as found in constricted, abnormally dilated, or tortuous vessels. Listen with the bell. Occurs with the following three conditions:

- *Aortic aneurysm:* Murmur is harsh, systolic, or continuous and accentuated with systole. Note in patient with hypertension.
- *Renal artery stenosis:* Murmur is midline or toward flank, soft, low-to-medium pitch.
- *Partial occlusion of femoral arteries:* Murmur is heard in the inguinal region (groin).

Venous Hum
Occurs rarely. Heard in periumbilical region. Originates from inferior vena cava. Medium pitch, continuous sound; pressure on bell may obliterate it. A palpable thrill may be present. Occurs with portal hypertension and cirrhotic liver.

TABLE 22-6   Abnormalities Detected on Palpation of Organs

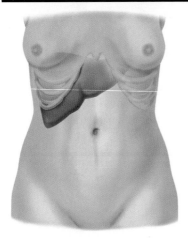

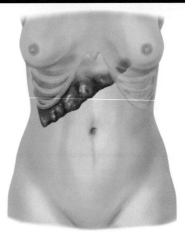

Enlarged Liver
The liver becomes enlarged, smooth, and nontender with fatty infiltration, portal obstruction or cirrhosis, obstruction high in the inferior vena cava, and lymphocytic leukemia. The liver feels enlarged and smooth but is tender to palpation with early heart failure, acute hepatitis, and hepatic abscess.

Enlarged Nodular Liver
The liver becomes enlarged and nodular with late portal cirrhosis, metastatic cancer, and tertiary syphilis.

TABLE 22-6	Abnormalities Detected on Palpation of Organs—cont'd

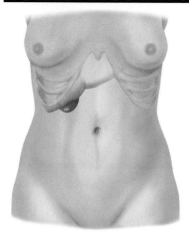

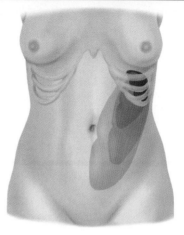

Enlarged Gallbladder

An enlarged, tender gallbladder is suggestive of acute cholecystitis. It is palpated behind the liver border as a smooth and firm mass like a sausage, although it may be difficult to palpate because of involuntary rigidity of abdominal muscles. The area is exquisitely painful to fist percussion, and inspiratory arrest (Murphy's sign) is present.

An enlarged, nontender gallbladder also feels like a smooth, sausage-like mass. This condition occurs when the gallbladder is filled with stones, as with obstruction of the common bile duct.

Enlarged Spleen

Because any enlargement superiorly is stopped by the diaphragm, the spleen enlarges downward and toward the midline. When enlargement is extreme, the spleen can extend down to the left aspect of the pelvis. It retains the splenic notch on the medial edge. When splenomegaly occurs with acute infections (mononucleosis), the spleen is moderately enlarged and soft, with rounded edges. When it is the result of a chronic cause, the enlargement is firm or hard, with sharp edges. An enlarged spleen is usually not tender to palpation; it is tender only if the peritoneum is also inflamed.

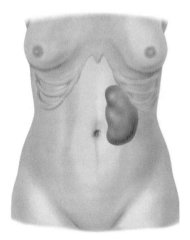

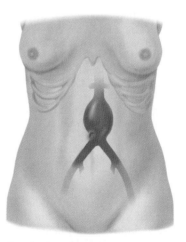

Enlarged Kidney

A kidney may become enlarged with hydronephrosis, cyst, or neoplasm. It may be difficult to distinguish an enlarged kidney from an enlarged spleen because they have a similar shape. Both extend forward and downward. However, the spleen may have a sharp edge, whereas the kidneys never do. The spleen retains the splenic notch, whereas the kidneys have no palpable notch. Percussion over the spleen yields dullness, whereas over the kidneys the sound is tympanitic because of the overriding bowel.

Aortic Aneurysm

Most aortic aneurysms (more than 95%) are located below the renal arteries and extend to the umbilicus. Approximately 80% of these are detectable during routine physical examination. You will hear a bruit. Femoral pulses are present but decreased. An aortic aneurysm has a high risk for rupture. If you hear a bruit, you should *not* palpate the area, to avoid rupturing the aneurysm.

Additional information on abdominal aneurysm is illustrated in Table 22-5.

Abnormal Findings

Summary Checklist: Abdomen Examination

For a PDA-downloadable version, go to *http://evolve.elsevier.com/Canada/Jarvis/examination/.*

1. Inspection
   Contour
   Symmetry
   Umbilicus
   Skin
   Pulsation or movement
   Hair distribution
   Demeanour

2. Auscultation
   Bowel sounds
   Any vascular sounds
3. Percussion
   All four quadrants
   Borders of liver, spleen
4. Palpation
   Light palpation in all four quadrants

Deeper palpation in all four quadrants
Palpation for liver, spleen, and kidneys
5. Health promotion and teaching

REFERENCES

American Celiac Disease Alliance. (2013). *What is celiac disease?* Retrieved from *http://americanceliac.org/celiac-disease/.*

Berry, J., & Malt, R. A. (1984). Appendicitis near its centenary. *Annals of Surgery, 200,* 567–575.

Canadian Digestive Health Foundation. (2012). *Digestive disorders: Statistics.* Retrieved from *http://www.cdhf.ca/digestive-disorders/statistics.shtml.*

Canadian Liver Foundation. (2011). *Gallstones.* Retrieved from *http://www.liver.ca/Liver_Disease/Adult_Liver_Diseases/Gallstones.aspx.*

Crohn's and Colitis Foundation of Canada. (2008). *The burden of inflammatory bowel disease (IBD) in Canada.* Retrieved from *http://www.ccfc.ca/atf/cf/%7B282e45d9-a03a-49d1-883c-39f4feaf7246%7D/BIBDC%20FINAL%20OCTOBER%2029TH%20EN.PDF.*

Fedorak, R. N., van Zanten, S. V., & Bridges, R. (2010). Canadian Digestive Health Foundation Public Impact Series: Gastroesophageal reflux disease in Canada: Incidence, prevalence, and direct and indirect economic impact. *Canadian Journal of Gastroenterology, 24*(7), 431–434.

Flaser, M. H., & Goldberg, E. (2006). Acute abdominal pain. *Medical Clinics of North America, 90,* 481–503. doi:10.1016/j.mcna.2005.11.005

Howland, R. H. (2009). Effects of aging on pharmacokinetic and pharmacodynamic drug processes. *Journal of Psychosocial Nursing, 47*(10), 15–18.

Keith, S. W., Redden, D. T., & Katzmarzyk, P. T. (2006). Putative contributors to the secular increase in obesity. *International Journal of Obesity, 30,* 1585–1594.

Khanna, R., Lakhanpaul, M., Burman-Roy, S., & Murphy, M. S. (2009). Diarrhoea and vomiting caused by gastroenteritis in children under 5 years: Summary of NICE guidelines. *British Medical Journal, 338,* 1009–1012. doi:10.1136/bmj.b1350

Majowicz, S. E., Horrocks, J., & Bocking, K. (2007). Demographic determinants of acute gastrointestinal illness in Canada: A population study. *BMC Public Health, 7*(162), 1–8. doi:10.1186/1471-2458-7-162

Mauk, K. L. (2005). Preventing constipation in older adults. *Nursing 2005, 35*(6), 22–23.

McGee, S. (2007). *Evidence-based physical diagnosis* (2nd ed.). Philadelphia: W. B. Saunders.

McGee, S. (2012). *Evidence-based physical diagnosis* (3rd ed.). Philadelphia: W. B. Saunders.

Miller, C. A. (2012). *Nursing for wellness in older adults* (6th ed.). Philadelphia: Lippincott Williams & Wilkins.

Moore, A. A., Whiteman, E. J., & Ward, K. T. (2007). Risks of combined alcohol/medication use in older adults. *American Journal of Geriatric Pharmacotherapy, 5*(1), 64–74. doi:10.1016/j.amjopharm.2007.03.006

Mourad, J., Elliott, J. P., Erickson, L., & Lisboa, L. (2000). Appendicitis in pregnancy: New information that contradicts long-held clinical beliefs. *American Journal of Obstetrics & Gynecology, 182*(5), 1027–1029.

Noël, A., & Larocque, F. (2009). *Aboriginal peoples and poverty in Canada: Can provincial governments make a difference?* Retrieved from *http://www.cccg.umontreal.ca/rc19/PDF/Noel-A_Rc192009.pdf.*

Oto, A., Srinivasan, P. N., Ernst, R. D., Koroglu, M., Cesani, F., Nishino, T., & Chaljub, G. (2006). Revisiting MRI for appendix location during pregnancy. *American Journal of Roentgenology, 186*(3), 883–887. doi:10.2214/AJR.05.0270

Pates, J. A., Avendanio, T. C., Zaretsky, M. V., McIntire, D. D., & Twickler, D. M. (2009). The appendix in pregnancy: Confirming historical observations with a contemporary modality. *Obstetrics & Gynecology, 114*(4), 805–808.

Registered Nurses Association of Ontario. (2005). *Nursing Best Practice Guideline: Prevention of constipation in the older adult population.* Retrieved from *http://rnao.ca/bpg/guidelines/prevention-constipation-older-adult-population.*

Anus, Rectum, and Prostate

Written by Carolyn Jarvis, PhD, APN, CNP
Adapted by Marian Luctkar-Flude, RN, MScN

⊖volve WEBSITE

OUTLINE

STRUCTURE AND FUNCTION

ANUS AND RECTUM

The **anal canal** is the outlet of the gastrointestinal tract, and it is about 3.8 cm long in adults. It is lined with modified skin (which has no hair or sebaceous glands) that merges with rectal mucosa at the anorectal junction. The canal slants forward toward the umbilicus, forming a distinct right angle with the rectum, which rests back in the hollow of the sacrum. Although the rectum contains only autonomic nerves, numerous somatic sensory nerves are present in the anal canal and external skin, and so any trauma to the anal area will cause sharp pain.

The anal canal is surrounded by two concentric layers of muscle called the **sphincters** (Figure 23-1). The internal sphincter is under involuntary control by the autonomic nervous system. The external sphincter surrounds the internal sphincter but also has a small section overriding the tip of the internal sphincter at the opening. It is under voluntary control. Except for the passing of feces and gas, the sphincters keep the anal canal tightly closed. The **intersphincteric**

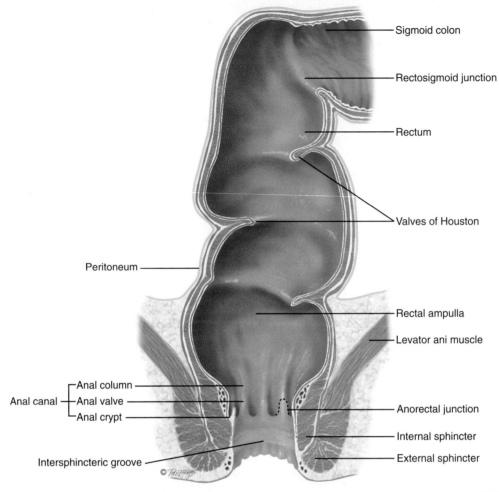

23-1 Anatomy of the anal sphincters.

© Pat Thomas, 2010.

groove separates the internal and external sphincters and is palpable.

The **anal columns** (or columns of Morgagni) are folds of mucosa. These extend vertically down from the rectum and end in the **anorectal junction** (also called the *mucocutaneous junction, pectinate line,* or *dentate line*). This junction is not palpable, but it is visible on proctoscopy. Each anal column contains an artery and a vein. Under conditions of chronic increased venous pressure, the vein may enlarge, forming a hemorrhoid. At the lower end of each column is a small crescent fold of mucous membrane called the **anal valve.** The space above the anal valve (between the columns) is a small recess called the **anal crypt.**

The **rectum,** which is 12 cm long, is the distal portion of the large intestine. It extends from the sigmoid colon, at the level of the third sacral vertebra, and ends at the anal canal. Just above the anal canal, the rectum dilates and turns posteriorly, forming the rectal ampulla. The rectal interior has three semilunar transverse folds called the **valves of Houston.** These cross half the circumference of the rectal lumen. Their function is unclear, but they may serve to hold feces as the flatus passes. The lowest is within reach of palpation, usually on the left side, and must not be mistaken for an intrarectal mass.

Peritoneal Reflection. The peritoneum covers only the upper two thirds of the rectum. In boys and men, the anterior part of the peritoneum reflects down to within 7.5 cm of the anal opening, forming the **rectovesical pouch** (Figure 23-2), and then covers the bladder. In girls and women, this area is termed the **rectouterine pouch,** and it extends down to within 5.5 cm of the anal opening.

PROSTATE

In boys and men, the **prostate gland** lies in front of the anterior wall of the rectum and 2 cm behind the symphysis pubis. It surrounds the bladder neck and the urethra and has 15 to 30 ducts that open into the urethra. The prostate secretes a thin, milky alkaline fluid that helps sperm viability. It is a bilobed structure that is round or heart-shaped. It measures 2.5 cm long and 4 cm in diameter. The two lateral lobes are separated by a shallow groove called the **median sulcus.**

The two **seminal vesicles** project like rabbit ears above the prostate. The seminal vesicles secrete a fluid that is rich in fructose, which nourishes the sperm, and contains prostaglandins. The two **bulbourethral** (Cowper's) glands are each the size of a pea and are located inferior to the prostate on

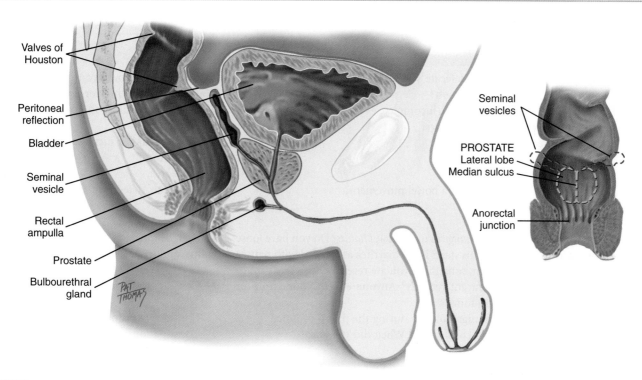

 23-2   Peritoneal reflection.

either side of the urethra (see Figure 23-5 on page 591). They secrete a clear, viscid mucus.

REGIONAL STRUCTURES

In girls and women, the uterine cervix lies in front of the anterior rectal wall and may be palpated through the wall.

The combined length of the anal canal and the rectum is about 16 cm in the adult. The average length of the examining finger is 6 to 10 cm, and so many rectal structures are within reach.

The sigmoid colon is named for its S-shaped course in the pelvic cavity. It extends from the iliac flexure of the descending colon and ends at the rectum. It is 40 cm long and is accessible to examination only through the colonoscope. The flexible fibreoptic colonoscope in current use provides a view of the entire mucosal surface of the sigmoid colon, as well as the colon itself.

DEVELOPMENTAL CONSIDERATIONS

The first stool passed by the newborn is dark green meconium; its occurrence, within 24 to 48 hours of birth, indicates anal patency. From that time on, the infant usually has a stool after each feeding. This response to eating is a wave of peristalsis called the *gastrocolic reflex*. It continues throughout life, although children and adults usually produce no more than one or two stools per day.

The infant passes stools by reflex. Voluntary control of the external anal sphincter cannot occur until the nerves supplying the area have become fully myelinated, usually around 1½ to 2 years of age. Toilet training usually starts after age 2 years.

At male puberty, the prostate gland undergoes a very rapid increase to more than twice its prepubertal size. During early adulthood, its size remains fairly constant.

The prostate gland commonly starts to enlarge during the middle adult years. This enlargement, **benign prostatic hypertrophy (BPH),** is present in 1 per 10 men at the age of 40 years and increases with age. The hypertrophy is thought to be caused by a hormonal imbalance that leads to the proliferation of benign adenomas. These gradually impede urine output because they obstruct the urethra. The risk of developing prostate cancer also increases with age (see the box Health Promotion: Screening for Prostate Cancer, p. 587).

SUBJECTIVE DATA

1. Usual bowel routine
2. Change in bowel habits
3. Rectal bleeding, blood in the stool
4. Medications (laxatives, stool softeners, iron)

5. Rectal conditions (pruritus, hemorrhoids, fissure, fistula)
6. Family history
7. Self-care behaviours (diet of high-fibre foods, most recent examinations)

HEALTH HISTORY QUESTIONS

Examiner Asks	Rationale
1. **Usual bowel routine.** Do you defecate regularly? How often? What is the usual colour? Is it usually hard or soft? • Do you have any straining at stool, incomplete evacuation, or urge to have bowel movement but nothing comes? • Do you eat breakfast? • Do you have pain while passing a bowel movement?	Assess usual bowel routine. Constipation is defined as three or fewer stools per week and is a common concern among older adults. Eating breakfast increases colon motility and prompts a bowel movement in many people. Pain with defecation (**dyschezia**) may be caused by a local condition (hemorrhoid, fissure) or constipation.
2. **Change in bowel habits.** Any *change* in usual *bowel habits?* Do you have loose stools or diarrhea? When did this start? Is the diarrhea associated with nausea and vomiting, abdominal pain, something you ate recently? • Have you eaten at a restaurant recently? Anyone else in your group or family have the same symptoms? • Have you travelled to a foreign country during the past 6 months? • Do your stools have a hard consistency? When did this start?	Diarrhea occurs with gastroenteritis, colitis, and irritable bowel syndrome. Consider food poisoning. Consider parasitic infection. Constipation is characterized by stool hardness.
3. **Rectal bleeding, blood in the stool.** Have you ever had? • When did you first notice blood in the stools? What is the colour: bright red or dark red-black? How much blood: spotting on the toilet paper or outright passing of blood with the stool? Do the bloody stools have a particular smell? • Have you ever had clay-coloured stools? • Have you ever had mucus or pus in stool? • Is your stool frothy? • Do you need to pass gas frequently?	Black or bloody stools (**melena**) should be investigated. Black stools may be tarry as a result of occult blood (melena) from gastrointestinal bleeding, or they may be nontarry as a result of ingestion of iron medications. Red blood in stools occurs with gastrointestinal bleeding or localized bleeding around the anus and also with colon and rectal cancer. Clay colour indicates absence of bile pigment. **Steatorrhea** is excessive fat in the stool, as occurs in malabsorption of fat. Excessive passing of gas (flatulence) should be investigated.
4. **Medications.** What **medications** do you take: prescription and over-the-counter? Laxatives or stool softeners? Which ones? How often? Iron pills? Do you ever use enemas to move your bowels? How often?	
5. **Rectal conditions.** Do you have any problems in rectal area: itching, pain or burning sensation, hemorrhoids? How do you treat these? Do you use any hemorrhoid preparations? Ever had a fissure or fistula? How was this treated? • Have you ever had a problem controlling your bowels?	Pruritus (itching) can be caused by hemorrhoids. Such a problem is known as *fecal incontinence.* Mucoid discharge and soiling of underwear occur with prolapsed hemorrhoids.
6. **Family history.** Any **family history** of polyps or cancer in the colon or rectum, inflammatory bowel disease, prostate cancer?	Assess risk factors for colon cancer, rectal cancer, prostate cancer.
7. **Self-care behaviours.** What is the usual amount of **high-fibre foods** in your daily diet: cereals, apples or other fruits, vegetables, whole-grain breads? How many glasses of water do you drink each day?	High-fibre foods of the soluble type (beans, prunes, barley, carrots, broccoli, cabbage) have been shown to lower cholesterol, and insoluble-fibre foods (cereals, wheat germ) reduce the risk of colon cancer. Also, high-fibre foods fight obesity, stabilize blood glucose levels, and help alleviate certain gastrointestinal disorders.

Examiner Asks	Rationale
• What were the dates of your most recent digital rectal examination, stool blood test, colonoscopy, PSA blood test (for men)?	For colon and prostate cancer screening guidelines for the early detection of cancer, refer to Table 23-1 and the Promoting Health boxes on the following pages.

Additional History for Infants and Children

1. **Skin problems.** Have you ever noticed any irritation in your child's anal area: redness, raised skin, frequent itching?

2. **Bowel movements.** How are your child's bowel movements (BMs)? Frequency? Any problems? Any pain or straining with BM?

In children, pinworms are a common cause of intense itching and irritation of the anal skin.

Assess usual stooling pattern. Constipation is a decrease in BM frequency, with difficult passing of very hard, dry stools. **Encopresis** is persistent passing of stools into clothing by a child older than age 4 years, at which age continence would be expected.

TABLE 23-1   Colon Cancer Screening Guidelines

Level of Risk*	Recommendations for Screening
Average risk: No affected family member	Begin screening at age 50. A decision to screen between ages 75–85 years should be made on an individual basis. Individuals older than age 85 should not be screened. Screening should include FOBT, or preferably FIT, at least every 2 years and may include flexible sigmoidoscopy. The interval between normal sigmoidoscopies should be 10 years or longer.
Higher risk: One first-degree relative with cancer or polyp at age <60, or two or more first-degree relatives affected with polyp or colon cancer at any age	Colonoscopy every 5 years, beginning at age 40 years or 10 years younger than the youngest age at diagnosis of polyp or cancer in the family, whichever comes first
One first-degree relative affected at age >60, or two or more second-degree relatives affected at any age	Average-risk screening but beginning at age 40
One second-degree relative or third-degree relative affected	Average-risk screening beginning at age 50
Special screening: Hereditary nonpolyposis colorectal cancer (HNPCC)	Colonoscopy every 1–2 years beginning at age 20 or 10 years younger than the youngest age at diagnosis of polyp or cancer in the family, whichever comes first
Familial adenomatous polyposis (FAP)	Sigmoidoscopy annually beginning at age 10–12 years
Attenuated adenomatous polyposis (AAPC)	Colonoscopy annually beginning at age 16–18 years

Source: Modified from Canadian Association of Gastroenterology and the Canadian Digestive Health Foundation. (2004). *Guidelines on colon cancer screening.*Retrieved from *http://www.cag-acg.org/uploads/guidelines/Colorectal%20cancer%20screening%202004.pdf*; and from Canadian Association of Gastroenterology. (2010). Position statement on screening individuals at average risk for developing colorectal cancer. Retrieved from *http://www.cag-acg.org/uploads/position_statement_colorectal_screening.pdf.*
*First-degree relative is a parent, child, or sibling; second-degree relative is a grandparent, aunt, uncle, nephew, niece, or grandchild; third-degree relative is a cousin, great-grandparent, or great-grandchild.
FIT, fecal immunochemical test; *FOBT,* fecal occult blood test.

PROMOTING HEALTH: SCREENING FOR COLORECTAL CANCER

Screening for Life

Colorectal cancer is the third most common cancer among Canadian men and women. It is expected that colorectal cancer will be diagnosed in 1 per 14 Canadians during their lifetime (Canadian Cancer Society & Statistics Canada, 2011). Some factors that appear to increase the risk of developing it are being of older age, particularly >50 years; having polyps; having a family history of colorectal cancer, especially a parent, sibling, or child who developed it before the age of 45; having familial adenomatous polyposis or hereditary nonpolyposis colon cancer; having inflammatory bowel disease (ulcerative colitis or Crohn's disease); eating a diet high in red and processed meats; consuming alcohol; smoking; being physically inactive; being obese; and having Ashkenazi (Eastern European) Jewish ancestry. However, colorectal cancer develops in some people who have none of

Continued

these risk factors. A diet high in vegetables and fruit is known to lower the risk, and research also suggests that a diet high in fibre and low in animal fats may also decrease the risk.

Colorectal cancer may not cause any symptoms in its early stages. Symptoms often appear once the tumour causes bleeding or blocks the bowel. Possible symptoms include a change in bowel habits, such as diarrhea or constipation; general abdominal discomfort (bloating, sensation of fullness, cramps); blood in the stool (either bright red or very dark); stools that are narrower than usual; a strong urge to defecate; a feeling that the bowel has not completely emptied; nausea or vomiting; fatigue; and weight loss.

Currently in Canada, screening for colorectal cancer with stool tests is recommended at least every 2 years for people aged 50 and over (see Table 23-1). There are two types of stool tests used in Canada. The guaiac-based fecal occult blood test (gFOBT) is the most common type of FOBT, and uses a chemical reaction on a paper card to find traces of blood in the stool from adenomatous polyps or tumours. The immunochemical-based fecal occult blood test (iFOBT) or fecal immunochemical test (FIT) is a

newer and more sensitive test that uses specific antibodies for human blood to find traces of blood in the stool. A positive FOBT or FIT result may be followed up with a colonoscopy, flexible sigmoidoscopy, or double-contrast barium enema (Canadian Cancer Society, 2013).

FIT is a more expensive test that is being used by some, but not all, colorectal screening programs in Canada. The Canadian Association of Gastroenterology (CAG) recommends FIT as the preferred screening test for individuals at average risk for developing colorectal cancer. The CAG also recommends that flexible sigmoidoscopy screening for colon cancer for all average-risk individuals with an interval of 10 years or longer between normal sigmoidoscopies (Leddin et al., 2010).

Individuals who are at higher than average risk of developing colorectal cancer may need to be tested more often and at an earlier age than people with average risk, and should talk to their doctor about a personal plan for testing. A personal plan for testing may include gFOBT or FIT, colonoscopy, flexible sigmoidoscopy, double-contrast barium enema, and genetic risk assessment/testing.

Sources: Data from Canadian Cancer Society. (2011). *Colorectal cancer: Understanding your diagnosis*. Retrieved from *http://www.cancer.ca/Canada-wide/Publications/Alphabetical%20list%20of%20publications/Colorectal%20cancer%20Understanding%20your%20diagnosis.aspx?sc_lang=en*; and from Canadian Cancer Society & Statistics Canada. (2011). *Canadian cancer statistics 2011: Featuring colorectal cancer.* Retrieved from *http://www.cancer.ca/Canada-wide/About%20cancer/~/media/CCS/Canada%20wide/Files%20List/English%20files%20heading/PDF%20-%20Policy%20-%20Canadian%20Cancer%20Statistics%20-%20English/Canadian%20Cancer%20Statistics%202011%20-%20English.ashx.*

PROMOTING HEALTH: SCREENING FOR PROSTATE CANCER

Understanding Prostate Changes

Prostate cancer is the most common cancer among Canadian men. A Canadian man has a 1 in 7 chance of receiving a diagnosis of prostate cancer during his lifetime (Izawa et al., 2011). Some factors that appear to increase the risk of developing it are being of older age, particularly >65 years; a family history of prostate cancer; a diet high in fat; and African ancestry. Obesity, physical inactivity, and exposure to cadmium are being studied as possible risk factors. Some men develop prostate cancer without any of these risk factors. Prostate cancer may not cause signs or symptoms, especially in the early stages. Symptoms may appear if the tumour enlarges the prostate and starts to press on the urethra, making the passage of urine difficult or painful or increasing the frequency of urination.

Throughout much of a man's life, the prostate gland is typically the size of a walnut. However, by the time a man is 40, it may grow slightly larger, to the size of an apricot. By age 60, it may be the size of a lemon. Although the size varies between individuals, this gradual enlargement is considered to be a normal part of aging. This enlargement is termed *benign prostatic hypertrophy* (BPH). It does not increase an individual's risk for prostate cancer, but the symptoms for BPH can be very similar to those of prostate cancer.

The risks and benefits of testing for prostate cancer should be discussed with men aged 50 years and older. Men who are at higher risk for prostate cancer because of family history or African ancestry should discuss the possibility of starting testing at a younger age. The digital rectal examination (DRE) and the prostate-specific antigen (PSA) blood test can help detect prostate cancer early, but they can also yield false-positive results or miss prostate cancer that is present (false-negative results). In some cases these tests can detect prostate cancer that may not

pose a serious threat to a man's health. There is very little evidence to support the widespread use of PSA screening among men who have no symptoms; some evidence exists to support its use among men in moderate- to high-risk groups; and there is no evidence to support its use among men with life expectancies of less than 10 years (O'Rourke, 2011). It is important to talk to men about their personal risk of developing prostate cancer and about the benefits and risks of testing.

PSA is a substance made by the normal prostate gland. When prostate cancer develops, the PSA level increases. However, benign or noncancerous enlargement of the prostate (e.g., BPH), age, and prostatitis can also cause PSA levels to increase. Ejaculation causes a temporary increase in PSA levels, and men need to be instructed to abstain from ejaculation for 2 days before having their PSA level tested. In addition, some medications, such as finasteride (Proscar) or dutasteride (Avodart), artificially lower PSA levels. If the PSA level is elevated, further laboratory work or transrectal ultrasonography and biopsy may be recommended.

In the DRE, the examiner inserts a gloved, lubricated finger into the patient's rectum. The prostate gland is located just in front of the rectum, and so it is possible to palpate the surface of the gland manually for bumps or hard areas that may represent developing cancer. Although the DRE is less effective than the PSA blood test in detecting prostate cancer, it can sometimes help detect cancers in men who have normal PSA levels. For this reason, it is recommended that PSA and DRE be performed together in screening for prostate cancer. A biopsy performed during transrectal ultrasonography is usually necessary to make a definitive diagnosis of cancer.

More details are available from the Canadian Cancer Society (2010).

Sources: Data from Canadian Cancer Society. (2007). *Prostate cancer: Understanding your diagnosis*. Retrieved from *http://www.cancer.ca/Canada-wide/Publications/Alphabetical%20list%20of%20publications/Prostate%20cancer%20Understanding%20your%20diagnosis.aspx?sc_lang=en;* and from Canadian Cancer Society. (2010). *Prostate cancer.* Retrieved from *http://www.cancer.ca/Canada-wide/Prevention/Getting%20checked/Prostate%20cancer%20NEW.aspx?sc_lang=en.*

OBJECTIVE DATA

PREPARATION

Perform a rectal examination on all adults and particularly for those in middle and older years. Help the patient assume one of the following positions (Figure 23-3): Examine a male patient in the left lateral decubitus or standing position. Instruct the standing male patient to point his toes together; this relaxes the regional muscles, making it easier to spread the buttocks.

Place the female patient in the lithotomy position if you are examining genitalia as well; use the left lateral decubitus position for examination of the rectal area alone.

These positions leave many patients feeling vulnerable and embarrassed. You can help the patient relax and retain a sense of control by using these measures:
- Ensure privacy.
- Explain each step in the examination before you perform it.
- Use a gentle, firm touch and gradual movements.
- Communicate throughout the examination. Maintain a dialogue to share information.

EQUIPMENT NEEDED

Penlight
Lubricating jelly
Glove
Guaiac test container

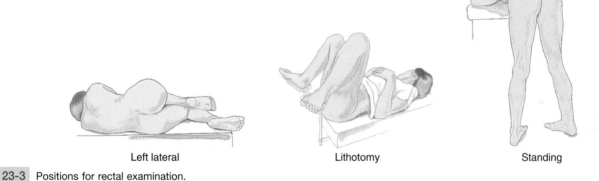

| Left lateral | Lithotomy | Standing |

23-3 Positions for rectal examination.

Normal Range of Findings	Abnormal Findings

INSPECT THE PERIANAL AREA

Spread the buttocks wide apart, and observe the perianal region. The anus normally looks moist and hairless, with coarse folded skin that is more pigmented than the perianal skin. The anal opening is tightly closed. No lesions are present.

Inflammation; lesions or scars.
Linear split: fissure.
Flabby skin sac: hemorrhoid.
Shiny blue skin sac: thrombosed hemorrhoid.
Small round opening in anal area: fistula (see Table 23-2 on p. 594).

Inspect the sacrococcygeal area. Normally, it appears smooth and even.

Inflammation or tenderness, swelling, tuft of hair, or dimple at tip of coccyx may indicate pilonidal cyst (see Table 23-2).
Appearance of fissure or hemorrhoids.

Instruct the patient to hold the breath and bear down (i.e., perform a Valsalva manoeuvre). No break in skin integrity or protrusion through the anal opening should be present. Describe any abnormality in clock face terms, with "12:00 position" as the anterior point toward the symphysis pubis and "6:00 position" toward the coccyx.

Circular red "doughnut" of tissue: rectal prolapse.

Normal Range of Findings	Abnormal Findings

 DEVELOPMENTAL CONSIDERATIONS

Infants and Children

To examine a newborn, hold the feet with one hand and flex the knees up onto the abdomen. Note the presence of the anus. Confirm patency of the rectum and anus by noting the first meconium stool passed within 24 to 48 hours of birth. To assess sphincter tone, check the *anal reflex:* Gently stroke the anal area and note a quick contraction of the sphincter.

In an infant or child, note that the buttocks are firm and rounded with no masses or lesions. Recall that the *mongolian spot* is a common variation of hyperpigmentation in newborns of African, Asian, Mediterranean, or Aboriginal descent (see Chapter 13).

The perianal skin is free of lesions. However, diaper rash is common in children younger than 1 year and manifests as a generalized reddened area with papules or vesicles.

Omit palpation unless the history or symptoms warrant. When internal palpation is needed, position the infant or child on the back with the legs flexed, and gently insert a gloved, well-lubricated finger into the rectum. Your fifth finger usually is long enough, and its smaller size is more comfortable for an infant or child. However, you may need to use the index finger because of its better control and increased tactile sensitivity. On withdrawing the finger, scant bleeding or protruding rectal mucosa may be evident.

Inspect the perianal region of a school-age child or adolescent during examination of the genitalia. Internal palpation is not performed routinely in patients of these ages.

Older Adults

As an older patient performs the Valsalva manoeuvre, you may note relaxation of the perianal musculature and decreased sphincter control. Otherwise, the full examination proceeds as described earlier for younger adults.

Abnormal Findings column:

Imperforate anus.

Flattened buttocks, as in cystic fibrosis or celiac syndrome.

Coccygeal mass.

Meningocele (sac containing meninges that protrude through a defect in the bony spine).

Tuft of hair or pilonidal dimple.

Pustules indicate secondary infection of diaper rash.

Signs of physical or sexual abuse include anal abrasions and perianal tears.

Fissure is a common cause of constipation or rectal bleeding in children. (Because it is painful, the child does not defecate.)

SPECIAL CONSIDERATIONS FOR ADVANCED PRACTICE

Normal Range of Findings	Abnormal Findings

PALPATE THE ANUS AND RECTUM

Drop lubricating jelly onto your gloved index finger. Inform the patient that palpation is not painful but that he or she may feel the need to move the bowels. Place the pad of your index finger gently against the anal verge (Figure 23-4). You will feel the sphincter tighten and then relax. As it relaxes, flex the tip of your finger and slowly insert it into the anal canal in a direction toward the umbilicus. *Never* approach the anus at right angles with your index finger extended. Such a jabbing motion does not promote sphincter relaxation and is painful.

Objective Data

Special Considerations for Advanced Practice

Normal Range of Findings	Abnormal Findings

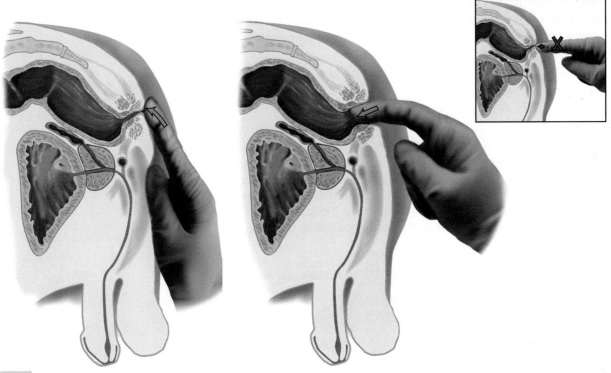

23-4   Palpating the anus and rectum.

Rotate your examining finger to palpate the entire muscular ring. The canal should feel smooth and even. Note the intersphincteric groove circling the canal wall. To assess tone, ask the patient to tighten the muscle. The sphincter should tighten evenly around your finger without causing pain for the patient.

Use a bidigital palpation technique, with your thumb against the perianal tissue (Figure 23-5). Press your examining finger toward it. This manoeuvre helps you detect any swelling or tenderness and helps you assess the bulboure-thral glands.

Decreased tone should be investi-gated.

Increased tone occurs with inflamma-tion and anxiety.

Tenderness should be investigated.

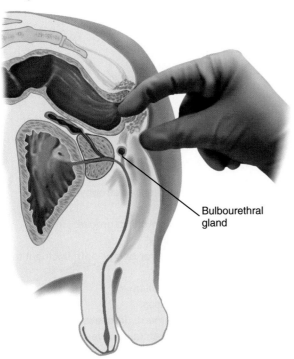

Bulbourethral
gland

23-5   Examiner's thumb against perianal tissue.

Normal Range of Findings	**Abnormal Findings**

Above the anal canal, the rectum turns posteriorly, following the curve of the coccyx and sacrum. Insert your finger farther, and explore all around the rectal wall. It normally feels smooth with no nodularity. Promptly report any mass you discover for further examination.

An internal hemorrhoid above the anorectal junction is not palpable unless it is thrombosed.

A soft, slightly movable mass may be a polyp.

A firm or hard mass with irregular shape or rolled edges may signify carcinoma (see Table 23-3, Abnormalities of the Rectum, p. 596).

Prostate Gland. On the anterior wall in a male patient, note the elastic, bulging prostate gland (Figure 23-6). Palpate the entire prostate in a systematic manner, but note that only the superior surface and part of the lateral surface are accessible to examination. Press *into* the gland at each location, because when a nodule is present, it does not project into the rectal lumen. The surface should feel smooth and muscular; search for any distinct nodule or diffuse firmness.

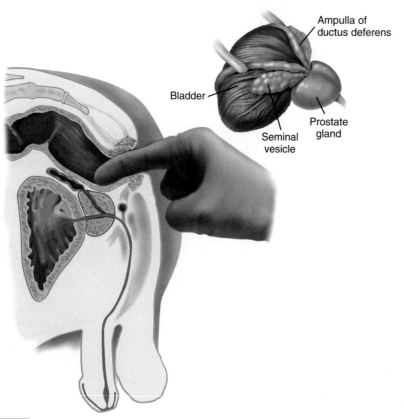

Ampulla of ductus deferens

Bladder

Seminal vesicle

Prostate gland

23-6 Palpating the prostate gland.

Note these characteristics:
Size: 2.5 cm long by 4 cm wide; should not protrude more than 1 cm into the rectum
Shape: heart shape, with palpable central groove
Surface: smooth
Consistency: elastic, rubbery
Mobility: slightly movable
Sensitivity: nontender to palpation

Enlargement or atrophy.

Flatness with no groove.
Nodularity.
Hardness or boggy, soft, fluctuant texture.
Fixed position.
Tenderness.
Enlargement, firmness, and smoothness with central groove obliterated: suggestive of BPH.

Normal Range of Findings	Abnormal Findings
	Swelling and exquisite tenderness: accompanies prostatitis. Any stone-hard, irregular, fixed nodule: indicates carcinoma (see Table 23-4).
In a female patient, palpate the cervix through the anterior rectal wall. It normally feels like a small round mass. You also may palpate a retroverted uterus or a tampon in the vagina. Do not mistake the cervix or a tampon for a tumour. Withdraw your examining finger; normally, no mucus or bright red blood is on the glove. To complete the examination, offer the patient tissues to remove the lubricant, and help the patient to a more comfortable position. **Examination of Stool.** Inspect any feces remaining on the glove. Normally, the colour is brown, and the consistency is soft.	
	Jelly-like shreds of mucus mixed in stool indicate inflammation. Bright red blood on stool surface indicates rectal bleeding. Bright red blood mixed with feces indicates possible colonic bleeding. Black tarry stool with distinct malodour indicates upper gastrointestinal bleeding with blood partially digested. (More than 50 mL of blood from upper gastrointestinal tract must be lost for this stool to be considered melena.) Black stool also occurs with ingesting iron or bismuth preparations. Grey, tan stool indicates the absence of bile pigment, as in obstructive jaundice. Pale yellow, greasy stool is indicative of increased fat content (steatorrhea), as occurs with malabsorption syndrome. Occult bleeding usually indicates cancer of the colon.
Test any stool on the glove for **occult blood;** use the specimen container that your agency directs. A negative response is normal. A positive *Hematest* result indicates occult blood. However, a false-positive finding may occur if the patient has ingested significant amounts of red meat within 3 days of the test.	

Documentation & Critical Thinking

DOCUMENTATION AND CRITICAL THINKING

Sample Charting

SUBJECTIVE

Has one BM daily, soft, brown; no pain, no change in bowel routine. Taking no medications. Has no history of pruritus, hemorrhoids, fissure, or fistula. Diet includes one to two servings daily each of fresh fruits and vegetables but no whole-grain cereals or breads.

OBJECTIVE

No fissure, hemorrhoids, fistula, or skin lesions in perianal area. Sphincter tone good, no prolapse. Rectal walls smooth, no masses or tenderness. Prostate not enlarged, no masses or tenderness. Stool brown, Hematest result negative.

ASSESSMENT

Rectal structures intact, no palpable lesions

Focused Assessment: Clinical Case Study

C.M. is a 62-year-old male with chronic obstructive pulmonary disease for 15 years, who today describes having had "diarrhea for 3 days."

SUBJECTIVE

- **7 days PTA:** C.M. seen at this agency for acute respiratory infection that was diagnosed as acute bronchitis and treated with oral ampicillin. Took medication as directed.
- **3 days PTA:** Symptoms of respiratory infection improved. Ingesting usual diet. Onset of four to five loose, unformed, brown stools a day. No abdominal pain or cramping. No nausea.
- **Now:** Diarrhea continues. No blood or mucus noticed in stool. No new foods or restaurant food in past 3 days. Wife not ill.

OBJECTIVE

Vital signs: Temp 37°C, HR 88, RR 18, BP 142/82.
Respiratory: Respirations unlaboured. Barrel chest. Hyperresonant to percussion. Lung sounds clear but diminished. No crackles or rhonchi today.
Abdomen: Flat. Bowel sounds present. No organomegaly or tenderness to palpation.
Rectal: No lesions in perianal area. Sphincter tone good. Rectal walls smooth, no mass or tenderness. Prostate smooth and firm, no median sulcus palpable, no masses or tenderness. Stool brown, Hematest result negative.

ASSESSMENT

Diarrhea R/T effects of antibiotic medication

ABNORMAL FINDINGS

TABLE 23-2   Abnormalities of the Anal Region

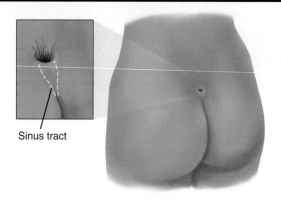

Sinus tract

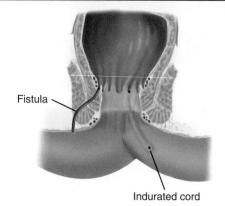

Fistula

Indurated cord

Pilonidal Cyst or Sinus

A hair-containing cyst or sinus located in the midline over the coccyx or lower sacrum. Often opens as a dimple with visible tuft of hair and, possibly, an erythematous halo, or may appear as a palpable cyst. When advanced, has a palpable sinus tract. Although congenital, the lesion is first diagnosed between the ages of 15 and 30 years.

Anorectal Fistula

A chronically inflamed gastrointestinal tract creates an abnormal passage from inner anus or rectum out to skin surrounding anus. Usually originates from a local abscess. The red, raised tract opening may drain serosanguineous or purulent matter when pressure is applied. Bidigital palpation may reveal an indurated spinal cord.

TABLE 23-2	Abnormalities of the Anal Region—cont'd

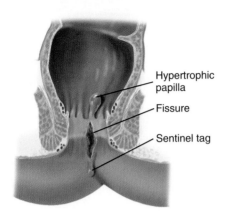

Hypertrophic papilla

Fissure

Sentinel tag

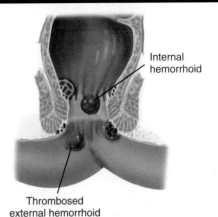

Internal hemorrhoid

Thrombosed external hemorrhoid

Fissure

A painful longitudinal tear in the superficial mucosa at the anal margin. Most fissures (>90%) occur in the posterior midline area. They are frequently accompanied by a papule of hyperplastic skin, called a *sentinel tag,* on the anal margin below. Fissures often result from trauma: for example, from passing a large, hard stool or from irritant diarrheal stools. Fissures cause itching, bleeding, and exquisite pain. A resulting spasm in the sphincters makes the area painful to examine; local anaesthesia may be indicated.

Hemorrhoids

These painless, flabby papules are varicose veins of the hemorrhoidal plexus. An *external hemorrhoid* originates below the anorectal junction and is covered by anal skin. When *thrombosed,* it contains clotted blood and becomes a painful, swollen, shiny blue mass that itches and bleeds with defecation. When it resolves, it leaves a painless, flabby skin sac around the anal orifice. An *internal hemorrhoid* originates above the anorectal junction and is covered by mucous membrane. When the patient performs a Valsalva manoeuvre, it may appear as a red mucosal mass. It is not palpable. All hemorrhoids result from increased portal venous pressure, as occurs with straining at stool, chronic constipation, pregnancy, obesity, chronic liver disease, or the low-fibre diet common in Western society.

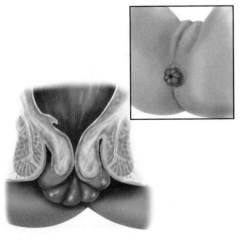

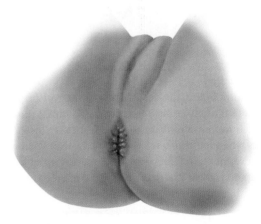

Rectal Prolapse

The rectal mucous membrane protrudes through the anus, appearing as a moist red doughnut with radiating lines. When prolapse is incomplete, only the mucosa bulges. When complete, the anal sphincters also bulge. Occurs after a Valsalva manoeuvre, such as straining at stool, or with exercise.

Pruritus Ani

Intense perianal itching is manifested by red, raised, thickened, excoriated skin around the anus. Common causes are pinworms in children and fungal infections in adults. The area is swollen and moist, and with a fungal infection, it appears dull greyish pink. The skin is dry and brittle with psychosomatic itching. Pruritus ani is classified as idiopathic when no cause can be found (Markell & Billingham, 2010).

TABLE 23-3   Abnormalities of the Rectum

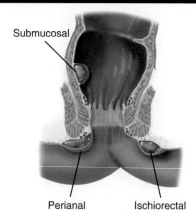

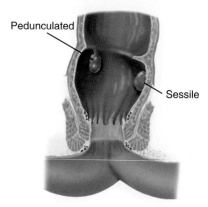

Abscess

A localized cavity of pus from infection in a pararectal space. Infection usually extends from an anal crypt. Characterized by persistent throbbing rectal pain. Termed according to the space it occupies (e.g., a perianal abscess is superficial around the anal skin) and appears red, hot, swollen, indurated, and tender. An ischiorectal abscess (lateral, between the anus and ischial tuberosity) is deep and tender to bidigital palpation. It is uncommon.

Rectal Polyp

A growth protruding from the rectal mucous membrane that is fairly common. The polyp may be *pedunculated* (on a stalk) or *sessile* (a mound on the surface, close to the mucosal wall). The soft nodule is difficult to palpate. Proctoscopy is needed, as is biopsy, to screen for malignancy.

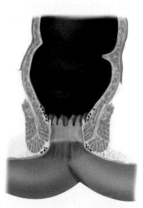

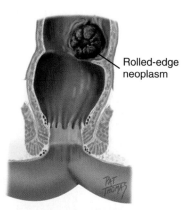

Fecal Impaction

A collection of hard, desiccated feces in the rectum. The obstruction often results from decreased bowel motility, in which more water is reabsorbed from the stool. Also occurs when barium is retained after gastrointestinal x-ray examination. The patient may complain of constipation or of diarrhea as a fecal stream passes around the impaction.

Carcinoma

A malignant neoplasm in the rectum is asymptomatic; thus routine rectal palpation is important. An early lesion may be a single firm nodule. You may palpate an ulcerated centre with rolled edges. As the lesion grows, its shape is irregular, like cauliflower, and it is fixed and stone hard. Refer a patient with any rectal lesion for further study because about half of such lesions are malignant.

TABLE 23-4   Abnormalities of the Prostate Gland

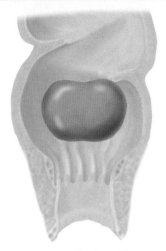

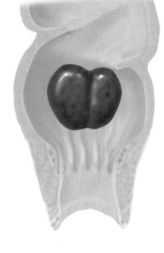

Benign Prostatic Hypertrophy (BPH)

S: Urinary frequency, urgency, hesitancy, straining to urinate, weak stream, intermittent stream, sensation of incomplete emptying, nocturia.

O: A symmetrical nontender enlargement, commonly occurs in men beginning in middle age. The prostate surface feels smooth, rubbery, or firm (like the consistency of the nose), and the median sulcus is obliterated.

Prostatitis

S: Fever, chills, malaise, urinary frequency and urgency, dysuria, urethral discharge; dull, aching pain in perineal and rectal area.

O: *Acute* inflammation of the prostate gland causes the gland to become swollen, slightly asymmetrical, and quite tender to palpation.

With a chronic inflammation, the signs can vary from tender enlargement with a boggy texture to isolated areas of firmness caused by fibrosis. Alternatively, the gland may feel normal.

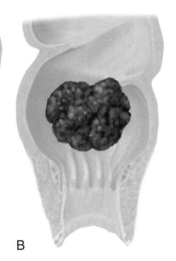

A   B

◄ Carcinoma

S: Frequency, nocturia, hematuria, weak stream, hesitancy, pain or burning sensation on urination, continuous pain in lower back, pelvis, thighs.

O: A malignant neoplasm often starts as a single hard nodule on the posterior surface (see diagram A), producing asymmetry and a change in consistency. As it invades normal tissue, multiple hard nodules appear, or the entire gland feels stone hard and fixed (see diagram B). The median sulcus is obliterated.

S, Subjective data; *O*, objective data.

Summary Checklist: Anus, Rectum, and Prostate Examination

For a PDA-downloadable version, go to *http://evolve.elsevier.com/Canada/Jarvis/examination/.*

1. Inspecting anus and perianal area
2. Inspecting during Valsalva manoeuvre
3. Palpating anal canal and rectum in all adults
4. Testing stool for occult blood
5. Teaching and health promotion

REFERENCES

Canadian Cancer Society. (2010). *Prostate cancer*. Retrieved from *http://www.cancer.ca/Canada-wide/Prevention/Getting%20 checked/Prostate%20cancer%20NEW.aspx?sc_lang=en.*

Canadian Cancer Society & Statistics Canada. (2011). *Canadian cancer statistics 2011*. Retrieved from *http://www.cancer.ca/ Canada-wide/About%20cancer/~/media/CCS/Canada%20wide/ Files%20List/English%20files%20heading/PDF%20-%20 Policy%20-%20Canadian%20Cancer%20Statistics%20-%20 English/Canadian%20Cancer%20Statistics%202011%20-%20 English.ashx.*

Canadian Cancer Society. (2013). *Screening for colorectal cancer*. Retrieved from *http://www.cancer.ca/en/cancer-information/ cancer-type/colorectal/screening/?region=on*

Izawa, J. I., Klotz, L., Siemens, D. R., Kassouf, W., So, A., Jordan, J., … & Iansavichene, A. E. (2011). Prostate cancer screening: Canadian guidelines 2011. *Canadian Urological Association Journal, 5*(4), 235–240. doi:10.5489/cuaj.11134

Leddin, D. J., Enns, R., Hilsden, R., Plourde, V., Rabaneck, L., Sadowski, D. C., & Singh, J. (2010). Canadian Association of Gastroenterology position statement on screening individuals at average risk for developing colorectal cancer: 2010. *Canadian Journal of Gastroenterology, 24*(12), 705–714.

Markell, K. W., & Billingham, R. P. (2010). Pruritis ani: Etiology and management. *Surgical Clinics of North America, 90*(1), 125–135. doi:10.1016/j.suc.2009.09.007

O'Rourke, M. E. (2011). The prostate-specific antigen screening conundrum: Examining the evidence. *Seminars in Oncology Nursing, 27*, 4, 251–259. doi:10.1016/j.soncn.2011.07.003

Musculoskeletal System

Written by Carolyn Jarvis, PhD, APN, CNP
Adapted by Marian Luctkar-Flude, RN, MScN

⊖volve WEBSITE

http://evolve.elsevier.com/Canada/Jarvis/examination/
- Animations
- Bedside Assessment Summary Checklist
- Case Study:
  - Joint Pain
  - Numbness in Hands
- Examination Review Questions
- Health Promotion Guide:
  - Osteoporosis

- Key Points
- Physical Examination Summary Checklist
- Quick Assessment for Common Conditions:
  - Degenerative Joint Disease (Osteoarthritis)
  - Fracture
  - Osteoporosis
- Video—Assessment:
  - Lower Extremities
  - Musculoskeletal and Neurological Systems

OUTLINE

STRUCTURE AND FUNCTION

The musculoskeletal system consists of the body's bones, joints, and muscles. Humans need this system (a) for *support* to stand erect and (b) for *movement*. The musculoskeletal system also functions (c) to encase and *protect* the inner vital organs (e.g., brain, spinal cord, heart), (d) to *produce* the red blood cells in the bone marrow (hematopoiesis), and (e) as a *reservoir* for storage of essential minerals such as calcium and phosphorus in the bones.

COMPONENTS OF THE MUSCULOSKELETAL SYSTEM

The skeleton is the bony framework of the body. It has 206 bones, which support the body like the posts and beams of a building. Bone and cartilage are specialized forms of connective tissue. **Bone** is hard, rigid, and very dense. Its cells are continually turning over and remodelling. The **joint** (or articulation) is the place of union of two or more bones.

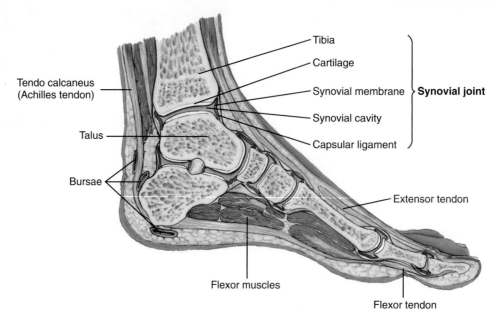

24-1 Synovial joints.

Joints are the functional units of the musculoskeletal system because they enable the mobility needed for activities of daily living (ADLs).

Nonsynovial or Synovial Joints

In **nonsynovial joints,** the bones are united by fibrous tissue or cartilage and are immovable (e.g., the sutures in the skull) or only slightly movable (e.g., the vertebrae). **Synovial joints** are freely movable because they have bones that are separated from each other and are enclosed in a joint cavity (Figure 24-1). This cavity is filled with a lubricant: synovial fluid. Just like grease on gears, synovial fluid allows sliding of opposing surfaces, and this sliding enables movement.

In synovial joints, a layer of resilient **cartilage** covers the surface of opposing bones. Cartilage is avascular; it receives nourishment from synovial fluid that circulates during joint movement. It is a very stable connective tissue with a slow cell turnover. It has a tough, firm consistency and yet is flexible. Cartilage cushions the bones and provides a smooth surface to facilitate movement.

Each joint is surrounded by a fibrous capsule and is supported by ligaments. **Ligaments** are fibrous bands running directly from one bone to another that strengthen the joint and help prevent movement in undesirable directions. A **bursa** is an enclosed sac filled with viscous synovial fluid, much like a joint. Bursae are located in areas of potential friction (e.g., subacromial bursa of the shoulder, prepatellar bursa of the knee) and help muscles and tendons glide smoothly over bone.

Muscles

Muscles account for 40% to 50% of the body's weight. When they contract, they produce movement. Muscles are of three types: skeletal, smooth, and cardiac. This chapter is concerned with skeletal, or voluntary, muscles, which are under conscious control.

Each **skeletal muscle** is composed of bundles of muscle fibres **(fasciculi).** The skeletal muscle is attached to bone by a **tendon,** a strong fibrous cord. Skeletal muscles produce the following movements (Figure 24-2):

1. Flexion: bending a limb at a joint
2. Extension: straightening a limb at a joint
3. Abduction: moving a limb away from the midline of the body
4. Adduction: moving a limb toward the midline of the body
5. Pronation: turning the forearm so that the palm is down
6. Supination: turning the forearm so that the palm is up
7. Circumduction: moving the arm in a circle around the shoulder
8. Inversion: moving the sole of the foot inward at the ankle
9. Eversion: moving the sole of the foot outward at the ankle
10. Rotation: moving the head around a central axis
11. Protraction: moving a body part forward and parallel to the ground
12. Retraction: moving a body part backward and parallel to the ground
13. Elevation: raising a body part
14. Depression: lowering a body part

Temporomandibular Joint

The temporomandibular joint is the articulation of the mandible and the temporal bone (Figure 24-3). You can feel it in the depression anterior to the tragus of the ear. The temporomandibular joint enables jaw function for speaking and

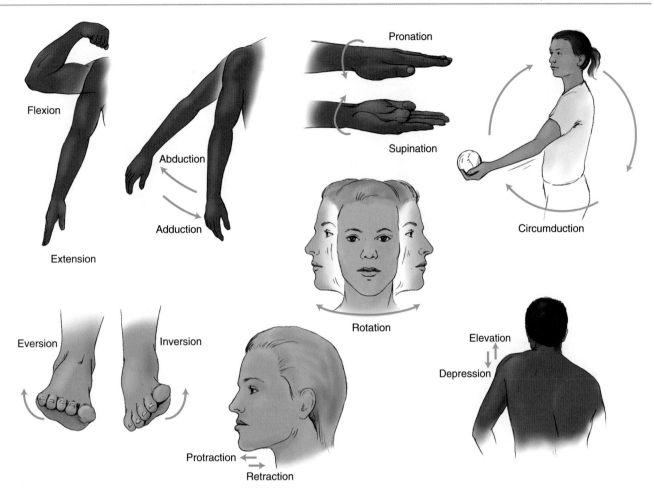

SKELETAL MUSCLE MOVEMENTS

24-2

© Pat Thomas, 2006.

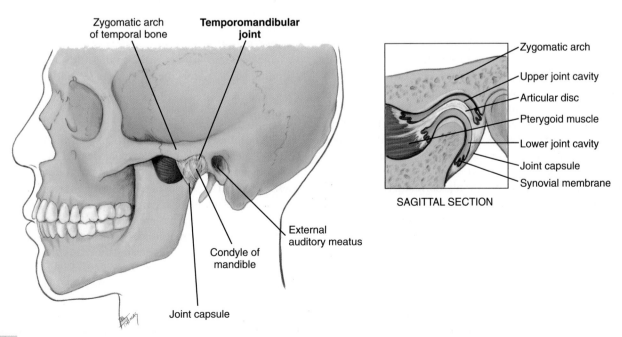

SAGITTAL SECTION

24-3

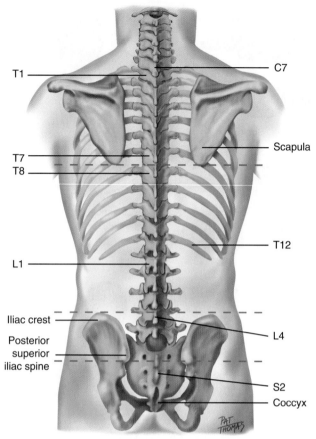

LANDMARKS OF THE SPINE

24-4

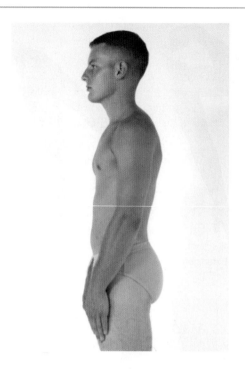

24-5

chewing. The joint allows three motions: (a) hinge action to open and close the jaws, (b) gliding action for protrusion and retraction, and (c) gliding action for side-to-side movement of the lower jaw.

Spine

The **vertebrae** are 33 connecting bones stacked in a vertical column (Figure 24-4). You can feel their spinous processes in a furrow down the midline of the back. The furrow has paravertebral muscles mounded on either side down to the sacrum, where it flattens. Humans have 7 cervical, 12 thoracic, 5 lumbar, 5 sacral, and 3 to 4 coccygeal vertebrae. The following surface landmarks will orient you to their levels:

- The spinous processes of C7 and T1 are prominent at the base of the neck.
- The inferior angle of the scapula normally is at the level of the interspace between T7 and T8.
- An imaginary line connecting the highest point on each iliac crest crosses L4.
- An imaginary line joining the two symmetrical dimples that overlie the posterior superior iliac spines crosses the sacrum.

A lateral view (Figure 24-5) shows that the vertebral column has four curves (a double S-shape). The cervical and lumbar curves are concave (inward or anterior), and the thoracic and sacrococcygeal curves are convex. The balanced or compensatory nature of these curves, together with the resilient intervertebral discs, allows the spine to absorb a great deal of shock.

The **intervertebral discs** are elastic fibrocartilaginous plates that constitute one fourth of the length of the column (Figure 24-6). Each disc centre has a **nucleus pulposus,** made of soft, semifluid, mucoid material that has the consistency of toothpaste in young adults. The discs cushion the spine like a shock absorber and help it move. As the spine moves, the elasticity of the discs allows compression on one side, with compensatory expansion on the other. If compression is too great, a disc can rupture, and the nucleus pulposus can herniate out of the vertebral column, compressing the spinal nerves and causing pain.

The unique structure of the spine enables both upright posture and flexibility for motion. The motions of the vertebral column are flexion (bending forward), extension (bending back), abduction (to either side), and rotation.

Shoulder

The **glenohumeral joint** is the articulation of the humerus with the glenoid fossa of the scapula (Figure 24-7). Its ball-and-socket action allows great mobility of the arm in many axes. The joint is enclosed by a group of four powerful muscles and tendons that support and stabilize it. Together, these muscles and tendons are called the **rotator cuff** of the shoulder. The large **subacromial bursa** helps during abduction of the arm so that the greater tubercle of the humerus moves easily under the acromion process of the scapula.

The bones of the shoulder have palpable landmarks to guide your examination (Figure 24-8). The scapula and the clavicle connect to form the shoulder girdle. You can feel the bump of the scapula's **acromion process** at the very top of the shoulder. Move your fingers in a small circle outward,

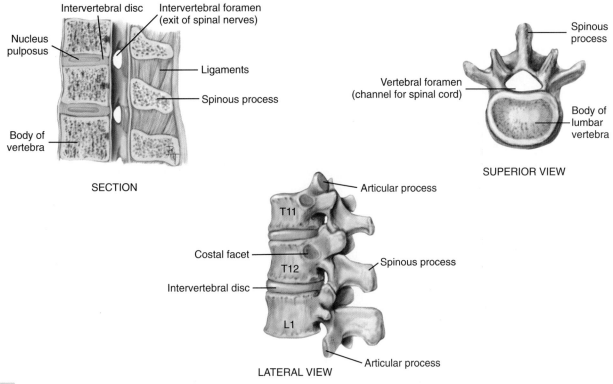

24-6   The vertebrae.

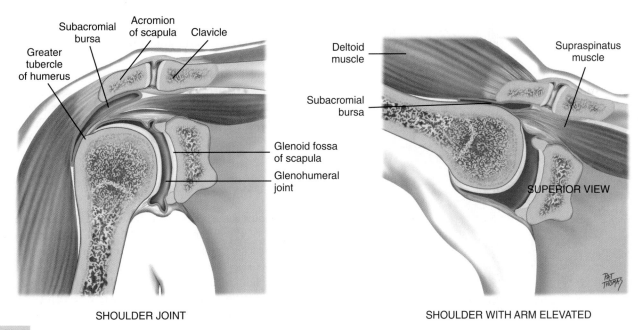

24-7

down, and around. The next bump is the **greater tubercle** of the humerus a few centimetres down and laterally, and from that the **coracoid process** of the scapula is a few centimetres medially. These surround the deeply situated joint.

Elbow

The elbow joint contains the three bony articulations of the humerus, radius, and ulna of the forearm (Figure 24-9). Its hinge action moves the forearm (radius and ulna) on one plane, allowing flexion and extension. The olecranon bursa lies between the olecranon process and the skin.

Palpable landmarks are the **medial** and **lateral epicondyles** of the humerus and the large **olecranon process** of the ulna in between them. The sensitive ulnar nerve runs between the olecranon process and the medial epicondyle.

The radius and ulna articulate with each other at two radioulnar joints, one at the elbow and one at the wrist. These

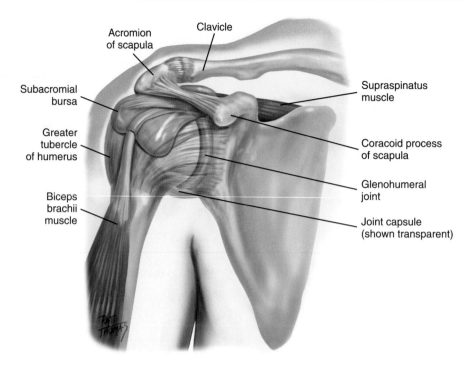

BONY LANDMARKS OF THE SHOULDER – ANTERIOR VIEW

24-8

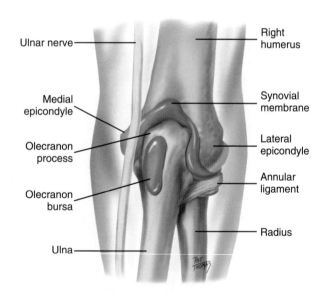

RIGHT ELBOW – POSTERIOR VIEW

24-9

move together to enable pronation and supination of the hand and forearm.

Wrist and Carpal Joints

Of the body's 206 bones, more than half are in the hands and feet. The wrist, or **radiocarpal joint,** is the articulation of the radius (on the thumb side) and a row of carpal bones (Figure 24-10). Its condyloid action enables movement in two planes at right angles: (a) flexion and extension and (b) side-to-side deviation. You can feel the groove of this joint on the dorsum of the wrist.

The **midcarpal joint** is the articulation between the two parallel rows of carpal bones. It allows flexion, extension, and some rotation. The **metacarpophalangeal** and the **interphalangeal joints** enable finger flexion and extension. The flexor tendons of the wrist and hand are enclosed in synovial sheaths.

Hip

The hip joint is the articulation between the acetabulum and the head of the femur (Figure 24-11). As in the shoulder, ball-and-socket action enables a wide range of motion (ROM) on many axes. The hip has somewhat less ROM than the shoulder, but it has more stability, which befits its weight-bearing function. Hip stability is enabled by powerful muscles that spread over the joint, by a strong fibrous articular capsule, and by the very deep insertion of the head of the femur. Three bursae facilitate movement.

Palpation of these bony landmarks will guide your examination: You can feel the entire iliac crest, from the **anterior superior iliac spine** to the posterior superior iliac spine. The **ischial tuberosity** lies under the gluteus maximus muscle and is palpable when the hip is flexed. The **greater trochanter** of the femur is normally the width of the person's palm below the iliac crest and halfway between the anterior superior iliac spine and the ischial tuberosity. You can palpate it, when the person is standing, in a flat depression on the upper lateral side of the thigh.

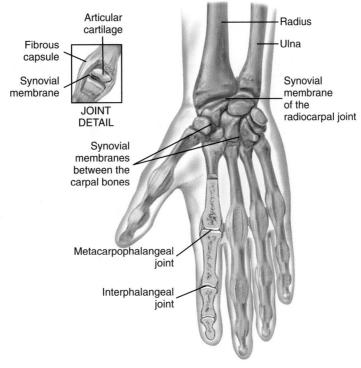

BONES OF THE HAND – PALMAR VIEW

24-10

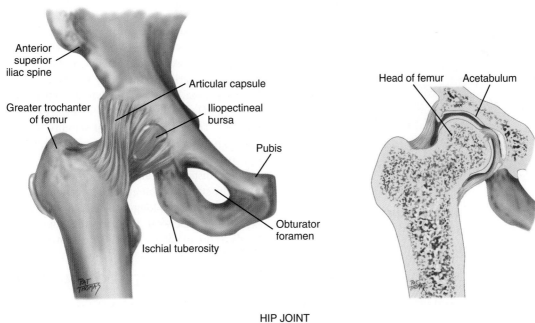

HIP JOINT

24-11

Knee

The knee joint is the articulation of three bones—the femur, the tibia, and the patella (kneecap)—in one common articular cavity (Figure 24-12). It is the largest joint in the body and is complex. It is a hinge joint, enabling flexion and extension of the lower leg on a single plane.

The knee's synovial membrane is the largest in the body. At the superior border of the patella, it forms a sac, called the **suprapatellar pouch,** that extends up as much as 6 cm behind the quadriceps muscle. Two wedge-shaped cartilages, the **medial** and **lateral menisci,** cushion the tibia and femur. The joint is stabilized by two sets of ligaments. The **cruciate ligaments** (not shown in Figure 24-12) crisscross within the

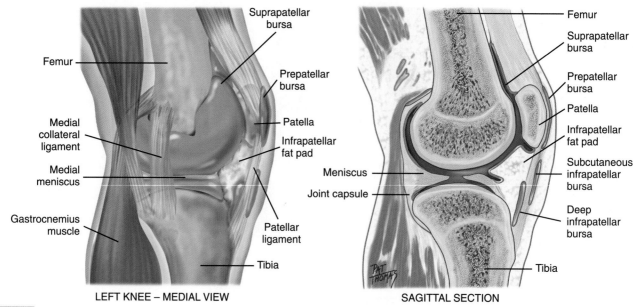

Femur

Suprapatellar bursa

Prepatellar bursa

Patella

Infrapatellar fat pad

Medial collateral ligament

Medial meniscus

Gastrocnemius muscle

Patellar ligament

Tibia

LEFT KNEE – MEDIAL VIEW

24-12

Femur

Suprapatellar bursa

Prepatellar bursa

Patella

Infrapatellar fat pad

Subcutaneous infrapatellar bursa

Deep infrapatellar bursa

Meniscus

Joint capsule

Tibia

SAGITTAL SECTION

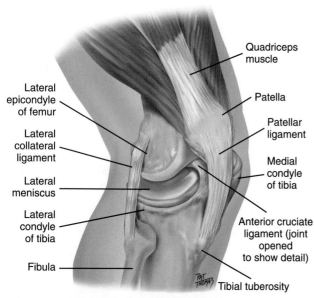

Quadriceps muscle

Patella

Patellar ligament

Medial condyle of tibia

Lateral epicondyle of femur

Lateral collateral ligament

Lateral meniscus

Lateral condyle of tibia

Fibula

Anterior cruciate ligament (joint opened to show detail)

Tibial tuberosity

LANDMARKS OF THE RIGHT KNEE JOINT

24-13

knee; they provide anterior and posterior stability and help control rotation. The **collateral ligaments** connect the joint at both sides; they provide medial and lateral stability and prevent dislocation. Numerous bursae prevent friction. One, the **prepatellar bursa,** lies between the patella and the skin. The **infrapatellar fat pad** is a small, triangular fat pad below the patella behind the patellar ligament.

Landmarks of the knee joint start with the large **quadriceps muscle,** which you can feel on your anterior and lateral thigh (Figure 24-13). The muscle's four heads merge into a common tendon that continues down to enclose the round bony patella. Then the tendon inserts down on the **tibial tuberosity,** which you can palpate as a bony prominence in

the midline. Move to the sides and a bit superiorly, and note the lateral and medial condyles of the tibia. Superior to these on either side of the patella are the medial and lateral epicondyles of the femur.

Ankle and Foot

The ankle, or **tibiotalar joint,** is the articulation of the tibia, fibula, and talus (Figure 24-14). It is a hinge joint, limited to flexion (dorsiflexion) and extension (plantar flexion) in one plane. Landmarks are two bony prominences on either side: the **medial malleolus** and the **lateral malleolus.** Strong, tight medial and lateral ligaments extend from each malleolus onto the foot. These help the lateral stability of the ankle joint, although they may be torn in eversion or inversion sprains of the ankle.

Joints distal to the ankle provide additional mobility in the foot. The subtalar joint enables inversion and eversion of the foot. The foot has a longitudinal arch, so that weight bearing is distributed between the parts that touch the ground: the heads of the metatarsals and the calcaneus (heel).

DEVELOPMENTAL CONSIDERATIONS

Infants and Children

By 3 months' gestation, a "scale model" of the skeleton that is made up of cartilage has formed. During succeeding months in utero, the cartilage ossifies into true bone and starts to grow. Bone growth continues after birth—rapidly during infancy and then steadily during childhood—and during adolescence, when both boys and girls undergo a rapid growth spurt.

Long bones grow in two dimensions. They increase in width or diameter by deposition of new bony tissue around the shafts. Lengthening occurs at the **epiphyses** (growth

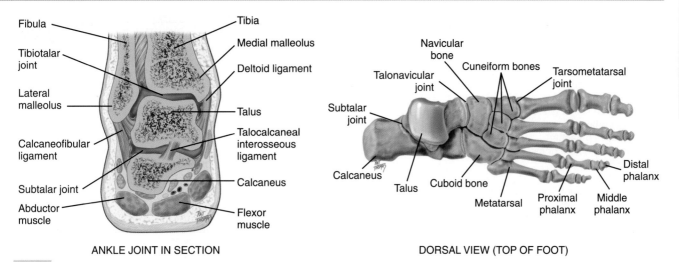

Fibula
Tibiotalar joint
Lateral malleolus
Calcaneofibular ligament
Subtalar joint
Abductor muscle

Tibia
Medial malleolus
Deltoid ligament
Talus
Talocalcaneal interosseous ligament
Calcaneus
Flexor muscle

ANKLE JOINT IN SECTION

Navicular bone
Talonavicular joint
Cuneiform bones
Tarsometatarsal joint
Subtalar joint
Calcaneus
Talus
Cuboid bone
Metatarsal
Proximal phalanx
Middle phalanx
Distal phalanx

DORSAL VIEW (TOP OF FOOT)

24-14

plates). These specialized growth centres are transverse discs located at the ends of long bones. Any trauma or infection at this location puts the growing child at risk for bone deformity. This longitudinal growth continues until closure of the epiphyses; the last closure occurs at about age 20 years.

Skeletal contour changes are apparent at the vertebral column. At birth the spine has a single C-shaped curve. At 3 to 4 months, when the baby can raise the head from the prone position, the anterior curve in the cervical neck region develops. From ages 1 year to 18 months, standing erect causes the development of the anterior curve in the lumbar region.

Although the skeleton contributes to linear growth, muscles and fat are significant for weight increase. Individual muscle fibres grow through childhood, but growth is marked during the adolescent growth spurt. At this time, muscles respond to increased secretion of growth hormone, to adrenal androgens, and, in boys, to further stimulation by testosterone. Muscles vary in size and strength in different people. This variation is attributable to genetic programming, nutrition, and exercise. All through life, muscles increase with use and atrophy with disuse.

The term *developmental dysplasia of the hip* (DDH) refers to a number of congenital abnormalities of the hip joint, including dislocated hip and subluxation of the hip. The Canadian Task Force on Preventive Health Care (Patel & Canadian Task Force on Preventive Health Care, 2001) recommends clinical examination of the hips by a trained clinician in the periodic health examination of all infants during the first week of life, during the first month, and then at 2, 4, 6, 9, and 12 months of age. Potential risk factors for DDH include having a first-degree relative with DDH, breech delivery, and clinical evidence of joint instability. Girls are more predisposed than boys to DDH, and Canadian Aboriginal people have a high risk for DDH.

The most common cause of childhood musculoskeletal pain is termed "growing pains," a noninflammatory pain syndrome affecting children mainly between the ages of 3 and 12 years (Uziel & Hashkes, 2007). The pain is usually nonarticular, bilateral, and located in the lower extremities; it occurs late in the day or is nocturnal, often awakening the child, and it frequently occurs on days of increased physical activity. The pain can be mild or very severe, lasting minutes to hours; is generally episodic but may occur daily; and usually resolves by late childhood.

Pregnant Women

Increased levels of circulating hormones (estrogen, relaxin from the corpus luteum, and corticosteroids) cause increases in mobility in the joints. Increased mobility in the sacroiliac, sacrococcygeal, and symphysis pubis joints in the pelvis contributes to the noticeable changes in maternal posture. The most characteristic change is progressive **lordosis,** which compensates for the enlarging fetus; otherwise, the centre of balance would shift forward. Lordosis compensates by shifting the weight farther back on the lower extremities. This shift in balance, in turn, creates strain on the low back muscles, which in some women is felt as low back pain during late pregnancy.

Anterior flexion of the neck and slumping of the shoulder girdle are other postural changes that compensate for the lordosis. These upper back changes may put pressure on the ulnar and median nerves during the third trimester. Nerve pressure creates aching, numbness, and weakness in the upper extremities in some women.

Older Adults

Bone remodelling is a cyclic process of loss of bone matrix (bone resorption) and new bone growth (deposition). Deposition predominates until skeletal maturity at 25 to 35 years, when bone mass reaches its peak (Pigozzi et al., 2009). After age 40, resorption occurs more rapidly than does deposition. The net effect is a loss of bone density **(osteoporosis).** Although some degree of osteoporosis is nearly universal, women are more affected than are men because for 5 years after menopause, the lack of estrogen causes bone loss to accelerate. People of European descent are also more affected

Structure & Function

TABLE 24-1	Indications for Measuring Bone Mineral Density to Assess for Osteoporosis	
Older Adults (Age ≥ 50 Years)		**Younger Adults (Age < 50 Years)**

Older Adults (Age ≥ 50 Years)	Younger Adults (Age < 50 Years)
Age ≥ 65 yr (both women and men) Clinical risk factors for fracture in men aged 50-64 yr and in menopausal women: • Fragility fracture after age 40 yr • Prolonged use of glucocorticoids* • Use of other high-risk medications† • Parental hip fracture • Vertebral fracture or osteopenia identified on radiography • Current smoking • High alcohol intake • Low body weight (<60 kg) or major weight loss (>10% of body weight at age 25 yr) • Rheumatoid arthritis • Other disorders strongly associated with osteoporosis	Fragility fracture Prolonged use of glucocorticoids* Use of other high-risk medication† Hypogonadism or premature menopause (age < 45 yr) Malabsorption syndrome Primary hyperparathyroidism Other disorders strongly associated with rapid bone loss and/or fracture

Source: From Papaioannou, A., Morin, S., Cheung, A. M., Atkinson, S., Brown, J. P., Feldman, S., … Scientific Advisory Council of Osteoporosis Canada. (2010). 2010 Clinical practice guidelines for the diagnosis and management of osteoporosis in Canada: Summary. *Canadian Medical Association Journal, 182*(17), 1864–1873. doi:10.1503/cmaj.100771
*At least 3 months of cumulative therapy in the previous year at a prednisone-equivalent dose of ≥7.5 mg daily.
†For example, aromatase inhibitors or androgen deprivation therapy.

than are people of African descent. Risk factors for fracture associated with osteoporosis are listed in Table 24-1.

Postural changes are evident with aging, and decreased height is the most noticeable. Long bones do not shorten with age; decrease in height is caused by shortening of the vertebral column. This is caused by loss of water content and thinning of the intervertebral discs, which occurs more in middle age. Also, the height of individual vertebrae decreases, which occurs in later years as a result of osteoporosis.

Both men and women can expect a progressive decrease in height beginning at age 30 years and accelerating with increasing age; cumulative height loss from ages 30 to 70 years averages about 3 cm for men and 5 cm for women, and by age 80 years, the cumulative height loss is 5 cm for men and 8 cm for women (Sorkin, Muller, & Andres, 1999). The decrease during the 70s and 80s is greater as a result of osteoporotic collapse of the vertebrae, which results in shortening of the trunk and the appearance of comparatively long extremities. Other postural changes are kyphosis, a backward head tilt to compensate for the kyphosis, and a slight flexion of hips and knees.

The distribution of subcutaneous fat changes through life. Usually, men and women gain weight in their 40s and 50s. The body contour is different, even if the weight is the same as when they were younger. They begin to lose fat in the face and deposit it in the abdomen and hips. In the 80s and 90s, fat further decreases in the periphery, noticeably in the forearms and over the abdomen and hips.

Loss of subcutaneous fat leaves bony prominences more marked (e.g., tips of vertebrae, ribs, iliac crests) and body hollows deeper (e.g., cheeks, axillae). An absolute loss in muscle mass occurs; some muscles decrease in size, and some atrophy, which causes weakness. The contour of muscles becomes more prominent, and muscle bundles and tendons feel more distinct.

Lifestyle affects musculoskeletal changes; a sedentary lifestyle hastens the musculoskeletal changes of aging. However, physical exercise increases skeletal mass. This helps prevent or delay bone loss and osteoporosis in postmenopausal women (Schmitt, Schmitt, & Doren, 2009), and in older men (Cousins et al., 2010; see the box Promoting Health: Preventing Osteoporosis). In 2009, only 52.5% of Canadians were at least moderately active during their leisure time; their activity was equivalent to walking at least 30 minutes a day or taking an hour-long exercise class at least three times a week (Statistics Canada, 2011b).

 CULTURAL AND SOCIAL CONSIDERATIONS

Arthritis is one of the most prevalent chronic health conditions and a leading cause of pain, physical disability, and health care utilization in Canada; in 2011, more than 4.7 million Canadians (14%) aged 15 and older reported that they had arthritis (Statistics Canada, 2012), and the number is expected to increase to 7 million (20%) by 2031, as a result of the aging of the population (Public Health Agency of Canada, 2010). Nearly two thirds of those affected were women. The prevalence of arthritis increases with age; however, of every five people with arthritis, nearly three were younger than 65 years, and their disability frequently resulted in loss of work and productivity. Prevalence of arthritis was higher among people with lower education and income level, and 1.3 to 1.6 times higher among First Nations and Métis adults.

Osteoarthritis is the most prevalent type of arthritis, affecting more than 3 million Canadians (Arthritis Society, 2011a). Risk factors for osteoarthritis include increasing age, family history, excess weight, and joint injury. About 300,000 Canadians have rheumatoid arthritis; three times more women than men are affected (Arthritis Society, 2011b). The cause of rheumatoid arthritis is unknown, and it can occur at any age, including childhood, but it usually appears between the ages of 25 and 50.

Hip fractures are a serious consequence of falls in older adults. More than 28,000 hospitalizations for hip fractures

PROMOTING HEALTH: PREVENTING OSTEOPOROSIS

Don't Overlook Osteoporosis

Bone is a living tissue that continually grows and changes. Every day old bone dissolves and is replaced with new, stronger bone. Until a person is 30 years old, new bone appears at a faster rate than the bone disappears. As people age, however, the opposite begins to occur. When this happens, bones can become "spongy," weak, and more likely to break with even the slightest of twists or bumps. This condition is called *osteoporosis*. The bones of the wrist, hip, and spine are most often affected.

Osteoporosis is more common in women, slender people, and individuals of European descent. It has been estimated that one per four women and one per eight men in Canada have osteoporosis. Postmenopausal women are especially vulnerable because of hormonal changes. Osteoporosis tends to run in families, but lifestyle choices can increase the risk even in individuals without a family history. A person whose calcium intake is low or who lacks exercise, smokes, or consumes large quantities of alcohol is at higher risk for developing osteoporosis. Long-term use of proton pump inhibitor medications to treat acid-related conditions such as stomach ulcers has also been associated with an increased risk of osteoporosis-related fractures (Targownik et al., 2008).

Osteoporosis Canada (Papaioannou et al., 2010) recommends that all women and men older than 50 be assessed for the presence of risk factors for osteoporosis and fracture. Bone mineral density (BMD) testing is used to diagnose osteoporosis and predict fracture risk. BMD testing is recommended for all women aged 65 and older and for those with clinical risk factors for fracture such as fragility fracture after age 40, prolonged use of glucocorticoids, or parental hip fracture (see Table 24-1).

Prevention of osteoporosis is important because there is no cure, only treatment, for osteoporosis. The gold standard for treatment of osteoporosis has traditionally been hormone replacement therapy (HRT), which has been shown to prevent bone loss and to improve bone mineralization. However, new research indicates that HRT may carry an increased risk for breast cancer and myocardial infarction in women. Alternative therapies that include exercise and diet provide similar, if not equal, benefits for women at risk for osteoporosis.

Recommendations for Bone Health

1. **Diet.** Adequate intake of calcium and vitamin D are necessary to maintain bone health.
   a. **Dine on dairy.** Low-fat and skim milk, nonfat yogourt, and reduced-fat cheese are healthy sources of calcium. Fortified milk products also contain vitamin D, which is needed to absorb calcium.
   b. **Go fish.** Salmon and sardines, which are canned with their bones, are also rich in calcium. Also, oily fish such as mackerel are rich in vitamin D.
   c. **Eat greens with gusto.** Leafy green vegetables have a lot of calcium. Fill up on broccoli, kale, Swiss chard, turnip greens, and bok choy. In addition to the calcium, these foods contain potassium and vitamin K, which help block calcium loss from bones.
   d. **Try soy.** Soy contains calcium and plant estrogens. Try substituting soy flour for regular flour in recipes, nibbling on soybean "nuts," or drinking soy milk.
   e. **Limit caffeine.** Caffeine causes the body to excrete calcium more readily. Caffeine is present in coffee, tea, hot chocolate, and many carbonated drinks (e.g., cola).
   f. **Eat onions.** Although onions are not known to have any nutritive value, they appear to reduce the bone breakdown process that can lead to osteoporosis.
2. **Exercise.** Participate in weight-bearing activities. Bones and muscles must work against gravity to have a bone-building effect. A regular program of weight-bearing exercise for at least 30 minutes three times a week is recommended as the minimum. Try walking, low-impact aerobics, dancing, or stationary cycling. Resistance training with light weights or resistance bands are also recommended, and exercises that focus on posture and balance, such as tai chi, can help reduce the risk of falls. Sunshine also helps the body produce vitamin D. About 15 minutes of exposure to sunshine a day is all that is needed to maintain a good vitamin D supply.
3. **Lifestyle.** Avoid smoking and excessive alcohol, and seek help for depression. People who smoke have twice the risk of spinal and hip fractures. Furthermore, fractures heal more slowly in people who smoke and are more apt to heal improperly. Too much alcohol prevents the body from absorbing calcium. In addition, seek help for depression. Research has shown that women with clinical depression have lower bone densities.
4. **Medical options.** Talk to a health care provider about bone health. Although many people consider osteoporosis prevention to be important, fewer than half discuss the topic with health care providers or undergo BMD screening. Ask that your height be measured on an annual basis. A loss of 2-5 cm is an early sign of undiagnosed vertebral fractures and osteoporosis. Seek treatment for conditions that can jeopardize BMD, including thyroid disease, certain intestinal and kidney diseases, and some cancers. Also, remember that some medications may contribute to bone loss: for example, corticosteroids, anticoagulants, thyroid supplements, and certain anticonvulsants.
5. **Supplements.** When it is appropriate, take supplemental calcium. Adults need 1000 mg of elemental calcium daily during middle age. The need rises to 1500 mg daily after menopause in women and after age 50 years in men. Most people do not get enough calcium in their diets, and supplements may help achieve the minimum dosage. Make sure the supplement contains vitamin D, which helps your body absorb the calcium. The recommended daily dose of vitamin D is 400-1000 IU daily for younger adults and those at low risk for osteoporosis and 800-2000 IU daily for older adults and those at high risk for osteoporosis (Hanley, Cranney, Jones, Whiting, & Leslie, 2010).

Sources: Data from Brown, J. P., Fortier, M., Frame, H., Lalonde, A., Papaioannou, A., Senikas, V., ... & Osteoporosis Guidelines Committee. (2006). Canadian Consensus Conference on Osteoporosis, 2006 update. *Journal of Obstetrics and Gynaecology Canada, 28*(2, Suppl. 1), S95–S112; and from Osteoporosis Canada. (2012). *Osteoporosis & You.* Retrieved from *http://www.osteoporosis.ca/osteoporosis-and-you/*.

occurred in Canada in the period 2005 to 2006; 88% of patients involved were aged 65 years and older (Canadian Institute for Health Information, 2007). Women are twice as likely as men to fracture a hip. Hip fractures can result in loss of mobility and independence, financial difficulties, and increased use of health care services. In a large Canadian study, adults aged 50 years and older with hip or vertebral fractures were more likely to die during the 5-year follow-up than were those without fractures (Ioannidis et al., 2009). Similarly, adults aged 65 or older accounted for the majority of joint replacements—63% of hip replacements and 64% of knee replacements—in Canada during the period 2006 to 2007 (Canadian Institute for Health Information, 2009). A high proportion of patients undergoing hip and knee replacement were obese, according to body mass index. Across the country, efforts have been initiated to reduce wait times for hip and joint replacement surgeries.

About 4.27 million Canadians aged 12 or older suffered an injury severe enough to limit their usual activities in the period 2009 to 2010 (Statistics Canada, 2011a). The most common types of injury were sprains and strains (51%), followed by fractures and broken bones (17%). Most adolescent patients were injured playing sports (66%), younger and middle-aged adults were injured playing sports or at work (47%), and more than half of older adults' injuries occurred while they were walking or performing household chores. Falls were the leading cause of injury among older adults (63%), adolescents (50%), and younger and middle-aged adults (35%).

SUBJECTIVE DATA

1. Joints:
   Pain
   Stiffness
   Swelling, heat, redness
   Limitation of movement
2. Muscles:
   Pain (cramps)
   Weakness
3. Bones:
   Pain
   Deformity
   Trauma (fractures, sprains, dislocations)
4. Functional assessment (activities of ADLs)
5. Self-care behaviours

HEALTH HISTORY QUESTIONS

Examiner Asks	Rationale
1. **Joints.** Any problems with your joints? Any **pain?**	**Joint pain** and loss of function are the most common musculoskeletal concerns that prompt a person to seek care.
• Location: Which joints? On one side or both sides?	Rheumatoid arthritis is symmetrical, involving the same joints on both sides; other musculoskeletal illnesses involve isolated or unilateral joints.
• Quality: What does the pain feel like: aching, stiff, sharp or dull, shooting?	Exquisite tenderness occurs with acute inflammation.
• Severity: How strong is the pain?	
• Onset: When did this pain start?	
• Timing: What time of day does the pain occur? How long does it last?	Rheumatoid arthritis pain is worse in the morning on arising; osteoarthritis is worse later in the day; tendinitis is worse in the morning and improves during the day.
• How often does it occur?	
• Is the pain aggravated by movement, rest, position, weather? Is the pain relieved by rest, medications, application of heat or ice?	Movement increases most joint pain except in rheumatoid arthritis, in which movement decreases pain.
• Is the pain associated with chills, fever, recent sore throat, trauma, repetitive activity?	Joint pain 10 to 14 days after an untreated streptococcal infection ("strep throat") is suggestive of rheumatic fever. Joint injury is caused by trauma and repetitive motion.

Examiner Asks	Rationale

- Any **stiffness** in your joints?

- Any swelling, heat, redness in the joints?

- Any **limitation of movement** in any joint? Which joint?
- Which activities give you problems? (See Functional Assessment below.)

2. Muscles. Any problems in the muscles, such as any **pain** or **cramping?** Which muscles?
   - If pain is widespread: How long have you had this pain? Is the pain associated with fatigue?

   - If pain is in calf muscles: Does the pain occur with walking? Does it go away with rest?
   - Are your muscle aches associated with fever, chills, the "flu"?

   - Any **weakness** in muscles?
   - Location: Where is the weakness? How long have you noticed weakness?
   - Do the muscles look smaller there?

3. Bones. Any **bone pain?** Is the pain affected by movement?
   - Any **deformity** of any bone or joint? Is the deformity caused by injury or trauma? Does the deformity affect ROM?
   - Have any **accidents** or **trauma** ever affected the bones or joints: fractures, joint strain, sprain, dislocation? Which ones?
   - When did this occur? What treatment was given? Any problems or limitations now as a result?
   - Any back pain? In which part of your back? Is pain felt anywhere else, such as shooting down your leg?
   - Any numbness and tingling? Any limping?

Rationale:

Rheumatoid arthritis stiffness occurs in morning and after rest periods.

These signs are suggestive of acute inflammation.

Decrease in ROM may be caused by joint injury to cartilage or the capsule, or it may result from muscle contracture.

Myalgia is usually felt as cramping or aching.

Widespread musculoskeletal pain lasting 3 months or longer and associated with fatigue is suggestive of fibromyalgia (see Table 24-10).

Calf pain may represent intermittent claudication (see Chapter 21).

Symptoms of viral illness often include myalgia.

Weakness may involve musculoskeletal or neurological systems (see Chapter 25).

Decrease in muscle size is indicative of atrophy.

CRITICAL FINDINGS

Fracture causes sharp pain that increases with movement (other bone pain usually feels "dull" and "deep" and is unrelated to movement). A fractured bone may also be misaligned. Report findings immediately. Never attempt to realign broken bones. Monitor vital signs and peripheral vascular circulation distal to the injury until the patient's care is transferred.

4. Functional assessment. Do problems with your joints (muscle, bone) impose any limits on your usual ADLs? Which ones? (Note: Ask about each category; if the patient answers "yes," ask specifically about each activity in category.)
   - Bathing: getting in and out of the tub, turning faucets
   - Toileting: urinating, defecating, ability to get self on and off toilet, wiping self
   - Dressing: manipulating buttons and zippers, fastening openings behind the neck, pulling dress or sweater over head, pulling up pants, tying shoes, wearing shoes that fit
   - Grooming: shaving, brushing teeth, brushing or fixing hair, applying makeup
   - Eating: preparing meals, pouring liquids, cutting up foods, bringing food to mouth, drinking
   - Mobility: walking, walking up or down stairs, getting in and out of bed, getting out of the home
   - Communicating: talking, using phone, writing

Functional assessment is used to assess the safety of independent living, the need for home health care services, and quality of life (see Chapter 31).

Assess any self-care deficit.

Assess for impairment in physical mobility.

Assess for impairment in verbal communication.

Subjective Data

Examiner Asks	Rationale

5. **Self-care behaviours.** Any occupational hazards that could affect the muscles and joints? Does your work involve heavy lifting? Or any repetitive motion or chronic stress to joints? Any efforts to alleviate these?

Assess risk for back pain or carpal tunnel syndrome.

- Tell me about your exercise program. Describe the type of exercise, frequency, the warm-up program.

Assess self-care behaviours.

- Any pain during exercise? How do you treat it?
- Have you had any recent weight gain? Please describe your usual daily diet. (Note the patient's usual caloric intake, all four food groups, daily amount of protein, calcium.)
- Are you taking any medications for musculoskeletal system: aspirin, anti-inflammatory, muscle relaxant, pain reliever?
- If patient has chronic disability or crippling illness: How has your illness affected the following:
  Your interaction with family?
  Your interaction with friends?
  The way you view yourself?

Assess for
- Self-esteem disturbance
- Loss of independence
- Body image disturbance
- Role performance disturbance
- Social isolation

Additional History for Infants and Children

1. **Birth trauma.** Were you told about any trauma to the infant during labour and delivery? Did the baby come out head first? Were forceps needed?
2. **Anoxia.** Did the baby need resuscitation?

Traumatic delivery increases risk for fractures (e.g., humerus, clavicle).
A period of anoxia may result in hypotonia of muscles.

3. **Milestones.** Were the baby's motor milestones achieved at about the same time as those of siblings or other children the same age?
4. **Bone injuries.** Has your child ever broken any bones? Any dislocations? How were these treated?
5. **Bone deformities.** Have you ever noticed any bone deformity? Spinal curvature? Unusual shape of toes or feet? At what age? Have you ever sought treatment for any of these?

Additional History for Adolescents

1. **Athletics.** Are you involved in any sports at school or after school? How frequently (times per week)?

Assess safety of sport for the child. Note whether the child's height and weight are adequate for the particular sport (e.g., football).

2. **Sports equipment.** Do you use any special equipment? Does any training program exist for your sport?

Use of safety equipment and presence of adult supervision decrease the risk for sports injuries.

3. **Warming up.** What is the nature of your daily warm-up?

Lack of adequate warm-up increases risk of sports injury.

4. **Injury.** What do you do if you get hurt?

Students may not report injury or pain for fear that their participation in the sport will be restricted.

5. **Time management.** How does your sport fit in with other school demands and other activities?

Additional History for the Older Adult

Use the functional assessment history questions in Chapter 5 (pp. 72 to 80) to elicit any loss of function, self-care deficit, or safety risk that may occur as a process of aging or musculoskeletal illness. (Review the complete functional assessment in Chapter 31.)

Age-related changes in the musculoskeletal, neurological, and sensory systems increase the probability of falls and fractures in older adults.

1. **Weakness.** Any change in weakness over the past months or years?
2. **Injury.** Any increase in falls or stumbling over the past months or years?
3. **Mobility.** Do you use any mobility aids to help you get around: cane, walker?

OBJECTIVE DATA

PREPARATION

The purpose of the musculoskeletal examination is to assess function for ADLs and to screen for any abnormalities. By documenting the history, you already will have considerable data regarding ADLs. Note additional ADL data as the patient goes through the motions necessary for an examination: gait, posture, how the patient sits in a chair, raises from chair, takes off jacket, manipulates small object such as a pen, raises from supine position.

A **screening musculoskeletal examination** suffices for most patients:

- Inspection and palpation of joints, integrated with inspection of each body region
- Observation of ROM as patient proceeds through motions described earlier
- Age-specific screening measures, such as the Ortolani manoeuvre for infants or scoliosis screening for adolescents

A **complete musculoskeletal examination,** as described in this chapter, is appropriate for patients with articular disease, a history of musculoskeletal symptoms, or any problems with ADLs. Nurses may work in collaboration with other health care providers (e.g., physiotherapists or occupational therapists) when performing these assessments in acute, rehabilitative, long-term, and home care settings.

Make the patient comfortable before and throughout the examination. Drape for full visualization of the body part you are examining without needlessly exposing the rest of the patient's body.

Use an orderly approach: head to toe, proximal to distal. The approach may need to be modified in patients with limitations in mobility, with pain, or with fatigue. Provide analgesics, rest periods, or both as required.

Support each joint at rest. Muscles must be soft and relaxed in order for you to assess the joints under them accurately. Take care when examining any inflamed area, where rough manipulation could cause pain and muscle spasm. To avoid pain and spasm, use firm support, gentle movement, and gentle return to a relaxed state. Compare corresponding paired joints. Expect symmetry of structure and function and normal parameters for each joint.

EQUIPMENT NEEDED
Tape measure
Skin marking pen

Normal Range of Findings	Abnormal Findings

ORDER OF THE EXAMINATION

Inspection

Note the *size* and *contour* of the joint. Inspect the skin and tissues over the joints for *colour, swelling,* and any *masses* or *deformity.* The presence of swelling is significant and signals joint irritation.

Swelling may be caused by excess joint fluid (effusion), thickening of the synovial lining, inflammation of surrounding soft tissue (bursae, tendons), or bony enlargement.

Deformities include **dislocation** (one or more bones in a joint being out of position), **subluxation** (partial dislocation of a joint), **contracture** (shortening of a muscle leading to limited ROM of joint), or **ankylosis** (stiffness or fixation of a joint).

Palpation

Palpate each joint, including its skin for temperature, its muscles, its bony articulations, and the area of the joint capsule. Note any heat, tenderness, swelling, or masses. Normally, joints are not tender to palpation. If any tenderness does occur, try to localize it to specific anatomical structures (e.g., skin, muscles, bursae, ligaments, tendons, fat pads, or joint capsule).

Warmth and tenderness signal inflammation.

Normal Range of Findings	Abnormal Findings

Normally, the synovial membrane is not palpable. When thickened, it feels doughy or boggy. A small amount of fluid is present in the normal joint, but it is not palpable.

Palpable fluid is abnormal. Fluid is contained in an enclosed sac; therefore, if you push on one side of the sac, the fluid will shift and cause a visible bulging on another side.

Range of Motion

Test for **active ROM** while stabilizing the body area proximal to that being moved. Familiarize yourself with each type of joint and its normal ROM so that you can recognize limitations. If you see a limitation, gently attempt **passive motion**: Anchor the joint with one hand while your other hand slowly moves it to its limit. The normal ranges of active and passive motions should be the same.

If any limitation or any increase in ROM is present, use a goniometer to measure the angles precisely (Fig. 24-15). First, extend the joint to neutral or 0 degrees. Centre the 0 point of the goniometer on the joint. Keep the fixed arm of the goniometer on the 0 line, and use the movable arm to measure; then flex the joint and measure through the goniometer to determine the angle of greatest flexion.

Limitation in ROM is the most sensitive sign of joint disease (McGee, 2007). The amount of limitation may alert you to the cause of disease. Articular disease (inside the joint capsule, such as arthritis) produces swelling and tenderness around the whole joint, and it limits both active and passive ROM in all planes. Extra-articular disease (injury to a specific tendon, ligament, nerve) produces swelling and tenderness to that one spot in the joint and affects ROM in only certain planes, especially during active (voluntary) motion.

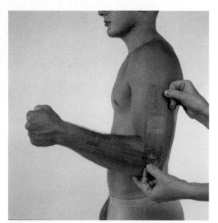

24-15

Joint motion normally causes no tenderness, pain, or crepitation. Do not confuse crepitation with the normal discrete "crack" heard as a tendon or ligament slips over bone during motion, such as a knee bend.

Crepitation is an audible and palpable crunching or grating that accompanies movement. It occurs when the articular surfaces in the joints are roughened, as in rheumatoid arthritis (see Table 24-2, p. 642).

Muscle Testing

Test the strength of the prime mover muscle groups for each joint. Instruct the patient to repeat the motions you tested for active ROM. Now ask the patient to flex the muscle and hold as you apply opposing force. Muscle strength should be equal bilaterally and should fully resist your opposing force. (Note: Muscle status and joint status are interdependent and should be interpreted together. Chapter 25 discusses the examination of muscles for size, strength, tone, and involuntary movements.)

Objective Data

Normal Range of Findings	Abnormal Findings

Strength varies widely among people. You may wish to use a system of grading from "no voluntary movement" to "full strength," such as the following:

GRADE	DESCRIPTION	% NORMAL	ASSESSMENT
5	Full ROM against gravity, full resistance	100	Normal
4	Full ROM against gravity, some resistance	75	Good
3	Full ROM with gravity	50	Fair
2	Full ROM with gravity eliminated (passive motion)	25	Poor
1	Slight contraction	10	Trace
0	No contraction	0	Zero

TEMPOROMANDIBULAR JOINT

With the patient seated, *inspect* the area just anterior to the ear. Place the tips of your first two fingers in front of each ear, and ask the patient to open and close the mouth. Drop your fingers into the depressed area over the joint, and note smooth motion of the mandible. An audible and palpable snap or click occurs in many healthy people as the mouth opens (Figure 24-16).

Test ROM as follows:

INSTRUCTIONS TO PATIENT

- Open mouth maximally.

- Partially open mouth, thrust lower jaw, and move it side to side.
- Stick out lower jaw.

MOTION AND EXPECTED RANGE

Vertical motion. You can measure the space between the upper and lower incisors. Normal space is 3 to 6 cm, or three fingers inserted sideways.
Lateral motion. Normal extent is 1 to 2 cm (Figure 24-17).
Protrusion without deviation.

Instruct the patient to clench the teeth, and palpate the patient's contracted temporalis and masseter muscles. Compare right and left sides for size, firmness, and strength. Ask the patient to move the jaw forward and laterally against your resistance, and to open mouth against your resistance. This is also a test of the integrity of cranial nerve V (trigeminal nerve).

Abnormal Findings:

Swelling looks like a round bulge over the joint, although it must be moderate or marked to be visible.

Crepitus and pain occur with temporomandibular joint dysfunction.

Lateral motion may be lost earlier and more significantly than vertical motion.

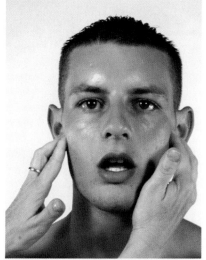

24-16

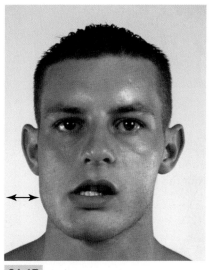

24-17

Objective Data

Normal Range of Findings	Abnormal Findings

CERVICAL SPINE

Inspect the alignment of the head and neck. The spine should be straight and the head erect. *Palpate* the spinous processes and the sternomastoid, trapezius, and paravertebral muscles. They should feel firm, with no muscle spasm or tenderness.

Test ROM as follows (Figure 24-18)*:

INSTRUCTIONS TO PATIENT

- Touch chin to chest.

- Lift the chin toward the ceiling.
- Move each ear toward the corresponding shoulder. Do not lift up the shoulder.
- Turn the chin toward each shoulder.

MOTION AND EXPECTED RANGE

Flexion of 45 degrees (see Figure 24-18, *A*)
Hyperextension of 55 degrees
Lateral bending of 40 degrees (see Figure 24-18, *B*)

Rotation of 70 degrees (see Figure 24-18, *C*)

Head tilted to one side.
Asymmetry of muscles.
Tenderness and hard muscles with muscle spasm.

Limited ROM.

Pain with movement.

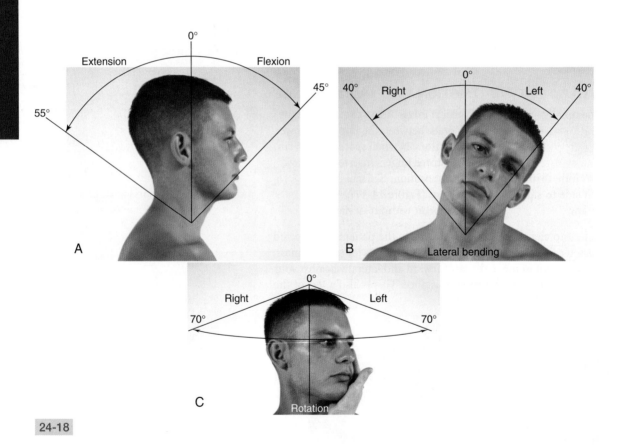

24-18

Ask the patient to repeat the motions while you apply opposing force. The patient normally can maintain flexion against your full resistance. This is also a test of the integrity of cranial nerve XI (spinal nerve).

The patient cannot maintain flexion.

*Do not attempt if you suspect neck trauma.

Normal Range of Findings	Abnormal Findings

UPPER EXTREMITY

Shoulders

Inspect and compare both shoulders posteriorly and anteriorly. Check the size and contour of the joint, and compare shoulders for equality of bony landmarks. Normally, no redness, muscular atrophy, deformity, or swelling is present. Check the anterior aspect of the joint capsule and the subacromial bursa for abnormal swelling.

Redness.
Inequality of bony landmarks.
Atrophy, manifesting as lack of fullness.
Dislocated shoulder: loses the normal rounded shape and looks flattened laterally.
Swelling from excess fluid: best seen anteriorly; considerable fluid must be present to cause a visible distension because the capsule is normally loose (see Table 24-3, p. 643).
Swelling of subacromial bursa is localized under the deltoid muscle and may be accentuated when the patient tries to abduct the arm.

If the patient reports any shoulder pain, ask that he or she point to the spot with the hand of the unaffected side. Be aware that shoulder pain may have local causes, or it may be referred pain from a hiatal hernia or a cardiac or pleural condition, which is potentially serious. Pain from a local cause is reproducible during the examination by palpation or motion.

While you stand in front of the patient, *palpate* both shoulders, noting any muscular spasm or atrophy, swelling, heat, or tenderness. Start at the clavicle and methodically explore the acromioclavicular joint, scapula, greater tubercle of the humerus, area of the subacromial bursa, the biceps groove, and the anterior aspect of the glenohumeral joint. Palpate the pyramid-shaped axilla; no adenopathy or masses should be present.

Swelling.
Hard muscles with muscle spasm.
Tenderness or pain.

Test ROM by asking the patient to perform four motions (Figure 24-19). Cup one hand over the shoulder during ROM to note any crepitation; normally, none is present.

INSTRUCTIONS TO PATIENT

- With arms at sides and elbows extended, move both arms forward and up in wide vertical arcs, and then move them back.

MOTION AND EXPECTED RANGE

Forward flexion of 180 degrees; hyperextension of up to 50 degrees (see Figure 24-19, *A*)

Limited ROM.
Asymmetry.
Pain with motion.

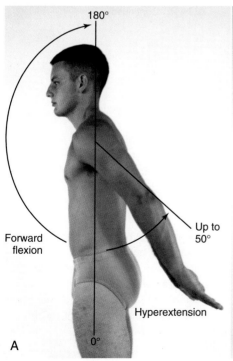

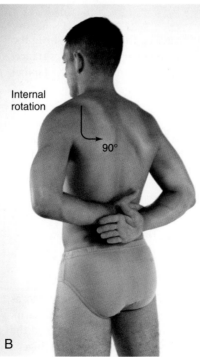

24-19

Objective Data

Normal Range of Findings		Abnormal Findings

Normal Range of Findings		**Abnormal Findings**
• Rotate arms internally behind back, and place back of hands as high as possible toward the scapulae.	Internal rotation of 90 degrees (see Figure 24-19, *B*)	Crepitus with motion. Rotator cuff lesions may cause limited ROM, pain, and muscle spasm during abduction, whereas forward flexion stays fairly normal.
• With arms at sides and elbows extended, raise both arms in wide arcs in the coronal plane. Touch palms together above head.	Abduction of 180 degrees Adduction of 50 degrees (see Figure 24-19, *C*)	
• Touch both hands behind the head with elbows flexed and rotated posteriorly.	External rotation of 90 degrees (see Figure 24-19, *D*).	

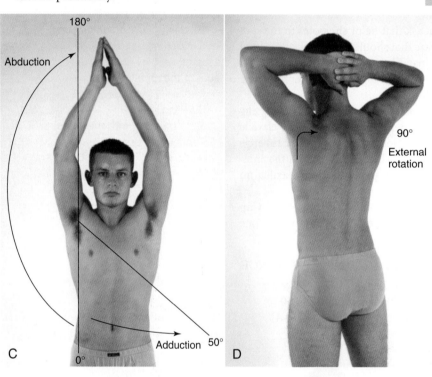

C   D   24-19   Continued

Test the strength of the shoulder muscles by asking the patient to shrug the shoulders, flex them forward and up, and abduct them against your resistance. The shoulder shrug is also a test of the integrity of cranial nerve XI (spinal nerve).

Elbow

Inspect the size and contour of the elbow in both flexed and extended positions. Look for any deformity, redness, or swelling. Check the olecranon bursa and the normally present hollows on either side of the olecranon process for abnormal swelling.

In subluxation of the elbow, the forearm is dislocated posteriorly.

Swelling and redness of olecranon bursa are localized and easy to observe because of the nearness of the bursa to skin.

Effusion or synovial thickening manifests first as a bulge or fullness in groove on either side of the olecranon process, and it occurs with gouty arthritis.

Epicondyles, head of radius, and tendons are common sites of inflammation and local tenderness, or "tennis elbow."

Palpate with the patient's elbow flexed about 70 degrees and as relaxed as possible (Figure 24-20). Use your left hand to support the patient's left forearm, and palpate the extensor surface of the elbow—the olecranon process and the medial and lateral epicondyles of humerus—with your right thumb and fingers.

Normal Range of Findings	Abnormal Findings

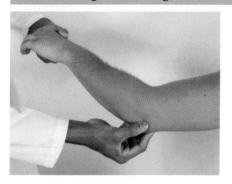

24-20

With your thumb in the lateral groove and your index and middle fingers in the medial groove, palpate either side of the olecranon process, using varying pressure. Normally, tissues and fat pads feel fairly solid. Check for any synovial thickening, swelling, nodules, or tenderness.

Palpate the area of the olecranon bursa for heat, swelling, tenderness, consistency, or nodules.

Soft, boggy, or fluctuant swelling in both grooves occurs with synovial thickening or effusion.

Local heat or redness (signs of inflammation) can extend beyond the synovial membrane.

Subcutaneous nodules are raised, firm, and nontender, and overlying skin moves freely. Common sites are in the olecranon bursa and along extensor surface of the ulna. These nodules occur with rheumatoid arthritis (see Table 24-4, p. 644).

Test ROM as follows:

INSTRUCTIONS TO PATIENT

• Bend and then straighten the elbow.

• Hold the hand midway; then touch the front and back sides of the hand to the table.

MOTION AND EXPECTED RANGE

Flexion of 150 to 160 degrees; extension at 0 (Figure 24-21)
Some healthy people lack 5 to 10 degrees of full extension, and others have 5 to 10 degrees of hyperextension.
Movement of 90 degrees in pronation and supination (Figure 24-22)

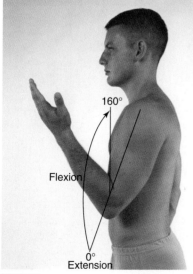

Flexion
160°
0°
Extension

24-21

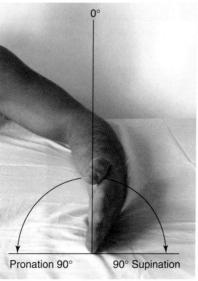

0°
Pronation 90°   90° Supination

24-22

Objective Data

| **Normal Range of Findings** | **Abnormal Findings** |

While you test *muscle strength,* stabilize the patient's arm with one hand (Figure 24-23). Apply resistance just proximal to the wrist , and instruct the patient to flex the elbow against your resistance. Then ask the patient to extend the elbow against your resistance.

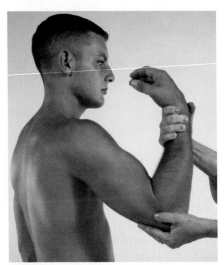

24-23

Wrist and Hand

Inspect the hands and wrists on the dorsal and palmar sides, noting position, contour, and shape. In the normal functional position of the hand, the wrist is in slight extension. This way the fingers can flex efficiently, and the thumb can oppose them for grip and manipulation. The fingers lie straight in the same axis as the forearm. Normally, no swelling or redness, deformity, or nodules are present.

The skin looks smooth, with knuckle wrinkles present and no swelling or lesions. Muscles are full, with the palm showing a rounded mound proximal to the thumb (the thenar eminence) and a smaller rounded mound proximal to the little finger.

Palpate each joint in the wrist and hands. Face the patient, support the patient's hand with your fingers under it, and palpate the wrist firmly with both your thumbs on its dorsum (Figure 24-24). Make sure the patient's wrist is relaxed and in straight alignment. Move your palpating thumbs side to side to identify the normal depressed areas that overlie the joint space. Use gentle but firm pressure. Normally, the joint surfaces feel smooth, with no swelling, bogginess, nodules, or tenderness.

Abnormal Findings

Subluxation of wrist.
Ulnar deviation; fingers list to ulnar side.
Ankylosis; wrist in extreme flexion.
Dupuytren's contracture: flexion contracture of one or more fingers (see Table 24-5).
Swan-neck or boutonnière deformity in fingers.
Atrophy of the thenar eminence (see Table 24-5, p. 645).
Ganglion cyst in wrist (see Table 24-5).
Synovial swelling on dorsum.
Generalized swelling.
Tenderness.

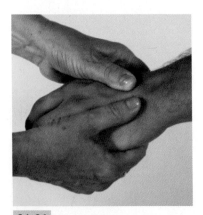

24-24

Normal Range of Findings	Abnormal Findings

Palpate the metacarpophalangeal joints with your thumbs, just distal to and on either side of the knuckle (Figure 24-25).

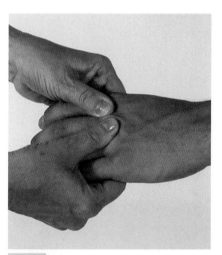

24-25

Use your thumb and index finger in a pinching motion to palpate the sides of the interphalangeal joints (Figure 24-26). Normally, no synovial thickening, tenderness, warmth, or nodules are present.

Heberden's and Bouchard's nodes are hard and nontender and occur with osteo-arthritis (see Table 24-5, p. 646).

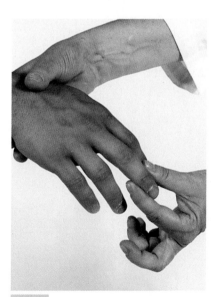

24-26

Normal Range of Findings	Abnormal Findings

Test ROM as follows (Figure 24-27):

INSTRUCTIONS TO PATIENT	**MOTION AND EXPECTED RANGE**
• Bend the hand up at the wrist.	Hyperextension of 70 degrees (see Figure 24-27, *A*)
• Bend hand down at the wrist.	Palmar flexion of 90 degrees
• Bend the fingers up and down at metacarpophalangeal joints.	Flexion of 90 degrees; hyperextension of 30 degrees (see Figure 24-27, *B*)
• With palms flat on table, turn them outward and in.	Ulnar deviation of 50 to 60 degrees; radial deviation of 20 degrees (see Figure 24-27, *C*)
• Spread fingers apart; then make a fist.	Abduction of 20 degrees; tight fist; equal bilateral responses (see Figure 24-27, *D, E*)
• Touch the thumb to each finger and to the base of little finger.	Ability to perform this manoeuvre, and equal bilateral responses (see Figure 24-27, *F*)

Loss of ROM (in this location, the most common and most significant functional loss in the wrist).
　Limited motion.
　Pain on movement.

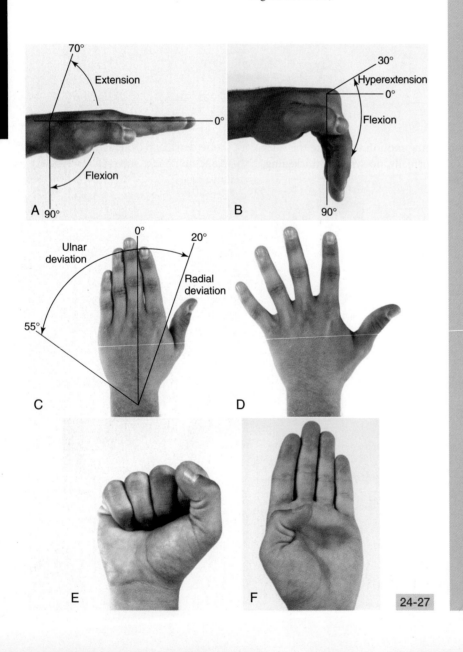

A
B
C
D
E
F

24-27

Normal Range of Findings	Abnormal Findings

For *muscle testing*, position the patient's forearm supinated (palm up) and resting on a table (Figure 24-28). Stabilize the patient's arm by holding your hand at the mid-forearm. Ask the patient to flex the wrist against your resistance at the palm.

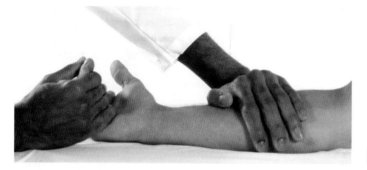

24-28

Phalen Test. Ask the patient to hold both hands back to back while flexing the wrists 90 degrees. Acute flexion of the wrist for 60 seconds produces no symptoms in the normal hand (Figure 24-29).

Tinel's Sign. Direct percussion of the location of the median nerve at the wrist produces no symptoms in the normal hand (Figure 24-30).

The Phalen test reproduces numbness and burning sensation in a patient with carpal tunnel syndrome (see Table 24-5, p. 645).

In carpal tunnel syndrome, percussion of the median nerve produces burning and tingling sensations along its distribution, which is Tinel's sign.

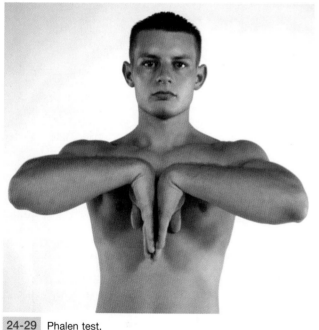

24-29   Phalen test.

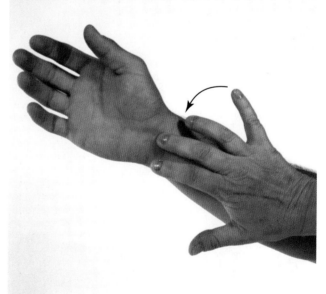

24-30

LOWER EXTREMITY

Hip

Inspect the hip joint together with the spine a bit later in the examination as the patient stands. At that time, note symmetrical levels of iliac crests, gluteal folds, and equal-sized buttocks. A smooth, even gait reflects equal leg lengths and functional hip motion.

Help the patient into the supine position, and *palpate* the hip joints. The joints should feel stable and symmetrical, with no tenderness or crepitation.

Pain with palpation.
Crepitation.

Normal Range of Findings	Abnormal Findings

Test ROM as follows (Figure 24-31):

INSTRUCTIONS TO PATIENT	**MOTION AND EXPECTED RANGE**
• Raise each leg with knee extended.	Hip flexion of 90 degrees (see Figure 24-31, *A*)
• Bend each knee up to the chest while keeping the other leg straight.	Hip flexion of 120 degrees; the opposite thigh should remain on the table (see Figure 24-31, *B*)
• Flex knee and hip to 90 degrees. (Examiner stabilizes by holding the thigh with one hand and the ankle with the other hand.) Swing the foot outward. Swing the foot inward. (Foot and thigh move in opposite directions.)	Internal rotation of 40 degrees External rotation of 45 degrees (see Figure 24-31, *C*)
• Swing leg laterally, then medially, with knee straight. Stabilize pelvis by pushing down on the opposite anterior superior iliac spine.	Abduction of 40 to 45 degrees Adduction of 20 to 30 degrees (see Figure 24-31, *D*)

Limited motion.
Pain with motion.
Flexion flattens the lumbar spine; if this reveals a flexion deformity in the opposite hip, it represents a positive sign of the *Thomas test.*
Limited internal rotation of hip is an early and reliable sign of hip disease.

Limitation of abduction of the hip in the supine position is the most common motion dysfunction in hip disease.

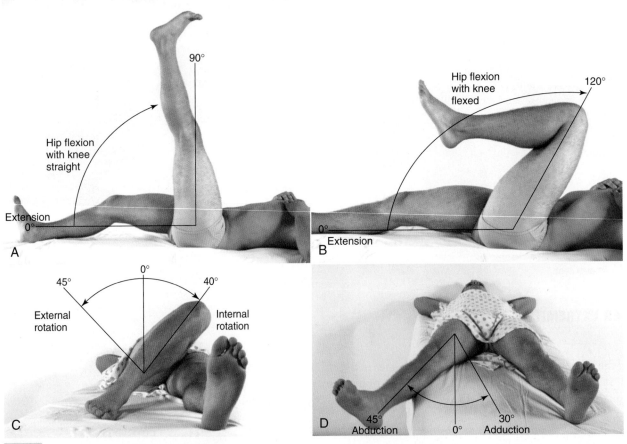

24-31

Normal Range of Findings	Abnormal Findings

- When standing (later in examination), swing straight leg back behind body. (Examiner stabilizes pelvis to eliminate exaggerated lumbar lordosis. The most efficient way is to ask patient to bend over the table and support the trunk on the table, or lie prone on the table.)

Hyperextension of 15 degrees when stabilized

Knee

The patient should remain supine with legs extended, although some examiners prefer the knees to be flexed and dangling for *inspection*. The skin normally looks smooth, with even colouring and no lesions.

Inspect lower leg alignment. The lower leg should extend in the same axis as the thigh.

Inspect the knee's shape and contour. Normally, distinct concavities (hollows) are present on either side of the patella. Check them for any sign of fullness or swelling. Check other locations, such as the prepatellar bursa and the suprapatellar pouch, for any abnormal swelling.

Check the quadriceps muscle in the anterior thigh for any atrophy. Because it is the prime mover of knee extension, this muscle is important for joint stability during weight bearing.

Palpate the patient's knee in the supine position with complete relaxation of the quadriceps muscle. Start high on the anterior thigh, about 10 cm above the patella. Palpate with your left thumb and fingers in a grasping manner (Figure 24-32). Proceed down toward the knee, exploring the region of the suprapatellar pouch. Note the consistency of the tissues. The muscles and soft tissues should feel solid, and the joint should feel smooth, with no warmth, tenderness, thickening, or nodularity.

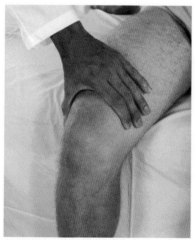

24-32

When swelling is present, you need to distinguish whether it represents soft tissue swelling or increased fluid in the joint. The tests for the bulge sign and ballottement of the patella aid in this assessment.

Shiny and atrophic skin.
Swelling or inflammation (see Table 24-6, p. 648).
Lesions (e.g., psoriasis).
Angulation deformity:
- Genu varum (bowlegs; see p. 636)
- Genu valgum (knock knees)
- Flexion contracture
With synovial thickening or effusion, hollows disappear; then they may bulge.

Atrophy occurs with disuse or chronic disorders. It first appears in the medial part of the muscle, although it is difficult to note because the vastus medialis is relatively small.
Fluctuant or boggy texture with synovitis of suprapatellar pouch.

Objective Data

SPECIAL CONSIDERATIONS FOR ADVANCED PRACTICE: KNEE

Normal Range of Findings	Abnormal Findings

Bulge Sign. The bulge sign confirms the presence of small amounts of fluid in the suprapatellar pouch as you try to move the fluid from one side of the joint to the other. Firmly stroke up on the medial aspect of the knee two or three times to displace any fluid (Figure 24-33, *A*). Tap the lateral aspect (see Figure 24-33, *B*). Watch the medial side in the hollow for a distinct bulge from a fluid wave. Normally, none is present.

The bulge sign occurs with very small amounts (4 to 8 mL) of fluid flowing across the joint (see Figure 24-33, *C*).

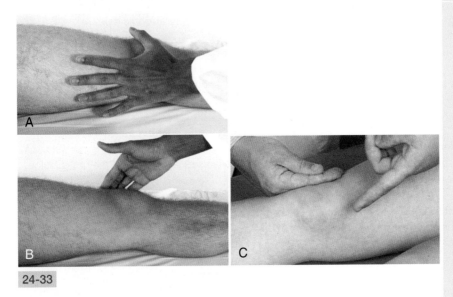

24-33

Ballottement of the Patella. This test is reliable when larger amounts of fluid are present. Use your left hand to compress the suprapatellar pouch to move any fluid into the knee joint. With your right hand, push the patella sharply against the femur. If no fluid is present, the patella is already snug against the femur (see Figure 24-34, *A*).

If fluid has collected, your tap on the patella moves it through the fluid, and you will hear a tap as the patella bumps up on the femoral condyles (see Figure 24-34, *B*).

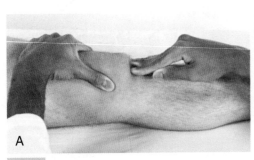 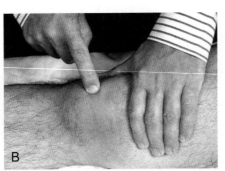

24-34

Continue assessment with palpation of the tibiofemoral joint (Figure 24-35). Note smooth joint margins and absence of pain. Palpate the infrapatellar fat pad and the patella. Check for crepitus by holding your hand on the patella as the knee is flexed and extended. Some crepitus in an otherwise symptom-free knee is not uncommon.

Irregular bony margins (present with osteoarthritis).
Pain at joint line.
Pronounced crepitus (a significant finding, occurs with degenerative diseases of the knee).

Normal Range of Findings	**Abnormal Findings**

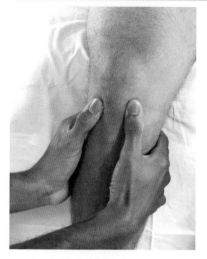

24-35

Test ROM as follows (Figure 24-36):

INSTRUCTIONS TO PATIENT
- Bend each knee.

- Extend each knee.

- Ambulate. (Examiner checks knee ROM during ambulation.)

MOTION AND EXPECTED RANGE

Flexion of 130 to 150 degrees

A straight line of 0 degrees in some persons; a hyperextension of 15 degrees in others

Limited ROM.
Contracture.
Pain with motion.
Limpness.

In sudden locking, the patient is unable to extend the knee fully. This usually occurs with a painful and audible "pop" or "click." Sudden buckling, or "giving way," occurs with ligament injury, which causes weakness and instability.

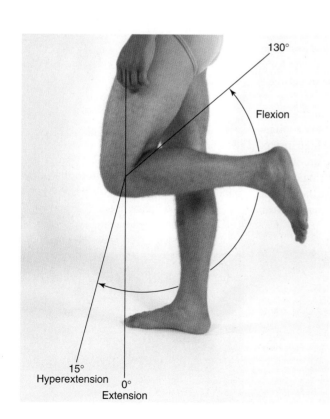

130°
Flexion
15°
Hyperextension
0°
Extension

24-36

Normal Range of Findings	Abnormal Findings

Check muscle strength by asking the patient to maintain knee flexion while you oppose by trying to pull the leg forward. The patient demonstrates muscle extension by successfully rising from a seated position in a low chair or rising from a squat without using the hands for support.

Special Test for Meniscal Tears

McMurray Test. Perform this test when a patient has reported a history of trauma followed by locking, giving way, or local pain in the knee. Position the patient supine as you stand next to the affected side. Hold the heel, and flex the knee and hip. Place your other hand on the knee with fingers on the medial side. Rotate the leg in and out to loosen the joint. Externally rotate the leg and push a valgus (inward) stress on the knee. Then slowly extend the knee. Normally, the leg extends smoothly with no pain (Figure 24-37).

A "click" is a positive result of the McMurray test that signifies a torn meniscus.

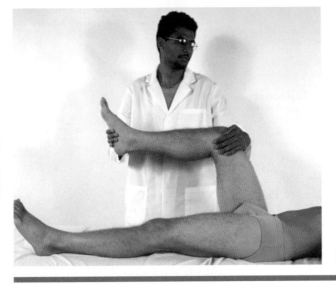

24-37

Ankle and Foot

Inspect while the patient is in a sitting, non–weight-bearing position, as well as when standing and walking. Compare both feet, noting position of feet and toes, contour of joints, and skin characteristics. The foot should align with the long axis of the lower leg; an imaginary line would fall from mid-patella to between the first and second toes.

Weight bearing should be borne on the middle of the foot, from the heel, along the midfoot, to between the second and third toes. Most feet have a longitudinal arch, although the arch can vary normally from "flat feet" to a high instep.

The toes point straight forward and lie flat. The ankles (malleoli) are smooth bony prominences. Normally, the skin is smooth, with even colouring and no lesions. Note the locations of any calluses or bursal reactions because they reveal areas of abnormal friction. Examining well-worn shoes helps assess areas of wear and accommodation.

In **hallux valgus,** the distal part of the great toe is directed *away* from the body midline (Figure 24-38).

Hammertoes; claw toes.
Swelling or inflammation.
Calluses; ulcers (see Table 24-7, p. 650).

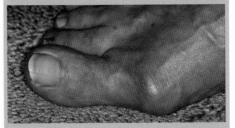

24-38

| **Normal Range of Findings** | **Abnormal Findings** |

Support the ankle by grasping the heel with your fingers while palpating with your thumbs (Figure 24-39). Explore the joint spaces. They should feel smooth and depressed, with no fullness, swelling, or tenderness.

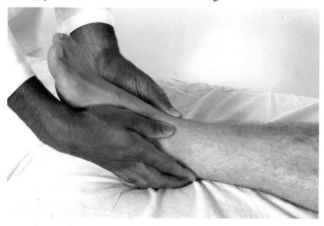

24-39

Palpate the metatarsophalangeal joints between your thumb on the dorsum and your fingers on the plantar surface (Figure 24-40).

Using a pinching motion of your thumb and forefinger, palpate the interphalangeal joints on the medial and lateral sides of the toes.

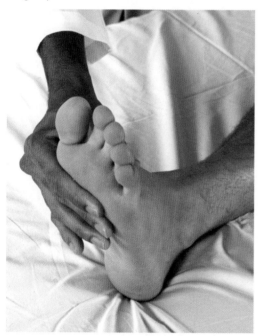

24-40

Test ROM as follows (Figure 24-41):

INSTRUCTIONS TO PATIENT	**MOTION AND EXPECTED RANGE**
• Point toes toward the floor.	Plantar flexion of 45 degrees
• Point toes toward your nose.	Dorsiflexion of 20 degrees (see Figure 24-41, *A*)
• Turn soles of feet out, then in. (Examiner stabilizes the ankle with one hand and holds heel with the other to test the subtalar joint.)	Eversion of 20 degrees Inversion of 30 degrees (see Figure 24-41, *B*)
• Flex and straighten toes.	

Assess muscle strength by asking the patient to maintain dorsiflexion and plantar flexion against your resistance.

Abnormal Findings column:

Swelling or inflammation.
Tenderness.

Swelling or inflammation; tenderness.

Limited ROM.
Pain with motion.

The patient cannot maintain flexion.

Objective Data

Normal Range of Findings	Abnormal Findings

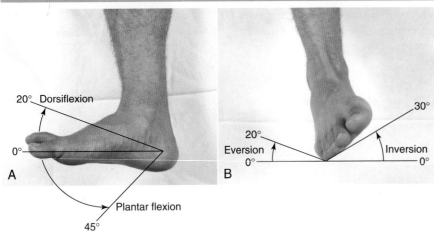

24-41

SPINE

The patient should be standing, draped in a gown open at the back. Place yourself far enough behind the patient so that you can see the entire back. *Inspect* and note whether the spine is straight by following an imaginary vertical line from the head through the spinous processes and down through the gluteal cleft; by noting equal horizontal positions for the shoulders, scapulae, iliac crests, and gluteal folds; and by noting equal spaces between the arm and lateral thorax on the two sides (Figure 24-42, *A*). The patient's knees and feet should be aligned with the trunk and should be pointing forward.

A difference in shoulder elevation and in level of scapulae and iliac crests occur with scoliosis (see Table 24-8, p. 651).

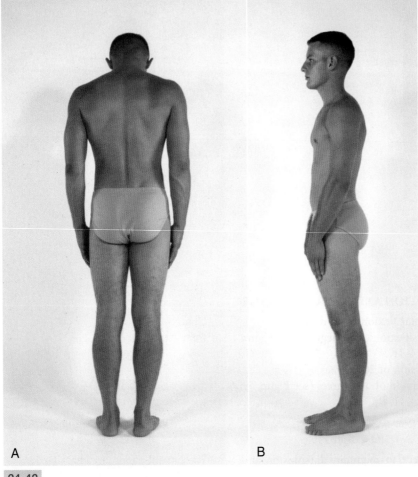

A   B

24-42

Normal Range of Findings	Abnormal Findings

From the side, note the normal convex thoracic curve and concave lumbar curve (see Figure 24-42, *B*). An enhanced thoracic curve, or kyphosis, is common in older adults. A pronounced lumbar curve, or lordosis, is common in obese people.

Palpate the spinous processes. Normally, they are straight and not tender. Palpate the paravertebral muscles; they should feel firm with no tenderness or spasm.

Test ROM of the spine by asking the patient to bend forward and touch the toes (Figure 24-43). Look for flexion of 75 to 90 degrees and smoothness and symmetry of movement. Note that the concave lumbar curve should disappear with this motion, and the back should have a single convex C-shaped curve.

Lateral tilting and forward bending occur with a herniated nucleus pulposus (see Table 24-8, p. 651).

Spinal curvature.
Tenderness; spasm of paravertebral muscles.
Chronic axial skeletal pain occurs with fibromyalgia syndrome (see Table 24-10, p. 654).

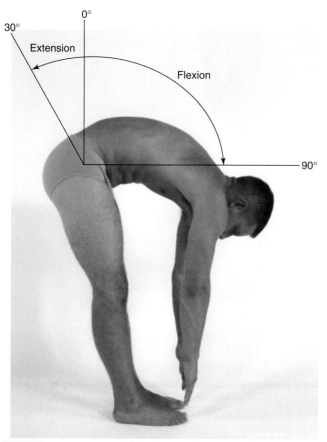

24-43

If you suspect a spinal curvature during inspection, this may be more clearly seen when the patient touches the toes. While the patient is bending over, mark a dot on each spinous process. When the patient resumes standing, the dots should form a straight vertical line.

If the dots form a slight S-shape when the patient stands, a spinal curve is present.

Normal Range of Findings	Abnormal Findings

Stabilize the pelvis with your hands. *Test ROM* as follows (Figure 24-44):

INSTRUCTIONS TO PATIENT

- Bend sideways.

- Bend backward.
- Twist shoulders to one side, then the other.

MOTION AND EXPECTED RANGE

Lateral bending of 35 degrees (see Figure 24-44, *A*)
Hyperextension of 30 degrees
Rotation of 30 degrees, bilaterally (see Figure 24-44, *B*)

Limited ROM.

Pain with motion.

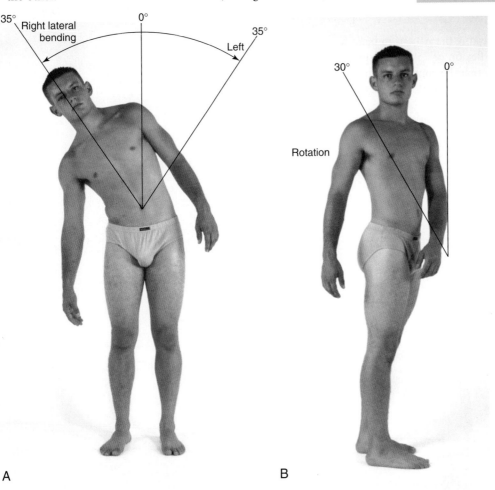

35° Right lateral bending   0°   35° Left   30°   0°

Rotation

A   B   24-44

These manoeuvres reveal only gross restriction. Movement is still possible even if some spinal fusion has occurred. Finally, ask the patient to walk on his or her toes for a few steps and then to walk on the heels.

SPECIAL CONSIDERATIONS FOR ADVANCED PRACTICE: SPINE

Normal Range of Findings	Abnormal Findings

Straight Leg Raising: LaSègue Test. These manoeuvres reproduce back and leg pain and help confirm the presence of a herniated nucleus pulposus. Straight leg raising while keeping the knee extended normally produces no pain. Raise the affected leg just short of the point where it produces pain. Then dorsiflex the foot (Figure 24-45).

Raise the unaffected leg while leaving the other leg flat. Inquire about the involved side.

The result of the LaSègue test is positive if it reproduces sciatic pain. If lifting the affected leg reproduces sciatic pain, it confirms the presence of a herniated nucleus pulposus.

If lifting the unaffected leg reproduces sciatic pain, it strongly suggests a herniated nucleus pulposus.

Normal Range of Findings	Abnormal Findings

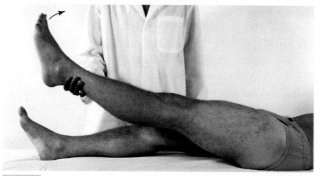

24-45

Measure Leg Length Discrepancy. Perform this measurement if you need to determine whether one leg is shorter than the other. For *true leg length,* measure between fixed points, from the anterior superior iliac spine to the medial malleolus, crossing the medial side of the knee (Figure 24-46). Normally, these measurements are equal or within 1 cm, indicating no true bone discrepancy.

Unequal leg lengths.

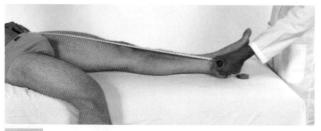

24-46

Sometimes the true leg length is equal, but the legs still look unequal. For *apparent leg length,* measure from a nonfixed point (the umbilicus) to a fixed point (medial malleolus) on each leg.

True leg lengths are equal, but leg lengths may appear unequal as a result of pelvic obliquity or adduction or flexion deformity in the hip.

DEVELOPMENTAL CONSIDERATIONS

Review the developmental milestones discussed on the Evolve Web site. Keep handy a concise chart of the usual sequence of motor development so that you can refer to expected findings for the age of each child you are examining. Use the Denver II test to identify the fine and gross motor skills expected for the child's age.

Because some aspects of the musculoskeletal and neurological examinations overlap, assessment of muscle tone, resting posture, and motor activity are discussed in the next chapter.

Infants

Examine an infant with the infant fully undressed and lying on the back. Take care to place the newborn on a warming table to maintain body temperature.

Feet and Legs. Start with the feet and work your way up the extremities. Note any *positional deformities,* a residual of fetal positioning. Often the newborn's feet are not held straight but in a varus (apart) or valgus (together) position. It is important to distinguish whether this position is flexible (and thus usually self-correctable) or fixed. Scratch the outside of the bottom of the foot. If the deformity is self-correctable, the foot assumes a normal right angle to the lower leg. Alternatively, immobilize the heel with one hand and gently push the forefoot to the neutral position with the other hand. If you can move it to neutral position, it is flexible.

A true deformity is fixed and assumes a right angle only with forced manipulation or not at all.

Objective Data

Normal Range of Findings

Note the relationship of the forefoot to the hindfoot. Commonly, the hindfoot is in alignment with the lower leg and just the forefoot angles inward. This forefoot adduction is *metatarsus adductus.* It is usually present at birth and usually resolves spontaneously by age 3 years.

Check for *tibial torsion,* a twisting of the tibia. Place the child's feet flat on the table, and push to flex up the knees. With the patella and the tibial tubercle in a straight line, place your fingers on the malleoli. In an infant, note whether an imaginary line connecting the four malleoli is parallel to the table.

Tibial torsion may originate from intrauterine positioning and then may be exacerbated at a later age by continuous sitting in a reverse tailor position, the "W" sitting position (sitting with the buttocks on the floor and the lower legs splayed back and out on either side).

Hips. Check the hips for *congenital dislocation.* The most reliable method is the **Ortolani manoeuvre,** which should be performed at every professional visit until the infant is 1 year old. With the infant supine, flex the knees by holding your thumbs on the inner mid-thighs and with your fingers outside on the hips, touching the greater trochanters. Adduct the legs until your thumbs touch (Figure 24-47, *A*). Then gently lift and *abduct* the legs, moving the knees apart and down so their lateral aspects touch the table (see Figure 24-47, *B*). This normally feels smooth and produces no sound.

Abnormal Findings

Metatarsus varus: adduction and inversion of forefoot.

Talipes equinovarus: inversion and adduction of forefoot, with downward pointing of foot (see Table 24-9, p. 653).

Tibial torsion: more than 20 degrees of deviation or location of lateral malleolus anterior to medial malleolus.

With a dislocated hip, the head of the femur is not cupped in the acetabulum but rests posterior to it.

Hip instability feels like a clunk as the head of the femur pops back into place. This is a *positive Ortolani sign* and warrants referral.

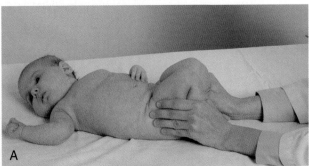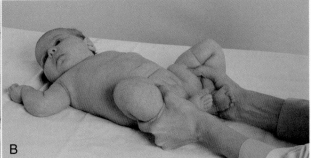

24-47   Ortolani manoeuvre.

The **Allis test** also is used to check for hip dislocation by comparing leg lengths (Figure 24-48). Place the baby's feet flat on the table, and flex the knees up. Scan the tops of the knees; normally, they are at the same elevation.

The finding that one knee is significantly lower than the other is a *positive Allis sign* and is suggestive of hip dislocation.

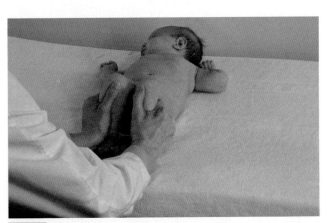

24-48   Allis test.

Normal Range of Findings	Abnormal Findings

Normal Range of Findings

Note the gluteal folds. Normally, they are equal on both sides. However, some asymmetry may be present in healthy children.

Hands and Arms. Inspect the hands, noting shape, number, and position of fingers and palmar creases. The palm usually has three strong horizontal lines (palmar flexion creases). A simian crease (single palmar crease) is often a normal finding, occurring in about 1 out of 30 people and twice as often in males (Kaneshiro, 2011).

Palpate the length of the clavicles because the clavicle is the bone most frequently fractured during birth. The clavicles should feel smooth, regular, and without crepitus. Also note equal ROM of arms during the Moro reflex (see Chapter 25 for description).

Back. Lift up the infant and examine the back. Note the normal single C-shaped curve of the newborn's spine (Figure 24-49). By 2 months of age, the infant can lift the head while prone. This builds the concave cervical spinal curve and indicates normal forearm strength. Inspect the length of the spine for any tuft of hair, dimple in midline, cyst, or mass. Normally, none are present. A sacral dimple is often normal.

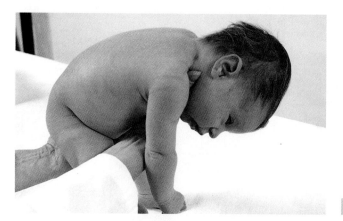

24-49

Observe ROM through spontaneous movement of extremities. Test muscle strength by lifting up the infant with your hands under the axillae (Figure 24-50). A baby with normal muscle strength wedges securely between your hands.

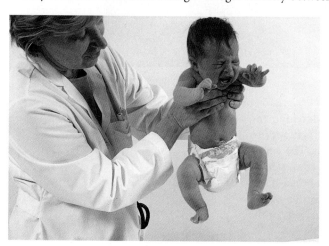

24-50

Abnormal Findings

Unequal gluteal folds may accompany hip dislocation after 2 to 3 months of age.

Polydactyly is the presence of extra fingers or toes. *Syndactyly* is webbing between adjacent fingers or toes (see Table 24-5, p. 647).

A simian crease frequently occurs with other conditions such as Down syndrome or fetal alcohol syndrome, and is accompanied by short broad fingers, incurving of little fingers, and low-set thumbs.

Fractured clavicle: Note irregularity at the fracture site, crepitus, and angulation. The site has rapid callus formation with a palpable lump within a few weeks. Observe limited arm ROM and unilateral response in the Moro reflex.

A small dimple in the midline—anywhere from the head to the coccyx—suggests dermoid sinus.

A tuft of hair, birthmark, or skin tag over a sacral dimple in the midline may indicate spina bifida.

Mass, such as meningocele, necessitates referral.

A baby who starts to "slip" between your hands shows weakness of the shoulder muscles.

Objective Data

Normal Range of Findings	Abnormal Findings

Preschool-Age and School-Age Children

Once the infant learns to crawl and then to walk, the waking hours are spent seemingly in perpetual motion. This is convenient for your musculoskeletal assessment; you can observe the muscles and joints during spontaneous play before a table-top examination. Most young children enjoy showing off their physical accomplishments. For specific motions, coax the toddler: "Show me how you can walk to Mom"; "Climb the step stool." Ask the preschooler to hop on one foot or to jump.

Back. While the child is standing, note the posture. From behind, you should note the plumb line from the back of the head, along the spine, to the middle of the sacrum. Shoulders are level within 1 cm, and scapulae are symmetrical. From the side, lordosis is common throughout childhood, appearing more pronounced in children with a protuberant abdomen.

Lordosis is marked in muscular dystrophy and rickets.

Legs and Feet. Anteriorly, note the leg position. A bowlegged stance (*genu varum*) is a lateral bowing of the legs (Figure 24-51, *A*). It is characterized by a persistent space of more than 2.5 cm between the knees when the medial malleoli are together. Genu varum is normal for 1 year after the child begins to walk. The child may walk with a waddling gait. Genu varum resolves with growth; no treatment is indicated.

Severe bowing or unilateral bowing also occurs with rickets.

Knock knees (*genu valgum*) are characterized by a span of more than 2.5 cm between the medial malleoli when the knees are together (see Figure 24-51, *B*). It occurs normally between 2 and 3½ years of age. Treatment is not indicated for genu valgum. (Note: A mnemonic for distinguishing the two conditions is to link the *r*s and *g*s: genu va*r*um—knees apa*r*t; genu val*g*um—knees to*g*ether.)

Genu valgum also occurs in rickets, poliomyelitis, and syphilis.

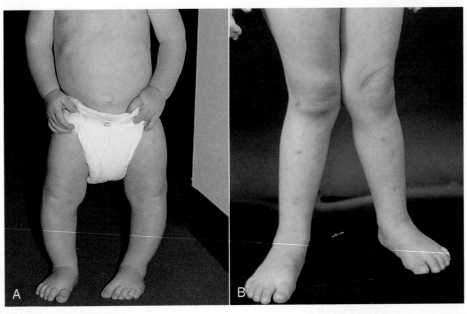

24-51   Leg position. **A,** Genu varum. **B,** Genu valgum.

Often, parents tell you they are concerned about the child's foot development. The most common questions are about "flatfeet" and "pigeon toes." Flatfoot (*pes planus*) is pronation, or turning in, of the medial side of the foot. The young child may look flatfooted because the normal longitudinal arch is concealed by a fat pad until age 3 years. When standing begins, the child takes a broad-based stance, which causes pronation. Thus pronation is common between 12 and 30 months. You can see it best from behind the child, where the medial side of the foot drops down and in.

Pronation beyond 30 months.

Normal Range of Findings	Abnormal Findings

Pigeon toes, or toeing in, are demonstrated when the child tends to walk on the lateral side of the foot, and the longitudinal arch looks higher than normal. It often starts as a forefoot adduction, which usually resolves spontaneously by age 3 years, as long as the foot is flexible.

Check the child's gait while the child walks away from and toward you. Let the child wear socks because a cold tile floor will distort the usual gait. In children 1 to 2 years of age, expect a broad-based gait, with arms out for balance. Weight bearing is borne on the inside of the foot. From 3 years of age, the base narrows, and the arms are kept closer to the sides. Inspect the shoes for spots of greatest wear to aid your judgement of the gait. Normally, the shoes show the most wear on the outside of the heel and the inside of the toe.

Check for the **Trendelenburg sign** to screen for progressive subluxation of the hip (Figure 24-52, *A*). As you watch from behind, ask the child to stand on one leg, then on the other. Note the iliac crests; they should stay level when weight is shifted.

The child may sit for the remainder of the examination. Start with the feet and hands of the child from 2 to 6 years of age because the child is happy to show these off, and proceed through the examination as described earlier.

Abnormal Findings:

Toeing in from forefoot adduction that is fixed or lasts beyond age 3 years.
Toeing in from tibial torsion.

Limp, usually caused by trauma, fatigue, or hip disease.
Abnormal gait patterns (see Chapter 25).

The *positive Trendelenburg sign* occurs with severe subluxation of one hip. When the child stands on the "good" leg, the pelvis looks level. When the child stands on the affected leg, the pelvis drops toward the "good" side. The hip abductors on the standing side are too weak to hold the pelvis level (see Figure 24-52, *B*).

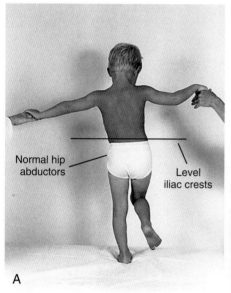

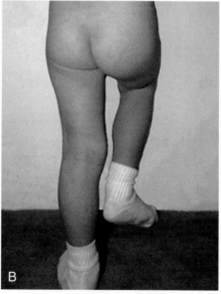

Normal hip abductors

Level iliac crests

A

B

24-52

In particular, check the arm for full ROM and presence of pain. Look for subluxation of the elbow (head of the radius). This occurs most often between 2 and 4 years of age as a result of forceful removal of clothing or dangling while adults suspend the child by the hands.

Palpate the bones, joints, and muscles of the extremities as described for the adult examination.

Inability to supinate the hand while the arm is flexed, together with pain in elbow, indicates subluxation of the head of the radius.

Pain or tenderness in extremities is usually caused by trauma or infection.

Fractures usually result from trauma and are exhibited as an inability to use the area, a deformity, or an excess motion in the involved bone with pain and crepitation.

Enlargement of the tibial tubercles with tenderness is suggestive of Osgood-Schlatter disease (see Table 24-6, p. 648).

Normal Range of Findings	Abnormal Findings

Adolescents

Proceed with the musculoskeletal examination as for adults, with special attention to spinal posture. Kyphosis is common during adolescence because of chronic poor posture. Be aware of the risk of sports-related injuries with adolescents because sports participation and competition often peak in this age group.

The Canadian Task Force on Preventive Health Care (Goldbloom, 1994) concluded that there was insufficient evidence to recommend the routine screening of symptom-free adolescents for idiopathic scoliosis; however, periodic visual inspection of the backs of adolescents seen for other reasons is reasonable.

Inspect for scoliosis with the *forward bend test* (Figure 24-53). Seat yourself behind the standing child, and ask the child to stand with the feet shoulder-width apart and to bend forward slowly to touch the toes. Expect a straight vertical spine while the child is both standing and bending forward. The posterior ribs should be symmetrical, with equal elevation of shoulders, scapulae, and iliac crests. You may wish to mark each spinous process with a felt marker. The lineup of ink dots highlights even a subtle curve.

Scoliosis is most apparent during the preadolescent growth spurt. Asymmetry is suggestive of scoliosis: The ribs "hump up" on one side as the child bends forward, and landmark elevation is unequal (see Table 24-8, p. 651).

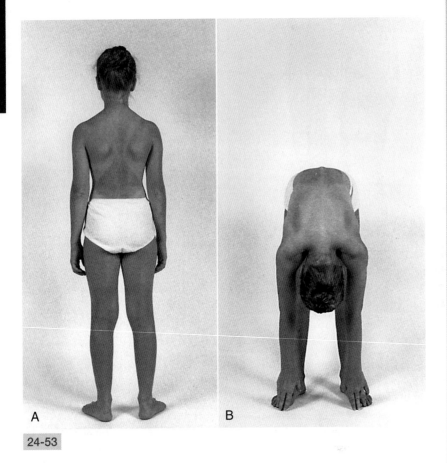

24-53

Pregnant Women

Proceed through the examination described for adults. Expected postural changes in pregnancy include progressive lordosis and, toward the third trimester, anterior cervical flexion, kyphosis, and slumped shoulders (Figure 24-54, *A*). At full term, the protuberant abdomen and the relaxed mobility in the joints create the characteristic waddling gait (see Figure 24-54, *B*).

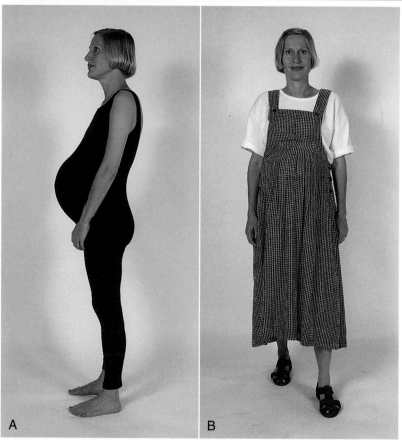

24-54

Objective Data

Older Adults

Postural changes include a decrease in height, which is more apparent in the eighth and ninth decades (Figure 24-55). "Lengthening of the arm–trunk axis" describes this shortening of the trunk with the appearance of comparatively long extremities. Kyphosis is common, with a backward head tilt to compensate. This creates the outline of a figure 3, as in the older adult pictured, viewed from the left side. Slight flexion of hips and knees is also common.

Contour changes include a decrease of fat in the body periphery and fat deposition over the abdomen and hips. The bony prominences become more marked.

With most older adults, ROM testing is performed as described earlier. ROM and muscle strength are much the same as in younger adults, provided that no musculoskeletal illnesses or arthritic changes are present.

Functional Assessment. For patients with changes caused by advanced aging or arthritis and those with musculoskeletal disability, perform a **functional assessment for ADLs.** In this assessment, ROM and muscle strength are tested with regard to the accomplishment of specific activities. You need to determine adequate and safe performance of functions essential for independent home life. See Chapter 31 for further assessments.

Objective Data

Normal Range of Findings	Abnormal Findings

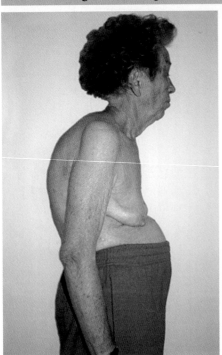

24-55

INSTRUCTIONS TO PATIENT

1. Walk (with shoes on).

2. Climb up stairs.

3. Walk down stairs.

4. Pick up object from floor.

5. Rise up from sitting in chair.

6. Rise up from lying in bed.

COMMON ADAPTATION FOR AGING CHANGES

Shuffling pattern; swaying; arms out to help balance; broader base of support; watching own feet

Holds tightly onto hand rail; may haul body up with arm; may lead with favoured (stronger) leg

Holds hand rail tightly, sometimes with both hands

With weakness, descending sideways, lowering the weaker leg first; with unsteadiness, watching the feet

Often bends at the waist instead of at the knees; holds onto furniture for support while bending or straightening

Uses arms to push off chair arms, upper trunk leans forward before body straightens, feet are planted wide in broad base of support

May roll to one side, pushes with arms to lift up torso, grabs bedside table to increase leverage

DOCUMENTATION AND CRITICAL THINKING

Sample Charting

SUBJECTIVE

Reports no joint pain, stiffness, swelling, or limitation. No muscle pain or weakness. No history of bone trauma or deformity. Able to manage all usual daily activities with no physical limitations. Occupation involves no musculoskeletal risk factors. Exercise pattern is brisk walk 1½ km (1 mile) 5×/week.

OBJECTIVE

Joints and muscles symmetrical; no swelling, masses, deformity; normal spinal curvature. No tenderness to palpation of joints; no heat, swelling, or masses. Full ROM; movement smooth, no crepitation, no tenderness. Muscle strength: able to maintain flexion against resistance and without tenderness.

ASSESSMENT

Muscles and joints: healthy and functional

Focused Assessment: Clinical Case Study

M.T. is a 45-year-old female salesperson with a diagnosis of rheumatoid arthritis 3 years PTA who seeks care now for "swelling and burning pain in my hands" for 1 day.

SUBJECTIVE

M.T. received a diagnosis of rheumatoid arthritis at age 41 years from staff at this agency. Since that time, her "flare-ups" seem to come every 6 to 8 months. Acute episodes involve hand joints and are treated with aspirin, which gives relief. Typically experiences morning stiffness, lasting ½ to 1 hour. Joints feel warm, swollen, tender. Has had weight loss of 7 kg (15 lb) over past 4 years and feels fatigued much of the time. States should rest more, but "I can't take the time." Daily exercises have been prescribed, but M.T. does not do them regularly. Takes aspirin for acute flare-ups, feels better in a few days, decreases dose herself.

OBJECTIVE

Body joints within normal limits except joints of wrist and hands. Radiocarpal, metacarpophalangeal, and proximal interphalangeal joints are red, swollen, tender to palpation. Spindle-shaped swelling of proximal interphalangeal joints of third digit right hand and second digit left hand; ulnar deviation of metacarpophalangeal joints.

ASSESSMENT

Acute pain R/T inflammation
Impaired physical mobility R/T inflammation
Deficient knowledge about aspirin treatment R/T lack of exposure
Noncompliance with exercise program R/T lack of perceived benefits of treatment
Noncompliance with advised rest periods R/T lack of perceived benefits of treatment

Documentation &
Critical Thinking

ABNORMAL FINDINGS

TABLE 24-2   Abnormalities Affecting Multiple Joints

Inflammatory Conditions

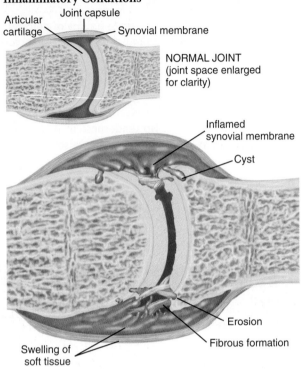

Articular cartilage — Joint capsule — Synovial membrane

NORMAL JOINT (joint space enlarged for clarity)

Inflamed synovial membrane

Cyst

Erosion

Fibrous formation

Swelling of soft tissue

Degenerative Conditions

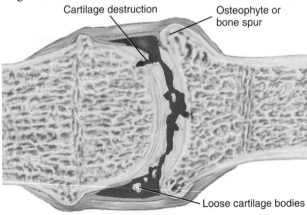

Cartilage destruction

Osteophyte or bone spur

Loose cartilage bodies

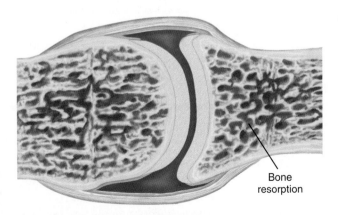

Bone resorption

◀ **Rheumatoid Arthritis**

This is a chronic, systemic inflammatory disease of joints and surrounding connective tissue. Inflammation of the synovial membrane leads to thickening; then to fibrosis, which limits motion; and finally to bony ankylosis. The disorder is symmetrical and bilateral and is characterized by heat, redness, swelling, and painful motion of the affected joints. Rheumatoid arthritis is associated with fatigue, weakness, anorexia, weight loss, low-grade fever, and lymphadenopathy. Associated signs are described in the following tables, especially Table 24-5, p. 646.

Ankylosing Spondylitis (Not Illustrated)

Chronic progressive inflammation of spine, sacroiliac, and larger joints of the extremities, leading to bony ankylosis and deformity. A form of rheumatoid arthritis, this affects primarily men by a 10:1 ratio, starting in late adolescence or early adulthood. Spasm of paraspinal muscles pulls the spine into forward flexion, obliterating cervical and lumbar curves. The thoracic curve is exaggerated into a single kyphotic rounding. Manifestations also include flexion deformities of the hips and knees.

◀ **Osteoarthritis (Degenerative Joint Disease)**

Noninflammatory, localized, progressive disorder involving deterioration of articular cartilages and subchondral bone and formation of new bone (osteophytes) at joint surfaces. Aging increases incidence; nearly all adults older than 60 years show some signs of osteoarthritis on radiographs. Asymmetrical joint involvement commonly affects hands, knees, hips, and lumbar and cervical segments of the spine. Affected joints have stiffness; swelling with hard, bony protuberances; pain with motion; and limitation of motion (see Table 24-5, p. 646).

◀ **Osteoporosis**

Decrease in skeletal bone mass occurring when rate of bone resorption is greater than that of bone formation. The weakened bone state increases risk for stress fractures, especially at wrist, hip, and vertebrae. Occurs primarily in postmenopausal women of European descent. Osteoporosis risk also is associated with smaller height and weight, younger age at menopause, lack of physical activity, and lack of estrogen replacement therapy.

TABLE 24-3   Abnormalities of the Shoulder

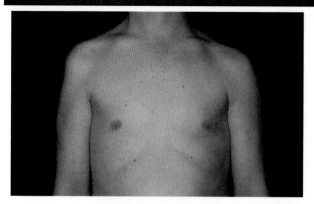

Atrophy

Loss of muscle mass is exhibited as a lack of fullness surrounding the deltoid muscle. In the case pictured (on the patient's left side), atrophy is caused by axillary nerve palsy. Atrophy also results from disuse, muscle tissue damage, or motor nerve damage.

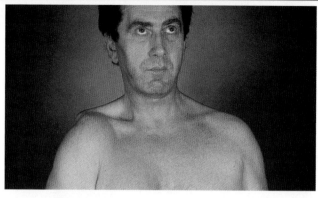

Dislocated Shoulder

Anterior dislocation (95%) is exhibited when the shoulder is hunched forward and the tip of the clavicle dislocates. It occurs with trauma involving abduction, extension, and rotation (e.g., falling on an outstretched arm or diving into a pool).

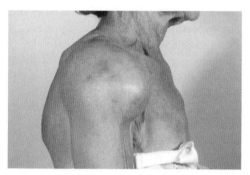

Joint Effusion

Swelling is caused by excess fluid in the joint capsule: in the case pictured, from rheumatoid arthritis. It is best observed anteriorly. It is fluctuant on palpation. Considerable fluid must be present to cause a visible distension because the capsule normally is loose.

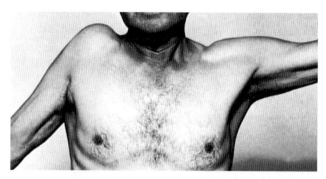

Tear of Rotator Cuff

Characteristics are a hunched position and limited abduction of arm (in the case pictured, on the patient's right side). Such tears are caused by traumatic adduction while the arm is held in abduction; by a fall on shoulder; by throwing; or by heavy lifting. In the *drop arm test,* the arm is passively abducted at the shoulder; a positive result is the patient's inability to sustain the position, and the arm falls to the side.

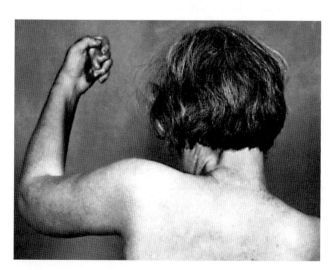

◄ Frozen Shoulder: Adhesive Capsulitis

Fibrous tissues form in the joint capsule, causing stiffness, progressive limitation of motion, and pain. Abduction and external rotation are limited; affected patients cannot reach overhead. It may lead to atrophy of shoulder girdle muscles. The onset is gradual, and the cause is unknown. It is associated with prolonged bed rest or shoulder immobility. It may resolve spontaneously.

Subacromial Bursitis (Not Illustrated)

Inflammation and swelling of the subacromial bursa over the shoulder cause both limitation in range of motion and pain with motion. Localized swelling under the deltoid muscle may increase with partial passive abduction of the arm. This condition is caused by direct trauma, strain during sports, local or systemic inflammatory process, or repetitive motion injury.

TABLE 24-4   **Abnormalities of the Elbow**

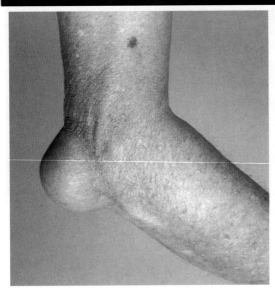

Olecranon Bursitis

Large soft knob, or "goose egg," and redness from inflammation of olecranon bursa. Localized and easy to see because bursa lies just under skin.

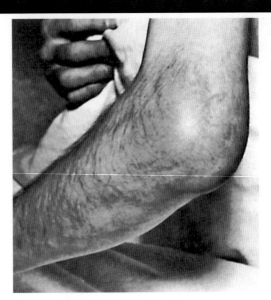

Gouty Arthritis

Joint effusion or synovial thickening, seen first as bulge or fullness in grooves on either side of olecranon process. Redness and heat can extend beyond area of synovial membrane. Soft, boggy, or fluctuant fullness to palpation. Limited extension of elbow.

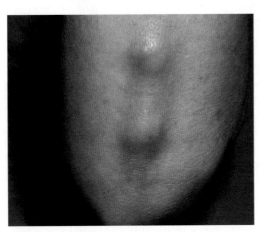

Subcutaneous Nodules

Raised, firm, nontender nodules that occur with rheumatoid arthritis. Common sites are in the olecranon bursa and along extensor surface of arm. The skin slides freely over the nodules.

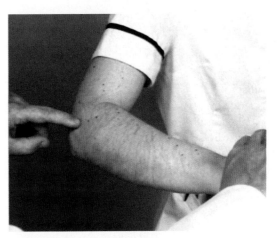

Epicondylitis: Tennis Elbow

Chronic, disabling pain at lateral epicondyle of humerus, radiates down extensor surface of forearm. Pain can be located by touching with one finger (as in illustration). Resisting extension of the hand will increase the pain. Occurs with activities combining excessive pronation and supination of forearm with an extended wrist (e.g., racket sports or using a screwdriver).

Medial epicondylitis is rarer and is caused by activity of forced palmar flexion of wrist against resistance.

TABLE 24-5   Abnormalities of the Wrist and Hand

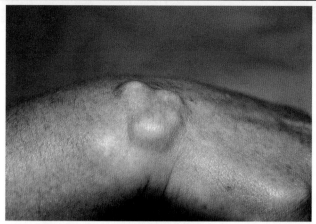

Ganglion Cyst

Round, cystic, nontender nodule overlying a tendon sheath or joint capsule, usually on dorsum of wrist. Flexion makes it more prominent. A common benign tumour; it does not become malignant.

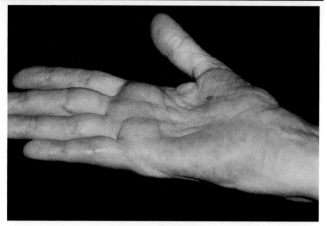

Reprinted from the Clinical Slide Collection on the Rheumatic Diseases, © 1991, 1995, 1997. Used by permission of the American College of Rheumatology.

Carpal Tunnel Syndrome with Atrophy of Thenar Eminence

Atrophy (pictured) is caused by interference with motor function as a result of compression of the median nerve inside the carpal tunnel. Caused by chronic repetitive motion; occurs between 30 and 60 years of age and is five times more common in women than in men. Symptoms of carpal tunnel syndrome include pain, burning sensation and numbness, positive findings on Phalen test, positive Tinel's sign, and often atrophy of thenar muscles.

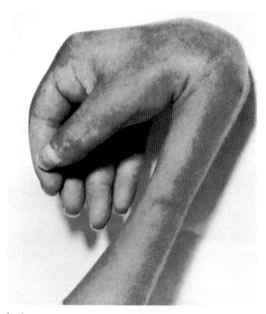

Ankylosis

Wrist in extreme flexion, as a result of severe rheumatoid arthritis. The affected hand is functionally useless because when the wrist is palmar flexed, a good deal of power is lost from the fingers, and the thumb cannot oppose the fingers.

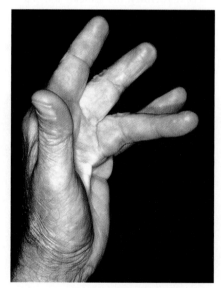

Reprinted from the Clinical Slide Collection on the Rheumatic Diseases, © 1991, 1995, 1997. Used by permission of the American College of Rheumatology.

Dupuytren's Contracture

Chronic hyperplasia of the palmar fascia causes flexion contractures of the digits, first in the fourth digit, then the fifth digit, and then the third digit. Note the bands that extend from the mid-palm to the digits and the puckering of palmar skin. The condition occurs commonly in men older than 40 years and is usually bilateral. It occurs with diabetes, epilepsy, and alcoholic liver disease and as an inherited trait. The contracture is painless but impairs hand function.

Colles' Fracture (Not Illustrated)

Nonarticular fracture of distal radius, with or without fracture of ulna at styloid process. Usually results from a fall on an outstretched hand; occurs most often in older women. Wrist looks puffy, with "silver fork" deformity, a characteristic hump when viewed from the side.

Continued

TABLE 24-5   Abnormalities of the Wrist and Hand—cont'd

Conditions Caused by Chronic Rheumatoid Arthritis

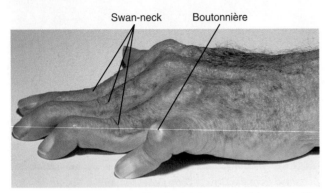

Reprinted from the Clinical Slide Collection on the Rheumatic Diseases, © 1991, 1995, 1997. Used by permission of the American College of Rheumatology.

Swan-Neck and Boutonnière Deformity

In **swan-neck deformity,** the flexion contracture resembles the curve of a swan's neck. Note flexion contracture of metacarpophalangeal joint, hyperextension of the proximal interphalangeal joint, and flexion of the distal interphalangeal joint. It occurs with chronic rheumatoid arthritis and is often accompanied by ulnar drift of the fingers.

In **boutonnière deformity,** the knuckle looks as if it is being pushed through a buttonhole. It is a relatively common deformity and includes flexion of proximal interphalangeal joint with compensatory hyperextension of distal interphalangeal joint.

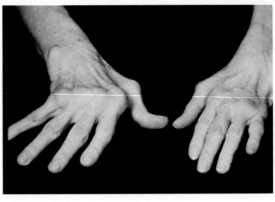

Ulnar Deviation or Drift

Fingers drift to the ulnar side because of stretching of the articular capsule and muscle imbalance (right hand in illustration). Also note subluxation and swelling in the joints and muscle atrophy on the dorsa of the hands. These are caused by chronic rheumatoid arthritis.

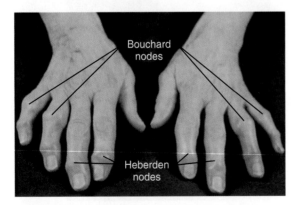

Degenerative Joint Disease or Osteoarthritis

Osteoarthritis is characterized by hard, nontender nodules (osteophytes, or bony overgrowths), 2 to 3 mm or more in diameter. The osteophytes of the distal interphalangeal joints are called **Heberden's nodes,** and those of the proximal interphalangeal joints are called **Bouchard's nodes.**

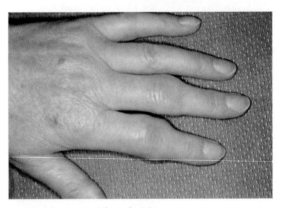

Acute Rheumatoid Arthritis

Painful swelling and stiffness of joints, with fusiform or spindle-shaped swelling of the soft tissue of proximal interphalangeal joints. Fusiform swelling is usually symmetrical, the hands are warm, and the veins are engorged. The inflamed joints have a limited range of motion.

TABLE 24-5   Abnormalities of the Wrist and Hand—cont'd

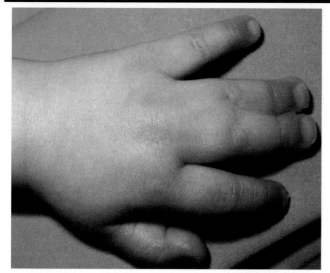

Syndactyly
Webbed fingers are a congenital deformity, usually
necessitating surgical separation. The metacarpals and
phalanges of the webbed fingers are different lengths, and
the joints do not line up. Not correcting fused fingers
would therefore limit their flexion and extension.

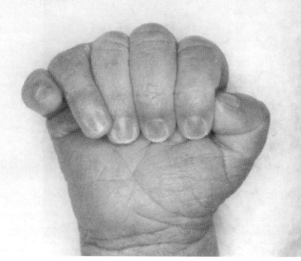

Polydactyly
Extra digits are a congenital deformity, usually occurring at
the fifth finger or the thumb. Surgical removal is
considered for cosmetic reasons. The sixth finger shown
here was not removed because it had full range of motion
and sensation and a normal appearance.

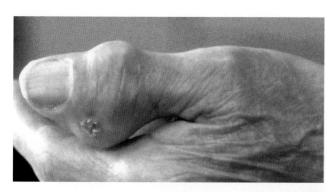

◄ *Gout in the Thumb*
See explanation of gout in Table 24-7.

TABLE 24-6   Abnormalities of the Knee

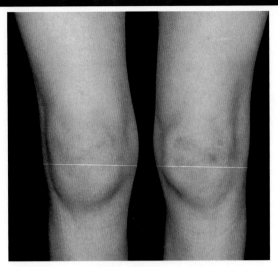

Mild Synovitis

Loss of normal hollows on either side of the patella, which are replaced by mild distension. Occurs with synovial thickening or effusion (excess fluid). Also note mild distension of the suprapatellar pouch.

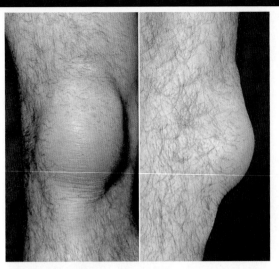

Prepatellar Bursitis

Localized swelling on anterior knee between patella and skin. A tender fluctuant mass indicates swelling; in some cases, infection spreads to surrounding soft tissue. The condition is limited to the bursa, and the knee joint itself is not involved. Overlying skin may be red, shiny, and either atrophic or coarse and thickened.

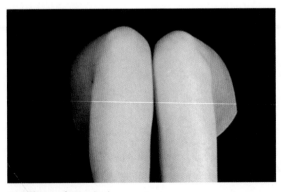

Swelling of Menisci

Localized soft swelling from cyst in lateral meniscus shows at the midpoint of the anterolateral joint line (right leg in illustration). Semiflexion of the knee makes swelling more prominent.

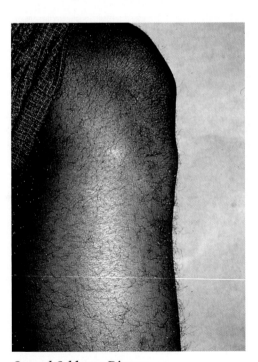

Osgood-Schlatter Disease

Painful swelling of the tibial tubercle just below the knee, probably from repeated stress on the patellar tendon. Occurs mostly in puberty during rapid growth and most often in boys. Pain increases with kicking, running, bicycling, stair climbing, or kneeling. The condition is usually self-limited, and symptoms resolve with rest.

TABLE 24-6   Abnormalities of the Knee—cont'd

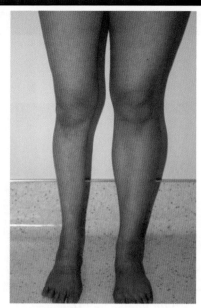

Chondromalacia Patellae (Not Illustrated)
Degeneration of articular surface of patellae. Occurs most often in girls and women, in adolescents, and in young adults. Cause is unknown, but condition is associated with overuse and injury. May produce mild effusion. Joint motion is painless, but crepitus may be present. Kneeling causes onset of pain.

Postpolio Muscle Atrophy
Leg and foot muscle atrophy as a result of childhood polio (in illustration, the patient's right leg and foot). Poliomyelitis epidemics peaked in North America in the 1940s and 1950s. The development of the oral polio vaccine (1962) has almost eradicated the disease. However, thousands of polio survivors have this muscle atrophy.

TABLE 24-7   Abnormalities of the Ankle and Foot

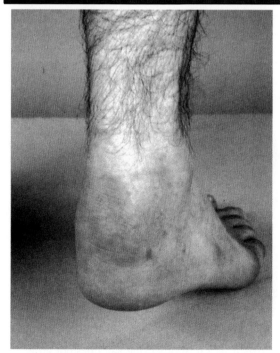

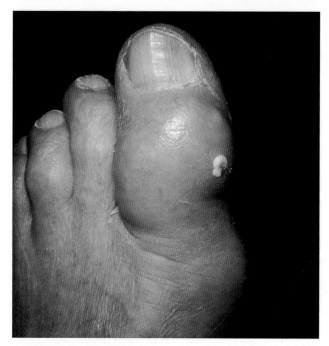

Achilles Tenosynovitis
Inflammation of a tendon sheath near the ankle (in illustration, the Achilles tendon) produces a superficial linear swelling and a localized tenderness along the route of the sheath. Movement of the involved tendon usually causes pain.

Tophi With Chronic Gout
In illustration, a hard, painless nodule (tophus) is over the metatarsophalangeal joint of the first toe. Tophi are collections of sodium urate crystals that develop in chronic gout in and around the joint that cause extreme swelling and joint deformity. They sometimes burst with a chalky discharge.

Continued

TABLE 24-7   Abnormalities of the Ankle and Foot—cont'd

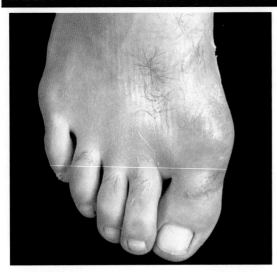

Acute Gout

Acute episode of gout usually involves first the metatarsophalangeal joint. Clinical findings consist of redness, swelling, heat, and extreme tenderness. Gout is a metabolic disorder of disturbed purine metabolism, associated with elevated serum levels of uric acid. It occurs primarily in men older than 40 years.

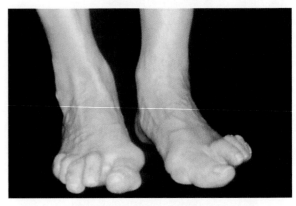

Hallux Valgus With Bunion and Hammertoes

Hallux valgus is a common deformity caused by rheumatoid arthritis. It is a lateral or outward deviation of the great toe with medial prominence of the head of the first metatarsal. The **bunion** is the inflamed bursa that forms at the pressure point. The great toe loses power to push off while walking; this stresses the second and third metatarsal heads, and they develop calluses and pain. Chronic sequelae include corns, calluses, hammertoes, and joint subluxation.

Note the **hammertoe** deformities in the second, third, fourth, and fifth toes. Often associated with hallux valgus, hammertoe includes hyperextension of the metatarsophalangeal joint and flexion of the proximal interphalangeal joint.

Corns (thickening of soft tissue) develop on the dorsum over the bony prominence as a result of prolonged pressure from shoes.

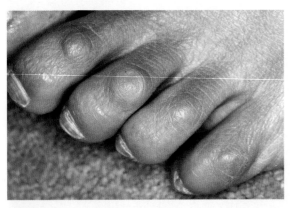

Callus

Hypertrophy of the epithelium develops because of prolonged pressure, commonly on the plantar surface of the first metatarsal head in the hallux valgus deformity. The condition is not painful.

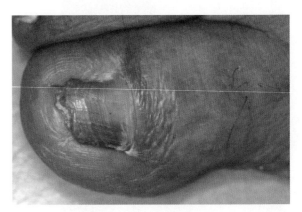

Ingrown Toenail

"Ingrown toenail" is a misnomer; the nail does not grow in, but the soft tissue grows over the nail and obliterates the groove. It occurs almost always on the great toe on the medial or lateral side. It is caused by trimming the nail too short or crowding of toes in tight shoes. The area becomes infected when the nail grows and its corner penetrates the soft tissue.

TABLE 24-7	Abnormalities of the Ankle and Foot—cont'd

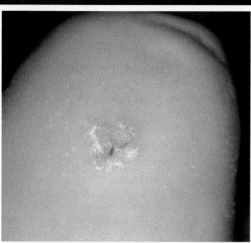

◄ *Plantar Wart*

Vascular papillomatous growth is probably caused by a virus and occurs on the sole of the foot, commonly at the ball. The condition is extremely painful.

TABLE 24-8	Abnormalities of the Spine

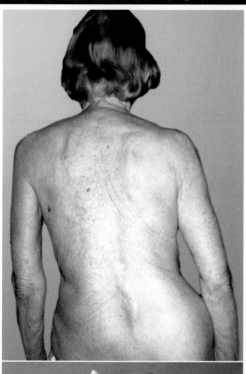

◄ *Scoliosis*

Lateral curvature of thoracic and lumbar segments of the spine, usually with some rotation of involved vertebral bodies.

Functional scoliosis is flexible; it is apparent on standing and disappears on forward bending. It may be compensatory for other abnormalities such as leg length discrepancy.

Structural scoliosis is fixed; the curvature shows both on standing and on bending forward. In illustration, note rib hump with forward flexion. When the patient is standing, note unequal shoulder elevation, unequal scapulae, obvious curvature, and unequal hip level. At greatest risk are girls aged 10 years through adolescence, during the peak of the growth spurt.

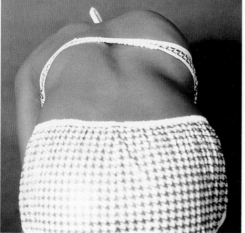

Continued

TABLE 24-8	**Abnormalities of the Spine—cont'd**

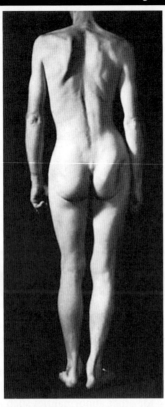

◄ *Herniated Nucleus Pulposus*

The nucleus pulposus (at the centre of the intervertebral disc) ruptures into the spinal canal and puts pressure on the local spinal nerve root. It is usually caused by stress, such as lifting, twisting, continuous flexion with lifting, or a fall onto the buttocks. It occurs mostly in men 20 to 45 years of age. Lumbar herniations occur mainly in interspaces L4-L5 and L5-S1. Note sciatic pain, numbness, and paraesthesia of involved dermatome; listing away from affected side; decreased mobility; low back tenderness; and decreased motor and sensory function in leg. Straight leg raising tests reproduce sciatic pain.

TABLE 24-9	**Common Congenital or Pediatric Abnormalities**

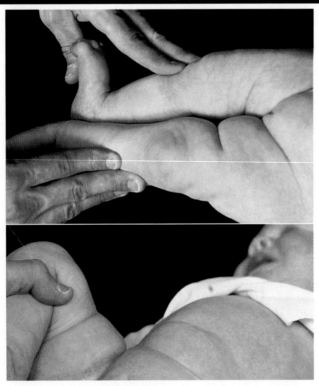

◄ *Congenital Dislocated Hip*

Head of the femur is displaced out of the cup-shaped acetabulum.

The degree of the condition varies; subluxation may occur as stretched ligaments allow partial displacement of the femoral head, and acetabular dysplasia may develop because of excessive laxity of the hip joint capsule.

Occurrence is 1:500 to 1:1000 births; more common in girls (7:1 ratio). Signs include limited abduction of flexed thigh, positive findings of Ortolani manoeuvre and positive Barlow's sign, asymmetrical skin creases or gluteal folds, limb length discrepancy, and positive indication of the Trendelenburg sign in older children.

TABLE 24-9   Common Congenital or Pediatric Abnormalities—cont'd

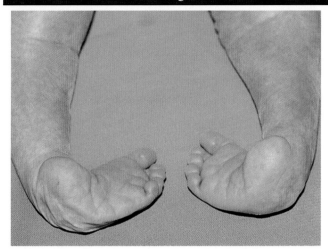

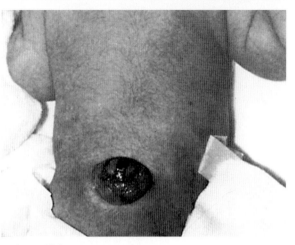

Talipes Equinovarus (Clubfoot)

Congenital, rigid, and fixed malposition of foot, including (a) inversion, (b) forefoot adduction, and (c) foot pointing downward (equinus). A common birth defect, with an incidence of 1:1000 to 3:1000 live births. Boys are affected twice as frequently as girls.

Coxa Plana (Legg-Calvé-Perthes Syndrome)
(Not Illustrated)

Avascular necrosis of the femoral head, occurring primarily in boys between 3 and 12 years of age, peaking at age 6 years. In the initial inflammatory stage, interruption of blood supply to femoral epiphysis occurs, halting growth. Revascularization and healing occur later, but significant residual deformity and dysfunction may be present.

Spina Bifida

Incomplete closure of posterior part of vertebrae results in a neural tube defect. Seriousness varies from skin defect along the spine to protrusion of the sac containing meninges, spinal fluid, or malformed spinal cord. The most serious type is myelomeningocele (shown in illustration), in which the meninges and neural tissue protrude. Most children with myelomeningocele are paralyzed below the level of the lesion.

TABLE 24-10	Fibromyalgia Syndrome

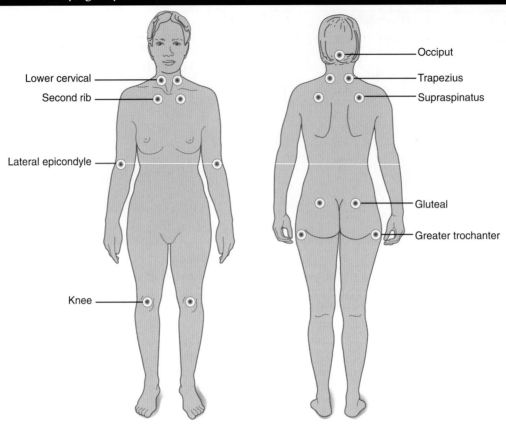

LOCATION OF TENDER POINTS

© Pat Thomas, 2010.

Chronic disorder of unknown cause characterized by widespread musculoskeletal pain lasting 3 months or longer, associated with fatigue, insomnia, and psychosocial distress. Most patients (90%) are women. There are two major diagnostic criteria (Wolfe et al., 1990): (a) pain on both sides of the body, above and below the waist, and axial skeletal pain (cervical, thoracic, lumbar spine, or anterior chest); and (b) point tenderness on digital palpation in 11 of 18 specific sites (shown in illustration). The examiner presses the thumb of the dominant hand with a force of 4 kg (same as needed to blanch or whiten the nail bed). The burden of illness is high: 25% to 33% of affected patients receive disability compensation.

Summary Checklist: Musculoskeletal Examination

For a PDA-downloadable version, go to *http://evolve.elsevier.com/Canada/Jarvis/examination/*.

For each joint to be examined:
1. Inspection:
   Size and contour of joint
   Skin colour and characteristics
2. Palpation of joint area:
   Skin

Muscles
Bony articulations
Joint capsule
3. Range of motion (ROM):
   Active
   Passive (if active ROM is limited)

Measure with goniometer (if ROM is abnormal)
4. Muscle testing:
5. Teaching and health promotion

REFERENCES

Arthritis Society. (2011a). *Osteoarthritis: Know your options.* Retrieved from *http://www.arthrite.ca/document.doc?id=82*.

Arthritis Society. (2011b). *Rheumatoid arthritis: Know your options.* Retrieved from *http://www.arthrite.ca/document. doc?id=87*.

Canadian Institute for Health Information. (2007). *Health indicators 2007.* Retrieved from *https://secure.cihi.ca/free_products/hi07_health_indicators_2007_e.pdf*.

Canadian Institute for Health Information. (2009). *Hip and knee replacements in Canada—Canadian Joint Replacement*

Abnormal Findings

Registry (CJRR) 2008-2009 annual report. Retrieved from https://secure.cihi.ca/free_products/2008_cjrr_annual_report_en.pdf.

Cousins, J. M., Petit, M. A., Paudel, M. L., Taylor, B. C., Hughes, J. M., Cauley, J. A., … Ensrud, K. E. (2010). Muscle power and physical activity are associated with bone strength in older men: The osteoporotic fractures in men study. Bone, 47(2), 205–211. doi:10.1016/j.bone.2010.05.003

Goldbloom, R. B. (1994). Screening for idiopathic adolescent scoliosis. In Canadian Task Force on the Periodic Health Examination (Ed.), Canadian guide to clinical preventive health care (pp. 346–354). Ottawa: Health Canada.

Hanley, D. A., Cranney, A., Jones, G., Whiting, S. J., & Leslie, W. D. (2010). Vitamin D in adult health and disease: A review and guideline statement from Osteoporosis Canada (summary). Canadian Medical Association Journal, 182(12), 1315–1319. doi:10.1503/cmaj.091062

Ioannidis, G., Papaioannou, A., Hopman, W. M., Akhtar-Danesh, N., Anastassiades, T., Pickard, L., … Adachi, J. D. (2009). Relation between fractures and mortality: Results from the Canadian Multicentre Osteoporosis Study. Canadian Medical Association Journal, 181(5), 265–271.

Kaneshiro, N. K. (2011). Simian crease. Retrieved from http://www.nlm.nih.gov/medlineplus/ency/article/003290.htm.

McGee, S. (2007). Evidence-based physical diagnosis (2nd ed.). St. Louis: W. B. Saunders.

Papaioannou, A., Morin, S., Cheung, A. M., Atkinson, S., Brown, J. P., Feldman, S., … Scientific Advisory Council of Osteoporosis Canada. (2010). 2010 Clinical practice guidelines for the diagnosis and management of osteoporosis in Canada: Summary. Canadian Medical Association Journal, 182(17): 1864–1873. doi:10.1503/cmaj.100771

Patel, H., & Canadian Task Force on Preventive Health Care. (2001). Preventive health care, 2001 update: Screening and management of developmental dysplasia of the hip in newborns. Canadian Medical Association Journal, 164(12), 1669–1677.

Pigozzi, E., Rizzo, M., Giombinin, A., Parisi, A., Fagnani, F., & Borrione, P. (2009). Bone mineral density and sport: Effect of physical activity. Journal of Sports Medicine and Physical Fitness, 49(2), 177–183.

Public Health Agency of Canada. (2010). Life with arthritis in Canada: A personal and public health challenge. Retrieved from http://www.phac-aspc.gc.ca/cd-mc/arthritis-arthrite/lwaic-vaaac-10/pdf/arthritis-2010-eng.pdf.

Schmitt, N. M., Schmitt, J., & Doren, M. (2009). The role of physical activity in the prevention of osteoporosis in postmenopausal women—An update. Maturitas, 63(1), 34–38. doi:10.1016/j.maturitas.2009.03.002

Sorkin, J. D., Muller, D. C., & Andres, R. (1999). Longitudinal change in height of men and women: Implications for interpretation of body mass index. American Journal of Epidemiology, 150(9), 969–977.

Statistics Canada. (2011a). Canadian community health survey: Injuries. Retrieved from http://www.statcan.gc.ca/daily-quotidien/110628/dq110628c-eng.htm.

Statistics Canada. (2011b). Physical activity during leisure time, 2009. Retrieved from http://www.statcan.gc.ca/pub/82-625-x/2010002/article/11267-eng.htm.

Statistics Canada. (2012). Arthritis, by sex, and by province and territory. Retrieved from http://www.statcan.gc.ca/tables-tableaux/sum-som/l01/cst01/health52a-eng.htm.

Targownik, L. E., Lix, L. M., Metge, C. J., Prior, H. J., Leung, S., & Leslie, W. D. (2008). Use of proton pump inhibitors and risk of osteoporosis-related fractures. Canadian Medical Association Journal, 179(4), 319–326. doi:10.1503/cmaj.071330

Uziel, Y., & Hashkes, P. J. (2007). Growing pains in children. Pediatric Rheumatology, 5(5), 1–4. doi:10.1186/1546-0096-5-5

Wolfe, F., Smythe, H. A., Yunus, M. B., Bennett, R. M., Bombardier, C., Goldenberg, D. L., … Sheon, R. P. (1990). The American College of Rheumatology 1990 criteria for the classification of fibromyalgia. Report of the Multicenter Criteria Committee. Arthritis and Rheumatism, 33(2), 160–172.

Written by Carolyn Jarvis, PhD, APN, CNP
Adapted by Annette J. Browne, PhD, RN

⊖volve WEBSITE

OUTLINE

STRUCTURE AND FUNCTION

The nervous system can be divided into two parts: central and peripheral. The **central nervous system (CNS)** includes the brain and spinal cord. The **peripheral nervous system** includes the 12 pairs of cranial nerves, the 31 pairs of spinal nerves, and all their branches. The peripheral nervous system carries sensory (*afferent*) messages *to* the CNS from sensory receptors, motor (*efferent*) messages *from* the CNS out to muscles and glands, and autonomic messages that govern the internal organs and blood vessels.

The meninges (dura, arachnoid, and pia mater) are the layers of membranes that envelope the CNS. The primary function of the meninges and of the cerebrospinal fluid is to protect the CNS.

THE CENTRAL NERVOUS SYSTEM

Cerebral Cortex

The cerebral cortex is the cerebrum's outer layer of nerve cell bodies; this layer looks like "grey matter" because it lacks myelin. Myelin is the white insulation on the axon that increases the conduction velocity of nerve impulses.

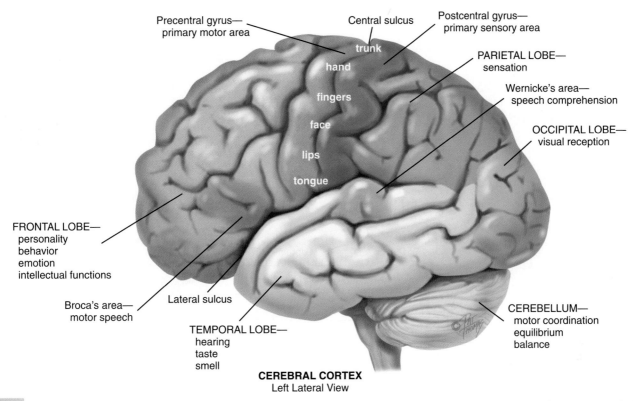

Precentral gyrus—
primary motor area

Central sulcus

Postcentral gyrus—
primary sensory area

trunk

hand

fingers

face

lips

tongue

PARIETAL LOBE—
sensation

Wernicke's area—
speech comprehension

OCCIPITAL LOBE—
visual reception

FRONTAL LOBE—
personality
behavior
emotion
intellectual functions

Broca's area—
motor speech

Lateral sulcus

TEMPORAL LOBE—
hearing
taste
smell

CEREBELLUM—
motor coordination
equilibrium
balance

CEREBRAL CORTEX
Left Lateral View

25-1

© Pat Thomas, 2006.

The cerebral cortex (cerebrum) is the centre for humans' highest functions, governing thought, memory, reasoning, sensation, and voluntary movement (Figure 25-1). Each half of the cerebrum is a **hemisphere;** the left hemisphere is dominant in ~ 95%) of right-handed people, and in many who are left-handed.

Each hemisphere is divided into four **lobes:** frontal, parietal, temporal, and occipital. The lobes have certain areas that mediate specific functions:

- The **frontal** lobe has areas concerned with personality, behaviour, emotions, and intellectual function.
- The precentral gyrus of the frontal lobe initiates voluntary movement.
- The **parietal** lobe contains the postcentral gyrus, which is the primary centre for sensation.
- The **occipital** lobe is the primary visual receptor centre.
- The portion of the **temporal** lobe behind the ear has the primary auditory reception centre.
- **Wernicke's area** in the temporal lobe is associated with language comprehension. When it is damaged in a person's dominant hemisphere, *receptive aphasia* results. The person hears sound, but it has no meaning, like hearing a foreign language.
- **Broca's area** in the frontal lobe mediates motor speech. When it is injured in the dominant hemisphere, *expressive aphasia* results; the person cannot talk. The person can understand language and knows what he or she wants to say but can produce only a garbled sound.

Damage to any of these specific cortical areas produces a corresponding loss of function: motor weakness, paralysis, loss of sensation, or impairment of the ability to understand and process language. Damage occurs when the highly specialized neurological cells are deprived of their blood supply, such as when a cerebral artery becomes occluded or when vascular bleeding or vasospasm occurs.

Basal Ganglia

The basal ganglia are additional bands of grey matter buried deep within the two cerebral hemispheres that form the subcortical associated motor system (the extrapyramidal system; Figure 25-2). They control automatic associated movements of the body, such as the arm swing that alternates with the leg movement during walking.

Thalamus

The thalamus is the main relay station for the nervous system. Sensory pathways of the spinal cord and brain stem form **synapses** (sites of contact between two neurons) on their way to the cerebral cortex.

Hypothalamus

The hypothalamus is a major control centre with many vital functions: controlling temperature, heart rate, and blood pressure; regulating sleep and the anterior and posterior pituitary gland; and coordinating autonomic nervous system activity and emotional status.

Cerebellum

The cerebellum is a coiled structure located under the occipital lobe that is concerned with motor coordination of voluntary movements, equilibrium (i.e., the postural balance of the body), and muscle tone. It does not initiate movement

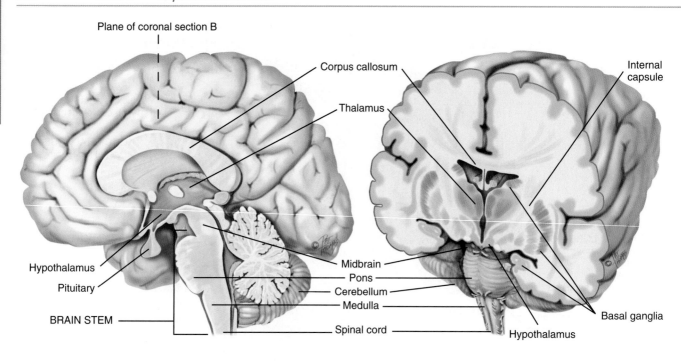

Plane of coronal section B

Corpus callosum

Thalamus

Internal capsule

Hypothalamus

Pituitary

BRAIN STEM

Midbrain

Pons

Cerebellum

Medulla

Spinal cord

Basal ganglia

Hypothalamus

A. Medial view of right hemisphere

B. Coronal section

COMPONENTS OF THE CENTRAL NERVOUS SYSTEM

25-2

© *Pat Thomas, 2006.*

but coordinates and smoothes it, such as the complex and quick coordination of many different muscles needed in playing the piano, swimming, or juggling. It is like the automatic pilot on an airplane in that it adjusts and corrects the voluntary movements but operates entirely below the conscious level.

Brain Stem

The brain stem is the central core of the brain consisting of mostly nerve fibres. It has three areas:

1. **Midbrain:** the most anterior part of the brain stem that still has the basic tubular structure of the spinal cord. It merges into the thalamus and hypothalamus. It contains many motor neurons and tracts.
2. **Pons:** the enlarged area containing ascending and descending fibre tracts.
3. **Medulla:** the continuation of the spinal cord in the brain that contains all ascending and descending fibre tracts connecting the brain and spinal cord. It has vital autonomic centres (respiratory, cardiac, gastrointestinal functions), as well as nuclei for cranial nerves VIII through XII. Pyramidal decussation (crossing of the motor fibres) occurs here (see p. 661).

Spinal Cord

The spinal cord is the long cylindrical structure of nervous tissue approximately as big around as the little finger. It occupies the upper two thirds of the vertebral canal from the medulla to lumbar vertebrae L1 and L2. It is the main pathway for ascending and descending fibre tracts that connect the brain to the spinal nerves, and it mediates reflexes. Its nerve

cell bodies, or grey matter, are arranged in a butterfly shape with anterior and posterior "horns."

Pathways of the Central Nervous System

Crossed representation is a notable feature of the nerve tracts; the *left* cerebral cortex receives sensory information from and controls motor function to the *right* side of the body, whereas the *right* cerebral cortex interacts with the *left* side of the body. Knowledge of where the fibres cross the midline helps you interpret clinical findings.

Sensory Pathways

Millions of sensory receptors are embroidered into the skin, mucous membranes, muscles, tendons, and viscera. They monitor conscious sensations, internal organ functions, body positions, and reflexes. Sensation travels in the afferent fibres in the peripheral nerve, then through the posterior (dorsal) root, and then into the spinal cord. In the spinal cord, it may take one of two routes: the spinothalamic tract or the posterior (dorsal) columns (Figure 25-3).

Spinothalamic Tract. The spinothalamic tract contains sensory fibres that transmit the sensations of pain, temperature, and crude or light touch (i.e., touch not precisely localized). The fibres enter the dorsal root of the spinal cord and synapse with a second sensory neuron. The second-order neuron fibres cross to the opposite side and ascend the spinothalamic tract to the thalamus. Fibres carrying pain and temperature sensations ascend the *lateral* spinothalamic tract, whereas those carrying sensations of crude touch form the *anterior* spinothalamic tract. At the thalamus, the fibres

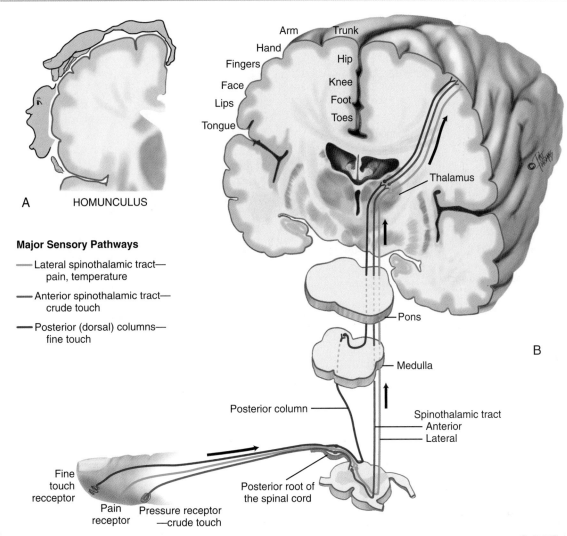

Major Sensory Pathways

—— Lateral spinothalamic tract—
pain, temperature

—— Anterior spinothalamic tract—
crude touch

—— Posterior (dorsal) columns—
fine touch

25-3 | Sensory pathways.

© *Pat Thomas, 2006.*

synapse with a third sensory neuron, which carries the message to the sensory cortex for full interpretation.

Posterior (Dorsal) Columns. These fibres conduct the sensations of position, vibration, and finely localized touch.

- **Position** (proprioception): the sense of where your body parts are in space and in relation to each other, without your looking
- **Vibration:** feeling vibrating objects
- **Finely localized touch** (stereognosis): the ability to identify familiar objects by touch, without looking

These fibres enter the dorsal root and proceed immediately up the same side of the spinal cord to the brain stem. At the medulla, they synapse with a second sensory neuron and then cross. They travel to the **thalamus,** synapse again, and proceed to the sensory cortex, which localizes the sensation and makes full discrimination.

The sensory cortex is arranged in a specific pattern forming a corresponding "map" of the body (see Figure 25-3, *A:* The *homunculus* [Latin for "little man"] is an illustration representing the proportion of the brain that is responsible for sensations in particular body parts). Pain in the right hand is perceived at its specific spot on the left cortex map. Some organs—such as the heart, liver, and spleen—are not

represented in the brain map. You know you have such organs, but you have no "felt image" of it. Pain originating in these organs is referred: that is, it is felt "by proxy" by another body part that does have a felt image. For example, pain in the heart is referred to the chest, shoulder, and left arm, which were its neighbours during fetal development. Pain originating in the spleen is felt on the top of the left shoulder.

Motor Pathways

Corticospinal or Pyramidal Tract. This area has been named *pyramidal* because it originates in pyramid-shaped cells in the motor cortex (Figure 25-4). Motor nerve fibres originate in the motor cortex and travel to the brain stem, where they cross to the opposite or contralateral side *(pyramidal decussation)* and then pass down in the lateral column of the spinal cord. At each cord level, they synapse with a lower motor neuron contained in the anterior horn of the spinal cord. Ten percent of corticospinal fibres do not cross, and these descend in the anterior column of the spinal cord. Corticospinal fibres mediate voluntary movement, particularly very skilled, discrete, purposeful movements, such as writing.

The corticospinal tract is a newer, "higher" motor system in humans that enables very skilled and purposeful

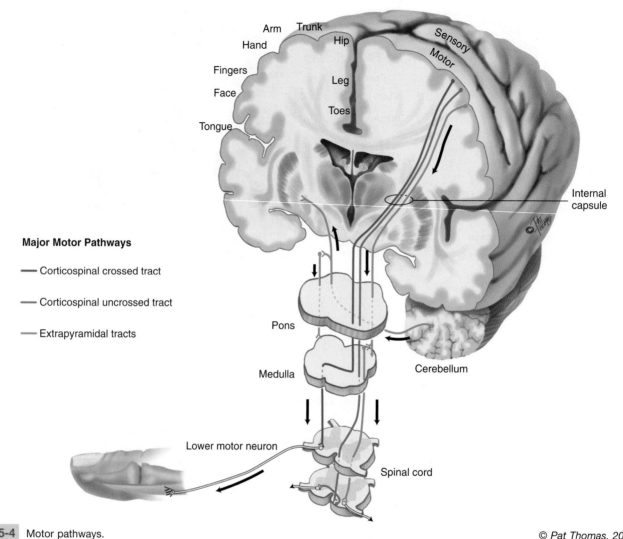

Major Motor Pathways

— Corticospinal crossed tract

— Corticospinal uncrossed tract

— Extrapyramidal tracts

25-4   Motor pathways.   © Pat Thomas, 2010.

movements. The origin of this tract in the motor cortex is arranged in a specific pattern called *somatotopic organization*. Another type of body map, a cortical *homunculus* (see Figure 25-3) shows the portion of the human brain directly responsible for the movement and exchange of sensory and motor information of the body; that is, body parts whose movements are relatively more important to humans (e.g., the hand) occupy proportionally more space on the brain map.

Extrapyramidal Tracts. The extrapyramidal tracts include all the motor nerve fibres originating in the motor cortex, basal ganglia, brain stem, and spinal cord that are *outside* the pyramidal tract. They constitute a phylogenetically older, more primitive motor system. These subcortical motor fibres maintain muscle tone and control body movements, especially gross automatic movements, such as walking.

Cerebellar System. This complex motor system coordinates movement, maintains equilibrium, and helps maintain posture. The cerebellum receives information about the position of muscles and joints—the body's equilibrium—and the kind of motor messages that are being sent from the cortex to the muscles. The information is integrated, and the cerebellum uses feedback pathways to exert its control back on the cortex or down to lower motor neurons in the spinal cord. This entire process occurs on a subconscious level.

Upper and Lower Motor Neurons

Upper motor neurons are a complex of all the descending motor fibres that can influence or modify the lower motor neurons. Upper motor neurons are located completely within the CNS. The neurons convey impulses from the motor areas of the cerebral cortex to the lower motor neurons in the anterior horn cells of the spinal cord (Figure 25-5).

Examples of upper motor neurons are corticospinal, corticobulbar, and extrapyramidal tracts. Examples of upper motor neuron diseases are cerebrovascular accident, cerebral palsy, and multiple sclerosis.

Lower motor neurons are located mostly in the peripheral nervous system. The cell body of the lower motor neuron is located in the anterior grey column of the spinal cord, but the nerve fibre extends from there to the muscle. The lower motor neuron is the "final common pathway" because it funnels many neural signals and it provides the final direct contact with the muscles. Any movement must be translated into action by lower motor neuron fibres. Examples of lower motor neurons are cranial nerves and spinal nerves of the peripheral nervous system. Examples of lower motor neuron diseases are spinal cord lesions, poliomyelitis, and amyotrophic lateral sclerosis.

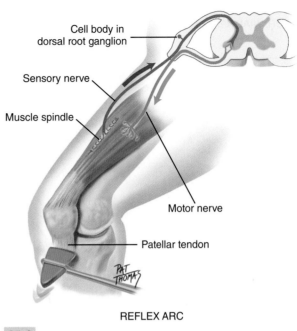

REFLEX ARC

25-6

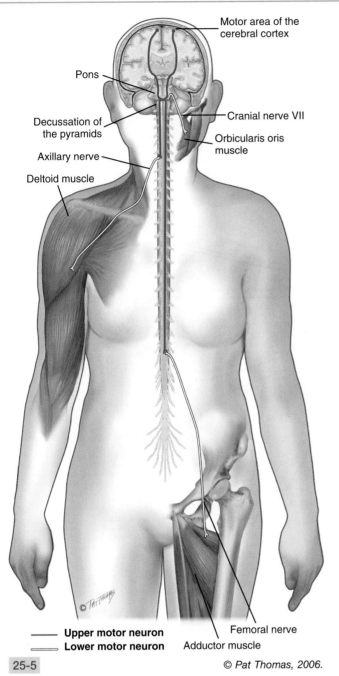

— Upper motor neuron
═ Lower motor neuron

25-5   © Pat Thomas, 2006.

THE PERIPHERAL NERVOUS SYSTEM

A **nerve** is a bundle of fibres *outside* the CNS. The peripheral nerves carry input to the CNS via their sensory afferent fibres and deliver output from the CNS via the efferent fibres.

Reflex Arc

Reflexes are basic defence mechanisms of the nervous system. They are involuntary, operating below the level of conscious control and enabling a quick reaction to potentially painful or damaging events. Reflexes also help the body maintain balance and appropriate muscle tone. There are four types of reflexes: (a) **deep tendon reflexes** (myotatic), such as patellar or knee jerk; (b) **superficial,** such as corneal reflex, abdominal reflex; (c) **visceral** (organic), such as pupillary response

to light and accommodation; and (d) **pathological** (abnormal), such as the Babinski (extensor plantar) reflex.

The fibres that mediate the reflex are carried by a specific spinal nerve. In the most simple reflex, tapping the tendon stretches the muscle spindles in the muscle, which activates the sensory afferent nerve. The sensory afferent fibres carry the message from the receptor and travel through the dorsal root into the spinal cord (Figure 25-6). They synapse directly in the cord with the motor neuron in the anterior horn. Motor efferent fibres leave via the ventral root and travel to the muscle, stimulating a sudden contraction.

The deep tendon (myotatic or stretch) reflex (DTR) has five components: (a) an intact sensory nerve (afferent); (b) a functional synapse in the cord; (c) an intact motor nerve fibre (efferent); (d) the neuromuscular junction; and (e) a competent muscle.

Cranial Nerves

Cranial nerves enter and exit the brain rather than the spinal cord (Figure 25-7). Cranial nerves I and II extend from the cerebrum; cranial nerves III to XII extend from the lower diencephalon and brain stem. The 12 pairs of cranial nerves supply primarily the head and neck, except the vagus nerve (from the Latin *vagus,* or wanderer, as in "vagabond"), which travels to the heart, respiratory muscles, stomach, and gallbladder.

Spinal Nerves

The 31 pairs of **spinal nerves** arise from the length of the spinal cord and supply the rest of the body. They are named for the region of the spine from which they exit: 8 cervical, 12 thoracic, 5 lumbar, 5 sacral, and 1 coccygeal. They are "mixed" nerves because they contain both sensory and motor fibres. The nerves enter and exit the spinal cord

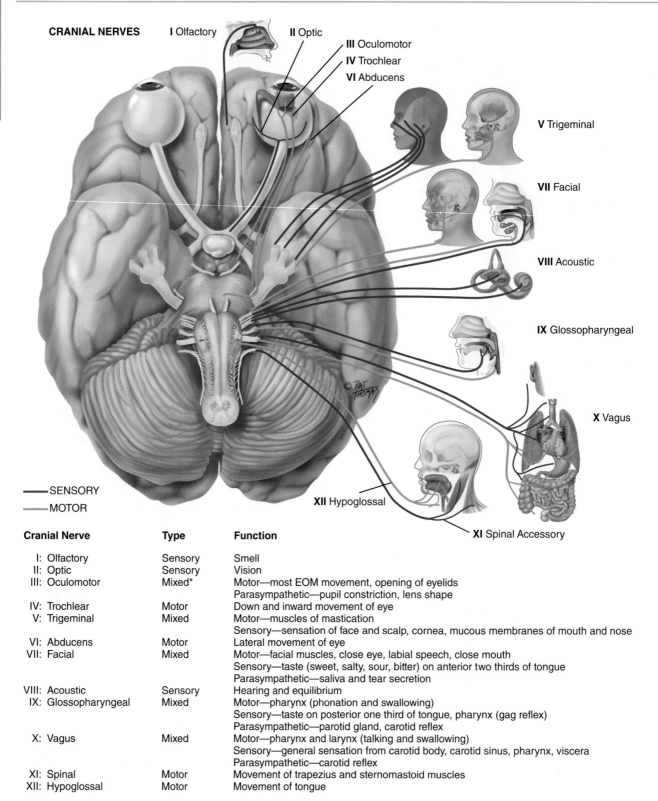

CRANIAL NERVES   I Olfactory   II Optic
III Oculomotor
IV Trochlear
VI Abducens
V Trigeminal
VII Facial
VIII Acoustic
IX Glossopharyngeal
X Vagus
XII Hypoglossal
XI Spinal Accessory

—— SENSORY
—— MOTOR

Cranial Nerve	Type	Function
I: Olfactory	Sensory	Smell
II: Optic	Sensory	Vision
III: Oculomotor	Mixed*	Motor—most EOM movement, opening of eyelids
		Parasympathetic—pupil constriction, lens shape
IV: Trochlear	Motor	Down and inward movement of eye
V: Trigeminal	Mixed	Motor—muscles of mastication
		Sensory—sensation of face and scalp, cornea, mucous membranes of mouth and nose
VI: Abducens	Motor	Lateral movement of eye
VII: Facial	Mixed	Motor—facial muscles, close eye, labial speech, close mouth
		Sensory—taste (sweet, salty, sour, bitter) on anterior two thirds of tongue
		Parasympathetic—saliva and tear secretion
VIII: Acoustic	Sensory	Hearing and equilibrium
IX: Glossopharyngeal	Mixed	Motor—pharynx (phonation and swallowing)
		Sensory—taste on posterior one third of tongue, pharynx (gag reflex)
		Parasympathetic—parotid gland, carotid reflex
X: Vagus	Mixed	Motor—pharynx and larynx (talking and swallowing)
		Sensory—general sensation from carotid body, carotid sinus, pharynx, viscera
		Parasympathetic—carotid reflex
XI: Spinal	Motor	Movement of trapezius and sternomastoid muscles
XII: Hypoglossal	Motor	Movement of tongue

*Mixed refers to a nerve carrying a combination of fibres: motor + sensory; motor + parasympathetic; or motor + sensory + parasympathetic.

25-7

© Pat Thomas, 2006.

through roots: sensory afferent fibres through the posterior (dorsal) roots, and motor efferent fibres through the anterior (ventral) roots.

The nerves exit the spinal cord in an orderly ladder shape. Each nerve innervates a particular segment of the body.

Dermal segmentation is the cutaneous distribution of the various spinal nerves.

A **dermatome** is a circumscribed skin area that is supplied mainly from one spinal cord segment through a particular spinal nerve (Figure 25-8). The dermatomes overlap, which

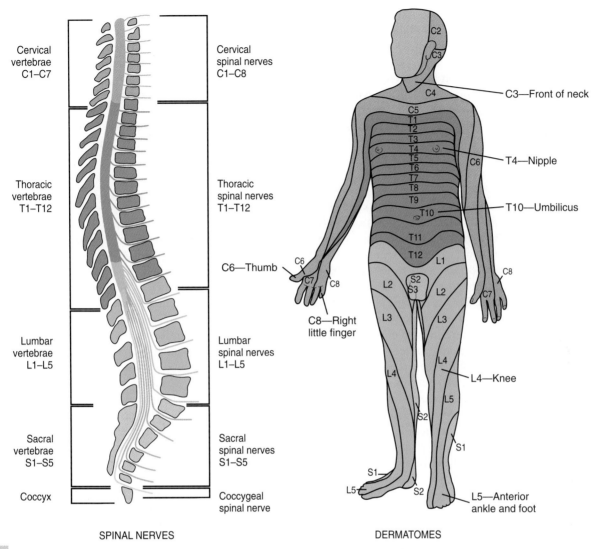

Cervical
vertebrae
C1–C7

Thoracic
vertebrae
T1–T12

Lumbar
vertebrae
L1–L5

Sacral
vertebrae
S1–S5

Coccyx

Cervical
spinal nerves
C1–C8

Thoracic
spinal nerves
T1–T12

C6—Thumb

C8—Right
little finger

Lumbar
spinal nerves
L1–L5

Sacral
spinal nerves
S1–S5

Coccygeal
spinal nerve

SPINAL NERVES

C2
C3
C4
C3—Front of neck
C5
T1
T2
T3
T4
T5
T6
T7
T8
T9
T10
T11
T12
C6
T4—Nipple
T10—Umbilicus
L1
C6
C7   C8
C8
C7
L2
S2
S3
L2
C8
L3
L3
L4
L4—Knee
L4
L5
S2
S1
S1
S2
L5
L5—Anterior
ankle and foot

DERMATOMES

25-8

is a form of biological insurance; that is, if one nerve is severed, most of the sensations will continue to be transmitted by the nerve above and the nerve below. Do not attempt to memorize all dermatome segments; focus on just the following as useful landmarks:

- The thumb, middle finger, and fifth finger are each in the dermatomes of C6, C7, and C8.
- The axilla is at the level of T1.
- The nipple is at the level of T4.
- The umbilicus is at the level of T10.
- The groin is in the region of L1.
- The knee is at the level of L4.

Peripheral Nervous System

The peripheral nervous system is composed of cranial nerves and spinal nerves. These nerves carry fibres that can be divided functionally into two parts: somatic and autonomic. The somatic fibres innervate the skeletal (voluntary) muscles; the autonomic fibres innervate smooth (involuntary) muscles, cardiac muscle, and glands. The autonomic system mediates unconscious activity. A detailed description of the autonomic system is beyond the scope of this book; its overall function is to maintain homeostasis of the body.

✦ DEVELOPMENTAL CONSIDERATIONS

Infants

The neurological system is not completely developed at birth. Motor activity in newborns is under the control of the spinal cord and medulla. Very little cortical control exists, and the neurons are not yet myelinated. Movements are directed primarily by primitive reflexes. As the cerebral cortex develops during the first year, it inhibits these reflexes, and they disappear at predictable times. Persistence of the primitive reflexes is an indication of CNS dysfunction.

Infants' sensory and motor development proceeds along with the gradual acquisition of myelin because myelin is needed to conduct most impulses. The process of myelinization follows a cephalocaudal order and a proximal-to-distal order (head, neck, trunk, and extremities). This is the order observed in infants as they gain motor control (lifting head, lifting head and shoulders, rolling over, moving whole arm, using hands, walking). As the milestones are achieved, each movement is more complex and coordinated. Milestones occur in an orderly sequence, although the exact age at occurrence may vary.

Sensation is also rudimentary at birth. Newborns need a strong stimulus and then respond by crying and with whole body movements. As myelinization develops, infants are able to localize the stimulus more precisely and to make a more accurate motor response.

Older Adults

The aging process causes a general atrophy with a steady loss of neurons in the brain and spinal cord. This causes a decrease in weight and volume with a thinning of the cerebral cortex, reduced subcortical brain structures, and expansion of the ventricles (Fjell, Walhovd, & Fennema-Notestine, 2009). Neuron loss leads many people over 65 to show signs that would be considered abnormal in the younger adult, such as general loss of muscle bulk; loss of muscle tone in the face, in the neck, and around the spine; decreased muscle strength; impaired fine coordination and agility; loss of vibratory sense at the ankle; decreased or absent Achilles reflex; loss of position sense at the big toe; and pupillary miosis, irregular pupil shape, and decreased pupillary reflexes.

The velocity of nerve conduction decreases between 5% and 10% with aging, which slows the reaction time in some older adults. An increased delay at the synapse also occurs, so that the impulse takes longer to travel. As a result, touch and pain sensation, taste, and smell may be diminished.

The motor system may show a general slowing down of movement. Muscle strength and agility decrease. A generalized decrease occurs in muscle bulk, which is most apparent in the dorsal hand muscles. Muscle tremors may occur in the hands, head, and jaw, along with possible repetitive facial grimacing (dyskinesias).

Aging involves a progressive decrease in cerebral blood flow and oxygen consumption. In some people, this causes dizziness and a loss of balance with position change. Older adults need to get up slowly; otherwise, they are at increased risk for falls and resulting injuries. In addition, older adults may forget that they fell, which makes it hard to diagnose the cause of an injury.

When they are in good health, older people walk about as well as they did during their middle and younger years, except more slowly and more deliberately. Some survey the ground for obstacles or uneven terrain. Some show hesitation and take a slightly wayward path.

CULTURAL AND SOCIAL CONSIDERATIONS

According to the Heart and Stroke Foundation of Canada (2012a), research has shown that in comparison with the general population, people of Aboriginal, African, or South Asian descent are more likely to have high blood pressure and diabetes and are at greater risk for heart disease and stroke. Reasons for this are complex and may relate to intersecting factors such as low socioeconomic status, poor access to health care and preventive services, and lack of opportunities for exercise. The foundation has translated and culturally adapted some health education resources into Ojibwe, Ojicree, Punjabi, Hindi, Mandarin, and Cantonese, among other languages, to help patients who speak those languages learn the risk factors and warning signs for heart disease and stroke.

People's social circumstances influence their ability to manage after a stroke. Social resources have been found to have a buffering effect in survivors, serving to reduce the adverse effects of physical disability on subjective well-being after stroke (Clarke, Marshall, Black, & Colantonio, 2002). Stroke survivors with higher levels of education report a greater sense of personal growth, purpose in life, and environmental mastery than do survivors with fewer years of education. In comparison with men, women who have had a stroke are more likely to live alone and less likely to have social supports (Heart and Stroke Foundation of Canada, 2012c). (See the box Promoting Health: Stroke Prevention.)

PROMOTING HEALTH: STROKE PREVENTION

Stroke is the third leading cause of death in Canada; 6% of all deaths in Canada are caused by stroke, and more women than men die of stroke (Heart and Stroke Foundation of Canada, 2012b). Almost 50,000 new cases of stroke occur in Canada each year, and the associated short-term mortality is approximately 20% to 25% (Côté et al., 2007). The prevalence of stroke increases with age and other risk factors, such as hypertension, smoking, and associated cardiac conditions such as atrial fibrillation. A stroke, or cerebrovascular accident, occurs when the blood flow is interrupted to a part of the brain, which is why it is often referred to as a "brain attack." The most common type is an ischemic stroke, in which a blood clot blocks a blood vessel in the brain. Less common is a hemorrhagic stroke, which occurs when a blood vessel in the brain ruptures and causes bleeding. The symptoms and aftereffects of a stroke depend on which area of the brain is affected and to what

extent. This can make a stroke difficult to diagnose. However, early recognition of symptoms and prompt treatment are essential so that appropriate treatments and interventions can be initiated as soon as possible. Only approximately 5% of patients with stroke receive appropriate therapy in a timely manner (Bergman, 2011).

Time from symptom onset is the most important piece of information in the initial assessment (Bergman, 2011, p. 660). Early assessment is particularly important because symptoms of stroke or transient ischemic attacks (TIAs) may be similar to those of other conditions, such as hypoglycemia, migraine, seizure, trauma, or medication overdose. The *most common* symptoms of stroke are as follows:

1. Sudden weakness or numbness in the face, arms, or legs, especially when it is on one side of the body

PROMOTING HEALTH: STROKE PREVENTION—cont'd

2. Sudden confusion, trouble speaking, or understanding speech
3. Sudden changes in vision, such as blurry vision or partial or complete loss of vision in one or both eyes
4. Sudden trouble walking, dizziness, or loss of balance or coordination
5. Sudden severe headache with no reason or explanation

Less common symptoms of stroke are as follows:

1. Sudden nausea or vomiting
2. Brief loss of consciousness, including fainting

Many Canadians continue to ignore, or fail to recognize, the symptoms of stroke. Stroke symptoms usually do not hurt, which is why many people ignore them or delay seeking medical attention. A "mini-stroke," or TIA, can also occur. In these cases, the stroke symptoms are only temporary and then disappear, often within an hour. Because the symptoms "go away," people too often do not report them or seek medical attention. However, a TIA is a warning sign that should not be ignored. The risk for an ischemic stroke is approximately 10% to 20% in the first year after an initial stroke or after a TIA (Côté et al., 2007). When people experience chest pain, they usually know to seek medical attention to rule out a heart attack. Having a TIA should also prompt people to seek medical attention to rule out the possibility of a future "brain attack." One significant reason for delay is that patients consult with their physician or relatives at the onset of symptoms (Bergman, 2011, p. 664). Patients must be instructed to call an ambulance for immediate transportation to a hospital instead.

Stroke can strike anyone without any warning. Preventing a stroke is still the best medicine. People need to be aware of their stroke risk and take steps to change the risk factors that they can control.

Most risk factors for stroke, such as high blood pressure, diabetes, smoking, inactivity, and high cholesterol are equivalent for men and women and are potentially modifiable, depending on personal and social contexts. Gender, however, is an important risk factor. In Canada, the risk for stroke is higher for men than for women, but the mortality rate is 45% higher for women at all ages (Heart and Stroke Foundation of Canada, 2012c), and the gap is widening. In part, this is because women live longer on average than do men, but new research suggests that there may exist some risk factors that are uniquely important for women. For example, women who have migraines with visual disturbances, such as flashing dots or blind spots, can be up to 10 times more likely to have a stroke than those without visual disturbances; women who develop preeclampsia in pregnancy may have a 60% greater risk of non–pregnancy-related ischemic stroke; and women who smoke and who are taking oral contraceptives or have high blood pressure, migraines, or blood clotting disorders have an increased risk of stroke.

The following modifiable risk factors for stroke have been well documented:

1. History of cardiovascular disease
   a. Coronary heart disease
   b. Cardiac failure
   c. Symptomatic peripheral artery disease (PAD)
2. Hypertension
3. Cigarette smoking or exposure to second-hand smoke
4. Diabetes
5. Atrial fibrillation
6. Other cardiac conditions
   a. Dilated cardiomyopathy
   b. Valvular heart disease (e.g., mitral valve prolapse, endocarditis, and prosthetic cardiac valves)
   c. Intracardiac congenital defects (e.g., patent foramen ovale, atrial septal defect, and atrial septal aneurysm)
7. Dyslipidemia
8. Asymptomatic carotid stenosis
9. Sickle cell disease
10. Postmenopausal hormone therapy
11. Diet and nutrition
12. Physical inactivity
13. Obesity and fat distribution
14. History of TIA

Nonmodifiable risk factors for stroke may still help identify people who, in conjunction with well-documented modifiable risks, are at highest risk for stroke and who may benefit from more rigorous treatment of modifiable risk factors.

Nonmodifiable risk factors for stroke include the following:

1. Age
2. Gender: Strokes are generally more prevalent in men than in women. However, the mortality rate for women is higher.
3. Low birth weight
4. Ethnocultural background: Aboriginal people and people of African or South Asian descent are more likely to have high blood pressure and diabetes and are therefore at greater risk for heart disease and stroke than is the general population.
5. Genetic factors, genetic disorders, such as Marfan's syndrome, Fabry's disease, and cerebral autosomal dominant arteriopathy with subcortical infarcts and leukoencephalopathy (CADASIL)

The *Canadian Best Practice Recommendations for Stroke Care (Update 2010)* (Lindsay et al., 2010) recommend that patients at risk for stroke and who have had a stroke focus on the following areas for prevention: eating a healthy balanced diet; adhering to the recommended daily limit of sodium intake, known as the Adequate Intake; moderate exercise; maintaining a healthy weight; smoking cessation or reduction; limiting alcohol intake; and managing underlying medical conditions, including hypertension, dyslipidemia, previous stroke or transient ischemic attack, atrial fibrillation and stroke, and carotid stenosis.

Resources

American Stroke Association. (2012). About stroke. *Retrieved from* http://www.strokeassociation.org/STROKEORG/.

Heart and Stroke Foundation of Canada. (2012b). Stroke. *Retrieved from* http://www.heartandstroke.com/site/c. iklQLcMWJtE/b.3483933/.

Lindsay, M. P., Gubitz, G., Bayley, M., Hill, M. D., Davies-Schinkel, C., Singh, S., & Phillips, S. (2010). Canadian Best Practice Recommendations for Stroke Care (Update 2010). *On behalf of the Canadian Stroke Strategy Best Practices and Standards Writing Group. 2010; Ottawa, Ontario Canada: Canadian Stroke Network. Retrieved from* http://www.strokebestpractices.ca/wp-content/uploads/2011/04/2010BPR_ENG.pdf.

Recommendations Will Prevent Stroke Patients From Falling Through Cracks. *Retrieved from* http://www.strokebestprac tices.ca/wp-content/uploads/2011/04/2010BPR_ENG.pdf.

SUBJECTIVE DATA

1. Headache	7. Incoordination
2. Head injury	8. Numbness or tingling sensation
3. Dizziness or vertigo	9. Difficulty swallowing
4. Seizures	10. Difficulty speaking
5. Tremors	11. Significant past history
6. Weakness	12. Environmental and occupational hazards

HEALTH HISTORY QUESTIONS

Examiner Asks	Rationale
1. Headache. Do you have any unusually frequent or severe headaches? • When did this start? How often does it occur? • Where in your head do you feel the headaches? Do the headaches seem to be associated with anything? (Headache history is fully discussed in Chapter 14.) **2. Head injury.** Have you ever had any **head injury?** Please describe. • What part of your head was hit? • Did you experience loss of consciousness? For how long? • Do you use a helmet consistently to prevent head injuries (e.g., helmet use with sports such as biking, skating, skiing, snowboarding)? **3. Dizziness/vertigo.** Do you ever feel lightheaded, a swimming sensation, like feeling faint? • When have you noticed this? How often does it occur? Does it occur with activity, change in position? • Do you ever feel a rotational spinning sensation? (Note: Distinguish vertigo from dizziness.) Do you feel as if the room spins (objective vertigo)? Or do you feel that you are spinning (subjective vertigo)? Did this come on suddenly or gradually? **4. Seizures.** Have you ever had any seizures? When did they start? How often do they occur? • Course and duration: When a seizure starts, do you have any warning sign? What type of sign? • Motor activity: Where in your body do the seizures begin? Do the seizures travel through your body? On one side or both? Does your muscle tone seem tense or limp? • Any associated signs, such as colour change in face or lips, loss of consciousness (for how long), automatisms (eyelid-fluttering, eye-rolling, lip smacking), incontinence? • Postictal phase: After the seizure, are you told that you spend time sleeping, or do you have any confusion, weakness, headache, or muscle ache? • Precipitating factors: Does anything seem to bring on the seizures: activity, discontinuing medication, fatigue, stress? • Are you taking any medication? • Coping strategies: How have the seizures affected daily life, your occupation?	**Syncope** is a sudden loss of strength and a temporary loss of consciousness (fainting), caused by lack of cerebral blood flow, as occurs with low blood pressure. True **vertigo** is the sensation of rotational spinning, caused by neurological disease in the vestibular apparatus in the ear or in the vestibular nuclei in the brain stem. **Seizures** occur with epilepsy, a paroxysmal disease characterized by altered or loss of consciousness, involuntary muscle movements, and sensory disturbances. *Aura* is a subjective sensation that precedes a seizure; it could be auditory, visual, or motor.

Examiner Asks	Rationale
5. **Tremors.** Do you have any shakes or tremors in the hands or face? When did these start? • Do they seem to grow worse with anxiety, intention (purposeful movement), or rest? • Are they relieved with rest, activity, alcohol? Do they affect daily activities?	Tremor is an involuntary shaking, vibrating, or trembling.
6. **Weakness.** Do you have any **weakness** in, or problem moving, any body part? Is this generalized or local? Does weakness occur with any particular movement, such as difficulty getting up out of a chair or reaching for an object (proximal or large muscle weakness) or difficulty opening a jar, writing, using scissors, or walking without tripping (with distal or small muscle weakness)?	*Paresis* refers to weakness of voluntary movements or impaired movement. *Paralysis* is a loss of motor function as a result of a lesion in the neurological or muscular system or loss of sensory innervation.
7. **Incoordination.** Do you have any problem with **coordination?** Any problem with balance when walking? Do you list to one side? Any falling? Which way? Do your legs seem to give way? Any clumsy movement?	*Dysmetria* is the inability to control range of motion of muscles.
8. **Numbness or tingling.** Do you have any **numbness** or **tingling** sensation in any body part? Does it feel like pins and needles? When did this start? Where do you feel it? Does it occur with activity?	*Paraesthesia* is an abnormal sensation, such as burning, tingling.
9. **Difficulty swallowing.** Do you have any problem **swallowing?** Does it occur with solids or liquids? Have you experienced excessive salivation, drooling?	Dysphagia refers to difficulty swallowing.
10. **Difficulty speaking.** Do you have any problem **speaking:** with forming words or with saying what you intended to say? When did you first notice this? How long did it last?	*Dysarthria* is difficulty forming words; *dysphasia* is difficulty with language comprehension or expression (see Table 25-12).
11. **Significant past history.** Have you ever had a stroke (cerebrovascular accident), spinal cord injury, meningitis or encephalitis, congenital defect, or alcoholism?	
12. **Environmental and occupational hazards.** Are you exposed to any environmental or occupational hazards: insecticides, organic solvents, lead? • Are you taking any medications now? • How much alcohol do you drink? Each week? Each day? • Do you take other mood-altering drugs, such as marijuana, cocaine, barbiturates, tranquilizers?	Review the patient's anticonvulsant, antitremor, antivertigo, and pain medications.

Additional History for Infants and Children

1. **Maternal health.** Did you (the mother) have any health problems during the pregnancy: any infections or illnesses, medications taken, toxemia, hypertension, alcohol or drug use, diabetes?	Prenatal history may affect an infant's neurological development.
2. **Neonatal period.** Please tell me about this baby's birth. Was the baby full term or premature? What was the birth weight? • Any birth trauma? Did the baby breathe immediately? • Were you told the baby's Apgar scores? • Any congenital defects?	
3. **Reflexes.** What have you noticed about the baby's behaviour? Do the baby's sucking and swallowing seem coordinated? When you touch the cheek, does the baby turn his or her head toward the touch? Is the baby startled by a loud noise or shake of the crib? Does the baby grasp your finger?	
4. **Weakness and balance.** Does the child seem to have any problem with balance? Have you noted any unexplained falling, clumsy or unsteady gait, progressive muscular weakness, problem with going up or down stairs, problem with getting up from lying position?	If any of these signs occurs, it may not be noticed until child starts to walk (in late infancy). Screen for muscular dystrophy.
5. **Seizures.** Has this child had any seizures? Please describe. Did the seizure occur with a high fever? Did any loss of consciousness occur? For how long? How many seizures occurred with this same illness (if occurred with high fever)?	In infants and toddlers, seizures may occur with high fever. Seizures may also be a sign of neurological disease.

Subjective Data

Examiner Asks	Rationale

6. **Physical development.** Did this child's motor or developmental milestones seem to occur at approximately the right age? Does this child seem to be growing and maturing normally to you? How does this child's development compare with that of siblings or other children the same age?

7. **Environmental hazards.** Do you know whether your child has had any environmental exposure to lead?

Chronically elevated lead levels may cause developmental delay or loss of a newly acquired skill, or no clinical signs may be present.

8. **Cognitive development.** Have you been told about any learning problems in school: whether the child has problems with attention span, cannot concentrate, is hyperactive?

9. **Family history.** Any family history of seizure disorder, cerebral palsy, muscular dystrophy?

Additional History for Older Adults

1. **Risk for falls.** Any problem with dizziness? Does this occur when you first sit or stand up, when you move your head, when you get up and walk just after eating? Does this occur with any of your medications?

Diminished cerebral blood flow and diminished vestibular response may produce staggering with position change, which increases risk of falls.

Micturition syncope

- (For men) Do you ever get up at night and then feel faint while standing to urinate?
- How does dizziness affect your daily activities? Are you able to drive safely and to manoeuvre within your house safely?
- What safety modifications have you applied at home?

2. **Cognitive function.** Have you noticed any decrease in memory, changes in mental function? Have you felt any confusion? Did this seem to come on suddenly or gradually?

3. **Tremor.** Have you ever noticed any tremor? Is this in your hands or face? Is this worse with anxiety, activity, rest? Does the tremor seem to be relieved with alcohol, activity, rest? Does the tremor interfere with daily or social activities?

Senile tremor is relieved by alcohol, although this is not a recommended treatment. Assess whether the patient is abusing alcohol in an effort to relieve tremor.

4. **Vision.** Have you ever had any sudden vision change, fleeting blindness? Did this occur along with weakness? Did you have any loss of consciousness?

Screen for symptoms of stroke. (See the box Critical Findings.)

CRITICAL FINDINGS

Critical findings that necessitate immediate medical intervention or immediate transport to a hospital include the following signs and symptoms:

- Sudden decline in alertness (loss of consciousness)
- Sudden change in speech or a new onset of speech difficulties
- Signs of stroke or transient ischemic attack (TIA)
- Sudden onset of severe headache
- Signs of raised intracranial pressure
- Sudden onset of weakness, numbness, eye movement problems, and double vision
- Seizures
- Lethargy that persists beyond appropriate times and circumstances

These signs and symptoms are described in Tables 25-2 to 25-12.

OBJECTIVE DATA

PREPARATION

Perform a **screening neurological examination** (items identified in the following sections) of seemingly healthy patients whose histories reveal no significant subjective findings.

Perform a **complete neurological examination** of patients who have neurological concerns (e.g., headache, weakness, loss of coordination) or who have shown signs of neurological dysfunction.

Perform a **neurological recheck examination** of patients with demonstrated neurological deficits who require periodic assessments (e.g., hospitalized patients or those in extended care), using the examination sequence beginning on p. 696.

Integrate the steps of the neurological examination with the examination of each particular part of the body, as much as you are able: For example, test cranial nerves while you assess the head and neck (recall Chapters 14 through 17) and superficial abdominal reflexes while you assess the abdomen (Chapter 22). When you record your findings, however, consider all neurological data as a functional unit, and record them all together.

Use the following sequence for the complete neurological examination:

1. Mental health (see Chapter 6)
2. Cranial nerves
3. Motor system
4. Sensory system
5. Reflexes

Ask the patient to sit up with the head at your eye level.

EQUIPMENT NEEDED

Penlight
Tongue blade
Cotton swab
Cotton ball
Tuning fork (128 Hz or 256 Hz)
Percussion hammer
(Possibly) familiar aromatic substances, such as peppermint, coffee, vanilla

Normal Range of Findings	Abnormal Findings

TEST CRANIAL NERVES

Cranial Nerve I: Olfactory Nerve

Do not test routinely. Test the sense of smell in patients who report loss of smell, those with head trauma, and those with abnormal mental status and when the presence of an intracranial lesion is suspected. First, assess patency by occluding one nostril at a time and asking the patient to sniff. Then, with the patient's eyes closed, occlude one nostril and present an aromatic substance. Use familiar, conveniently obtainable, and nonnoxious smells, such as coffee, toothpaste, orange, vanilla, soap, or peppermint. Alcohol wipes smell familiar and are easy to find but are irritating.

Anosmia (decrease or loss of smell) occurs bilaterally with tobacco smoking, allergic rhinitis, and cocaine use.

Normally, a person can identify an odour through each side of the nose. The sense of smell normally decreases bilaterally with aging. Any asymmetry in the sense of smell is important.

Unilateral loss of smell in the absence of nasal disease is *neurogenic anosmia* (see Table 25-2 on p. 703).

> Smell cannot be tested when air passages are occluded, as in upper respiratory infection or sinusitis.

Cranial Nerve II: Optic Nerve

Test visual acuity, and test visual fields by confrontation (see Chapter 15).

Using the ophthalmoscope, examine the ocular fundus to determine the colour, size, and shape of the optic disc (see Chapter 15).

> Visual field loss (see Table 15-5, p. 334).
>
> Papilledema with increased intracranial pressure; optic atrophy (see Table 15-9, p. 337).

Objective Data

Normal Range of Findings	Abnormal Findings

Cranial Nerves III, IV, and VI: Oculomotor, Trochlear, and Abducens Nerves

Palpebral fissures are usually equal, or nearly so, in width.

Check pupils for size, regularity, equality, direct and consensual light reactions, and accommodation (see Chapter 15).

Assess extraocular movements with the cardinal positions of gaze (see Chapter 15).

Nystagmus is a back-and-forth oscillation of the eyes. Endpoint nystagmus—a few beats of horizontal nystagmus at extreme lateral gaze—is normal.

Assess any other nystagmus carefully, noting the following:

- Presence of nystagmus: Document whether it is in one or both eyes.
- *Pendular* movement (oscillations move equally left to right) or *jerk* (a quick phase in one direction, then a slow phase in the other): Classify the jerk nystagmus in the direction of the quick phase.
- Amplitude: Judge whether the degree of movement is fine, medium, or coarse.
- Frequency: Note whether the nystagmus is constant or whether it fades after a few beats.
- Plane of movement: Note whether the nystagmus is horizontal, vertical, rotary, or a combination.

Cranial Nerve V: Trigeminal Nerve

Motor Function. Assess the muscles of mastication by palpating the temporal and masseter muscles as the patient clenches the teeth (Figure 25-9). Muscles should feel equally strong on both sides. Next, try to separate the jaws by pushing down on the chin; normally, you cannot.

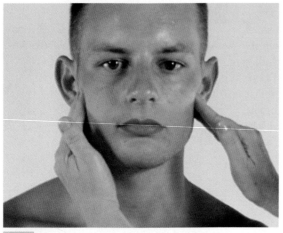

25-9

Sensory Function. With the patient's eyes closed, test light touch sensation by brushing a cotton wisp on designated areas of the patient's face: forehead, cheeks, and chin (Figure 25-10). Ask the patient to say "Now" whenever the touch is felt. This tests all three divisions of the nerve: (a) ophthalmic, (b) maxillary, and (c) mandibular.

Abnormal Findings (column):

Ptosis (drooping) occurs with myasthenia gravis, dysfunction of cranial nerve III, or Horner's syndrome (see Table 15-2, p. 330).

Increasing intracranial pressure causes sudden, unilateral dilation and nonreactivity of a pupil.

Strabismus (deviated gaze) or limited movement (see Table 15-1, p. 328).

Nystagmus occurs with disease of the vestibular system, cerebellum, or brain stem.

Decreased strength on one or both sides.

Asymmetry in jaw movement.

Pain with clenching of teeth.

Decreased or unequal sensation.

Normal Range of Findings	Abnormal Findings

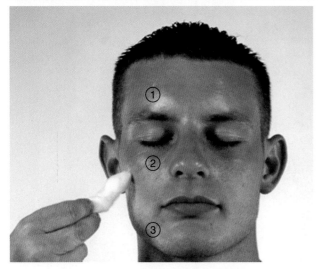

25-10

Corneal Reflex. (Omit this test, unless the patient has abnormal facial sensation or abnormalities of facial movement.) Ask the patient to remove any contact lenses. With the patient looking forward, bring a wisp of cotton in from the side (to minimize defensive blinking) and lightly touch the cornea, not the conjunctiva (Figure 25-11). Normally, a person will blink bilaterally. The corneal reflex may be decreased or absent in people who have worn contact lenses. This procedure tests the sensory afferent fibres in cranial nerve V and the motor efferent fibres in cranial nerve VII (muscles that close the eye).

No blink occurs with a lesion of cranial nerve V or with cranial nerve VII paralysis.

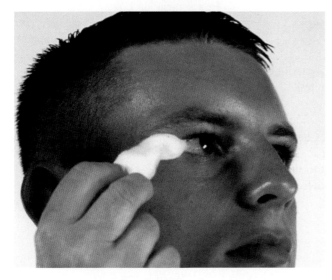

25-11

Cranial Nerve VII: Facial Nerve

Motor Function. Note mobility and facial symmetry as the patient responds to your requests to smile (Figure 25-12), frown, close eyes tightly (against your attempt to open them), lift eyebrows, show teeth, and puff cheeks (Figure 25-13). Then, press the patient's puffed cheeks in, and note whether the air escapes equally from both sides.

Sensory Function. Do not test routinely. Test only when you suspect facial nerve injury. When it is indicated, test sense of taste by applying to the tongue a cotton applicator soaked in a solution of sugar, salt, or lemon juice (sour). Ask the patient to identify the taste.

Muscle weakness is demonstrated by flattening of the nasolabial fold, drooping of one side of the face, lower eyelid sagging, and escape of air from only one cheek that is pressed in.

Loss of movement and asymmetry of movement occur both with CNS lesions (e.g., cerebrovascular accident that affects the lower face on one side) and with lesions of the peripheral nervous system (e.g., cases of Bell's palsy that affect the upper *and* lower portions of one side of the face).

Normal Range of Findings | **Abnormal Findings**

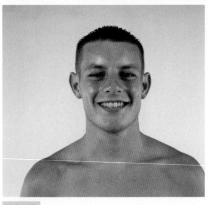

25-12

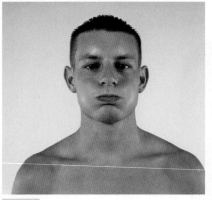

25-13

Cranial Nerve VIII: Acoustic (Vestibulocochlear) Nerve

Test hearing acuity by determining the patient's ability to hear normal conversation, by the whispered voice test (see Chapter 16).

Cranial Nerves IX and X: Glossopharyngeal and Vagus Nerves

Motor Function. Depress the tongue with a tongue blade, and note pharyngeal movement as the patient says "ahhh" or yawns; the uvula and soft palate should rise in the midline, and the tonsillar pillars should move medially.

Absence or asymmetry of soft palate movement.
Deviation of uvula to side.
Asymmetry of tonsillar pillar movement.

Touch the posterior pharyngeal wall with a tongue blade, and note the gag reflex. Also note that the voice sounds smooth and not strained.

Hoarseness or brassy quality of the voice occurs with vocal cord dysfunction; nasal twang occurs with weakness of soft palate.

Sensory Function. Cranial nerve IX does mediate taste on the posterior one third of the tongue, but technically this sensation is too difficult to test.

Cranial Nerve XI: Spinal Accessory Nerve

Examine the sternomastoid and trapezius muscles for equal size. Check equal strength by asking the patient to rotate the head forcibly against resistance applied to the side of the chin (Figure 25-14). Then ask the patient to shrug the shoulders against resistance (Figure 25-15). These movements should feel equally strong on both sides.

Atrophy.
Muscle weakness or paralysis.

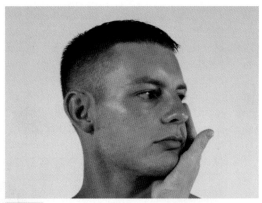

25-14

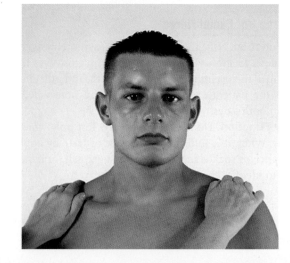

25-15

Normal Range of Findings	Abnormal Findings

Cranial Nerve XII: Hypoglossal Nerve

Inspect the tongue. No wasting or tremors should be present. Note the forward thrust in the midline as the patient sticks out the tongue. Also ask the patient to say "light, tight, dynamite," and note that lingual speech (sounds of letters *l, t, d, n*) is clear and distinct.

Atrophy; fasciculations.

Tongue deviates to side with lesions of the hypoglossal nerve. (When this occurs, deviation is toward the paralyzed side.)

INSPECT AND PALPATE THE MOTOR SYSTEM

Muscles

Size. As you proceed through the examination, inspect all muscle groups for size. Compare the right side with the left. Muscle groups should be within the normal size limits for age and should be symmetric bilaterally. When muscles in the extremities look asymmetrical, measure each in centimetres, and record the difference. A difference of 1 cm or less is not significant. Note that it is difficult to assess muscle mass in very obese patients.

Strength. (See Chapter 24.) Test the power of homologous muscles simultaneously. Test muscle groups of the extremities, neck, and trunk.

Atrophy: abnormally small muscle with a wasted appearance; occurs with disuse, injury, lower motor neuron disease such as polio, diabetic neuropathy.

Hypertrophy: increased size and strength; occurs with isometric exercise.

Paresis (weakness) is diminished strength; paralysis (plegia) is absence of strength.

Limited range of motion.

Pain with motion.

Tone. Tone is the normal degree of tension (contraction) in voluntarily relaxed muscles. It is demonstrated as mild resistance to passive stretch. To test muscle tone, move the extremities through a passive range of motion. First, persuade the patient to relax completely, to "go limp like a rag doll." Move each extremity smoothly through a full range of motion. Support the arm at the elbow and the leg at the knee (Figure 25-16). Normally, you will note a mild, even resistance to movement.

Flaccidity: decreased resistance, hypotonicity.

Spasticity and rigidity: types of increased resistance (see Table 25-3, p. 704).

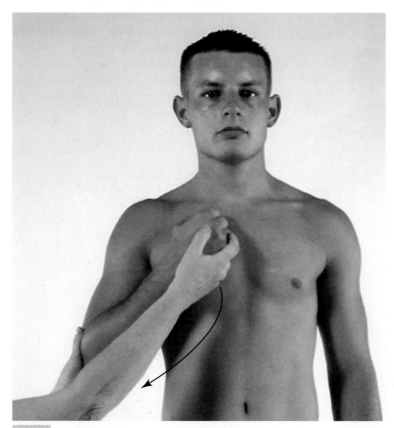

25-16

Involuntary Movements. Normally, no involuntary movements occur. If they are present, note their location, frequency, rate, and amplitude. Note whether the movements can be controlled at will.

Tic, tremor, fasciculation, myoclonus, chorea, and athetosis (see Table 25-4, p. 705).

Normal Range of Findings	Abnormal Findings

Cerebellar Function

Balance Tests

Gait. Observe as the patient walks 3 to 6 m, turns, and returns to the starting point. Normally, a person moves with a sense of freedom. The gait is smooth, rhythmic, and effortless; the opposing arm swing is coordinated; the turns are smooth. The step length is approximately 30 cm from heel to heel.

Ask the patient to walk a straight line in a heel-to-toe manner (tandem walking; Figure 25-17). This decreases the base of support and accentuates any problem with coordination. Normally, a person can walk straight and stay balanced.

You may also test for balance by asking the patient to walk on the toes and then on the heels for a few steps.

The Romberg Test. Ask the patient to stand up with feet together and arms at the sides. Once he or she is in a stable position, ask the patient to close the eyes and to hold the position (Figure 25-18). Wait approximately 20 seconds. Normally, a person can maintain posture and balance even with the visual orienting information blocked, although slight swaying may occur. (Stand close to catch the patient in case he or she falls.)

Stiff, immobile posture; staggering or reeling; wide base of support.

Lack of arm swing or rigid arms.

Unequal rhythm of steps; slapping of foot; scraping of toe of shoe.

Ataxia: uncoordinated or unsteady gait (see Table 25-5, p. 707).

Crooked line of walk.

Widening of base to maintain balance.

Staggering, reeling, loss of balance.

An ataxia that did not appear with regular gait may appear now. Inability to tandem walk is indicative of an upper motor neuron lesion, such as multiple sclerosis, or acute cerebellar dysfunction, as with alcohol intoxication.

Muscle weakness in the legs makes toe and heel walking difficult.

Swaying, falling, widening base of feet to avoid falling.

Positive Romberg sign is loss of balance that occurs when the eyes are closed. You eliminate the advantage of orientation with the eyes, which had compensated for sensory loss. A positive Romberg sign occurs with cerebellar ataxia (caused by multiple sclerosis, alcohol intoxication), loss of proprioception, and loss of vestibular function.

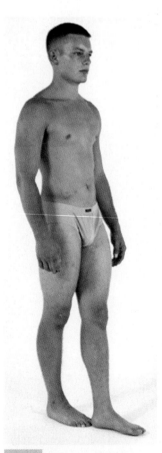

25-17 Tandem walking.

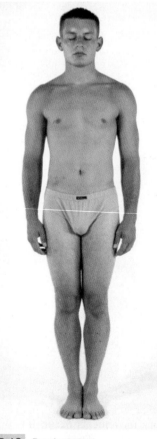

25-18 Romberg test.

Normal Range of Findings	**Abnormal Findings**

Ask the patient to perform a shallow knee bend or to hop in place, first on one leg, then the other (Figure 25-19). This demonstrates normal position sense, muscle strength, and cerebellar function. Note that some individuals cannot hop because of aging or obesity.

Inability to perform knee bend because of weakness in quadriceps muscle or hip extensors.

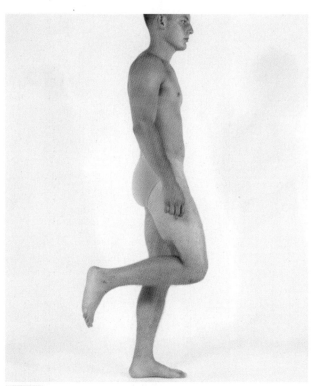

25-19

Coordination and Skilled Movements

Rapid Alternating Movements. Ask the patient to pat the knees with both hands, lift up and turn over the hands, and pat the knees with the backs of the hands (Figure 25-20). Then ask the patient to do this faster. Normally, this is done with equal turning and a quick rhythmic pace.

Alternatively, ask the patient to touch the thumb to each finger on the same hand, starting with the index finger, then reverse direction (Figure 25-21). Normally, this can be done quickly and accurately.

Lack of coordination.
Slow, clumsy, and sloppy response is termed *dysdiadochokinesia* and occurs with cerebellar disease.
Lack of coordination.

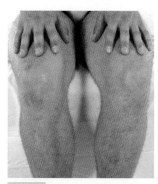

25-20

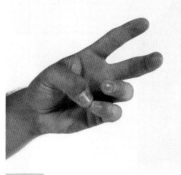

25-21

Objective Data

Normal Range of Findings	Abnormal Findings

Finger-to-Finger Test. With the patient's eyes open, ask that he or she use the index finger to touch your finger and then his or her own nose (Figure 25-22). After a few times, move your finger to a different spot. The patient's movement should be smooth and accurate.

Dysmetria is clumsy movement with overshooting of the mark; it occurs with cerebellar disorders and acute alcohol intoxication.

Past-pointing is a constant deviation to one side.

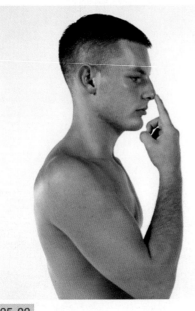
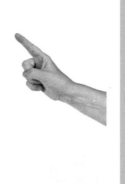

25-22

Finger-to-Nose Test. Ask the patient to close the eyes and to stretch out the arms. Ask the patient to touch the tip of his or her nose with each index finger, alternating hands and increasing speed. Normally, this movement is accurate and smooth.

Heel-to-Shin Test. Test lower extremity coordination by asking the patient to assume a supine position, to place the heel on the opposite knee, and run it down the shin from the knee to the ankle (Figure 25-23). Normally, a person moves the heel in a straight line down the shin.

The patient's finger misses the nose.

Worsening of coordination when the eyes are closed occurs with cerebellar disease or alcohol intoxication.

Lack of coordination (heel falls off shin) occurs with cerebellar disease.

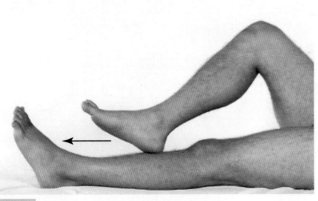

25-23

Normal Range of Findings	Abnormal Findings

ASSESS THE SENSORY SYSTEM

To test the intactness of the peripheral nerve fibres, the sensory tracts, and higher cortical discrimination, ask the patient to identify various sensory stimuli.

Ensure the validity of sensory system testing by making sure the patient is alert, cooperative, and comfortable and has an adequate attention span; otherwise, you may get misleading and invalid results. Testing of the sensory system can be fatiguing. You may need to repeat the examination later or to conduct only parts of it when the patient is tired.

You do not need to test the entire skin surface for every sensation. Routine screening procedures include testing superficial pain, light touch, and vibration in a few distal locations, and testing stereognosis. This will suffice for all patients who have not demonstrated any neurological symptoms or signs. Complete testing of the sensory system is warranted in patients with neurological symptoms (e.g., localized pain, numbness, and tingling sensation) or when you discover abnormalities (e.g., motor deficit). In those cases, test all sensory modalities, and cover most dermatomes of the body.

Compare sensations on symmetrical parts of the body. When you find a definite decrease in sensation, map it out by systematic testing in that area. Proceed from the point of decreased sensation toward the sensitive area. By asking the patient to tell you where the sensation changes, you can map the exact borders of the deficient area. Note your results on a diagram.

Avoid asking leading questions, such as "Can you feel this pinprick?" This creates an expectation of how the patient should feel the sensation, which is called *suggestion*. Instead, use unbiased directions.

Note whether the topographical pattern of sensory loss is distal—that is, over the hands and feet in a "glove and stocking" distribution—or whether it is over a specific dermatome.

The patient's eyes should be closed during each of the tests. Take time to explain what will be happening and exactly how you expect the patient to respond.

Spinothalamic Tract

Pain. Pain is tested by the patient's ability to perceive a pinprick. Break a tongue blade lengthwise, forming a sharp point at the fractured end and a dull spot at the rounded end. Lightly apply the sharp point or the dull end to the patient's body in a random, unpredictable order (Figure 25-24). Ask the patient to say "sharp" or "dull," depending on the sensation felt. (Note that the sharp edge is used to test for pain; the dull edge is used as a general test of the patient's responses.)

Let at least 2 seconds elapse after each stimulus, to avoid *summation*. With summation, frequent consecutive stimuli are perceived as one strong stimulus. When you are done, discard tongue blade.

Hypoalgesia: decreased pain sensation.

Analgesia: absence of pain sensation.

Hyperalgesia: increased pain sensation.

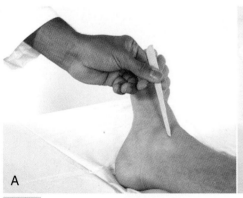
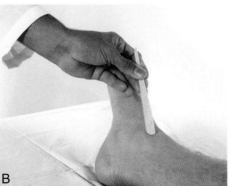

A   B

25-24

Normal Range of Findings	Abnormal Findings

Temperature. Test temperature sensation only when pain sensation is abnormal; otherwise, you may omit it because the fibre tracts are much the same. Fill two test tubes, one with hot water and one with cold water, and apply the bottom ends to the patient's skin in a random order. Ask the patient to say which temperature is felt. Alternatively, you could place the flat side of a tuning fork on the skin; its metal always feels cool.

Light Touch. Apply a wisp of cotton to the skin. Stretch a cotton ball to lengthen it, and brush it over the skin in a random order of sites and at irregular intervals (Figure 25-25). This prevents the patient from responding just from repetition. Include the arms, forearms, hands, chest, thighs, and legs. Ask the patient to say "now" or "yes" when touch is felt. Compare symmetrical points.

Hypoaesthesia: decreased touch sensation.

Anaesthesia: absent touch sensation.

Hyperaesthesia: increased touch sensation.

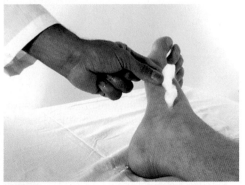

25-25

Posterior Column Tract

Vibration. Test the patient's ability to feel vibrations of a tuning fork over bony prominences. Use a low-pitch tuning fork (128 or 256 Hz) because its vibration has a slower decay. Strike the tuning fork on the heel of your hand, and hold the base on a bony surface of the patient's fingers and great toe (Figure 25-26). Ask the patient to indicate when the vibration starts and stops. If the patient feels the normal vibration or buzzing sensation on these distal areas, you may assume that the proximal spots are normal, too, and proceed no further. If no vibrations are felt, move proximally and test ulnar processes, ankles, patellae, and iliac crests. Compare responses on the right side with those on the left side. If you find a deficit, note whether it is gradual or abrupt.

Inability to feel vibration: Loss of vibration sense occurs in peripheral neuropathy such as diabetes and alcoholism. Often, this is the first sensation lost.

Peripheral neuropathy is worst at the feet, and sensation gradually improves up the leg, whereas a specific nerve lesion produces a clear zone of deficit for its dermatome.

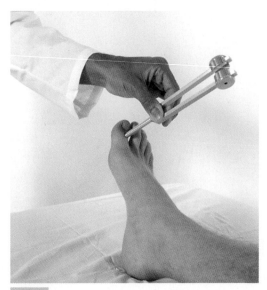

25-26

Objective Data

Normal Range of Findings	Abnormal Findings

Position (Kinaesthesia). Test the patient's ability to perceive passive movements of the extremities. Move a finger or the big toe up and down, and ask the patient to tell you which way it is moved (Figure 25-27). The test is done with the patient's eyes closed, but to be sure it is understood, have the patient watch a few trials first. Vary the order of movement up or down. Hold the digit by the sides because upward or downward pressure on the skin may provide a clue as to how it has been moved. Normally, a person can detect movement of a few millimetres.

Loss of position sense.

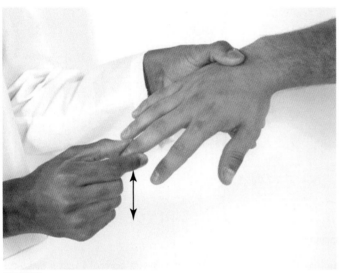

25-27

Tactile Discrimination (Fine Touch). The following tests also measure the discrimination ability of the sensory cortex. As a prerequisite, the patient needs a normal or near-normal sense of touch and a normal position sense.

Stereognosis. Test the patient's ability to recognize objects by feeling their forms, sizes, and weights, with the eyes closed. Place a familiar object (paper clip, key, coin, cotton ball, or pencil) in the patient's hand, and ask the patient to identify it (Figure 25-28). Normally, a person's fingers explore the object, and then the person correctly names it. Test a different object in each hand; testing the left hand helps you assess functioning of the right parietal lobe.

Problems with tactile discrimination occur with lesions of the sensory cortex or posterior column.

Astereognosis (inability to identify object correctly) occurs with sensory cortex lesions such as cerebrovascular attack (stroke).

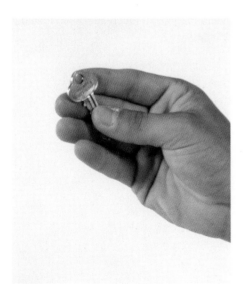

25-28

Objective Data

Normal Range of Findings	Abnormal Findings

Graphaesthesia. Graphaesthesia is the ability to "read" a number by having it traced on the skin. Ask the patient to close the eyes, and use a blunt instrument to trace a single-digit number or a letter on the patient's palm (Figure 25-29). Ask the patient to tell you what the character is. Graphaesthesia is a good measure of sensory loss if the patient cannot make the hand movements needed for stereognosis, as occurs in arthritis.

Inability to distinguish number occurs with lesions of the sensory cortex.

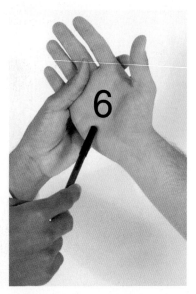

25-29 Testing for graphaesthesia.

Two-Point Discrimination. Test the patient's ability to distinguish the separation of two simultaneous pinpoints on the skin. Apply the two points of an opened paper clip lightly to the skin in ever-closing distances. Note the distance at which the patient no longer perceives two separate points. The level of perception varies considerably with the region tested; it is most sensitive in the fingertips (2 to 8 mm) and least sensitive on the upper arms, thighs, and back (40 to 75 mm).

The distance it normally takes to identify two separate points is increased with sensory cortex lesions.

Extinction. Simultaneously touch both sides of the body at the same point. Ask the patient to state how many sensations are felt and where they are. Normally, both sensations are felt.

The ability to recognize only one of the stimuli occurs with sensory cortex lesion; the stimulus is extinguished on the side *opposite* the cortex lesion.

Point Location. Touch the skin, and withdraw the stimulus promptly. Tell the patient, "Put your finger where I touched you." You can perform this test simultaneously with light touch sensation.

With a sensory cortex lesion, the sensation cannot be localized accurately, even though light touch sensation may be retained.

TEST THE REFLEXES

Stretch (Deep Tendon) Reflexes

Measurement of the stretch reflexes reveals the intactness of the reflex arc at specific spinal levels, as well as the normal override on the reflex of the higher cortical levels.

For an adequate response, the limb should be relaxed and the muscle partially stretched. Stimulate the reflex by directing a short, snappy blow of the reflex hammer onto the muscle's insertion tendon. Use a relaxed hold on the hammer. As with the percussion technique, the action takes place at the wrist. Strike a brief, well-aimed blow, and bounce up promptly; do not let the hammer rest on the tendon. Use the pointed end of the reflex hammer when aiming at a smaller target, such as your thumb, on the tendon site; use the flat end when the target is wider or to diffuse the impact and prevent pain.

Use just enough force to get a response. Compare responses on the right and left sides; they should be equal. The reflex response is graded on a five-point scale:

Normal Range of Findings

4+: Very brisk, hyperactive with clonus, indicative of disease

3+: Brisker than average, may indicate disease

2+: Average, normal

1+: Diminished, low normal

0: No response

This is a subjective scale, and its use requires some clinical practice. Even then the scale is not completely reliable because no standard exists to say *how* brisk a reflex should be to warrant a grade of 3+. Also, normality in reflex responses has a wide range. Healthy people may have diminished or brisk reflexes. Your best plan is to interpret the DTRs *only* within the context of the other results of the neurological examination.

Sometimes the reflex response fails to appear. Try further encouragement of relaxation, varying the patient's position, or increasing the strength of the blow. **Reinforcement** is another technique to relax the muscles and enhance the response (Figure 25-30). Ask the patient to perform an isometric exercise in a muscle group somewhat distant from the one being tested. For example, to enhance a patellar reflex, ask the patient to lock the fingers together and "pull." Then strike the tendon. To enhance a biceps response, ask the patient to clench the teeth or to grasp the thigh with the opposite hand.

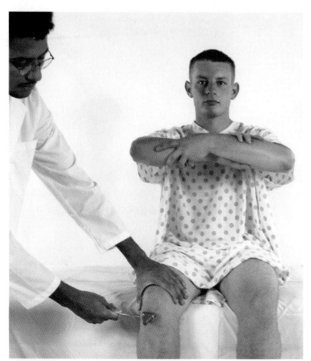

25-30 Reinforcement.

Biceps Reflex (C5 to C6). Support the patient's forearm on yours; this position relaxes, as well as partially flexes, the patient's arm. Place your thumb on the biceps tendon, and strike a blow on your thumb. You can feel as well as see the normal response, which is contraction of the biceps muscle and flexion of the forearm (Figure 25-31).

Abnormal Findings

Clonus is a set of rapid, rhythmic contractions of the same muscle.

Hyperreflexia is the exaggerated reflex that occurs when the monosynaptic reflex arc is released from the usually inhibiting influence of higher cortical levels. This occurs with upper motor neuron lesions, such as a cerebrovascular accident.

Hyporeflexia is the reduced functioning of a reflex. In some cases, the reflex may be absent. Hyporeflexia is a lower motor neuron problem. It results from interruption of sensory afferent pathways or destruction of motor efferent fibres and anterior horn cells, as in spinal cord injury.

Objective Data

Normal Range of Findings	Abnormal Findings

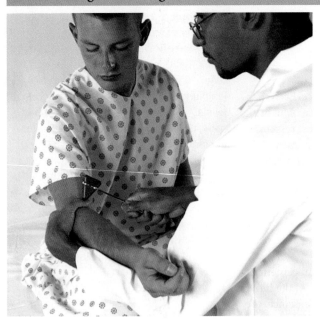

25-31   Biceps reflex.

Triceps Reflex (C7 to C8). Tell the patient to let the arm "just go limp" as you suspend it by holding the upper arm. Strike the triceps tendon directly just above the elbow (Figure 25-32). The normal response is extension of the forearm. Alternatively, hold the patient's wrist across the chest to flex the arm at the elbow, and tap the tendon.

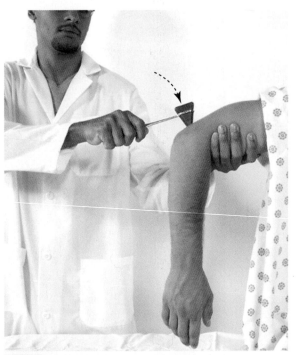

25-32   Triceps reflex.

Brachioradialis Reflex (C5 to C6). Hold the patient's thumbs to suspend the forearms in relaxation. Strike the forearm directly, approximately 2 to 3 cm above the radial styloid process (Figure 25-33). The normal response is flexion and supination of the forearm.

Normal Range of Findings	**Abnormal Findings**

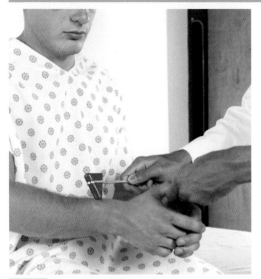

25-33 Brachioradialis reflex.

Quadriceps or Patellar ("Knee Jerk") Reflex (L2 to L4). Let the patient's lower legs dangle freely to flex the knee and stretch the tendons. Strike the tendon directly just below the patella (Figure 25-34). Extension of the lower leg is the expected response. Contraction of the quadriceps will also be palpable.

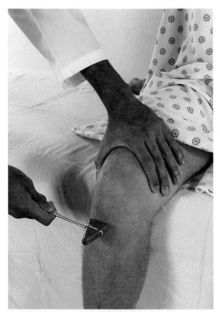

25-34 Quadriceps reflex.

To test this reflex with the patient in the supine position, use your own arm as a lever to support the weight of one of the patient's legs against the other leg (Figure 25-35). This manoeuvre also flexes the knee.

Objective Data

Objective Data

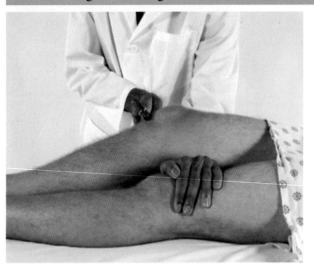

25-35   Supine quadriceps reflex.

Achilles ("Ankle Jerk") Reflex (L5 to S2). Position the patient with the knee flexed and the hip externally rotated. Hold the patient's foot in dorsiflexion, and strike the Achilles tendon directly (Figure 25-36). Feel the normal response as the foot plantar flexes against your hand.

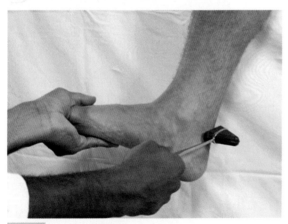

25-36   Achilles reflex.

To test this reflex with the patient in the supine position, flex one of the patient's knees and support that lower leg against the other leg so that it falls "open." Dorsiflex the foot, and tap the tendon (Figure 25-37).

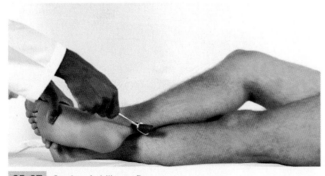

25-37   Supine Achilles reflex.

Normal Range of Findings	Abnormal Findings

Clonus. Test for clonus, particularly when the reflexes are hyperactive. Support one of the patient's lower legs in one of your hands. With your other hand, move the foot up and down a few times to relax the muscle. Then stretch the muscle by briskly dorsiflexing the foot. Hold the stretch (Figure 25-38). A normal response is no further movement. When clonus is present, rapid rhythmic contractions of the calf muscle and movement of the foot are visible and palpable.

Clonus is repeated reflex muscular movements. A hyperactive reflex with sustained clonus (lasting as long as the stretch is held) occurs with upper motor neuron disease.

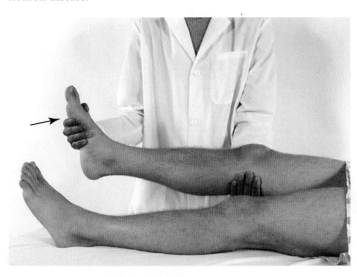

25-38

Superficial (Cutaneous) Reflexes

For cutaneous reflexes, the sensory receptors are in the skin rather than in the muscles. The motor response is a localized muscle contraction.

Abdominal Reflexes: Upper (T8 to T10) and Lower (T10 to T12). Have the patient assume a supine position, with the knees slightly bent. Use the handle end of the reflex hammer, a wood applicator tip, or the end of a split tongue blade to stroke the skin. Move from the side of the abdomen toward the midline at both the upper and lower abdominal levels (Figure 25-39). The normal response is ipsilateral contraction of the abdominal muscle, with an observed deviation of the umbilicus toward the stroke. When the abdominal wall is very thick, pull the skin to the opposite side; the muscle palpably contracts toward the stimulus.

Superficial reflexes are absent with diseases of the pyramidal tract (e.g., they are absent on the contralateral side with cerebrovascular accident).

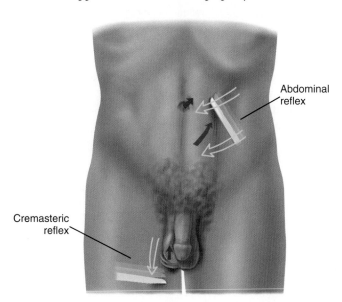

Abdominal reflex

Cremasteric reflex

25-39

Normal Range of Findings	Abnormal Findings

Cremasteric Reflex (L1 to L2). This reflex is not routinely tested. On a male patient, lightly stroke the inner aspect of the thigh with the reflex hammer or tongue blade (see Figure 25-39). Note the elevation of the ipsilateral testicle.

This reflex is absent in both upper and lower motor neuron lesions.

Plantar Reflex (L4 to S2). Position the thigh in slight external rotation. With the reflex hammer, stroke lightly up the lateral side of the sole of the foot and inward across the ball of the foot, in an upside-down J shape (Figure 25-40, *A*). The normal response is plantar flexion of the toes and inversion and flexion of the forefoot.

Except in infancy, the abnormal response is dorsiflexion of the big toe and fanning of all toes, which is a positive Babinski sign, also called *upgoing toes* (see Figure 25-40, *B*). This occurs with upper motor neuron disease of the corticospinal (or pyramidal) tract.

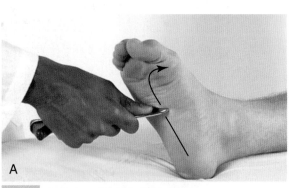 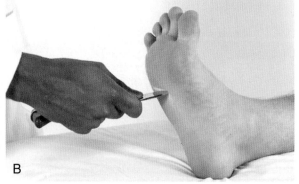

A   B

25-40   **A**, Plantar reflex. **B**, Babinski sign.

❖ DEVELOPMENTAL CONSIDERATIONS

Infants (Birth to Age 12 Months)

The neurological system undergoes dramatic growth and development during the first year of life. Assessment includes noting that milestones you normally would expect for each month have indeed been achieved and that the early, more primitive reflexes are eliminated from the baby's repertory when they are supposed to be.

At birth, the newborn is very alert, with the eyes open, and demonstrates strong, urgent sucking. The normal cry is loud and lusty and may even sound angry. The next 2 or 3 days may be spent mostly sleeping as the baby recovers from the birth process. After that, the pattern of sleep and waking activity is highly variable; it depends on the baby's individual body rhythm, as well as external stimuli.

The behavioural assessment should include your observations of the infant's spontaneous waking activity, responses to environmental stimuli, and social interaction with the parents and others.

By 2 months of age, the baby smiles responsively and recognizes the parent's face. Babbling begins at 4 months, and one or two words (mama, dada) are used nonspecifically after 9 months.

The cranial nerves cannot be tested directly, but you can infer their proper functioning by the manoeuvres shown in Table 25-1.

Failure to attain a skill by expected time.

Persistence of reflex behaviour beyond the normal time.

With CNS damage, the cry may be high-pitched or shrill or sound like a feline screech.

With respiratory distress, the cry may be weak or groaning, or an expiratory grunt occurs.

Lethargy, hyporeactivity, hyperirritability, and parent's report of significant change in behaviour all warrant referral.

Normal Range of Findings	Abnormal Findings

TABLE 25-1	Testing Cranial Nerve Function of Infants
Cranial Nerve	**Response**
II, III, IV, VI	Optical blink reflex: shine light in open eyes, note rapid closure Size, shape, equal-sized pupils Looking at face or close object Eyes follow movement
V	Rooting reflex, sucking reflex
VII	Facial movements (e.g., wrinkling forehead and nasolabial folds) symmetrical when crying or smiling
VIII	Moro reflex (until age 4 mo): elicited by loud noise Acoustic blink reflex: infant blinks in response to a loud hand clap 30 cm (12 in.) from head (avoid creating air current) Eyes follow direction of sound
IX, X	Swallowing, gag reflex Coordinated sucking and swallowing
XII	In response to pinching of nose, infant's mouth opens and tongue rises in midline

The Motor System

Observe spontaneous motor activity for smoothness and symmetry. Smoothness of movement suggests proper cerebellar function, as does the coordination involved in sucking and swallowing. To screen gross and fine motor coordination, use the Nipissing District Developmental Screen (NDDS), or other parent-report screening tool (as discussed in Chapter 2), with its age-specific developmental milestones. You also can assess movement by testing the reflexes listed in the following section. Note their smoothness of response and symmetry. Also, note whether their presence or absence is appropriate for the infant's age.

Assess muscle tone by first observing resting posture. The newborn favours a flexed position; extremities are symmetrically folded inward, the hips are slightly abducted, and the fists are tightly flexed (Figure 25-41). Infants born by breech delivery, however, will not immediately demonstrate flexion in the lower extremities.

Motor activity is delayed with brain damage, intellectual disability, peripheral neuromuscular damage, prolonged illness, and parental neglect.

Frog position: hips abducted and almost flat against the table, externally rotated (normal only after breech delivery).

Opisthotonos: head arched back, stiffness of neck, and extension of arms and legs; occurs with meningeal or brain stem irritation and kernicterus (see Table 25-10, p. 712).

Extension of limbs: may occur with intracranial hemorrhage.

Continual asymmetry of any type (e.g., asymmetry of upper limbs, which occurs with brachial plexus palsy).

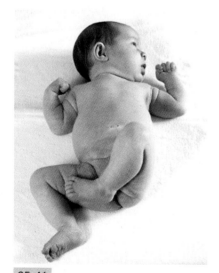

25-41

Objective Data

Objective Data

Normal Range of Findings

After 2 months of age, flexion gives way to gradual extension, beginning with the head and continuing in a cephalocaudal direction. Now is the time to check for spasticity; none should be present. Test for spasticity by flexing the infant's knees onto the abdomen and then quickly releasing them. They will unfold but not too quickly. Also, gently push the head forward; the baby should comply.

The fists normally are held in tight flexion for the first 3 months. Then the fists open for part of the time. A purposeful reach for an object with both hands occurs at approximately 4 months of age; a transfer of an object from one hand to the other hand, at 7 months of age; a grasp with fingers and opposing thumb, at 9 months of age; and a purposeful release, at 10 months of age. Babies are normally ambidextrous for the first 18 months.

Head control is an important milestone in motor development. You can incorporate the following two movements into every infant assessment to check the muscle tone necessary for head control.

First, holding the wrists, pull the baby up to the sitting position, and note head control (Figure 25-42). The newborn will hold the head almost in the same plane as the body; the head will balance briefly when the baby reaches the sitting position and then flop forward. (Even premature infants demonstrate this.) At 4 months of age, the head stays in line with the body and does not flop.

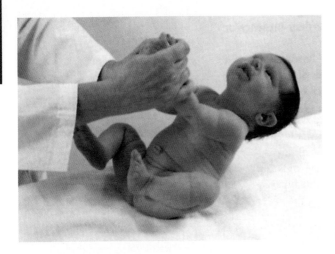

25-42

Second, lift up the baby in a prone position, with one of your hands supporting the baby's chest (Figure 25-43). The full-term newborn holds the head at an angle of 45 degrees or less from horizontal, the back is straight or slightly arched, and the elbows and knees are partly flexed.

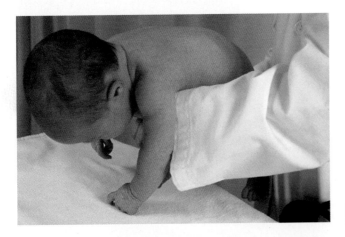

25-43

Abnormal Findings

Spasticity is an early sign of cerebral palsy. In affected infants, after you release the flexed knees, the legs quickly extend and adduct, even to a "scissoring" motion. Also, affected infants often resist head flexion and extend back against your hand.

Note persistent one-hand preference in baby younger than 18 months of age, which may indicate a motor deficit on the opposite side.

Because development progresses in a cephalocaudal direction, a lag in head control is an early sign of brain damage.

Any baby who cannot hold the head in midline when sitting after 6 months of age should be referred for neurological evaluation.

Normal Range of Findings	Abnormal Findings

At 3 months of age, the baby raises the head and arches the back, as in a swan dive. This is the *Landau reflex,* which persists until 1½ years of age (Figure 25-44).

Head lag, a limp floppy trunk, and dangling arms and legs are abnormal signs.

Absence of the Landau reflex indicates motor weakness, upper motor neuron disease, or intellectual disability.

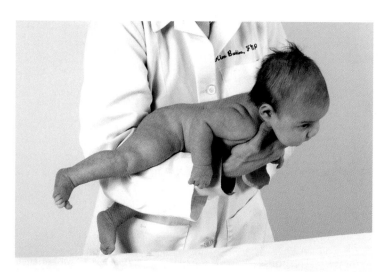

25-44

Assess muscle strength by noting the strength of sucking and of spontaneous motor activity. Normally, no tremors are present, and in a baby aged 4 months or older, no continual overshooting of the mark occurs when the baby reaches for an object.

The Sensory System

You will perform very little sensory testing with infants and toddlers. The newborn normally has hypoaesthesia, and a stimulus must be strong to elicit a response. The baby responds to pain by crying and a general reflex withdrawal of all limbs. By 7 to 9 months of age, the infant can localize the stimulus and shows more specific signs of withdrawal. Other sensory modalities are not tested.

Unusually rapid withdrawal is *hyperaesthesia,* which occurs with spinal cord lesions, CNS infections, increased intracranial pressure, and peritonitis.

No withdrawal is indicative of decreased sensation, which occurs with decreased consciousness, mental disability, and lesions of the spinal cord or peripheral nerves.

Reflexes

Infantile automatisms are reflexes that have a predictable timetable of appearance and disappearance. The reflexes most commonly tested are listed in the following section. For the screening examination, you need check only the rooting, grasp (palmar and plantar), tonic neck, and Moro reflexes.

Rooting Reflex. Brush the infant's cheek near the mouth. Note whether the infant turns the head toward that side and opens the mouth (Figure 25-45). This reflex is present at birth and disappears at ages 3 to 4 months.

Sucking Reflex. Touch the lips and offer your gloved little finger to suck. Note strong sucking reflex. This reflex is present at birth and disappears at ages 10 to 12 months.

Objective Data

Normal Range of Findings	Abnormal Findings

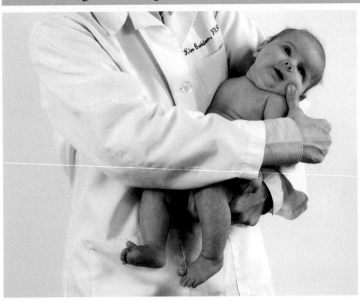

25-45

Palmar Grasp. Place the baby's head midline to ensure symmetrical response. Offer your finger from the baby's ulnar side, away from the thumb. Note tight grasp of all the baby's fingers (Figure 25-46). Sucking enhances grasp. Often, you can pull the baby to a sit with the palmar grasp. This reflex is present at birth, is strongest at ages 1 to 2 months, and disappears at ages 3 to 4 months.

The palmar grasp reflex is absent at birth with brain damage and with local muscle or nerve injury.

The palmar grasp reflex persists after 4 months of age with frontal lobe lesion.

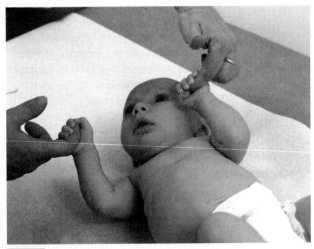

25-46

Plantar Grasp. Touch your thumb at the ball of the baby's foot. Note that the toes curl down tightly (Figure 25-47). This reflex is present at birth and disappears at ages 8 to 10 months.

Normal Range of Findings	Abnormal Findings

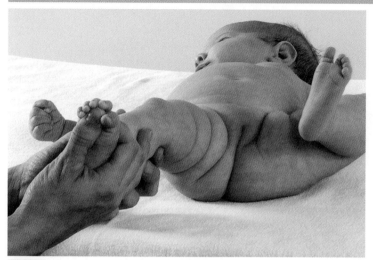

25-47

Babinski Reflex. Stroke your finger up the lateral edge and across the ball of the infant's foot. Note fanning of toes (positive Babinski reflex; Figure 25-48). The reflex is present at birth and disappears (changes to the adult response) by approximately 24 months of age (variable).

The Babinski reflex persists after 2 or 2½ years of age with pyramidal tract disease.

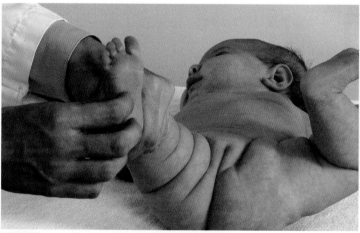

25-48

Tonic Neck Reflex. With the baby supine, relaxed, or sleeping, turn the head to one side with the chin over the shoulder. Note ipsilateral extension of the arm and leg, and flexion of the opposite arm and leg; this is the "fencing" position (Figure 25-49). If you turn the infant's head to the opposite side, arm and leg positions will switch sides. This reflex appears by ages 2 to 3 months, decreases at ages 3 to 4 months, and disappears by ages 4 to 6 months.

This reflex persists in later infancy with brain damage.

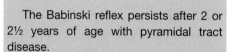
Objective Data

Normal Range of Findings	Abnormal Findings

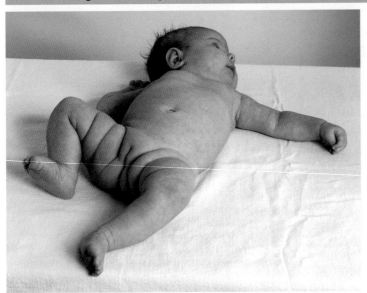

25-49   Tonic neck reflex.

Moro Reflex. Startle the infant by jarring the crib, making a loud noise, or supporting the head and back in a semisitting position and quickly lowering the infant to 30 degrees. The baby looks as if he or she is hugging a tree; that is, symmetrical abduction and extension of the arms and legs, fanning of fingers, and curling of the index finger and thumb to a C-shape position occur (Figure 25-50). The infant then brings in both arms and legs. This reflex is present at birth and disappears at ages 1 to 4 months.

Absence of the Moro reflex in the newborn or its persistence after 5 months of age indicates severe CNS injury.

Absence of movement in just one arm occurs with fracture of the humerus or clavicle and with brachial nerve palsy.

Absence of movement in one leg occurs with a lower spinal cord problem or a dislocated hip.

The Moro reflex appears hyperactive with tetany or CNS infection.

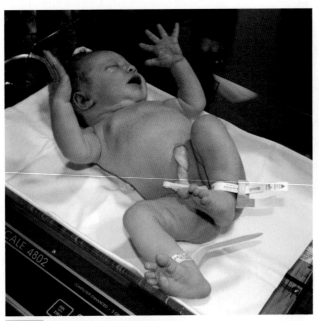

25-50   Moro reflex.

Placing Reflex. Hold the infant upright under the arms, close to a table. Let the dorsal aspect (top) of the foot touch the underside of table. Note flexing of hip and knee, followed by extension at the hip, to place foot on table (Figure 25-51). This reflex appears 4 days after birth.

Normal Range of Findings	**Abnormal Findings**

Stepping Reflex. Hold the infant upright under the arms, with the feet on a flat surface. Note regular alternating steps (Figure 25-52). This reflex disappears before voluntary walking begins.

Extensor thrust, or "scissoring"; crossing of lower extremities.

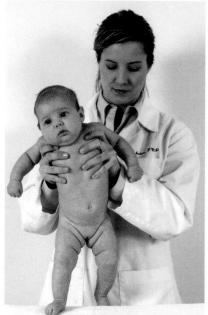

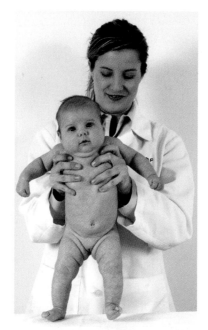

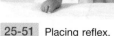 25-51   Placing reflex.

25-52   Stepping reflex.

Preschool- and School-Age Children

Use the same sequence of neurological assessment as with adults, except for the omissions and modifications mentioned in the following sections.

Assess the child's general behaviour during play activities, reaction to parent, and cooperation with parent and with you.

Smell and taste are almost never tested, but if you need to test the child's sense of smell (cranial nerve I), use a scent familiar to the child, such as, perhaps, orange peel. When testing visual fields (cranial nerve II) and cardinal positions of gaze (cranial nerves III, IV, VI), you often need to gently immobilize the head, or else the child will track with the whole head. Make a game out of asking the child to imitate your "funny faces" (cranial nerve VII); thus, the child has fun, and you have the child's friendship.

Much of the motor assessment can be derived from watching the child undress and dress and manipulate buttons. This indicates muscle strength, symmetry, joint range of motion, and fine motor skills. Use the Nipissing District Developmental Screen (NDDS) or other parent-report screening tool to screen gross and fine motor skills that are appropriate for the child's specific age. Be familiar with developmental milestones (examples are provided on the Evolve Web site).

Note the child's gait during both walking and running. A wide-based gate is normal in toddlers, and a knock-kneed walk is normal in preschoolers. Normally, children can balance on one foot for approximately 5 seconds by 4 years of age, can balance for 8 to 10 seconds at 5 years of age, and can hop at 4 years. Children enjoy participating in these tests (Figure 25-53).

Muscle hypertrophy or atrophy occurs with muscular dystrophy.

Muscle weakness should be investigated.

Incoordination should be investigated.

Causes of motor delay are listed earlier in the infant section.

Staggering and falling should be investigated.

Weakness climbing up or down stairs occurs with muscular dystrophy.

Broad-based gait beyond toddlerhood and scissor gait should be investigated (see Table 25-5, p. 707).

Failure to hop after 5 years of age indicates incoordination of gross motor skill.

Objective Data

Normal Range of Findings	Abnormal Findings

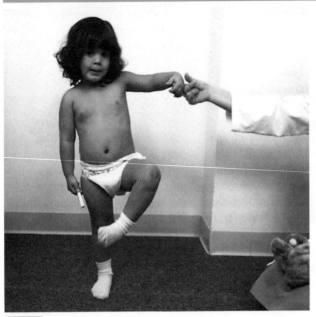

25-53

Observe the child as he or she rises from the supine position on the floor to the sitting position and then to the standing position. Note the muscles of the neck, abdomen, arms, and legs. Normally, the child curls up in the midline to sit up and then pushes off with both hands against the floor to stand (Figure 25-54, *A*).

Assess fine coordination by using the finger-to-nose test if you can be sure the young child understands your directions. Demonstrate the procedure first, then ask the child to do the test with the eyes open, then with the eyes closed. Fine coordination is not fully developed until the child has reached 4 or 6 years of age. If a younger child can bring the finger to within 2 to 5 cm of the nose, consider the result normal.

Weak pelvic muscles are a sign of muscular dystrophy; from the supine position, affected children roll to one side, bend forward to all four extremities, plant hands on legs, and literally "climb" up themselves. This is *Gower's sign* (see Figure 25-54, *B*).

Failure of the finger-to-nose test with the eyes open indicates gross incoordination; failure of the test with the eyes closed indicates minor incoordination or lack of position sense.

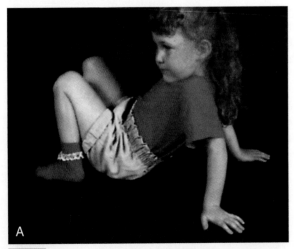

A

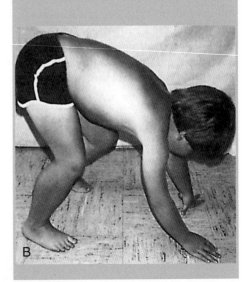

B

25-54

Normal Range of Findings

Testing sensation is very unreliable in toddlers and preschoolers. You may test the sense of light touch by asking the child to close the eyes and then to point to the spot where you touch or tickle. Senses of vibration, position, stereognosis, graphaesthesia, and two-point discrimination are usually not tested in children younger than 6 years of age. Also, do not test for perception of superficial pain. In children older than 6 years of age, you may perform sensory testing as with adults. Use a broken tongue blade if you need to test superficial pain.

The DTRs usually are not tested in children younger than 5 years of age because they cannot be relied upon to cooperate in relaxation. When you need to test DTRs in a young child, use your finger to percuss the tendon. Use a reflex hammer only with older children. Coax the child to relax, or distract and percuss discreetly when the child is not paying attention. The knee jerk is present at birth, then the ankle jerk and brachial reflex appear, and the triceps reflex is present at 6 months.

Older Adults

Use the same examination as used with younger adults. Be aware that some older adults show a slower response to your requests, especially to those involving coordination of movements. The conditions discussed in the following sections are normal variants related to aging.

Although the cranial nerves mediating taste and smell are not usually tested, they may show some decline in function.

Any decrease in muscle bulk is most apparent in the hand, as seen by guttering between the metacarpals. These dorsal hand muscles often look wasted, even with no apparent arthropathy. The grip strength remains relatively good.

Senile tremors occasionally occur. These benign tremors include an intention tremor of the hands, head nodding (as if saying yes or no), and tongue protrusion. *Dyskinesias* are the repetitive stereotyped movements in the jaw, lips, or tongue that may accompany senile tremors. No associated rigidity is present.

The gait may be slower and more deliberate than that in younger adults, and it may deviate slightly from a midline path.

The rapid alternating movements, such as pronating and supinating the hands on the thigh, may be more difficult to perform by an older adult.

After 65 years of age, loss of the sensation of vibration at the ankle malleolus is common and is usually accompanied by loss of the ankle jerk reflex. Position sense in the big toe may be lost, although this is less common than vibration loss. Tactile sensation may be impaired. Older adults may need stronger stimuli for light touch and especially for pain.

The DTRs are less brisk. Those in the upper extremities are usually present, but the ankle jerk reflex is commonly lost. The knee jerk reflex may be lost, but this occurs less often. Because older adults find it difficult to relax their limbs, always encourage relaxation when eliciting the DTRs.

The plantar reflex may be absent or difficult to interpret. A definite normal flexor response is often not apparent. However, a definite extensor response should be considered abnormal.

The superficial abdominal reflexes may be absent, probably because of stretching of the musculature through pregnancy or obesity.

Abnormal Findings

Sensory loss occurs with decreased consciousness, mental deficiency, or spinal cord or peripheral nerve dysfunction.

Hyperactivity of DTRs occurs with upper motor neuron lesion, hypocalcemia, and hyperthyroidism and with muscle spasm associated with early poliomyelitis.

Reflexes are decreased or absent with a lower motor neuron lesion, muscular dystrophy, and flaccidity or flaccid paralysis.

Clonus may occur with fatigue, but it usually indicates hyperreflexia.

Hand muscle atrophy is worsened with disuse and degenerative arthropathy.

Distinguish senile tremors from tremors of parkinsonism. The latter include rigidity, slowness, and weakness of voluntary movement.

The rhythmic reciprocal gait pattern may be absent in parkinsonism and hemiparesis (see Table 25-5, p. 707).

Note any difference in sensation between right and left sides, which may indicate a neurological deficit.

Normal Range of Findings	Abnormal Findings

NEUROLOGICAL RECHECK

Some hospitalized patients have a neurological deficit caused by head trauma or a systemic disease process. These patients must be monitored closely for any improvement or deterioration in neurological status and for any indication of increasing intracranial pressure. Signs of increasing intracranial pressure signal impending cerebral disaster and death and necessitate early and prompt intervention.

Conduct an abbreviated neurological examination in the following sequence:

1. Level of consciousness
2. Motor function
3. Pupillary response
4. Vital signs

Level of Consciousness. A *change* in the level of consciousness is the most important factor in this examination. It is the earliest and most sensitive index of change in neurological status. Note the ease of *arousal* and the state of awareness, or *orientation.* Assess orientation by asking questions about the following:

- Person: own name, occupation, names of workers around person, their occupations
- Place: where person is, nature of building, city, province
- Time: day of week, month, year

Vary the questions during repeat assessments to ensure that the patient is not merely memorizing and recalling answers. Note the quality and the content of the verbal response; articulation, fluency, manner of thinking; and any deficit in language comprehension or production (see Chapter 6).

When a patient is intubated and cannot speak, you will have to ask questions that require a nod or shake of the head: "Is this a hospital?" "Are you at home?" "Are we in Alberta?"

A patient is fully alert when his or her eyes open at your approach or spontaneously; when he or she is oriented to person, place, and time; and when he or she is able to follow verbal commands appropriately.

If the patient is not fully alert, increase the amount of stimulus used in this order:

1. Calling of name
2. Light touch on patient's arm
3. Vigorous shake of patient's shoulder
4. Pain applied (pinch the patient's nail bed, pinch the patient's trapezius muscle, rub your knuckles on the patient's sternum)

Record the stimulus used, as well as the patient's response to it.

Motor Function. Check the voluntary movement of each extremity by giving the patient specific commands. (With this procedure, you also test level of consciousness by noting the patient's ability to follow commands.)

Ask the patient to lift the eyebrows, frown, and bare teeth. Note symmetrical facial movements and bilateral nasolabial folds (cranial nerve VII).

You can check upper arm strength by testing hand grasps. Ask the patient to squeeze your fingers. Offer your two fingers, one on top of the other, so that a strong hand grasp does not hurt your knuckles (Figure 25-55). Be judicious about asking the patient to squeeze your hands; in some patients with diffuse brain damage, especially frontal lobe injury, the grasp is only a reflex.

Abnormal Findings column:

A change in consciousness may be subtle. Note any decreasing level of consciousness, disorientation, memory loss, uncooperative behaviour, or even complacency in a previously combative patient.

Review Table 6-2: Levels of Consciousness, p. 98.

Normal Range of Findings

Abnormal Findings

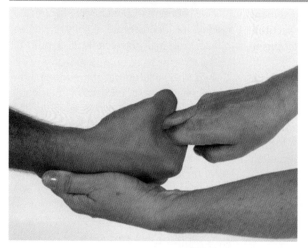

25-55

Alternatively, ask the patient to lift each hand or to hold up one finger. You also can check upper extremity strength by palmar drift. Ask the patient to extend both arms forward or halfway up, palms up, eyes closed, and hold for 10 to 20 seconds (Figure 25-56). Normally, the arms stay steady with no downward drift.

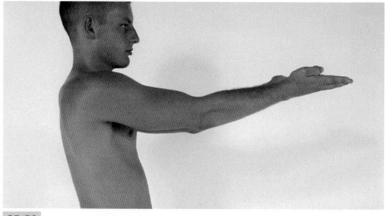

25-56

Check lower extremities by asking the patient to perform straight leg raises, in which the supine patient lifts one leg at a time straight up off the bed (Figure 25-57). Full strength enables the patient to lift the leg 90 degrees. If multiple trauma, pain, or equipment preclude this motion, ask the patient to push one foot at a time against your hand's resistance, "like putting your foot on the gas pedal of your car" (Figure 25-58).

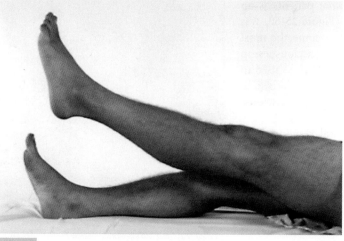

25-57

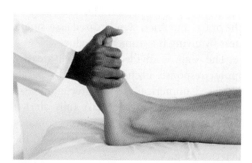

25-58

Normal Range of Findings	Abnormal Findings

In a patient with decreased level of consciousness, note whether movement occurs spontaneously and as a result of noxious stimuli such as pain or suctioning. An attempt to push away your hand after such stimuli is called *localizing* and is characterized as purposeful movement.

Pupillary Response. Note the size, shape, and symmetry of both pupils. Shine a light into each pupil and note the direct and consensual light reflex. Both pupils should constrict briskly. (Allow for the effects of any medication that could affect pupil size and reactivity.) When you record pupil size, express the value in millimetres. Tape a millimetre scale onto a tongue blade and hold it next to the patient's eyes for the most accurate measurement (Figure 25-59).

Any abnormal posturing, decorticate rigidity, or decerebrate rigidity indicates diffuse brain injury (see Table 25-9, p. 711).

In a brain-injured patient, sudden, unilateral dilation and nonreactivity of a pupil is an ominous sign. Cranial nerve III runs parallel to the brain stem. When increasing intracranial pressure pushes the brain stem down (uncal herniation), it puts pressure on cranial nerve III, causing pupil dilatation.

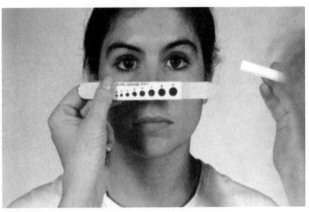

25-59

Vital Signs. Measure the temperature, pulse, respiration, and blood pressure as often as the patient's condition warrants. Although they are vital to the overall assessment of the critically ill patient, pulse and blood pressure are notoriously unreliable parameters of CNS deficit. Any changes are late consequences of rising intracranial pressure.

The Cushing reflex consists of signs of increasing intracranial pressure: sudden elevation of blood pressure with widening pulse pressure and decreased pulse rate or slow and bounding pulse.

Assessment of Unconscious and Brain-Damaged Patients

The Glasgow Coma Scale. The assessment of *comatose* patients is an important aspect of critical care. The Glasgow Coma Scale (Figure 25-60) was originally designed for patients with head trauma and has become the most widely used scoring system for patients with an altered level of consciousness in the critical care unit (Fischer et al., 2010). The Glasgow Coma Scale is used to assess the functional state of the brain as a whole, not of any particular site in the brain, and it is a standardized assessment that defines the level of consciousness by giving it a numerical value.

The scale is divided into three areas: eye opening, verbal response, and motor response. Each area is rated separately, and the patient's best response is scored numerically. The three numbers are added; the total score reflects the brain's functional level. A fully alert, normal patient has a score of 15, whereas a score of 7 or less reflects coma. Serial assessments can be plotted on a graph to illustrate visually whether the patient is stable, improving, or deteriorating.

Normal Range of Findings			Abnormal Findings

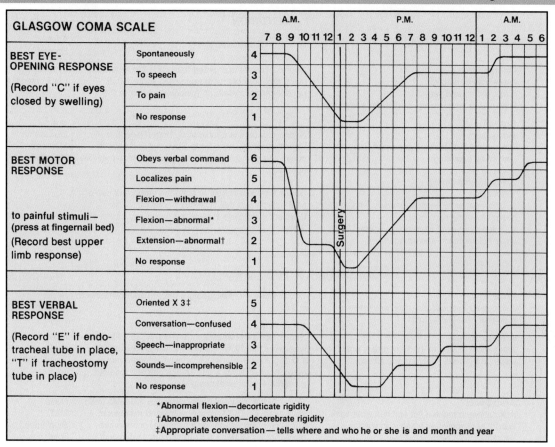

GLASGOW COMA SCALE			A.M. 7 8 9 10 11 12	P.M. 1 2 3 4 5 6 7 8 9 10 11 12	A.M. 1 2 3 4 5 6
BEST EYE-OPENING RESPONSE (Record "C" if eyes closed by swelling)	Spontaneously	4			
	To speech	3			
	To pain	2			
	No response	1			
BEST MOTOR RESPONSE to painful stimuli—(press at fingernail bed) (Record best upper limb response)	Obeys verbal command	6			
	Localizes pain	5			
	Flexion—withdrawal	4			
	Flexion—abnormal*	3			
	Extension—abnormal†	2			
	No response	1			
BEST VERBAL RESPONSE (Record "E" if endotracheal tube in place, "T" if tracheostomy tube in place)	Oriented X 3‡	5			
	Conversation—confused	4			
	Speech—inappropriate	3			
	Sounds—incomprehensible	2			
	No response	1			

*Abnormal flexion—decorticate rigidity
†Abnormal extension—decerebrate rigidity
‡Appropriate conversation—tells where and who he or she is and month and year

25-60

Limitations of the Glasgow Coma Scale include inconsistent interrater reliability and the impossibility of assessing the verbal score in intubated or aphasic patients (Fischer et al., 2010; Kornbluth & Bhardwaj, 2011). Since 2000, alternative scoring systems have been developed, including new coma scales that are not reliant on verbal responses, such as the Full Outline of UnResponsiveness (FOUR; Wijdicks, Bamlet, Maramattom, Manno, & McClelland, 2005).

The Canadian Neurological Scale. The Canadian Neurological Scale is a valid, reliable, standardized neurological assessment tool that is used to evaluate and monitor both mentation (level of consciousness, orientation, and speech) and motor function (face, arm, and leg) in patients with *stroke* (Côté et al., 1989, 2007; Côté, Hachinski, Shurvell, Norris, & Wolfson, 1986; O'Farrell & Zou, 2008). An advantage is that it is a short, simple assessment that does not need to be administered by a neurologist (Teasell, McClure, Salter, & Krugger, n.d.). The Canadian Neurological Scale can be used to monitor change and predict patient outcomes, such as length of stay, death, and dependency. The Canadian Neurological Scale Reference Card is shown in Figure 25-61.

Normal Range of Findings	Abnormal Findings

Objective Data

SECTION A	MENTATION			*SCORE*
	Level of consciousness		Alert Drowsy	3.0 1.5
	Orientation Place: city or hospital Time: month and year Patient can speak, write, or gesture a response.	*Score:* If patient is oriented (can correctly state both place and correct month and year), score 1.0. If patient cannot state both (disoriented), score 0.0.	Oriented Disoriented/NA	1.0 0.0
	Speech *Receptive:* Ask patient the following separately (do not prompt by gesturing): 1. Close your eyes 2. Point to the ceiling *Expressive:* 1. Show patient 3 items separately, and ask patient to name each object 2. Ask patient what each object is used for, while holding each one up again	*Score:* If patient is unable to do both (Receptive Deficit), score 0.0 and go to Section A2. If patient obeys commands, leave blank and assess expressive speech. *Score:* If patient is able to state the name and use of all 3 objects (Normal Speech), score 1.0. If patient is not able to state the name and use of all 3 objects (Expressive Deficit), score 0.5.	Normal Expressive Deficit Receptive Deficit	1.0 0.5 0.0
			TOTAL:	

SECTION A1	MOTOR FUNCTIONS: WEAKNESS		WEAKNESS	
NO COMPREHENSION DEFICIT	**Face** Ask patient to smile/grin, note weakness in mouth or nasal/labial folds.	*Score:* None (no weakness) = 0.5; Present (weakness) = 0.0	None Present	0.5 0.0
	Arm: Proximal Ask patient to lift arm 45-90 degrees; apply resistance between shoulder and elbow.	*Score:* None (no weakness present) = 1.5; Mild (mild weakness, full ROM, cannot withstand resistance) = 1.0; Significant (moderate weakness, some movement, not full ROM) = 0.5; Total (complete loss of movement; total weakness) = 0	None Mild Significant Total	1.5 1.0 0.5 0
	Arm: Distal Ask patient to make a fist and flex wrist backwards; apply resistance between wrist and knuckles.	*Score:* None (no weakness present) = 1.5; Mild (mild weakness, full ROM, cannot withstand resistance) = 1.0; Significant (moderate weakness, some movement, not full ROM) = 0.5; Total (complete loss of movement; total weakness) = 0	None Mild Significant Total	1.5 1.0 0.5 0
	Leg: Proximal With patient in supine position, ask patient to flex hip to 90 degrees; apply pressure to mid-thigh.	*Score:* None (no weakness present) = 1.5; Mild (mild weakness, full ROM, cannot withstand resistance) = 1.0; Significant (moderate weakness, some movement, not full ROM) = 0.5; Total (complete loss of movement; total weakness) = 0	None Mild Significant Total	1.5 1.0 0.5 0
	Leg: Distal Ask patient to dorsiflex foot; apply resistance to top of foot	*Score:* None (no weakness present) = 1.5; Mild (mild weakness, full ROM, cannot withstand resistance) = 1.0; Significant (moderate weakness, some movement, not full ROM) = 0.5; Total (complete loss of movement; total weakness) = 0	None Mild Significant Total	1.5 1.0 0.5 0
			TOTAL:	

SECTION A2	MOTOR FUNCTIONS: MOTOR RESPONSE			
COMPREHENSION DEFICIT	**Face** Have patient mimic your smile. If patient is unable, note facial expression while applying sternal pressure.		Symmetrical Asymmetrical	0.5 0.0
	Arms Demonstrate or lift patient's arms to 90 degrees; score ability to maintain raised arms; apply nail bed pressure to assess reflex response.		Equal Unequal	1.5 0.0
	Legs Lift patient's hip to 90 degrees; score ability to maintain equal levels (>5 seconds). If patient is unable to maintain raised position, apply nail bed pressure to assess reflex response.		Equal Unequal	1.5 0.0
			TOTAL:	

25-61   The Canadian Neurological Scale. *NA,* not applicable; *ROM,* range of motion.

DOCUMENTATION AND CRITICAL THINKING

Sample Charting

SUBJECTIVE

No unusually frequent or severe headaches; no head injury, dizziness or vertigo, seizures, or tremors. No weakness, numbness, or tingling; no difficulty swallowing or speaking. Has no past history of stroke, spinal cord injury, meningitis, or alcoholism.

OBJECTIVE

Mental Status: Appearance, behaviour, and speech appropriate; alert and oriented to person, place, and time; recent and remote memory intact.

Cranial Nerves:

I: Identifies coffee and peppermint.

II: Vision 20/20 O.S. [left eye], 20/20 O.D. [right eye], peripheral fields intact by confrontation, fundi normal.

III, IV, VI: EOMs [extraocular movements] intact, no ptosis or nystagmus; PERRLA [pupils equal, round, react to light and accommodation].

V: Sensation intact and equal bilaterally, jaw strength equal bilaterally.

VII: Facial muscles intact and symmetrical.

VIII: Hearing: whispered words heard bilaterally.

IX, X: Swallowing intact, gag reflex present, uvula rises in midline on phonation.

XI: Shoulder shrug, head movement intact and equal bilaterally.

XII: Tongue protrudes midline, no tremors.

Motor: No atrophy, weakness, or tremors. Gait smooth and coordinated, able to tandem walk, negative Romberg reflex. Rapid alternating movements: finger-to-nose smoothly intact.

Sensory: Pinprick, light touch, vibration intact. Stereognosis: able to identify key.

Reflexes: Normal abdominal, no Babinski sign, DTRs 2+ and = bilaterally with downgoing toes; see drawing below:

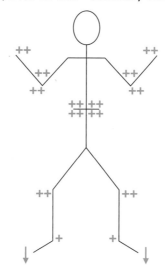

ASSESSMENT

Neurological system intact, normal function

Focused Assessment: Clinical Case Study

J.T. is a 61-year-old male carpenter at a large building firm; he is admitted to the Rehabilitation Institute with a diagnosis of right hemiplegia and aphasia after a "brain attack" (cerebrovascular accident [CVA]) 4 weeks PTA.

SUBJECTIVE

- Because of J.T.'s speech dysfunction, history was provided by wife.
- 4 weeks PTA: complaint of severe headache, then sudden onset of collapse and loss of consciousness while at work. Did not strike head as fell. Transported by ambulance to Memorial Hospital where admitting physician said J.T. "probably had

a stroke." Right arm and leg were limp, and he remained unconscious. Admitted to CCU [critical care unit]. Regained consciousness day 3 after admission, unable to move right side, unable to speak clearly or write. Remained in CCU 4 more days until "doctors were sure heart and breathing were steady."

- 3 weeks PTA: transferred to medical floor where care included physical therapy 2×/day and passive ROM 4×/day.
- Now: some improvement in right motor function. Bowel control achieved with use of commode same time each day (after breakfast). Bladder control improved. Some occasional incontinence, usually when unable to tell people he needs to urinate.

OBJECTIVE

Mental Status: Dressed in jogging suit, sitting in wheelchair, appears alert with appropriate eye contact, listening intently to history. Speech is slow, requires great effort, able to give one-word answers that are appropriate but lack normal tone. Seems to understand all language spoken to him. Follows requests appropriately, within limits of motor weakness.

Cranial Nerves:

II: Acuity normal, fields by confrontation: right homonymous hemianopsia, fundi normal.

III, IV, VI: EOMs intact, no ptosis or nystagmus, PERRLA.

V: Sensation intact to pinprick and light touch. Jaw strength weak on right.

VII: Flat nasolabial fold on right, motor weakness on right lower face. Able to wrinkle forehead bilaterally, but unable to smile or bare teeth on right.

VIII: Hearing intact.

IX, X: Swallowing intact, gag reflex present, uvula rises midline on phonation.

XI: Shoulder shrug, head movement weaker on right.

XII: Tongue protrudes midline, no tremors.

Sensory: Pinprick and light touch present but diminished on right arm and leg. Vibration intact. Position sense impaired on right side. Stereognosis intact.

Motor: Right hand grip weak, right arm drifts, right leg weak, unable to support weight. Spasticity in right arm and leg muscles, limited range of motion on passive motion. Unable to stand up and walk unassisted. Unable to perform finger-to-nose or heel-to-shin on right side; left side smoothly intact.

Reflexes: Hyperactive 4+ with clonus, and upgoing toes in right leg. Abdominal and cremasteric reflexes absent on right.

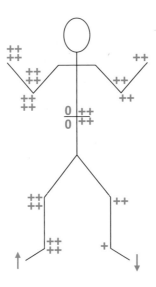

ASSESSMENT

Impaired verbal communication R/T effects of CVA
Impaired physical mobility R/T neuromuscular impairment
Disturbed body image R/T effects of loss of body function
Self-care deficits: feeding, bathing, toileting, dressing/grooming R/T muscular weakness
Disturbed sensory perception (absent right visual fields) R/T neurological impairment
Risk for injury R/T visual field deficit

ABNORMAL FINDINGS

TABLE 25-2	**Abnormalities in Cranial Nerves**		
Nerve	Test	Abnormal Findings	Possible Causes
I: Olfactory	Identifying familiar odours	Anosmia	Upper respiratory infection (temporary); tobacco or cocaine use; fracture of cribriform plate or ethmoid area; frontal lobe lesion; tumour in olfactory bulb or tract
II: Optic	Visual acuity Visual fields Shining light in eye	Defect in or absence of central vision Defect in peripheral vision, hemianopsia Absence of light reflex	Congenital blindness, refractive error, acquired vision loss as result of numerous diseases (e.g., cerebrovascular accident, diabetes), trauma to globe or orbit (see discussion of cranial nerve III)
	Direct inspection	Papilledema Optic atrophy Retinal lesions	Increased intracranial pressure Glaucoma Diabetes
III: Oculomotor	Inspection	Dilated pupil, ptosis, eye turns out and slightly down	Paralysis in cranial nerve III from internal carotid aneurysm, tumour, inflammatory lesions, uncal herniation with increased intracranial pressure
	Extraocular muscle movement Shining light in eye	Failure to move eye up, in, down Absence of light reflex	Ptosis from myasthenia gravis, oculomotor nerve palsy, Horner's syndrome Blindness, drug influence, increased intracranial pressure, CNS injury, circulatory arrest, CNS sequelae of syphilis
IV: Trochlear	Extraocular muscle movement	Failure to turn eye down or out	Fracture of orbit, brain stem tumour
V: Trigeminal	Superficial touch: three divisions Corneal reflex Clenching teeth	Absence of sense of touch and pain, paraesthesias No blink Weakness of masseter or temporalis muscles	Trauma, tumour, pressure from aneurysm, inflammation, sequelae of alcohol injection for trigeminal neuralgia Unilateral weakness with cranial nerve V lesion; bilateral weakness with upper or lower motor neuron disorder
VI: Abducens	Extraocular muscle movement to right and left sides	Failure to move laterally, diplopia on lateral gaze	Brain stem tumour or trauma, fracture of orbit
VII: Facial	Wrinkling forehead, closing eyes tightly	Absence of or asymmetrical facial movement	Bell's palsy (lower motor neuron lesion), which causes paralysis of entire half of face
	Smiling, puffing cheeks Identifying tastes	Loss of taste	Upper motor neuron lesions (cerebrovascular accident, tumour, inflammatory), which cause paralysis of lower half of face, leaving forehead intact; lower motor neuron lesions that cause paralysis: swelling from ear or meningeal infections

Continued

TABLE 25-2	Abnormalities in Cranial Nerves—cont'd		
Nerve	Test	Abnormal Findings	Possible Causes
VIII: Acoustic	Hearing acuity	Decrease or loss of hearing	Inflammation, occlusion of ear canal, otosclerosis, presbycusis, drug toxicity, tumour
IX: Glossopharyngeal	Gag reflex	See cranial nerve X	
X: Vagus	Phonating "ahh"	Deviation of uvula to side	Brain stem tumour, neck injury, cranial nerve X lesion
	Gag reflex	No gag reflex	Vocal cord weakness
	Voice quality	Hoarse or brassy voice	Soft palate weakness
		Nasal twang	Unilateral cranial nerve X lesion
		Husky voice	
	Swallowing	Dysphagia, regurgitation of fluids through nose	Bilateral cranial nerve X lesion
XI: Spinal accessory	Turning head, shrugging shoulders against resistance	Absence of movement of sternomastoid or trapezius muscles	Neck injury, torticollis
XII: Hypoglossal	Protruding tongue	Deviation to side	Lower motor neuron lesion
	Wiggling tongue from side to side	Slowed rate of movement	Bilateral upper motor neuron lesion

CNS, central nervous system.

TABLE 25-3	Abnormalities in Muscle Tone	
Condition	Description	Associated With
Flaccidity	Decreased muscle tone *(hypotonia)*; muscle feels limp, soft, and flabby; muscle is weak and easily fatigued	Lower motor neuron injury anywhere from the anterior horn cell in the spinal cord to the peripheral nerve (peripheral neuritis, poliomyelitis, Guillain-Barré syndrome) Early cerebrovascular accident and spinal cord injury: flaccidity at first
Spasticity	Increased tone *(hypertonia)*; increased resistance to passive lengthening and then suddenly giving way (clasp-knife phenomenon)	Upper motor neuron injury to corticospinal motor tract, such as paralysis with cerebrovascular accident (chronic stage)
Rigidity	Constant state of resistance (lead-pipe rigidity); resistance to passive movement in any direction; dystonia	Injury to extrapyramidal motor tracts: for example, basal ganglia with parkinsonism
Cogwheel rigidity	Type of rigidity in which the increased tone lessens by degrees during passive range of motion so that it feels like small, regular jerks	Parkinsonism

TABLE 25-4   Abnormalities in Muscle Movement

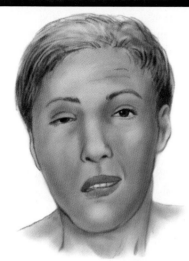

Paralysis

Decrease in or loss of motor power caused by problem
with motor nerve or muscle fibres. Acute causes: trauma,
spinal cord injury, cerebrovascular accident, poliomyelitis,
polyneuritis, Bell's palsy; chronic causes: muscular
dystrophy, diabetic neuropathy, multiple sclerosis;
episodic causes: myasthenia gravis

Patterns of paralysis: *hemiplegia* (spastic or flaccid paralysis
of one [right or left] side of body and extremities);
paraplegia (symmetrical paralysis of both lower
extremities); *quadriplegia* (paralysis in all four
extremities); *paresis* (weakness of muscles rather than
paralysis)

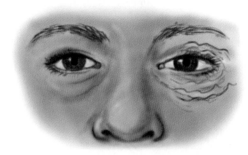

Fasciculation

Rapid, continuous twitching of resting muscle or part of
muscle, without movement of limb, that can be seen or
palpated. Types: fine (occurs with lower motor neuron
disease, associated with atrophy and weakness) and
coarse (occurs with cold exposure or fatigue and is not
significant)

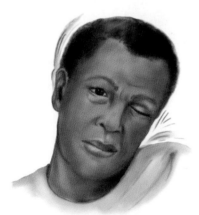

Tic

Involuntary, compulsive, repetitive twitching of a muscle
group, such as wink, grimace, head movement, shoulder
shrug; has a neurological cause, such as tardive
dyskinesias and Tourette's syndrome, or a psychogenic
cause (habit tic).

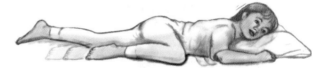

Myoclonus

Rapid, sudden jerk or a short series of jerks at fairly
regular intervals. A hiccup is a myoclonus of the
diaphragm. Single myoclonic arm or leg jerk is normal
when a person is falling asleep; myoclonic jerks are severe
with grand mal seizures.

Continued

TABLE 25-4	Abnormalities in Muscle Movement—cont'd

Tremor

Involuntary contraction of opposing muscle groups. Results in rhythmic, back-and-forth movement of one or more joints. May occur at rest or with voluntary movement. All tremors disappear during sleep. Tremors may be slow (3 to 6 per second) or rapid (10 to 20 per second).

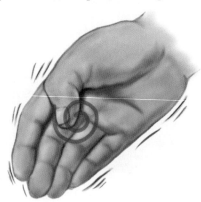

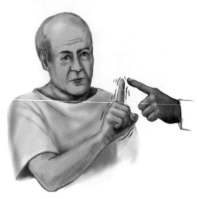

Rest Tremor

Coarse and slow (3 to 6 per second); partly or completely disappears with voluntary movement (e.g., "pill rolling" tremor of parkinsonism, with thumb and opposing fingers).

Intention Tremor

Rate varies; worse with voluntary movement. Occurs with cerebellar disease and multiple sclerosis.

Essential tremor (familial): a type of intention tremor; most common tremor in older adults. Benign (no associated disease) but causes emotional stress in work or social situations. Improves with the administration of sedatives, propranolol, and alcohol, but use of alcohol is discouraged because of the risk for addiction.

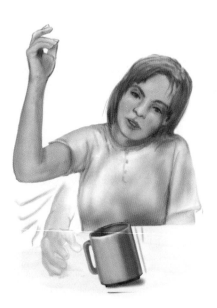

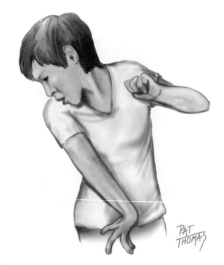

Chorea

Sudden, rapid, jerky, purposeless movement involving limbs, trunk, or face.

Occurs at irregular intervals, not rhythmic or repetitive, more convulsive than a tic. Some are spontaneous, and some are initiated; all are accentuated by voluntary acts. Disappears with sleep. Common with Sydenham's chorea and Huntington's disease.

Athetosis

Slow, twisting, writhing, continuous movement, resembling a snake or worm. Involves distal part of limb more than the proximal part. Occurs with cerebral palsy. Disappears with sleep. "Athetoid" hand: some fingers are flexed and some are extended.

TABLE 25-5   Abnormal Gaits

Type	Characteristic Appearance	Possible Causes
Spastic Hemiparesis 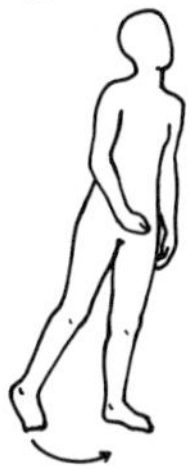	Arm is immobile against the body, with flexion of the shoulder, elbow, wrist, and fingers and adduction of shoulder. The leg is stiff and extended and circumducts with each step (patient drags toe in a semicircle).	Upper motor neuron lesion of the corticospinal tract, such as those caused by cerebrovascular accident, trauma
Cerebellar Ataxia 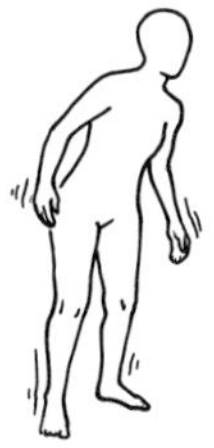	Patient has staggering, wide-based gait; difficulty with turns; uncoordinated movement with positive Romberg sign.	Alcohol or barbiturate effect on cerebellum; cerebellar tumour; multiple sclerosis
Parkinsonian (Festinating) 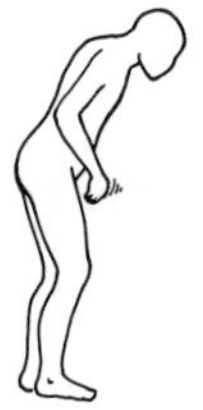	Posture is stooped; trunk is pitched forward; elbows, hips, and knees are flexed. Steps are short and shuffling. Patient hesitates to begin walking and has difficulty stopping suddenly. Patient holds the body rigid, walks and turns body as one fixed unit and has difficulty with any change in direction.	Parkinsonism
Scissors 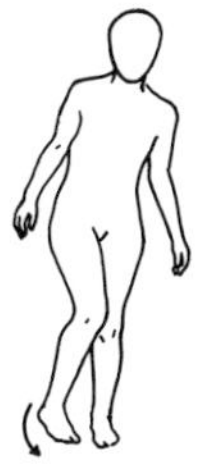	Knees cross or are in contact, like holding an orange between the thighs. The patient uses short steps, and walking requires effort.	Paraparesis of legs, multiple sclerosis
Steppage or Footdrop 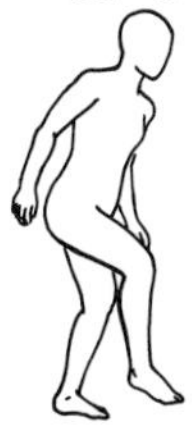	Slapping quality: Gait looks as if patient is walking up stairs and finding no stair there. Patient lifts knee and foot high and slaps it down hard and flat to compensate for footdrop.	Weakness of peroneal and anterior tibial muscles; caused by lower motor neuron lesion at the spinal cord, such as poliomyelitis, Charcot-Marie-Tooth disease (an inherited peripheral neuropathy)

Continued

Abnormal Findings

TABLE 25-5	Abnormal Gaits—cont'd	
Type	**Characteristic Appearance**	**Possible Causes**
Waddling	Weak hip muscles: When the patient takes a step, the opposite hip drops, which allows compensatory lateral movement of pelvis. Often, the patient also has marked lumbar lordosis and a protruding abdomen.	Hip girdle muscle weakness, caused by muscular dystrophy, dislocation of hips
Short Leg	Leg length discrepancy > 2.5 cm. Vertical telescoping of affected side, which dips as the patient walks. Appearance of gait varies, depending on amount of accompanying muscle dysfunction.	Congenital dislocated hip; acquired shortening as a result of disease, trauma

TABLE 25-6	Characteristics of Upper and Lower Motor Neuron Lesions	
Characteristic	**Upper Motor Neuron Lesion**	**Lower Motor Neuron Lesion**
Weakness or paralysis	In muscles that correspond to distribution of damage in pyramidal tract lesion; usually in hand grip, arm extensors, leg flexors	In specific muscles served by damaged spinal segment, ventral root, or peripheral nerve
Location	Descending motor pathways that originate in the motor areas of cerebral cortex and carry impulses to the anterior horn cells of the spinal cord	Nerve cells that originate in the anterior horn of spinal cord or in brain stem and carry impulses by the spinal nerves or cranial nerves to the muscles, the "final common pathway"
Example	Cerebrovascular accident	Poliomyelitis, herniated intervertebral disc
Muscle tone	Increased tone; spasticity	Loss of tone, flaccidity
Bulk	Some atrophy from disuse; otherwise normal	Atrophy (wasting), may be marked
Abnormal movements	None	Fasciculations
Reflexes	Hyperreflexia, ankle clonus; diminished or absent superficial abdominal reflexes; positive Babinski sign	Hyporeflexia or areflexia; no Babinski sign, no pathological reflexes
Possible nursing diagnoses	Risk for contractures; impairment in physical mobility	Impairment in physical mobility

TABLE 25-7   Patterns of Motor System Dysfunction

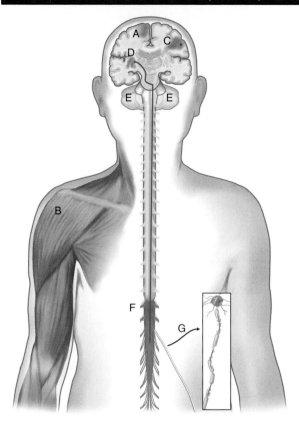

A: Cerebral Palsy

Mixed group of paralytic neuromotor disorders of infancy and childhood; results from damage to cerebral cortex caused by a developmental defect, intrauterine meningitis or encephalitis, birth trauma, anoxia, or kernicterus.

B: Muscular Dystrophy

Chronic, progressive wasting of skeletal musculature, which produces weakness, contractures, and in severe cases, respiratory dysfunction and death. Onset of symptoms occurs in childhood. Many types exist; the most severe is Duchenne's muscular dystrophy, characterized by the waddling gait described in Table 25-5.

C: Hemiplegia

Damage to corticospinal tract (e.g., cerebrovascular accident). Upper motor neuron damage occurs above the pyramidal decussation crossover; thus motor impairment is on contralateral (opposite) side. Affected muscles are initially flaccid when the lesion is acute; later, the muscles become spastic, and abnormal reflexes appear. Characteristic posture of arm: shoulder adducted, elbow flexed, wrist pronated, leg extended; characteristic facies: weakness only in lower muscles. Hyperreflexia and sometimes clonus occur on the involved side; loss of corneal, abdominal, and cremasteric reflexes; positive Babinski and Hoffman reflexes.

D: Parkinsonism

Defect of extrapyramidal tracts, in the region of the basal ganglia, with loss of the neurotransmitter dopamine. Classic triad of symptoms: tremor, rigidity, akinesia. Also slower monotonous speech and diminutive writing. Body tends to stay immobile; facial expression is flat, staring, expressionless; excessive salivation occurs; eye blinking is reduced. Posture is stooped; equilibrium is impaired; balance is easily lost; gait is as described in Table 25-5. Parkinsonian tremor; cogwheel rigidity on passive range of motion.

E: Cerebellar

A lesion in one hemisphere produces motor abnormalities on the ipsilateral side. Characterized by ataxia, lurching forward of affected side during walking, rapid alternating movements that are slow and arrhythmic; finger-to-nose test reveals ataxia and tremor with overshoot or undershoot, and eyes display coarse nystagmus.

F: Paraplegia

Lower motor neuron damage caused by spinal cord injury. A severe injury or complete transection initially produces "spinal shock" (no movement or reflex activity below the level of the lesion). Gradually, deep tendon reflexes reappear and become increased, flexor spasms of legs occur, and then extensor spasms of legs occur; these spasms lead to prevailing extensor tone.

G: Multiple Sclerosis

Chronic, progressive, immune-mediated disease in which axons undergo inflammation, demyelination, degeneration, and sclerosis (Courtney, Treadaway, Remington, & Frohman, 2009). Structures most frequently involved are the optic nerve, oculomotor nerve, corticospinal tract, posterior column tract, and cerebellum. Thus symptoms are varied but include blurred vision, diplopia, extreme fatigue, weakness, spasticity, numbness and tingling sensation, and loss of balance.

TABLE 25-8   Common Patterns of Sensory Loss

Type	Characteristics	Possible Causes
Peripheral Neuropathy	Loss of sensation involves all modalities. Loss is most severe distally (feet and hands); response improves as stimulus is moved proximally (glove-and-stocking anaesthesia). Zone of anaesthesia gradually merges into a hypoaesthesia zone, then gradually becomes normal.	Diabetes, chronic alcoholism, nutritional deficiency
Individual Nerves or Roots	Decrease in or loss of all sensory modalities. Area of sensory loss corresponds to distribution of the involved nerve.	Trauma, vascular occlusion
Spinal Cord Hemisection (Brown-Séquard Syndrome)	Loss of pain and temperature sensation on the contralateral side, starting one to two segments below the level of the lesion. Loss of vibration sensation and position discrimination on the ipsilateral side, below the level of the lesion.	Meningioma, neurofibroma, cervical spondylosis, multiple sclerosis
Complete Transection of the Spinal Cord	Complete loss of *all* sensory modalities below the level of the lesion. Condition is associated with motor paralysis and loss of sphincter control.	Spinal cord trauma, demyelinating disorders, tumour

TABLE 25-8 Common Patterns of Sensory Loss—cont'd

Type	Characteristics	Possible Causes
Thalamus 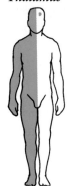	Loss of *all* sensory modalities on the face, arm, and leg on the side contralateral to the lesion.	Vascular occlusion
Cortex 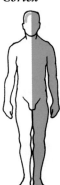	Because pain, vibration sensation, and crude touch sensation are mediated by the thalamus, little loss of these sensory functions occurs with a cortex lesion. Loss of discrimination occurs on the contralateral side. Loss of graphaesthesia, stereognosis, recognition of shapes and weights, finger finding.	Cerebral cortex, parietal lobe lesion (e.g., cerebrovascular accident)

TABLE 25-9 Abnormal Postures

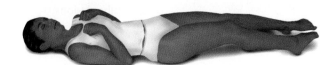

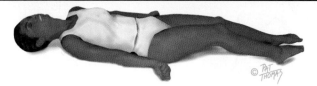

Decorticate Rigidity

Upper extremities: flexion of arm, wrist, and fingers; adduction of arm (i.e., tight against thorax). Lower extremities: extension, internal rotation, plantar flexion. This type of rigidity indicates hemispheric lesion of cerebral cortex.

Decerebrate Rigidity

Upper extremities: stiffly extended, adducted, and internally rotated; palms pronated. Lower extremities: stiffly extended; plantar flexion. Other areas: teeth clenched; back hyperextended. More ominous than decorticate rigidity; indicates lesion in brain stem at midbrain or upper pons.

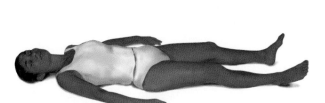

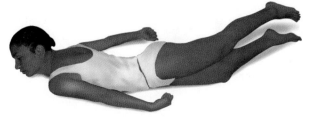

Flaccid Quadriplegia

Complete loss of muscle tone and paralysis of all four extremities, indicating completely nonfunctional brain stem.

Opisthotonos

Prolonged arching of the back, with head and heels bent backward. This indicates meningeal irritation.

TABLE 25-10   Pathological Reflexes

Reflex	Method of Testing	Abnormal Response (Reflex Is Present)	Indications
Babinski	Stroke lateral aspect and across ball of foot.	Extension of great toe, fanning of toes	Corticospinal (pyramidal) tract disease (e.g., stroke, trauma)
Oppenheim	Using heavy pressure with your thumb and index finger, stroke anterior medial tibial muscle.	Same as for Babinski reflex	Same as for Babinski reflex
Gordon	Firmly squeeze calf muscles.	Same as for Babinski reflex	Same as for Babinski reflex
Hoffman	With patient's hand relaxed, wrist dorsiflexed, fingers slightly flexed, sharply flick nail of distal phalanx of middle or index finger.	Clawing of fingers and thumb	Same as for Babinski reflex
Kernig	With patient in flat-lying supine position, raise leg straight or flex thigh on abdomen, then extend knee.	Resistance to straightening (because of hamstring spasm), pain down posterior thigh	Meningeal irritation (e.g., meningitis, infections)
Brudzinski	With one hand under patient's neck and other hand on patient's chest, sharply flex chin on chest, and watch hips and knees.	Resistance and pain in neck with flexion of hips and knees	Meningeal irritation (e.g., meningitis, infections)

TABLE 25-11   Frontal Release Signs

Reflex	Method of Testing	Abnormal Response (Reflex Is Present)	Indications
Snout Snout	Gently percuss patient's oral region	Puckering of lips	Frontal lobe disease, cerebral degenerative disease (Alzheimer's disease), amyotrophic sclerosis, corticobulbar lesions
Sucking Sucking	Touch patient's oral region	Sucking movement of lips, tongue, and jaw; swallowing	Same as for snout reflex

TABLE 25-11   Frontal Release Signs—cont'd

Reflex	Method of Testing	Abnormal Response (Reflex Is Present)	Indications
Grasp Grasp	Touch patient's palm with your finger	Uncontrolled, forced grasping (grasp is usually last of these signs to appear, so its presence indicates severe disease)	When grasping is unilateral: frontal lobe lesion on contralateral side When grasping is bilateral: diffuse bifrontal lobe disease

Images © Pat Thomas, 2006.

TABLE 25-12   Speech Disorders

Condition	Function Affected	Description
Dysphonia	Voice	Difficulty or discomfort in talking, with abnormal pitch or volume, caused by laryngeal disease. Voice sounds hoarse or whispered, but articulation and language are intact.
Dysarthria	Articulation	Distorted speech sounds; speech may sound unintelligible; basic language (word choice, grammar, comprehension) is intact.
Aphasia	Language comprehension and production	True language disturbance, defect in word choice and grammar or defect in comprehension; defect is in *higher* integrative language processing and is secondary to brain damage.
Types of aphasia*		
	Speech production	An earlier dichotomy classified aphasias as expressive (difficulty producing language) or receptive (difficulty understanding language). Because all people with aphasia have some difficulty with expression, beginning examiners tend to classify all types as expressive. The following system is more descriptive.
• Global aphasia		The most common and severe form. Spontaneous speech is absent or reduced to a few stereotyped words or sounds. Comprehension is absent or reduced to only the patient's own name and a few select words. Repetition, reading, and writing are severely impaired. Prognosis for language recovery is poor. Caused by a large lesion that damages most of combined anterior and posterior language areas.
• Broca's aphasia		Expressive aphasia. The patient can understand language but cannot express himself or herself with language. This is characterized by nonfluent, dysarthric, and effortful speech. The speech is mostly nouns and verbs (high-content words) with few grammatical fillers ("agrammatic" or "telegraphic" speech). Repetition and reading aloud are severely impaired. Auditory and reading comprehensions are surprisingly intact. Lesion is in anterior language area called the *motor speech cortex* or *Broca's area*.
• Wernicke's aphasia		Receptive aphasia. The linguistic opposite of Broca's aphasia. The person can hear sounds and words but cannot relate them to previous experiences. Speech is fluent, effortless, and well articulated but has many paraphasias (word substitutions that are malformed or wrong) and neologisms (made-up words) and often lacks substantive words. Speech can be totally incomprehensible. Often, there is a great urge to speak. Repetition, reading, and writing also are impaired. Lesion is in posterior language area called the *association auditory cortex* or *Wernicke's area*.

*For a discussion of other types of aphasia (e.g., conduction, anomic, transcortical, and so on), please consult a neurology text.

Abstract Findings (sidebar)

Summary Checklist: Neurological Examination

For a PDA-downloadable version, go to *http://evolve.elsevier.com/Canada/Jarvis/examination/*.

Neurological Screening Examination

1. Mental status
2. Cranial nerves
   II: Optic
   III, IV, VI: Extraocular muscles
   V: Trigeminal
   VII: Facial mobility
3. Motor function
   Gait and balance
   Knee flexion: hop or shallow knee bend
4. Sensory function
   Superficial pain and light touch: arms and legs
   Vibration: arms and legs

5. Reflexes
   Biceps
   Triceps
   Patellar
   Achilles

Neurological Complete Examination

1. Mental status
2. Cranial nerves II through XII
3. Motor system
   Muscle size, strength, tone
   Gait and balance
   Rapid alternating movements
4. Sensory function
   Superficial pain and light touch

Vibration
Position sense
Stereognosis, graphaesthesia, two-point discrimination

5. Reflexes
   Deep tendon: biceps, triceps, brachioradialis, patellar, Achilles
   Superficial: abdominal, plantar

REFERENCES

American Stroke Association. (2012). *About stroke*. Retrieved from *http://www.strokeassociation.org/STROKEORG/*.

Bergman, D. (2011). Preventing recurrent cerebrovascular events in patients with stroke or transient ischemic attack: The current data. *Journal of the American Academy of Nurse Practitioners, 23*(12), 659–666. doi:10.1111/j.1745-7599.2011.00650.x

Clarke, P., Marshall, V., Black, S., & Colantonio, A. (2002). Well-being after stroke in Canadian seniors: Findings from the Canadian study of health and aging. *Stroke, 33*, 1016–1021. doi:10.1161/01.STR.0000013066.24300.F9

Côté, R., Battista, R. N., Wolfson, C., Boucher, J., Adam, J., & Hachinski, V. (1989). The Canadian Neurological Scale: Validation and reliability assessment. *Neurology, 39*, 638–643.

Côté, R., David, M., Deveber, G., Teal, P., Roussin, A., & Sharma, M. (2007). *Stroke prevention*. The Thrombosis Interest Group of Canada. Retrieved from *http://www.tigc.org/eguidelines/previschemstroke05.htm*.

Côté, R., Hachinski, V. C., Shurvell, B. L., Norris, J. W., & Wolfson, C. (1986). The Canadian Neurological Scale: A preliminary study in acute stroke. *Stroke, 17*, 731–737. doi:10.1161/01.STR.17.4.731

Courtney, A. M., Treadaway, K., Remington, G., & Frohman, E. (2009). Multiple sclerosis. *Medical Clinics of North America, 93*(2), 451–476. doi:10.1016/j.mcna.2008.09.014

Fischer, M., Rüegg, S., Czaplinski, A., Strohmeier, M., Lehmann, A., Tschan, F., ... Marsch, S. C. (2010). Inter-rater reliability of the Full Outline of UnResponsiveness score and the Glasgow Coma Scale in critically ill patients: A prospective observational study. *Critical Care* (London, England), *14*(2), R64. Retrieved from *http://ccforum.com/content/14/2/R64*.

Fjell, A. M., Walhovd, K. B., & Fennema-Notestine, C. (2009). One-year brain atrophy evident in healthy aging. *Journal of Neuroscience, 29*(48), 1523–1531. doi:10.1523/JNEUROSCI.3252-09.2009

Heart and Stroke Foundation of Canada. (2012a). *Multilingual and multicultural resources*. Retrieved from *http://www.heartandstroke.com/site/c.ikIQLcMWJtE/b.3532103/apps/s/content.asp?ct=4512409*.

Heart and Stroke Foundation of Canada. (2012b). *Statistics*. Retrieved *http://www.heartandstroke.com/site/c.ikIQLcMWJtE/b.3483991/k.34A8/Statistics.htm*.

Heart and Stroke Foundation of Canada. (2012c). *Women and stroke special risks, worse prognosis*. Retrieved from *http://www.heartandstroke.com/site/c.ikIQLcMWJtE/b.3532103/apps/s/content.asp?ct=4512777*.

Kornbluth, J., & Bhardwaj, A. (2011). Evaluation of coma: A critical appraisal of popular scoring systems. *Neurocritical Care, 14*(1), 134–143. doi:10.1007/s12028-010-9409-3

Lindsay, M. P., Gubitz, G., Bayley, M., Hill, M. D., Davies-Schinkel, C., Singh, S., & Phillips, S. (2010). *Canadian Best Practice Recommendations for Stroke Care (Update 2010)*. On behalf of the Canadian Stroke Strategy Best Practices and Standards Writing Group. 2010; Ottawa, Ontario Canada: Canadian Stroke Network. Retrieved from: *http://www.strokebestpractices.ca/wp-content/uploads/2011/04/2010BPR_ENG.pdf*

O'Farrell, B., & Zou, G. Y. (2008). Implementation of the Canadian Neurological Scale on an acute care neuroscience unit: A program evaluation. *Journal of Neuroscience Nursing, 40*(4), 201–211.

Teasell, R., McClure, A., Salter, K., & Krugger, H. (n.d.). *Clinical assessment tools*. Retrieved from *http://www.ebrsr.com/~ebrsr/uploads/H_Clinical_Assessment_Tools.pdf*.

Wijdicks, E., Bamlet, W., Maramattom, B., Manno, E., & McClelland, R. (2005). Validation of a new coma scale: The FOUR score. *Annals of Neurology, 58*(4), 585–593. doi:10.1002/ana.20611

Male Genitourinary System

Written by Carolyn Jarvis, PhD, APN, CNP
Adapted by Marian Luctkar-Flude, RN, MScN

evolve WEBSITE

OUTLINE

STRUCTURE AND FUNCTION

THE MALE GENITALIA

The male genital structures include the penis and scrotum externally and the testis, epididymis, and vas deferens internally. Glandular structures accessory to the genital organs (the prostate, seminal vesicles, and bulbourethral glands) are discussed in Chapter 23.

Penis

The **penis** is composed of three cylindrical columns of erectile tissue: the two corpora cavernosa on the dorsal side and the corpus spongiosum ventrally (Figure 26-1). At the distal end of the shaft, the corpus spongiosum expands into a cone of erectile tissue, the **glans.** The area where the glans joins the shaft is the **corona.** The **urethra** transverses the corpus spongiosum, and its meatus forms a slit at the glans tip. Over the glans, the skin folds in and back on itself, forming a hood or flap. This is the **foreskin,** or **prepuce.** Sometimes, it is surgically removed shortly after birth by circumcision. The **frenulum** is a fold of the foreskin extending from the urethral meatus ventrally.

Scrotum

The **scrotum** is a loose protective sac that is a continuation of the abdominal wall (Figure 26-2). After adolescence, the scrotal skin is deeply pigmented and has large sebaceous

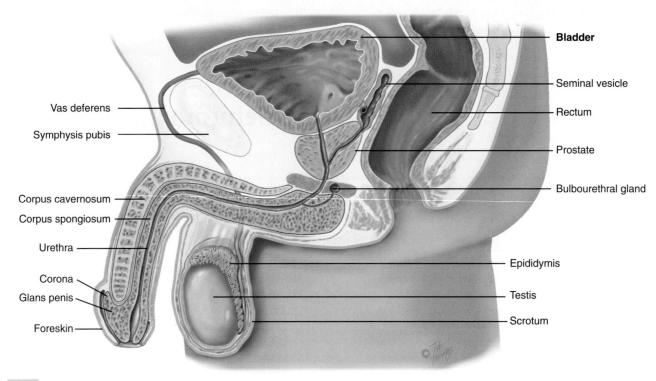

Vas deferens

Symphysis pubis

Corpus cavernosum

Corpus spongiosum

Urethra

Corona

Glans penis

Foreskin

Bladder

Seminal vesicle

Rectum

Prostate

Bulbourethral gland

Epididymis

Testis

Scrotum

26-1

© Pat Thomas, 2010.

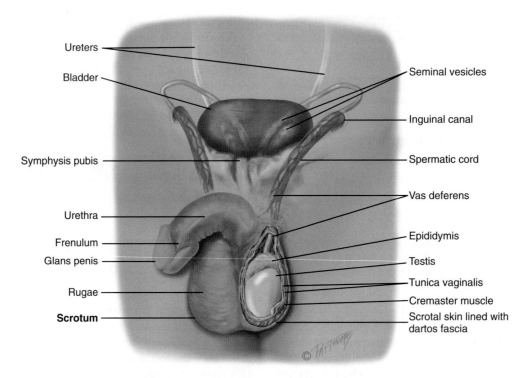

Ureters

Bladder

Symphysis pubis

Urethra

Frenulum

Glans penis

Rugae

Scrotum

Seminal vesicles

Inguinal canal

Spermatic cord

Vas deferens

Epididymis

Testis

Tunica vaginalis

Cremaster muscle

Scrotal skin lined with dartos fascia

26-2   Male genital structures.

© Pat Thomas, 2010.

follicles. The scrotal wall consists of thin skin lying in folds, or **rugae,** and the underlying cremaster muscle. The **cremaster** and **dartos muscles** control the size of the scrotum by responding to ambient temperature. This is to keep the testes at the best temperature for producing sperm: 3°C below

abdominal temperature. When it is cold, the cremaster muscle contracts, raising the sac and bringing the testes closer to the body to absorb heat necessary for sperm viability. The dartos muscle, located within the dartos fascia, also contracts, causing the scrotal skin to wrinkle. When it is warmer, these

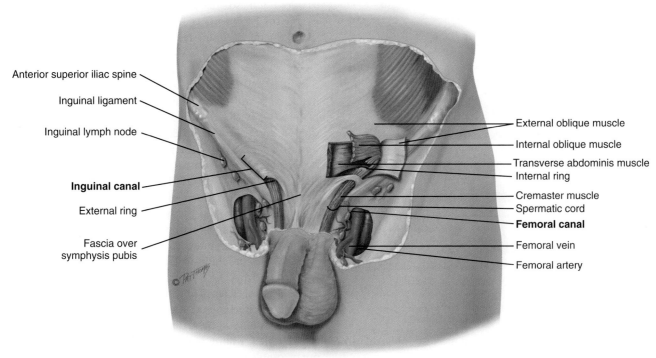

Anterior superior iliac spine

Inguinal ligament

Inguinal lymph node

Inguinal canal

External ring

Fascia over
symphysis pubis

External oblique muscle

Internal oblique muscle

Transverse abdominis muscle

Internal ring

Cremaster muscle

Spermatic cord

Femoral canal

Femoral vein

Femoral artery

STRUCTURES OF INGUINAL AREA

26-3

© Pat Thomas, 2010.

muscles relax, the scrotum lowers, and the skin looks smoother.

Inside, a septum separates the sac into two halves. In each scrotal half is a **testis,** which produces sperm. Each testis is a solid oval structure that is compressed laterally and measures 4 to 5 cm long by 3 cm wide in adults. The testis is suspended vertically by the spermatic cord (see Figure 26-2). The left testis is lower than the right because the left spermatic cord is longer. Each testis is covered by a double-layered membrane, the tunica vaginalis, which separates it from the scrotal wall. The two layers are lubricated by fluid so that the testis can slide a little within the scrotum; this helps prevent injury.

Sperm are transported along a series of ducts. First, the testis is capped by the **epididymis,** which is a markedly coiled duct system and the main storage site of sperm. It is a comma-shaped structure, curved over the top and the posterior surface of the testis. In 6% to 7% of boys and men, the epididymis is anterior to the testis.

The lower part of the epididymis is continuous with a muscular duct, the **vas deferens.** This duct approximates with other vessels (arteries and veins, lymphatic vessels, nerves) to form the **spermatic cord.** The spermatic cord ascends along the posterior border of the testis and runs through the tunnel of the inguinal canal into the abdomen. At that point, the vas deferens continues back and down behind the bladder, where it joins the duct of the seminal vesicle to form the **ejaculatory duct.** This duct empties into the urethra.

The **lymphatic vessels** of the penis and scrotal surface drain into the inguinal lymph nodes, whereas those of the testes drain into the abdomen. Abdominal lymph nodes are not accessible to clinical examination.

Inguinal Area

The **inguinal area,** or groin, is the juncture of the lower abdominal wall and the thigh (Figure 26-3). Its diagonal borders are the anterior superior iliac spine and the symphysis pubis. Between these landmarks lies the **inguinal ligament** (Poupart's ligament). Superior to the ligament lies the **inguinal canal,** a narrow tunnel passing obliquely between layers of abdominal muscle. It is 4 to 6 cm long in the adult. Its openings are an internal ring, located 1 to 2 cm above the midpoint of the inguinal ligament, and an external ring, located just above and lateral to the pubis.

Inferior to the inguinal ligament is the **femoral canal.** It is a potential space located 3 cm medial to and parallel with the femoral artery. You can use the artery as a landmark to find this space.

Knowledge of these anatomical areas in the groin is useful because they are potential sites for a hernia, which is a loop of bowel protruding through a weak spot in the musculature.

 DEVELOPMENTAL CONSIDERATIONS

Infants

During gestation, the testes develop in the abdominal cavity near the kidneys. During the later months of gestation, the testes migrate, pushing the abdominal wall in front of them and dragging the vas deferens, the blood vessels, and nerves behind. The testes descend along the inguinal canal into the scrotum before birth. At birth, each testis measures 1.5 to

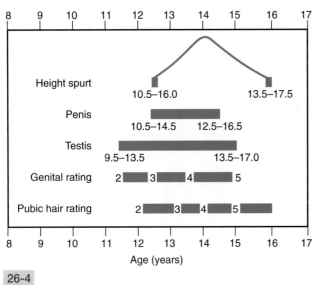

26-4

2 cm long and 1 cm wide. Their size increases only slightly during the prepubertal years.

Adolescents

Puberty begins sometime between the ages of 9½ and 13½. The first sign is enlargement of the testes. Next, pubic hair appears, and then penis size increases. The stages of development are documented in Tanner's sexual maturity rating (Table 26-1).

The complete change in development from a preadolescent to an adult takes approximately 3 years; the normal range is 2 to 5 years (Figure 26-4). The chart shown in Figure 26-4 is useful in teaching a boy the expected sequence of events and in reassuring him about the wide range of ages when these events normally occur.

Adults and Older Adults

The level of sexual development at the end of puberty remains constant through early and middle adulthood, with no further genital growth and no change in circulating sex hormone.

Men do not experience a definite end to fertility, as women do. At approximately age 40 years, the production of sperm begins to decrease, although production continues into the 80s and 90s. After age 55 to 60 years, testosterone production declines very gradually so that resulting physical changes are not evident until later in life. Aging changes also result from decreased muscle tone, decreased subcutaneous fat, and decreased cellular metabolism.

In older men, the amount of pubic hair decreases, and the remaining hair turns grey. Penis size decreases. Because of decreased tone of the dartos muscle, the scrotal contents hang lower, the rugae decrease, and the scrotum looks pendulous. The testes decrease in size and are less firm to palpation. Increased connective tissue is present in the tubules, and so these become thickened and produce less sperm.

In general, declining testosterone production leaves older men with a slower and less intense sexual response. Although a wide range of individual differences can occur, an older man may find that an erection takes longer to develop and that it is less full or firm. Once obtained, the erection may be maintained for longer periods without ejaculation. Ejaculation is shorter and less forceful, and the volume of seminal fluid is less than when the man was younger. After ejaculation, detumescence (return to the flaccid state) is rapid, especially after 60 years of age. This occurs in a few seconds, in comparison with minutes or hours in a younger man. The refractory state—when the man is physiologically unable to ejaculate—lasts longer (from 12 to 24 hours) than in a younger man (2 minutes).

Sexual Expression in Later Life. Chronological age by itself should not halt sexual activity. The aforementioned physical changes need not interfere with libido or pleasure from sexual intercourse. An older man is capable of sexual function as long as he is in reasonably good health and has an interested, willing partner. Even chronic illness does not put a complete end to sexual desire or activity.

An older man may misinterpret normal age changes as sexual failure. Once this idea occurs, it may demoralize the man and place undue emphasis on performance rather than on pleasure. In the absence of disease, older men may withdraw from sexual activity for various reasons: loss of spouse; depression; preoccupation with work; marital or family conflict; side effects of medications such as antihypertensives, psychotropics, antidepressants, antispasmodics, sedatives, tranquilizers or narcotics, and estrogens; heavy use of alcohol; lack of privacy (living with adult children or in a nursing home); economic or emotional stress; poor nutrition; or fatigue.

CULTURAL AND SOCIAL CONSIDERATIONS

On occasion, parents ask about whether to circumcise an infant boy. Common reasons given in favour of circumcision are hygiene, avoidance of a later need for circumcision, medical indications, the father's circumcision status, and religious and cultural values. Since 1975, the policy of the Canadian Paediatric Society is that there is no medical indication for male neonatal circumcision. A statement issued by the Canadian Paediatric Society in 1996 and reaffirmed in 2002 strongly recommended that nontherapeutic neonatal circumcision not be routinely performed, and the procedure is no longer covered by provincial health insurance plans. Neonatal circumcision rates in Canada declined from about 48% in 1970 to about 31.99% in the period 2006 to 2007 (Public Health Agency of Canada, 2009).

Research has demonstrated, however, that circumcision reduces acquisition of the human immunodeficiency virus (HIV) in men by 53% to 60% (Gray, Wawer, Serwadda, & Kigozi, 2009; Viscidi & Shah, 2010) and reduces HIV transmission to uninfected female sexual partners (Wawer et al.,

TABLE 26-1	Sexual Maturity Ratings in Boys		
Developmental Stage	Pubic Hair	Penis	Scrotum
1	No pubic hair; fine body hair on abdomen (vellus hair) continues over pubic area	Preadolescent; size and proportion are the same as during childhood	Preadolescent; size and proportion are the same as during childhood
2	Few straight, slightly darker hairs at base of penis are long and downy	Little or no enlargement	Enlargement of testes and scrotum; scrotal skin reddens and changes in texture
3	Sparse growth over entire pubis; hair is darker, coarser, and curly	Enlargement, especially in length	Further enlargement
4	Thick growth over pubic area but not on thighs; hair coarse and curly, as in adult	Continued enlargement in length and diameter, with development of glans	Testes almost fully grown; scrotum darker
5	Growth spread over medial thighs, although not yet up toward umbilicus; after puberty, pubic hair growth continues until the mid-20s, extending up the abdomen toward the umbilicus	Adult size and shape	Adult size and shape

Source: Adapted from Tanner, J. M. (1962). *Growth at adolescence.* Oxford, UK: Blackwell Scientific Publications.

2009). Circumcision also significantly reduces the incidence of herpes simplex virus type 2 (HSV-2) acquisition; the prevalence of human papillomavirus (HPV) (Tobian et al., 2009); and the risk for other sexually transmitted infections (STIs), such as *Trichomonas vaginalis* and bacterial vaginosis, in women with circumcised partners (Sobngwi-Tambekou et al., 2009). Circumcision carries a very small risk of complications. Most are minor and treatable: pain, bleeding, swelling, or inadequate skin removal. Serious complications are rare and include excess bleeding, wound infections, and urinary retention (Weiss, Larke, Halperin, & Schenker, 2010). Neonates are capable of perceiving pain; therefore, parents need to be apprised of pain-relief measures for the circumcision procedure, including oral and transdermal pain medication, dorsal penile nerve block, and comfort measures such as sucrose pacifier, stroking the infant, talking, and rocking (Stratman-Lucey & Caldwell, 2006).

For an uncircumcised newborn, assess parental knowledge about care of the uncircumcised penis. The infant's penis should be cleansed with soap and water, but the foreskin should not be forcibly retracted. When the foreskin retracts easily, the area under the foreskin should be cleansed occasionally. By the age of 3 or 4 years, a boy can be taught to clean under his foreskin. When a boy reaches puberty, he needs to clean under his foreskin daily.

Infection with HPV is common in boys and men, causes most cases of genital warts, and is associated with cancers of the penis, anus, and head and neck. The quadrivalent HPV vaccine previously approved for the prevention of cervical cancer in girls and women (see p. 753) has demonstrated efficacy in preventing HPV infection and diseases in boys and men (Giuliano et al., 2011). The vaccine has been approved for the prevention of genital warts in boys and men aged 9 to 26 in Canada (Public Health Agency of Canada, 2011).

SUBJECTIVE DATA

1. Frequency, urgency, and nocturia
2. Dysuria
3. Hesitancy and straining
4. Urine colour
5. Past genitourinary history

6. Penis: pain, lesion, discharge
7. Scrotum: self-care behaviours, lump
8. Sexual activity and contraceptive use
9. STI contact

HEALTH HISTORY QUESTIONS

Examiner Asks	Rationale
1. Frequency, urgency, and nocturia. Are you urinating more often than usual?	The average adult voids five to six times per day; this amount varies with fluid intake, individual habits. Polyuria: excessive quantity Oliguria: diminished quantity, <400 mL/ 24 hr
• When you need to urinate, do you feel as if you cannot wait?	**Urgency** may be indicative of infection or conditions causing irritation or obstruction.
• Do you awaken during the night because you need to urinate? How often? Is this a recent change?	**Nocturia** occurs together with frequency and urgency in urinary tract disorders. Other origins: cardiovascular, habitual, diuretic medication.
2. Dysuria. Any pain or burning sensation with urinating?	**Dysuria:** Burning sensation is common with acute cystitis, prostatitis, and urethritis.
3. Hesitancy and straining. Any trouble starting the urine stream?	**Hesitancy** may be indicative of prostate enlargement.
• Do you need to strain to start or maintain the stream?	Straining may be indicative of prostate enlargement.
• Any change in force of stream: narrowing, becoming weaker?	Loss of force and decreased calibre should be investigated.
• Do you experience dribbling, so that you must stand closer to the toilet?	Terminal dribbling should be investigated.
• Afterward, do you still feel you need to urinate?	Sense of residual urine should be investigated.
• Have you ever had any urinary tract infections?	Recurrent episodes of acute cystitis should be investigated. Aforementioned symptoms (i.e., hesitancy and so on) suggest progressive prostatic obstruction.

Examiner Asks	Rationale

4. **Urine colour.** Is the usual urine clear or discoloured, cloudy, foul-smelling, bloody (Figure 26-5)?

Urine is cloudy in urinary tract infection.

Some colour changes are temporary or harmless. However, for blood in urine or for a colour change lasting more than 1 day, the patient should seek health care. For a complete description, see Table 26-2, p. 734.

CRITICAL FINDINGS

Hematuria (blood in the urine)—a danger sign that warrants further workup—is the most common symptom of cancers of the bladder and kidney. Hematuria is also associated with disease, inflammation, infection, or trauma within the urinary tract.

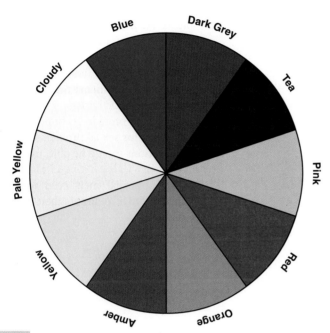

26-5 Urine colour chart.

5. **Past genitourinary history.** Do you have any difficulty controlling your urine?

True incontinence: loss of urine without warning

Urge incontinence: involuntary urine loss from overactive detrusor muscle in bladder; bladder contracts, causing urgent need to void

- Do you accidentally urinate when you sneeze, laugh, cough, or bear down?
- Any *history* of kidney disease, kidney stones, flank pain, urinary tract infections, prostate trouble?

Stress incontinence: involuntary loss of urine with physical strain, sneezing, or coughing; caused by weakness in pelvic floor

6. **Penis.** Any problem with your penis: **pain, lesions?**
- Any **discharge?** How much? Has that increased or decreased since it started?
- What is the colour of the urine? Any odour? Is the discharge associated with pain or with urination?

Urethral discharge occurs with infection.

7. **Scrotum, self-care behaviours.** Any problem with the scrotum or testicles?
- Do you perform testicular self-examination (TSE)?
- Have you noticed any **lump** or **swelling** on your testes?
- Have you noted any change in size of the scrotum?

Assess self-care behaviours.

Concern about any self-discovered mass (spermatocele, hydrocele, varicocele, rarely testicular cancer) alerts you to careful exploration during examination.

- Have you noted any bulge or swelling in the scrotum? For how long? Have you ever been told you have a hernia? Any dragging, heavy feeling in scrotum?

Assess for possible hernia.

8. **Sexual activity and contraceptive use.** Are you now in a relationship involving sexual intercourse?
- Are aspects of sex satisfactory to you and your partner?

Questions about **sexual activity** should be routine in review of body systems for these reasons:

Examiner Asks	Rationale
• Are you satisfied with the way you and your partner communicate about sex?	• This question communicates your acceptance of the patient's sexual activity and belief it is important.
• Occasionally a man notices a change in ability to have an erection when aroused. Have you noticed any changes?*	• Your comfort with discussion prompts patient's interest and possibly relief that topic has been introduced and gives the patient permission to talk about sexual health.
• Do you and your partner use a contraceptive? Which method? Is this satisfactory? Any questions about this method?	
• How many sexual partners have you had in the past 6 months?	• With these data, you establish a database for comparisons with any future sexual activities.
	• These data provide an opportunity to screen for sexual problems.
	Your questions should be objective and matter-of-fact.
• What is your sexual preference: relationship with a woman, a man, both?	Gay and bisexual men need to feel acceptance in order to discuss their health concerns.
9. **STI contact.** Any sexual contact with a partner who has an STI, such as gonorrhea, herpes, HIV, *Chlamydia* infection, genital warts, syphilis?	
• When was this contact? Did you become infected?	
• How was it treated? Any complications?	
• Do you use condoms to help prevent STIs?	
• Any questions or concerns about any of these infections?	

Additional History for Infants and Children

1. **Urination.** Does your child have any problem urinating? Does the urine stream look straight?
   - Any pain, crying, or holding the genitals when your child urinates?
   - Has your child had any urinary tract infection?
2. **Toilet training.** (If child is older than 2½ years) Has toilet training started? How is it progressing?

(If child 5 years or older) Does he wet the bed at night? Is this a problem for the child or for you (parents)? What have you done? How does the child feel about it?	**Nocturnal enuresis:** involuntary passing of urine after an age at which continence is expected.

3. **Abnormalities.** Any problem with child's penis or scrotum: sores, swelling, discoloration?
   - Have you been told whether his testes are descended or undescended?
   - Has he ever had a hernia or hydrocele?
   - Have you seen swelling in his scrotum during crying or coughing?

4. **Molestation.** (Ask directly of preschooler or young school-age child) "Has anyone ever touched your penis or in between your legs and you did not want them to? Sometimes that happens to children, and it's not okay." The patient should be reminded that he has not been "bad" and that he should try to tell an adult about it. "Can you tell me three different big people you trust who you could talk to?"	Screen for sexual abuse. For prevention, teach the child that it is not "okay" for someone to look at or touch their private parts while telling them it is a secret. Being asked to name three trusted adults will help the child include someone outside the family: This is important because most molestation is performed by a parent.

Additional History for Preadolescents and Adolescents

Use the following questions regarding sexual growth and development and sexual behaviour. First:

*Phrase your questions so that the patient is comfortable acknowledging a problem.

Examiner Asks	Rationale

- Ask questions appropriate for a boy's age, but be aware that norms vary widely. When you are in doubt, it is better to ask too many questions than to omit something. Children obtain information, often misinformation, from the media and from peers at surprisingly early ages. Your information will be more thoughtful and accurate.
- Ask direct, matter-of-fact questions. Avoid sounding judgemental.
- Start with a *permission statement.* "Often boys your age experience…." This conveys that it is normal and all right to think or feel a certain way.
- Try the *ubiquity approach.* "When did you…." rather than "Do you…." This method is less threatening because it implies that the topic is normal and unexceptional.
- Do not be concerned if a boy will not discuss sexuality with you or respond to offers for information. He may not feel comfortable letting on that he needs or wants more information. You should convey your willingness to talk when the boy is ready. The adolescent may come back at a future time.

1. **Puberty.** At approximately ages 12 to 13 years, but sometimes earlier, boys start to change and grow around the penis and scrotum. What changes have you noticed? Have you ever seen charts and pictures of normal growth patterns for boys? Let us go over these now.
   - Whom can you talk to about your body changes and about sex information? How do these talks go? Do you think you get enough information? What about sex education classes at school? How about your parents? Is there a favourite teacher, nurse, doctor, minister, or counsellor to whom you can talk?

2. **Nocturnal emission.** Boys approximately 12 to 13 years old (sexual maturity rating 3) have a normal experience of fluid coming out of the penis at night, called a *nocturnal emission,* or "wet dream." Have you had this?

   On occasion, a boy confuses this with a sign of STI or feels guilty.

3. **Erotic feelings.** Teenage boys have other normal experiences and wonder if they are the only ones who ever had them, like having an erection at embarrassing times, having sexual fantasies, or masturbating. Also, a boy might have a thought about touching another boy's genitals and wonder whether this means he might be homosexual. Would you like to talk about any of these things?

   A boy may feel guilty about experiencing these feelings if he is not informed that they are normal.

4. **Sexual activity.** Often boys your age have questions about sexual activity. What questions do you have? How about things such as birth control, or STIs such as gonorrhea or herpes? Any questions about these?
   - Are you dating? Someone steady? Have you had intercourse? Are you using birth control? What kind?

   Assess level of knowledge. Many boys do not admit that they need more knowledge.

   Avoid the term "having sex." It is ambiguous, and teenagers can take it to mean anything from foreplay to intercourse. Use behaviour-specific words.

   - What kind of birth control did you use the *last* time you had intercourse?

   This particular question often elicits the information that the teenager is not using any method of birth control.

5. **Self-examination.** Has a nurse or doctor ever taught you how to examine your own testicles to make sure they are healthy?

   Assess knowledge of TSE.

6. **Molestation.** Has anyone ever touched your genitals when you did not want him or her to? Another boy, or an adult, even a relative? Sometimes that happens to teenagers. They should remember it is not their fault. They should tell another adult about it.

Additional History for Older Adults

1. **Prostate enlargement.** Do you have any difficulty urinating? Any hesitancy and straining? Is the force of stream weaker? Any dribbling? Or any incomplete emptying?

   Early symptoms of enlarging prostate may be tolerated or ignored. Later symptoms are more dramatic: hematuria, urinary tract infection.

2. **Incontinence.** Do you ever leak water/urine when you do not want to? Do you use pads or tissue to catch urine in your underwear?

   Incontinence is any involuntary leaking of urine.

Examiner Asks	Rationale

3. **Nocturia.** Do you need to get up at night to urinate? What medications are you taking? What fluids do you drink in the evening?

Nocturia may be habitual, or it may be caused by diuretic medication or fluid ingestion 3 hours before bedtime; coffee and alcohol in particular have a diuretic effect. Also, fluid retention from mild heart failure or varicose veins produces nocturia because recumbency at night mobilizes fluid.

4. **Sexual function.** A man in his 70s, 80s, or 90s may experience changes in his sexual relationship or in his sexual response; have you noticed this? Have you wondered whether it is normal? For example, it is normal for an erection to develop slowly at this age. This is not a sign of impotence, but a man might wonder if it is. Except in cases of physical illness, older men are fully capable of sexual function.

Some older men assume normal changes mean they are "old men" and withdraw from sexual activity. Older men are not reluctant to discuss sexual activity, and most welcome the opportunity.

Substances that depress sexual desire and function include antihypertensives, sedatives, tranquilizers, estrogens, and alcohol. Alcohol decreases the sexual response even more dramatically in older men.

OBJECTIVE DATA

PREPARATION

Position the male patient standing with undershorts down. Appropriate draping protects the modesty of the patient. This is important for male patients of all ethnocultural backgrounds. The examiner should be sitting. Alternatively, the patient may be supine for the first part of the examination and stand to be checked for a hernia.

It is normal for a male patient to feel apprehensive about having his genitalia examined, especially by a female examiner. Younger adolescents usually have more anxiety than do older adolescents. But any male patient may have difficulty dissociating a necessary, matter-of-fact step in the physical examination from the feeling that this is an invasion of his privacy. His concerns are similar to those experienced by the female patient during the examination of the genitalia: modesty, fear of pain, cold hands, negative judgement, or memory of previously uncomfortable examinations. In addition, he may fear comparison with other male patients, or he may fear having an erection during the examination and that this would be misinterpreted by the examiner.

This normal apprehension becomes manifested in different behaviours. Many patients act resigned and embarrassed and avoid eye contact. On occasion, a man will laugh and make jokes to cover embarrassment. Also, a man may refuse examination by a female examiner and insist on a male examiner.

Take time to consider these feelings, as well as to explore your own. It is normal for you to feel embarrassed and apprehensive, too. You may worry about your age, lack of clinical experience, causing pain, or even that your movements might "cause" an erection. Some examiners feel guilty when this occurs. You need to accept these feelings and work through them so that you can examine the male patient in a professional way. Discuss these concerns with an experienced examiner. Your unresolved discomfort magnifies any discomfort that the patient may have.

Your demeanour should be *confident* and relaxed, unhurried and yet businesslike. Do not discuss genitourinary history or sexual practices while you are performing the examination; this may be perceived as judgemental. Use a firm, deliberate touch, not a soft, stroking one. If an erection does occur, do *not* stop the examination or leave the room. This only focuses more attention on the erection and increases embarrassment. Reassure the male patient that this is only a normal physiological response to touch, just as when the pupil constricts in response to bright light. Proceed with the rest of the examination.

EQUIPMENT NEEDED

Gloves: wear gloves during every examination of male genitalia
Occasionally: glass slide for urethral specimen
Materials for cytological study
Flashlight

Normal Range of Findings	Abnormal Findings

INSPECT AND PALPATE THE PENIS

The skin normally looks wrinkled, hairless, and without lesions (Figure 26-6). The dorsal vein may be apparent.

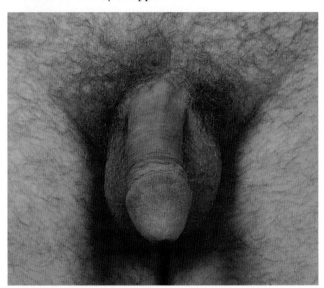

26-6

The glans looks smooth and without lesions. Ask the uncircumcised male patient to retract the foreskin, or you retract it. It should move easily. Some cheesy smegma may have collected under the foreskin. After inspection, slide the foreskin back to the original position.

The urethral meatus is positioned just about centrally.

At the base of the penis, pubic hair distribution is consistent with age. Hair is without infestations.

Compress the glans anteroposteriorly between your thumb and forefinger (Figure 26-7). The meatus edge should appear pink, smooth, and without discharge.

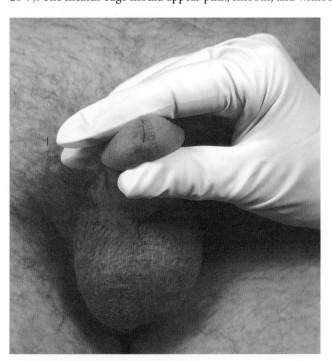

26-7

Abnormal Findings

Inflammation.
Lesions: nodules, solitary ulcer (chancre), grouped vesicles or superficial ulcers, wartlike papules (see Table 26-4, p. 736).

Inflammation; lesions on glans or corona
Phimosis: inability to retract the foreskin
Paraphimosis: inability to return foreskin to original position
Hypospadias: ventral location of meatus
Epispadias: dorsal location of meatus (see Table 26-5, p. 737)
Pubic lice or nits can be seen with the unaided eye. Excoriated skin usually accompanies their presence.
Stricture: narrowed opening.
Edges that are red, everted, and edematous, along with purulent discharge, are suggestive of urethritis (see Table 26-4, p. 735).

Objective Data

Normal Range of Findings	Abnormal Findings

If you note urethral discharge, collect a smear for microscopic examination and a culture. If no discharge shows but the person gives a history of it, ask him to milk the shaft of the penis. This should produce a drop of discharge.

Urethral discharge occurs with infection.

Palpate the shaft of the penis between your thumb and first two fingers. Normally, the penis feels smooth, semifirm, and nontender.

Nodule or induration.
Tenderness.

INSPECT AND PALPATE THE SCROTUM

Inspect the scrotum as the patient holds the penis out of the way. Alternatively, you hold the penis out of the way with the back of your hand (Figure 26-8). Scrotal size varies with ambient room temperature. Asymmetry is normal; the left scrotal half is usually lower than the right half.

Scrotal swelling (edema) may be taut and pitting. This occurs with heart failure, renal failure, and local inflammation.
Lesions should be investigated.

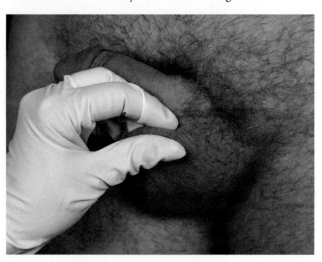

26-8

Spread rugae out between your fingers. Lift the sac to inspect the posterior surface. Normally, no scrotal lesions are present, except for sebaceous cysts, which are commonly found. These are yellowish, 1-cm nodules and are firm, nontender, and often multiple.

Inflammation.

Palpate gently each scrotal half between your thumb and first two fingers (Figure 26-9). The scrotal contents should slide easily. Testes normally feel oval, firm and rubbery, smooth, and equal bilaterally, and they are freely movable and slightly tender to moderate pressure. Each epididymis normally feels discrete, softer than the testis, smooth, and nontender.

Absence of testis: may be a temporary migration or true cryptorchidism (see Table 26-6, p. 738).
Atrophied testes: small and soft.
Fixed testes.
Nodules on testes or epididymides.
Marked tenderness.
An indurated, swollen, and tender epididymis: indicative of epididymitis.

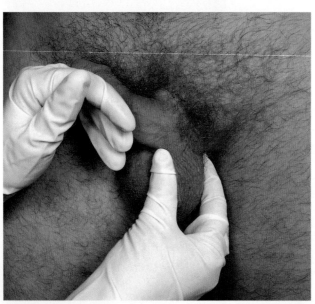

26-9

Normal Range of Findings	Abnormal Findings

Palpate each spermatic cord between your thumb and forefinger, along its length from the epididymis up to the external inguinal ring (Figure 26-10, *A*). You should feel a smooth, nontender cord.

Normally, no other scrotal contents are present. If you do find a mass, note the following:

- Is there any tenderness?
- Is the mass distal or proximal to testis?
- Can you place your fingers over it?
- Is it reduced when the patient lies down?
- Can you auscultate bowel sounds over it?

Thickened cord.

Soft, swollen, and tortuous cord: see varicocele (see Figure 26-10, *B*).

Abnormalities in the scrotum: hernia, tumour, orchitis, epididymitis, hydrocele, spermatocele, varicocele (see Table 26-6, pp. 738–740).

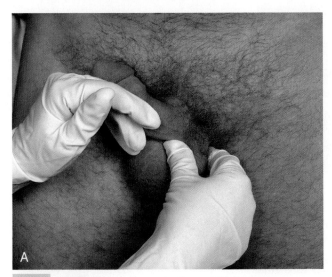

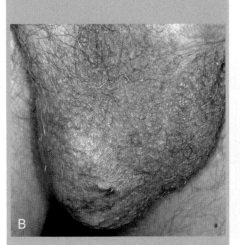

26-10   **A,** Palpating each spermatic cord. **B,** Varicocele.

Transillumination. Perform this manoeuvre only if you note a swelling or mass. Darken the room. Shine a strong flashlight from behind the scrotal contents. Normal scrotal contents cannot be transilluminated.

Serous fluid (e.g., hydrocele or spermatocele) can be transilluminated and glows red. Solid tissue (e.g., hernia, epididymitis, or tumour) and blood cannot be transilluminated (see Table 26-6, p. 738).

INSPECT AND PALPATE FOR HERNIA

Inspect the inguinal region for a bulge as the patient stands and as he strains down. Normally, none is present.

Bulge at external inguinal ring or at femoral canal should be investigated. (A hernia may be present but is easily reduced and may appear only intermittently with an increase in intra-abdominal pressure.)

A palpable herniating mass bumps your fingertip or pushes against the side of your finger (see Table 26-7, p. 742).

Palpate the inguinal canal (Figure 26-11). For the right side, ask the patient to shift his weight onto the left (unexamined) leg. Place your right index finger low on the right scrotal half. Palpate up the length of the spermatic cord, invaginating the scrotal skin as you go, to the external inguinal ring. It feels like a triangular slitlike opening, and it may or may not admit your finger. If it will admit your finger, gently insert it into the canal and ask the person to "bear down."* Normally, you feel no change. Repeat the procedure on the left side.

Palpate the femoral area for a bulge. Normally, you feel none.

*Avoid the old instruction to "turn your head and cough." For one thing, a brief cough does not produce the steady, increased intra-abdominal pressure you need. For another, the patient might cough right in your face.

Normal Range of Findings	Abnormal Findings

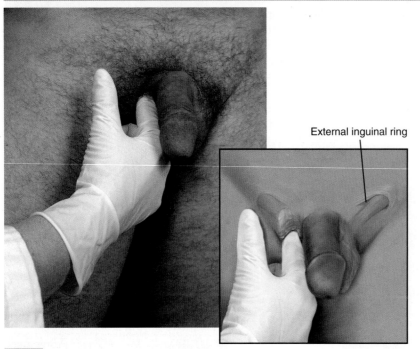

External inguinal ring

26-11

PALPATE THE INGUINAL LYMPH NODES

Palpate the horizontal chain along the groin inferior to the inguinal ligament and the vertical chain along the upper inner thigh.

It is normal to palpate an isolated node on occasion; it then feels small (<1 cm), soft, discrete, and movable (Figure 26-12).

Enlarged, hard, matted, fixed nodes.

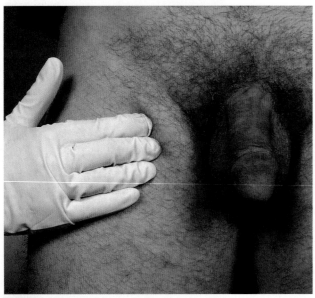

26-12

ASSESSMENT OF URINE OUTPUT

Normal adult urine output is 1500 mL per day, which varies with food and fluid intake, and normal bladder capacity ranges from 600 to 1000 mL. Most people urinate five to six times during the day and occasionally at night. On average, 200 to 250 mL of urine in the bladder causes moderate distension and the urge to urinate; 400 to 600 mL causes discomfort (Lewis et al., 2010).

CRITICAL FINDINGS

Acute urinary retention is an inability to pass urine, characterized by lower abdominal pain and bladder distension. It may be confirmed by bladder scan. Report acute urinary retention immediately; management involves bladder decompression by intermittent or indwelling urinary catheter.

Objective Data

Normal Range of Findings

Abnormal Findings

ASSESSMENT OF PATIENT WITH INDWELLING URINARY CATHETER

Monitor catheterized patients for signs and symptoms of catheter-acquired urinary tract infection, the most common infection in acute and long-term care settings. Risk factors include prolonged catheterization (>6 days), female gender, diabetes, malnutrition, old age, and impaired immunity.

Catheter should be properly anchored; tubing should be free from kinking; collecting bag should be below bladder level (Figure 26-13); urethral meatus is pink, smooth, and without discharge.

Assess urine output.

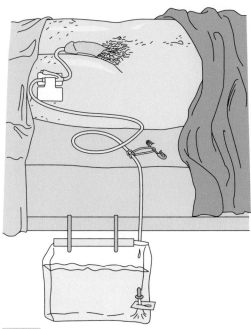

26-13 Indwelling urinary catheter.

Urgency, suprapubic tenderness, costovertebral angle pain or tenderness, fever >38°C, change in character of urine (bloody, foul smell, increased sediment), positive dipstick for leukocytes, worsening of mental or functional status.

Drainage or excoriation of urethral orifice.

CRITICAL FINDINGS

Decreased urine output may be a sign of renal or systemic problems such as dehydration, renal failure or hypovolemic shock. In an adult, urine output of less than 30 mL/hour can indicate decreased renal perfusion and should be reported (Perry & Potter, 2010, p. 168).

SELF-CARE: TESTICULAR SELF-EXAMINATION

The overall incidence is rare, but testicular cancer occurs most commonly in men aged 15 to 49. Other risk factors include delayed descent of the testicles (if not corrected early), family or personal history of testicular cancer, and abnormal development of the testicle. Some men develop testicular cancer without having any of these risk factors. Some authorities consider teaching TSE controversial because the harm of causing anxiety and unwarranted medical costs exceed benefits of detection of a relatively rare lesion (Joffe, 2009). If detected early by palpation and treated, the cure rate is almost 100%; therefore, all men aged 15 years and older should be aware of how their testicles normally look and feel and should report any of the following changes (Canadian Cancer Society, 2011) to a doctor:
- A lump on the testicle
- A painful testicle
- A feeling of heaviness or dragging in the lower abdomen or scrotum
- A dull ache in the lower abdomen and groin
  Points to include during health teaching are as follows:
- *T* = timing, once a month
- *S* = showering; warm water relaxes scrotal sac
- *E* = examining, checking for changes, reporting changes immediately

Objective Data

Normal Range of Findings	**Abnormal Findings**

Phrase your teaching something like this (Figure 26-14):

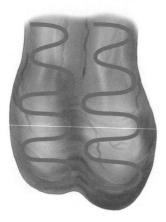

26-14 Instruct patients to check each testicle by feeling it in a systematic pattern, such as the one shown.

A good time to examine the testicles is during the shower or bath, when your hands are warm and soapy and the scrotum is warm. Cold hands stimulate a muscle (cremasteric) reflex, which causes the the scrotal contents to retract. The procedure is simple. Hold the scrotum in the palm of your hand and gently feel each testicle, using your thumb and first two fingers. If it hurts, you are using too much pressure. The testicle is egg-shaped and movable. It feels rubbery with a smooth surface, like a peeled hard-boiled egg. The epididymis is on top and behind the testicle; it feels a bit softer. If you ever notice a firm, painless lump, a hard area, or an overall enlarged testicle, call your physician for a further check.

 DEVELOPMENTAL CONSIDERATIONS

Infants and Children

For an infant or toddler, perform this procedure right after the abdominal examination. In preschool-age and young school-age children (3 to 8 years of age), leave underpants on until just before the examination. In an older school-age child or adolescent, offer an extra drape, as with an adult. Reassure the child and parents of normal findings.

Inspect the penis and scrotum. Penis size is usually small in infants (2 to 3 cm; Figure 26-15) and in young boys until puberty. In obese boys, the penis looks even smaller because of folds of skin covering the base.

In rare cases, a very small penis may be an enlarged clitoris in a genetically female infant.

Enlarged penis is indicative of precocious puberty.

Redness, swelling, and lesions should be investigated.

Urethral discharge occurs with infection.

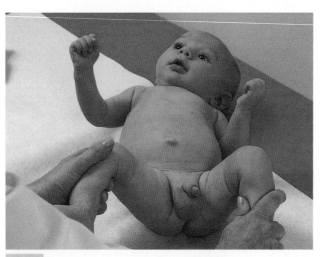

26-15

Normal Range of Findings	Abnormal Findings

Normal Range of Findings

In the circumcised infant, the glans looks smooth with the meatus centred at the tip. During the diaper-wearing stage, the meatus may become ulcerated from ammonia irritation. This is more common in circumcised infants.

If possible, observe the newborn's first voiding to assess strength and direction of stream.

If the infant is uncircumcised, the foreskin is normally tight during the first 3 months and should *not* be retracted because of the risk of tearing the membrane attaching the foreskin to the shaft. This leads to scarring and, possibly, to adhesions later in life. In infants older than 3 months of age, retract the foreskin gently to check the glans and meatus. It should return to its original position easily.

The scrotum looks pink in light-skinned infants and dark brown in dark-skinned infants. Rugae are well formed in full-term infants. Size varies with ambient temperature, but overall, the infant's scrotum looks large in relation to the penis. No bulges, either constant or intermittent, are present.

Palpate the scrotum and testes. The cremasteric reflex is strong in the infant, pulling the testes up into the inguinal canal and abdomen from exposure to cold, touch, exercise, or emotion. Take care not to elicit the reflex; to prevent it, (a) keep your hands warm and palpate from the external inguinal ring down, and (b) block the inguinal canals with the thumb and forefinger of your other hand to prevent the testes from retracting (Figure 26-16).

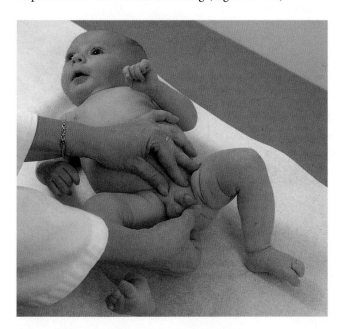

26-16

Normally, the testes are descended and equal in size bilaterally (1.5 to 2 cm until puberty). It is important to document that you have palpated the testes. Once palpated, they are considered descended, even if they have retracted momentarily at the next visit.

If the scrotal half feels empty, search for the testes along the inguinal canal and try to milk them down. Ask the toddler or child to squat with the knees flexed up; this pressure may force the testes down. Another manoeuvre is have the young child sit cross-legged to relax the reflex (Figure 26-17).

Abnormal Findings

Hypospadias, epispadias (see Table 26-5, p. 737) should be corrected.

Stricture is a narrowed opening.

On occasion, ulceration may produce a stricture, evidenced by a pinpoint meatus and a narrow stream. This increases the risk of urine obstruction.

Poor stream is significant because it may indicate a stricture or neurogenic bladder.

In phimosis, the foreskin is tight and cannot be retracted.

In paraphimosis, the foreskin cannot be slipped forward once it is retracted.

Dirt and smegma may collect under the foreskin.

Cryptorchidism: undescended testes (those that have never descended). Undescended testes are common in premature infants. They occur in 3% to 4% of full-term infants, although in most cases, they have descended by 3 months of age. Physicians have different opinions concerning the age at which an affected child should be referred (see Table 26-6, p. 738).

Objective Data

Normal Range of Findings	Abnormal Findings

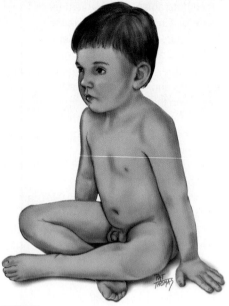

26-17

Objective Data

Migratory testes (physiological cryptorchidism) are common because of the strength of the cremasteric reflex and the small mass of the prepubertal testes. Note that the affected side has a normally developed scrotum (with true cryptorchidism, the scrotum is atrophic) and the testis can be milked down. These testes descend at puberty and are normal.

Palpate the epididymis and spermatic cord as described for adults. A common scrotal finding in the boy younger than 2 years is a **hydrocele** (fluid in the scrotum). It appears as enlargement of the scrotum and glows faint pink under transillumination. It usually disappears spontaneously.

Inspect the inguinal area for a bulge. If you do not see a bulge but the parent gives a positive history of one, try to elicit it by increasing intra-abdominal pressure. Ask the boy to hold his breath and strain down, or have him blow up a balloon.

If a hernia is suspected, palpate the inguinal area. Use your little finger to reach the external inguinal ring.

A hydrocele is a cystic collection of serous fluid in the tunica vaginalis, surrounding the testis (see Table 26-6, p. 740).

Adolescents

Adolescents show wide variation in normal development of the genitals. Using the sexual maturity rating charts, note (a) enlargement of the testes and scrotum; (b) pubic hair growth; (c) darkening of scrotal colour; (d) roughening of scrotal skin; (e) increase in penis length and width; and (f) axillary hair growth.

Be familiar with the normal sequence of growth.

Older Adults

In older men, you may note thinner, greying pubic hair and decreased size of the penis. Testes may decrease in size and feel less firm. The scrotal sac is pendulous, with fewer rugae. The scrotal skin may become excoriated if the man continually sits on it.

DOCUMENTATION AND CRITICAL THINKING

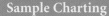

Sample Charting

SUBJECTIVE

Urinates four to five times per day; urine clear, straw-coloured. No nocturia, dysuria, or hesitancy. No pain, lesions, or discharge from penis. Does not perform TSE. No history of genitourinary disease. Sexually active in a monogamous relationship. Sexual life satisfactory to self and partner. Uses birth control via barrier method (partner uses diaphragm). No known STI contact.

OBJECTIVE

No lesions, inflammation, or discharge from penis. Scrotum: testes descended, symmetrical, no masses. No inguinal hernia.

ASSESSMENT

Genital structures normal.

Focused Assessment: Clinical Case Study

R.C. is a 19-year-old student who 2 days PTA noted acute onset of painful urination, frequency, and urgency. Noted some thick penile discharge.

SUBJECTIVE

States has no side pain, no abdominal pain, no fever, no genital skin rash. R.C. is concerned he has an STI because of episode of unprotected intercourse with a new partner 6 days PTA. Has no known allergies.

OBJECTIVE

Vital signs: Temp 37°C; HR72; RR-16. No lesions or inflammation around penis or scrotum. Urethral meatus has mild edema with purulent urethral discharge. No pain on palpation of genitalia. Testes symmetrical with no masses. No lymphadenopathy.

ASSESSMENT

Urethral discharge
Deficient knowledge about STI prevention R/T lack of information recall

Documentation &
Critical Thinking

ABNORMAL FINDINGS

TABLE 26-2   Urine Colour and Discolorations

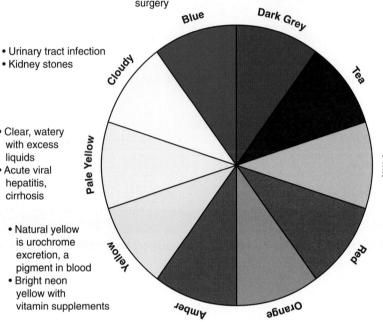

- Medication side effect: amitriptyline, indomethacin (Indocin)
- Foods: asparagus
- Dye after prostate surgery

- Urine contains melanin, melaninuria

- Liver disease, especially with pale stools, jaundice
- Myoglobinuria
- Some medications or food dyes
- Blood in urine

- Urinary tract infection
- Kidney stones

- Clear, watery with excess liquids
- Acute viral hepatitis, cirrhosis

- Some foods: beets, berries, food dyes
- Some laxatives
- Kidney stones
- Urinary tract infection

- Natural yellow is urochrome excretion, a pigment in blood
- Bright neon yellow with vitamin supplements

- Blood in urine
- Nephritis, cystitis
- Cancer
- Following prostate surgery

Blue
Dark Grey
Cloudy
Tea
Pale Yellow
Pink
Yellow
Red
Amber
Orange

- Gold coloured or concentrated with dehydration
- Some laxatives
- Food or supplements with B-complex vitamins

- Medication side effect: rifampin for meningitis, phenazopyridine (Pyridium), warfarin (Coumadin)
- Some foods, food dyes, laxatives
- Dehydration
- Jaundice (bilirubinemia)

TABLE 26-3   Urinary Problems

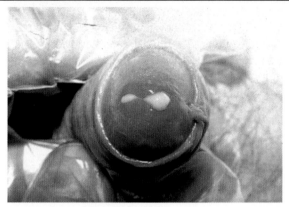

Reprinted from Emond, R. (1995). Colour atlas of infectious diseases (3rd ed., p. 161). St. Louis: Mosby.

◀ *Urethritis (Urethral Discharge and Dysuria)*
Infection of urethra causes painful burning urination or pruritus. Meatus edges are reddened, everted, and swollen with purulent discharge. Urine is cloudy with discharge and mucous shreds. Cause determined by culture: (a) In gonococcal urethritis, discharge is thick, profuse, and yellow or grey-brown; (b) in nonspecific urethritis, discharge may be similar but often is scanty and mucoid. Of these infections, about 50% are caused by *Chlamydia* organisms. This is important to differentiate because antibiotic treatment is different.

Renal Calculi (Not Illustrated)
Renal stones (crystals of calcium oxalate or uric acid) form in kidney tubules and then migrate. Their presence becomes an emergency when they pass into the ureter, become lodged, and obstruct urine flow. They cause abrupt, severe flank pain, which radiates to the groin or abdomen; nausea and vomiting; restlessness; and gross or microscopic hematuria.

Acute Urinary Retention (Not Illustrated)
Affected patients experience abrupt inability to pass urine, with bladder distension and lower abdominal pain. This is much more common in men than in women because of bladder outlet obstruction, such as benign prostatic hyperplasia (see Chapter 23). Catheterization must be performed to relieve acute discomfort; then the underlying problem must be managed.

TABLE 26-4   Male Genital Lesions

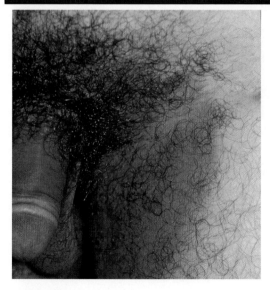

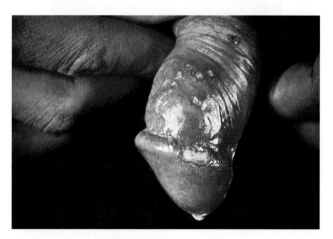

Tinea Cruris
A fungal infection in the crural fold, not extending to scrotum, occurring in postpubertal boys and men ("jock itch") after sweating or wearing layers of occlusive clothing. It forms a red-brown half-moon shape with well-defined borders.

Genital Herpes: HSV-2 Infection
Clusters of small vesicles with surrounding erythema, which are often painful, erupt on the glans or foreskin. These rupture to form superficial ulcers. Genital herpes is a sexually transmitted infection (STI); the initial manifestation lasts 7–10 days. The virus remains dormant indefinitely; recurrent manifestations last 3–10 days with milder symptoms.

Continued

TABLE 26-4   Male Genital Lesions—cont'd

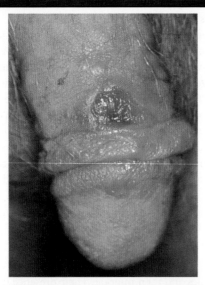

◄ *Syphilitic Chancre*

Manifests within 2–4 weeks of infection as a small, solitary, silvery papule that erodes to a red, round or oval, superficial ulcer with a yellowish serous discharge. Palpation reveals a nontender, indurated base that can be lifted like a button between the thumb and the finger. Lymph nodes enlarge early but are nontender. Syphilis, an STI, is easily treated with penicillin G, but if untreated, it leads to cardiac problems, neurological problems, and blindness.

Reprinted from Emond, R. (1995). Colour atlas of infectious diseases (3rd ed., p. 173). St. Louis: Mosby, by permission of the publisher.

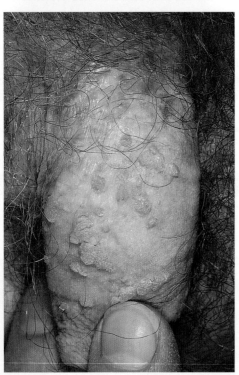

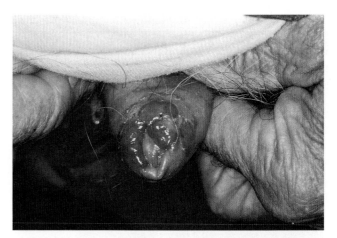

Genital Warts

Soft, pointed, moist, fleshy, painless papules may be single or multiple in a cauliflower-like patch. Colour may be grey, pale yellow, or pink in White men and black or translucent grey-black in Black men. They occur on the shaft of the penis, behind the corona, or around the anus, where they may grow into large grapelike clusters.

These are caused by the human papillomavirus (HPV), which is one of the most common STIs. The HPV infection is correlated with early onset of sexual activity, infrequent use of contraception, and multiple sexual partners.

Carcinoma

Begins as red, raised warty growth or as an ulcer, with watery discharge. As it grows, it may necrose and slough. It is usually painless. It almost always appears on the glans or inner lip of the foreskin and after chronic inflammation. Enlarged lymph nodes are common.

TABLE 26-5   Abnormalities of the Penis

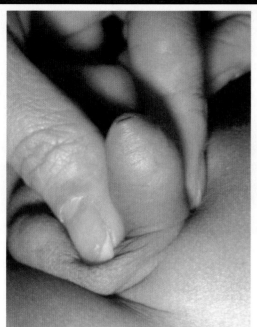

◄ *Phimosis*

Nonretractable foreskin forms a pointy tip with a tiny orifice. Foreskin is advanced and so tight that it is impossible to retract over glans. May be congenital or acquired from adhesions secondary to infection. Poor hygiene leads to retained dirt and smegma, which increases risk of inflammation, calculus formation, and obstructive uropathy.

Paraphimosis (Not Illustrated)

Foreskin is retracted and fixed. Once retracted behind glans, a tight or inflamed foreskin cannot return to its original position. Constriction impedes circulation, and so glans swells. A medical emergency; the constricting band prevents venous and lymphatic return from the glans and compromises arterial circulation.

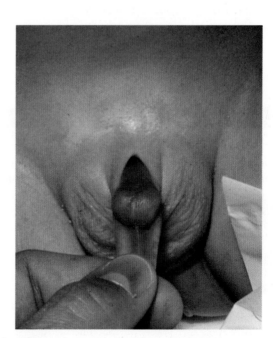

Hypospadias

Urethral meatus opens on the ventral aspect (underside) of glans or shaft or at the penoscrotal junction. A groove extends from the meatus to the normal location at the tip. This congenital defect should be recognized at birth. Affected newborns should not be circumcised because surgical correction may entail use of foreskin tissue to extend urethral length.

Epispadias

Meatus opens on the dorsal (upper) side of glans or shaft above a broad, spadelike penis. Rare; less common than hypospadias but more disabling because of associated urinary incontinence and separation of pubic bones. Corrective surgery is usually done in early childhood.

Continued

Abnormal Findings

TABLE 26-5   Abnormalities of the Penis—cont'd

Urethral Stricture (Not Illustrated)
Pinpoint, constricted opening at meatus or inside along urethra. Occurs congenitally or secondary to urethral injury. Gradual decrease in force and calibre of urine stream is the most common symptom. Shaft feels indurated along ventral aspect at the site of the stricture.

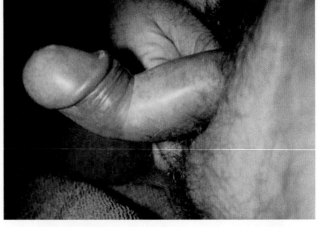

Priapism (Not Illustrated)
Prolonged painful erection of penis without sexual stimulation and unrelieved by intercourse or masturbation, most common in men in 30s and 40s. This condition is rare, but when it lasts 4 hours or longer, it can cause ischemia of penis, fibrosis of tissue, and erectile dysfunction. Can occur as a side effect of some medications and street drugs and with sickle cell trait or disease; with leukemia, when increased numbers of white blood cells produce engorgement; with malignancy; and as a result of local trauma or spinal cord injuries with autonomic nervous system dysfunction.

Peyronie's Disease
Hard, nontender, subcutaneous plaques palpated on dorsal or lateral surface of penis. May be single or multiple and asymmetrical. They are associated with painful bending of the penis during erection. Plaques are fibrosis of covering of corpora cavernosa. Usually occurs after age 45 years. Its cause is trauma to the erect penis, such as an unexpected change in angle during intercourse. More common in men with diabetes, gout, and Dupuytren's contracture of the palm.

TABLE 26-6   Abnormalities in the Scrotum

Disorder	Clinical Findings	Discussion
Absence of Testis (Cryptorchidism) 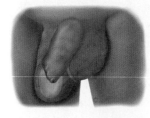	S: Empty scrotal half. O: Inspection: in true maldescent, atrophic scrotum on affected side. Palpation: no testis. A: Absence of testis.	True cryptorchidism: testes that have never descended. Incidence at birth is 3%–4%; in half these cases, the testes descend in first month. Incidence in premature infants is 30%; in adults, 0.7%–0.8%. True undescended testes undergo a histological change by 6 years, causing decreased spermatogenesis and infertility.
Small Testis 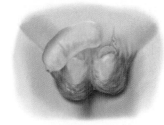	S: None. O (palpation): small and soft (in rare cases, may be firm). A: Small testis.	Smallness with softness (<3.5 cm) indicates atrophy, as with cirrhosis, hypopituitarism, after estrogen therapy, or as a sequelae of orchitis. Smallness with firmness (<2 cm) occurs with Klinefelter's syndrome (hypogonadism).

TABLE 26-6	Abnormalities in the Scrotum—cont'd	
Disorder	Clinical Findings	Discussion
Testicular Torsion 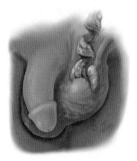	S: Excruciating pain in testicle; of sudden onset, often during sleep or after trauma. May be accompanied by lower abdominal pain, nausea, and vomiting, but no fever. O: • Inspection: red, swollen scrotum, one testis (usually left) higher as a result of rotation and shortening. • Palpation: cord feels thick, swollen, tender; epididymis may be anterior; cremasteric reflex is absent on side of torsion. A: Acute, painful swelling of spermatic cord, with elevation of one testis.	Sudden twisting of spermatic cord. Occurs in late childhood and early adolescence; rare after age 20 years. Torsion usually occurs on the left side. Faulty anchoring of testis on wall of scrotum allows testis to rotate. The anterior part of the testis rotates medially toward the other testis. Blood supply is cut off, which results in ischemia and engorgement. This is an emergency necessitating surgery; testis can become gangrenous in a few hours.
Epididymitis 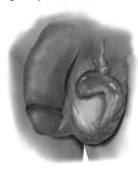	S: Severe pain of sudden onset in scrotum, somewhat relieved by elevation (a positive Phren sign); also rapid swelling, fever. O: • Inspection: enlarged scrotum; reddened. • Palpation: exquisitely tender; epididymis enlarged, indurated; may be hard to distinguish from testis. Overlying scrotal skin may be thick and edematous. • Laboratory: white blood cells and bacteria in urine. A: Tender swelling of epididymis.	Acute infection of epididymis is commonly caused by prostatitis; occurs after prostatectomy because of trauma of urethral instrumentation; or is caused by *Chlamydia*, gonorrhea, or other bacterial infection. Distinguishing between epididymitis and testicular torsion is often difficult.
Varicocele 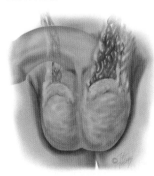	S: Dull pain; constant pulling or dragging sensation; or may be asymptomatic. O: • Inspection: usually no sign. Bluish colour may show through light scrotal skin. • Palpation: when patient is standing, a soft, irregular mass is palpable posterior to and above testis; collapses when patient is supine, refills when patient is upright. Feels distinctive, like a "bag of worms." • The testis on the side of the varicocele may be smaller because of impaired circulation. A: Soft mass on spermatic cord.	A varicocele is a collection of dilated, tortuous varicose veins in the spermatic cord as a result of incompetent valves within the vein, which enable reflux of blood. It occurs most often on left side, perhaps because left spermatic vein is longer and inserts at a right angle into left renal vein. Common in boys and young men. Screen at early adolescence; early treatment is important to prevent potential infertility in adulthood.

Continued

TABLE 26-6	Abnormalities in the Scrotum—cont'd	
Disorder	**Clinical Findings**	**Discussion**
Spermatocele 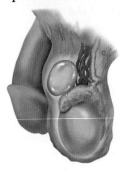	S: Painless, usually found on examination. O: • Inspection: can be transilluminated higher in the scrotum than a hydrocele, and the sperm may be fluorescent. • Palpation: round, freely movable mass lying above and behind testis. If large, feels like a third testis. A: Free cystic mass on epididymis.	Retention cyst in epididymis. Cause unclear but may be obstruction of tubules. Filled with thin, milky fluid that contains sperm. Most spermatoceles are small (<1 cm); occasionally are larger and then may be mistaken for hydrocele.
Early Testicular Tumour 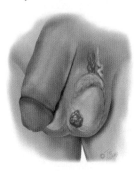	S: Painless, found on examination. O (palpation): firm nodule or harder than normal section of testicle. A: Solitary nodule.	Most testicular tumours occur in men between the ages of 15 and 49. Practically all are malignant and occur most often in men of European descent. Biopsy is necessary to confirm malignancy. Most important risk factor is undescended testis, even those surgically corrected. Early detection is important in prognosis, but practice of testicular self-examination is currently low.
Diffuse Tumour 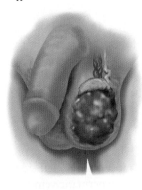	S: Enlarging testis (most common symptom). When enlarges, has feel of increased weight. O: • Inspection: enlarged, cannot be transilluminated. • Palpation: enlarged, smooth, ovoid, firm. • Important: firm palpation does *not* cause usual sickening discomfort as with normal testis. A: Nontender swelling of testis.	Diffuse tumour maintains shape of testis.
Hydrocele 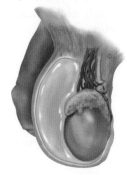	S: Painless swelling, although affected patient may complain of weight and bulk in scrotum. O: • Inspection: enlargement; mass can be transilluminated, glows pink or red (in contrast to a hernia). • Palpation: nontender mass, fingers can reach above mass (in contrast to scrotal hernia). A: Nontender swelling of testis.	Cystic. Circumscribed collection of serous fluid in tunica vaginalis, surrounding testis. May occur after epididymitis, trauma, hernia, tumour of testis, or spontaneously in a newborn.

TABLE 26-6   Abnormalities in the Scrotum—cont'd

Disorder	Clinical Findings	Discussion
Scrotal Hernia 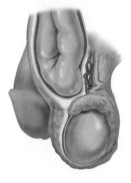	S: Swelling; pain may occur with straining. O: • Inspection: enlargement; may be reduced when patient is supine; cannot be transilluminated. • Palpation: soft mushy mass; palpating fingers cannot reach above mass; mass is distinct from testicle that is normal. A: Nontender swelling of scrotum.	Scrotal hernia is usually a result of indirect inguinal hernia (see Table 26-7).
Orchitis 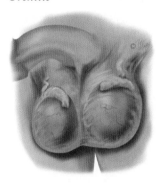	S: Acute or moderate pain of sudden onset, swollen testis, feeling of weight, fever. O: • Inspection: enlarged, edematous, reddened; cannot be transilluminated. • Palpation: swollen, congested, tense, and tender; hard to distinguish testis from epididymis. A: Tender swelling of testis.	Acute inflammation of testis. Most common cause is mumps; can occur with any infectious disease. May be associated with hydrocele, which can be transilluminated.
Scrotal Edema 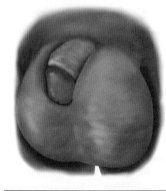	S: Tenderness. O: • Inspection: enlarged, may be reddened (with local irritation). • Palpation: taut with pitting; scrotal contents probably cannot be palpated. A: Scrotal edema.	Accompanies marked edema in lower half of body (e.g., in heart failure, renal failure, and portal vein obstruction). Occurs with local inflammation: epididymitis, torsion of spermatic cord. Also, obstruction of inguinal lymphatic vessels produces lymphedema of scrotum.

S, subjective data; *O,* objective data; *A,* assessment.

Images © Pat Thomas, 2006.

Abnormal Findings

TABLE 26-7   Inguinal and Femoral Hernias

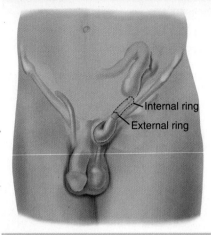
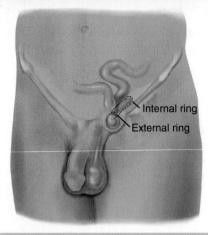
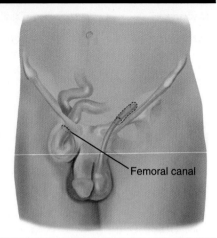

Characteristic	Indirect Inguinal	Direct Inguinal	Femoral
Course	Sac herniates through internal inguinal ring; can remain in canal or pass into scrotum	Directly behind and through external inguinal ring, above inguinal ligament; rarely enters scrotum	Through femoral ring and canal, below inguinal ligament, more often on right side
Clinical symptoms and signs	Pain with straining; soft swelling that increases with increased intra-abdominal pressure; swelling may decrease when patient is lying down	Usually painless; round swelling close to the pubis in area of internal inguinal ring; easily reduced when patient is supine*	Pain may be severe; hernia may become strangulated
Frequency	Most common; 60% of all hernias More common in infants <1 year old and in boys and men 16 to 20 years of age	Less common, occurs most often in men >40 years, rare in women	Least common, 4% of all hernias; more common in women
Cause	Congenital or acquired	Acquired weakness; brought on by heavy lifting, muscle atrophy, obesity, chronic cough, or ascites	Acquired; caused by increased abdominal pressure, muscle weakness, or frequent stooping

*Reducible: contents return to abdominal cavity by gentle pressure or when patient is supine. Incarcerated: herniated bowel cannot be returned to abdominal cavity. Strangulated: blood supply to hernia is shut off; accompanied by nausea, vomiting, and tenderness.

Images © Pat Thomas, 2006.

Summary Checklist: Examination of Male Genitalia

 For a PDA-downloadable version, go to *http://evolve.elsevier.com/Canada/Jarvis/examination/*

1. Inspect and palpate the penis.
2. Inspect and palpate the scrotum.
3. If a mass exists, transilluminate the scrotum.
4. Palpate for an inguinal hernia.
5. Palpate the inguinal lymph nodes.
6. Teaching and health promotion.

REFERENCES

Canadian Cancer Society. (2011). *What is testicular cancer?* Retrieved from *http://www.cancer.ca/Canada-wide/About%20 cancer/Types%20of%20cancer/What%20is%20testicular%20 cancer.aspx.*

Giuliano, A. R., Palefsky, J. M., Goldstone, S., Moreira, E. D., Penny, M. E., Aranda, C., … Guris, E. (2011). Efficacy of quadrivalent HPV vaccine against HPV infection and diseases in males. *New England Journal of Medicine, 364*(5), 401–411. doi:10.1056/NEJMoa0909537

Gray, R. H., Wawer, M. J., Serwadda, D., & Kigozi, G. (2009). The role of male circumcision in the prevention of human papillomavirus and HIV infection. *Journal of Infectious Diseases, 199*, 1–3. doi:10.1086/595568

Joffe, A. (2009). Should we teach testicular self-exam? *Contemporary Pediatrics, 26*(8), 33–34.

Lewis, S. L., Heitkemper, M. M., Dirksen, S. R., O'Brien, P. G., Bucher, L., Barry, M. A., … & Goodridge, D. (Eds.). (2010). *Medical-surgical nursing in Canada* (2nd Canadian ed.). Toronto: Elsevier.

Perry, A. G., & Potter, P. A. (2010). *Clinical nursing skills and techniques* (7th ed.). St. Louis: Elsevier.

Public Health Agency of Canada. (2009). *What mothers say: The Canadian Maternity Experiences Survey.* Retrieved from *http:// www.phac-aspc.gc.ca/rhs-ssg/pdf/survey-eng.pdf.*

Public Health Agency of Canada. (2011). *Human papillomavirus (HPV) prevention and HPV vaccines: Questions and answers.* Retrieved from *http://www.phac-aspc.gc.ca/std-mts/hpv-vph/pdf/ hpv-vph-vac-eng.pdf.*

Sobngwi-Tambekou, J., Taljaard, D., Nieuwoudt, M., Lissouba, P., Puren, A., & Auvert, B. (2009). Male circumcision and *Neisseria gonorrhoeae, Chlamydia trachomatis* and *Trichomonas vaginalis:* Observations after a randomised controlled trial for HIV prevention. *Sexually Transmitted Infections, 85*, 116–120. doi:10.1136/sti.2008.032334

Stratman-Lucey, D., & Caldwell, D. (2006, August-September). Pain management protocol with infant circumcision. *The Illinois Nurse, 13*.

Tobian, A. R., Serwadda, D., Quinn, T. C., Kigozi, G., Gravitt, P. E., Laeyendeck, O., … Gray, R. H. (2009). Male circumcision for the prevention of HSV-2 and HPV infections and syphilis. *New England Journal of Medicine, 360*(13), 1298–1309. doi:10.1056/ NEJMoa0802556

Viscidi, R. P., & Shah, K. V. (2010). Adult male circumcision: Will it reduce disease caused by human papillomavirus? *Journal of Infectious Diseases, 201*(10), 1447–1449. doi:10.1086/652186

Wawer, M. J., Makumbi, F., Kigozi, G., Serwadda, D., Watya, S., Nalugoda, F., … Gray, R. H. (2009). Circumcision in HIV-infected men and its effect on HIV transmission to female partners in Rakai, Uganda: A randomised controlled trial. *Lancet, 374*, 229–237.

Weiss, H. A., Larke, N., Halperin, D., & Schenker, I. (2010). Complications of circumcision in male neonates, infants and children: A systematic review. *BMC Urology, 10*, 2. doi:10.1186/1471-2490-10-2 or *http://www.biomedcentral. com/1471-2490/10/2.*

CHAPTER

27

Female Genitourinary System

Written by Carolyn Jarvis, PhD, APN, CNP
Adapted by Marian Luctkar-Flude, RN, MScN

⊖volve WEBSITE

OUTLINE

STRUCTURE AND FUNCTION

EXTERNAL GENITALIA

The external genitalia are called the **vulva,** or pudendum (Figure 27-1). The **mons pubis** is a round, firm pad of adipose tissue covering the **symphysis pubis,** the cartilaginous joint between the two pubic bones. After puberty, it is covered with hair in the pattern of an inverted triangle. The **labia majora** are two rounded folds of adipose tissue extending from the mons pubis down and around to the perineum. After puberty, hair covers the outer surfaces of the labia, whereas the inner folds are smooth and moist and contain sebaceous follicles.

Inside the labia majora are two smaller, darker folds of skin, the **labia minora.** These are joined anteriorly at the clitoris, where they form a hood *(prepuce).* The labia minora are joined posteriorly by a transverse fold, the **frenulum** (or *fourchette).* The **clitoris** is a small, pea-shaped erectile body, homologous with the male penis and highly sensitive to tactile stimulation.

The labial structures encircle a boat-shaped space, or cleft, termed the **vestibule.** Within it are numerous openings. The **urethral meatus** appears as a dimple 2.5 cm posterior to the clitoris. Surrounding the urethral meatus are the tiny,

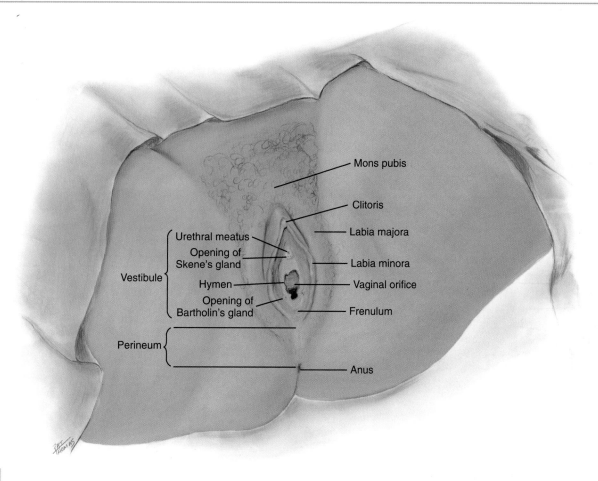

Mons pubis

Clitoris

Labia majora

Labia minora

Vaginal orifice

Frenulum

Anus

Vestibule

Urethral meatus

Opening of Skene's gland

Hymen

Opening of Bartholin's gland

Perineum

27-1

multiple **paraurethral (Skene's) glands.** Their ducts are not visible, but they open posterior to the urethra at the 5:00 and 7:00 positions.

The **vaginal orifice** is posterior to the urethral meatus. It appears either as a thin median slit or as a large opening with irregular edges, depending on the presentation of the membranous hymen. The **hymen** is a thin, circular or crescent-shaped fold that may cover part of the vaginal orifice or may be absent completely. On either side, and posterior to the vaginal orifice, are two **vestibular (Bartholin's) glands,** which secrete clear lubricating mucus during intercourse. Their ducts are not visible, but they open in the groove between the labia minora and the hymen.

INTERNAL GENITALIA

The internal genitalia include the **vagina,** a flattened, tubular canal extending from the orifice up and backward into the pelvis (Figure 27-2). It is 9 cm long and sits between the rectum posteriorly and the bladder and urethra anteriorly. Its walls are in thick transverse folds, or **rugae,** which enable the vagina to dilate widely during childbirth.

At the end of the canal, the uterine **cervix** projects into the vagina. In nulliparous women, the cervix appears as a smooth, doughnut-shaped area with a small circular hole (the **os**).

After childbirth, the os is slightly enlarged and irregular. The cervical epithelium is of two distinct types. The vagina and cervix are covered with smooth, pink, stratified squamous epithelium. Inside the os, the endocervical canal is lined with columnar epithelium that looks red and rough. The point where these two tissues meet is the **squamocolumnar junction** and is not visible.

A continuous recess is present around the cervix; the front part is the **anterior fornix,** and the rear aspect is the **posterior fornix.** Behind the posterior fornix, another deep recess is formed by the peritoneum. It dips down between the rectum and cervix to form the **rectouterine pouch,** or **cul-de-sac of Douglas.**

The **uterus** is a pear-shaped, thick-walled, muscular organ. It is flattened anteroposteriorly, measuring 5.5 to 8 cm long by 3.5 to 4 cm wide and 2 to 2.5 cm thick. It is freely movable, not fixed, and usually tilts forward and superior to the bladder (an anteverted and anteflexed position; see p. 764).

The **fallopian tubes** are two pliable, trumpet-shaped tubes, 10 cm in length, extending from the uterine fundus laterally to the brim of the pelvis. There they curve posteriorly, their fimbriated ends located near the **ovaries.** The two ovaries are located one on each side of the uterus at the level of the anterior superior iliac spine. Each is oval, 3 cm long by 2 cm wide by 1 cm thick, and serves to develop ova (eggs) and the female hormones.

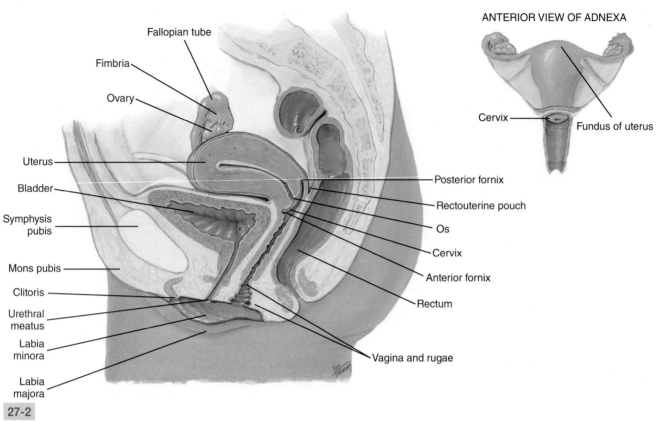

27-2

◈ DEVELOPMENTAL CONSIDERATIONS

Infants and Adolescents

At birth, the external genitalia are engorged because of the presence of maternal estrogen. The structures recede in a few weeks, remaining small until puberty. The ovaries are located in the abdomen during childhood. The uterus is small with a straight axis and no anteflexion.

At puberty, estrogens stimulate the growth of cells in the reproductive tract and the development of secondary sex characteristics. The first signs of puberty are breast and pubic hair development, beginning between the ages of 8½ and 13 years. These signs are usually concurrent, but it is not abnormal if they do not develop together. They take about 3 years to complete.

Menarche occurs during the latter half of this sequence, just after the peak of growth velocity. Irregularity of the menstrual cycle is common during adolescence because of occasional failure to ovulate. With menarche, the uterine body flexes on the cervix, and the ovaries have migrated to the pelvic cavity.

Tanner's table on the five stages of pubic hair development (sexual maturity rating) is helpful in teaching girls the expected sequence of sexual development (Table 27-1).

Pregnant Women

Pregnancy is discussed in detail in Chapter 30. In summary, shortly after the first missed menstrual period, the genitalia show signs of the presence of a growing fetus. The cervix softens *(Goodell's sign)* at 4 to 6 weeks, and the vaginal mucosa and cervix look cyanotic *(Chadwick's sign)* at 6 to 8 weeks. These changes occur because of increased vascularity and edema of the cervix and hypertrophy and hyperplasia of the cervical glands. The isthmus of the uterus softens *(Hegar's sign)* at 6 to 8 weeks.

The greatest change is in the uterus itself. Its capacity increases by 500 to 1000 times its nonpregnant state, at first because of hormone stimulation and then because of the increasing size of its contents (Cunningham et al., 2005). The nonpregnant uterus has a flattened pear shape. In early pregnancy, its growth encroaches on the space occupied by the bladder, producing the symptom of urinary frequency. By 10 to 12 weeks' gestation, the uterus becomes globular in shape and is too large to stay in the pelvis. At 20 to 24 weeks, the uterus has an oval shape. It rises almost to the liver, displacing the intestines superiorly and laterally.

A clot of thick, tenacious mucus (the mucous plug) forms in the spaces of the cervical canal, which protects the fetus from infection. The mucous plug dislodges when labour begins at the end of term, producing a sign of labour called the "bloody show." Cervical and vaginal secretions increase during pregnancy and are thick, white, and more acidic. The acidity is increased because of the action of *Lactobacillus acidophilus,* which changes glycogen into lactic acid. The acidic pH keeps pathogenic bacteria from multiplying in the vagina, but the increase in glycogen increases the risk of candidiasis (commonly called a *yeast infection)* during pregnancy.

TABLE 27-1	Sexual Maturity Ratings in Girls

Stage 1

Preadolescent. No pubic hair. Mons and labia covered with fine vellus hair, as on abdomen.

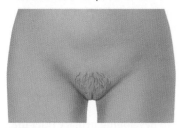

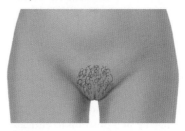

Stage 2

Growth sparse and mostly on labia. Long, downy hair, slightly pigmented, straight or only slightly curly.

Stage 3

Growth sparse but spreading over mons pubis. Hair is darker, coarser, curlier.

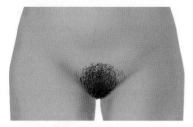

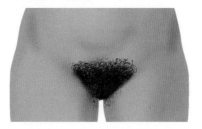

Stage 4

Hair is adult in type but over smaller area; none on medial thigh.

Stage 5

Adult in type and pattern; inverse triangle. Also on medial thigh surface.

Adapted from Tanner, J. M. (1962). *Growth at adolescence.* Oxford, UK: Blackwell Scientific.

Older Women

In contrast to the slowly declining levels of hormones in aging men, the hormonal levels in women decrease rapidly. *Menopause* is cessation of the menses. Usually this occurs at approximately 48 to 51 years of age, although the variation in ages is wide (from 35 to 60 years). The stage of menopause includes the preceding 1 to 2 years of decline in ovarian function, shown by irregular menses that gradually become farther apart and whose flow is lighter. Ovaries stop producing progesterone and estrogen. Because cells in the reproductive tract are estrogen dependent, decreased estrogen levels during menopause bring dramatic physical changes.

The uterus shrinks in size because of decreased myometrium. The ovaries atrophy to 1 to 2 cm and are not palpable after menopause. Ovulation still may occur sporadically after menopause. The sacral ligaments relax and the pelvic musculature weakens, and so the uterus droops. Sometimes it may protrude, or prolapse, into the vagina. The cervix shrinks and looks paler, with a thick, glistening epithelium.

The vagina becomes shorter, narrower, and less elastic because of increased connective tissue. Without sexual activity, the vagina atrophies to one half of its former length and width. The vaginal epithelium atrophies, becoming thinner, drier, and itchy. This results in a fragile mucosal surface that is at risk for bleeding and vaginitis. Decreased vaginal secretions leave the vagina dry and at risk for irritation and pain with intercourse (dyspareunia). The vaginal pH becomes more alkaline, and glycogen content decreases as a result of the decreased estrogen. These factors also increase the risk of vaginitis because they result in conditions suitable for pathogens.

Externally, the mons pubis looks smaller because the fat pad atrophies. The labia and clitoris gradually decrease in size. Pubic hair becomes thin and sparse.

Declining estrogen levels produce some physiological changes in the female sexual response cycle: reduced amount of vaginal secretion and lubrication during excitement; shorter duration of orgasm; and rapid resolution.

However, these changes do not affect sexual pleasure and function. Sexual desire and the need for full sexual expression continue. Like older men, older women are capable of sexual function if they are in reasonably good health and have an interested partner. The problem for many older women is the availability of an acceptable sexual partner. Older women greatly outnumber their male counterparts and are more likely to be single, whereas men of the same age are more likely to be married.

CULTURAL AND SOCIAL CONSIDERATIONS

Female circumcision, or *female genital mutilation* (FGM), is the ritual removal of part or all of the external female genitalia, usually performed on prepubertal girls. FGM is an ancient cultural practice, most common in Africa but also practised in parts of southeast Asia, the Middle East, and Central and South America; an estimated 120 to 140 million girls have undergone the procedure. The health implications of FGM include both (a) immediate effects, such as severe pain, hemorrhage, urinary retention, infection, sepsis, and death, and (b) long-term effects, such as urinary tract and genital tract dysfunction, painful menstruation, sexual and birth control difficulties, infertility, difficulties during pregnancy and childbirth, and psychological difficulties. FGM is illegal in Canada and most Western countries; however, an increasing number of immigrant women who have undergone these procedures are now living in Canada. Affected women may be reluctant to seek health care, and when they do, they may find it difficult and at times traumatic. Health care providers may be in a position to educate immigrants from practising communities about the health considerations and legal consequences of FGM.

Sexually transmitted infections (STIs) are a major health concern. Chlamydia continues to be the most commonly reported STI in Canada; reported rates increased by 80% from 1999 to 2008; women accounted for almost twice as many cases as did men; and the highest rates were reported in Nunavut, the Northwest Territories, and Yukon (Public Health Agency of Canada, 2008). Consequences of untreated chlamydia for women include pelvic inflammatory disease, which can lead to chronic pelvic pain, ectopic pregnancy, and infertility. Women represent an increasing proportion of Canadians living with human immunodeficiency virus (HIV) infection and acquired immune deficiency syndrome (AIDS), accounting for 26.2% of positive test results in 2008 (Public Health Agency of Canada, 2010). The two main risk factors for HIV infection in women are heterosexual contact and injection drug use; Aboriginal women account for 42.9% of reported cases.

Women are more prone to developing urinary tract infections than are men because of the shortness of the female urethra, which makes it easier for bacteria to reach the bladder. Canadian women make about 500,000 visits to doctors per year because of such infections (Kidney Foundation of Canada, 2007). Risk factors for the development of urinary tract infection include abnormalities of the urinary tract, pregnancy, postmenopausal status, diabetes, and the presence of an indwelling urinary catheter.

SUBJECTIVE DATA

1. Menstrual history
2. Obstetrical history
3. Menopause
4. Self-care behaviours
5. Urinary symptoms
6. Vaginal discharge

7. Past history
8. Sexual activity
9. Contraceptive use
10. STI contact
11. STI risk reduction

HEALTH HISTORY QUESTIONS

Examiner Asks	Rationale
1. **Menstrual history.** Tell me about your menstrual periods:	Documentation of the menstrual history is usually nonthreatening; thus it is a good topic to start recording the history.
• What was the date of your most recent menstrual period?	This is referred to as the last menstrual period (LMP).
• What was your age at the time of your first period?	Menarche: Mean age at onset is 12 to 13; delayed onset suggests endocrine or underweight problem.
• How often are your periods?	Cycle: normally every 18 to 45 days Amenorrhea: absence of menses
• How many days does your period last?	Duration: average of 3 to 7 days
• What is the usual amount of flow: light, medium, heavy? How many pads or tampons do you use each day or hour?	Menorrhagia: heavy menses
• Have you noted any clotting?	Clotting indicates heavy flow or vaginal pooling.
• Do you have any pain or cramps before or during your period? How do you treat it? Does it interfere with daily activities? Any other associated symptoms: bloating, breast tenderness, moodiness? Any spotting between periods?	Dysmenorrhea

Examiner Asks	Rationale

2. Obstetrical history. Have you ever been pregnant?

- How many times?
- How many babies have you had?
- Any miscarriage or abortion?

- For each pregnancy, describe the duration, any complication, labour and delivery, baby's sex, baby's birth weight, and baby's condition.
- Do you think you may be pregnant now? What symptoms have you noticed?

3. Menopause. Have your periods slowed down or stopped?

- Any associated symptoms of menopause (e.g., hot flash, numbness and tingling sensation, headache, palpitations, drenching sweats, mood swings, vaginal dryness, itching)? Any treatment?

- If you are taking hormone replacement, how much? How is it working? Any side effects?

- How do you feel about going through menopause?

4. Self-care behaviours. How often do you have a gynecological checkup?
- When was your most recent Papanicolaou (Pap) smear? What were the results?
- Has your mother ever mentioned taking hormones while pregnant with you?

5. Urinary symptoms. Any problems with urinating? Do you urinate frequently and in small amounts? When you feel the need to urinate, is it impossible to wait?
- Do you have any burning sensation or pain on urinating?
- Do you awaken during the night to urinate?
- Have you seen blood in the urine?
- Is urine dark, cloudy, foul smelling?
- Do you have any difficulty controlling urine or wetting yourself?

- Do you urinate when you sneeze, laugh, cough, or bear down?

6. Vaginal discharge. Have you noticed any unusual vaginal discharge? Has the amount increased?
- What is the character or colour: white, yellow-green, grey, curdlike, foul smelling?

- When did this begin?

Record the obstetrical history. (see Chapter 30, Pregnancy p. 817 for details).
Gravida (G): number of pregnancies
Para (P): number of births
Abortions (A): interrupted pregnancies, including elective abortions and spontaneous miscarriages

Menopause is the cessation of menstruation.
Perimenopausal period from ages 40 to 55 years is characterized by hormone shifts, which result in vasomotor instability.
Side effects of hormone replacement therapy include fluid retention, breast pain or enlargement, vaginal bleeding, possibly breast cancer risk.
Although this is a normal life stage, reaction varies from acceptance to feelings of loss.
Assess self-care behaviours.

Maternal ingestion of diethylstilbestrol (DES) causes cervical and vaginal abnormalities in female offspring, which necessitates frequent follow-up.
Frequency
Urgency

Dysuria
Nocturia
Hematuria
Bile in urine or urinary tract infection
True incontinence: loss of urine without warning
Urgency incontinence: sudden loss of urine, as with acute cystitis.
Functional incontinence: loss of urine in association with inability to access the toilet because of impairment in cognitive or physical functioning, or both, or because of an environmental barrier
Stress incontinence: loss of urine with physical strain from muscle weakness
Normal discharge is small, clear or cloudy, and always nonirritating.
With vaginal infection, character of discharge often suggests causative organism (see Table 27-5 on pp. 775–776).
Determine whether problem is acute or chronic.

Examiner Asks	Rationale
• Is the discharge associated with vaginal itching, rash, pain with intercourse?	Itching or rash may occur as a result of irritation from discharge. Dyspareunia occurs with vaginitis of any cause.
• Are you taking any medications?	Factors that increase risk of vaginitis: • Oral contraceptives increase glycogen content of vaginal epithelium, which renders epithelium conducive to the growth of some organisms. • Broad-spectrum antibiotics alter the balance of normal flora.
• Do you have a family history of diabetes? • What part of your menstrual cycle are you in now?	• Diabetes increases glycogen content. • Menses, postpartum status, and menopause cause vaginal pH to be more alkaline.
• Do you use a vaginal douche? How often? • Do you use feminine hygiene spray?	• Frequent douching alters vaginal pH. • Use of such sprays increases risk of contact dermatitis.
• Do you use talcum powder in the genital area? Cornstarch powder?	• Talcum powder use is associated with a higher risk for ovarian cancer. Cornstarch powder is not.
• Do you wear nonventilating underpants, pantyhose? • Have you treated the discharge with anything? What was the result?	• Local irritation
7. **History.** Any other problems in the genital area? Sores or lesions: now or in the past? How were these treated? • Any abdominal or pelvic pain? • Any past surgery on uterus, ovaries, vagina?	Assess the patient's feelings. Some women fear loss of sexual response after hysterectomy, which may cause problems in intimate relationships.
8. **Sexual activity.** Often women have a question about their sexual relationship and how it affects their health. Do you? • Are you in a relationship involving intercourse now? • Are aspects of your sexual relationship satisfactory to you and your partner? • Are you satisfied with the way you and your partner communicate about sex? • Are you satisfied with your ability to respond sexually? • Do you have more than one sexual partner?	Begin with open-ended question to assess individual needs. Include appropriate questions as a routine: • Such questions communicate your acceptance of the patient's sexual activity and your belief that it is important. • Your comfort with discussion prompts the patient's interest and possibly relief that the topic has been introduced. • This question helps establishes a database for comparison with any future sexual activities. • It also provides opportunity to screen for sexual problems.
• What is your sexual preference: relationship with a man, with a woman, both?	Lesbians and bisexual women need to feel acceptance to discuss their health concerns.
9. **Contraceptive use.** Are you currently planning a pregnancy or avoiding pregnancy? • Do you and your partner use a **contraceptive?** Which method? Is this satisfactory? Do you have any questions about method? • Which methods have you used in the past? Have you and your partner discussed having children? • Have you ever had any problems becoming pregnant?	Assess smoking history. Oral contraceptives, together with cigarette smoking, increase the risk of vascular problems. Infertility is considered after 1 year of engaging in unprotected sexual intercourse without conceiving.

Examiner Asks	Rationale
10. **Sexually transmitted infection (STI) contact.** Have you had any sexual contact with a partner who had an STI, such as gonorrhea, herpes, HIV, chlamydial infection, venereal warts, syphilis? When? How was this treated? Were there any complications?	An STI is any condition that can be transmitted during intercourse or intimate sexual contact with an infected partner.
11. **STI risk reduction.** Do you take any precautions to reduce risk of STIs? Do you use condoms every time you have sexual intercourse?	

Additional History for Infants and Children

Examiner Asks	Rationale
1. **Urination problems.** Does your child have any problem urinating? Does the child have pain with urinating? Does the child cry or hold the genitals while urinating? Has the child ever had a urinary tract infection? • (If the child is older than 2 to 2½ years of age) Has toilet training started? How is it progressing? • Does the child wet the bed at night? Is this a problem for the child or you (parents)? What have you (parents) done?	
2. **Genital problems.** Does the child have a problem with the genital area: itching, rash, vaginal discharge?	Such problems occur with poor perineal hygiene or insertion of a foreign body in the vagina.
3. **Molestation.** (To child) "Has anyone ever touched you in between your legs and you did not want them to? Sometimes that happens to children, and it's not okay."	Screen for sexual abuse (see Chapter 8). For prevention, teach the child that it is not "okay" for someone to look at or touch her private parts while telling her it is a secret. The patient who has been abused should be told that she has not been "bad" and that she should try to tell an adult about it: "Can you tell me three different big people you trust who you could talk to?" Being asked to name three trusted adults will help the child include someone outside the family: This is important because most molestation is performed by a parent.

Additional History for Preadolescents and Adolescents

Use the following questions, as appropriate, to assess sexual growth and development and sexual behaviour:

- Ask questions that seem appropriate for girl's age, but be aware that norms vary widely. When in doubt, it is better to ask too many questions than to omit something. Children obtain information, often misinformation, from the media and from peers at surprisingly early ages. You can be sure your information will be more thoughtful and accurate.
- Ask direct, matter-of-fact questions. Avoid sounding judgemental.
- Start with a *permission statement:* "Often girls your age experience…." This conveys that it is normal to think or feel a certain way.
- Try the *open-ended:* "When did you…?" rather than "Do you…?" This is less threatening because it implies that the topic is normal and unexceptional.

Examiner Asks	Rationale
1. **Puberty.** At approximately age 9 or 10, girls start to develop breasts and pubic hair. Have you ever seen charts and pictures of normal growth patterns for girls? Let us go over these now.	
2. **Menstruation.** Have your periods started? How did you feel? Were you prepared or surprised?	Assess attitude of girl and parents. Note inadequate preparation or attitude of distaste.

Subjective Data

Examiner Asks	Rationale
3. **Information.** Who in your family do you talk to about your body changes and about sex information? How do these talks go? Do you think you get enough information? What about sex education classes at school? Is there a teacher, a nurse or doctor, a minister, a counsellor to whom you can talk? • Often girls your age have questions about sexual activity. Do you have questions? Are you dating? Someone steady? • Do you and your boyfriend have intercourse? Are you using condoms? What kind of protection did you use the last time you had intercourse?	
4. **Disease.** Has anyone ever talked to you about STIs, such as chlamydia, herpes, gonorrhea, or AIDS?	Avoid the term "sexually active," which is ambiguous. Teach STI risk reduction.
5. **Immunization.** Have you and your parents discussed the human papillomavirus (HPV) vaccine (Gardasil, Cervarix)? It is recommended before girls become sexually active.	The HPV vaccines are approved for girls and women aged 9 to 45 for prevention of cervical cancer. See the box Promoting Health: HPV Vaccine.
6. **Molestation.** Sometimes a person touches a girl in a way that she does not want to be touched. Has that ever happened to you?	Screen for sexual abuse. If abuse has occurred, the patient should be reminded that it is not her fault and that she should tell another adult about it.

PROMOTING HEALTH: HPV VACCINE

Vaccine to Prevent Cervical Cancer: A Breakthrough in Cancer Prevention

Human papillomavirus (HPV) is estimated to be the most prevalent sexually transmitted infection (STI) in Canada, and HPV is responsible for most cases of cervical cancer, the second most common malignancy in women. In 2006 the first HPV vaccine was approved for use in Canada. The National Advisory Committee on Immunization (2007) has recommended the vaccine for (a) girls between 9 and 13 years of age, as this is before the onset of sexual intercourse for most Canadian girls; (b) girls and women between the ages of 14 and 26 years, even if they are already sexually active, because they may not yet have HPV infection and are very unlikely to have been infected with all four HPV types present in the vaccine; and (c) girls and women between the ages of 14 and 26 who have had previous abnormalities on a Papanicolaou (Pap) smear test, including cervical cancer, or have had genital warts or known HPV, because they are very unlikely to have been infected with all four HPV types in the vaccine. The vaccine is given in three separate injections over a 6-month period. Some Canadian provinces have introduced HPV immunization programs. More recently, HPV vaccination has been approved by Health Canada for use in boys and men aged 9 to 26, and in women up to age 45 years.

Canadian women who are older, immigrant women, Aboriginal women, and women who have a low socioeconomic status are at higher risk for developing cervical cancer, primarily as a result of lower participation rates in regular screening schedules. Reluctance to undergo screening may be attributable to reasons such as lack of knowledge, lack of access, or failure of the clinician to offer screening. Other factors that appear to increase the risk of developing cervical cancer are becoming sexually active at a young age; having many sexual partners or a sexual partner who has had many partners; being a smoker; having a weakened immune system (e.g., from taking drugs after organ transplantation or having a disease such as acquired immune deficiency syndrome); using oral contraceptives; giving birth to many children; and having taken diethylstilbestrol (DES) or being the biological daughter of a mother who took DES (Canadian Cancer Society, 2010).

Overall, cervical cancer incidence and mortality rates have been declining as a result of widespread Pap test screening. The Canadian Task Force on Preventive Health Care (2013) recently released new recommendations on screening for cervical cancer for women with no symptoms of cervical cancer who are or who have been sexually active regardless of sexual orientation. Routine Pap test screening is no longer recommended for women under the age of 25 years. Screening every three years with cervical cytology is recommended for women aged 25 to 69 years. For women aged 70 years and older, screening with cervical cytology every three years is recommended if previous screening was inadequate and until three negative results have been received; otherwise screening may stop. More frequent testing may be considered for women at high risk. Women who have received the HPV vaccine should still take part in the currently recommended cervical cancer screening programs. As more girls and women receive the vaccine, the recommended type or frequency of screening may be modified.

Sources: From Canadian Cancer Society. (2010). *Causes of cervical cancer.* Retrieved from *http://www.cancer.ca/Alberta-NWT/About%20cancer/Types%20of%20cancer/Causes%20of%20cervical%20cancer.aspx?sc_lang=en;* Canadian Task Force on Preventive Health Care. (2013). Recommendations on screening for cervical cancer. *Canadian Medical Association Journal, 185*(1), 35–45; Canadian Paediatric Society. (2007). Position statement (ID 2007-01): Human papillomavirus vaccine for children and adolescents. *Paediatrics and Child Health, 12,* 599–603. Also available at *http://www.cps.ca/documents/position/hpv-vaccine;* National Advisory Committee on Immunization. (2007). Statement on human papillomavirus vaccine. *Canada Communicable Disease Report, 33*(ACS-2), 1–32; Public Health Agency of Canada. (2007). *What everyone should know about human papillomavirus.* Retrieved from *http://www.phac-aspc.gc.ca/std-mts/hpv-vph/hpv-vphqaqr_e.html;* and Society of Obstetricians and Gynaecologists of Canada. (2008). *HPV info.* Retrieved from *http://www.hpvinfo.ca/hpvinfo/home.aspx.*

Examiner Asks	Rationale

Additional History for Older Women

1. **Bleeding.** Since menopause, have you noted any vaginal bleeding?

    Postmenopausal bleeding warrants further workup and referral.

2. **Vaginal problems.** Any vaginal itching, dryness, discharge, pain with intercourse? Do you use a vaginal lubricant?

    These problems are associated with atrophic vaginitis related to decreased estrogen levels. Lubricant may relieve vaginal dryness and decrease discomfort with intercourse.

3. **Incontinence.** Have you experienced any pressure in the genital area, back pain, constipation, or loss of urine when you cough or sneeze?

    These problems occur with weakened pelvic musculature and uterine prolapse.

4. **Sexuality.** During and after menopause, a woman may notice changes in her sexual relationship or in her sexual response and wonder whether it is normal. Are you in a relationship involving intercourse now? Are aspects of intercourse satisfactory to you and your partner? Is there adequate privacy for a sexual relationship?

    Most older adults are not reluctant to discuss sexual activity, and most welcome the opportunity. A decline in libido and difficulty in maintaining arousal and achieving orgasm are normal changes that may occur with aging. In the absence of physical illness, an older woman is fully capable of sexual function.

Subjective Data

Objective Data

OBJECTIVE DATA

PREPARATION

Examination of the internal genitalia is an advanced assessment; however, the generalist nurse may be asked to assist with the procedure, particularly if the physician or nurse practitioner who is performing the examination is male. Assemble the equipment before helping the patient into position. Arrange equipment within easy reach. Familiarize yourself with the vaginal speculum before the examination. Practise opening and closing the blades, locking them into position, and releasing them. Try both metal and plastic types. Note that the plastic speculum locks and unlocks with a resounding click that can be alarming to the uninformed patient.

EQUIPMENT NEEDED

Gloves
Goose-necked lamp with a strong light
Vaginal speculum of appropriate size (Figure 27-3)
Graves speculum: useful for most women, available in varying lengths and widths
Pederson speculum: narrow blades, useful for young or postmenopausal women with narrowed introitus
Large cotton-tipped applicators (rectal swabs)
Materials for cytological study as specified within your region or facility:
- Glass slide with frosted end
- Specimen container for liquid-based cytological study
- Sterile Cytobrush or cotton-tipped applicator
- Ayre spatula
- Spray fixative
- Specimen container for gonorrhea/*Chlamydia* culture
- Small bottle of normal saline solution, potassium hydroxide (KOH), and acetic acid (white vinegar)
- Lubricant

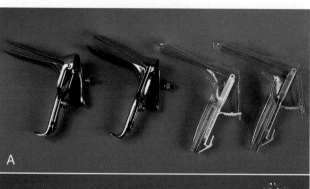
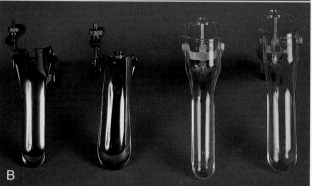

27-3 Vaginal specula.

POSITION

Initially, the patient should be sitting up. An equal-status position is important for establishing trust and rapport before the vaginal examination.

For the examination, the patient should be placed in the lithotomy position; the examiner sits on a stool. Help the patient into the lithotomy position, with the body supine, feet in stirrups and knees apart, and buttocks at edge of examining table (Figure 27-4). Ask the woman to lift her hips as you guide them to the edge of the table. Some women prefer to leave their shoes or socks on; alternatively, you can place an examination glove over each of the stirrups to warm the stirrups and keep the patient's feet from slipping.

Place the patient's arms at her sides or across the chest and not over the head (because this position tightens the abdominal muscles). Appropriate draping protects the modesty of the patient. This is important for female patients of all ethnocultural backgrounds. The traditional mode is to drape the patient fully, covering the stomach and legs, exposing only the vulva to your view. Be sure to push down the drape between the woman's legs, and elevate her head so that you can see her face.

The lithotomy position leaves many patients feeling helpless and vulnerable. Indeed, many women tolerate the pelvic examination because they consider it basic for health care, but they find it embarrassing and uncomfortable. Previous examinations may have been painful, or the previous examiner's attitude was hurried and patronizing.

The examination need not be this way. You can help the patient relax, decrease her anxiety, and help her retain a sense of control by using these measures:

- Have her empty the bladder before the examination.
- Position the examination table so that her perineum is not exposed to an inadvertent open door.

- Ask whether she would like a friend, family member, or chaperone present. Position this person by the patient's head to maintain privacy.
- Elevate the patient's head and shoulders to a semi-sitting position to maintain eye contact.
- Place the stirrups so that the legs are not abducted too far.
- Explain each step in the examination before you do it.
- Assure the patient that she can stop the examination at any point if she feels any discomfort.
- Use a gentle, firm touch and gradual movements.
- Communicate throughout the examination. Maintain a dialogue to share information, answer questions, and provide health teaching.
- Use the techniques of the *educational* or *mirror pelvic examination* (Figure 27-5). This is a routine examination with some modifications in attitude, position, and communication. First, the patient is considered an active participant who is interested in learning and in sharing decisions about her own health care. The patient props herself up on one elbow, or the head of the table is raised. Her other hand holds a mirror between her legs, above the examiner's hands. The woman can see all that the examiner is doing and has a full view of her genitalia.

The mirror works well for teaching normal anatomy and its relation to sexual behaviour. Even women who are in a sexual relationship or who have had children may be surprisingly uninformed about their own anatomy. This is an ideal opportunity to provide teaching and to clarify any misconceptions. Most patients respond enthusiastically on seeing their own cervix, which is rewarding, too.

The mirror pelvic examination also works well when abnormalities arise because the patient can see the rationale for treatment and can monitor progress at the next appointment. Patients are more willing to comply with treatment when they share in the decision.

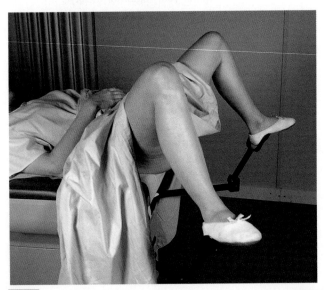

27-4

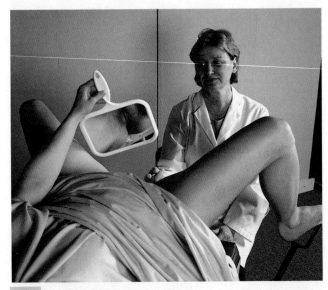

27-5

| **Normal Range of Findings** | **Abnormal Findings** |

EXTERNAL GENITALIA

Inspection

Note the following characteristics:
- Skin colour (Figure 27-6).

Refer any suspect pigmented lesion for biopsy.

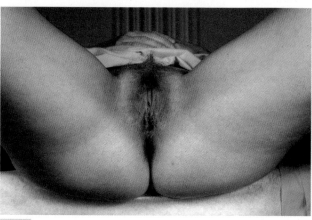

27-6

- Hair distribution. The usual female pattern is an inverted triangle, although it may trail up the abdomen toward the umbilicus; this is normal.

Consider puberty delayed if no pubic hair or breast development has occurred by age 13 years.

Nits or lice at the base of pubic hair should be eradicated.

Swelling.

- Labia majora. Normally the labia are symmetrical, plump, and well formed. In nulliparous women, labia meet in the midline; after a vaginal delivery, the labia are no longer meet in the midline, and appear slightly shrunken and less defined.
- Skin texture. No lesions should be present, except for occasional sebaceous cysts. These are yellowish, 1-cm nodules that are firm, nontender, and often multiple.

With your gloved hand, separate the labia majora to inspect the following anatomical features:
- Clitoris (Figure 27-7).

Excoriation, nodules, rash, or lesions (see Table 27-2, p. 771).

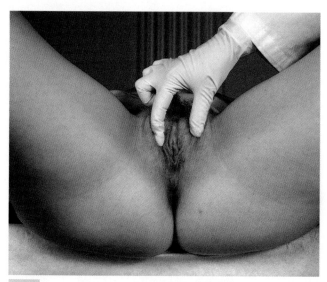

27-7

Normal Range of Findings	Abnormal Findings
• Labia minora. The labia minora are dark pink, moist, and usually symmetrical.	Inflammation or lesions.
• Urethral opening. This appears stellate or slitlike and is midline.	
• Vaginal opening, or introitus. This may appear as a narrow vertical slit or as a larger opening.	Polyp. Foul-smelling, irritating discharge.
• Perineum. The perineum is normally smooth. A well-healed episiotomy scar, midline or mediolateral, may be present after a vaginal birth.	
• Anus. The skin of the anus is coarse and has increased pigmentation (see Chapter 23 for assessment).	

SPECIAL CONSIDERATIONS FOR ADVANCED PRACTICE: EXTERNAL AND INTERNAL GENITALIA

Palpation

Assess the urethra and Skene's glands (Figure 27-8). Dip your gloved finger in a bowl of warm water to lubricate. Then insert your index finger into the vagina, and gently milk the urethra by applying pressure up and out. This procedure should produce no pain. If any discharge appears, culture it.

Tenderness.
Induration along urethra.
Urethral discharge.

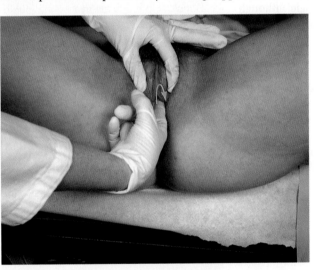

27-8

Assess Bartholin's glands. Palpate the posterior parts of the labia majora with your index finger in the vagina and your thumb outside (Figure 27-9). Normally, the labia feel soft and homogeneous.

Swelling (see Table 27-2, p. 772).
Induration.
Pain with palpation.
Erythema around or discharge from duct opening.

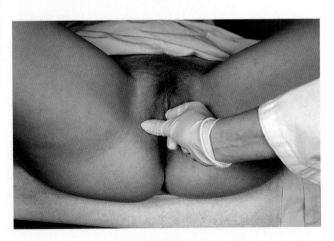

27-9

Assess the support of pelvic musculature by using these manoeuvres:

1. Palpate the perineum. Normally, it feels thick, smooth, and muscular in a nulliparous woman but thin and rigid in a multiparous woman.
2. Ask the woman to squeeze the vaginal opening around your fingers; it should feel tight in a nulliparous woman and should have less tone in a multiparous woman.
3. Using your index and middle fingers, separate the vaginal orifice and ask the woman to strain down. Normally, no bulging of vaginal walls or urinary incontinence occurs.

Internal Genitalia

Speculum Examination

Select the proper-sized speculum. Warm and lubricate the speculum under warm running water. In many Canadian provinces, small amounts of water-soluble lubricants are allowable for speculum exams for PAP smears, as research indicates there is no effect on cervical cytology results (Amies, et al., 2002; Pawlik & Martin, 2009).

A good technique is to dedicate one hand to the patient and the other hand to picking up equipment in the room. For example, hold the speculum in your left hand (the equipment hand), with the index and the middle fingers surrounding the blades and your thumb under the thumbscrew. This prevents the blades from opening painfully during insertion. With your right index and middle fingers (the hand on the patient), push the introitus down and open to relax the pubococcygeal muscle (Figure 27-10). Tilt the width of the blades obliquely and insert the speculum past your right fingers, applying any pressure *downward*. This avoids pressure on the sensitive urethra above it.

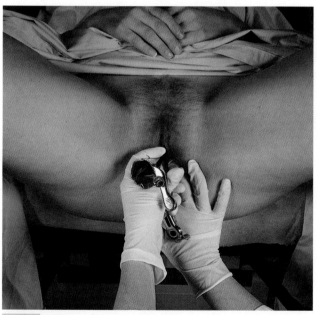

27-10

Ease insertion by asking the patient to bear down. This method relaxes the perineal muscles and opens the introitus. (With experience, you can combine speculum insertion with assessing the support of the vaginal muscles.) As the blades pass your right fingers, withdraw your fingers. Now change the hand holding the speculum to your right hand, and turn the width of the blades horizontally. Continue to insert in a 45-degree angle *downward* toward the small of the woman's back (Figure 27-11). This matches the natural slope of the vagina.

Tenderness.

Paper-thin perineum.

Absence or decrease of tone may diminish sexual satisfaction.

Bulging of the vaginal wall indicates cystocele, rectocele, or uterine prolapse (see Table 27-3, p. 773).

Urinary incontinence should be investigated.

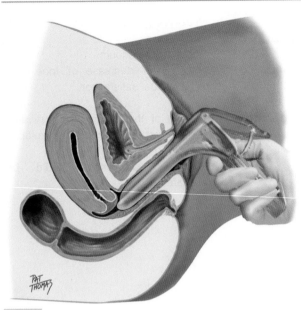

27-11

After the blades are fully inserted, open them by squeezing the handles together (Figure 27-12). The cervix should be in full view. Sometimes this does not occur (especially for novice examiners), because the blades are angled above the location of the cervix. Try closing the blades, withdrawing about halfway, and reinserting in a more *downward* plane. Then slowly sweep upward. Once you have the cervix in full view, lock the blades open by tightening the thumbscrew.

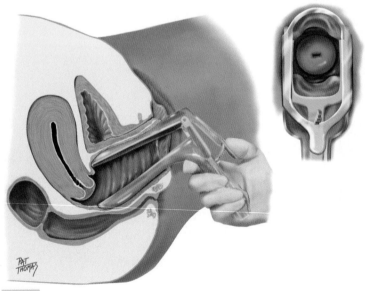

27-12

Inspect the Cervix and Its Os

Note the following characteristics:

- Colour. The cervical mucosa is normally pink and even. During the second month of pregnancy it looks blue (Chadwick's sign), and after menopause it is pale.

- Position. The cervix is midline, either anterior or posterior. It projects 1 to 3 cm into the vagina.

Redness, inflammation.
Pallor with anemia.
Cyanotic other than with pregnancy (see Table 27-4, p. 774).

Lateral position may result from adhesion or tumour. Projection of more than 3 cm may be a prolapse.

- Size. Diameter is 2.5 cm (1 in).
- Os. This is small and round in nulliparous women. In parous women, it is a horizontal irregular slit, and healed lacerations may be visible on the sides (Figure 27-13, *A* and *B*).

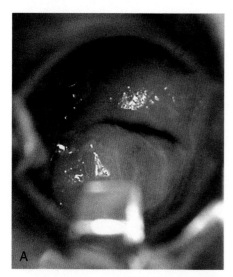

A

NORMAL VARIATIONS OF THE CERVIX

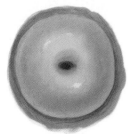

Nulliparous

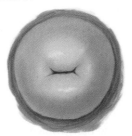

Parous (after childbirth)

LACERATIONS

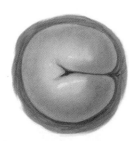

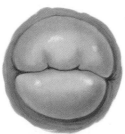

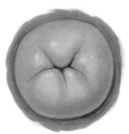

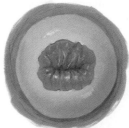

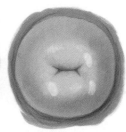

B   Unilateral transverse   Bilateral transverse   Stellate   Cervical eversion   Nabothian cysts

27-13   Cervix. **A,** View of os. **B,** Normal variations.

- Surface. This is normally smooth, but **cervical eversion,** or ectropion, may occur normally after vaginal deliveries. The endocervical canal is everted or "rolled out." It looks like a red, beefy halo inside the pink cervix surrounding the os. It is difficult to distinguish this normal variation from an abnormal condition (e.g., erosion or carcinoma), and biopsy may be needed.

Reddened, granular, and asymmetrical surface, particularly around os.

Friable, bleeding easily.

Any lesions: white patch on cervix; strawberry spot.

Refer any suspect red, white, or pigmented lesion for biopsy (see erosion, ulceration, and carcinoma, Table 27-4, pp. 774–775).

Special Considerations for Advanced Practice

- **Nabothian cysts** are benign growths that commonly appear on the cervix after childbirth. They are small, smooth, yellow nodules that may be single or multiple and are less than 1 cm in diameter. They are retention cysts caused by obstruction of cervical glands.
- Cervical secretions. Depending on the day of the menstrual cycle, secretions may be clear and thin, or they may be thick, opaque, and stringy. They are always odourless and nonirritating.

If secretions are copious, swab the area with a thickly tipped rectal swab. This method sponges away secretions, and you have a better view of the structures.

Obtain Cervical Smears and Cultures

The Papanicolaou (Pap) smear is a screen for cervical cancer. Screening recommendations vary by province. Previously, guidelines recommended annual screening starting at early ages, but now all provinces have increased the starting age and intervals between screens (Canadian Task Force on Preventive Health Care, 2013). See the Promoting Health Box on the HPV Vaccine on page 752 for the updated screening guidelines. Do not obtain a Pap smear during the woman's menses or if a heavy infectious discharge is present. Instruct the woman not to douche, have intercourse, or put anything into the vagina within 24 hours before the specimens are collected. Obtain the Pap smear before other specimens so that you will not disrupt or remove cells.

Conventional glass slide cytological study remains the most common screening test for cervical cancer available to women in Canada. A single slide is sufficient for the entire specimen. When fixative is to be used, as in most regions in Canada other than British Columbia, it should be applied to the slide immediately after the cells are spread from both sides of the brush or spatula in a thin layer (Murphy, 2007).

Cervical Scrape. Insert the bifid end of the Ayre spatula into the vagina with the more pointed bump into the cervical os. Rotate it 360 to 720 degrees, using firm pressure (Figure 27-14). The rounded cervix fits snugly into the spatula's groove. The spatula scrapes the surface of the squamocolumnar junction and cervix as you turn the instrument. After you withdraw the spatula, spread the specimen from both sides of the spatula onto a glass slide. Use a single stroke to thin out the specimen, not a back-and-forth motion. Spray with a fixative (or not) according to the procedures required at your agency. This specimen is important for an adolescent whose endocervical cells have not yet migrated into the endocervical canal.

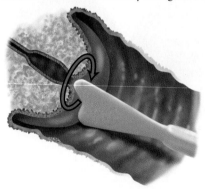

27-14

Endocervical Specimen. Insert a Cytobrush (instead of a cotton applicator) into the os (Figure 27-15). With a Cytobrush, you obtain a higher yield of endocervical cells at the squamocolumnar junction (SCJ), and it is safe for use during pregnancy (Stillson, Knight, & Elswick, 1997). The transformation zone (T zone) is generally located at the external cervical os, at the junction of squamous and glandular cells, and is the area at greatest risk for development of cervical cancers (Schiffman et al., 2007). The patient may feel a slight pinch with the brush, and scant bleeding may occur. For this reason, collect the endocervical specimen last so that bleeding does not obscure cytological evaluation.

Cervical polyp: bright red growth protruding from the os (see Table 27-4, p. 774).

Foul-smelling, irritating, with yellow, green, white, or grey discharge (see Table 27-5, pp. 775–776).

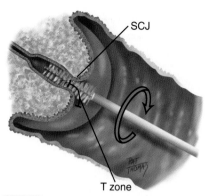

SCJ

T zone

27-15

Rotate the brush 720 degrees in *one* direction in the endocervical canal, either clockwise or counterclockwise. Then withdraw the brush and rotate it gently on a slide to deposit all the cells. Rotate in the direction opposite the one you used to obtain the specimen. Avoid leaving a thick specimen, which would be hard to analyze under the microscope.

Immediately (within 2 seconds) spray the slide with fixative to avoid drying, if procedures require this step.

For a patient after hysterectomy whose cervix has been removed, collect a scrape from the end of the vagina and a vaginal pool.

Immediately spray the slides with fixative. The frosted ends of the slides should be labelled with the patient's name. Send the slides to the laboratory with the following necessary data:
- Date of specimen
- Patient's date of birth
- Date of most recent menstrual period
- Any hormone medication
- If the patient is pregnant, estimated date examination of delivery
- Known infections
- Prior surgery or radiation treatment
- Prior abnormal cytological findings
- Abnormal findings on physical examination

These data are important for accurate interpretation; for example, a specimen may be interpreted as abnormal unless the laboratory technicians know that the patient has had prior radiation treatment.

Newer methods of cervical screening entail **liquid-based cytology (LBC).** The sample is collected with a cervical spatula or an endocervical brush but is placed in a vial containing cell-preserving fluid. Since June 2011, LBC has been used in cancer screening programs in Newfoundland, Northwest Territories, and Nunavut, and both conventional and LBC screening tests are being used in Ontario, Alberta and New Brunswick (Canadian Partnership against Cancer, 2011). To screen for STIs, and if you note any abnormal vaginal discharge, obtain the **gonorrhea/chlamydia culture.** Insert a sterile cotton applicator into the os, rotate it 360 degrees, and leave it in place 10 to 20 seconds for complete saturation. Withdraw the applicator, and insert it into a labelled specimen container.

On occasion, you need the following samples:

Saline Mount, or "Wet Preparation." Spread a sample of the discharge onto a glass slide, and add one drop of normal saline solution and a coverslip.

Potassium Hydroxide Preparation. To a sample of the discharge on a glass slide, add one drop of KOH and a coverslip.

Anal Culture. Insert a sterile cotton swab into the anal canal about 1 cm. Rotate it, and move it side to side. Leave in place 10 to 20 seconds. If the swab collects feces, discard it and begin again. Withdraw the swab, and insert the culture sample into a labelled specimen container.

Acetic Acid Wash. Acetic acid (white vinegar) wash is a method of screening for asymptomatic HPV infection, which causes genital warts. This is not a common practice in Canada, as ready access to PAP testing is available across the country. However, if desired or indicated, after all other specimens are gathered, soak a thick-tipped cotton rectal swab with acetic acid, and "paint" the cervix. Acetic acid dissolves mucus and temporarily causes intracellular dehydration and coagulation of protein. A normal response (indicating no HPV infection) is no change in the cervical epithelium.

Rapid acetowhitening or blanching, especially with irregular borders, is suggestive of HPV infection (see Table 27-2, p. 771).

Inspect the Vaginal Wall

Loosen the thumbscrew but continue to hold the speculum blades open. Slowly withdraw the speculum, rotating it as you go, to fully inspect the vaginal wall. Normally, the wall looks pink, deeply rugated, moist, and smooth and is free of inflammation or lesions. Normal discharge is thin and clear, or opaque and stringy, but always odourless.

Inflammation or lesions should be investigated.

Leukoplakia appears as a spot of dried white paint.

Vaginal discharge is abnormal when it has the following characteristics: thick, white, and curdlike (with candidiasis); profuse, watery, grey-green, and frothy (with trichomoniasis); or any grey, green-yellow, white, or foul-smelling discharge (see Table 27-5, p. 776).

When the blade ends of the speculum near the vaginal opening, let them close, but be careful not to pinch the mucosa or catch any hairs. Turn the blades obliquely to avoid stretching the opening. Place a metal speculum in a basin to be cleaned later and soaked in a sterilizing and disinfecting solution; discard the plastic variety. Discard your gloves, and wash hands.

Bimanual Examination

Rise to a stand, and have the patient remain in lithotomy position. Drop lubricant onto the first two fingers of the gloved hand that will be inserted intravaginally (Figure 27-16). Assume the "obstetrical" position with the first two fingers extended, the last two flexed onto the palm, and the thumb abducted. Insert your lubricated fingers into the vagina, with any pressure directed posteriorly. Wait until the vaginal walls relax, then insert your fingers fully.

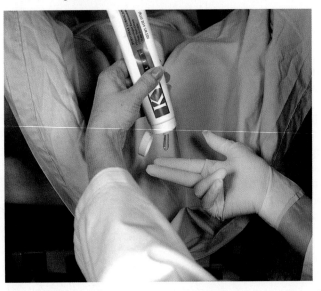

27-16

Use both hands to palpate the internal genitalia to assess their location, size, and mobility and to screen for any tenderness or mass. One hand is on the abdomen (the "abdominal" hand), and the other (often the dominant, more sensitive hand) inserts two fingers into the vagina (the "intravaginal" hand; Figure 27-17). It does not matter which hand you choose to be inserted intravaginally; try each way (on different patients), and settle on the method most comfortable for you.

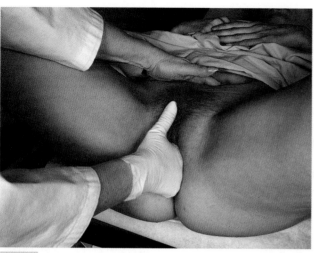

27-17

Palpate the vaginal wall. Normally, it feels smooth and has no area of induration or tenderness.

Cervix. Locate the cervix in the midline, often near the anterior vaginal wall. The cervix points in the opposite direction of the fundus of the uterus. Palpate, using the palmar surface of your fingers. Note the following characteristics of a normal cervix:

- Consistency: smooth and firm, like the consistency of the tip of the nose. It softens and feels velvety at 5 to 6 weeks of pregnancy (Goodell's sign).
- Contour: evenly rounded
- Mobility—With a finger on either side, move the cervix gently from side to side. Normally, this produces no pain (Figure 27-18).

Nodule.
Tenderness.

Hard with malignancy.
Nodular.
Irregular.
Immobile with malignancy.

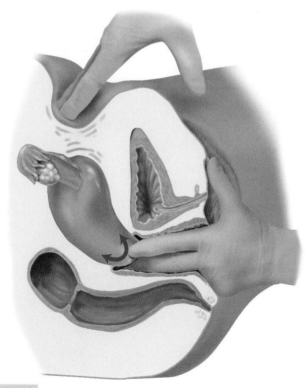

27-18

Palpate all around the fornices; the wall should feel smooth.

Painful with inflammation or ectopic pregnancy.

Next, use your "abdominal" hand to push the pelvic organs closer for your intravaginal fingers to palpate. Place your "abdominal" hand midway between the umbilicus and the symphysis; push down in a slow, firm manner, fingers together and slightly flexed. Brace the elbow of your "intravaginal" arm against your hip, and keep it horizontal. The patient must be relaxed.

Uterus. With your "intravaginal" fingers in the anterior fornix, assess the uterus. Determine the position, or *version,* of the uterus (Figure 27-19). This compares the long axis of the uterus with the long axis of the body. In many women, the uterus is anteverted; you palpate it at the level of the pubis with the cervix pointing posteriorly. Two other positions are also normal (midposition and retroverted), as are two aspects of flexion, in which the long axis of the uterus is not straight but is flexed.

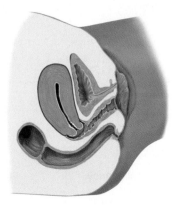

Anteverted

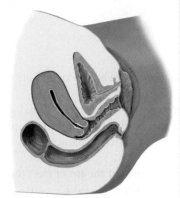

Midposition

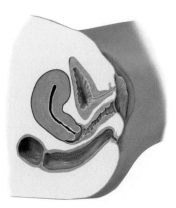

Anteflexed

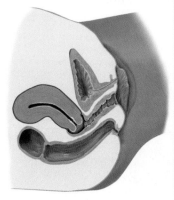

Retroflexed

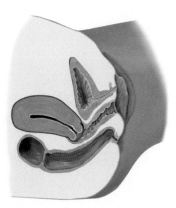

Retroverted

27-19

Palpate the uterine wall with your fingers in the fornices. Normally, it feels firm and smooth, with the contour of the fundus rounded. It softens during pregnancy. Bounce the uterus gently between your abdominal and intravaginal hands. It should be freely movable and nontender.

Adnexa. Move both hands to the right to explore the adnexa. Place your abdominal hand on the lower quadrant just inside the anterior iliac spine and your "intravaginal" fingers in the lateral fornix (Figure 27-20). Push the "abdominal" hand down, and try to palpate the ovary. In many patients, you cannot palpate the ovary. When you can, it normally feels smooth, firm, and almond-shaped and is highly movable, sliding through the fingers. It is slightly sensitive but not painful. The fallopian tube is normally not palpable. No other mass or pulsation should be felt.

Enlarged uterus (see Table 27-6, p. 777).
Lateral displacement.
Nodular mass.
Irregular, asymmetrical uterus.
Fixed and immobile uterus.
Tenderness.
Enlarged adnexa; nodules or mass in adnexa.
Immobile adnexa.
Marked tenderness (see Table 27-7, p. 778).

CRITICAL FINDINGS

Pulsation or palpable fallopian tube suggests ectopic pregnancy; this warrants immediate referral (see Table 27-7).

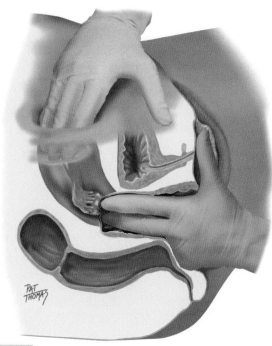

27-20

A note of caution: Normal adnexal structures often are not palpable. Be careful not to mistake an abnormality for a normal structure. To be safe, consider abnormal any mass that you cannot *positively* identify, and refer the patient for further study.

Move to the left to palpate the other side. Then, withdraw your hand and check secretions on the gloved fingers before you discard the glove. Normal secretions are clear or cloudy and odourless.

Rectovaginal Examination

Use this technique to assess the rectovaginal septum, posterior uterine wall, cul-de-sac, and rectum. Change gloves to avoid spreading any possible infection. Lubricate the first two fingers. Instruct the woman that this may feel uncomfortable and will mimic the feeling of moving her bowels. Ask her to bear down as you insert your index finger into the vagina and your middle finger gently into the rectum (Figure 27-21).

Special Considerations for Advanced Practice

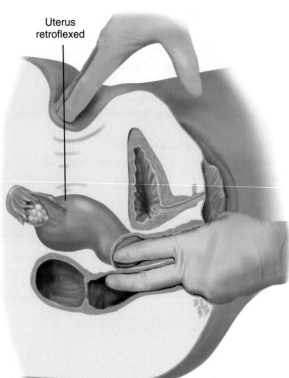

Uterus retroflexed

RECTOVAGINAL PALPATION

27-21

While pushing with the "abdominal" hand, repeat the steps of the bimanual examination. Try to keep the "intravaginal" finger on the cervix so that the finger in the rectum does not mistake the cervix for a mass. Note the following characteristics:

- The rectovaginal septum should feel smooth, thin, firm, and pliable.
- The rectovaginal pouch, or cul-de-sac, is a potential space and usually not palpable.
- The uterine wall and fundus feel firm and smooth.

Rotate the "intrarectal" finger to check the rectal wall and anal sphincter tone. (See Chapter 23 for assessment of anus and rectum.) Check your gloved finger as you withdraw it; test any adherent stool for occult blood.

Give the patient tissues to wipe the area, and help her up. Remind her to slide her hips back from the edge before sitting up so that she does not fall.

Nodular or thickened.

❖ DEVELOPMENTAL CONSIDERATIONS

Infants and Children

Preparation

- Infant: Place on examination table.
- Toddler or preschooler: Place on parent's lap in the frog-leg position: hips flexed and soles of feet together and touching the child's buttocks. A preschool-age child may want to separate her own labia. Do not use drapes; a young girl wants to see what you are doing.
- School-age child: place on examination table, frog-leg position, no drapes. During childhood, a routine screening is limited to inspection of the external genitalia to determine that (a) the structures are intact, (b) the vagina is present, and (c) the hymen is patent.

The newborn's genitalia are somewhat engorged. The labia majora are swollen; the labia minora are prominent and protrude beyond the labia majora; the clitoris looks relatively large; and the hymen appears thick. Because of transient engorgement, the vaginal opening is more difficult to see now than it will be later. Place your thumbs on the labia majora. Push laterally while pushing the perineum down, and try to note the vaginal opening above the hymenal ring. Do not palpate the clitoris because it is very sensitive.

A sanguineous vaginal discharge or leukorrhea (mucoid discharge) are normal during the first few weeks because of the maternal estrogen effect. (This also may cause transient breast engorgement and secretion.) During the early weeks, the genital engorgement resolves, and the labia minora atrophy and remain small until puberty (Figure 27-22).

Ambiguous genitalia are rare. The appearance is of a markedly enlarged clitoris, fusion of the labia (resembling scrotum), and palpable mass in fused labia (resembling testes; see Table 27-8, p. 780).

Imperforate hymen warrants referral. Lesions, rash.

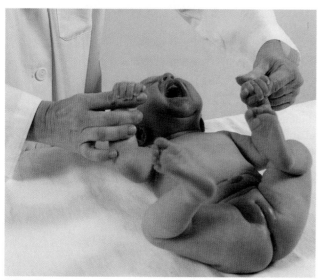

27-22

Between the ages of 2 months and 7 years, the labia majora are flat, the labia minora are thin, the clitoris is relatively small, and the hymen is tissue-paper thin. Normally, no irritation or foul-smelling discharge is present.

In young school-age girls (7 to 10 years), the mons pubis thickens, the labia majora thicken, and the labia minora become slightly rounded. Pubic hair begins to appear at approximately age 11 years, although sparse pubic hair may appear as early as age 8 years. Normally, the hymen is perforate.

Almost always in these age groups, an external examination will suffice. An internal pelvic examination, if needed, is best performed by a pediatric gynecologist with the use of specialized instruments.

Poor perineal hygiene.

Pest inhabitants; excoriations.

During and after toddler age, foul-smelling discharge occurs with lodging of foreign body, pinworms, or infection.

Absence of pubic hair by 13 years indicates delayed puberty.

Amenorrhea in an adolescent, together with bluish and bulging hymen, indicates imperforate hymen and warrants referral.

Adolescents

Adolescent girls have special needs during the genitalia examination. Examine such a patient alone, without the mother present. Assure her of privacy and confidentiality. Allow plenty of time for health education and discussion of pubertal progress. Assess the patient's growth velocity and menstrual history, and use the sexual maturity rating charts to teach breast and pubic hair development. Assure her that increased vaginal fluid (physiological *leukorrhea*) is normal because of the estrogen effect.

Objective Data

Perform pelvic examination when contraception is desired, when the girl's sexual activity includes intercourse, or at age 18 years in virgins. Start periodic Pap smears when intercourse begins. Although the techniques of the examination are listed in the section for adults, you will need to provide additional time and psychological support for an adolescent undergoing her first pelvic examination.

The experience of the first pelvic examination determines how the adolescent will approach future care. Your accepting attitude and gentle, unhurried approach are important. You have a unique teaching opportunity here. Take the time to teach, using the girl's own body as illustration. Your frank discussion of anatomy and sexual behaviour communicates that these topics are not taboo and are acceptable to discuss with health care providers. This affirms the girl's self-concept and helps the girl understand that her body is normal.

During the bimanual examination, note that the adnexa are not palpable in an adolescent.

Pelvic or adnexal mass.

Pregnant Women

Depending on the week of the pregnancy, inspection reveals the enlarging abdomen (see Figure 30-1 on p. 813). The height of the fundus ascends gradually as the fetus grows. At 16 weeks, the fundus is palpable halfway between the symphysis and umbilicus; at 20 weeks, at the lower edge of the umbilicus; at 28 weeks, halfway between the umbilicus and the xiphoid process; and at 34 to 36 weeks, almost to the xiphoid process. Close to term, the fundus drops as the fetal head engages in the pelvis.

The external genitalia exhibit hyperemia of the perineum and vulva because of increased vascularity. Varicose veins may be visible in the labia or legs, and hemorrhoids may be visible around the anus. Both are caused by interruption in venous return from the pressure of the fetus.

Internally, the walls of the vagina appear violet or blue (Chadwick's sign) because of hyperemia. The vaginal walls are deeply rugated, and the vaginal mucosa thickens. The cervix looks blue, feels velvety, and feels softer than in the nonpregnant state; thus it is a bit more difficult to differentiate from the vaginal walls.

During bimanual examination, the isthmus of the uterus feels softer and is more easily compressed between your two hands (Hegar's sign). The fundus balloons between your two hands; it feels connected to, but distinct from, the cervix because the isthmus is so soft.

Search the adnexal area carefully during early pregnancy. Normally, the adnexal structures are not palpable.

An ectopic pregnancy has serious consequences (see Table 27-7, p. 779).

Older Women

Natural lubrication is decreased; to avoid a painful examination, take care to lubricate instruments and the examining hand adequately. Use the Pedersen speculum (rather than the Graves) because its narrower, flatter blades are more comfortable in women with vaginal stenosis or dryness.

Menopause and the resulting decrease in estrogen production cause numerous physical changes. Pubic hair gradually decreases, becoming thin and sparse in later years. The skin is thinner, and fat deposits decrease, leaving the mons pubis smaller and the labia flatter. Clitoris size also decreases after age 60 years.

Internally, the rugae of the vaginal walls decrease, and the walls look pale pink because of the thinned epithelium. The cervix shrinks and looks pale and glistening. It may retract, appearing to be flush with the vaginal wall. In some women, it is hard to distinguish the cervix from the surrounding vaginal mucosa. Alternately, the cervix may protrude into the vagina if the uterus has prolapsed.

Refer any suspect red, white, or pigmented lesion for biopsy.

Vaginal atrophy increases the risk of infection and trauma.

With the bimanual examination, you may need to insert only one gloved finger if vaginal stenosis exists. The uterus feels smaller and firmer, and the ovaries are normally not palpable.

Cervical cancer screening is not required after total hysterectomy for benign conditions in women who do not have a history of cervical dysplasia and have had a negative and adequate screening history (Murphy, 2007); however, recommendations may vary by region. Be aware that older women may have special needs and will appreciate the following plans of care: For example, advise those with arthritis to take a mild analgesic or anti-inflammatory agent before the appointment to ease joint pain in positioning; schedule appointment times when joint pain or stiffness is at its least; allow extra time for positioning and "unpositioning" after the examination; and be careful to maintain dignity and privacy.

> Refer any mass for prompt evaluation.

DOCUMENTATION AND CRITICAL THINKING

Sample Charting

SUBJECTIVE

Menarche age 12 years, cycle usually q28d, duration 5 days, flow moderate, no dysmenorrhea, LMP [last menstrual period] April 3. Grav 0/Para 0/Ab 0. Gynecological checkups yearly. Last Pap test 1 year PTA, negative.

No urinary problems, no irritating or foul-smelling vaginal discharge, no sores or lesions, no history of pelvic surgery. Satisfied with sexual relationship with husband, uses vaginal diaphragm for birth control, no plans for pregnancy at this time. Aware of no contact by self or husband with STIs.

OBJECTIVE

External genitalia: No swelling, lesions, or discharge. No urethral swelling or discharge.
Internal: Vaginal walls have no bulging or lesions; cervix is pink with no lesions; scant clear mucoid discharge.
Bimanual: No pain on moving cervix; uterus anteflexed and anteverted; no enlargement or irregularity.
Adnexa: Ovaries not enlarged.
Rectal: No hemorrhoids, fissures, or lesions; no masses or tenderness; stool brown with guaiac test result negative.

ASSESSMENT

Genital structures intact and appear healthy

Focused Assessment: Clinical Case Study 1

J.K., 27-year-old, married newspaper reporter, Grav 0/Para 0/Ab 0. Presents at clinic with "urinary burning, vaginal itching, and discharge" × 4 days.

SUBJECTIVE

- 3 weeks PTA: treated at clinic for bronchitis with erythromycin. Improved within 5 days.
- 4 to 5 days PTA: noted burning sensation on urination; intense vaginal itching; thick, white, "smelly" discharge. Warm water douche; no relief.
- No previous history vaginal infection, urinary tract infection, or pelvic surgery. Monogamous sexual relationship, has used low-estrogen birth control pills for 3 years with no side effects.

Objective Data

Documentation &
Critical Thinking

OBJECTIVE

Vulva and vagina erythematous and edematous. Thick, white, curdlike discharge clinging to vaginal walls. Cervix pink, no lesions.

Bimanual examination: No pain on palpating cervix, uterus not enlarged, ovaries not enlarged.

Specimens: Pap smear, gonorrhea/chlamydia culture to laboratory. KOH preparation shows mycelia and spores of *Candida albicans.*

ASSESSMENT

Candida vaginitis
Pain R/T infectious process

Focused Assessment: Clinical Case Study 2

Brenda, a 17-year-old high school student, comes to clinic for pelvic examination.

SUBJECTIVE

- Menarche 12 years, cycle q30d, duration 6 days, mild cramps relieved by acetaminophen. LMP March 10. No dysuria, vaginal discharge, vaginal itching. Relationship involving intercourse with one boyfriend for 8 months PTA. For birth control, boyfriend uses condoms "sometimes." Brenda wants to start birth control pills. Never had pelvic examination. No knowledge of breast self-examination. No knowledge of STIs except AIDS. Smokes cigarettes, ½ PPD, started age 11 years.

OBJECTIVE

Breasts: Symmetrical, no lesions or discharge, palpation reveals no mass or tenderness.

External genitalia: No redness, lesions, or discharge.

Internal genitalia: Vaginal walls and cervix pink with no lesions or discharge. Specimens obtained. Acetic acid wash shows no acetowhitening.

Bimanual: No tenderness to palpation, uterus anteverted with no enlargement, ovaries not enlarged.

Rectum: No masses, fissure, or tenderness. Stool brown, and guaiac test result negative.

Specimens: gonorrhea/*Chlamydia* culture, Pap smear to laboratory.

ASSESSMENT

Breast and pelvic structures appear healthy

Deficient knowledge regarding: breast self-examination; birth control measures; STI prevention; cigarette smoking R/T lack of education

ABNORMAL FINDINGS

TABLE 27-2	Abnormalities of the External Genitalia

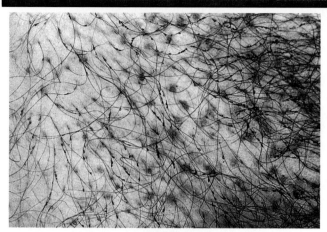

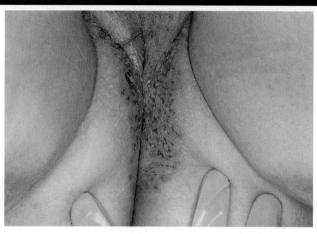

Pediculosis Pubis (Crab Lice)

S: Severe perineal itching.

O: Excoriations and erythematous areas. Little dark spots (lice are small), nits (eggs) adherent to pubic hair near roots may be visible. Usually localized in pubic hair, occasionally in eyebrows or eyelashes.

Herpes Simplex Virus Type 2 (Herpes Genitalis)

S: Episodes of local pain, dysuria, fever.

O: Clusters of small, shallow vesicles with surrounding erythema; erupt on genital areas and inner thigh. Also, inguinal adenopathy, edema. Vesicles on labia rupture in 1–3 days, leaving painful ulcers. Initial manifestation lasts 7–10 days. Virus remains dormant indefinitely; recurrent manifestations last 3–10 days with milder symptoms.

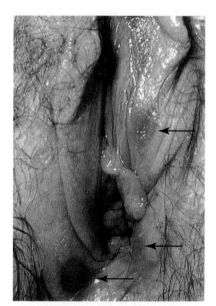

Reprinted from Emond, R. (1995). Colour atlas of infectious diseases (3rd ed., p. 173). St. Louis: Mosby, by permission of the publisher Mosby.

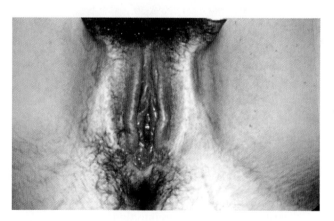

Syphilitic Chancre

O: Begins as a small, solitary silvery papule that erodes to a red, round or oval, superficial ulcer with a yellowish serous discharge. Palpation: nontender indurated base; can be lifted like a button between thumb and finger. Nontender inguinal lymphadenopathy.

Red Rash: Contact Dermatitis

S: History of skin contact with allergenic substance in environment; intense pruritus.

O: Primary lesion: red, swollen vesicles, which may then weep; crusts, scales, thickening of skin, excoriations from scratching may be present. Rash may result from reaction to feminine hygiene spray or synthetic underclothing.

Continued

TABLE 27-2   Abnormalities of the External Genitalia—cont'd

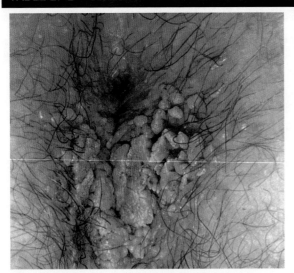

Human Papillomavirus (HPV) Genital Warts

S: Painless warty growths, may be unnoticed by woman.

O: Pink or flesh-coloured, soft, pointed, moist, warty papules. Single or multiple in a cauliflower-like patch. Occur around vulva, introitus, anus, vagina, cervix.

HPV infection is common among sexually active women, especially adolescents, regardless of ethnicity or socioeconomic status. Risk factors include early age at menarche and multiple sexual partners. The long incubation period (6 weeks to 8 months) makes it difficult to establish history of exposure. HPV infection is strongly associated with abnormal cervical cytological findings.

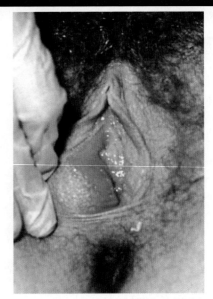

Reprinted from Emond, R. (1995). Colour atlas of infectious diseases (3rd ed., p. 161). St. Louis: Mosby, by permission of the publisher Mosby.

Abscess of Bartholin's Gland

S: Local pain, can be severe.

O: Overlying skin red and hot. Posterior part of labia swollen; palpable fluctuant mass and tenderness. Red spot is visible on mucosa at site of duct opening; can express purulent discharge. Often secondary to gonococcal infection.

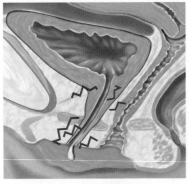

Urethritis

Urethritis

S: Dysuria.

O: Palpation of anterior vaginal wall reveals erythema, tenderness, induration along urethra, purulent discharge from meatus. Caused by *Neisseria gonorrhoeae*, *Chlamydia*, or *Staphylococcus* infection.

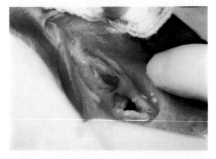

Urethral Caruncle

S: Tenderness, pain with urination, urinary frequency, hematuria, dyspareunia, or no symptoms.

O: Small, deep red mass protruding from meatus; usually secondary to urethritis or skenitis; lesion may bleed on contact.

S, Subjective data; *O,* objective data.

TABLE 27-3   Abnormalities of the Pelvic Musculature

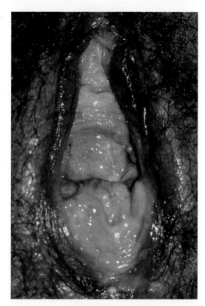

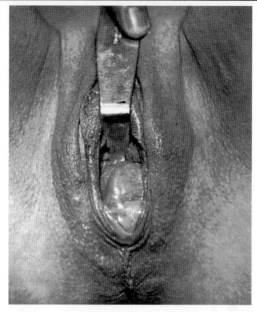

Cystocele (With Bladder Prolapse)

S: Sensation of pressure in vagina, stress incontinence.

O: With straining or standing, introitus widens, and a soft, round anterior bulge is evident. The bladder, covered by vaginal mucosa, prolapses into vagina; in the case illustrated, it is accompanied by an extreme uterine prolapse.

Rectocele

S: Sensation of pressure in vagina, possibly constipation.

O: With straining or standing, note introitus widening and the presence of a soft, round bulge from posterior. Here, part of the rectum, covered by vaginal mucosa, prolapses into vagina.

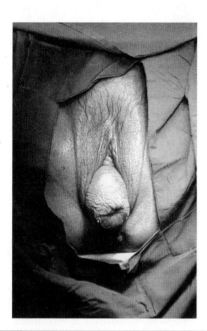

◄ Uterine Prolapse

O: With straining or standing, uterus protrudes into vagina. Prolapse is graded as follows:

- First degree: Cervix appears at introitus with straining.
- Second degree: Cervix bulges outside introitus with straining.
- Third degree (in illustration): Whole uterus protrudes even without straining; in essence, uterus is inside out.

S, Subjective data; O, objective data.

TABLE 27-4	Abnormalities of the Cervix

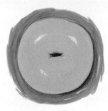

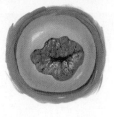

Bluish Cervix: Cyanosis

O: Bluish discoloration of the mucosa is normal during pregnancy (Chadwick's sign at 6–8 weeks) and with any other condition causing hypoxia or venous congestion (e.g., heart failure, pelvic tumour).

Erosion

O: Cervical lips are inflamed and eroded. Reddened granular surface is superficial inflammation, with no ulceration (loss of tissue). It is usually secondary to purulent or mucopurulent cervical discharge. Biopsy is needed to distinguish erosion from carcinoma; clinician cannot rely on inspection.

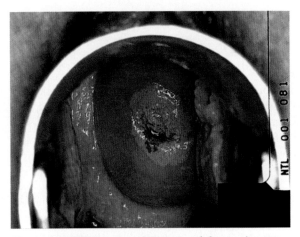

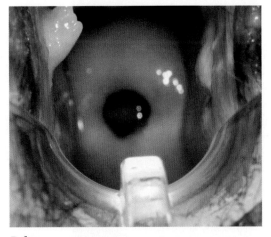

Human Papillomavirus (HPV, Condylomata)

O: Virus can appear in various forms when affecting cervical epithelium. In illustration, warty growth appears as abnormal thickened white epithelium. Visibility of lesion is enhanced by acetic acid (vinegar) wash, which dissolves mucus and temporarily causes intracellular dehydration and coagulation of protein.

Polyp

S: Mucoid discharge or bleeding may occur.

O: Bright red, soft, pedunculated growth emerges from os. It is a benign lesion, but this must be determined through biopsy. It may be lined with squamous or columnar epithelium.

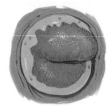

◄ Diethylstilbestrol (DES) Syndrome

S: Prenatal exposure to DES causes cervical and vaginal abnormalities.

O: Red, granular patches of columnar epithelium extend beyond normal squamocolumnar junction onto cervix and into fornices (vaginal adenosis). Cervical abnormalities may also be present: circular groove, transverse ridge, protuberant anterior lip, "cock's-comb" formation. Frequent monitoring is warranted.

TABLE 27-4   Abnormalities of the Cervix—cont'd

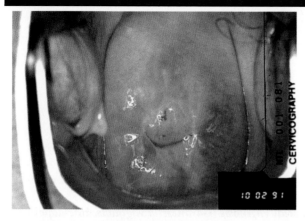

◄ *Carcinoma*

S: Carcinoma may manifest as bleeding between menstrual periods or after menopause or as unusual vaginal discharge.

O: Chronic ulcer and induration are early signs of carcinoma, although the lesion may or may not show on the exocervix. (In illustration, lesion is mostly around the external os.) It is diagnosed through Pap smear and biopsy. Risk factors for cervical cancer are early age at first intercourse, multiple sex partners, cigarette smoking, and certain sexually transmitted infections.

S, Subjective data; *O,* objective data.

TABLE 27-5   Vulvovaginal Inflammations

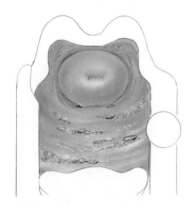

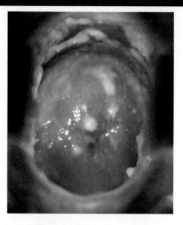

Atrophic Vaginitis

S: Postmenopausal vaginal itching, dryness, burning sensation, dyspareunia, mucoid discharge (may be flecked with blood).

O: Mucosa is pale, with abraded areas that bleed easily; bloody discharge may be present.

This is an opportunistic infection related to chronic estrogen deficiency.

Candidiasis (Moniliasis)

S: Intense pruritus; thick, whitish discharge.

O: Vulva and vagina are erythematous and edematous. Discharge is usually thick, white, curdy, "like cottage cheese." Infection is diagnosed through microscopic examination of discharge on potassium hydroxide wet mount.

Predisposing causes include use of oral contraceptives or antibiotics, more alkaline vaginal pH (as with menstrual periods, postpartum, menopause), and pregnancy (because of increased glycogen and diabetes).

Continued

TABLE 27-5   **Vulvovaginal Inflammations—cont'd**

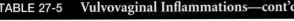

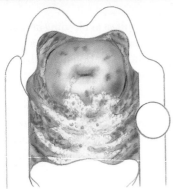

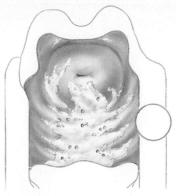

Trichomoniasis

S: Pruritus, watery and often malodorous vaginal discharge, urinary frequency, terminal dysuria. Symptoms are worse during menstruation, when the pH becomes optimal for the organism's growth.

O: Vulva may be erythematous. Vagina is diffusely red, granular, occasionally with red raised papules and petechiae ("strawberry" appearance). Discharge is frothy, yellow-green, and foul-smelling. Microscopic examination of saline wet mount specimen reveals characteristic flagellated cells.

Bacterial Vaginosis (Gardnerella vaginalis, Haemophilus vaginalis, or Nonspecific Vaginitis)

S: Profuse discharge, "constant wetness" with "foul, fishy, rotten" odour.

O: Discharge is thin, creamy, grey-white, and malodorous. No inflammation is present on vaginal wall or cervix because the pathogen is a surface parasite. Microscopic view of saline wet mount specimen reveals typical "clue cells."

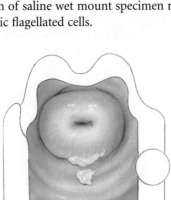

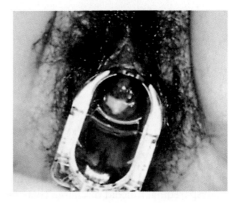

Chlamydia

S: (Mimics gonorrhea.) Of infected women, 75% have no symptoms. Symptoms may include urinary frequency, dysuria, vaginal discharge, or postcoital bleeding.

O: Affected patients may have yellow or green mucopurulent discharge, friable cervix, cervical motion tenderness. Signs are subtle, easily mistaken for gonorrhea. The two are important to distinguish because antibiotic treatment is different; if the wrong drug is given or if the condition is untreated, *Chlamydia* can ascend the reproductive tract to cause pelvic inflammatory disease (PID) and result in infertility. This is the most common sexually transmitted infection in Canada; nearly 70% of all reported cases occur in the 15- to 24-year-old age cohort. Clinicians are urged to screen all sexually active girls and young women every 6 months, regardless of symptoms or risk.

Gonorrhea

S: Variable: vaginal discharge, dysuria, abnormal uterine bleeding, abscess in Bartholin's or Skene's glands; the majority of cases are asymptomatic.

O: Often no signs are apparent. Purulent vaginal discharge may be present. The disease is diagnosed through positive culture of organism. If the condition is untreated, it may progress to acute salpingitis, PID.

S, Subjective data; *O,* objective data.

TABLE 27-6   Uterine Enlargement

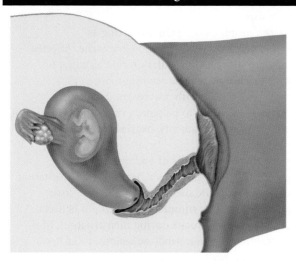

◄ *Pregnancy*

Obviously a normal condition; included here for comparison.

S: Amenorrhea, fatigue, breast engorgement, nausea, change in food tolerance, weight gain.

O: Early signs include cyanosis of vaginal mucosa and cervix (Chadwick's sign). Palpation reveals soft consistency of cervix, enlarging uterus with compressible fundus and isthmus (Hegar's sign) at 10–12 weeks.

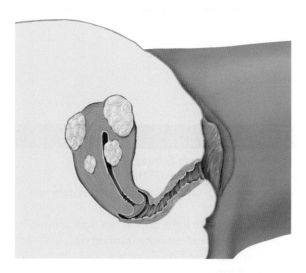

◄ *Myomas (Leiomyomas, Uterine Fibroids)*

S: Varies, depending on size and location. Often no symptoms. Symptoms that do occur include vague discomfort, bloating, heaviness, pelvic pressure, dyspareunia, urinary frequency, backache, or hypermenorrhea if myoma disturbs endometrium. Heavy bleeding produces anemia.

O: Uterus irregularly enlarged, firm, mobile, and nodular with hard, painless nodules in the uterine wall.

Myomas are usually benign. Incidence is highest between the ages of 30 and 45 years and in women of African descent. Myomas are estrogen dependent; after menopause, the lesions usually regress but do not disappear. Surgery may be indicated.

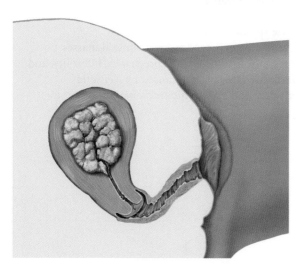

◄ *Carcinoma of the Endometrium*

S: Abnormal and intermenstrual bleeding before menopause; postmenopausal bleeding or mucosanguineous discharge. Pain and weight loss occur late in the disease.

O: Uterus may be enlarged.

The Pap smear is rarely effective in detecting endometrial cancer. Women with abnormal vaginal bleeding or at high risk for endometrial cancer should undergo biopsy of an endometrial tissue sample. Risk factors for endometrial cancer are early menarche, late menopause, history of infertility, failure to ovulate, use of tamoxifen, unopposed estrogen therapy (which continually stimulates the endometrium, causing hyperplasia), and obesity (which increases endogenous estrogen).

Continued

Abnormal Findings

TABLE 27-6	Uterine Enlargement—cont'd

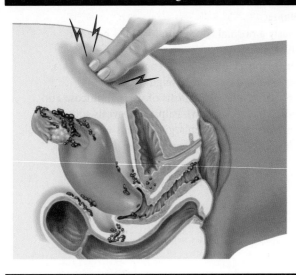

◀ *Endometriosis*

S: Cyclic or chronic pelvic pain, occurring as dysmenorrhea, dyspareunia, or low backache. Affected patients may also have irregular uterine bleeding or hypermenorrhea or may be asymptomatic.

O: Uterus fixed, tender with movement. Small, firm nodular masses tender to palpation on posterior aspect of fundus, uterosacral ligaments, ovaries, sigmoid colon. Ovaries often enlarged.

Masses are aberrant growths of endometrial tissue scattered throughout pelvis as a result of transplantation of tissue by retrograde menstruation. Ectopic tissue responds to hormone stimulation: builds up between menstrual periods, sloughs during menstruation. May cause infertility through pelvic adhesions, tubal obstruction, decreased ovarian function.

S, Subjective data; *O,* objective data.

TABLE 27-7	Adnexal Enlargement

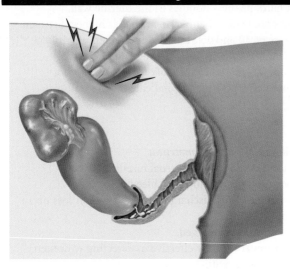

◀ *Fallopian Tube Mass: Acute Salpingitis (Pelvic Inflammatory Disease [PID])*

S: Sudden fever >38°C, suprapubic pain and tenderness.

O:

• Acute: Rigid boardlike lower abdominal musculature. Purulent discharge may emanate from cervix. Movement of uterus and cervix causes intense pain. Pain in lateral fornices and adnexa. Bilateral adnexal masses are difficult to palpate because of pain and muscle spasm.

• Chronic: Bilateral, tender, fixed adnexal masses.

Complications include ectopic pregnancy, infertility, and reinfection. PID is usually caused by *Neisseria gonorrhoeae* and *Chlamydia trachomatis.*

TABLE 27-7   Adnexal Enlargement—cont'd

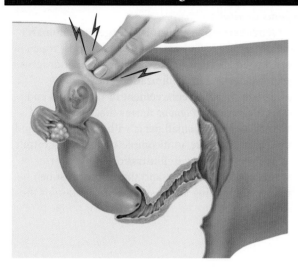

◄ *Fallopian Tube Mass: Ectopic Pregnancy*

S: Amenorrhea or irregular vaginal bleeding, pelvic pain.

O: Softening of cervix and fundus; movement of cervix and uterus causes pain; palpable tender pelvic mass, which is solid, mobile, unilateral.

This condition has potential for serious sequelae; seek gynecological consultation immediately before the mass ruptures or the patient shows signs of acute peritonitis.

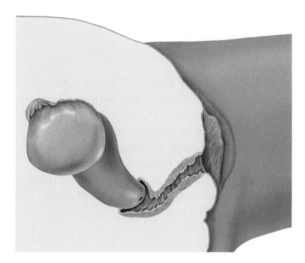

◄ *Fluctuant Ovarian Mass: Ovarian Cyst*

S: Usually asymptomatic.

O: Smooth, round, fluctuant, mobile, nontender mass on ovary. Some cysts resolve spontaneously within 60 days but must be monitored closely.

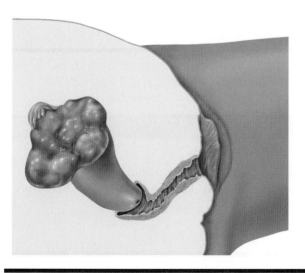

◄ *Solid Ovarian Mass: Ovarian Cancer*

S: Usually asymptomatic. Abdomen may enlarge from fluid accumulation.

O: Solid tumour palpated on ovary. Heavy, solid, fixed, poorly defined mass suggests malignancy; benign mass may feel mobile and solid.

Biopsy necessary to distinguish the two types of masses. The Pap smear does not detect ovarian cancer. Women older than 40 years should have a thorough pelvic examination every year.

S, Subjective data; *O,* objective data.

TABLE 27-8 Abnormalities in Pediatric Genitalia

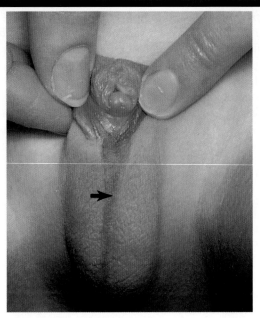

◄ **Ambiguous Genitalia**

Female pseudohermaphroditism is a congenital anomaly resulting from hyperplasia of the adrenal glands, which exposes the female fetus to excess amounts of androgens. This exposure causes masculinization of external genitalia, here shown as enlargement of the clitoris and fusion of the labia. *Ambiguous* means that the enlarged clitoris may look like a small penis with hypospadias, and the fused labia look like an incompletely formed scrotum with absent testes (*arrow* in illustration). Other forms of intersexual conditions occur, and the family must be referred for counselling and diagnostic evaluation of the child.

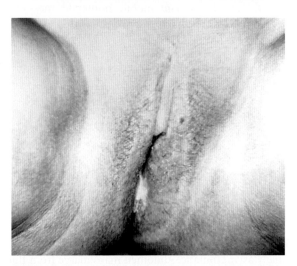

◄ **Vulvovaginitis in Child**

This infection is caused by *Candida albicans* in a diabetic child. Symptoms include pruritus and burning when urine touches excoriated area. Examination reveals red, shiny, edematous vulva; vaginal discharge; and area that has become excoriated from scratching.

Other, more common causes of vulvovaginitis in prepubertal children include infection from a respiratory or bowel pathogen, sexually transmitted infection, or presence of a foreign body.

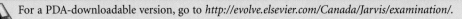

Summary Checklist: Female Genitalia Examination

For a PDA-downloadable version, go to *http://evolve.elsevier.com/Canada/Jarvis/examination/*.

1. Inspect external genitalia.
2. Palpate labia, Skene's, and Bartholin's glands.
3. Using vaginal speculum, inspect cervix and vagina.
4. Obtain specimens for cytological study.
5. Perform bimanual examination: cervix, uterus, adnexa.
6. Perform rectovaginal examination.
7. Test stool for occult blood.
8. Perform teaching and health promotion.

REFERENCES

Amies, A. M., Miller, L., Lee, S. K., & Koutsky, L. (2002). The effect of vaginal speculum lubrication on the rate of unsatisfactory cervical cytology diagnosis. *Obstetrics & Gynecology*, 100(5), 889–892.

Canadian Partnership Against Cancer. (2011). *Cervical cancer screening in Canada: Monitoring program performance 2006–2008*. Retrieved from *http://www.cancerview.ca/idc/groups/public/documents/webcontent/cccic_cervical_cs_report.pdf*.

Canadian Task Force on Preventive Health Care. (2013). Recommendations on screening for cervical cancer. *Canadian Medical Association Journal*, 185(1), 35–45.

Cunningham, F. G., Leveno, K. J., Bloom, S. L., Hauth, J. C., Gilstrap, L. C., & Wenstrom, K. D. (2005). *Williams' obstetrics* (22nd ed.). New York: McGraw-Hill Professional.

Kidney Foundation of Canada. (2007). *Urinary tract infections*. Retrieved from *http://www.kidney.ca/document.doc?id=316*.

Murphy, K. J. (2007). Screening for cervical cancer. *Journal of Obstetrics and Gynaecology Canada*, 29(8), S27–S36.

Pawlik, M., & Martin, F.J. (2009). Does a water-based lubricant affect Pap smear and cervical microbiology results? *Canadian Family Physician*, 55(4), 376–377.

Public Health Agency of Canada. (2008). *Report on sexually transmitted infections in Canada: 2008*. Retrieved from *http://www.phac-aspc.gc.ca/std-mts/report/sti-its2008/PDF/10-047-STI_report_eng-r1.pdf*.

Public Health Agency of Canada (2010). *HIV/AIDS among women in Canada*. Retrieved from *http://www.phac-aspc.gc.ca/aids-sida/publication/epi/2010/pdf/EN_Chapter5_Web.pdf*.

Schiffman, M., Castle, P. E., Jeronimo, J., Rodriguez, A. C., & Wacholder, S. (2007). Human papillomavirus and cervical cancer. *Lancet*, 370(9590), 890–907.

Stillson, T., Knight, A. L., & Elswick, R. K. (1997). The effectiveness and safety of two cervical cytologic techniques during pregnancy. *Journal of Family Practice*, 45, 159–163.

The Complete Health Assessment: Putting It All Together

Written by Carolyn Jarvis, PhD, APN, CNP
Adapted by Marian Luctkar-Flude, RN, MScN

evolve WEBSITE

http://evolve.elsevier.com/Canada/Jarvis/examination/

OUTLINE

The choreography of the complete history and physical examination is the art of arranging all the separate steps you have learned so far. Your first examination may seem awkward and contrived; you may have to pause and think of what comes next rather than just gather data. Repeated rehearsals make the choreography smoother. You will come to the point at which the procedure flows naturally, and even if you forget a step, you will be able to insert it gracefully at the next logical time. Continue to engage the patient in a dialogue at appropriate moments during the physical examination to collect additional subjective data. Abnormal findings in the physical assessment will prompt you to explore further. Remain attentive to physical signs suggestive of abuse. If abuse is suspected, ask the patient directly, in a nonjudgemental manner, about the presence of interpersonal violence. The following examination sequence is one suggested route. It is intended to minimize the number of position changes for the patient and for you. With experience, you may wish to rearrange this sequence in a way that feels natural for you.

A complete examination is performed at a patient's first entry in an outpatient setting or initial admission to the hospital. Perform all the steps listed here for a complete examination. With experience, you will learn to strike a balance between the steps you must retain to be thorough and those that you may safely omit when time is pressing. The steps for the follow-up or shift assessment are described in the next chapter.

Review Chapter 9 for preparing the setting, preparing the patient, and your approach with regard to his or her age.

Have all equipment prepared and accessible before the examination. Refer to the following list of equipment usually needed for a screening physical examination.

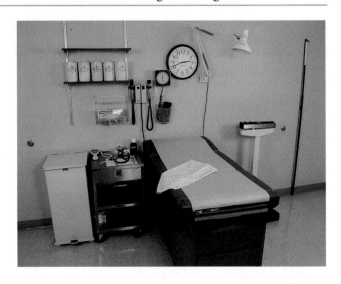

EQUIPMENT LIST

Platform scale with height attachment	Tongue depressor
Skinfold calipers (if necessary)	Snellen eye chart or pocket vision screener
Flexible measuring tape	Skin-marking pen
Sphygmomanometer	Ruler marked in centimetres
Stethoscope with bell and diaphragm	Reflex hammer
Thermometer	Sharp object (split tongue blade)
Pulse oximeter (if necessary)	Cotton balls
Flashlight or penlight	Bivalve vaginal speculum
Otoscope/ophthalmoscope	Clean gloves
Tuning fork	Materials for cytological study
Nasal speculum (if a short, broad speculum is not included with the otoscope)	Lubricant
	Fecal occult blood test materials

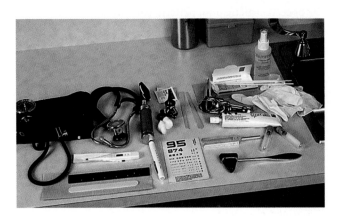

SUBJECTIVE DATA

Sequence   **Selected Photos**

The patient walks into the room, sits; the examiner sits facing the patient; the patient is in street clothes. (Note: Position changes are noted in *italics*.)

THE HEALTH HISTORY

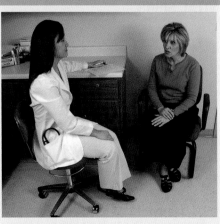

Collect the history, complete or limited as visit warrants (refer to Chapter 5):
1. Biographical data
2. Reason for seeking care
3. Present health or history of present illness
4. Past history
5. Family history
6. Review of systems
7. Functional assessment or activities of daily living (ADLs)

While you obtain the history and throughout the examination, note data on the patient's general appearance.

OBJECTIVE DATA

GENERAL APPEARANCE

1. Whether patient appears stated age
2. Level of consciousness
3. Skin colour
4. Nutritional status
5. Posture and position; comfortably erect
6. Obvious physical deformities
7. Mobility:
   Gait
   Use of assistive devices
   Range of motion (ROM) of joints
   No involuntary movement
   Ability to rise from a seated position easily
8. Facial expression
9. Mood and affect
10. Speech: articulation, pattern, content appropriate, first language
11. Hearing
12. Personal hygiene

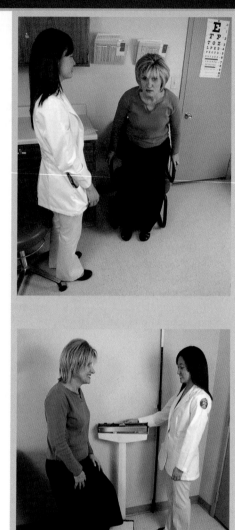

MEASUREMENT

1. Weight
2. Height
3. Body mass index
4. Vision (with Snellen eye chart)
5. Skinfold measurements (if they are necessary)
6. Waist and hip measurements (not indicated for patients younger than 18 years or for pregnant or lactating women)

Ask the patient to empty the bladder (save urine specimen, if needed), to disrobe except for underpants, and to put on a gown. The patient *sits with legs dangling* off side of the bed or table; you stand in front of the patient.

VITAL SIGNS

1. Radial pulse
2. Respirations
3. Blood pressure in arms
4. Blood pressure in lower leg; compute ankle/brachial index (if this is necessary)
5. Temperature (if this is necessary)
6. Oxygen saturation (if this is necessary)
7. Patient's rating of pain level on a scale of 0 to 10; note location of pain

SKIN

1. Examine both hands and inspect the nails.
2. For the rest of the examination, examine the skin of the corresponding region.

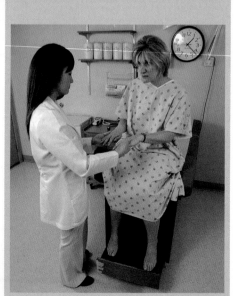

Objective Data

HEAD AND FACE

1. Inspect and palpate scalp, hair, and cranium.
2. Inspect face: expression, symmetry (cranial nerve VII).
3. Palpate the temporal artery and then the temporomandibular joint as the patient opens and closes the mouth.
4. Palpate the maxillary sinuses and the frontal sinuses.

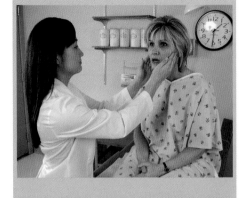

EYE

1. Test visual fields by confrontation (cranial nerve II).
2. Test extraocular muscles: corneal light reflex, six cardinal positions of gaze (cranial nerves III, IV, VI).
3. Inspect external eye structures.
4. Inspect conjunctivae, sclerae, corneas, irides.
5. Test pupil: size, response to light and accommodation.
6. Darken room. Using an ophthalmoscope, inspect ocular fundus: red reflex, disc, vessels, and retinal background.

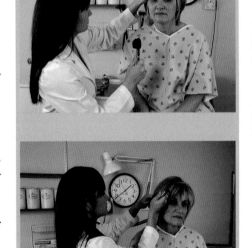

EAR

1. Inspect the external ear: position and alignment, skin condition, and auditory meatus.
2. Move auricle, and push tragus for tenderness.
3. With an otoscope, inspect the canal and then the tympanic membrane for colour, position, landmarks, and integrity.
4. Assess hearing with the whispered voice test.

NOSE

1. Inspect the external nose: symmetry, lesions.
2. Inspect facial symmetry (cranial nerve VII).
3. Test the patency of each nostril.
4. With a speculum, inspect the nares: nasal mucosa, septum, and turbinates.

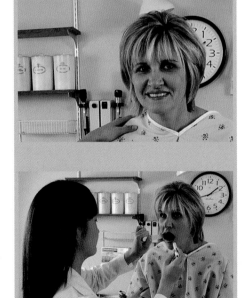

MOUTH AND THROAT

1. With a penlight, inspect the mouth: buccal mucosa, teeth and gums, tongue, floor of mouth, palate, and uvula.
2. Grade tonsils, if they are present.
3. Note mobility of uvula as the patient phonates "ahh," and test gag reflex (cranial nerves IX, X).
4. Ask the patient to stick out the tongue (cranial nerve XII).
5. With a gloved hand, bimanually palpate the mouth, if this is necessary.

Objective Data

NECK

1. Inspect the neck: symmetry, lumps, and pulsations.
2. Palpate the cervical lymph nodes.
3. Inspect and palpate the carotid pulse, one side at a time. Listen for carotid bruits, if this is necessary.
4. Palpate the trachea in midline.
5. Test ROM and muscle strength against your resistance: head forward and back, head turned to each side, and shoulder shrug (cranial nerve XI).

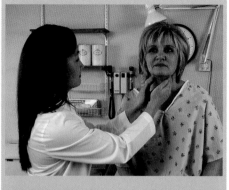

Step behind the patient, taking your stethoscope, ruler, and marking pen with you.
6. Palpate thyroid gland, posterior approach.
   Open the patient's gown to expose all of the back for examination of the thorax, but leave gown on shoulders and chest.

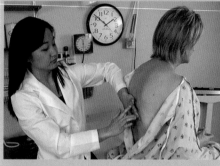

CHEST, POSTERIOR AND LATERAL

1. Inspect the posterior chest: configuration of the thoracic cage, skin characteristics, and symmetry of shoulders and muscles.
2. Palpate for symmetrical expansion; tactile fremitus; lumps or tenderness.
3. Palpate length of spinous processes.
4. Percuss over all lung fields; percuss diaphragmatic excursion.
5. Percuss costovertebral angle, noting tenderness.
6. Auscultate breath sounds, comparing side with side in upper and lateral lung fields; note any adventitious sounds.

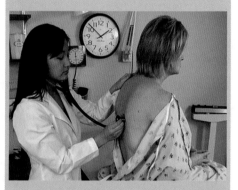

Move around to face the patient; the patient remains sitting. For a female breast examination, ask permission to lift gown to drape on the shoulders, exposing the chest; for a male patient, lower the gown to the lap.

CHEST, ANTERIOR

1. Inspect respirations and skin characteristics.
2. Palpate for tactile fremitus, lumps, or tenderness.
3. Percuss anterior lung fields.
4. Auscultate breath sounds, comparing side to side in upper and lower lung fields; note any adventitious sounds.

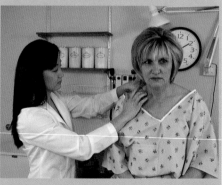

HEART

1. Ask the patient to lean forward and exhale briefly; auscultate the cardiac base for any murmurs.

UPPER EXTREMITIES

1. Test ROM and muscle strength of hands, arms, and shoulders.
2. Palpate the epitrochlear nodes.

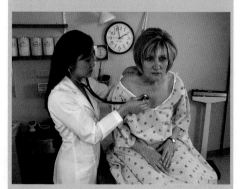

FEMALE BREASTS

1. Inspect for symmetry, mobility, and dimpling as the woman lifts her arms over her head, pushes her hands on her hips, and leans forward.
2. Inspect supraclavicular and infraclavicular areas.
   Help the woman *lie supine with her head flat or up to a 30-degree angle.* Stand at the patient's right side. Drape the gown up across her shoulders to expose the anterior chest, and place an extra sheet across her lower abdomen.
3. Palpate each breast, lifting the same-side arm up over her head. As you palpate, include the tail of Spence and areola.
4. Palpate each nipple for discharge.
5. Support the patient's arm, and palpate the axilla and regional lymph nodes.
6. Teach breast self-examination, if the patient asks to learn it.

MALE BREASTS

1. Inspect and palpate the chest wall.
2. Supporting each arm, palpate the axilla and regional nodes.

NECK VESSELS

1. Inspect each side of the patient's neck for a jugular venous pulse, turning the patient's head slightly to the other side.
2. Estimate jugular venous pressure, if this is necessary.

HEART

1. Inspect the precordium for any pulsations or heave (lift).
2. Palpate the apical impulse, and note the location.
3. Palpate the precordium for any abnormal thrill.
4. Auscultate apical rate and rhythm.
5. Auscultate with the diaphragm of the stethoscope to study heart sounds, inching from the apex up to the base, or vice versa.
6. Auscultate the heart sounds with the bell of the stethoscope, again inching through all locations.
7. Turn the patient over to the left side while you again auscultate the apex with the bell.

ABDOMEN

The patient should be *supine,* with the bed or table flat; arrange drapes to expose the abdomen from the chest to the pubis.

1. Inspect contour, symmetry, skin characteristics, umbilicus, and pulsations.
2. Auscultate bowel sounds.
3. Auscultate for vascular sounds over the aorta and renal arteries.
4. Percuss all quadrants.
5. Percuss the height of the liver span at the right midclavicular line.
6. Percuss the location of the spleen.
7. Lightly palpate in all quadrants; then palpate deeply in all quadrants.

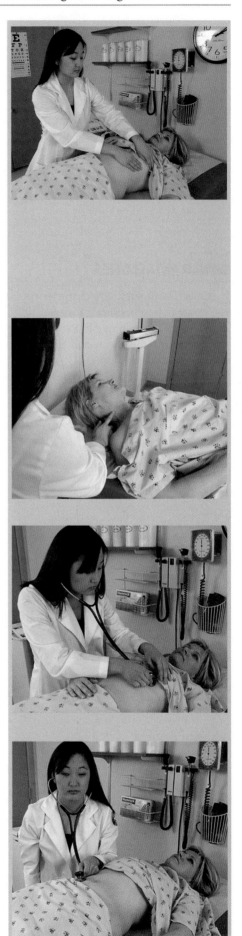

Objective Data

8. Palpate for liver, spleen, kidneys, and aorta.
9. Test the abdominal reflexes, if this is necessary.

INGUINAL AREA

1. Palpate each side of the groin for the femoral pulse and the inguinal nodes. Lift the drape to expose the legs.

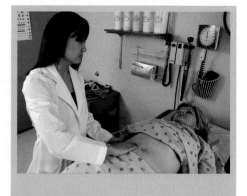

LOWER EXTREMITIES

1. Inspect: symmetry, skin characteristics, and hair distribution.
2. Palpate pulses: popliteal, posterior tibial, dorsalis pedis.
3. Use Doppler technique to locate peripheral pulses (if this is necessary).
4. Palpate for temperature and pretibial edema.
5. Separate toes and inspect.
6. Test ROM and muscle strength of hips, knees, ankles, and feet.

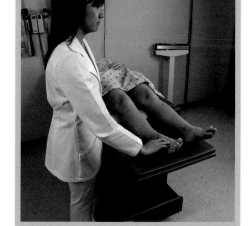

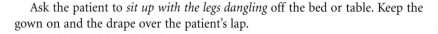

Ask the patient to *sit up with the legs dangling* off the bed or table. Keep the gown on and the drape over the patient's lap.

MUSCULOSKELETAL

1. Note muscle strength as the patient sits up.

NEUROLOGICAL

1. Test sensation in selected areas on face, arms, hands, legs, and feet: superficial pain, light touch, and vibration.
2. Test position sense of finger, one hand.
3. Test stereognosis, using a familiar object.
4. Evaluate cerebellar function of the upper extremities with the finger-to-nose test or the test of rapid alternating movements.

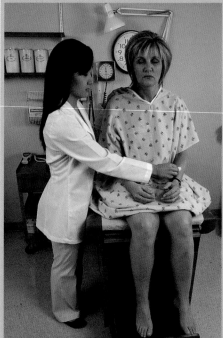

5. Elicit deep tendon reflexes of the upper extremities: biceps, triceps, and brachioradialis.

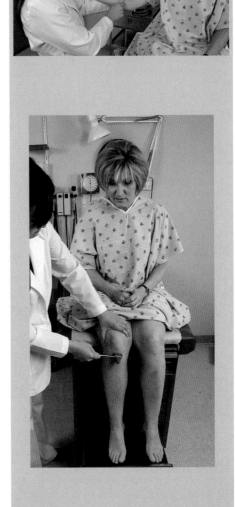

6. Test the cerebellar function of the lower extremities by asking the patient to run each heel down the opposite shin.
7. Elicit deep tendon reflexes of the lower extremities: patellar and Achilles.
8. Test for the Babinski reflex.

Ask the patient to *stand* with the gown on. Stand close to the patient.

LOWER EXTREMITIES

1. Inspect the patient's legs for varicose veins.

MUSCULOSKELETAL

1. Ask the patient to *walk* across the room in his or her regular gait, turn, and then walk back toward you in heel-to-toe manner.
2. Ask the patient to walk on the toes for a few steps and then to walk on the heels for a few steps.
3. Stand close and check for the Romberg sign.

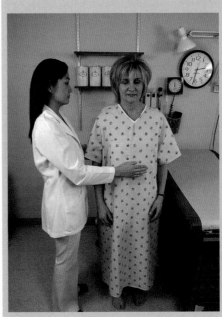

4. Ask the patient to hold the edge of the bed and to stand on one leg and perform a shallow knee bend, one for each leg.
5. Stand behind the patient, and check the spine as the patient touches the toes.
6. Stabilize the patient's pelvis and test the ROM of the spine as the patient hyperextends, rotates, and laterally bends.

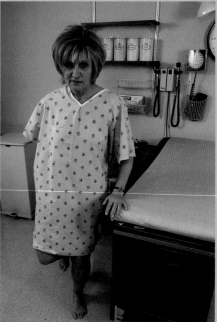

MALE GENITALIA

For a male patient, sit on a stool in front of him. The patient stands.
1. Inspect the penis and scrotum.
2. Palpate the scrotal contents. If a mass exists, transilluminate the scrotum.
3. Check for inguinal hernia.
4. Teach testicular self-examination.

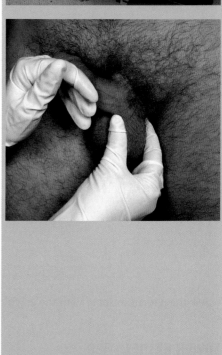

MALE RECTUM

For a male adult, ask him to bend over the examination table, supporting his torso with his forearms on the table. Assist a bedridden man to a left lateral position, with his right leg drawn up.
1. Inspect the perianal area.
2. With a gloved lubricated finger, palpate the rectal walls and prostate gland.
3. Save a stool specimen for an occult blood test.

FEMALE GENITALIA

Assist the female patient back to the examination table, and help her *assume the lithotomy position.* Drape her appropriately. For the speculum examination, sit on a stool at the foot of the table; for the bimanual examination, stand.

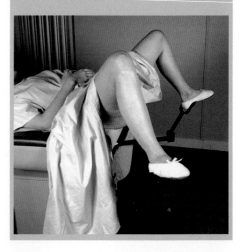

1. Inspect the perineal and perianal areas.
2. With a vaginal speculum, inspect the cervix and vaginal walls.
3. Procure specimens.
4. Perform a bimanual examination; cervix, uterus, and adnexa.
5. Continue the bimanual examination, checking the rectum and rectovaginal walls.
6. Save a stool specimen for an occult blood test.
7. Provide tissues for the patient to wipe the perineal area, and help her up to a *sitting position.*

Tell the patient that you are finished with the examination and that you will leave the room as he or she gets dressed. Return to discuss the examination and further plans and to answer any questions. Thank the patient for his or her time.

For a hospitalized patient, return the bed and any room equipment to the way you found it. Make sure the call bell and telephone are within easy reach.

NEWBORNS AND INFANTS

Review Chapter 9 for the steps on preparation and positioning and on developmental principles of the infant. The 1-minute and 5-minute Apgar results are important data about the newborn's immediate response to extrauterine life. The following sequence expands these data. You may reorder this sequence as the infant's sleep and wakefulness state or physical condition warrants.

The infant is *supine* on a warming table or examination table with an overhead heating element. The infant may be nude except for a diaper over a boy.

Vital Signs

Note pulse, respirations, and temperature.

Measurement

Weight, length, and head circumference are measured and plotted on growth curves for the infant's age.

General Appearance

1. Body symmetry, spontaneous position, flexion of head and extremities, and spontaneous movement
2. Skin colour and characteristics; any obvious deformities
3. Symmetry and positioning of the facial features
4. Alert, responsive affect
5. Strong, lusty cry

Chest and Heart

1. Inspect the condition of the skin over the chest and abdomen; chest configuration; and nipples and breast tissue.
2. Note movement of the abdomen with respirations and any chest retraction.
3. Palpate the apical impulse and note its location; palpate the chest wall for thrills; assess tactile fremitus if the infant is crying.
4. Auscultate breath sounds, heart sounds in all locations, and bowel sounds in the abdomen and in the chest.

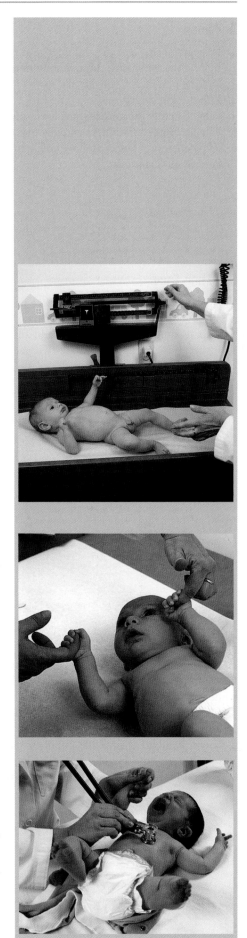

Objective Data

Abdomen

1. Inspect the shape of the abdomen and skin condition.
2. Inspect the umbilicus; count vessels; note the condition of the cord or stump and the presence of any hernia.
3. Palpate skin turgor.
4. Palpate lightly for muscle tone, liver, spleen tip, and bladder.
5. Palpate deeply for kidneys and any mass.
6. Palpate femoral pulses and inguinal lymph nodes.
7. Percuss all quadrants.

Head and Face

1. Note moulding of the cranium after delivery, any swelling on the cranium, and bulging of fontanelle with crying or at rest.
2. Palpate fontanelles, suture lines, and any swellings.
3. Inspect positioning and symmetry of facial features while the infant is at rest and during crying.

Eyes

To open the newborn's eyes, support the head and shoulders and gently lower the baby backward, or ask the parent to hold the baby over his or her shoulder while you stand behind the parent.

1. Inspect the eyelids (edematous in newborns), palpebral slant, conjunctivae, any nystagmus, and any discharge.
2. Use a penlight to elicit the pupillary reflex, blink reflex, and corneal light reflex; assess tracking of a moving light.
3. Using an ophthalmoscope, elicit the red reflex.

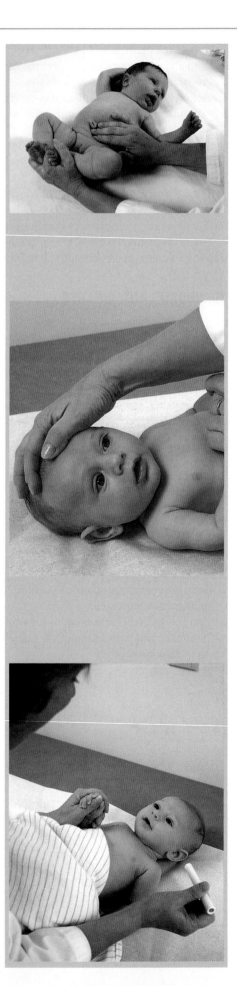

Objective Data

Ears

(Defer otoscopic examination until the end of the complete examination.)

1. Inspect size, shape, alignment of auricles; patency of auditory canals; and any extra skin tags or pits.
2. Note the startle reflex in response to a loud noise.
3. Palpate flexible auricles.

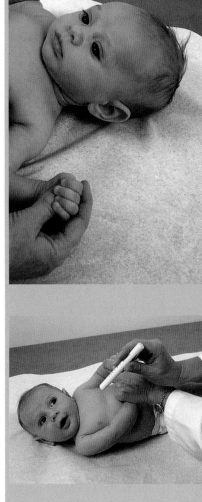

Nose

1. Determine the patency of the nares.
2. Note the nasal discharge, sneezing, and any flaring with respirations.

Mouth and Throat

1. Inspect the lips and gums, high-arched intact palate, buccal mucosa, tongue size, and frenulum of tongue; in a newborn, note absence of or minimal salivation.
2. Note the rooting reflex.
3. Insert a gloved little finger, note the sucking reflex, and palpate palate.

Neck

1. Lift the infant's shoulders, and let the head lag to inspect the neck: Note midline trachea, any skinfolds, and any lumps.
2. Palpate the lymph nodes, the thyroid, and any masses.
3. While the infant is supine, elicit the tonic neck reflex; note suppleness of the neck with movement.

Upper Extremities

1. Inspect and manipulate, noting ROM, muscle tone, and absence of the scarf sign (elbow should not reach midline).
2. Count fingers, count palmar creases, and note colour of hands and nail beds.
3. Place your thumbs in the infant's palms to note the grasp reflex; then wrap your hands around infant's hands to pull up, and note the head lag.

Objective Data

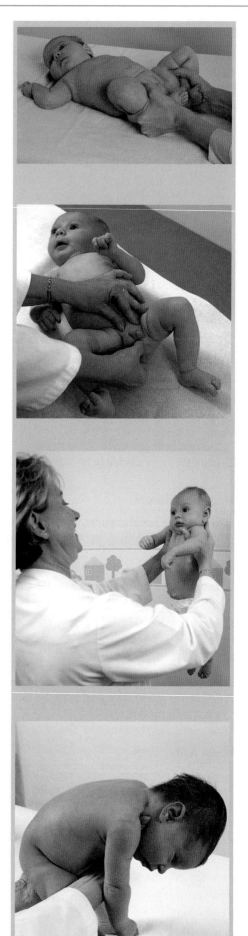

Lower Extremities

1. Inspect and manipulate the legs and feet, noting ROM, muscle tone, and skin condition.
2. Note alignment of feet and toes, look for flat soles, and count toes; note any syndactyly.
3. Perform the Ortolani manoeuvre to test for hip stability.

Genitalia

Girls: Inspect labia and clitoris (edematous in the newborn), vernix caseosa between labia, and patent vagina.

Boys:

1. Inspect position of urethral meatus (do not retract the foreskin); strength of urine stream, if possible; and rugae on scrotum.
2. Palpate the testes in the scrotum.

Lift the infant under the axillae, and hold the infant so that he is facing you at eye level.

Neuromuscular

1. Note shoulder muscle tone and the infant's ability to stay in your hands without slipping.
2. Rotate the newborn slowly side to side; note the doll's eye reflex.
3. Turn the infant around so his or her back is to you; elicit the stepping reflex and the placing reflex against the edge of the examination table.

Spine and Rectum

Turn the infant over, and hold him or her prone in your hands, or place the infant prone on the examination table.

1. Inspect the length of the spine, trunk incurvation reflex, and symmetry of gluteal folds.
2. Inspect skin; note any sinus openings, protrusions, or tufts of hair.
3. Note patent anal opening. In a newborn, check for passage of meconium stool during the first 24 to 48 hours.

Objective Data

Final Procedures

1. With an otoscope, inspect the auditory canals and the tympanic membranes.
2. Elicit the Moro reflex by letting the infant's head and trunk drop back a short way, by jarring crib sides, or by making a loud noise.

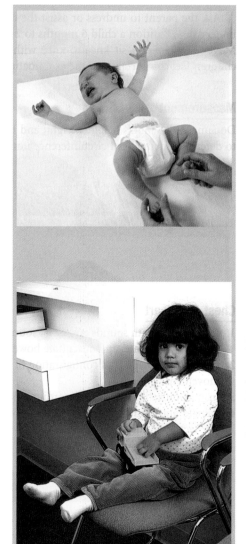

YOUNG CHILDREN

Review the developmental considerations in preparing for an examination of a toddler and a young child in Chapter 9. During this time, the young child's desire for independence conflicts with his or her basic dependence. Also, the child is aware of and fearful of a new environment, has a fear of invasive procedures, dislikes being restrained, and may be emotionally attached to a security object.

Focus on the parent as the child plays with a toy.

The Health History

1. Collect the history, including developmental data. During the history, note data on general appearance.

General Appearance

1. Note child's ability to amuse himself or herself while the parent speaks.
2. Note interaction between parent and child.
3. Note gross motor and fine motor skills as the child plays with toys. Gradually focus on and involve yourself with the child, at first in a "play" period.
4. Evaluate developmental milestones by using an age-appropriate Nipissing District Developmental Screen (see example in Chapter 2, Figure 2-3).
5. Evaluate posture while the child is sitting and standing. Evaluate alignment of the legs and feet while the child is walking.
6. Evaluate speech acquisition.
7. Evaluate vision and hearing ability.
8. Evaluate social interaction.

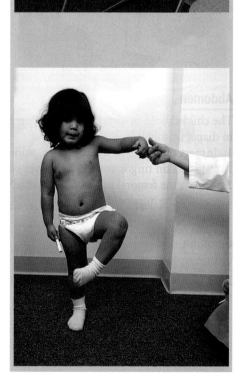

Objective Data

Subjective and Objective Data

ABDOMEN

1. Assess contour of abdomen: flat, rounded, or protuberant.
2. Listen to bowel sounds in all four quadrants.
3. Perform light palpation in all four quadrants.
4. Inquire whether nauseated or vomiting.
5. Inquire whether the patient is passing flatus or stool, or experiencing constipation or diarrhea. Note date of most recent bowel movement.
6. Check any drainage tube placement for colour, consistency, odour, and amount of drainage, and evaluate the integrity of the insertion site. Assess all tubes from site to source for kinks, leaks, and disconnections.
7. Check any stoma for colour, moisture, excoriation, and bleeding, and evaluate the integrity of the stomal appliance. Check stomal drainage for colour, consistency, odour, and amount.
8. With regard to diet orders, determine whether the patient is tolerating ice chips, liquids, or solids. Order the correct diet as it is advanced. Note whether the patient is at high risk for nutrition deficit.

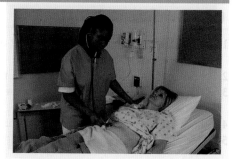

GENITOURINARY SYSTEM

1. Inquire whether the patient is voiding regularly, or assess the indwelling urinary catheter if indicated.
2. Check urine for colour and clarity.
3. If a Foley catheter is in place, check colour, quantity, and clarity of urine with every check of vital signs.
4. If urine output is less than the expected amount, perform a bladder scan according to agency protocol. Determine whether the problem is associated with the production of urine or its retention.

ACTIVITY

1. With regard to activity orders, if the patient is on bed rest, the head of bed should be angled at 15 degrees or higher. Note whether the patient is at high risk for skin breakdown.
2. If the patient is ambulatory, assist the patient to a sitting position, and move him or her to a chair. Increase activity as tolerated.
3. Note any assistance needed, how the patient tolerates movement, the distance walked to the chair, and the patient's ability to turn.
4. Note any need for ambulatory aid or equipment.
5. Complete any standardized scales used to quantify the patient's risk for falling.
6. If antiembolism compression (T.E.D.) stockings and sequential compression devices (SCDs) are ordered, the patient needs to use them 22 of 24 hours. SCDs must be hooked up and turned on, except during ambulation.

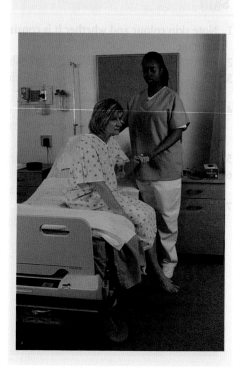

Sequence	Selected Photos

REPORT CRITICAL FINDINGS

Note examination findings that necessitate immediate attention:

1. Systolic BP ≤ 90 or ≥160 mmHg
2. Temperature ≥ 38°C
3. Heart rate ≤ 60 or ≥ 100 bpm
4. Respiratory rate ≤ 10/minute or ≥ 28/minute
5. Oxygen saturation ≤ 92%
6. Urine output < 30 mL/hour for 2 hours
7. Dark amber urine or bloody urine (except for urology patients)
8. Postoperative nausea or vomiting not relieved with medication
9. Surgical pain not controlled with medication; any other unusual pain, such as chest pain
10. Bleeding
11. Altered level of consciousness, confusion
12. Sudden restlessness or anxiety

Subjective and Objective Data

DOCUMENTATION AND CRITICAL THINKING

ELECTRONIC CHARTING

Charting in most hospitals is at least partially computerized. Although use of computers for charting can be intimidating at first, it has several advantages. First, for novice clinicians, the structure imposed by the computerized database can serve as a prompt to guide them through a complete assessment. Second, it decreases the chances that you will waste time waiting for access to a paper chart or searching for it when it is not in the proper location. Finally, charting in a computer system is rarely dependent on writing or typing in narrative form; check boxes and drop-down menus are much more common. If you avoid the temptation to write everything on paper first and, instead, learn to use all the functions programmed into the hospital's system, you will find that computer charting is faster than its paper equivalent. The following illustrations show the equipment used for computerized charting and two examples of a patient's computerized chart.

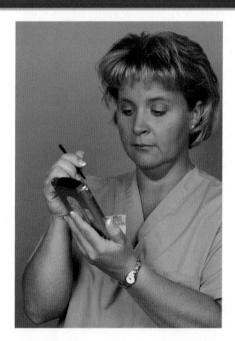

Documentation & Critical Thinking

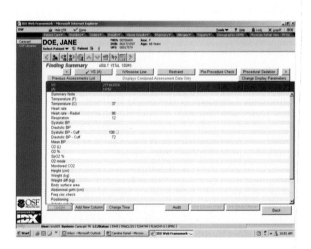

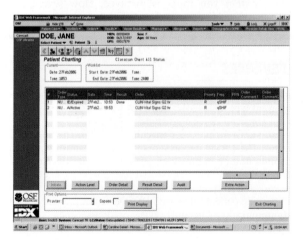

USING THE SBAR TECHNIQUE FOR STAFF COMMUNICATION

Throughout this text we have used the SOAP acronym (*subjective, objective, assessment, plan*) to organize assessment findings into written or charted communication. To organize assessment data for *verbal* communication (e.g., calls to physicians, nursing shift reports, patient transfers to other units), we use the SBAR framework: *situation, background, assessment, recommendation*.

The SBAR is a structured communication technique to standardize communication and prevent misunderstandings. Communication errors contribute to most patient safety incidents and medical errors in health care (Leonard, Graham & Bonacum (2004). The U.S. Joint Commission (2013) data from 2010 to 2012 indicated that communication failures contributed to between 59% and 76% of sentinel events; however, reporting is voluntary and represents only a small proportion of actual events. With the incidence of patient safety incidents in Canada as high as 7.5%, communication tools such as the SBAR technique are recommended to improve verbal communication and reduce medical errors (Teamwork and Communication Working Group, 2011; Thomas, Bertram, & Johnson, 2009; Trentham, Andreoli, Boaro, Velji, & Fancott, 2010). The SBAR technique is a standardized framework to transmit important in-the-moment information. Using the SBAR technique will keep your message concise and focused on the immediate problem and yet give your colleagues enough information to understand the current situation and make a decision. To formulate your verbal message, use these four points:

Situation: What is happening right now? What are you calling about? State your name, your unit, patient's name, room number, patient's problem, when the problem happened or when it started, and how severe it is.

Background: Do not recite the patient's full history since admission. Do state the data pertinent to this moment's problem: admitting diagnosis, time of admission, and appropriate immediate assessment data (e.g., vital signs, pulse oximetry, change in mental status, allergies, current medications, IV fluids, laboratory results).

Assessment: What do *you* think is happening in regard to the current problem? If you do not know, at least state which body system you think is involved. How severe is the problem?

Recommendation: What do you want the physician to do to improve the patient's situation? Offer probable solutions: Order more pain medication? Come and assess the patient?

Review the following examples of SBAR communication.

Situation 1

S: This is Bill on the Oncology Unit. I'm calling about Daniel Meyers in room 8417. He is refusing all oral medications as of now.

B: Daniel is a 59-year-old male with multiple myeloma. He was admitted for an autologous stem cell transplant and received chemotherapy 10 days ago. Now he is 5 days post transplantation. Vital signs are stable, he is alert and oriented, IV fluids are D_5W [5% dextrose in water]. As of 1 hour ago, he has been feeling extreme nausea and vomiting, refusing all food and oral meds.

A: I think the chemo he had before transplantation is hitting him now. His uncontrolled nausea isn't going away in the next few days.

R: I'm concerned that he cannot stay hydrated, and he needs his meds. I need you to please change the IV rate and change all scheduled oral meds to IV. I also think we need to add an additional PRN [as needed] antiemetic. If he continues to refuse food, we may have to consider starting him on TPN [total parenteral nutrition]/lipids.

Situation 2

S: This is Andrea. I'm the nurse taking care of Max Goodson in 6443. His condition has changed, and his most recent vital signs show a significant drop in BP.

B: Max is 40 years old with a history of alcoholism. He was admitted through the ED last night with abdominal pain and a suspected GI [gastrointestinal] bleeding. His BPs have been running in the 130s/80s. He just produced a large amount of liquid maroon stool and reported feeling dizzy. I rechecked his vitals, and his BP is 88/50 and heart rate is 104.

A: I'm worried his GI bleed is getting worse.

R: Will you order a stat. CBC [complete blood cell count] and place an order to transfuse RBCs [red blood cells] if his Hgb [hemoglobin] is below 8 g? Also, can you please come and assess? I think we may need to drop an NG [nasogastric] tube and do lavage.

REFERENCES

Joint Commission, The. (2013). Sentinel Event Data—Root causes by event type 2004–2012. Retrieved from: *http://www.jointcommission.org/sentinel_event.aspx*.

Leonard, M., Graham, S., & Bonacum, D. (2004). The human factor: The critical importance of effective teamwork and communication in providing safe care. *Quality and Safety in Health Care, 13*(Suppl 1), i85–i90.

Teamwork and Communication Working Group. (2011). Improving patient safety with effective teamwork and communication: Literature review needs assessment, evaluation of training tools and expert consultations.

Edmonton: Canadian Patient Safety Institute. *http://www.patientsafetyinstitute.ca/English/toolsResources/teamworkCommunication/Documents/Canadian%20Framework%20for%20Teamwork%20and%20Communications%20Lit%20Review.pdf*.

Thomas, C. M., Bertram, E., & Johnson, D. (2009). The SBAR communication technique. *Nurse Educator, 34*(4), 176–180.

Trentham, B., Andreoli, A., Boaro, N., Velji, K., & Fancott, C. (2010). *SBAR: A shared structure for effective team communication: An implementation toolkit* (2nd ed.). Toronto Rehabilitation Institute: Toronto.

Written by Deborah E. Swenson, MSN, ARNP, C-WHCNP
Adapted by Nancy Watts, RN, MN

⊖volve WEBSITE

http://evolve.elsevier.com/Canada/Jarvis/examination/

OUTLINE

STRUCTURE AND FUNCTION

PREGNANCY AND THE ENDOCRINE PLACENTA

The first day of menses is day 1 of the menstrual cycle. For the first 14 days of the cycle, one or more follicles in the ovaries develop and mature. One follicle grows faster than the others, and on approximately day 14 of the menstrual cycle, this dominant follicle ruptures, and ovulation occurs. If the ovum meets viable sperm, fertilization occurs somewhere in the oviduct (fallopian tube). The remaining cells in the follicle form the **corpus luteum,** or "yellow body," which makes important hormones. Chief among these is progesterone, which prevents the sloughing of the endometrial wall, thereby ensuring a rich vascular network into which the fertilized ovum will become implanted.

The fertilized ovum, now called the **blastocyst,** continues to divide, differentiate, and grow rapidly. Specialized cells in the blastocyst produce human chorionic gonadotropin (hCG), which stimulates the corpus luteum to continue making progesterone. Between days 20 and 24 the blastocyst becomes implanted into the wall of the uterus, which may cause a small amount of vaginal bleeding. A specialized layer of cells around that blastocyst becomes the **placenta.** The placenta starts to produce progesterone to support the pregnancy at 7 weeks and takes over this function completely from the corpus luteum at approximately 10 weeks.

The placenta functions as an endocrine organ and produces several hormones. These hormones help in the growth and development of the fetus and direct changes in the woman's body in preparation for birth and lactation. The hCG stimulates the rise in progesterone levels during pregnancy. Progesterone maintains the endometrium around the fetus, increases the alveoli in the breast, and keeps the uterus in a quiescent state. Estrogen stimulates the duct formation in the breast, increases the weight of the uterus, and increases the amount of certain receptors in the uterus that are important at birth.

The average length of pregnancy is 280 days from the first day of the last menstrual period (LMP), which is equal to 40 weeks, 10 lunar months, or 9 calendar months. Note that this includes the 2 weeks when the follicle was maturing but before conception actually occurred. Pregnancy is divided into three trimesters: (a) the first 12 weeks, (b) from 13 to 27 weeks, and (c) from 28 weeks to birth.

Any woman who has ever been pregnant, regardless of the outcome, is described as a *gravida* (G). In the first pregnancy she is a **primigravida.** With subsequent pregnancies she is a **multigravida.** *Parity* (P) refers to a pregnancy that has led to birth at a minimum of 20 weeks' gestation (often referred to as the *age of viability*). A nulliparous woman is pregnant for the first time (notation: G1 P0). She becomes a primipara after she has given birth once at 20 weeks' gestation or more (G1 P1). A **multipara** has given birth more than once (e.g., for a woman who has given birth twice, G2 P2). Preterm labour or preterm birth occurs at least 20 weeks' gestation but before 37 weeks' gestation. Pregnancy loss at less than 20 weeks is an abortion (A) that can be spontaneous (miscarriage) or induced (therapeutic). It is common to document pregnancy history with the notations G (gravida), T (term), P (preterm), A (abortion), and L (living children). If a woman is now pregnant for the sixth time, has given birth three times at 37 weeks' gestation or later, has had one miscarriage and one therapeutic abortion, and has three living children, her pregnancy history may be written "G6 T3 P0 A2 L3" (or "G6 TPAL 3023").

CHANGES DURING NORMAL PREGNANCY

Pregnancy is diagnosed by three types of signs and symptoms. **Presumptive signs** are those that the woman experiences, such as amenorrhea, breast tenderness, nausea, fatigue, and increased urinary frequency. **Probable signs** are those detected by the examiner, such as enlargement of the uterus. **Positive signs** of pregnancy are those that are direct evidence of the fetus, such as fetal heart tones (FHTs) detected through auscultation or positive cardiac activity detected through ultrasonography.

First Trimester

Conception occurs on approximately the fourteenth day of the menstrual cycle. The blastocyst (developing fertilized ovum) becomes implanted in the uterus 6 to 10 days after conception; implantation is sometimes accompanied by a small amount of painless bleeding, which may be interpreted as a menstrual period (Cunningham, Leveno, Bloom, & Hauth, 2010). The serum hCG test result becomes positive after implantation when hCG is first detectable in maternal serum, at approximately 8 to 11 days after conception.

The following menstrual period is missed. At the time of the missed menses, hCG can be detected in the urine. Tingling sensation and tenderness in the breasts begin as the rising estrogen levels promote mammary growth and development of the ductal system; progesterone stimulates the alveolar system, as well as the mammary growth. Chorionic somatomammotropin (also called *human placental lactogen* [*hPL*]), also produced by the placenta, stimulates breast growth and exerts lactogenic properties (DeCherney, Goodwin, Nathan, & Laufer, 2007). Up to 80% of all pregnant women experience nausea and vomiting, which usually subsides by the sixteenth week but may continue throughout pregnancy in as many as 20% of women (Einarson, Maltepe, Boskovic, & Koren, 2007). The cause is unclear but may involve the hormonal changes of pregnancy, hypoglycemia, gastric overloading, slowed peristalsis, enlargement of the uterus, and psychosocial factors. Fatigue is common and may be related to the initial fall in metabolic rate that occurs in early pregnancy (Kriebs & Gegor, 2005).

Estrogen, and possibly progesterone, causes hypertrophy of the uterine muscle cells, and the uterine blood vessels and lymphatic vessels enlarge. The uterus becomes globular in shape, softens, and flexes easily over the cervix (**Hegar's sign).** This causes compression of the bladder, which results in urinary frequency. Increased vascularity, congestion, and edema cause the cervix to soften (**Goodell's sign**) and become bluish purple in the primiparous woman (**Chadwick's sign).**

Early in the first trimester, the blood pressure (BP) reflects prepregnancy values. In the seventh gestational week, BP begins to drop until midpregnancy as a result of falling peripheral vascular resistance. The BP gradually returns to the nonpregnant baseline value by term. Systemic vascular resistance decreases from the vasodilatory effect of progesterone and prostaglandins and possibly because of the low resistance of the placental bed (Blackburn, 2007; Creasy, Resnick, Iams, Lockwood, & Moore, 2009).

At the end of 9 weeks, the embryonic period ends, and the fetal period begins, at which time major structures are present (DeCherney et al., 2007). FHTs can be heard through Doppler ultrasonography beginning between 9 and 10 weeks (Blackburn, 2007). The uterus may be palpated just above the symphysis pubis at approximately 12 weeks. Figure 30-1 depicts the growth of the uterine fundus during the first trimester.

When the pregnancy is viable, a gestational sac should be visible on transvaginal ultrasonography by 5 weeks' gestation or when the maternal serum hCG level is between 1100 and 1500 mU/mL (Creasy et al., 2009). When a fertilized egg develops a placenta and membranes but no embryo, this is called a *blighted ovum.* In this situation, the hCG levels rise early on and then begin to drop, and vaginal bleeding ensues.

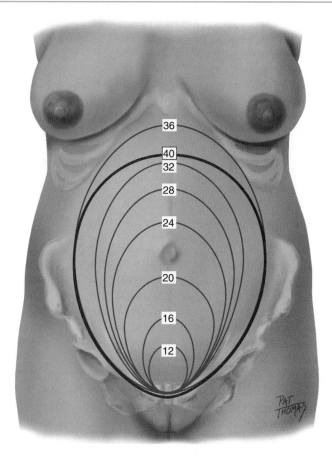

HEIGHT OF FUNDUS AT WEEKS OF GESTATION

30-1

Some women with blighted ovum are not aware that they were pregnant.

Second Trimester

By weeks 12 to 16, the nausea, vomiting, fatigue, and urinary frequency of the first trimester decrease. The woman recognizes fetal movement ("quickening") at approximately 18 to 20 weeks (a multigravida is aware of fetal movement earlier). As breast enlargement continues, the veins of the breast enlarge and are more visible through the skin. **Colostrum,** or first milk, is yellow and contains more minerals and protein but less carbohydrate and fat than mature milk. Colostrum is rich in antibodies, which protect the newborn during the first weeks of life (Blackburn, 2007; Cunningham et al., 2010). Colostrum may be expressed or may leak from the breast during pregnancy.

The areolae and nipples darken because, it is thought, estrogen and progesterone have a melanocyte-stimulating effect, and melanocyte-stimulating hormone levels escalate from the second month of pregnancy until birth. For the same reason, the midline of the abdominal skin becomes pigmented; the dark area is called the **linea nigra.** You may note **striae gravidarum** ("stretch marks") on the breast, abdomen, and areas where enlargement has occurred.

During the second trimester, systolic BP may be 2 to 8 mm Hg lower and diastolic BP 5 to 15 mm Hg lower than

prepregnancy levels (Blackburn, 2007; Cunningham et al., 2010). This drop is most pronounced at 20 weeks and may cause dizziness and faintness, particularly after the woman rises quickly. The enlargement of the uterus causes displacement of the stomach, and progesterone causes alterations in esophageal sphincter and gastric tone; these changes predispose the woman to heartburn. The intestines are also displaced by the growing uterus, and tone and motility are decreased because of the action of progesterone, which often results in constipation. The gallbladder empties sluggishly and may become distended, possibly as a result of the action of progesterone on its smooth muscle. The stasis of bile, together with the increased cholesterol saturation of pregnancy, predisposes some women to gallstone formation.

Progesterone and, to a lesser degree, estrogen cause increased respiratory effort during pregnancy by increasing tidal volume. Hemoglobin, and therefore oxygen-carrying capacity, also increases. Increased tidal volume causes a slight drop in partial pressure of arterial carbon dioxide, which in turn causes pregnant women to have occasional dyspnea (Cunningham et al., 2010).

The high level of estrogen during pregnancy causes an increase in the major thyroxine transport protein, thyroxine-binding globulin. Several thyroid-stimulating factors of placental origin are produced. The thyroid gland enlarges as a result of hyperplasia and increased vascularity. Thyroid function plays a vital role in maternal–fetal morbidity and mortality, inasmuch as 2.5% to 5% of pregnant women demonstrate some dysfunction. Maternal hypothyroidism increases the risk of miscarriage, pre-eclampsia, low birth weight, preterm birth, and placental abruption (Vane, Lazarus, & Chan, 2011). Even mild maternal hypothyroidism adversely affects the fetus, leading to neurodevelopmental changes with potential to decrease mental function (Vane et al., 2011).

Cutaneous blood flow is augmented during pregnancy as a result of decreased vascular resistance, which presumably helps dissipate heat generated by increased metabolism. This may cause nosebleeds to occur more frequently than usual. Gums may also hypertrophy and bleed easily in 30% to 80% of pregnant women. This condition is called **gingivitis of pregnancy,** and it occurs as a result of growth of the capillaries of the gums (Cunningham et al., 2010). Pregnant women with periodontal disease, which is a chronic local oral infection, are at risk for preterm birth, and their babies are at risk for low birth weight. Untreated, this condition may lead to a systemic infection that affects the maternal levels of prostaglandin E_2 (Stevens, Iida, & Ingersoll, 2007).

FHTs are audible on fetoscopy (as opposed to Doppler imaging) at approximately 17 to 19 weeks' gestation. The fetal outline is palpable through the abdominal wall at approximately 20 weeks. See Figure 30-1 for the growth of the uterine fundus during the second trimester.

Third Trimester

Blood volume, which increases rapidly during the second trimester, peaks in the middle of the third trimester to approximately 30% to 45% higher than the prepregnancy level, and it plateaus thereafter. This volume is greater with multiple gestations: up to 65% for twins and even more for higher-order multiple fetuses (Blackburn, 2007; Creasy et al., 2009). Erythrocyte mass increases by 20% to 30% (as a result of an increase in erythropoiesis, mediated by progesterone, estrogen, and placental chorionic somatomammotropin). However, plasma volume increases slightly more, causing a slight hemodilution and a small drop in hematocrit. BP slowly rises again to approximately the prepregnancy level (Blackburn, 2007; Cunningham et al., 2010).

Uterine enlargement causes the diaphragm to rise and the shape of the rib cage to widen at the base. The decrease in space for lung expansion may cause a sense of shortness of breath. The rising diaphragm displaces the heart up and to the left. Cardiac output, stroke volume, and force of contraction are increased. The pulse rate rises 15 to 20 beats per minute (Creasy et al., 2009). Because of the increase in blood volume, a functional systolic murmur, grade II/IV or less, can be heard in more than 95% of pregnant women (Creasy et al., 2009).

Edema of the lower extremities may occur (a) because the enlargement of the uterus impedes venous return and (b) because of lower colloid osmotic pressure. The edema worsens with dependency, such as that caused by prolonged standing. Varicosities, which have a familial tendency, may form or enlarge as a result of progesterone-induced vascular relaxation. Also causing varicosities is the engorgement that results when the weight of the full uterus compresses the inferior vena cava and the vessels of the pelvic area, which causes venous congestion in the legs, vulva, and rectum. Hemorrhoids are varicosities of the rectum that are worsened by constipation, which is caused by relaxation of the large bowel by progesterone.

Progressive lordosis (an inward curvature of the lumbar spine) occurs to compensate for the shifting centre of balance caused by the anteriorly enlarging uterus; this development predisposes pregnant women to backaches. Slumping of the shoulders and anterior flexion of the neck from the increasing weight of the breasts causes compression of the median and ulnar nerves in the arm, which may result in aching and numbness of the arms and hands (DeCherney et al., 2007); this condition is commonly referred to as *carpal tunnel syndrome.*

Approximately 2 weeks before going into labour, a primigravida experiences engagement (also called "lightening" or "dropping"), when the presenting part of the fetus, most often the fetal head, moves down into the pelvis. The fundus appears to be lower, and its measurement is smaller; other symptoms include urinary frequency, increased vaginal secretions as a result of increased pelvic congestion, and increased lung capacity. In a multigravida, the fetus may move down at any time in late pregnancy or, often, not until labour. The cervix, in preparation for labour, begins to thin (efface) and open (dilate). A thick **mucus plug,** formed in the cervix as a mechanical barrier during pregnancy, is expelled at variable times before or during labour. Between 37 and 42 weeks, the pregnancy is considered full term. After 42 weeks, the pregnancy is considered *post-term.*

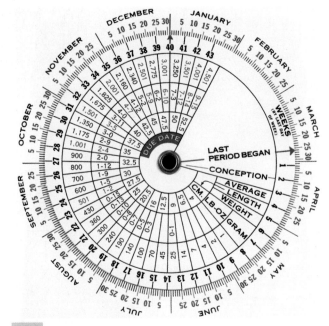

30-2 Pregnancy wheel.

Determining Gestational Age

The *expected date of birth* (EDB)—also known as *expected date of delivery* or *due date*—occurs 266 days after conception or 280 days (40 weeks) after the first day of the LMP. The LMP can only be reliable to determine EDB with a history of spontaneous regular 28- to 30-day cycles with normal flow and duration. Implantation of the fertilized egg can cause some light bleeding and may be wrongly noted as the LMP. The EDB may be calculated according to **Nägele's rule:** by adding 7 days to the LMP and subtracting 3 months. Pregnancy wheels or calculators can also be used (Figure 30-2): On the wheel, move day 1 of the LMP on the outer wheel to align with the LMP line on the inner wheel; the EDB is the date at the 40-week mark. Gestational age is similarly identified by the corresponding date on the wheel. Because Nägele's rule and the pregnancy wheels are based on regular 28-day cycles, adjustments must be made for longer or shorter menstrual cycles. Accurate history of coitus, ovulation, and fertility treatments, combined with physical findings (pelvic and bimanual, auscultation of the fetal heart rate [FHR], β–human chorionic gonadotropin [β-hCG] levels, and perceived fetal movement), aid in estimation of EDB. The most reliable method of dating a pregnancy in the absence of a reliable history is first trimester ultrasonography. (See Table 30-4 on p. 843 for notes on inconsistencies between fetal size and dates.)

Weight Gain During Pregnancy

The amount of weight gained by term accounts for fetal weight, amniotic fluid, placenta, increased uterine size, increased blood volume, increased extravascular fluid, maternal fat stores, and increased breast size. Weight gain during pregnancy reflects the gain in both the mother and the fetus and represents approximately 62% water gain, 30% fat gain,

TABLE 30-1	Guidelines for Gestational Weight Gain Ranges				
	Mean Rate of Weight Gain in the Second and Third Trimesters			Recommended Range of Total Weight Gain	
Prepregnancy BMI Category	Kilograms/Week	Pounds/Week		Kilograms	Pounds
BMI < 18.5 (underweight)	0.5	1.0		12.5-18	28-40
BMI 18.5-24.9 (normal weight)	0.4	1.0		11.5-16	25-35
BMI 25.0-29.9 (overweight)	0.3	0.6		7-11.5	15-25
BMI ≥ 30 (obese)	0.2	0.5		5-9	11-20

Source: Health Canada. (2010). *Canadian gestational weight gain recommendations*. Retrieved from *http://www.hc-sc.gc.ca/fn-an/nutrition/prenatal/qa-gest-gros-qr-eng.php*.

Notes: Values are rounded. Calculations assume a total weight gain of 0.5 to 2 kg in the first trimester. A narrower range of weight gain may be advised for women with a prepregnancy BMI of 35 or greater. Individualized advice is recommended for these women. Health Canada (2010) has adapted the Institute of Medicine's 2009 guidelines.

BMI, body mass index.

and 8% protein. Approximately 25% of the total gain is attributable to the fetus, 11% to the placenta and amniotic fluid, and the remainder to the mother (Blackburn, 2007). A healthy outcome may be expected within a great range of weight gain (Cunningham et al., 2010), as indicated in Table 30-1.

 ## DEVELOPMENTAL CONSIDERATIONS

In Canada, the rate of adolescent pregnancy is decreasing (4.6% of all births; Barrett & McKay, 2010; Public Health Agency of Canada, 2012). However, the potential complications for pregnancy in teenagers include psychosocial as well as medical risks. Most often in Canada, such young women live in a rural area, belong to a lower socioeconomic group, have little family support, have limited access to prenatal care, or may be part of an Aboriginal community (Maticka-Tyndale, 2008). Their education may not be complete, and this may lead to failure to establish a vocation and become independent. Medical risks for pregnant adolescents are generally related to poverty, inadequate nutrition, substance use, increased rate of sexually transmitted infections (STIs), poor health before pregnancy, and emotional and physical abuse from their partners (up to 35% reported by teenaged women).

Pregnant adolescents are also at risk for pre-eclampsia, and their infants are at risk for low birth weight; it is unclear whether these two outcomes are related to biological or psychosocial factors (Cunningham et al., 2010). Pregnant adolescents, for social reasons, seek health care later in the pregnancy than do other pregnant patients, although early prenatal care has been shown to provide optimal management. In developing countries, rates of maternal mortality among pregnant teenagers are higher because of poorer access to care for hypertension, embolism, and ectopic pregnancy, as well as complications from illegal abortions (Cunningham et al., 2010).

More women are delaying pregnancy. The average age of women who give birth in Canada is currently 29 years of age; 11% of first births are in women who are 35 years of age or older (Society of Obstetricians and Gynaecologists of Canada

[SOGC], 2012). Fertility declines as women age, partly because of decreases both in viable eggs and in ovulation and partly because of other conditions, including endometriosis, early-onset menopause, and an increase in pregnancy loss. Advanced paternal age is also a concern because quantity and quality of sperm may be decreased (SOGC, 2012). Pregnancy in women of advanced maternal age is related to an increase in congenital anomalies. The incidence of Down syndrome (trisomy 21) in an infant increases from 1 per 1250 among mothers aged 25 years to 1 per 365 among mothers aged 35 years; 1 per 109 among those aged 40 years; and 1 per 32 among those aged 45 years (March of Dimes, 2009a). Pregnant adolescents and older pregnant woman are at increased risk for multiple fetuses. In Canada, such pregnancies account for 3.0% of all births, and a large percentage occur as preterm births.

Women of advanced age are more likely than younger women to have coexisting medical conditions—such as hypertension, diabetes, and obesity—that further complicate any pregnancy (Cunningham et al., 2010). Hypertension and diabetes are associated with intrauterine growth restriction (IUGR) and pre-eclampsia, which, in turn, are associated with oligohydramnios, placental abruption, and preterm birth. Older women are also more likely to experience multiple pregnancy and complications, including the need for Caesarean birth and, although rare in Canada, maternal death.

 ## CULTURAL AND SOCIAL CONSIDERATIONS

Pregnancy is a state of health; however, some complications of pregnancy occur more frequently in particular populations. In Canada, immigration has resulted in a complex mix of hereditary and genetic factors that may not always be discernible. Certain population groups are known to have an increased risk for carrying particular genetic disorders (SOGC, 2011). For example, mutations for hemoglobinopathies (e.g., sickle cell anemia, β-thalassemia, α-thalassemia) are common among people whose ancestors were from areas where malaria is endemic, including Africa, the Mediterranean basin, the Middle East, the Indian subcontinent, Southeast Asia, and southern China. In practice, it has been recommended that everyone whose ancestors do not come from northern Europe should be considered at high risk for these genetically linked disorders. The carrier frequency for Tay-Sachs disease, another genetic disorder, is 1 per 30 among Ashkenazi Jews and 1 per 14 among French Canadians in Eastern Quebec. The frequency outside Eastern Quebec, however, is much lower (1 per 41 to 1 per 98).

Pregnancy and breastfeeding outcomes are significantly affected not only by maternal and fetal health but also by the social determinants of health, such as educational levels, income, and social support systems. Many contributing factors, including knowledge and beliefs, can affect a woman's decision to seek prenatal care. Other factors can include work environment, transportation, caring for other family members, and support of a partner or friends.

All families, regardless of ethnocultural background, recognize the birth of a child as a significant moment for women, families, and communities. It marks a psychological, social, and spiritual moment in people's lives. Complex and important rituals, customs, and beliefs are integrated into this experience. The spiritual practices and beliefs that underlie women's lives are unique to each woman and her family. A relational approach to nursing (see Chapter 1) enables you to provide compassionate care in a culturally competent way as women deal with emotionally charged issues such as sexuality, relationships, contraception, maternal weight gain, and, in some cases, spontaneous or therapeutic abortion. You may begin by inquiring whether the patient or her significant other have any special requests. Sensitivity and dialogue that communicate respect for people's preferences and differences are essential components of developing rapport and enable the patient and her family to share concerns as they develop. Use your skill to understand such preferences within a sociocultural context and to convey acceptance of the patient and her family. Whenever their preferences are safe and possible, respect them. This enhances the success of childbirth in its psychological and social dimensions and demonstrates value of the diversity of women and families (Registered Nurses' Association of Ontario, 2007).

Safe Motherhood: Global Pregnancy Outcomes

The World Health Organization (WHO) defines **maternal death** as any death that occurs during pregnancy or within 42 days after termination of any pregnancy. It must be a direct or indirect result of the pregnancy or any condition aggravated by the pregnancy. It does not include deaths that result from accidental or incidental causes. The **maternal mortality rate** is the number of maternal deaths per 100,000 live births. The maternal mortality rate represents the risk of dying that a pregnant woman faces with each pregnancy. In 2008, the WHO estimated that there were 358,000 maternal deaths in the world. Developing nations account for 99% of these deaths. From 2008 to 2010, Canada had a maternal mortality rate of 7.8 per 100,000 (Public Health Agency of Canada, 2012). In contrast, women in developing nations have a lifetime risk of 1 per 4300 (WHO, 2010). More than 80% of maternal deaths worldwide are caused by postpartum hemorrhage, sepsis, unsafe abortion, obstructed labour, and hypertensive disorders (WHO, 2010).

SUBJECTIVE DATA

1. Menstrual history
2. Gynecological history
3. Obstetrical history
4. History of current pregnancy
5. Medical history

6. Family history
7. Review of systems
8. Nutritional history
9. Environment and hazards

HEALTH HISTORY QUESTIONS

Examiner Asks	Rationale
1. **Menstrual history.** When was the first day of your most recent menstrual period that was normal in timing? • Did you have premenstrual symptoms? How long was your period? What was the amount of flow? Did you have cramping? • What is the number of days in a normal cycle for you? • What was your age at menarche?	Using Nägele's rule, calculate the EDB with the LMP. Using a pregnancy wheel, determine the current number of weeks of gestation.

|

2. **Gynecological history.** Have you ever had surgery of the cervix or uterus?

Cervical surgery may affect the integrity of the cervix during pregnancy and may impede cervical dilation during labour. Uterine surgery increases risk for cervical insufficiency and uterine rupture during pregnancy and labour. Uterine surgery also increases the risk of abnormal placental implantation, such as placenta accreta or placenta percreta, particularly with placenta previa.

- Any known history of or exposure to genital herpes?

Onset of this disease during pregnancy is potentially *teratogenic* (i.e., causing physical defects in the developing fetus), and a lesion at time of birth precludes vaginal birth.

- Papanicolaou (Pap) test: When was your most recent one? Any history of abnormality? If so, when? Have you ever had a colposcopy? Cervical biopsy?

Because more women delay childbearing, gynecological cancers may be increasingly diagnosed during pregnancy. Approximately one third of recorded maternal deaths are the result of a coexisting malignancy (Gabbe et al., 2007).

- Any history of infertility, fibroids, or uterine abnormalities?

These conditions may increase risk for ectopic pregnancy, miscarriage, and preterm labour/preterm birth.

- Any history of gonorrhea, chlamydia, syphilis, trichomoniasis, bacterial vaginitis, or pelvic inflammatory disease (PID)?

STIs increase the risk of premature rupture of membranes, preterm labour/preterm birth, and postpartum maternal and fetal infections.

- Do you or does your partner have more than one sexual partner?

Intercourse with multiple partners increases the risk of STIs and human immunodeficiency virus (HIV) infection.

- Were you a preterm infant?

Women who themselves were preterm infants are at increased risk for preterm birth.

- Have you had a mammogram, breast biopsy, breast implants, lumpectomy, or mastectomy?

Approximately 2% to 3% of all breast cancers in women younger than 40 years occur concurrently with pregnancy or lactation (Gabbe et al., 2007).

3. **Obstetrical history.** In earlier pregnancies, did you experience hypertension, pre-eclampsia, eclampsia, the HELLP (**h**emolysis, **e**levated **l**iver enzyme levels, **l**ow **p**latelet count) syndrome, diabetes, β-hemolytic *Streptococcus* infection, IUGR, congenital anomalies, preterm labour, postpartum hemorrhage, or postpartum depression?

A patient who has experienced any of these complications in the past is at increased risk for them in subsequent pregnancies.

- How did you experience previous pregnancies and births?

The subjective quality of previous experiences has an effect on emotions regarding the current pregnancy.

- Have you ever had a Caesarean section? If so, what was the indication? At how many centimetres of dilation, if any, was the surgery performed? What type of uterine incision was made? (Confirming records of this surgery must be obtained.) Have you ever had a vaginal birth after a Caesarean section?

A patient who has undergone uterine surgery is at risk for uterine rupture during pregnancy and labour. The vertical ("classic") incision increases the risk for rupture; in women with this incision, all subsequent births must be by Caesarean section. The pfannenstiel ("low transverse") horizontal incision carries a low risk, and subsequent births may be vaginal. Note that the direction of the scar does not indicate how the uterus was incised.

Examiner Asks	Rationale
• How many times have you been pregnant? How many full-term or preterm births have you delivered? • How many spontaneous miscarriages, elective abortions, or ectopic pregnancies have you experienced? Any fetal or neonatal deaths? Any losses? • Do you have any history of infertility? Have you used assisted reproductive technology? • Do you have any history of preterm labour or preterm rupture of membranes? • Have you been told that you have cervical insufficiency or incompetence? Have you had a cervical cerclage placed in previous pregnancies? • What were the gestational ages and weights of your babies at birth?	Establishing an obstetrical history is beneficial in providing care during the current pregnancy. In the case of donor eggs, the age of the egg donor is used in calculating genetic testing. A patient with such a history requires close observation during the current pregnancy. Previous preterm birth is associated with recurrence. A cervical cerclage is a stitch placed surgically to hold the cervix closed during the pregnancy and is normally placed between weeks 12 and 15. Smallness of an infant may indicate prematurity or IUGR; these complications are repeatable. Largeness of an infant may indicate gestational diabetes mellitus (also repeatable). Conversely, birth weights of other children may indicate a "constitutional size" (e.g., the tendency of a couple to conceive small but normal children). Also, a patient's pelvis has accommodated to the weight of the largest baby born vaginally; bear this number in mind as labour begins, estimating and comparing the weight of the baby about to be born.
• Have you breastfed before? How was that experience for you? • Do you have any history of mastitis?	A patient's experience and knowledge base will shape your teaching and support. A poor or painful previous experience increases the need for breastfeeding support after this pregnancy.
4. **History of current pregnancy.** (Having calculated the current number of weeks of gestation, you can reassess the probable accuracy of that date when eliciting the following history.) • What method of contraceptive did you use most recently, and when did you discontinue it? • Was the pregnancy planned? How do you feel about it?	Recent use of birth control pills or other hormonal contraceptives may cause delays in ovulation and irregular menses; consider this when establishing the EDB. An intrauterine device that is still in place must be removed; it threatens the pregnancy. Also, the presence of this device raises question of whether the pregnancy was planned. Even a planned pregnancy represents loss for a patient: perhaps a loss of freedom, compromise of goals, loss of time with other children or partner. The first trimester is known as the "trimester of ambivalence," and encouraging acceptance and expression of these feelings facilitates resolution. Up to 50% of pregnancies are thought to be unplanned, and so discussion is helpful.

Examiner Asks	Rationale
• How does the baby's father or your support person feel about the pregnancy? How do other family members feel about it?	Women may need assistance in gathering support groups. Your patient may have a female partner, or the baby's father may not be involved. Inviting significant others to future office visits affirms their importance and supports involvement of whomever this woman wishes to include in her support group.
• Have you experienced any vaginal bleeding? When? How much? What colour? Was it accompanied by any pain? (Determine the patient's Rh status.)	Vaginal bleeding may indicate threatened abortion, cervicitis, or other complications and must be investigated. Rh-negative women should receive Rho(D) immune globulin within 72 hours of an episode of antepartum bleeding.
• Are you experiencing any nausea, vomiting, or both?	Nausea and vomiting are symptoms of pregnancy that usually begin between weeks 4 and 5, peak between weeks 8 and 12, and resolve between weeks 14 and 16. Persistent and severe nausea and vomiting lead to hyperemesis.
• Have you experienced abdominal pain? When? Where in your abdomen? Was it accompanied by vaginal bleeding?	The most common causes of abdominal pain in early pregnancy are spontaneous abortion (see Table 30-5, p. 845), ectopic pregnancy, urinary tract infection (UTI), and round ligament discomfort. Late in pregnancy, causes of pain are premature labour, placental abruption, and the HELLP syndrome (see Table 30-3, p. 842). Also consider other medical and surgical causes of abdominal pain.
• Have you experienced any contractions? How painful? How often? How long do they last?	Uterine contractions associated with true labour are painful, occur regularly at least every 5 minutes, last 30 to 60 seconds and increase steadily in intensity and duration. *Braxton Hicks* contractions (false labour) are generally painless, irregular, occur every 10 to 20 minutes and last less than 30 seconds.
• Have you experienced any illnesses since being pregnant? Any recent fever, unexplained rash, or infections?	These questions helps document any possible exposures to infectious agents.
• Since becoming pregnant, have you had any x-ray studies? Taken any medications? Used any recreational drugs or alcohol? Do you smoke cigarettes?	Discuss the potential effect of any teratogenic exposure. Refer the patient for expert counselling if necessary.

CRITICAL FINDINGS

Historically, women were advised not to seek dental health during pregnancy and not to have radiographs of any kind. Current thinking stresses the importance of good oral hygiene, including dental care for any dental problems.

Gingivitis has been associated with preterm birth and low weight for gestational age in infants. In addition, poor maternal oral health increases the risk for childhood caries, inasmuch as the mother's saliva is the primary source of cariogenic bacteria in children's oral flora (Stevens et al., 2007).

Examiner Asks	Rationale
• Are you experiencing any vision changes, such as the new onset of blurred vision or seeing spots before your eyes?	In the third trimester, vision changes may be a sign of pre-eclampsia. Evaluate the patient for other signs and symptoms of pre-eclampsia (see Table 30-3, p. 842).
• Are you experiencing any edema? In what parts of your body, and under what circumstances?	In the third trimester, differentiate the normal weight-dependent edema of pregnancy from the edema of pre-eclampsia.
• Are you experiencing any unusual frequency or burning sensation with urination? Any blood in your urine? Do you void in small amounts? Do you have any history of UTIs, pyelonephritis, or kidney stones?	Differentiate the normal urinary frequency of the first and third trimesters from UTI, for which pregnant women are at increased risk. Confirm UTI by urinalysis. UTIs increase the rate of preterm birth.
• Are you experiencing any vaginal burning sensation or itching? Any foul-smelling or coloured discharge?	Check for vaginal infection. If symptoms exist, obtain specimens for cultures or a wet mount during the pelvic examination. Discuss partner treatment if necessary. Explain the normal increase in vaginal secretions during pregnancy.
• Do you have cats in the home?	Explain toxoplasmosis, a teratogenic disease transmitted through cat feces. To avoid exposure, someone other than the pregnant patient should empty cat litter at frequent intervals.
• On what date did you first feel the baby move?	This sign is compared to the EDB to evaluate the accuracy of that date. Tell a patient who has not felt movement to note and report that event at the following prenatal visit.
• How does the baby move on a daily basis?	Fetal movement is an excellent indicator of fetal health. Clinicians assign women to count fetal movements starting at 26 to 28 weeks of pregnancy.
• Do you plan to breastfeed this baby?	Arrange for reading materials, classes, and other support for a patient who is breastfeeding for the first time or for a patient who had an unsuccessful earlier experience.
5. **Medical history.** Do you have allergies to medications or foods? If so, what type of reaction?	Document such allergies to prevent prescription errors. A "penicillin allergy" should be explored to understand the reaction (e.g., rash versus nausea and vomiting). Group B streptococcal infection is best treated with penicillin in patients without a true allergy.
• What is your blood group and type?	Rh-negative women should be identified early in pregnancy so that Rho(D) immune globulin can be given to prevent antibody stimulation in the event of an antepartum, intrapartum, or postpartum uptake of fetal blood.
• Any personal or family history of cancer?	Advanced maternal age increases risk of breast, ovarian, uterine, and colon cancers.
• Do you have a history of asthma? If yes, have you ever been intubated?	Poor control and frequent exacerbations of asthma during pregnancy may result in maternal hypoxia and a decrease in fetal oxygenation.

Subjective Data

Examiner Asks	Rationale
• Have you ever had German measles (rubella)?	This disease, which has mild effects in children, is highly teratogenic in fetuses, especially during the first trimester. Instruct a patient who has not had rubella to avoid small children who are ill. Check immunity status in the serum prenatal panel. A nonimmune patient will be offered immunization after birth while in hospital.
• Have you ever had chicken pox?	In rare cases, varicella causes congenital anomalies. A nonimmune patient should avoid exposure. Offer postpartum immunization.
• Have you had any injury to the back or another weight-bearing part?	The localized and overall weight gain of pregnancy and the joint-softening effects of progesterone cause lordosis and aggravate such injuries with increasing gestational age.
• Have you been tested for HIV infection? When? What was the result? Have you ever had a blood transfusion? Used intravenous drugs? Had a sexual partner at risk for HIV infection? Are both you and your partner monogamous?	Address HIV status to promote the health of the gravida and to decrease the risk of transmission of the virus across the placenta to the fetus. Breastfeeding is contraindicated in HIV-positive mothers because the virus is present in the breast milk. Provide information on "safer sex" to a patient who describes engaging in high-risk sexual behaviour, and consider retesting in each trimester.
• Do you smoke cigarettes? How many? For how many years? Have you ever tried to quit? Do you drink any alcohol? How many times per week? Do you use any street drugs?	Explain the danger of using these substances during pregnancy. Smoking increases the risk of ectopic pregnancy, spontaneous abortion, low birth weight, prematurity, preterm rupture of membranes, hypertensive disorders, placental abruption, and sudden infant death syndrome. Alcohol increases the fetus's risk for fetal alcohol syndrome (see Table 14-3, p. 291). Cocaine use during pregnancy is associated with congenital anomalies, a fourfold increased risk for placental abruption, and the risk for withdrawal symptoms in newborns. Infants exposed during pregnancy to problematic substances may have developmental delays or behavioural disturbances (Cunningham et al., 2010). Refer such patients to a counselling or support program and for periodic toxicology screening. Refer patients who smoke to a smoking cessation program.
• Do you take any prescribed, over-the-counter, or herbal medications?	Screen all medications to establish safety during pregnancy.
• Do you participate in a regular exercise program? What type?	Regular exercise during pregnancy may reduce risk for hypertension and helps control weight gain.

Subjective Data

Subjective Data

Examiner Asks	Rationale
• Has your vitamin D level been checked?	Vitamin D is essential for maternal response to the calcium demands of the fetus for growth and bone development. Maternal anorexia and malaise are often associated with vitamin D deficiency (Hollis & Wagner, 2004), and the vitamin D should be evaluated when these symptoms occur.
6. **Family history.** Does anyone in your family have hypertension?	Hypertension increases the risk for chronic hypertension and for pre-eclampsia.
• Does anyone in your family have diabetes? If so, is it of juvenile or adult onset? Is the relative insulin dependent?	If a first-degree relative has type 2 diabetes, a pregnant patient is at higher risk for gestational diabetes mellitus. Counsel on risk, and offer a nutrition and exercise program, plus screening.
• Has anyone in your family had a mental illness such as anxiety, depression, or schizophrenia?	Mental illness increases risk for postpartum depression (Cunningham et al., 2010).
• Do you have kidney disease?	Kidney disease increases risk for renal disease, hypertension, and pre-eclampsia.
• Has anyone in your family had fraternal twins?	The tendency to ovulate twice in 1 month is familial, and thus the incidence of twinning is increased in families of such women.
• Has anyone in your family, or in the family of the baby's father, had congenital anomalies?	Some anomalies, such as certain heart conditions, are familial. Offer genetic counselling if it is needed.
• Are you of Mediterranean descent?	Risk for β-thalassemia is increased.
• Are you of African descent?	Risk for sickle-cell anemia is increased.
• Are you of Ashkenazi Jewish descent?	Risk for Tay-Sachs disease is increased.
• Are you of Irish descent?	Risk for spinal malformations is increased.
7. **Review of systems**	
• What was your weight before pregnancy?	Baseline weight is needed to evaluate changes. Calculating the body mass index (BMI) with prepregnancy weight is helpful for determining risks for various conditions, such as gestational diabetes.
• Do you wear glasses?	A transient change in vision correction may occur during pregnancy.
• When did you most recently see the dentist? Do you need any dental work?	Gums may be puffy and bleed easily during pregnancy, predisposing to caries. Poor dental hygiene can lead to preterm birth, low birth weight, and neonatal death. Encourage dental hygiene. Suggest that any dental work be performed during the second trimester and that the dentist be notified that the patient is pregnant.
• Have you been exposed to tuberculosis or had a positive tuberculin test result or chest x-ray study?	Consider tuberculosis screening with the tuberculin skin test.
• Do you have any cardiovascular disease, such as coronary artery disease, heart failure, or disease of a heart valve?	A patient with cardiac disease who becomes pregnant must be monitored carefully for signs of cardiac compromise. Blood volume increases by 40%, and the demand on the heart is significantly increased.

Examiner Asks	Rationale
• Have you had anemia? What kind? When? Was it treated? How? Did it improve?	Pregnancy worsens any preexisting anemia because iron in the mother's body is used up extensively by the fetus. Identify the need for early supplementation. Sickle cell disease may worsen during pregnancy, whereas sickle cell carriers have more UTIs. Screen the latter periodically for bacteriuria.
• Have you had thrombophlebitis, pulmonary embolus, or deep venous thrombosis?	Pregnancy itself is a hypercoagulable state because of increases in coagulation factors I, VII, VIII, IX, and X. This increases the risk for phlebitis (Cunningham et al., 2010).
• Have you had hypertension or kidney disease?	A pregnant patient with renal disease or with chronic hypertension is at increased risk for pre-eclampsia. Document the baseline BP and renal function to evaluate any changes.
• Do you have any history of hepatitis B or C?	Confirm this with serum testing. Perinatal transmission to the infant usually occurs through exposure to infected blood and genital secretions during birth and through cracked and bleeding nipples during breastfeeding.
• Do you have any history of thyroid disease?	Uncontrolled hypothyroidism is associated with increased neonatal morbidity that results from preterm birth and low birth weight. Uncontrolled hypothyroidism is related to delayed mental development in children.
• Do you have any history of seizures? Are you taking any medications for seizures?	Maternal seizure disorders are associated with increased incidences of stillbirths and IUGR.
• Have you had a UTI?	The hormonal levels during pregnancy predispose women to UTI, and so a history of UTIs before pregnancy is an indication for periodic screening. Pregnancy may also mask the symptoms of UTI. Furthermore, a serious UTI may cause irritability of the uterus, posing a risk for preterm labour. Educate patients about measures to prevent UTI.
• Have you had a mental illness such as anxiety, depression, or schizophrenia? Were you treated? Are you still being treated?	Such a patient is at risk for postpartum depression. Assist her to prepare a support network. Counselling may help her navigate the developmental challenges of becoming a mother. If a patient was taking antidepressants before pregnancy, it is important to establish whether she should continue taking them or be gradually weaned. If she has a condition such as schizophrenia, it is very important to continue with medication, and the patient should be encouraged to have regular care for this.

Subjective Data

Examiner Asks	Rationale
• Do you feel safe in your relationship or home environment?	Interpersonal violence during pregnancy is common. Questioning the safety of the patient is part of prenatal care.
• Are you in a relationship with someone who physically or emotionally abuses or threatens you?	Most abused patients do not freely offer this information. You must ask these questions at the appropriate time, privately, and without causing distress, by framing them as follows: "I ask everyone these questions because of my concern for all women."
• Has anyone forced you to perform sexual activities against your will?	Women who have been subjected to incest or other abuse are candidates for dysfunctional labour and subsequent Caesarean delivery.
• Do you have diabetes? Did you have diabetes during a previous pregnancy?	Diabetes is carefully managed during pregnancy to avoid serious complications, such as macrosomia in the infant and operative delivery. Consider early screening and nutritional interventions.

9. Nutritional history.
   • Are you taking a folic acid–fortified multivitamin every day?

A daily multivitamin with at least 0.4 to 1.0 mg of folic acid is recommended for all women who could become pregnant, for 3 months or longer before conception through the first 3 months of pregnancy, to prevent neural tube defects in the baby.

CRITICAL FINDINGS

For pregnant women with high medical risks, such as diabetic women taking insulin, women with epilepsy, those with a family history of neural tube defect, or those with body mass index exceeding 35 kg/m², a supplement of 5 mg of folic acid is encouraged 3 months before and up to 10 to 12 weeks of pregnancy (Genetics Committee of the Society of Obstetricians and Gynecologists of Canada and Motherisk Program, 2007).

Examiner Asks	Rationale
• Do you follow a special diet? Are you vegetarian?	A special diet may put the patient at nutritional risk. Help achieve adequate nutrition within the confines of her diet.
• Any food intolerance?	A food intolerance might affect the woman's and fetus's nutrition (e.g., lactose intolerance limits calcium intake).
• Do you crave nonfoods such as ice, paint chips, dirt, or clay?	Craving for nonfood items is called *pica* and is associated with anemia.
10. **Environment and hazards.** What is your occupation? What are the physical demands of the work? Are you exposed to any strong odours, chemicals, radiation, or other harmful substances?	Environmental hazards represent possible teratogens. A patient who is not immune to rubella may be advised not to continue working in a day care centre. A patient whose job requires long hours of standing may be required to stop work early in her pregnancy if signs of preterm labour occur.

Examiner Asks	Rationale
• Do you consider your food and housing adequate?	If it is appropriate, refer the patient for provincial and federal programs to assist with food, housing, or other needs.
• How do you wear your seatbelt when driving?	For maternal and fetal safety, instruct the patient to place the lap belt below the abdomen.
• Do you have other questions or concerns?	Encourage the patient to write down questions that may come up between visits.

OBJECTIVE DATA

PREPARATION

The initial examination for pregnancy may be a patient's first pelvic examination, and many women become extremely anxious about it. Moreover, the patient may not know for certain whether she is pregnant and may be anxious about the findings. Before touching the patient, explain to her what will happen during the examination. Save the pelvic examination for last; by that time the patient will have become more comfortable with your gentle, informative approach. Communicate all findings as you proceed, to demonstrate your respectful affirmation of her control and responsibility in her own health and health care and that of her child's.

Ask the patient to empty her bladder before the examination; reserve a specimen for protein and glucose testing and, if necessary, for urinalysis. Before the examination, ask her to weigh herself on the office scale. Provide the patient with a chaperone if desired. Some clinics require an escort or chaperone during examinations.

Give the patient a gown and a drape, and give her time to undress and put on the gown. Begin the examination with the patient sitting on the examination table, wearing the gown, her lap covered by the drape. Measure and record vital signs, including BP, pulse, temperature, and fetal heart rate. Before beginning the breast examination, help her lie down. She remains recumbent for the abdominal and extremity examination. She must be placed in the lithotomy position for the pelvic examination (see Chapter 27). Help her to the sitting position. Recheck after the examination if BP was previously elevated.

EQUIPMENT NEEDED

Stethoscope, BP cuff
Centimetre measuring tape
Fetoscope and Doppler sonometer
Reflex hammer
Urine collection containers
Urinalysis test strips to check urine for glucose and protein
Equipment needed for pelvic examination as noted in Chapter 27

Normal Range of Finding	Abnormal Findings
GENERAL SURVEY	
Observe the patient's state of nourishment, and her grooming, posture, mood, and affect, which reflect her mental state. Throughout the examination, observe her maturity and ability to pay attention and to learn in order to plan how to provide the information she needs to successfully complete a healthy pregnancy.	Undernourished or obese. Poor grooming, a slumped posture, and a flat affect may be signs of depression and risk for postpartum depression. Poor grooming may reflect a lack of resources and a need for a social service referral. A lack of attention may indicate a preoccupation with some concern. The patient who has had learning difficulties may benefit from printed and oral information, special classes, and a support person to accompany her. A flat, unfocused affect may indicate depression or the influence of drugs.

Subjective Data

Objective Data

Normal Range of Finding	Abnormal Findings

SKIN

Note any scars (particularly those of previous Caesarean delivery). Many pregnant women exhibit skin changes, such as acne or skin tags, that may resolve spontaneously after the pregnancy. Vascular spiders may be present on the upper body. Some women have **chloasma,** known as the "mask of pregnancy," which is a butterfly-shaped pigmentation of the face. Note the presence of the linea nigra, a hyperpigmented line that begins at the sternal notch and extends down the abdomen through the umbilicus to the pubis (Figure 30-3). Also note striae, or stretch marks, in areas of enlargement, particularly on the abdomen and breasts of multiparous women. These marks are bright red when they first form, but they shrink and lighten to a silvery colour (in light-skinned women) after the pregnancy (see Figure 30-3). In dark-skinned women the straie will appear lighter than the surrounding skin.

Multiple bruises may suggest physical abuse.

Tracks (scars along easily accessed veins) may indicate intravenous drug use.

Complaints of nasal irritation, nasal crusting, nasal stuffiness, or recurrent nose bleeds may indicate drug sniffing.

Palmar erythema in the first trimester may indicate hepatitis, but thereafter it is not clinically significant (Kriebs & Gegor, 2005).

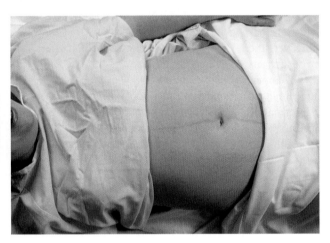

30-3

MOUTH

Mucous membranes should be red and moist. Gum hypertrophy (surface looks smooth, and stippling disappears) may occur normally during pregnancy (pregnancy gingivitis). Gums may bleed as a result of estrogen stimulation, which increases vascularity and causes fragility.

Pale mucous membranes are indicative of anemia.

Poor dental hygiene during pregnancy may lead to preterm birth or low birth weight.

NECK

The thyroid may be palpable and feel full but smooth during the normal pregnancy of a euthyroid patient.

Solitary nodules indicate neoplasm; multiple nodules usually indicate inflammation or a multinodular goitre. Significant diffuse enlargement occurs with hyperthyroidism, thyroiditis, and hypothyroidism.

BREASTS

The breasts are enlarged (Figure 30-4), perhaps with resulting striae, and may be very tender. The areolae and nipples enlarge and darken in pigmentation, the nipples become more erect, and "secondary areolae" (mottling around the areolae) may develop. The blood vessels of the breast enlarge; the chest wall may seem more translucent than usual, with blue veins visible just below the skin. When you auscultate, you can hear blood flow through these blood vessels, and the sound may be mistaken for a cardiac murmur. This sound is called the *mammary souffle* (pronounced *soof'fl*). Montgomery's tubercles, located around the areola and responsible for skin integrity of the areola, enlarge. Colostrum, a thick yellow fluid, may be expressed from the nipples.

Objective Data

Normal Range of Finding	Abnormal Findings

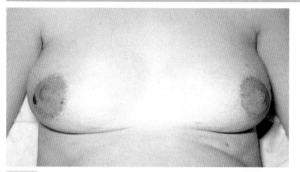

30-4

The breast tissue feels nodular as the mammary alveoli hypertrophy. Take this opportunity to teach or reinforce breast self-examination. For more information on teaching and advising about breast self-examination, review Chapter 18. The patient should expect changes in the breast tissue during pregnancy. Because of the lack of menses, instruct her to palpate over her breasts in a circular motion to feel for any changes (e.g., hardened, hot, or reddened areas that are painful to the touch).

Recall that some women have an embryological remnant called a *supernumerary nipple*, which may or may not have breast tissue beneath it. These remnants, which may have been mistaken previously for moles, appear under the arm or in a line directly underneath each nipple on the abdominal wall (see Chapter 18). Such nipples and breast tissue may show the same changes of pregnancy. Instruct the patient to check these areas as well during breast self-examination.

For any unusual breast lump, refer the patient for further study. Ultrasonography of the breasts is used in lieu of mammography during pregnancy and lactation.

HEART

Many pregnant patients have a functional, soft, blowing, systolic murmur that occurs as a result of increased volume. The murmur necessitates no treatment and resolves after pregnancy.

If you note any other murmur, refer the patient for further evaluation. Valvular disease may necessitate the use of prophylactic antibiotics at delivery. Pregnancy places a large hemodynamic burden on the heart, and a pregnant patient with cardiac disease must be managed closely.

LUNGS

The lungs are clear bilaterally to auscultation with no crackles or wheezing. Shortness of breath is common in the third trimester as a result of pressure on the diaphragm from the enlarged uterus.

Women with asthma exacerbations during pregnancy may have expiratory (and possibly inspiratory) wheeze.

PERIPHERAL VASCULATURE

Diffuse, bilateral pitting edema may be observed on the legs, particularly during the third trimester and if the examination occurs later in the day, when the patient has been on her feet. Varicose veins in the legs are common in the third trimester. Nondependent edema is no longer a criterion for diagnosing pre-eclampsia.

Pregnant patients are at risk for thrombophlebitis. Carefully evaluate any redness or red, hot, tender swelling to rule out phlebitis. Varicosities increase the risk of thrombophlebitis, and such patients should not wear restrictive clothing or sit for a long period without moving the legs. Varicosities worsen with the weight and volume of pregnancy, and support hose helps minimize them.

Objective Data

Normal Range of Finding	Abnormal Findings

NEUROLOGICAL SYSTEM

Using the reflex hammer, check the biceps, patellar, and ankle deep tendon reflexes (DTRs). Normally these are graded 1+ to 2+ and are equal bilaterally.

> DTRs that are brisk or greater than grade 2+ and clonus may be associated with elevated BP and cerebral edema in preeclamptic women.

INSPECT AND PALPATE THE ABDOMEN

Observe the shape and contours of the abdomen to discern signs of fetal position. Note the linea nigra and any bruises or cuts. As the patient lifts her head, you may see the **diastasis recti,** the separation of the abdominal muscles, which occurs during pregnancy. The muscles return together after pregnancy with abdominal exercise. When palpating, note the abdominal muscle tone, which grows more relaxed with each subsequent pregnancy. Note any tenderness; the uterus is normally nontender.

> Suspect multiple gestation if uterine size is greater than expected for gestational age, if multiple fetal heart tones are auscultated, if multiple fetal parts are felt, or if the patient describes use of assisted reproductive technologies (Hurt, Guile, Bienstock, Fox, & Wallach, 2011).

The fundus should be palpable abdominally after 12 weeks' gestation. Using the side of your hand, begin palpating centrally on the abdomen higher than you expect the uterus to be. Palpate down until you feel the fundus (the top of the uterus). Alternatively, stand at the patient's right side, facing her head (Figure 30-5). Place the palm of your right hand on the curve of the uterus in the left lower quadrant and your left palm on the curve of the uterus in the right lower quadrant. Moving from hand to hand, allowing the curve of the uterus to guide you, move your hands to where they meet centrally at the fundus.

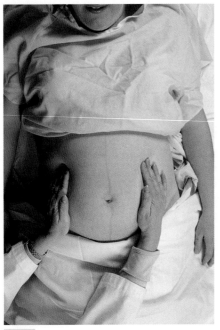

30-5

Note the fundal location by landmarks and fingerbreadths, as described in Figure 30-1 (p. 813). Because of individual women's variations in location of landmarks and examiners' variations in fingerbreadth, this measurement is inexact. From 20 weeks' gestation, measurement is more accurate with the use of the centimetre measuring tape; measure the height of the fundus in centimetres from the superior border of the symphysis to the fundus (Figure 30-6). After 20 weeks, the number of centimetres should approximate the number of weeks of gestation.

> A lag in fundal height of more than 2 cm may indicate IUGR, transverse lie, oligohydramnios, inaccurate calculation of gestational age, or oblique presentation of the fetus.
>
> An increase in fundal height of more than 2 cm may indicate multiple gestation, macrosomia, polyhydramnios, or inaccurate calculation of gestational age.

Objective Data

| **Normal Range of Finding** | **Abnormal Findings** |

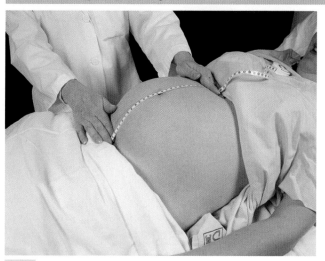

30-6

Beginning at 20 weeks, you may feel fetal movement, and the fetus's head can be palpated with ballottement. A gentle, quick palpation with the fingertips can locate the head, which is hard not only when you push it away but also as it bobs or bounces back against your fingers.

If you suspect the patient to be in labour, palpate for uterine contractions. Palpate the uterus over its entire surface to familiarize yourself with its "indentability." Then rest your hand lightly on the uterine fundus with fingers opened. When the uterus contracts, it rises and pulls together, drawing your fingers closer together.

During the contraction, notice that the uterus is less "indentable." When the uterus relaxes, your fingers relax open again. In this way, contractions can be monitored for frequency (from the beginning of one contraction to the beginning of the next), length, and quality. Note that a mild contraction feels like the firmness of the tip of your nose; a moderate contraction feels like your chin; and a hard contraction feels like a forehead. (Make allowance for the amount of soft tissue between your fingers and the uterus.)

True labour is characterized by painful, repetitive uterine contractions that increase steadily in intensity and duration and lead to progressive effacement and dilatation of the cervix (VanRooyen & Scott, 2011). True labour pains typically begin in the fundal region and upper abdomen and radiate into the pelvis and the lower back whereas false labour is characterized by brief, irregular contractions, commonly called Braxton Hicks contractions, that are usually confined to the lower abdomen and do not lead to cervical changes.

An abnormal uterine contraction is dystonic in nature; the contraction begins in the lower uterine segment and may delay cervical dilation.

An inadequate resting tone can indicate uterine irritability or tachysystole associated with placental abruption. Tenderness of the uterus may indicate chorioamnionitis or placental abruption.

Leopold's Manoeuvres

In the patient's third trimester, perform Leopold's manoeuvres to determine fetal lie, presentation, attitude, position, variety, and engagement. **Fetal lie** is the orientation of the fetal spine to the maternal spine and may be longitudinal, transverse, or oblique. **Presentation** describes the part of the fetus that is entering the pelvis first. **Attitude,** the position of fetal parts in relation to each other, may be flexed, military (straight), or extended. **Position** designates the location of a fetal part to the right or left of the maternal pelvis. **Variety** is the location of the fetal back to the anterior, lateral, or posterior part of the maternal pelvis. **Engagement** occurs when the widest diameter of the presenting part has passed through the pelvic inlet. In a full-term pregnancy, engagement usually occurs at the same time that the leading point of the presenting part reaches the level of the ischial spines (Kriebs & Gegor, 2005).

Multiple gestational presentations (common) are illustrated in Table 30-6, p. 846. The most common presentation is vertex.

Objective Data

Normal Range of Finding	Abnormal Findings

To perform **Leopold's first manoeuvre,** face the patient's head and place your fingertips around the top of the fundus (Figure 30-7). Note its size, consistency, and shape. Imagine which fetal part is in the fundus. When a fetus is in the breech position, the fetal part at the top feels large and firm. Moving it between the thumb and fingers of the hand, because it is attached to the fetus at the waist, results in moving it slowly and with difficulty. In contrast, the fetal head feels large, round, hard, and mobile. When it is in ballottement, it feels hard as you push it away and hard again as it bobs back against your fingers in response. Note that the bobbing movement occurs because the head is attached at the neck and moves easily. If you palpate no part in the fundus, the fetus is in the transverse lie.

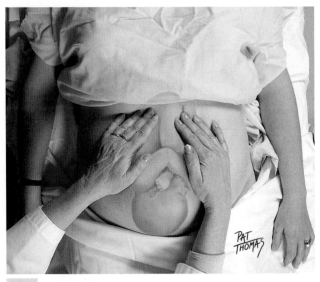

30-7 Leopold's first manoeuvre.

For **Leopold's second manoeuvre,** move your hands to the sides of the uterus (Figure 30-8). Note whether small parts or a long, firm surface are palpable on the patient's left or right side. The long, firm surface is the fetal back. Note whether the back is anterior, lateral, or out of reach (posterior). The small parts, or limbs, indicate a posterior position when they are palpable all over the abdomen.

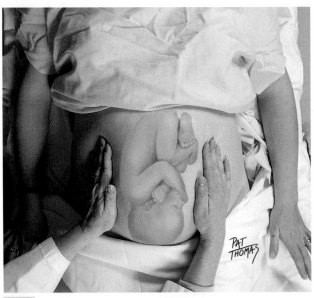

30-8 Leopold's second manoeuvre.

Normal Range of Finding	Abnormal Findings

Leopold's third manoeuvre, also called *Pawlik's manoeuvre,* requires the patient to bend her knees up slightly (Figure 30-9). Grasp the patient's lower abdomen just above the symphysis pubis between the thumb and fingers of one hand and, as you did at the fundus during the first manoeuvre, to determine what part of the fetus is there. If the presenting part is beginning to engage, it will feel "fixed." With this manoeuvre alone, it may be difficult to differentiate the shoulder from the vertex.

By 36 weeks of gestation, the presenting part should be cephalic. If a breech or transverse presentation is detected, referral to an obstetrician is indicated. The patient should be offered external cephalic version in the absence of contraindications.

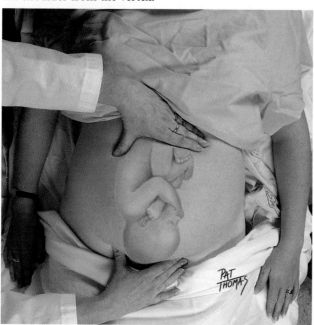

30-9 Leopold's third manoeuvre.

Leopold's fourth manoeuvre assists in determining engagement and, in the vertex presentation, to differentiate shoulder from vertex (Figure 30-10). The patient's knees are still bent. Face her feet, and place your palms, with fingers pointing toward the feet, on either side of the lower abdomen. Pressing your fingers firmly, move slowly down toward the pelvic inlet. If your fingers meet, the presenting part is not engaged. If your fingers diverge at the pelvic rim, meeting a hard prominence on one side, this prominence is the fetal occiput. This indicates vertex presentation with a deflexed head (the face presenting). If your fingers meet hard prominences on both sides, the vertex is engaged in either a military or a flexed position. If your fingers come to the pelvic brim diverged but with no prominences palpable, the vertex is "dipping" into the pelvis, or is engaged. In this case, the firm object felt above the symphysis pubis in the third manoeuvre is the fetal shoulder.

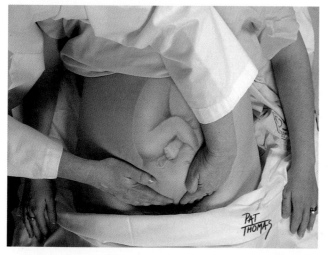

30-10 Leopold's fourth manoeuvre.

Objective Data

Figure 30-11 depicts various fetal positions and where to auscultate the FHTs for each. At the end of pregnancy, 96% of fetal presentations are vertex, 3.5% are breech, 0.3% are face, and 0.4% are shoulder (Cunningham et al., 2001).

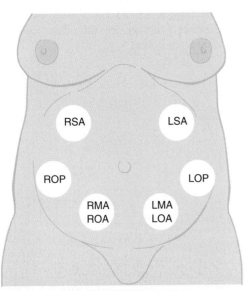

RSA and LSA = right and left sacral anterior (breech)
RMA and LMA = right and left mentum anterior (face)
ROA and LOA = right and left occiput anterior (vertex)
ROP and LOP = right and left occiput posterior (vertex)

30-11 Location of fetal heart tones (FHTs) for various fetal positions.

AUSCULTATE THE FETAL HEART TONES

FHTs are a positive sign of pregnancy. A fetal heartbeat should be heard on Doppler ultrasonography by 12 to 13 weeks' gestation and as early at 8 to 10 weeks in some women. This use of the fetoscope assists in dating the pregnancy. FHTs are auscultated best over the fetal back. After you identify the position of the fetus (see Figure 30-11), use the heart tones to confirm your findings. Count the FHTs for 15 seconds and multiply by 4 to obtain the rate (Figure 30-12). The normal rate is between 110 and 160 beats per minute (SOGC, 2007b). Spontaneous accelerations of FHTs indicate fetal well-being.

If no FHTs are heard, verify fetal cardiac activity with ultrasonography.

Further investigate any decelerations of FHTs because they can be an abnormal finding. Abrupt and brief decelerations are common in preterm fetuses. Decelerations cannot be classified by type unless the fetal heart is assessed by electronic fetal monitoring.

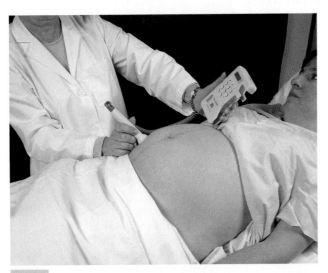

30-12

Normal Range of Finding	Abnormal Findings

Differentiate the FHTs from the slower rate of the maternal pulse and the uterine souffle (the soft, swishing sound of the placenta receiving the pulse of maternal arterial blood) by palpating the mother's pulse while you listen. Also, distinguish FHTs from the funic souffle (blood rushing through the umbilical arteries at the same rate as the FHTs). The FHTs are a double sound, like the tick-tock of a watch under a pillow, whereas the funic souffle is a sharp, whistling sound that is heard in only 15% of cases (Cunningham et al., 2010).

All the abdominal findings are of interest to the patient. Share them with her. Often she will want to listen to FHTs with her significant other. For a hearing-impaired pregnant patient, place her hand on the fetal monitor to feel the fetal heart vibrating.

PELVIC EXAMINATION

Genitalia

Use the procedure for the pelvic examination described in Chapter 27. Note the following characteristics. The enlargement of the labia minora is common in multiparous women. Labial varicosities may be present. The perineum may be scarred from a previous episiotomy or from lacerations. Note the presence of any hemorrhoids of the rectum. Note any lesions on the symphysis pubis, labia, or perianal area.

Lesions may indicate an infection, condyloma, or herpes simplex virus.

Speculum Examination

When examining the vagina, you may see Chadwick's sign, the bluish purple discoloration and congested look of the vaginal wall and cervix that results from increased vascularity and engorgement (Figure 30-13). Note the vaginal discharge. Vaginal discharge in pregnancy may be heavier in amount but should be similar in description to the patient's nonpregnant discharge and should not be accompanied by itching, burning sensation, or an unusual odour (except that, occasionally, chapping of the vaginal area may result from excessive moisture). Perform a wet mount or culture of the discharge when you are uncertain of its normality.

Many cervical infections or STIs are asymptomatic. Any cervical secretions that are purulent or mucopurulent (chlamydia or gonorrhea); yellow or green frothy (trichomoniasis); thin, white, grey, or milky, with a "fishy" odour (bacterial vaginosis); or thick, white, and clumpy (candidiasis) should be treated appropriately during pregnancy. Bacterial vaginosis can lead to preterm labour and rupture of membranes.

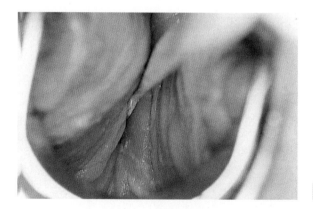

30-13

Note whether the cervix appears open. Note whether it is smooth and round with a dotlike external os (in a nulliparous patient) or irregular with an external os that appears more like a crooked line (in a multiparous patient; the result of cervical dilation and possibly lacerations during a previous pregnancy).

A friable cervix bleeds easily when touched with a cotton swab, Cytobrush, or speculum; friability may be caused by cervicitis. Obtain cultures. Any lesions should be investigated.

CRITICAL FINDINGS

Cervical cancer is the most common cancer in pregnancy. Most women with cervical cancer have a visible cervical lesion.

Bleeding on contact is common. Investigate any concerns related to the speculum examination (Hurt et al., 2011).

Objective Data

Normal Range of Finding	Abnormal Findings

Bimanual Examination

As described in Chapter 27, palpate the uterus between the hand that is performing the internal examination and the hand placed on the abdomen. Note the position of the uterus. The pregnant uterus may be rotated toward the right side as it rises out of the pelvis because of the presence of the descending colon on the left. This positioning is called **dextrorotation.** Irregular enlargement of the uterus may be noted at 8 to 10 weeks and occurs when implantation occurs close to a corneal area of the uterus. This appearance is called **Piskacek's sign.** You may also note Hegar's sign, when the enlarged uterus bends forward on its softened isthmus between the fourth and sixth weeks of pregnancy.

Note the size and consistency of the uterus. When the embryo is at 6 weeks of gestation, the uterus may seem only slightly enlarged and softened. At 8 weeks, the uterus is approximately the size of an avocado, approximately 7 to 8 cm across the fundus. At 10 weeks, the uterus is approximately the size of a grapefruit and may reach to the pelvic brim, but it is narrow and does not fill the pelvis from side to side; at 12 weeks, the uterus does fill the pelvis. After 12 weeks, the uterus is sized from the abdomen. A multigravid uterus may be larger initially, and early sizing of such a uterus may be less reliable for dating.

Softening of the cervix is called *Goodell's sign.* When examining the cervix, note its position (anterior, midposition, or posterior), the degree of effacement (or thinning, expressed in percentages, if the cervix is at least 2 cm long initially), dilation (opening, expressed in centimetres), the consistency (soft or firm), and the station of the presenting part (centimetres above or below the ischial plane; Figure 30-14).

The ovaries rise with the growing uterus. Always examine the adnexa to rule out the presence of a mass, such as an ectopic pregnancy.

Abnormal Findings

Uterine fibroids (leiomyomas) may also be palpated during a bimanual examination.

A shortened cervix is less than 2 cm long.

Adnexal enlargement and pain with palpation occur with ectopic pregnancy or ovarian mass.

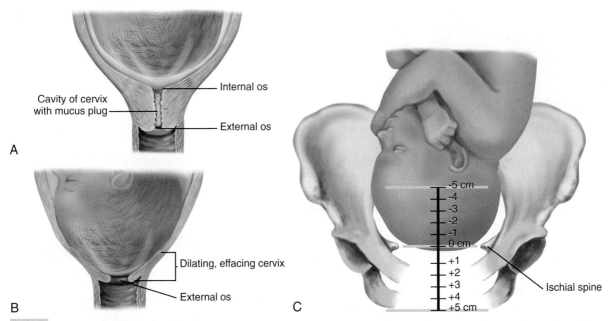

30-14   A, Cervix before labour. **B,** Beginning of cervical effacement and dilatation. **C,** Station height of presenting part in relation to maternal ischial spines.

Normal Range of Finding	Abnormal Findings

To determine tone, ask the patient to squeeze your fingers as they rest in the vagina. Take this opportunity to teach Kegel exercises, with the aim of strengthening the pubococcygeus muscles to prevent, reduce, or improve pelvic floor issues such as urinary incontinence, uterine prolapse, and sexual function. Women can identify the muscle by inserting a finger into the vagina. Alternatively, these muscles can be identified by stopping the flow of urine midstream. The patient should perform this manoeuvre only once to help confirm the function of the muscle group. There are several variations of Kegel exercises, including use of biofeedback. Patients should be encouraged to consider a strategy that will work for them. The patient contracts and relaxes the muscle group in sets of 10 or more, several times a day.

Pelvimetry

Assess the bones of the pelvis for shape and size. The dimensions may indicate the amenability of the bony structure for vaginal birth but are no longer considered a reliable indicator of pelvic capacity. The relaxation of the pelvic joints, the widening of the pelvis in the squatting position, and the capacity of the fetal head to mould to the shape of the pelvis may enable a vaginal birth despite seemingly unfavourable measurements.

To aid in visualizing the pelvis, imagine three planes: the pelvic inlet (from the sacral promontory to the upper edge of the pubis), the midpelvis, and the pelvic outlet (from the coccyx to the lower edge of the pubis; Figure 30-15). Assessment of each of these pelvic planes, as described in the following techniques, allows you to estimate the adequacy of the pelvis for vaginal delivery.

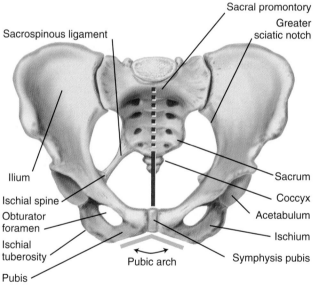

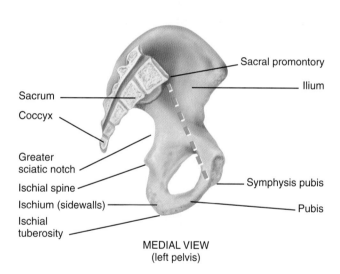

■ ■ ■ ■ ■ ■ Sagittal diameter, posterior portion
━━━━━━ Sagittal diameter, anterior portion
▬ ▬ ▬ ▬ Diagonal conjugate

30-15 Planes of the pelvis.

You may postpone examination of the bony pelvis until the third trimester, when the vagina is more distensible.

There are four general types of pelves: gynecoid, anthropoid, android, and platypelloid (Table 30-2). With your two fingers still in the vagina, note the shape and width of the pubic arch (a 90-degree arch, or 2 fingerbreadths, is desirable). If you are right-handed, move your hand to the right side of the patient's pelvis. If you are left-handed, move it to the left side of the patient's pelvis. Assess the inclination and curve of the side walls and the prominence of the ischial spine (refer to Figure 30-15 for location of these landmarks).

Normal Range of Findings	Abnormal Findings

TABLE 30-2   The Four Pelvic Types

Objective Data

GYNECOID PELVIS

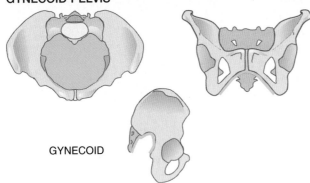

GYNECOID

Inlet: round or oval

Posterior sagittal diameter of inlet: only slightly less than anterior sagittal diameter

Pubic arch: wide (≥90 degrees)

Ischial spines: not prominent; allowing a transverse diameter of 10 cm or more

Sacrosciatic notch: round and wide

Straight side walls

Posterior pelvis: round and wide

Sacrum: parallel with the symphysis pubis; hollow and concave

Favourable for vaginal delivery

Observed in 50% of all women

ANDROID PELVIS

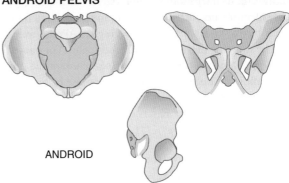

ANDROID

Inlet: heart-shaped

Posterior sagittal diameter of inlet: less than the anterior sagittal diameter

Pubic arch: narrow (<90 degrees)

Ischial spines: prominent; transverse diameter decreases

Sacrosciatic notch: narrow and highly arched

Convergent side walls

Posterior sagittal diameter: decreases from inlet to outlet as sacrum inclines forward
Anterior of pelvis: narrow and triangular; the "male" pelvis

Sacrum: straight and prominent; coccyx may be prominent

Unfavourable for vaginal delivery

ANTHROPOID PELVIS

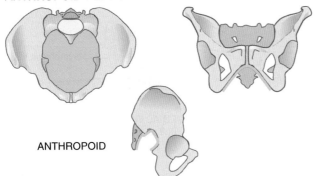

ANTHROPOID

Inlet: oval

Pubic arch: may be somewhat narrow

Ischial spines: usually prominent but not encroaching because of the spaciousness of the posterior segment

Sacrosciatic notch: average height but wide (approximately 4 fingerbreadths)

Side walls: somewhat convergent

Sacrum: posteriorly inclined, with posterior sagittal diameters long throughout the pelvis

If pelvis is somewhat large, adequate for vaginal birth because posterior pelvis is generous

PLATYPELLOID PELVIS

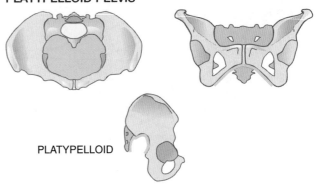

PLATYPELLOID

Inlet: shaped like a flattened gynecoid pelvis

Pubic arch: wide

Ischial spines usually prominent but not encroaching because of the already wide interspinous diameter

Sacrosciatic notch: wide and flat

Side walls: slightly convergent

Sacrum: posteriorly inclined and hollow, rendering pelvis short and shallow
Observed in fewer than 3% of all women

Unfavourable for vaginal birth

Data from Varney, H. (1997). *Varney's midwifery* (3rd ed.) Sudbury, MA: Jones & Bartlett.

Normal Range of Finding	Abnormal Findings

Move your fingers back and forth between the ischial spines to get an impression of the transverse diameter; 10 cm is desirable. Sweep your fingers down the sacrum, noting its shape and inclination (hollow, J-shaped, or straight). Assess the coccyx for prominence and mobility. From the sacrum, locate the sacrospinous ligament. Assess the length of the ligament; 2½ to 3 fingerbreadths is adequate. Assess the shape and width of the sacrospinous notch. Shift to the other side of the pelvis and assess it for similarity to the first side.

The pelvic inlet cannot be palpated, but you can estimate its shape by the measure of the **diagonal conjugate,** which indicates the anteroposterior diameter of the pelvic inlet. Having measured the length of the second and third fingers of your examining hand, with your fingers still in the vagina, point these fingers toward the sacral promontory (Figure 30-16). If you cannot reach the promontory, note the measurement as being greater than the centimetres of length of your examining fingers. A measurement of 11.5 to 12.0 cm is desirable.

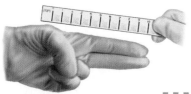

■ ■ ■ Diagonal conjugate

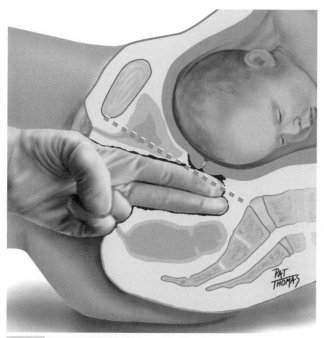

30-16   Diagonal conjugate.

Remove your fingers from the vagina. Having previously measured the width of your own hand across the knuckles, form your hand into a closed fist and place it across the perineum between the ischial tuberosities. Estimate this diameter, which is the **bi-ischial diameter** (also known as the *bituburous* or *intertuberous diameter* and the *transverse diameter of the pelvic outlet*). A measurement greater than 8 cm is generally adequate (Figure 30-17).

Objective Data

Normal Range of Finding	Abnormal Findings

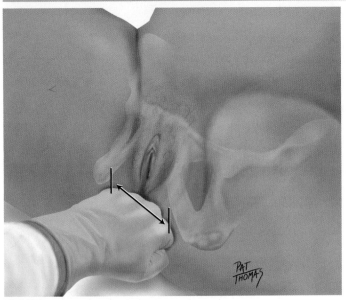

30-17   Bi-ischial diameter.

When describing pelvimetry, note all the aforementioned measurements, and state the pelvic type. The pelvis may be described as being "proven" (accommodated) to the weight of the largest vaginally born infant. Alternatively, to describe a small pelvis, you may make the assessment such as "adequate for a 3-kg baby."

Blood Pressure

Measure the BP after the patient has been sitting quietly and before the physical examination, when the patient is most relaxed. With the patient sitting upright and her arm at heart level, check for an elevated BP. The fifth Korotkoff sound implies diastolic BP. Hypertension in pregnancy is defined by a diastolic BP of at least 90 mm Hg as an average of two readings taken in the same arm (SOGC, 2008). "White coat" hypertension is recognized and can be confirmed by a home BP of less than 135/85 mm Hg.

Hypertension is considered chronic if a patient has a documented history of high BP before pregnancy or a persistent elevation of at least 140/90 mm Hg on two occasions more than 24 hours apart before the twentieth week after conception (Gabbe et al., 2007).

ROUTINE LABORATORY AND RADIOLOGICAL IMAGING STUDIES

At the first prenatal encounter, discuss options for screening and diagnostic tests. In the first trimester or at booking, all pregnant patients should be offered the following tests: a complete blood cell count, measurement of rubella antibody titre, blood typing, Rhesus (Rh) factor determination with antibody screen, syphilis serological study, hepatitis B surface antigen determination, and HIV screen with full counselling and consent. Special populations identified by history can be offered screening for hepatitis C, thyroid-stimulating hormone, ferritin, vitamin B_{12}, and TORCH infection.* Screen for sickle cell anemia, β-thalassemia, α-thalassemia, Tay-Sachs disease, and cystic fibrosis in at-risk populations. Women who work with children benefit from screening for varicella (because immunization is safe) and parvovirus.

---

*TORCH is an acronym for a special group of infections that can be transmitted to the fetus: **t**oxoplasmosis; **o**ther infections, namely, hepatitis B, syphilis, and herpes zoster, the virus that causes chicken pox; **r**ubella (formerly known as German measles); **c**ytomegalovirus; and **h**erpes simplex virus, the cause of genital herpes.

Normal Range of Finding	Abnormal Findings

A midstream urine culture should be obtained to screen for asymptomatic bacteriuria at 12 to 16 weeks. The value of testing urine for protein at every prenatal visit in women without hypertension is debated (British Columbia Perinatal Health Program, 2005; SOGC, 2008).

A pelvic examination should be offered to screen for cervical cancer. Consent should be obtained for a cervical culture for chlamydia and gonorrhea. If the patient has a history of preterm birth or symptoms of infection or bacterial vaginosis, add a vaginal screen for culture and sensitivity. Perform a bimanual examination to confirm uterine size for gestational age.

Genetic counselling programs vary across Canada. All women should receive timely counselling and be offered appropriate screening and diagnostic procedures per regional availability. It is essential that nurses responsible for preconception and prenatal care be aware of screening options and their optimal timing during pregnancy. The SOGC recommends that all pregnant women be offered noninvasive screening for Down syndrome, trisomy 18, and open neural tube defects (SOGC, 2007a). Invasive diagnostic procedures should be reserved for women whose findings exceed the set screen risk cutoff and for women who will be 40 years old by the EDB; they should also receive counselling about the risks of pregnancy loss with the procedures. Age alone is no longer recommended as an appropriate risk assessment tool (SOGC, 2007a). Screening programs offer risk assessment that is based on biochemical and ultrasound markers. Noninvasive options include (a) maternal age combined with first trimester serum markers and ultrasonography for nuchal translucency, plus second trimester serum testing; (b) second trimester serum screening alone; and (c) a two-step integrated approach with first and second trimester serum testing with or without ultrasonography for nuchal translucency. Invasive procedures (amniocentesis and chorionic villi sampling) enable diagnosis of a number of chromosomal abnormalities.

Screening ultrasonography should be offered to all women at 18 to 20 weeks, including a discussion about the risks and benefits, as well as limitations, of ultrasound technology. First trimester ultrasonography for dating is recommended when the history is unclear or complicated by irregular menstrual cycles. Ultrasound studies may also be part of a provincial or regional integrated genetic screening program. Nuchal translucency can be assessed by ultrasonography between 11 and 14 weeks. The single recommended ultrasound study at 18 to 20 weeks provides gestational age assessment that is accurate within 7 to 10 days, describes fetal number, fetal anatomy (including open neural tube defects, soft markers of fetal aneuploidy), amniotic fluid volume, and placental location, in addition to uterine and umbilical arterial blood flow.

Ultrasonography can also help visualize fetal presentation, position, activity, tone, breathing, gender, interval growth, estimated fetal weight, and maternal anatomy, including cervical length and dilation. Additional scans may be indicated at any time for complications such as bleeding, pain, suspected ectopic or molar pregnancy, trauma, fetal concerns, inappropriate fundal height measures, medical complications (including hypertension disorders and diabetes), preterm premature rupture of membranes, and noncephalic presentation.

Additional screening during the second and third trimesters includes an antibody screen for Rh-negative women (at 26 to 28 weeks), hemoglobin (at 28 weeks), gestational diabetes screen (at 24 to 28 weeks), and single vaginal anal swab for group B streptococcus (at 35 to 37 weeks).

Objective Data

DOCUMENTATION AND CRITICAL THINKING

Rosa G. is a 27-year-old woman, Grav 2/Para 1, who presents with her husband and daughter for her first prenatal visit.

SUBJECTIVE

Rosa G. is a full-time homemaker who completed 2 years of postsecondary education. LMP was April 4 of this year (certain of date), with an EDB of January 11 of next year; thus she is at 10 weeks' gestation today. Her obstetrical history includes a normal spontaneous vaginal birth 3 years ago of a viable 3.5-kg female infant after an 8-hour labour without anaesthesia, intact perineum. No complications of pregnancy, birth, or post partum. She breastfed this daughter, Ana, for 1 year. Current pregnancy was planned, and Rosa and her husband are pleased. Rosa is having breast tenderness, and nausea on occasion, which resolves with crackers. No past medical or surgical conditions are present. She denies allergies. Family history is significant only for diet-controlled adult-onset diabetes in two maternal aunts.

OBJECTIVE

General: Appears well nourished and is carefully groomed. English is second language, and Rosa is fluent.
Skin: Light tan in colour, surface smooth with no lesions, small tattoo noted on left forearm.
Mouth: Good dentition and oral hygiene. Oral mucosa pink, no gum hypertrophy. Thyroid gland small and smooth.
Chest: Expansion equal, respirations effortless. Lung sounds clear bilaterally with no adventitious sounds. No CVA [costovertebral angle] tenderness.
Heart: Rate 76 bpm, regular rhythm; S_1 and S_2 are normal, not accentuated or diminished, with soft, blowing systolic murmur grade II/VI at second left interspace.
Breasts: Tender, without masses, with supple, everted nipples. Breast self-examination reviewed.
Abdomen: No masses; bowel sounds present. No hepatosplenomegaly. Uterus nonpalpable. No inguinal lymphadenopathy noted.
Extremities: No varicosities, redness, or edema. DTRs 2+ and equal bilaterally. BP 110/68 sitting.
Pelvic: Bartholin's glands, urethra, and Skene's glands negative for discharge. Vagina: pink, with white, creamy, nonodorous discharge. Cervix: pink, closed, multiparous, 5 cm long, firm.
Uterus: 10-week size, consistent with dates, nontender, dextrorotated. FHTs heard with Doppler fetoscope, rate 140s.
Pelvis: Pubic arch wide; side walls straight, spines blunt, interspinous diameter >10 cm. Sacrum hollow; coccyx mobile. Sacrospinous ligament 3 fingerbreadths wide. Diagonal conjugate >12 cm, bituberous diameter >8 cm. Spacious gynecoid pelvis proven to 3.5 kg.

ASSESSMENT

Intrauterine pregnancy 10 weeks by good dates, size = dates
Rosa and husband happy with pregnancy; she feels well

PLAN

Prenatal vitamins to begin
Prenatal blood screen and urinalysis
HIV screen offered and accepted
Reviewed comfort measures for nausea
Reviewed warning signs: vaginal bleeding and abdominal pain
Informed of genetic screening options
Return visit in 4 weeks

Kadija is a 30-year-old Ethiopian woman, Grav 5 TPAL 3204, who presents with an interpreter and her eldest daughter for her first prenatal visit.

SUBJECTIVE

Kadija runs a daycare facility within her home. She immigrated to Canada with her family 5 years ago. Her husband is employed. She lives in a three-bedroom townhouse in a subsidized housing complex with her family. Her LMP was May 28th of this year, with an EDB of March 5th next year; thus she is at 11 weeks' gestation today. She finds it challenging to remember details of her births in Ethiopia, other than the fact that one child "died in childbirth." She gave birth to her youngest child after coming to Canada; she delivered vaginally, without complications, after 5 hours of labour. She is unsure of the baby's weight at birth. She had a female circumcision as a child, so has scarring from her previous births. She is having nausea with occasional vomiting, has breast tenderness, and 1 week ago experienced "pink" vaginal spotting. She is unsure of her family health history. Both parents are deceased, as are all but one of her seven siblings. This pregnancy is unplanned, but she accepts it. She is concerned about transportation to her appointments because her husband works days and she does not drive.

OBJECTIVE

General: Appears well nourished and is carefully groomed. English is her second language, but she understands some. Daughter who is present is well groomed and speaks English.

Skin: Dark tan in colour, smooth surface, small scarring on left arm and both legs. No lesions or tattoos.

Mouth: Poor dentition. Oral mucosa pink, some gum hypertrophy. Thyroid gland small and smooth.

Chest: Expansion equal, respiration effortless. Lung sounds clear bilaterally with no adventitious sounds. No CVA tenderness.

Heart: Rate 84 bpm, regular rhythm; S_1 and S_2 are normal, not accentuated or diminished, with soft, blowing systolic murmur grade II/VI at second left interspace.

Breasts: Tender, no masses; large everted nipples. No drainage present. Breast self-examination reviewed.

Abdomen: No masses; bowel sounds present in four quadrants. No hepatomegaly or splenomegaly. Uterus nonpalpable. No inguinal lymphadenopathy noted. No healed incisions noted.

Extremities: No lower extremity varicosities, edema, or redness noted. Negative Homan's sign. 1+ DTRs. BP 124/76 mm Hg.

Pelvic: Female circumcision present with scarring noted. Bartholin's glands, urethra, and Skene's glands negative for discharge. Vagina pink, with white, creamy, nonodorous discharge. Cervix pink, not friable, closed, and approximately 3 cm long and soft. Vaginal wall muscles lax. No evidence of a cystocele or rectocele.

Uterus: Approximately 11-week size and nontender. Dextrorotated. FHTs not heard with Doppler. Confirmed on ultrasound studies along with dating.

Pelvis: Pubic arch wide; side walls straight, spines blunt, interspinous diameter >12 cm, bituberous diameter >8 cm. Spacious, proven, gynecoid pelvis to ≈8 pounds.

ASSESSMENT

Intrauterine pregnancy at 11 weeks' gestation by ultrasonography today with positive fetal cardiac activity. Size = dates. Mother aware of potential language and cultural issues. Via interpreter, understands advised prenatal testing, clinic routine, and warning signs and symptoms in pregnancy. Physical examination findings within normal limits.

PLAN

Prenatal vitamins to begin

Routine prenatal blood screening, plus thyroid function tests, vitamin D level, sickle cell screen, and thalassemia screen

HIV, hepatitis B, and rubella screening discussed, offered, and accepted

Reviewed integrated prenatal screening with US [ultrasonography] for NT [nuchal translucency] understands need to complete within 2 weeks and will discuss with her husband and let us know

Reviewed clinic routines and whom to contact after hours

Reviewed comfort measures for nausea and vomiting; offered medication; declined at this time

Reviewed warning signs: vaginal bleeding, abdominal pain, pain with urination

Will return to clinic within 2 weeks if desires prenatal screening, or 4 weeks if does not

Refer to social worker for financial planning and transportation services

Obtain records from previous pregnancy and birth

ABNORMAL FINDINGS

TABLE 30-3   Pre-eclampsia

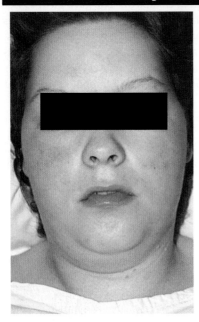

Pre-eclampsia is a condition specific to pregnancy that rarely occurs before 20 weeks' gestation except in the presence of a molar (gestational trophoblastic) pregnancy. The cause remains unknown, but theories include coagulation abnormalities, vascular endothelial damage, cardiovascular maladaptation, immunological phenomena, dietary deficiencies or excess, and genetic predisposition. Predisposing conditions include a family or personal history of pre-eclampsia; nulliparity; obesity; multifetal gestation; and preexisting medical genetic conditions such as chronic hypertension, renal disease, type 1 (insulin-dependent) diabetes, factor V Leiden, and thrombophilias such as antiphospholipid antibody syndrome (Gabbe et al., 2007).

The classic symptoms of pre-eclampsia are elevated BP and proteinuria. Edema is common in pregnancy and is no longer considered a part of the diagnosis of pre-eclampsia (Gabbe et al., 2007). However, when edema of the face (see photo) is of sudden onset and is associated with sudden weight gain, the diagnosis of pre-eclampsia should be considered. Proteinuria is a late development in pre-eclampsia and is an indicator of the severity of the disease. The Canadian guidelines for managing hypertension in pregnancy (SOGC, 2008) define hypertension as a diastolic BP of >90 mm Hg, by office measurement, with the patient sitting and her arm at the level of the heart according to the fifth Korotkoff sound. The presence of hypertension is necessary for the diagnosis of pre-eclampsia, but pre-eclampsia may occur without the edema or proteinuria.

Onset and worsening of symptoms may be sudden. Subjective signs may include headaches and vision changes (seeing spots, blurring, or seeing flashing lights), caused by cerebral edema, and right upper quadrant or epigastric pain, caused by liver enlargement in which the liver also becomes necrotic and hemorrhagic. Liver enzyme levels become elevated. Hematocrit usually increases, and the platelet levels drop. Serum creatinine and blood urea nitrogen levels become elevated. Hemolysis occurs, at least partly as a result of vasospasm. A serious variant of pre-eclampsia, the HELLP syndrome, involves **h**emolysis, **e**levated **l**iver enzyme levels, and **l**ow **p**latelet count, and represents an ominous clinical picture.

Untreated pre-eclampsia may progress to eclampsia, which is manifested by generalized tonic-clonic seizures. Eclampsia may develop as late as 10 days post partum. Before the syndrome becomes clinically manifested, it affects the placenta through vasospasm and a series of small infarctions. The placenta's capacity to deliver oxygen and nutrients to the fetus may be seriously diminished, and fetal growth may be restricted.

BP, blood pressure.

TABLE 30-4	Fetal Size Inconsistent With Dates
Size	Fundal Height Measures Smaller Than Expected for Dates.
Small for Dates	Fundal height measures less than expected for dates.
Inaccuracy of dates	Conception may have occurred later than originally thought. Reconsider the woman's menstrual history, sexual history, contraceptive use, early pregnancy testing, early measurement of the uterus, ultrasonography results, timing of pregnancy symptoms (including the date of quickening), and the fundal height measurements. If, after this review, the EDB is correct, then further investigation is required.
Preterm labour and birth	Preterm birth occurs before 37 weeks' gestation; it affected 7.9% of pregnancies in Canada in 2008 (Public Health Agency of Canada, 2012). The cause of preterm labour is not known, and 50% of preterm births occur in the absence of any known risk factors. The following preexisting factors are associated with preterm birth: maternal history of previous preterm birth, three of more pregnancy losses in the first trimester (habitual abortion), second trimester loss, uterine anomalies, and cervical conization. Current pregnancy risks include multiple pregnancy, preterm rupture of membranes, polyhydramnios, antepartum hemorrhage, intra-abdominal surgery, urinary tract infection, tobacco or cocaine use, serious maternal infection, and physical or emotional trauma (Public Health Agency of Canada, 2012). Prevention strategies include bed rest, tocolysis, home uterine monitoring, and hydration. Group prenatal care known as "centring pregnancy" facilitated by midwives has decreased rates of preterm birth in a high-risk population in the United States (Ickovics et al., 2007). Serial ultrasonographic assessments of cervical effacement and the use of fetal fibronectin sometimes reassure women who present with threatened preterm labour that they are not likely to give birth immediately; however, the ability to predict who will proceed to have a preterm birth is not yet possible.
Intrauterine growth restriction (IUGR) or fetal growth restriction	IUGR, a syndrome in which the fetus fails to meet its growth potential, is associated with an increase in fetal and neonatal mortality and morbidity. Its origin may be fetoplacental, as with chromosomal abnormalities, genetic syndromes, congenital malformations, infectious diseases, and placental disorders; or its origin may be maternal, as with decreased uteroplacental blood flow (as occurs with hypertensive disorders), poor maternal weight gain, poor maternal nutrition, and a previous pregnancy with an IUGR infant. Other contributing factors include infectious diseases (rubella, cytomegalovirus); multiple gestation; and environmental toxins such as cigarette smoke and maternal drug and alcohol use.
Fetal position	Fetal position varies until approximately 34 weeks, when the vertex should settle into the pelvis and remain there. The position of the fetus in a transverse lie, or shoulder presentation, results in a widening of the maternal abdomen from side to side and a decrease in fundal height. Fetal malposition may occur with lax maternal abdominal musculature (inability to hold the baby in close), an abnormality in the fetus (e.g., the enlarged head of the hydrocephalic infant), placenta previa (implantation of the placenta over the cervix, blocking fetal descent), or a restricted maternal pelvis.
Large for Dates	Fundal height measures more than expected for dates.
Inaccuracy of Dates	Review the same findings as listed for "Small for Dates."
Hydatidiform mole	Also termed *gestational trophoblastic neoplasia,* this condition is a result of abnormal proliferation of trophoblastic tissue associated with pregnancy. In 50% of cases, uterine size is excessive; in these cases, the gestational age and uterine size do not coincide.

Continued

Abnormal Findings

TABLE 30-4	Fetal Size Inconsistent With Dates—cont'd
Size	Fundal Height Measures Smaller Than Expected for Dates.
Multiple gestation	The incidence of multiple gestations is rising in Canada (≈20% since 1995) and other developed countries, mostly because of assisted reproductive technologies and advanced maternal age (Blackburn, 2007; Schuurmans, Senikas, & Lalonde, 2009). Up to 12% of twin pregnancies become singletons by the loss of one embryo without symptoms early in the pregnancy (Blackburn, 2007). Twin gestations are either monozygotic (division of a single ovum after fertilization) or dizygotic (simultaneous fertilization of two ova). Higher order multiple gestations are rarer; they can be monozygotic or dizygotic or a combination (Blackburn, 2007). The placenta and fetal membranes also differ according to the type of twin pregnancy: (a) monoamniotic or diamniotic and (b) monochorionic or dichorionic. The placentas may be separate or fused. Multifetal pregnancies have many risks: preterm birth and increased risks for congenital anomalies, maternal anemia, or placenta previa. Prenatal care includes more frequent visits to assess fetal growth and development, maternal coping, and amniotic fluid volume. More frequent ultrasound studies are used to determine fetal health (Lowdermilk, Perry, Cashion, & Alden, 2012). Mothers and families need support to cope with the need for more prenatal care and increased needs of their infants after birth. Breastfeeding support by a lactational consultant is beneficial if this is the woman's choice.
Polyhydramnios	An amniotic fluid volume is a maximum volume pocket >8.0 cm or an amniotic fluid index (AFI) >95th percentile or ≥20 cm. The cause is usually idiopathic but may result from fetal anomalies, diabetes in pregnancy, or the presence of multiple fetuses (Creasy et al., 2009).
Oligohydramnios	Oligohydramnios is a reduction in amniotic fluid volume (i.e., an AFI <5 or a single deepest pocket <2 cm).
Leiomyoma (myoma or "fibroid")	This is a preexisting benign tumour of the uterine wall, which then is stimulated to enlarge by the estrogen levels of pregnancy. Myomata may be located anywhere in the uterine wall (see Table 27-6). When they grow in the outer uterine wall, the myometrium, they may affect the clinician's judgement of where the fundus of the uterus should be measured. A myoma may grow just underneath the endometrial surface into the uterine cavity, displacing the fetus or preventing its descent into the pelvis.
Fetal macrosomia 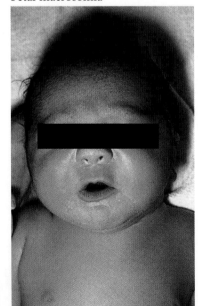	The definition of macrosomia varies between 4000 and 4500 g at birth. Maternal risk factors for macrosomia include a history of a macrosomic infant, maternal obesity, increased weight gain during pregnancy, multiparity, male fetus, gestational age >40 weeks, ethnicity, maternal birth weight, maternal height, maternal age <17 years, and gestational diabetes and glucose intolerance. Birth risks to the mother include labour abnormalities, an increased incidence of the need for Caesarean delivery, bladder trauma, and vaginal tissue trauma. Fetal risks include birth trauma such as fractured clavicle and brachial plexus nerve damage from shoulder dystocia, decreased Apgar scores, extended hospitalizations, and possible fetal or neonatal mortality.

TABLE 30-5	**Disorders of Pregnancy**
Disorder/Condition	Description
Anemia	The most common cause of anemia in pregnancy is iron deficiency. Women should be tested at their first prenatal visit and again between 24 and 28 weeks' gestation (March of Dimes Foundation, 2009b). This testing is usually performed at the same time as the gestational diabetes screening. The fetus uses maternal red blood cells for growth and development, and this use increases around week 20. Women at risk for iron deficiency anemia are those with persistent nausea and vomiting who are unable to eat a healthy diet rich in iron, those with multiple gestation, those who have two pregnancies relatively close together, and those with poor nutrition before pregnancy. Iron deficiency anemia during pregnancy increases risk for low birth weight, preterm birth, maternal infections, and perinatal mortality. Severe anemia with maternal hemoglobin (Hgb) less than 120 g/L is associated with abnormal fetal oxygenation, which may manifest as an atypical or abnormal fetal heart rate pattern during fetal monitoring (American College of Obstetricians and Gynecologists, 2008; Coad & Conlon, 2011). Oral iron supplementation is usually sufficient, but some women cannot tolerate this and require intravenous iron administration.
Vaginal Bleeding	Some women have bright red, pink, or dark brown spotting at some time during the first trimester. This is not always a sign of pending pregnancy loss, but it may be caused by a blighted ovum, friable cervix, ectopic pregnancy, perigestational hemorrhage, or cervical lesions. In the second and third trimesters, vaginal bleeding may be indicative of placental abruption, placenta previa, uterine rupture, cervical dilation, cervical lesion, or a friable cervix. Risk factors for increased risk of vaginal bleeding include gestational or chronic hypertension, cocaine use, abdominal trauma, uterine anomalies, prolonged preterm rupture of membranes, prior placental abruption, and cervical cancer.
Spontaneous Abortion	An estimated 50% of all pregnancies end in spontaneous abortion (the lay term is miscarriage) with many not recognized clinically (McLaughlin Centre for Population Health Risk Assessment, 2013). Spontaneous abortion is defined as loss of a fetus weighing less than 500 g before 20 weeks' gestation. Most first trimester losses are attributed to chromosomal abnormalities while those occurring in the second trimester are often attributed to uterine abnormalities. Risk factors for spontaneous abortion include advanced maternal or paternal age, increasing parity, maternal heavy lifting, and maternal and paternal exposure to environmental toxicants. Other risk factors are exposure to tobacco, ethanol, cocaine, and other drugs as well as to therapeutic agents such as chemotherapy, radiation, and anaesthetics.
Incompetent Cervix	Cervical incompetence is marked by gradual and painless premature dilation and effacement of the cervix that can lead to fetal loss if not detected in time to have a cervical cerclage placed. Its cause may be congenital, or it may be acquired after cervical trauma or a cone biopsy.
Hyperemesis	Hyperemesis is excessive vomiting in pregnancy that may last well into the second trimester and beyond. It can interfere with electrolyte levels, acid–base balance, and nutritional status. Dehydration and starvation may ensue and lead to fetal IUGR. Nausea and vomiting are not uncommon in pregnancy; they usually resolve between weeks 16 and 20 and may be controlled with dietary and lifestyle changes. Vitamin B_6, ginger, acupuncture, acupressure, or Diclectin can be used with some effectiveness. Diclectin is a delayed-release formulation of doxylamine succinate, 10 mg, with pyridoxine hydrochloride (vitamin B_6), 10 mg. This effective treatment can be offered to alleviate nausea and vomiting. It has a pregnancy risk factor rating of A−. There is no risk to the fetus (Briggs, Freeman, & Yaffe, 2008). Risk factors for hyperemesis include a history of previous hyperemesis, molar pregnancy, multiple gestation, emotional stress, history of gastrointestinal reflux, uncontrolled thyroid disease, primigravid status, and obesity.
Preterm Labour	Preterm labour is labour that occurs after 20 weeks' gestation and before completion of 37 weeks' gestation. Preterm labour is a major factor in fetal morbidity and mortality. Some risk factors are chronic urinary tract infections, polyhydramnios, multiple gestation, previous preterm labour or preterm birth, smoking, problematic substance use, limited or irregular prenatal care, poor weight gain after 20 weeks' gestation, history of cervical conization, low socioeconomic status, being of non-European descent, uterine infections, and cases in which the woman herself was a preterm infant.

Continued

Abnormal Findings

TABLE 30-5	Disorders of Pregnancy—cont'd
Disorder/Condition	**Description**
Decreased Fetal Movement	Fetal movement is one indicator of fetal well-being. Various methods of fetal movement counting have been described in the literature. Maternal awareness of fetal movement during the third trimester is important; formal counting should be performed in women at risk for adverse perinatal outcome between 26 and 28 weeks' gestation.
Psychological Illness	Mental illness during pregnancy has significant effects on fetal well-being. According to research reports, as many as 18% of pregnant women experience depression during pregnancy. Depression is a risk factor for low fetal birth weight and premature birth. Anxiety disorders, eating disorders, and psychotic illness that are present during pregnancy are additional predictors of adverse perinatal outcomes. It is important to understand these disorders and their effect on pregnancy in order to weigh the potential risks from psychiatric medications used to treat these disorders (Gold & Marcus, 2008).

TABLE 30-6	Malpresentations

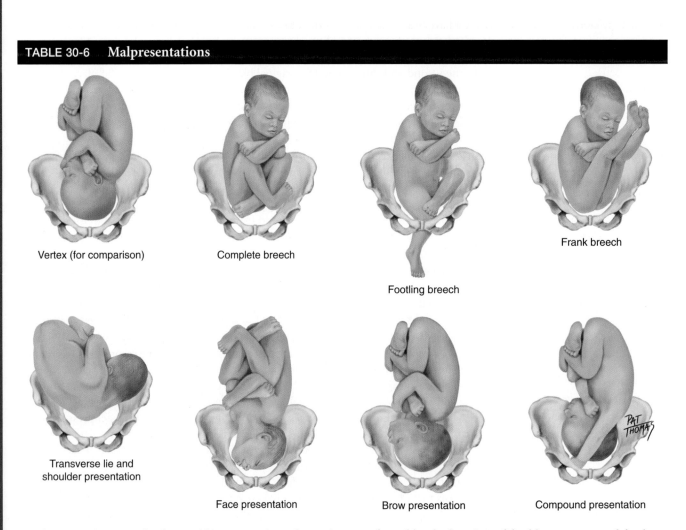

Vertex (for comparison)   Complete breech   Footling breech   Frank breech

Transverse lie and shoulder presentation   Face presentation   Brow presentation   Compound presentation

Malpresentations may be detected by an experienced examiner, confirmed by the location of fetal heart tones, and further confirmed by ultrasonography. Before 34 weeks' gestation, any position is normal. The vertex presentation is desirable thereafter because spontaneous turning becomes less likely as the fetus grows in proportion to the amount of space and fluid available in the uterus and pelvis.

Abnormal Findings

Summary Checklist: Pregnancy

For a PDA-downloadable version, go to *http://evolve.elsevier.com/Canada/Jarvis/examination/*

1. Collect historical information.
2. Determine EDB and current number of weeks of gestation.
3. Ask the patient to undress and empty her bladder, saving her urine for it to be tested for protein and glucose.
4. Measure weight and height. Calculate prepregnancy BMI, and monitor ongoing weight gain.
5. Perform a physical examination, starting with general survey.
6. Inspect skin for pigment changes and scars.
7. Check oral mucous membranes.
8. Palpate thyroid gland.
9. Inspect breast changes and palpate for masses.
10. Auscultate breath sounds, heart sounds, heart rate, and any murmurs.
11. Check lower extremities for edema, varicosities, and reflexes.
12. The abdomen: Measure fundal height, perform Leopold's manoeuvres, auscultate fetal heart tones.
13. The pelvic examination: Note signs of pregnancy, the condition of the cervix, and the size and position of the uterus.
14. Perform pelvimetry.
15. Measure the BP.
16. Obtain appropriate laboratory work.
17. Perform teaching and health promotion.

REFERENCES

American College of Obstetricians and Gynecologists. (2008). *Anemia in pregnancy* (Practice Bulletin No. 95). Washington, DC: Author.

Barrett, M., & McKay, A. (2010). Trends in teen pregnancy rates from 1996–2006: A comparison between Canada, Sweden, U.S.A. and England/Wales. *Canadian Journal of Human Sexuality, 19*(1-2), 43.

Blackburn, S. T. (2007). *Maternal, fetal, & neonatal physiology: A clinical perspective* (3rd ed.). St. Louis: W. B. Saunders.

Briggs, G., Freeman, R., & Yaffe, S. (2008). *Drugs in pregnancy and lactation: A reference guide to fetal and neonatal risk* (8th ed.). Baltimore: Lippincott Williams & Wilkins.

British Columbia Perinatal Health Program. (2005). *Obstetrics guideline 17: Antenatal screening and diagnostic tests for singleton pregnancies.* Vancouver, BC: Author.

Coad, J., & Conlon, C. (2011). Iron deficiency in women: Assessment, causes, and consequences. *Current Opinion in Clinical Nutrition and Metabolic Care, 14,* 625–634.

Creasy, R. K., Resnick, R., Iams, J.D., Lockwood, C. J., & Moore, T. R. (2009). *Creasy & Resnick's maternal–fetal medicine: Principles and practice* (6th ed.). Philadelphia: W. B. Saunders.

Cunningham, F. G., Leveno, K. J., Bloom, S. L., & Hauth, J. (2010). *Williams' obstetrics* (23rd ed.). Stamford, CT: Appleton & Lange.

DeCherney, A., Goodwin, T., Nathan, L., & Laufer, N. (2007). *Current diagnosis and treatment: Obstetrics & gynecology* (10th ed.). New York: McGraw-Hill.

Einarson, A., Maltepe, C., Boskovic, R., & Koren, G. (2007). *Treatment of nausea and vomiting in pregnancy—An updated algorithm.* Retrieved from *http://www.motherisk.org/prof/updatesDetail.jsp?content_id=875.*

Gabbe, S. G., Niebyl, J. R., Galan, H., Jauniaux, E. R. M., Landon, M., Simpson, J. L., & Driscoll, D. (2007). *Obstetrics: Normal and problem pregnancies* (5th ed.). New York: Churchill Livingstone.

Genetics Committee of the Society of Obstetricians and Gynecologists of Canada and Motherisk Program. (2007). Pre-conceptual vitamin/folic acid supplement: 2007: The use of folic acid in combination with a multivitamin supplement for prevention of neural tube defects and other congenital anomalies. *Journal of Obstetricians and Gynecologists of Canada, 201,* 1003–1013.

Gold, K. J., & Marcus, S. M. (2008). Effect of maternal mental illness on pregnancy outcomes. *Expert Review of Obstetrics & Gynecology, 3*(3), 391–401. Retrieved from *http://www.medscape.com/viewarticle/573947.*

Hollis, B. W., & Wagner, C. L. (2004). Assessment of dietary vitamin D requirements during pregnancy and lactation. *American Journal of Clinical Nutrition, 79,* 717–726.

Hurt, K., Guile, M., Bienstock, J., Fox, H., & Wallach, E. (2011). *The Johns Hopkins manual of gynecology and obstetrics* (4th ed.). Philadelphia: Wolters Kluwer/Lippincott Williams & Wilkins.

Ickovics, J. R., Kershaw, T. S., Westdahl, C., Magriples, U., Massey, Z., Reynolds, H., & Rising, S. S. (2007). Group prenatal care and perinatal outcomes: A randomized controlled trial. *Obstetrics and Gynecology, 110,* 330–339.

Kriebs, J., & Gegor, C. (2005). *Varney's pocket midwife* (2nd ed.). Sudbury, MA: Jones & Bartlett.

Lowdermilk, D., Perry, S., Cashion, K., & Alden, K. (2012). *Maternity & women's health care* (10th ed.). St. Louis: Elsevier/Mosby.

March of Dimes. (2009a). *Birth defects, Down syndrome.* White Plains, NY: March of Dimes Birth Defects Foundation.

March of Dimes Foundation. (2009b). *Pregnancy complications: Anemia.* Retrieved from *http://www.marchofdimes.com/pregnancy/complications_anemia.html.*

Maticka-Tyndale, E. (2008). Sexuality and sexual health of Canadian adolescents: Yesterday, today and tomorrow. *Canadian Journal of Human Sexuality, 17*(3), 85–95.

McLaughlin Centre for Population Health Risk Assessment. (2013). *Spontaneous Abortion.* Ottawa: Institute for Population Health, University of Ottawa. Retrieved from *http://www.emcom.ca/health/abortion.shtml.*

Public Health Agency of Canada. (2012). *Perinatal health indicators for Canada 2011.* Ottawa: Author.

Registered Nurses Association of Ontario. (2007). *Embracing cultural diversity in health care: Developing cultural competence.* Retrieved from *http://rnao.ca/bpg/guidelines/embracing-cultural-diversity-health-care-developing-cultural-competence.*

Schuurmans, N., Senikas, V., & Lalonde, A. (2009). *Healthy beginnings* (4th ed.). Ottawa: Society of Obstetricians and Gynaecologists of Canada.

Society of Obstetricians and Gynaecologists of Canada. (2007a). Clinical practice guideline: Prenatal screening for fetal aneuploidy. *Journal of Obstetrics and Gynaecology Canada, 29*(2), 146–161.

Society of Obstetricians and Gynaecologists of Canada. (2007b). Fetal health surveillance: Antenatal and intrapartum consensus guideline. *Journal of Obstetrics and Gynaecology Canada, 29*(9, Suppl. 4), S3–S56.

Society of Obstetricians and Gynaecologists of Canada. (2008). Clinical practice guideline: Diagnosis, evaluation and management of the hypertensive disorders of pregnancy. *Journal of Obstetrics and Gynaecology Canada, 30*(3), S1–S48.

Society of Obstetricians and Gynaecologists of Canada. (2011). Genetic considerations for a woman's pre-conception evaluation. *Journal of Obstetrics and Gynaecology Canada, 33*(1), 57–64.

Society of Obstetricians and Gynaecologists of Canada. (2012). Clinical practice guideline: Delayed child-bearing. *Journal of Obstetrics and Gynaecology Canada, 34*(1), 80–93.

Stevens, J., Iida, H., & Ingersoll, G. (2007). Implementing an oral health program in a group prenatal practice. *Journal of Obstetrical, Gynecological and Neonatal Nurses, 36*(6), 581–590.

VanRooyen, M. J., & Scott, J. A. (2011). Emergency delivery. In J. E. Tintinalli, J. S. Stapczynski, D. M. Cline, O. J. Ma, R. K. Cydulka, & G. D. Meckler (Eds.), *Tintinalli's emergency medicine: A comprehensive study guide, 7e (section 11, chapter 105)*. New York: McGraw Hill Medical.

Vane, N., Lazarus, J., & Chan, S. (2011). Thyroid function in pregnancy: Maternal and fetal outcomes with hypothyroidism and subclinical thyroid dysfunction. *Fetal and Maternal Medicine Review, 22*(3), 169–187.

World Health Organization. (2010). *Trends in maternal mortality: 1990 to 2008*. Retrieved from *http://whqlibdoc.who.int/publications/2010/9789241500265_eng.pdf*.

Functional Assessment of the Older Adult

Written by Carla Graf, MS, RN, CNS-BC, and Melissa A. Lee, MS, RN, CNS-BC

Adapted by Dianne Groll, RN, BA, BScH, MScH, PhD

⊖volve WEBSITE

OUTLINE

Canada has a large and growing population of older adults. In 2012, 16.3% of Canadians were 65 years of age or older (Statistics Canada, 2012a). Many older adults lead fulfilling lives without significant physical or cognitive changes. They welcome the opportunity to pursue interests and activities that were previously restricted by the responsibilities of work and family (Figure 31-1). In a 2009 survey, respondents were asked to rate, on a scale from 0 ("very dissatisfied") to 10 ("very satisfied"), how they felt about their life as a whole. More than 85% of people older than 65 reported being "satisfied" or "very satisfied" (Statistics Canada, 2009).

Despite being healthier than ever before, the 2008/2009 Canadian Community Health Survey (Statistics Canada, 2011) revealed that 81.3% of older adults living at home had at least one diagnosed chronic condition, whereas only 54% of individuals aged 30 to 64 reported a chronic illness.

The comprehensive assessment of an older adult requires knowledge not only of normal aging changes but also of the effects of chronic diseases, heredity, and lifestyle. A comprehensive geriatric assessment incorporates both the physical examination and assessments of the patient's mental, functional, social, and economic status; pain; and the physical environment for safety concerns.

Professionals from multiple disciplines—including physicians; nurses; physical, occupational, and speech therapists; social workers; case managers; nutritionists; and pharmacists—may participate in the assessment. Early recognition of disabilities and treatable conditions is instrumental in preserving function and quality of life for older adults.

The normal process of aging does not necessarily represent disease; however, normal aging changes and disease may precipitate transitions from home to settings in which nursing-focused assessments are performed. Care may be provided in hospitals, skilled nursing facilities, long-term care facilities, assisted living facilities, acute rehabilitation centres, hospice, senior centres, the home, and clinics. The care setting usually determines the types of assessment and instruments used. However, the goal of the functional assessment remains the same (i.e., to identify an older adult's strengths and any limitations) so that appropriate interventions will promote independence and prevent functional decline.

FUNCTIONAL ABILITY

Functional ability refers to a person's ability to perform activities necessary to live in modern society; it can include driving, using the telephone, or performing personal tasks such as bathing and toileting. Functional ability also incorporates the person's physiological and psychological status and the physical and social environments (Pearson, 2000). Functional status, as defined by Richmond, Tang, Tulman, Fawcett, and McCorkle (2004), is "the individuals' actual performance of activities and tasks associated with their current life roles" and is dependent on motivation, sensory capacity such as

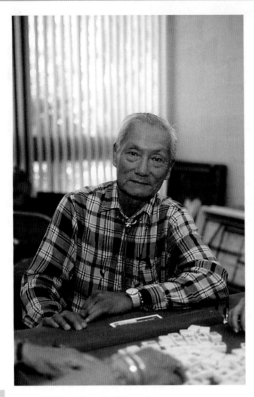

31-1

vision and hearing, degree of assistance needed to accomplish the tasks, and cognition (Kresevic & Mezey, 2003). For example, the effect that arthritis might have on a person's ability to exercise may affect physical function. A condition such as Alzheimer's disease may affect problem solving, safety concerns, and motivation, which in turn affect function. Presence or lack of social support and the safety of the physical setting are environmental issues that affect functional status and possibly the ability to live independently. The interaction of these components provides a "snapshot" of an older adult's functional status at a given point (Pearson, 2000). Functional status is not static; older adults may move continuously through varying stages of independence and disability.

The assessment of function is important for comparison, prognosis, and objective data to determine efficacy of treatments. Medical diagnosis is not sufficient to predict functional abilities. Older adults may not experience the usual symptoms of an acute illness. A decline in functional status may indicate another process, such as an infection.

A functional assessment of an older adult is the basis for care planning, goal setting, and discharge planning. A functional assessment also is needed to determine eligibility for obtaining many services, such as durable medical equipment, home modifications, and inpatient or outpatient rehabilitation services. For an older adult and the family, a functional assessment can identify areas for current and future planning, such as the most appropriate living situation.

A functional assessment includes three overarching domains: **activities of daily living (ADLs), instrumental activities of daily living (IADLs),** and **mobility** (Pearson, 2000). A functional evaluation should be systematic, with attention paid to the particular needs of the patient, such as

the presence of pain, fatigue, shortness of breath, or memory problems. There are two approaches to use for performing a functional assessment: *asking individuals* about their abilities to perform the tasks (using self-reports) or actually *observing* their ability to perform the tasks. For patients with memory problems, the use of surrogate reporters (proxy reports) such as family members or caregivers may be necessary; the examiner should note that they may either overestimate or underestimate the actual abilities.

Activities of Daily Living

ADLs are the tasks necessary for self-care. Typically, ADLs encompass domains of eating/feeding, bathing, grooming (the individual tasks of washing face, combing hair, shaving, cleaning teeth), dressing (lower body and upper body), toileting (bowel and bladder), walking (including propelling a wheelchair), using stairs (ascending and descending), and transferring (such as bed to chair). The ADL instruments are designed as self-report, observation of tasks, or proxy/surrogate report.

ADL dependency in both sexes has been related to the presence of chronic disease such as arthritis and rheumatism; diabetes; urinary incontinence; bronchitis, emphysema, or chronic obstructive pulmonary disease; the effects of stroke; and Alzheimer's disease or other dementia (Rotermann, 2006). Therefore, chronic illness must be considered when ADLs and IADLs are assessed, and instruments such as the Functional Comorbidity Index have been designed specifically for this purpose (Groll, To, Bombardier, & Wright, 2005).

The Katz Index of ADL

The Katz Index of ADL (Katz, Ford, Moskowitz, Jackson, & Jaffe, 1963) is based on the concept of physical disability and was intended to measure physical function in older adults and chronically ill patients. It is one of the few functional assessment instruments to provide a theoretical framework for its domains of measurement (McDowell, 2006), and it is the foundation for most of the newer functional assessment instruments (Pearson, 2000). It is widely used in both clinical practice and research to measure performance, evaluate treatment outcomes, and predict the need for continuing supervised care.

The Katz Index of ADL was developed as a hierarchical structure. Katz and colleagues (1963) believed that loss of physical function occurred in the most complex activities first, that these functions were lost in descending order of complexity, and that they were regained in ascending order (McDowell, 2006). Activities assessed are bathing, dressing, toileting, transferring from bed to chair, continence, and feeding. This instrument has been modified over the years. A simplified scoring method involves a dichotomous rating of "independent" or "dependent" in the six activities (Figure 31-2). Only activities that can be performed without help are rated as independent. One point is given for each item rated independent.

The Katz Index of ADL is a useful instrument in many settings. The tool takes approximately 5 minutes to

---

Katz Activities of Daily Living

Activities

Points (1 or 0)

Independence
(1 Point)
NO supervision, direction, or personal assistance

Dependence
(0 Points)
WITH supervision, direction, personal assistance, or total care

Bathing
Points _____
(1 Point) Bathes self completely or needs help in bathing only a single part of the body such as the back, genital area, or disabled extremity
(0 Point) Needs help with bathing more than one part of the body or with getting in or out of the tub or shower; requires total bathing

Dressing
Points _____
(1 Point) Gets clothes from closet and drawers and puts on clothes and outer garments complete with fasteners; may have help tying shoes
(0 Point) Needs help with dressing self or needs to be completely dressed

Toileting
Points _____
(1 Point) Gets to toilet, gets on and off, arranges clothes, cleans genital area without help
(0 Point) Needs help transferring to the toilet or cleaning self, or uses bedpan or commode

Transferring
Points _____
(1 Point) Moves into and out of bed or chair unassisted; mechanical transferring aids are acceptable
(0 Point) Needs help in moving from bed to chair or requires a complete transfer

Continence
Points _____
(1 Point) Exercises complete self-control over urination and defecation
(0 Point) Is partially or totally incontinent of bowel or bladder

Feeding
Points _____
(1 Point) Gets food from plate into mouth without help; preparation of food may be done by another person
(0 Point) Needs partial or total help with feeding or requires parenteral feeding

Total Points = _____
6 = High (patient independent)
0 = Low (patient very dependent)

Adapted from Gerontological Society of America. Katz S., et al. (1970). Progress in the development of the index of ADL. *Gerontologist, 10* (1, Part 1), 20-30.

31-2

---

administer, but its use has limitations. In a hospital setting, a patient cannot demonstrate all of the activities and may need to adjust the degree of dependence or independence. The patient's function may be overestimated or underestimated, and small changes in the activities may not be identified.

Because the instrument helps measure current function, it is valuable for planning specific types of assistance. For example, a patient may be unable to bathe independently on hospital discharge but can feed himself or herself and transfer to a commode safely and independently. In this case, plan for a home health aide to visit twice weekly to assist with bathing.

Additional Activity of Daily Living Instruments

Additional tools used to assess ADL ability are the Barthel Index (Mahoney & Barthel, 1965), the Functional Independence Measure (Hamilton, Granger, Sherwin, Zielezny, & Tashman, 1987), and the Rapid Disability Rating Scale-2

(Linn, 1988; Linn & Linn, 1982). The Barthel Index includes definitions of each task to facilitate ease of scoring and has a more comprehensive assessment of mobility than the Index of ADL. The Barthel Index is often used to follow progress in rehabilitation settings (Pearson, 2000).

The Functional Independence Measure was developed by a consensus panel of physical medicine and rehabilitation staff and has been widely tested on older adults. It can be administered three ways: by telephone, by in-person interview, and by proxy. It is more sensitive to change than the other ADL instruments, but formal training in its use is necessary, and it is more time consuming (Pearson, 2000).

The Rapid Disability Rating Scale-2 is completed by a family member or professional caregiver who is familiar with the abilities of the older adult. It is designed to measure what the patient *actually can do* versus what he or she might be able to do. You should conduct a session to train the observer in the use of this instrument.

Instrumental Activities of Daily Living

Many IADL instruments have been developed since the 1960s, with the goal of measuring functional abilities necessary for independent community living. IADL tasks typically include shopping, meal preparation, housekeeping, laundry, managing finances, taking medications, and using transportation. These instruments may have cultural and gender biases, especially in older cohorts (Pearson, 2000). IADL instruments focus on tasks historically performed by women (doing laundry, cooking, housework), and most do not address activities traditionally performed primarily by men, such as home repairs, car maintenance, and yard work.

Lawton Instrumental Activities of Daily Living

IADL measures were first developed by Lawton and Brody in 1969 to address higher order components of the Katz Index of ADL and to measure the more complex ADLs required for a person to adapt to the environment (Pearson, 2000). The instrument was originally developed to determine the most suitable living situation for an older adult. The theory was that competence and maintenance of life skills such as shopping, cooking, and managing finances are a meaningful way to assess function because these abilities are prerequisites for independent living. As with the Katz Index of ADL, the IADL instrument assumes a hierarchical nature of skill acquisition and loss. The Lawton IADL scale contains eight items (Figure 31-3); women's functions are scored in all eight domains, whereas men's are scored in five (laundry, housekeeping, and preparing food are omitted).

The Lawton IADL instrument is designed as a self-report measure of performance rather than ability. Direct testing is often not feasible; for example, a hospital inpatient cannot demonstrate the ability to prepare food. Attention to the final score is less important than identifying a patient's strengths and areas in which assistance is needed. The instrument is useful in acute hospital settings for discharge planning and for ongoing assessment in outpatient settings. It would not be useful for residents in institutional settings because many of these tasks are already being managed for the residents.

Additional IADL Instruments

Other IADL instruments available are the Older Americans Resources and Services Multidimensional Functional Assessment Questionnaire-IADL (OARS-IADL; Fillenbaum & Smyer, 1981) and the Direct Assessment of Functional Abilities (DAFA; Karagiozis, Gray, Sacco, Shapiro, & Kawas, 1998). The OARS-IADL is an assessment of five areas of personal function: social, economic, mental health, physical health, and self-care capacity; it is administered either as a self-report instrument or by trained observer. The questions are the same for men and women. The DAFA is a 10-item observational instrument for use with adults with dementia. It requires the patient to demonstrate tasks of money management, shopping, hobbies, meal preparation, awareness, reading, and transportation (Pearson, 2000). The obvious strength of this instrument is the direct observation versus self- or proxy reporting; however, it can take up to an hour

and a half to complete, so it would not be feasible to use in an acute-care hospital setting.

Advanced Activities of Daily Living

Advanced activities of daily living (AADLs) are activities that an older adult performs as a family member and a member of society and community; they include occupational and recreational activities (Guse, 2006). Various AADL instruments commonly include items concerning self-care, mobility, work (either paid or volunteer), recreational activities/hobbies, and socialization.

A disadvantage of many of the ADL and IADL instruments is the self- or proxy report of functional activities. Incorporating an objective standardized measure of performance prevents overestimation or underestimation of abilities. Many of the physical performance measures also incorporate balance, gait, motor coordination, and endurance. Many of the tests are timed.

Although direct observation of the older adult performing the activities has clear advantages, there are some disadvantages. The instruments can be very time consuming; administering them may require training and special equipment; and performing certain activities entails the possibility that the individual might fall or sustain an injury during the testing. Commonly used physical performance measures include the **Physical Performance Test** (Reuben & Siu, 1990), the **performance activities of daily living** (Kuriansky & Gurland, 1976), and the **Timed Up and Go Test** (Mathias, Nayak, & Isaacs, 1986). In a review of 17 functional balance tests, Langley and Mackintosh (2007) recommended the Timed Up and Go Test as valid and reliable for the older adult population.

Assessment of Cognition

The assessment of cognitive status in older adults is an important part of the functional assessment. In general, a gradual and mild to moderate decline in short-term memory may be attributable to aging; an older adult may need more time to learn new material or a new task or may need a system for reminders. However, although some decline in memory is a normal part of aging, sudden or severe cognitive decline is not. Altered cognition in older adults is commonly attributed to three disorders: delirium, dementia, and depression. However, other factors, such as certain medications or infection, also may be contributory.

Delirium is a common, life-threatening disordered mental state that, when recognized and treated promptly, is often reversible. Delirium is characterized by an acute decline in attention and cognition that usually develops over a period of hours or days. It occurs in as many as 24% of individuals at the time of hospital admission, and the 1-year mortality rate is 35% to 40% (Inouye, 2006). National guidelines for the assessment and treatment of delirium have been developed and can be downloaded free from the Canadian Coalition for Seniors' Mental Health (CCSMH) Web site (CCSMH, 2006).

The Lawton Instrumental Activities of Daily Living Scale

A. Ability to Use Telephone
   1. Operates telephone on own initiative; looks up and dials numbers   1
   2. Dials a few well-known numbers   1
   3. Answers telephone, but does not dial   1
   4. Does not use telephone at all   0

B. Shopping
   1. Takes care of all shopping needs independently   1
   2. Shops independently for small purchases   0
   3. Needs to be accompanied on any shopping trip   0
   4. Completely unable to shop   0

C. Food Preparation
   1. Plans, prepares, and serves adequate meals independently   1
   2. Prepares adequate meals if supplied with ingredients   0
   3. Heats and serves prepared meals or prepares meals, but does not
   maintain adequate diet   0
   4. Needs to have meals prepared and served   0

D. Housekeeping
   1. Maintains house alone with occasional assistance (heavy work)   1
   2. Performs light daily tasks such as dishwashing, bed making   1
   3. Performs light daily tasks, but cannot maintain acceptable level of
   cleanliness   1
   4. Needs help with all home maintenance tasks   1
   5. Does not participate in any housekeeping tasks   0

E. Laundry
   1. Does personal laundry completely   1
   2. Launders small items, rinses socks, stockings, etc   1
   3. All laundry must be done by others   0

F. Mode of Transportation
   1. Travels independently on public transportation or drives own car   1
   2. Arranges own travel via taxi, but does not otherwise use public
   transportation   1
   3. Travels on public transportation when assisted or accompanied by
   another   1
   4. Travel limited to taxi or automobile with assistance of another   0
   5. Does not travel at all   0

G. Responsibility for Own Medications
   1. Is responsible for taking medication in correct dosages at correct time   1
   2. Takes responsibility if medication is prepared in advance in
   separate dosages   0
   3. Is not capable of dispensing own medication   0

H. Ability to Handle Finances
   1. Manages financial matters independently (budgets, writes checks,
   pays rent and bills, goes to bank); collects and keeps track of income   1
   2. Manages day-to-day purchases, but needs help with banking, major
   purchases, etc.   1
   3. Incapable of handling money   0

Scoring: For each category, circle the item description that most closely resembles the client's
highest functional level (either 0 or 1).

From Lawton, M. P., & Brody, E. M. (1969). Assessment of older people: Self-maintaining and instrumental activities of daily living. *Gerontologist, 9* (3, Part 1), 179-186. Copyright © The Gerontological Society of America.

TABLE 31-1	Common Cognitive Assessment Instruments		
Name of Instrument	Type of Test	Domains Covered	Administration Time
Mini-Mental State Examination (Folstein, Folstein, & McHugh, 1975)	Mental status	Orientation, immediate and delayed recall, working memory, language, visuospatial ability	10 minutes
Northern Cultural Assessment of Memory (N-CAM; Crossley et al., 2012)	Mental status	Mental status examination designed for Aboriginal individuals	
The Montreal Cognitive Assessment (MOCA; Nasreddine et al., 2005)	Mental status	Orientation, general/personal information, working memory	5–10 minutes
Mini-Cog (Borson, Scanlan, Chen, & Ganguli, 2003)	Mental status	Immediate and delayed recall, visuospatial ability	5–10 minutes
Cornell Scale for Depression (Alexopoulos, Abrams, Young, & Shamoian, 1988)	Depression with concomitant dementia	Signs and symptoms of major depression in patients with dementia	20 minutes
Geriatric Depression Scale, Short Form (Yesavage et al., 1983)	Depression	Depression and changes in level of depression	5–10 minutes
Confusion Assessment Method (Inouye et al., 1990)	Delirium	Acute onset or fluctuating course, inattention, disorganized thinking, altered level of consciousness	Less than 5 minutes
Neecham Confusion Scale (Neelon, Champagne, Carlson, & Funk, 1996)	Delirium	Processing (attention, command, orientation), behaviour (appearance, motor, verbal), vital function stability	10 minutes
Clock Drawing Test (Shulman, Shedletsky, & Silver, 1986)	Mental status	Cognitive and adaptive functioning, memory, ability to process information	2–5 minutes

Dementia is a progressive loss of brain function that can occur with several different diseases such as stroke and brain injury. The most common form of dementia in Canada is Alzheimer's disease. Individuals with dementia have alterations in short-term and long-term memory, difficulty in finding words and naming objects, problems with judgement and reasoning, and changes in mood and behaviour. As the Canadian population ages, the proportion of individuals with dementia is expected to increase from 1.5% of the population in 2008 to 2.8% in 2038; the resulting economic burden is estimated to be $153 billion by 2038 (Alzheimer Society of Canada, 2010).

Mild cognitive impairment, in which very mild symptoms of memory impairment become apparent, may or may not progress to a form of dementia, such as Alzheimer's disease (Visser, Kester, Jolles, & Verhey, 2006). There is growing evidence that some kinds of mental exercises, such as computer-assisted training programs, may significantly improve cognitive function in individuals with mild cognitive impairment (Jean, Bergeron, Thivierge, & Simard, 2010).

The Physical, Intellectual, Emotional, Capabilities, Environment and Social (P.I.E.C.E.S.) program was developed for all health care providers to enhance understanding of and care for patients with complex physical and cognitive/mental health needs and behavioural changes. The P.I.E.C.E.S. Web site (*www.piecescanada.com*) offers resources such as videos and learning packages about how to administer and score the Mini-Mental Status Examination and how to use the Cornell Scale for Depression in Dementia.

For nurses in various settings, cognitive assessments provide continuing comparisons to the individual's baseline to detect any acute changes. The assessments are not diagnostic but are for screening purposes and identify the need for a more comprehensive workup. As with screening for ADLs and IADLs, assessment of cognition helps with determining the best discharge plan. Common assessment instruments are listed in Table 31-1.

Depression and Function

Many older adults live with multiple chronic health conditions (Rotermann, 2006); therefore, medical comorbidity is more likely in this age group. In the presence of comorbid conditions, accurate diagnosis of mental illnesses is much more challenging: untangling symptoms of physical illnesses from somatic presentations of mental illnesses such as depression can be difficult and, without proper training and attention, treatable illnesses can, and do, go unnoticed by health care providers.

As an illness, **depression** (or clinical depression) usually includes persistent feelings of sadness or hopelessness, a loss of interest or pleasure in previously enjoyable activities, or a combination of these. It also includes cognitive and physical changes, such as trouble with concentration (which leads to memory problems), disturbed sleep, decreased energy or excessive tiredness, and decreased appetite. These changes are present for at least 2 weeks and are not just ascribable to a "passing mood" or a normal reaction to a sad event. Depression is the most common mental health problem among older adults, and substantial depressive symptoms affect an estimated 15% of those living in the community (MacCourt, Wilson, & Tourigny-Rivard, 2011). Rates of depression are higher in long-term care facilities; up to 44% of residents have an established diagnosis of depression or significant (three or more) depressive symptoms (Canadian Institute for Health Information, 2010).

The most tragic consequence of mood disorders is death by suicide. Although research shows that older men have the highest suicide rate in Canada, it is widely believed that published suicide rates still underestimate the total number of deaths by suicide among older men and women, partly because of the stigma of suicide. Currently, men aged 80 and older are the population with the highest suicide rates in Canada (MacCourt et al., 2011).

Nursing guidelines incorporating best practices related to caregiving strategies for adults aged 65 years and older with delirium, dementia, and depression have been developed by the Registered Nurses' Association of Ontario (2004) and are available free of charge on the organization's Web site (*http://www.rnao.org*).

Social Domain

For older adults, the quality of life is closely linked to the success of social function. The social domain focuses on relationships within family, social groups, and the community and is composed of multiple dimensions, including the sources of formal and informal assistance available from those relationships. A health care provider's knowledge of a patient's day-to-day routines can provide baseline health information and serve as a reference point for detecting functional decline during future encounters.

A comprehensive social assessment is typically spread over several evaluation periods. Because more than 80% of all care is provided by family members, the social assessment also addresses assessment of caregivers (Hollander, Liu, & Chappell, 2009). Using a multidimensional approach may help to identify potential risks, such as elder abuse (Box 31-1).

Social networks consist of informal supports that are accessible to the older adult (Morano & Morano, 2006). Informal support is based on cultural beliefs regarding who should be providing care, prior relationships, and location and availability of the caregiver. Informal support includes family and close long-time friends and is usually provided free of charge. According to one analysis, informal caregiving saved the Canadian health care system $25 billion in 2007 (Hollander et al., 2009). Such caregiving includes domestic work (e.g., cooking, cleaning, shopping) and care of other household members.

Formal supports include programs such as social welfare and other social service and health care delivery agencies, such as those that provide home health care. Semiformal supports such as church societies, neighbourhood groups, and senior centres also play an important role in social support (Zarit & Pearlin, 1993).

The availability of assistance from family or friends frequently determines whether a functionally dependent older adult remains at home or is placed in residential care. It is important to know which people would be available to help the older adult if he or she becomes ill, even for healthy older adults.

Several standardized assessment instruments are available to provide structured assessment. The Duke Social Support and Stress Scale (Parkerson, Broadhead, & Tse, 1991) is a measure of a patient's perceptions of support and stress in family and nonfamily relationships.* It allows the individual to rate perceived support and stress associated with specific social relationships and to further identify the relationship that provide the most support and stress.

CAREGIVER ASSESSMENT

According to Statistics Canada's General Social Survey (Cranswick & Dosman, 2007), most care for older adults (75%) was provided by people between 45 and 64 years of age. That also means that of the people who were providing care to older adults, 25% were themselves older adults. Nearly 16% of caregivers were 65 to 74 years of age, and 8% of caregivers were 75 and older. Approximately one third of all caregivers were friends (14%), extended family (11%), and neighbours (5%; Cranswick & Dosman, 2007). As the number of older adults grows (to 27% by 2050), so will the need for families to provide care to them (Butler-Jones, 2010).

Many caregivers value providing care and experience positive benefits from doing so. However, caregiving is also associated with physical and psychosocial symptoms (including depression; stress; sense of burden; fatigue; feelings of anger, guilt, grief, and loss; frustration; loneliness; isolation; and decreased well-being and life satisfaction) that may diminish the physical and mental health of the caregiver and the caregiver's ability to continue to provide care (Keating, Fast, Frederick, Cranswick, & Perrier, 1999). Caregivers also face "increased financial expenses such as fees for home care services, transportation costs for medical appointments, drug dispensing, technical aids and equipment, and home modification" (Maytree Policy in Focus, 2010, p. 2), which can cause further strain.

Assessment of Caregiver Burden

The health and well-being of the patient and caregiver are closely linked. For these reasons, part of caring for a frail older adult involves paying attention to the well-being of the caregiver, and all caregivers should be screened for caregiver

---

BOX 31-1 **COMPONENTS OF SOCIAL ASSESSMENT**
• Social network (formal, semiformal, informal)
• Caregiver assessment
• Potential for elder abuse
• Environment
• Spiritual needs

---

*The Duke Social Support and Stress Scale (DUSOCS) is available online at *http://healthmeasures.mc.duke.edu/images/DUSOCS.pdf*.

Modified Caregiver Strain Index

Directions: Here is a list of things that other caregivers have found to be difficult. Please put a checkmark in the columns that apply to you. We have included some examples that are common caregiver experiences to help you think about each item. Your situation may be slightly different, but the item could still apply.

	Yes, on a regular basis = 2	Yes, sometimes = 1	No = 0
My sleep is disturbed (For example, *the person I care for* is in and out of bed or wanders around at night)			
Caregiving is inconvenient (For example, helping takes so much time or it's a long drive over to help)			
Caregiving is a physical strain (For example, lifting in or out of a chair; effort or concentration is required)			
Caregiving is confining (For example, helping restricts free time or *I* cannot go visiting)			
There have been family adjustments (For example, helping has disrupted *my* routine; there has been no privacy)			
There have been changes in personal plans (For example, *I* had to turn down a job; *I* could not go on vacation)			
There have been other demands on my time (For example, other family members *need me*)			
There have been emotional adjustments (For example, severe arguments *about caregiving*)			
Some behaviour is upsetting (For example, incontinence; *the person cared for* has trouble remembering things; or *the person I care for* accuses people of taking things)			
It is upsetting to find the person I care for has changed so much from his or her former self (For example, he or she is a different person than he or she used to be)			
There have been work adjustments (For example, *I* have to take time off *for caregiving duties*)			
Caregiving is a financial strain			
I feel completely overwhelmed (For example, *I* worry about *the person I care for; I* have concerns about how *I* will manage)			

Total Score =

Words appearing in *italics* represent modifications from the original Caregiver Strain Index from Robinson, B. C. (1983). Validation of a caregiver strain index. *J Gerontol 38*:344-348. Copyright © The Gerontological Society of America.

31-4

burden. One formal screening tool is the Modified Caregiver Strain Questionnaire (Figure 31-4), which is used to identify caregivers of any age who need a more comprehensive assessment. It is a brief tool with 13 questions addressing potential strain in employment, financial, physical, social, and time domains (Thornton & Travis, 2003).

Elder Abuse

The World Health Organization (2002) defines elder abuse as "a single or repeated act, or lack of appropriate action, occurring within a relationship where there is an expectation of trust, which causes harm or distress to an older person." *Elder abuse* is an umbrella term used to describe one or more of the following situations: physical abuse, sexual abuse, emotional or psychological abuse, financial or material exploitation, abandonment, neglect, or a combination of these (Box 31-2).

A study conducted for Human Resources and Social Development Canada (Environics Group, 2008) revealed that 5% of the older adults surveyed had experienced abuse. According to the Statistics Canada (2012b) family violence report, in 2010 there were 2800 police-reported incidents of family violence against older adults aged 65 and older. The data also showed that older adults had the highest risk for being victimized by friends and acquaintances (73 victims per 100,000 older adults), followed by victimization by family (61 victims per 100,000 older adults) and strangers (51 victims per 100,000 older adults). Thus more than two thirds of the abuse of older adults was not committed by a stranger (Statistics Canada, 2012b).

Canada has four major categories of laws to protect older adults from abuse and neglect: family violence laws, the *Criminal Code of Canada,* adult protection laws, and adult guardianship laws.

BOX 31-2 DEFINITIONS OF THE TYPES OF ELDER ABUSE

- Psychological abuse: Anything that diminishes a person's sense of dignity, self-worth, or identity
- Financial or material abuse: Theft or misuse of the older person's money or property
- Neglect
  - Active (intentional withholding of basic necessities of life)
  - Passive (not providing basic necessities because of lack of experience, information, or ability)
- Physical abuse: Nonaccidental use of force to coerce or harm; does not have to result in injury
- Sexual abuse: Any nonconsensual sexual behaviour, either physical or psychological
- Violation of rights: Disregard of basic human and legal rights of the individual
- Systemic abuse: Rules, regulations, or policies that harm or discriminate against older adults

Source: Data from Canadian Network for the Prevention of Elder Abuse. (2012). *What is senior abuse?* Retrieved from *http://www.cnpea.ca/what_is_abuse.htm*.

BOX 31-3 CANADIAN MEDICAL ASSOCIATION SCREENING QUESTIONS

1. Has anyone ever hurt you?
2. Has anyone ever touched you without your consent?
3. Has anyone ever made you do things you didn't want to do?
4. Has anyone taken anything of yours without asking?
5. Has anyone ever scolded or threatened you?
6. Have you signed any papers that you didn't understand?
7. Is there anyone at home you are fearful of?
8. Has anyone ever refused to help you take care of yourself when you needed help?

Source: From Patterson, C. (1994). Secondary prevention of elder abuse. In Canadian Task Force on the Periodic Health Examination (Ed.), *Canadian guide to clinical preventive health care* (pp. 922–999). Ottawa: Health Canada.

Family violence laws, which can vary slightly from province to province or from territory to territory, focus primarily on physical protection and protecting the patient's safety, although some also cover threats or intimidation. The laws tend to come into effect after the fact and usually do not deal with other forms of abuse such as financial abuse. The *Criminal Code of Canada* covers abuses such as physical and sexual assault, intimidation and harassment, and crimes such as theft of property, fraud, or theft by power of attorney. Adult protection laws assign specific provincial health or social service departments the responsibility to respond to the abuse or neglect cases that are brought to their attention. Adult guardianship laws are used when people are mentally incapable of protecting themselves or their property. An excellent guide to elder abuse and neglect law in Canada can be found at the Canadian Centre for Elder Law (2011).

It is important to note that older adults may be reluctant to press charges or to cooperate with criminal prosecutions if the perpetrator is a friend or relative (often an adult child) or if they believe that they themselves will suffer some form of retribution (Canadian Network for the Prevention of Elder Abuse, 2008).

Assessing for Elder Abuse

In interviews of older adults, a general guideline is to ask direct and simple questions (Box 31-3). Structure your assessment questions in a nonjudgemental and nonthreatening manner.

Start with general questions and become progressively more specific if the patient's responses indicate elder abuse (Lachs & Pillemer, 1995). Arrange time to interview the patient and caregiver together and separately. This is done not only to detect abusive behaviour but to detect disparities in stories or to assess for caregiver stress. Caregivers may be reluctant to discuss their personal problems in the presence of the person who depends on their care.

Although there is no set marker of abuse, several clinical situations are suggestive of abuse and warrant further assessment. Clues to elder abuse include observations that the caregiver is reluctant to leave the older adult alone with health care providers, the patient defers excessively to the caregiver to answer questions, there are delays between injuries and when treatment is sought, and inconsistencies are noted between an observed injury and the explanation for it (Beers & Berkow, 2000; Lachs & Pillemer, 1995). A positive finding of these clinical situations does not necessarily mean that abuse has occurred. Instead, treat such findings as signs that further assessment is needed. To learn more about recognizing the signs of elder abuse and how to interact with older adults at risk, see the *ONPEA Core Curriculum & Resource Guide* (Ontario Network for Prevention of Elder Abuse, 2008).

Risk Factors for Abuse

Older women are at greater risk of abuse because of increased social isolation, cultural norms, familial status, disadvantage, or disability (Carstairs & Keon, 2009). In a study of older adults, as well as formal and informal caregivers, Walsh and colleagues (2007) found that gender, ageism, and cultural factors play important roles in elder abuse experiences. Study participants revealed that (a) abuse is cyclical and occurs from generation to generation; (b) abuse occurs throughout the lifespan; (c) exposure to multiple forms of elder abuse is common; and (d) spousal abuse continues in older life.

Documentation

Proper and precise documentation is important in recording suspected cases of elder abuse because medical records may become part of the legal record. If possible, document verbatim descriptions of events, and draw or photograph physical findings. Box 31-4 lists a mnemonic (STOP HARM) to help detect, diagnose, and manage elder abuse. For more information on elder abuse, see Chapter 8, Interpersonal Violence Assessment.

MAINTAINING INDEPENDENCE

Exercise

Staying physically active is key to remaining in good health and remaining independent. Fitness is crucial for preventing or delaying the onset of chronic diseases of aging and for reducing the period of disability and dependent living. The important role of physical activity in maintaining physical and psychological health, in reducing the risk of chronic disease, and in management of pain in chronic disease needs to be actively promoted to all older adults (Carstairs & Keon, 2009). According to the Active Living Coalition for Older Adults, it is estimated that 60% of older Canadians are "inactive." Older women are significantly less likely than older men to be physically active, as are individuals older than 80, older adults with low incomes or low education levels, older adults with disabilities or chronic health conditions, older adults who live in institutions or in isolation, and older adults who are members of ethnocultural and ethnolinguistic minority population groups (Carstairs & Keon, 2009).

Canada's Physical Activity Guidelines for Older Adults—65 Years & Older (Canadian Society for Exercise Physiology, 2013) recommends levels of activity that will help reduce the risk of developing chronic illnesses such as diabetes, heart disease, and depression, and help to maintain mobility and functional independence. Older adults should aim to accumulate at least 150 minutes of moderate to vigorous-intensity aerobic physical activity per week. These activities may be performed in bouts of 10 minutes or more. In addition to endurance activities, older adults should try to include muscle and bone strengthening activities at least 2 days per week as well as physical activities to enhance balance and prevent falls.

Older adults can remain healthy and live independently longer by maintaining and improving their aerobic fitness and endurance. *Aerobic fitness* is a person's ability to perform a physical activity for 2 minutes or longer. Research has shown that adults who are less active lose 16% of their existing level of aerobic fitness every 10 years (Public Health Agency of Canada, 2011). Experts also recommend that older adults perform strength training to maintain their strength, muscle mass, and balance. Loss of muscle mass and inactivity result in an increased risk for disability, falls, and diseases such as diabetes.

Health care practitioners should encourage older adults to maintain their physical fitness and mobility by continuing or initiating an exercise program.

ENVIRONMENTAL ASSESSMENT

The physical environment of the older adult includes the home environment and community system and is crucial for maintaining independence. Environmental hazards within the home can be a potential constraint on the older adult's day-to-day functioning. Common environmental hazards include inadequate lighting, loose throw rugs, curled carpet edges, obstructed hallways, cords in walkways, lack of grab bars in tub and shower, and low and loose toilet seats (Chu, 1998b; Eliopoulis, 1997; Kim & Dyer, 2006). These hazards increase the risk for falls and fractures. Environmental modification can promote mobility and reduce the likelihood of an older adult's falling. The *Inventory of Fall Prevention Initiatives in Canada* (Health Canada, 2005) provides a current overview of fall prevention activities across the country.

In the functional assessment, the examiner should inquire about the safety of the neighbourhood and whether older patients have transportation or transportation services readily available near where they live (Figure 31-5). The older adult

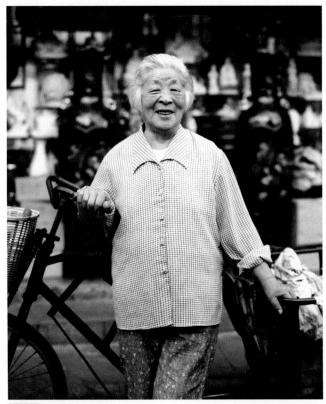

31-5

BOX 31-4 STOP HARM: A MNEMONIC TO HELP DETECT, DIAGNOSE, AND MANAGE ELDER ABUSE

Screen for abuse in all older adult patients
Think about risk factors
Ominous danger signs present?
Physical findings
History
Address issue of elder abuse
Report to adult protective services
Manage with prevention and risk factor modification

Source: From Kruger, R. M., & Moon, C. H. (1999). Can you spot the signs of elder mistreatment? *Postgraduate Medicine, 106*(2), 169–183.

needs access to basic services such as food and clothing stores, pharmacists, financial institutions, health care facilities, and social service agencies. The environment must be safe and must include street lamps, sidewalks, and police and fire protection (Chu, 1998a). Both the home and community environment affect the safety of the older adult (Carol, 1996). Safety is especially important for older adults dependent in IADLs and still living within the community.

Older patients often have problems not easily detected during an office visit. A home visit can reveal problems in the living situation, such as household and bathing hazards, social isolation, family/caregiver stress, and nutrition issues (Kim & Dyer, 2006). The Canadian Consumer Product Safety Bureau with Health Canada (*http://www.hc-sc.gc.ca/cps-spc/index-eng.php*) provides publications that contain injury data and information about the safe handling and design of products, as does the Public Health Agency of Canada (Box 31-5).

SPIRITUAL ASSESSMENT

Spirituality provides personal answers about the meaning and purpose of one's own life (Heriot, 1992) and how to interpret life events and regard them as "bigger than oneself." Spiritual health may improve with age, even as physical and mental health deteriorate. The aging process is a part of a person's spiritual journey, with capability for growth (Berggren-Thomas & Griggs, 1995). Views on spirituality vary greatly from one adult to another and between people of the same faith or belief system. It is important to acknowledge spirituality as a powerful coping mechanism during stressful life events, during illness, and to the end of life (Moore, 1998).

Spiritual assessment is highly individual and may be delayed until a professional–patient relationship has been developed. Open-ended questions provide a foundation for future dialogue. A sample question posed during the initial assessment may be "Do you consider yourself to be a spiritual person?" If the patient says yes, a follow-up question could be "How does that spirituality relate to your health or health care decisions?" Involving chaplains or clergy members, when possible and appropriate, can provide the older adult with support and can serve as a resource for the clinician.

SEX, DRUGS, AND DISEASE

Sexual health assessment in older adults is often overlooked; however, sexual activity is reported by more than 50% of adults aged 65 to 74 and by more than 25% of adults aged 75 to 84 (Lindau et al., 2007). Although the topic can be uncomfortable, it is important to assess older adults for sexual health to ensure that they are practising safe behaviours and able to express their sexuality as they desire.

Older adults may be at higher risk for sexually transmitted infections such as human immunodeficiency virus (HIV) infection and acquired immune deficiency syndrome (AIDS). Some older adults are recently divorced or widowed and may enter into new relationships without considering safer sex practices.

Polypharmacy is the prescription and use of multiple drugs (usually five or more) to deal with concomitant multiple diseases. Polypharmacy may lead to an increased risk of inappropriate drug use, underuse of effective treatments, medication errors, poor adherence to regimens, drug–drug and drug–disease interactions, and potentially dangerous drug reactions (Nobili, Garattini, & Mannucci, 2011). In a report for Statistics Canada, Ramage-Morin (2009) found that polypharmacy "was reported for 53% of older adults in health care institutions and 13% of those in private households."

Because many older adult patients require prescription medications, it is very important to assess for inappropriate use of these medications, such as combinations of medications that cancel out each other's effects or concurrent use of other drugs, including alcohol. The Beers Criteria for Potentially Inappropriate Medication Use in Older Adults (Fick et al., 2003) and the Canadian criteria (McLeod, Huang, & Tamblyn, 1997) are two commonly used guides to inappropriate prescribing practices and potential complications and interactions regarding specific medications commonly taken by older adults. ConsultGeriRN, the Web site of the Hartford

Institute for Geriatric Nursing *(www.consultgerirn.org)* provides links to several useful tools, including the Beers criteria.

While you ask about prescription medications, take the opportunity to ask about any other nonprescription or over-the-counter medications, alternative medications or preparations, and alcohol use.

Immunizations and vaccines are an important part of health promotion for people of all ages, including the older adult population. Of Ontarians aged 65 and older, those who have received the influenza vaccine have a significantly lower rate of mortality during influenza season than do those who did not receive the vaccine (Campitelli, Rosella, Stukel, & Kwong, 2010). Therefore, it is important to check the immunization history, ensure that it is both complete and up-to-date, and encourage seasonal vaccinations.

SPECIAL CONSIDERATIONS

Assessment of the functional status of an older adult can be more time consuming than for younger adults (Table 31-2). It may take longer for an older adult to understand and process the questions and to respond. The presence of physical disabilities, anxiety, depression, pain, or fatigue may necessitate several sessions to complete the assessment. An older adult may need assistance with clothing and may prefer that a family member be present for all or parts of the examination. For older adults who are hospitalized or placed in residential care, consider assessing function during normal activities such as grooming, at mealtime, or during toileting.

A patient with multiple medical problems may tire early and easily, and many medications have side effects that contribute to fatigue or affect the attention span. Again, assessments may need to be performed incrementally, such as positioning for comfort and clustering similar tasks to prevent fatigue. Having the patient use glasses or hearing aids can mitigate communication difficulties resulting from vision or hearing loss. Provide directions in written format if necessary, and have hearing amplifiers and page magnifiers available. Face the patient as much as possible, speak slowly in a low-pitched voice, and enunciate words clearly. For non–English-speaking patients, be prepared to use the services of interpreters rather than family members.

Older adults are a heterogeneous population. You must be aware of your own attitudes and beliefs about older adults to ensure that the functional assessment is truly reflecting abilities and not rely on the myth that functional decline is a normal outcome of aging. Demonstrating respect and interest and treating the patient as an individual is imperative. Ask how the older adult would like to be addressed. Maximize communication by using terms understandable to the patient, rather than medical jargon. Include the older adult in decision making about how the interview or testing is to be performed; such inclusion establishes rapport and promotes self-esteem. Be aware of body language and behaviours, and be prepared to modify your approach. Touch can also help in establishing rapport and can reduce anxiety, but may not be appropriate for certain cultures.

A functional assessment can be intimidating for older adults. Frustration or embarrassment may arise if some physical manoeuvres cannot be performed or questions cannot be answered during cognitive testing. Older adults may also be fearful about the consequences of functional testing, such as losing independence or having a caregiver move into the home. Try to provide reassurance that not everyone can complete all of the tasks or answer all of the questions and that, to the extent possible, confidentiality will be honoured.

Ensure adequate space if you are performing tests of mobility. An older adult may need room to manoeuvre an assistive device. When testing mobility, stand close to him or her to prevent a fall. The environment should be well-lit; avoid high-gloss, shiny, slippery surfaces. Minimize extraneous noises such as those from intercoms, televisions, or high-traffic areas. Warm rooms, access to fluids, proximity to a bathroom, and privacy are important.

CULTURAL CONSIDERATIONS

Be aware that culture influences all parts of each patient's life (review Chapter 3). Food habits and dietary beliefs may conflict with dietary recommendations made by health care providers. The response to pain—including how it is perceived, how much is considered tolerable, and the reaction to pain experienced—varies among and within different cultures. How the patient interprets the symptoms, meaning, and causes of illness can be defined by his or her culture. It also plays a part in the older adult's choice of when to seek care and may influence how the illness is treated (Jett, 2011). He or she may want to try traditional or alternative practices to prevent or treat certain conditions.

Wide differences appear among individuals in every culture. Learn how the patient's culture fits together with suggested interventions. Culture influences whether an older adult relies on family for care or the approach to decision making (e.g., involvement of family and friends), disclosure of medical information (e.g., cancer diagnosis), and end-of-life care (e.g., advance directives, resuscitation preferences, and nutrition; Chu, 1998b; Reuben et al., 2003; Jett, 2011).

Assessing Older Adults in Pain

Pain is not a normal part of aging. If the older adult is feeling pain or discomfort, the knowledge gathered through the assessments will be deficient. Alleviating pain should be a priority over other aspects of the assessment. It may be necessary to administer premedication before portions of the assessment, especially if the assessment requires movement. Another strategy is to use positioning to decrease pain. Ask what position is most comfortable. Providing comfort can help maximize the information gathered. It is paramount to remember that older adults with cognitive impairment do *not* experience less pain. See Chapter 11, Pain Assessment, for more information about pain in older adults.

Various pain assessment scales are available for use in cognitively impaired older adults. Studies have demonstrated that in assessments of patients with cognitive impairment, both self-report and observational–behavioural measures should be used; however, an emphasis should be placed on self-report measures because they have been shown to be the most accurate assessments of pain (Kaasalainen, 2007).

Assessing Older Adults with Altered Cognition

Cognitive impairment poses unique challenges. The older adult may not be able to actively participate in the evaluation or provide consistent answers. Cognitive impairment may severely restrict the ability for expression. Gathering information from an older adult firsthand is always best but not

TABLE 31-2	Comprehensive Older Person's Evaluation

Name (print): _____
Date of Visit: _____
Chief complaint: _____
_____

Today I will ask you about your overall health and function and will be using a questionnaire to help me obtain this information. The first few questions are to check your memory.

Preliminary Cognition Questionnaire:

Record if answer is correct with (+); if answer is incorrect, with (–). Record total number of errors.

	(+, –)
1. What is the date today?	_____
2. What day of the week is it?	_____
3. What is the name of this place?	_____
4. What is your telephone number or room number? *(Record answer: _____)* *If subject does not have phone, ask:* What is your street address?	_____
5. How old are you? *(Record answer: _____)*	_____
6. When were you born? *(Record answer from records if patient cannot answer: _____)*	_____
7. Who is the prime minister of Canada now?	_____
8. Who was the previous prime minister?	_____
9. What was your mother's maiden name?	_____
10. Subtract 3 from 20, and keep subtracting from each new number you get, all the way down.	_____
Total errors	_____

If patient makes more than 4 errors, ask #11. If more than 6 errors, complete questionnaire from informant.

11. Do you think you would benefit from a legal guardian, someone who would be responsible for your legal and financial matters?
    a. No
    b. Has functioning legal guardian for sole purpose of managing money (describe: _____)
    c. Has legal guardian
    d. Yes
    Do you have a living will? Would you like one?
    a. No
    b. Yes

	Yes	No
12. Is your daily life full of things that keep you interested?	_____	_____
13. Have you, at times, very much wanted to leave home?	_____	_____
14. Does it seem that no one understands you?	_____	_____
15. Are you happy most of the time?	_____	_____
16. Do you feel weak all over much of the time?	_____	_____
17. Is your sleep fitful and disturbed?	_____	_____

18. Taking everything into consideration, how would you describe your satisfaction with your life in general at the present time: good, fair, or poor?
    a. Good
    b. Fair
    c. Poor

19. Do you feel you now need help with your mental health: for example, a counsellor or psychiatrist?
    a. No
    b. Has such help *(specify: _____)*
    c. Yes

Continued

TABLE 31-2	**Comprehensive Older Person's Evaluation—cont'd**

Physical Health Section:

The next few questions are about your health.

20. During the past month (30 days), how many days were you so sick that you couldn't do your usual activities, such as working around the house or visiting with friends?

21. Relative to other people your age, how would you rate your overall health at the present time: excellent, good, fair, poor, or very poor?
   a. Excellent (*Skip to #22*)
   b. Very good (*Skip to #22*)
   c. Good (*Ask #i*)
   d. Fair (*Ask #i*)
   e. Poor (*Ask #i*)
      i. Do you feel you need additional medical services such as a doctor, nurse, visiting nurse, or physical therapist? (*Circle all that apply*)
         A. Doctor
         B. Nurse
         C. Visiting nurse
         D. Physiotherapist
         E. None

22. Do you use an aid for walking, such as a wheelchair, walker, cane, or anything else? (*Circle aid usually used*)
   a. Wheelchair
   b. Other (*specify:* _____)
   c. Visiting nurse
   d. Walker
   e. None

23. How much do your health troubles stand in the way of your doing things you want to do: not at all, a little, or a great deal?
   a. Not at all (*Skip to #24*)
   b. A little (*Ask #i*)
   c. A great deal (*Ask #i*)
      i. Do you think you need assistance to do your daily activities? For example, do you need a live-in aide or chore worker?
         A. Live-in aide
         B. Chore worker
         C. Has aide, chore worker, or other assistance (*describe:* _____)
         D. None needed

24. Have you had, or do you currently have, any of the following health problems? (*If yes, place an "X" in appropriate box and describe; medical record information may be used to help complete this section*)

	History	Current	Describe
a. Arthritis or rheumatism?			
b. Lung or breathing problem?			
c. Hypertension?			
d. Heart trouble?			
e. Phlebitis or poor circulation problems in arms or legs?			
f. Diabetes or low blood glucose level?			
g. Digestive ulcers?			
h. Other digestive problem?			
i. Cancer?			
j. Anemia?			
k. Effects of stroke?			
l. Other neurological problem? (*Specify:* _____)			
m. Thyroid or other glandular problem? (*Specify:* _____)			
n. Skin disorders such as pressure sores, leg ulcers, burns?			
o. Speech problem?			
p. Hearing problem?			
q. Vision or eye problem?			
r. Kidney or bladder problems or incontinence?			
s. A problem of falls?			
t. Problem with eating or your weight? (*Specify:* _____)			

TABLE 31-2 Comprehensive Older Person's Evaluation—cont'd

u. Problem with depression or your nerves? *(Specify: _____)*

v. Problem with your behaviour? *(Specify: _____)*

w. Problem with your sexual activity?

x. Problem with alcohol?

y. Problem with pain?

z. Other health problems? *(Specify: _____)*

Immunizations: _____

_____

25. What medications are you currently taking, or have been taking, in the past month? May I see your medication bottles? *(If patient cannot list, ask categories a-r below, and note dosage and schedule, or obtain information from medical or pharmacy records and verify accuracy with the patient.)*

Allergies:	Prescription (Dosage and Schedule)
a. Arthritis medication	
b. Pain medication	
c. Blood pressure medication	
d. Water pills or pills for fluid	
e. Medication for your heart	
f. Medication for your lungs	
g. Blood thinners	
h. Medication for your circulation	
i. Insulin or diabetes medication	
j. Seizure medication	
k. Thyroid pills	
l. Steroids	
m. Hormones	
n. Antibiotics	
o. Medicine for nerves or depression	
p. Prescription sleeping pills	
q. Other prescription drugs	
r. Other nonprescription drugs	

26. Many people have problems remembering to take their medications, especially ones they need to take on a regular basis. How often do you forget to take your medications? Would you say you forget often, sometimes, rarely, or never?
    a. Never
    b. Rarely
    c. Sometimes
    d. Often

Activities of Daily Living:

The next set of questions asks whether you need help with any of the following activities of daily living.

27. I would like to know whether you can do these activities without any help at all, or if you need assistance to do them. *(If yes, describe, including patient's needs.)* Do you need help to:

	Yes	No	Describe (Include Needs)
a. Use the telephone?			
b. Get to places out of walking distance (using transportation)?			
c. Shop for clothes and food?			
d. Do your housework?			
e. Handle your money?			
f. Feed yourself?			
g. Dress and undress yourself?			
h. Take care of your appearance?			

Continued

TABLE 31-2	Comprehensive Older Person's Evaluation—cont'd

   i. Get in and out of bed?

   j. Take a bath or shower?

   k. Prepare your meals?

   l. Do you have any problem getting to the bathroom on time?

28. During the past 6 months, have you had any help with such things as shopping, housework, bathing, dressing, and getting around?

   a. Yes *(specify:* _____ *)*

   b. No

Signature of person completing the form: _____

Source: Adapted with permission from Pearlman, R. (1987). Development of a functional assessment questionnaire for geriatric patients: COPE. *Journal of Chronic Diseases, 40*(1), 85S–94S.

always feasible. To ensure that the information collected is reliable, one strategy is to interview the caregiver or family for subjective assessment data. Another is to arrange opportunities to assess the patient during different times of the day, when he or she may be more clear-headed. If possible, split the assessment into smaller sections at a time. Be flexible.

Adults with cognitive impairment may need questions or directions broken down into single commands, repeated word for word, ongoing verbal cueing, or a physical cue. For example, after getting the patient's attention, you might say, "Sit here" and pat the chair. Never assume that the patient cannot respond to questions even when he or she is known to have cognitive impairment. Using yes-or-no questions may prevent frustration. Be relaxed and patient, because an older adult with dementia may mirror your emotions. If a family member or caregiver does need to provide collateral information, avoid collecting it in front of the patient.

Assessment at the End of Life

Ideally, all aspects of the social assessment are completed before the approach to the end of life. If this is not the case,

the depth and completeness of the assessment are dependent on the plan of care. If interviewing is not possible, gather all available data to formulate interventions. Use information from caregivers and other existing sources. Be aware that caregiver stress may be increased during this time of added strain.

The Canadian Researchers at the End of Life Network (CARENET) is a group of health care providers from across the country who research care at the end of life *(http://www.thecarenet.ca)* and provide excellent resources for people caring for individuals at the end of life.

CONCLUSION

This chapter highlights the importance and components of a functional assessment of older adults in a variety of settings. Additional resources for nurses and nursing students can be found at the National Initiative for the Care of the Elderly (NICE; *http://www.nicenet.ca*) and the Canadian Gerontological Nursing Association *(http://www.cgna.net/Home_Page.html)*.

REFERENCES

Alexopoulos, G. A., Abrams, R. C., Young, R. C., & Shamoian, C. A. (1988). Cornell scale for depression in dementia. *Biological Psychiatry, 23*, 271–284.

Alzheimer Society of Canada. (2010). *Rising tide: The impact of dementia on Canadian society.* Toronto: Author. Retrieved from http://www.alzheimer.ca/~/media/Files/national/Advocacy/ASC_Rising%20Tide_Full%20Report_Eng.ashx.

Beers, M. H., & Berkow, R. (Eds.). (2000). *The Merck manual of geriatrics* (3rd ed.). Whitehouse Station, NJ: Merck Research Laboratories.

Berggren-Thomas, P., & Griggs, M. J. (1995). Spirituality in aging: Spiritual need or spiritual journey? *Journal of Gerontological Nursing, 21*(3), 5–10.

Borson, S., Scanlan, J. M., Chen, P., & Ganguli, M. (2003). The Mini Cog as a screen for dementia: Validation in a population-based sample. *Journal of the American Geriatric Society, 51*, 1451.

Butler-Jones, D. (2010). *The Chief Public Health Officer's Report on the State of Public Health in Canada 2010: Growing older—adding life to years.* Ottawa: Public Health Agency of Canada.

Campitelli, M. A., Rosella, L. C., Stukel, T. A., & Kwong, J. C. (2010). Influenza vaccinations and all-cause mortality in community dwelling elderly in Ontario, Canada, a cohort study. *Vaccine, 29*, 240–246.

Canadian Centre for Elder Law. (2011). *A practical guide to elder abuse and neglect laws in Canada.* Retrieved from http://www.bcli.org/sites/default/files/Practical_Guide_English_Rev_JULY_2011_0.pdf.

Canadian Coalition for Seniors' Mental Health. (2006). *National guidelines for seniors' mental health: The assessment and treatment of delirium.* Retrieved from http://www.ccsmh.ca/en/natlGuidelines/delirium.cfm.

Canadian Institute for Health Information. (2010). *Depression among seniors in residential care.* Retrieved from https://secure.cihi.ca/free_products/ccrs_depression_among_seniors_e.pdf.

Canadian Network for the Prevention of Elder Abuse. (2008). *What is senior abuse?* Retrieved from http://www.cnpea.ca/what_is_abuse.htm.

Canadian Society for Exercise Physiology. (2013). *Canada's physical activity guidelines for older adults-65 years & older.*

Retrieved from *http://www.csep.ca/CMFiles/Guidelines/ CSEP_PAGuidelines_older-adults_en.pdf.*

Carol, W. (1996). Socioeconomic and environmental influences. In A. G. Lueckenotte (Ed.), *Gerontological nursing* (pp. 180–191). St. Louis: Mosby.

Carstairs, S., & Keon, W. J. K. (2009). *Special Senate Committee on Aging Final Report. Canada's Aging Population: Seizing the opportunity.* Retrieved from *http://www.parl.gc.ca/Content/SEN/ Committee/402/agei/rep/AgingFinalReport-e.pdf.*

Chu, N. L. (1998a). Culture, race, and ethnicity. In A. S. Luggen, S. S. Travis, & S. Meiner (Eds.), *NGNA core curriculum for gerontological advanced practice nurses* (pp. 390–393). Thousand Oaks, CA: Sage.

Chu, N. (1998b). Environment/home. In A. S. Luggen, S. S. Travis, & S. Meiner (Eds.), *NGNA core curriculum for gerontological advanced practice nurses* (pp. 385–389). Thousand Oaks, CA: Sage.

Cranswick, K., & Dosman, D. (2007). *Eldercare: What we know today* (Cat. no. 86 2008002). Ottawa: Statistics Canada. Retrieved from *http://www.statcan.gc.ca/pub/11-008-x/2008002/ article/10689-eng.htm#footnote8.*

Crossley, M., Lanting, S., St. Denis-Katz, H., O'Connell, M.E., Haugrud, N., & Morgan, D.G. (2012). The Northern Cultural Assessment of Memory (N-CAM): Normative data from an inner-city clinic supports efficacy and validity of a cognitive screen for Aboriginal adults. In *Final Program, Fortieth Annual Meeting, International Neuropsychological Society*, February 15–18, 2012, Montreal, Quebec, Canada. Retrieved from: *http:// www.the-ins.org/includes/ckfinder/userfiles/files/Linked%20 Program_abstracts.pdf.*

Eliopoulis, C. (1997). *Gerontological nursing* (4th ed.). Philadelphia: J. B. Lippincott.

Environics Group. (2008). *Awareness and perceptions of Canadians toward elder abuse.* Prepared for Human Resources and Social Development Canada. Contract number: G9178-070030 001 CY. Retrieved from *http://epe.lac-bac.gc.ca/100/200/301/ pwgsc-tpsgc/por-ef/human_resources_social_development_ canada/2008/001-08-e/report.pdf.*

Fick, D. M., Cooper, J. W., Wade, W. E., Waller, J. L., MacLean, J. R., & Beers, M. H. (2003). Updating the Beers Criteria for Potentially Inappropriate Medication Use in Older Adults. Results of a US consensus panel of experts. *Archives of Internal Medicine, 163*(22), 2716–2724.

Fillenbaum, G. C., & Smyer, M. (1981). The development, validity, and reliability of the ORS, multidimensional functional assessment questionnaire. *Journal of Gerontology, 36,* 428–434.

Folstein, M. F., Folstein, S. E., & McHugh, P. R. (1975). "Mini-mental state": A practical method for grading the cognitive state of patients for the clinician. *Journal of Psychiatric Research, 12*(3), 189–198.

Groll, D. L., To, T., Bombardier, C., & Wright, J. G. (2005). The development of a comorbidity index with physical function as the outcome. *Journal of Clinical Epidemiology, 58,* 595–602.

Guse, L. W. (2006). Assessment of the older adult. In K. L. Mauk (Ed.), *Gerontological nursing competencies for care* (pp. 265–292). Sudbury, MA: Jones & Bartlett.

Hamilton, B., Granger, C. V., Sherwin, F. S., Zielezny, M., & Tashman, J. S. (1987). A uniform national data system for medical rehabilitation. In M. J. Fuher (Ed.), *Rehabilitation outcomes: Analysis and measurement* (pp. 137–147). Baltimore: Brooks.

Health Canada. (2005). *Inventory of fall prevention initiatives in Canada.* Retrieved from *http://www.saskatoonhealthregion.ca/ pdf/fp-InventoryofCdafpinitiatives05.pdf.*

Heriot, C. S. (1992). Spirituality and aging. *Holistic Nursing Practice, 7,* 22–31.

Hollander, M. J., Liu, G., & Chappell, N. L. (2009). Who cares and how much? The imputed economic contribution to the Canadian healthcare system of middle-aged and older unpaid caregivers providing care to the elderly. *Health Care Quarterly, 12*(2), 42–49.

Inouye, S. K. (2006). Delirium in older persons. *New England Journal of Medicine, 354*(11), 1157–1165.

Inouye, S. K., van Dyck, C. H., Alessi, C. A., Balkin, S., Siegal, A. P., & Horowitz, R. I. (1990). Clarifying confusion: The confusion assessment method. *Annals of Internal Medicine, 113,* 941–948.

Jean, L., Bergeron, M. E., Thivierge, S., & Simard, M. (2010). Cognitive intervention programs for individuals with mild cognitive impairment: Systematic review of the literature. *American Journal of Geriatric Psychiatry, 18*(4), 281–296.

Jett, K. F. (2011). Cultural influences. In S. E. Meiner (Ed.), *Gerontological nursing* (4th ed.) (pp. 81–93). St. Louis: Mosby.

Kaasalainen, S. (2007). Pain assessment in older adults with dementia: Using behavioral observation methods in clinical practice. *Journal of Gerontological Nursing, 33*(6), 6–10.

Karagiozis, H., Gray, S., Sacco, J., Shapiro, M., & Kawas, C. (1998). The Direct Assessment of Functional Abilities (DAFA): A comparison to an indirect measure of instrumental activities of daily living. *Gerontologist, 38,* 113–121.

Katz, S., Ford, A. B., Moskowitz, R. W., Jackson, B. A., & Jaffe, M. W. (1963). Studies of illness in the aged. The Index of ADL: A standardized measure of biological and psychosocial functioning. *Journal of the American Medical Association, 185*(12), 914–919.

Keating, N., Fast, J., Frederick, J., Cranswick, K., & Perrier, C. (1999). *Eldercare in Canada: Context, content and consequences (Statistics Canada Cat. no. 89-570-XPE).* Ottawa: Statistics Canada.

Kim, L. C., & Dyer, C. B. (2006). Assessment of older adults in their homes. In J. J. Gallo (Ed.), *Handbook of geriatric assessment* (4th ed.). Sudbury, MA: Jones & Bartlett.

Kresevic, D. M., & Mezey, M. (2003). Assessment of function. In M. Mezey et al. (Eds.), *Geriatric nursing protocols for best practice* (2nd ed., pp. 31–46). New York: Springer Publishing Company.

Kuriansky, J. B., & Gurland, B. (1976). Performance test of activities of daily living. *International Journal of Aging and Human Development, 7,* 343–352.

Lachs, M., & Pillemer, K. (1995). Abuse and neglect of elderly persons. *New England Journal of Medicine, 332,* 437–443.

Langley, F. A., & Mackintosh, S. F. H. (2007). Functional balance assessment of older community dwelling adults: A systematic review of the literature. *Internet Journal of Allied Health Sciences and Practice, 5*(4). Retrieved from *http:// ijahsp.nova.edu/articles/vol5num4/pdf/langley.pdf.*

Lawton, M. P., & Brody, E. M. (1969). Assessment of older people: Self-maintaining and instrumental activities of daily living. *Gerontologist, 9,* 179–186.

Lindau, S. T., Schumm, L. P., Laumann, E. O., Levinson, W., O'Muircheartaigh, C. A., & Waite, L. J. (2007). A study of sexuality and health among older adults in the United States. *New England Journal of Medicine, 357,* 762–744.

Linn, M. (1988). Rapid Disability Rating Scale-2 (RDRS-2). *Psychopharmacology Bulletin, 24,* 799–800.

Linn, M., & Linn, B. (1982). The Rapid Disability Rating Scale-2. *Journal of the American Geriatric Society, 30,* 378–382.

MacCourt, P., Wilson, K., & Tourigny-Rivard, M.-F. (2011). *Guidelines for comprehensive mental health services for older adults in Canada.* Calgary: Mental Health Commission of Canada. Retrieved from *http://www.akeresourcecentre.org/files/ BSOResources/Mental%20Health%20Commission%20of%20 Canada%20Guidelines.pdf.*

Mahoney, F. I., & Barthel, D. W. (1965). Functional evaluation: The Barthel index. *Maryland State Medical Journal, 14,* 61–65.

Mathias, S., Nayak, U. S., & Isaacs, B. (1986). Balance in the elderly patient: The "Get Up and Go" test. *Archives of Physical Medicine and Rehabilitation, 67,* 387–389.

Maytree Policy in Focus. (2010, March). *Protect caregivers from financial ruin as population ages* (Issue 11). Retrieved from *http://maytree.com/policyPDF/MaytreePolicyInFocusIssue11.pdf*.

McDowell, I. (2006). Physical disability and handicap. In *Measuring health: A guide to rating scales and questionnaires* (3rd ed.), pp. 55–149. New York: Oxford University Press.

McLeod, J. P., Huang, A. R., & Tamblyn, R. M. (1997). Defining inappropriate practices in prescribing for elderly people: A national consensus panel. *Canadian Medical Association Journal, 156*(3), 385–391.

Moore, S. (1998). Spirituality. In A. S. Luggen, S. S. Travis, & S. Meiner (Eds.), *NGNA core curriculum for gerontological advanced practice nurses* (pp. 415–419). Thousand Oaks, CA: Sage.

Morano, C., & Morano, B. (2006). Social assessment. In J. J. Gallo, H. R. Bogner, T. Fulmer, & G. J. Paveza (Eds.), *Handbook of geriatric assessment* (4th ed.). Sudbury, MA: Jones & Bartlett.

Nasreddine, Z. S., Phillips, N. A., Bédirian, V., Charbonneau, S., Whitehead, V., Collin, I., Cummings, J. L., & Chertkow, H. (2005). The Montreal Cognitive Assessment, MoCA: A brief screening tool for mild cognitive impairment. *Journal of the American Geriatrics Society, 53*, 695–699. doi:10.1111/j.1532-5415.2005.53221.x

Neelon, V. J., Champagne, M. T., Carlson, J. R., & Funk, S. G. (1996). The NEECHAM Confusion Scale: Construction, validation, and clinical testing. *Nursing Research, 45*, 324–330.

Nobili, A., Garattini, S., & Mannucci, P. M. (2011). Multiple diseases and polypharmacy in the elderly: Challenges for the internist of the third millennium. *Journal of Comorbidity, 1*, 28–44.

Ontario Network for Prevention of Elder Abuse. (2008). *ONPEA core curriculum & resource guide.* Toronto: Author. Retrieved from *http://www.onpea.org/english/trainingtools/corecurriculum.html*.

Parkerson, G. R., Jr., Broadhead, W. E., & Tse, C.-K. J. (1991). Validation of the Duke Social Support and Stress Scale. *Family Medicine, 23*(5), 357–360.

Pearson, V. (2000). Assessment of function. In R. Kane & R. Kane (Eds.), *Assessing older persons: Measures, meaning and practical applications* (pp. 17–48). New York: Oxford University Press.

Public Health Agency of Canada. (2011). *Tips to get active: Physical activity tips for older adults (65 years and older).* Ottawa: Author. Retrieved from *http://www.phac-aspc.gc.ca/hp-ps/hl-mvs/pa-ap/assets/pdfs/08paap-eng.pdf*.

Ramage-Morin, P. L. (2009, March). *Medication use among senior Canadians* (Statistics Canada Cat. no. 82-003-XPE). *Health Reports, 20*(1). Retrieved from *http://www.statcan.gc.ca/pub/82-003-x/2009001/article/10801-eng.pdf*.

Registered Nurses' Association of Ontario. (2004). *Caregiving strategies for older adults with delirium, dementia and depression.* Toronto: Author.

Reuben, D. B., Herr, K. A., Pacala, J. T., Pollock, B. G., Potter, J. F., & Semla, T. P. (Eds.). (2003). *Geriatrics at your fingertips* (5th ed). Boston: Blackwell/American Geriatrics Society.

Reuben, D. B., & Siu, A. L. (1990). An objective measure of physical function of elderly outpatients: The physical performance test. *Journal of the American Geriatrics Society, 38*(10), 1105–1112.

Richmond, T., Tang, S. T., Tulman, L., Fawcett, J., & McCorkle, R. (2004). Measuring function. In M. Frank-Stromberg & S. J. Olsen (Eds.), *Instruments for clinical health-care research* (3rd ed.), pp. 83–99. Sudbury, MA: Jones & Bartlett.

Rotermann, M. (2006). Seniors' health care use. *Health Reports, 16*(Suppl.), 33–45.

Shulman, K., Shedletsky, R., & Silver, I. (1986). The challenge of time: Clock drawing and cognitive function in the elderly. *International Journal of Geriatric Psychiatry, 1*, 135–140.

Statistics Canada. (2009). *Life satisfaction (Cat. no. 82-625-X).* Ottawa: Author. Retrieved from *http://www.statcan.gc.ca/pub/82-625-x/2010002/article/11264-eng.htm*.

Statistics Canada. (2011). *Healthy aging indicators, by age group and sex, household population aged 45 and over, Canada and provinces, occasional* (CANSIM Table 105-1200). Ottawa: Author. Retrieved from *http://www5.statcan.gc.ca/cansim/a26?lang=eng&retrLang=eng&id=1051200&paSer=&pattern=&stByVal=1&p1=1&p2=-1&tabMode=dataTable&csid=*.

Statistics Canada. (2012a). *Family violence in Canada: A statistical profile (Cat. no. 85-002-X).* Ottawa: Author. Retrieved from *http://www5.statcan.gc.ca/bsolc/olc-cel/olc-cel?catno=85-224-xie&lang=eng*.

Statistics Canada. (2012b). *Population by sex and age groups, by province and territory (CANSIM Table 051-0001).* Ottawa: Author. Retrieved from *http://www.statcan.gc.ca/tables-tableaux/sum-som/l01/cst01/demo31c-eng.htm*.

Thornton, M., & Travis, S. S. (2003). Analysis of the reliability of the Modified Caregiver Strain Index. *The Journal of Gerontology, Series B, Psychological Sciences and Social Sciences, 58*(2), S129.

Visser, P. J., Kester, A., Jolles, J., & Verhey, F. (2006). Ten-year risk of dementia in subjects with mild cognitive impairment. *Neurology, 67*(7), 1201–1207.

Walsh, C. A., Ploeg, J., Lohfeld, L., Horne, J., MacMillan, H., & Lai, D. (2007). Violence across the lifespan: Interconnections among forms of abuse as described by marginalized Canadian elders and their caregivers. *British Journal of Social Work, 37*, 491–514.

World Health Organization. (2002). *Prevention of elder maltreatment (elder abuse).* Retrieved from *http://www.who.int/violence_injury_prevention/violence/elder_abuse/en/*.

Yesavage, J. A., Brink, T. L., Rose, T. L., Lum, O., Huang, V., Adey, M., & Leirer, V. O. (1983). Development and validation of a geriatric depression rating scale: A preliminary report. *Journal of Psychiatric Research, 17*, 37–49.

Zarit, S., & Pearlin, L. (1993). Family caregiving: Integrating informal and formal systems for care. In S. Zarit, L. Pearlin, & K. Schaie (Eds.), *Caregiving systems: Informal and formal helpers* (pp. 303–316). Hillsdale, NJ: Erlbaum.

CREDITS

Inside Back Cover

"Key Laboratory Values" listing: Excerpted from Lewis, S. L., Dirksen, S. R., Heitkemper, M. M., Bucher, L., Camera, I., et al. (2014). *Medical-surgical nursing in Canada* (3rd Canadian ed., pp. 2061–2072). Toronto: Elsevier Canada.

Chapter 1

Figure 1-1: Aleksandra Yakovleva/iStockphoto.
Figure 1-2: Alfaro-LeFevre, R. (2009). *Critical thinking and clinical judgment: A practical approach* (4th ed.). St. Louis: W.B. Saunders.
Figure 1-3: Alfaro-LeFevre, R. (1999). *Critical thinking in nursing: A practical approach* (2nd ed.). Philadelphia: W.B. Saunders.
Figure 1-4: blackwaterimages/iStockphoto.

Chapter 2

Unnumbered photo: © Annette J. Browne.
Figure 2-2: World Health Organization (WHO). (2012). *Health promotion: The Ottawa Charter for Health Promotion.* Retrieved from *http://www.who.int/healthpromotion/conferences/previous/ottawa/en/index4.html.*
Figure 2-3: The Nipissing District Developmental Screen. Reprinted with permission. The Nipissing, Nipissing District Developmental Screen, and NDDS are trademarks of NDDS Intellectual Property Association, used under license. All rights reserved.
Figure 2-4: Pender, N., Murdaugh, C. L., & Parsons, M. A. (2006). *Health promotion in nursing practice* (5th ed, p. 50). Upper Saddle River, NJ: Pearson–Prentice Hall.

Chapter 3 (updated)

Unnum photo: © Annette J. Browne.
Figure 3-1: © Colleen Varcoe.
Figure 3-2: © Annette J. Browne.
Figure 3-3: © Mary Zhang.
Figures 3-4 and 3-5: © Colleen Varcoe.
Figure 3-6: © Annette J. Browne.
Figure 3-7: © Access Alliance Multicultural Health and Community Services, Toronto, Ontario. Reprinted with permission.
Figure 3-8: © Karol Ghuman.
Figure 3-9: Kirby, M. J. L. (2002). *The health of Canadians—The federal role. Final report. Volume 6: Recommendations for reform* (Chapter 13). Retrieved from *http://www.parl.gc.ca/37/2/parlbus/commbus/senate/Com-e/soci-e/rep-e/repoct02vol6-e.htm#ORDER%20OF%20REFERENCE.* Reprinted with permission.
Figure 3-10: From *The Georgia Straight* (March 6–13, 2008, p. 13). Reprinted with permission.
Figure 3-11: Raphael, D. (2011). *Poverty in Canada: Implications for health and quality of life* (2nd ed., p. 64). Toronto: Canadian Scholars' Press.
Figure 3-12: Courtesy Rachel E. Spector, 2006. From Jarvis, C. (2008). *Physical examination & health assessment* (5th ed., p. 39, Figure 3-3). St. Louis: W.B. Saunders.
Figure 3-13: sack/iStockphoto.
Figure 3-14: © Hospital Employees Union, British Columbia. Reprinted with permission.
Figure 3-15: © Mark Richards/PhotoEdit.
Figure 3-16: © Colleen Varcoe.

Chapter 4

Figure 4-2: Potter, P. A., & Perry, A. G. (2005). *Fundamentals of nursing* (6th ed., p. 286, Figure 15-4). St. Louis: Mosby.
Figure 4-5: © Photawa/Dreamstime.com.
Figure 4-6: © Tony Freeman/PhotoEdit.

Chapter 5

Figure 5-2: Adapted from American Society of Human Genetics. (2004). Retrieved from *http://www.ashg.org.*
Figure 5-4: Goldenring J. M., & Rosen, D. S. (2004). Getting into adolescent heads: An essential update. *Contemporary Pediatrics, 21*(1), 64–68, 70, 73–74. Copyright © 2013, Advanstar Communications Inc. 100328:613JM.

Chapter 6

Figure 6-1: Retrieved from *http://www.mocatest.org/pdf_files/test/MoCA-Test-English_7_1.pdf.* Copyright © Dr. Z. Nasreddine, 2003 to 2012: *The Montreal Cognitive Assessment* (MoCA). All rights reserved. Reprinted with permission.

Chapter 8

Figure 8-1: © Colleen Varcoe.
Figure 8-2: Cory, J., & Dechief, L. (2007). *SHE framework: Safety and health enhancement for women experiencing abuse. A toolkit for health care providers and planners.* Vancouver: BC Women's Hospital and Health Centre. Reprinted with permission. Retrieved from *http://www.bcwomens.ca/NR/rdonlyres/8D65CADE-8541-4398-B264-7C28CED7D208/37000/SHE_Framework_May20091.pdf.*
Figure 8-3: Department of Health. (2000). *Framework for the assessment of children in need and their families.* Norwich, UK: Her Majesty's Stationery Office (HMSO). Retrieved from *https://www.education.gov.uk/publications/standard/publicationDetail/Page1/DH-4014430.* © Crown copyright material is reproduced with the permission of the Controller of HMSO and Queen's Printer for Scotland.
Figures 8-4, 8-5, and 8-6: Courtesy Daniel J. Sheridan, PhD, RN, CNS, Hanover, MD. From Sheridan, D. J. (2001). Treating survivors of intimate partner abuse: Forensic, identification and documentation. In J. S. Olshaker, M. C., Jackson, & W. S. Smock (Eds.), *Forensic emergency medicine.* Philadelphia: Lippincott, Williams, & Wilkins.
Figure 8-7: Courtesy Jacquelyn C. Campbell, PhD, RN © 1985, 1988, 2001.

Chapter 9

Figure 9-14: Courtesy of *The Pantagraph* (August 10, 1998). Bloomington, IL.

Chapter 10

Figure 10-1: Health Canada. (2003). *Canadian guidelines for body weight classifications in adults* (Catalogue No. H49-179/2003E; p. 37). Ottawa: Author. Retrieved from *http://www.hc-sc.gc.ca/fn-an/alt_formats/hpfb-dgpsa/pdf/nutrition/weight_book-livres_des_poids_e.pdf.*
Figure 10-4: © Pat Thomas, 2006.
Figure 10-8: Potter, P. A., & Perry, A. G. (2005). *Fundamentals of nursing* (6th ed., p. 650, Figure 31-10). St. Louis: Mosby.
Figure 10-21: Canadian Hypertension Education Program. (2013). The expedited assessment and diagnosis of patients with hypertension: Focus on validated technologies for blood pressure assessment (Figure 1). Retrieved from *http://www.hypertension.ca/images/CHEP_2013/2013_CHEP_Booklet_EN.pdf.* Reprinted with permission of the Canadian Hypertension Education Program.
Art for Table 10-5: (hypopituitary dwarfism; gigantism) from Hall, R., & Evered, D. C. (1990). *Colour atlas of endocrinology* (2nd ed.). London: Mosby; (acromegaly [hyperpituitarism]) Reprinted from the Clinical Slide Collection on the Rheumatic Diseases ©

1991, 1995, 1997. Used by permission of the American College of Rheumatology; (anorexia nervosa) Courtesy of George, D. Comerci, M. D.; (Marfan's syndrome) from Manusov, E. G., & Martucci, E. (1994). The Marfan syndrome. *Archives of Family Medicine, 3,* 824. Copyrighted 1994, American Medical Association; (endogenous obesity—Cushing's syndrome) from Wenig, B. M., Heffess, C. S., & Adair, C. F. (1997). *Atlas of endocrine pathology.* Philadelphia: W.B. Saunders; (achondroplastic dwarfism) Jones, A., & Owen, R. (1995). Color atlas of clinical orthopaedics (2nd ed., p. 10, Fig. 3). London, England: Mosby.

Chapter 11

Figure 11-3: Adapted from McCaffery, M., & Pasero, C. (1999). *Pain: Clinical manual* (2nd ed., p. 61, Form 3.2). St. Louis: Mosby.

Figure 11-4: McCaffery M., & Pasero, C. (1999). *Pain: Clinical manual* (2nd ed., p. 63, Figure 3-2). St. Louis: Mosby.

Figure 11-5 [FACES Pain Rating Scale]: Hicks, C.L., von Baeyer, C.L., Spafford, P., van Korlaar, I., Goodenough, B. (2001). The Faces Pain Scale—Revised: Toward a common metric in pediatric pain measurement. *Pain, 93,* 173–183; and Bieri, D., Reeve, R., Champion, G.D., Addicoat, L., Ziegler, J. (1990). The Faces Pain Scale for the self-assessment of the severity of pain experienced by children: Development, initial validation and preliminary investigation for ratio scale properties. *Pain, 41,* 139–150.

Unnumbered figure in Promoting Health box (WHO Pain Ladder): Adapted from World Health Organization. (1996). *Cancer pain relief with a guide to opioid availability.* Geneva, Switzerland: Author. Retrieved from *http://whqlibdoc.who.int/publications/ 9241544821.pdf.* Figure also available at *http://www.who.int/ cancer/palliative/painladder/en/.*

Chapter 12

Unnumbered photo: © Annette J. Browne.

Figure 12-1: Excerpts from Health Canada. (2007). *Eating well with Canada's food guide.* © Her Majesty the Queen in Right of Canada, represented by the Minister of Health Canada. Cat No. H164-38/1-2007E. Retrieved from *http://www.hc-sc.gc.ca/fn-an/ alt_formats/hpfb-dgpsa/pdf/food-guide-aliment/print_eatwell_ bienmang_e.pdf.*

Figure 12-2: Adapted from Canadian Food Inspection Agency. (2009). *Nutrition labelling.* Retrieved from *http://www.inspection. gc.ca/english/fssa/labeti/guide/ch5e.shtml#a5_4.* Adapted with the permission of the Minister of Public Works and Government Services Canada, 2012.

Chapter 13

Figure 13-1: Lewis, S. L., Dirksen, S. R., Heitkemper, M. M., Bucher, L., & Camera, I. M. (2011). *Medical-surgical nursing: Assessment and management of clinical problems* (8th ed., p. 437, Figure 23-1). St. Louis: Mosby.

Figure 13-3, B: Marks, J.G., & Miller, J.J. (2006). *Lookingbill & Marks' principles of dermatology* (4th ed., p. 191, Figure 13.8) Philadelphia: W.B. Saunders.

Figure 13-4, A & B: Hurwitz, S. (1993). *Clinical pediatric dermatology: A textbook of skin disorders of childhood and adolescence* (2nd ed., pp. 200, 212). Philadelphia: W.B. Saunders.

Figure 13-4, C: Lookingbill, D. P., & Marks, J. G. (1993). *Principles of dermatology* (2nd ed., p. 91). Philadelphia: W.B. Saunders.

Figure 13-5: Images retrieved from the National Cancer Institute database (*http://visualsonline.cancer.gov/*) and used with permission.

Figure 13-6: Bloom, A., Watkins, P. H., & Ireland, J. (1992). *Color atlas of diabetes* (2nd ed.). St. Louis: Mosby.

Figure 13-7: Lookingbill, D. P., & Marks, J. G. (1993). *Principles of dermatology* (2nd ed.). Philadelphia: W.B. Saunders.

Figure 13-10: Courtesy Lemmi & Lemmi, 2011.

Figure 13-11: Courtesy Lemmi & Lemmi, 2011.

Figure 13-13: Courtesy Jane Deacon, RNC, MS, NNP, The Children's Hospital, Denver, CO.

Figure 13-14: Bowden, V. R., Dickey, S. B., & Greenburg, C. S. (1998). *Children and their families: The continuum of care.* Philadelphia: W.B. Saunders.

Figures 13-15 and 13-16: Hurwitz, S. (1993). *Clinical pediatric dermatology: A textbook of skin disorders of childhood and adolescence* (2nd ed.). Philadelphia: W.B. Saunders.

Figure 13-17: Courtesy Lemmi & Lemmi, 2011.

Figure 13-18: Hurwitz, S. (1993). *Clinical pediatric dermatology: A textbook of skin disorders of childhood and adolescence* (2nd ed.). Philadelphia: W.B. Saunders.

Figure 13-19: Murray, S. S., & McKinney, E. S. (2010). *Foundations of maternal–newborn nursing and women's health nursing* (5th ed., p. 536, Figure 20-13). St. Louis: W.B. Saunders.

Figure 13-20, A & B: Habif, T. P., Campbell, J. L., Jr., Chapman, M. S., Dinulos, J. G. H., & Zug, K. A. (2005). *Skin disease: Diagnosis and treatment* (3rd ed., p. 73). St. Louis: Mosby.

Figure 13-21: Lookingbill, D. P., & Marks, J. G. (1993). *Principles of dermatology* (2nd ed., p. 89). Philadelphia: W.B. Saunders.

Figure 13-22: Lookingbill, D. P., & Marks, J. G. (1993). *Principles of dermatology* (2nd ed.). Philadelphia: W.B. Saunders.

Figure 13-23: Lookingbill, D. P., & Marks, J. G. (1993). *Principles of dermatology* (2nd ed.). Philadelphia: W. B. Saunders.

Figure 13-24: Lookingbill, D. P., & Marks, J. G. (1993). *Principles of dermatology* (2nd ed., p. 75). Philadelphia: W.B. Saunders.

Figure 13-25: Callen, J. P., & Greer K. E. (1993). *Color atlas of dermatology* (p. 103, Figure 3.118). Philadelphia: W.B. Saunders.

Art for Table 13-4: Line drawings © Pat Thomas, 2010; (photos of macule, patch, papule, plaque, nodule, tumour, wheal, vesicle, bulla, cyst, and pustule): Courtesy Lemmi & Lemmi, 2011; (photo of urticaria [hives]) from Fireman, P. (1996). *Atlas of allergies* (2nd ed., p. 250, Figure 16-2). London: Mosby.

Art for Table 13-5: Line drawings © Pat Thomas, 2010; (photos of crust, scale, fissure, erosion, ulcer, excoriation, scar, atrophic scar, lichenification, and keloid): Courtesy Lemmi & Lemmi, 2011.

Art for Table 13-6: (photos of pressure ulcers): Potter, P. A., & Perry, A. G. (2009). *Fundamentals of nursing* (7th ed., p. 1283, Figure 48-6). St. Louis: Mosby.

Art for Table 13-8: (port-wine stain [nevus flammeus]) from Hurwitz, S. (1993). *Clinical pediatric dermatology: a textbook of skin disorders of childhood and adolescence* (2nd ed.). Philadelphia: W.B. Saunders; (strawberry mark [immature hemangioma]) from Lookingbill, D. P., & Marks, J. G. (1993). *Principles of dermatology* (2nd ed.). Philadelphia: W.B. Saunders; (cavernous hemangioma [mature]) from Habif, T. P., Campbell, J. L., Jr., Chapman, M. S., Dinulos, J. G. H., & Zug, K. A. (2005). *Skin disease: Diagnosis and treatment* (3rd ed., p. 437). St. Louis: Mosby; (telangiectasis spider or star angioma) Courtesy Lemmi & Lemmi, 2011; (venous lake) from Habif, T. P., Campbell, J. L., Jr., Chapman, M. S., Dinulos, J. G. H., & Zug, K. A. (2001). *Skin disease: Diagnosis and treatment* (2nd ed.). St. Louis: Mosby; (petechiae) from Dockery, G. L. (1997). *Cutaneous disorders of the lower extremity* (p. 119, Figure 9-47). Philadelphia: W.B. Saunders. Reprinted with the permission of the author; (purpura) from Hurwitz, S. (1993). *Clinical pediatric dermatology: a textbook of skin disorders of childhood and adolescence* (2nd ed.). Philadelphia: W.B. Saunders; (ecchymosis) Courtesy Lemmi & Lemmi, 2011.

Art for Table 13-9: (diaper dermatitis) from Hurwitz, S. (1993). *Clinical pediatric dermatology: a textbook of skin disorders of childhood and adolescence* (2nd ed.). Philadelphia: W.B. Saunders; (intertrigo [candidiasis]) and (impetigo) Courtesy Lemmi & Lemmi, 2011; (atopic dermatitis [eczema]) from Hurwitz, S. (1993). *Clinical pediatric dermatology: a textbook of skin disorders of childhood and adolescence* (2nd ed.). Philadelphia: W.B. Saunders; (measles [rubeola] in dark skin) from Feigin, R. D., & Cherry, J. D. (1998). *Textbook of pediatric infectious diseases* (4th ed.). Philadelphia: Saunders; (measles [rubeola] in light skin) Courtesy Lemmi & Lemmi, 2011; (German measles [rubella]) from Hurwitz, S. (1993). *Clinical pediatric dermatology: a textbook of skin disorders of childhood and adolescence* (2nd ed.). Philadelphia: W.B. Saunders; (chickenpox [varicella]) from Callen, J. P., & Greer K. E. (1993). *Color atlas of dermatology* (p. 170, Figure 5.34). Philadelphia: W.B. Saunders.

Art for Table 13-10: (primary contact dermatitis) from Lookingbill, D. P., & Marks, J. G. (1993). *Principles of dermatology* (2nd ed., p. 124). Philadelphia: W.B. Saunders; (allergic drug reaction) from Lookingbill, D. P., & Marks, J. G. (1993). *Principles of dermatology* (2nd ed., p. 218). Philadelphia: W.B. Saunders; (tinea corporis [ringworm of the body]) from Hurwitz, S. (1993). *Clinical pediatric dermatology: a textbook of skin disorders of childhood and adolescence* (2nd ed.). Philadelphia: W. B. Saunders; (tinea pedis [ringworm of the foot], labial herpes simplex [cold sores], tinea versicolor, and herpes zoster [shingles]) from Lemmi & Lemmi, 2011; (psoriasis) from Lookingbill, D. P., & Marks, J. G. (1993). *Principles of dermatology* (2nd ed.). Philadelphia: W.B. Saunders; (erythema migrans of Lyme disease) from Swartz, M. H. (2006). *Textbook of physical diagnosis: History and examination* (5th ed.). Philadelphia: W.B. Saunders.

Art for Table 13-11: (basal cell carcinoma; malignant melanoma) from Lookingbill, D. P., & Marks, J. G. (1993). *Principles of dermatology* (2nd ed.). Philadelphia: W.B. Saunders; (squamous cell carcinoma) from Habif, T. P., Campbell, J. L., & Quitadamo, M. J. (2001). *Skin disease: Diagnosis and treatment.* St. Louis: Mosby; (metastatic malignant melanoma) courtesy Lemmi & Lemmi, 2011.

Art for Table 13-12: (AIDS-related Kaposi's sarcoma: patch stage) from Friedman-Kien, A. E. (1989). *Color atlas of AIDS.* Philadelphia: W.B. Saunders.

Art for Table 13-13: (tinea capitis [scalp ringworm]; furuncle and abscess) from Lookingbill, D. P., & Marks, J. G. (1993). *Principles of dermatology* (2nd ed.). Philadelphia: W.B. Saunders; (toxic alopecia) from Hurwitz, S. (1993). *Clinical pediatric dermatology: A textbook of skin disorders of childhood and adolescence* (2nd ed.). Philadelphia: W.B. Saunders; (alopecia areata; traumatic alopecia: traction alopecia; and seborrheic dermatitis [cradle cap]) from Hurwitz, S. (1993). *Clinical pediatric dermatology: A textbook of skin disorders of childhood and adolescence* (2nd ed.). Philadelphia: W.B. Saunders; (pediculosis capitis [head lice]; and trichotillomania) from Callen, J. P., & Greer, K. E. (1993). *Color atlas of dermatology.* Philadelphia: W.B. Saunders; (hirsutism) from Wenig, B. M., Heffess, C. S., & Adair, C. F. (1997). *Atlas of endocrine pathology* (p. 282, Figure 13-25). Philadelphia: W.B. Saunders.

Art for Table 13-14: (scabies; paronychia; onycholysis; pitting; habittic dystrophy) courtesy Lemmi & Lemmi, 2011; (Beau's line; splinter hemorrhages) from Callen, J. P., & Greer, K. E. (1993). *Color atlas of dermatology.* Philadelphia: W. B. Saunders; (late clubbing) Reprinted from the Clinical Slide Collection on the Rheumatic Diseases. © 1991, 1995, 1997. Used by permission of the American College of Rheumatology.

Chapter 14

Figure 14-8: © Pat Thomas, 2006.

Figure 14-14, B: Courtesy Lemmi & Lemmi, 2011.

Figures 14-16 and 14-17, A: Murray, S. S., & McKinney, E. S. (2010). *Foundations of maternal–newborn and women's health nursing* (5th ed., pp. 514–15). St. Louis: W.B. Saunders.

Art for Table 14-1: (hydrocephalus) from Bowden, V. R., Dickey, S. B., & Greenburg, C. S. (1998). *Children and their families: The continuum of care.* Philadelphia: W.B. Saunders; (Paget's disease of bone [osteitis deformans]) Reprinted from the Clinical Slide Collection on the Rheumatic Diseases. © 1991, 1995, 1997. Used by permission of the American College of Rheumatology; (acromegaly) from Damjanov, I. (1996). *Pathology for the health-related professions.* Philadelphia: Saunders.

Art for Table 14-2: (torticollis [wryneck]) from Zitelli, B. J., McIntire, S.C., & Nowalk, A.J. (2012). *Zitelli & Davis' atlas of pediatric physical diagnosis* (6th ed., p. 648, Figure 17-15). St. Louis: Mosby; (thyroid: multiple nodules) from Swartz, M. H. (2006). *Textbook of physical diagnosis: History and examination* (5th ed.). Philadelphia: W.B. Saunders; (pilar cyst [wen]) from Callen, J. P., & Greer K. E. (1993). *Color atlas of dermatology.* Philadelphia: Saunders; (parotid gland enlargement) from Swartz, M. H. (2009). *Textbook of physical diagnosis: History and examination* (6th ed., p. 347, Figure 12-39). Philadelphia: W.B. Saunders.

Art for Table 14-3: (fetal alcohol syndrome) Photo from Streissguth, A. P., Landesman-Dwyer, S., Martin, J. C., & Smith, D. W. (1980). Teratogenic effects of alcohol in humans and laboratory animals. *Science, 209,* 353–361; illustration © Pat Thomas, 2006; (congenital hypothyroidism) from Zitelli, B. J., McIntire, S.C., & Nowalk, A.J. (2012). *Zitelli & Davis' atlas of pediatric physical diagnosis* (6th ed., p. 381, Figure 9-17) St. Louis: Mosby. Courtesy Dr. Thomas P. Foley, Jr., Pittsburgh, PA; (Down's syndrome): from Zitelli, B. J., & Davis, H. W. (2007). *Atlas of pediatric physical diagnosis* (5th ed., p. 81, Figure 3-36). St. Louis: Mosby; (atopic [allergic] facies; allergic salute and crease) from Zitelli, B. J., McIntire, S.C., & Nowalk, A.J. (2012). *Zitelli & Davis' atlas of pediatric physical diagnosis* (6th ed., Figures 4-14 and 4-16). St. Louis: Mosby.

Art for Table 14-4: (Cushing's syndrome) from Zitelli, B. J., & Davis, H. W. (2007). *Atlas of pediatric physical diagnosis* (5th ed.). St. Louis: Mosby; (hyperthyroidism) from Swartz, M. H. (2006). *Textbook of physical diagnosis: History and examination* (5th ed.). Philadelphia: W.B. Saunders; (myxedema [hypothyroidism]) from Hall, R., & Evered, D. C. (1990). *Colour atlas of endocrinology* (2nd ed.). London: Mosby; (Bell's palsy [right side]) from Swartz, M. H. (2009). *Textbook of physical diagnosis: History and examination* (6th ed., p. 666, Figure 21-17). Philadelphia: W.B. Saunders; (scleroderma) Reprinted from the Clinical Slide Collection on the Rheumatic Diseases. © 1991, 1995, 1997. Used by permission of the American College of Rheumatology.

Chapter 15

Figure 15-1, 15-2, 15-3, 15-4, 15-18: © Pat Thomas, 2006.

Figure 15-23: Courtesy Heather Boyd-Monk and Wills Eye Hospital, Philadelphia, PA.

Figures 15-24 and 15-25: Courtesy Lemmi & Lemmi, 2011.

Figure 15-30: Zitelli, B. J., McIntire, S.C., & Nowalk, A.J. (2012). *Zitelli & Davis' atlas of pediatric physical diagnosis* (6th ed., p. 739, Figure 19-18).St. Louis: Mosby.

Figure 15-31: Albert, D. M., & Jakobiec, F. A. (1994). *Principles and practice of ophthalmology.* Philadelphia: Saunders.

Figures 15-32 and 15-34: Courtesy Lemmi & Lemmi, 2011.

Figure 15-33: Swartz, M. H. (2009). *Textbook of physical diagnosis: History and examination* (6th ed., p. 244, Figure 10-54). Philadelphia: W.B. Saunders.

Figure 15-35: Friedman, N., & Pineda, R. (1998). *The Massachusetts Eye and Ear Infirmary illustrated manual of ophthalmology.* Philadelphia: W.B. Saunders (p. 535).

Art in Table 15-1: (**A,** pseudostrabismus; **B,** esotropia; **C,** exotropia) from Zitelli, B. J., McIntire, S.C., & Nowalk, A.J. (2012). *Zitelli & Davis' atlas of pediatric physical diagnosis* (6th ed., pp. 737–40, Figures 19-12, 19-18, 19-20). St. Louis: Mosby.

Art in Table 15-2: (periorbital edema) from Ibsen, O. A. C., & Phelan, J. A. (1996). *Oral pathology for the dental hygienist* (2nd ed.). Philadelphia: W.B. Saunders; (exophthalmos [protruding eye]) from Scheie, H. G., & Albert, D. M. (1977). *Textbook of ophthalmology* (9th ed.). Philadelphia: W.B. Saunders; (ptosis [drooping upper lid]) Courtesy Lemmi & Lemmi, 2011; (upward palpebral slant) from Zitelli, B. J., McIntire, S.C., & Nowalk, A.J. (2012). *Zitelli & Davis' atlas of pediatric physical diagnosis* (6th ed., p. 101, Figure 3-37) St. Louis: Mosby; (ectropion; entropion) from Albert, D. M., & Jakobiec, F. A. (1994). *Principles and practice of ophthalmology* (vol. 3, p. 1849). Philadelphia: W.B. Saunders.

Art in Table 15-3: (blepharitis [inflammation of the eyelids]; dacryocystitis [inflammation of the lacrimal sac]) from Friedman, N., & Pineda, R. (1998). *The Massachusetts Eye and Ear Infirmary illustrated manual of ophthalmology.* Philadelphia: W.B. Saunders; (chalazion) Courtesy Heather Boyd-Monk and Wills Eye Hospital, Philadelphia, PA; (hordeolum [stye]) Courtesy Lemmi & Lemmi, 2011; (basal cell carcinoma) from Scheie, H. G., & Albert, D. M. (1977). *Textbook of ophthalmology* (9th ed., p. 449). Philadelphia: W.B. Saunders.

Art in Table 15-6: (conjunctivitis; subconjunctival hemorrhage) courtesy Lemmi & Lemmi, 2011; (iritis [circumcorneal redness]; acute glaucoma) from Scheie, H. G., & Albert, D. M. (1977). *Textbook of ophthalmology* (9th ed., pp. 13, 536). Philadelphia: W. B. Saunders.

Art in Table 15-7: (pterygium) from Albert, D. M., & Jakobiec, F. A. (1994). *Principles and practice of ophthalmology* (vol. 1). Philadelphia: W. B. Saunders; (corneal abrasion) Courtesy Heather Boyd-Monk and Wills Eye Hospital, Philadelphia, PA; (hyphema) from Scheie, H. G., & Albert, D. M. (1977). *Textbook of ophthalmology* (9th ed.). Philadelphia: W. B. Saunders; (hypopyon) from Scheie, H. G., & Albert, D. M. (1977). *Textbook of ophthalmology* (9th ed., p. 391). Philadelphia: W. B. Saunders.

Art in Table 15-8: (central grey opacity: nuclear cataract; star-shaped opacity: cortical cataract) from Friedman, N., & Pineda, R. (1998). *The Massachusetts Eye and Ear Infirmary illustrated manual of ophthalmology.* Philadelphia: W. B. Saunders (pp. 220–21, Figures 8-4 and 8-6).

Art in Table 15-9: (optic atrophy [disc pallor]; papilledema [choked disc]; excessive cup-disc ratio) from Friedman, N., Kaiser, P.K., & Pineda, R. (2009). *The Massachusetts Eye and Ear Infirmary illustrated manual of ophthalmology.* Philadelphia: W. B. Saunders.

Art in Table 15-10: (arteriovenous crossing [nicking]) from Friedman, N., Kaiser, P. K., & Pineda, R. (2009). *The Massachusetts Eye and Ear Infirmary illustrated manual of ophthalmology* (3rd ed., p. 268, Figure 10-35). Philadelphia: W. B. Saunders; (narrowed [attenuated] arteries; microaneurysms; exudates) courtesy Lemmi & Lemmi, 2011; (intraretinal hemorrhages) from Friedman, N., Kaiser, P. K., & Pineda, R. (2009). *The Massachusetts Eye and Ear Infirmary illustrated manual of ophthalmology* (3rd ed.). Philadelphia: W. B. Saunders.

Chapter 16

Figure 16-1: Courtesy Lemmi & Lemmi, 2011.

Figure 16-2: © Pat Thomas, 2010.

Figure 16-4: © Pat Thomas, 2006.

Figure 16-9: Adams, G. L., Boies, L. R., & Hilger, P. A. (1989). *Boies fundamentals of otolaryngology: A textbook of ear, nose, and throat diseases* (6th ed.). Philadelphia: W. B. Saunders.

Figure 16-10: © Pat Thomas, 2006.

Art for Table 16-1: (frostbite) Reprinted from the Clinical Slide Collection on the Rheumatic Diseases. © 1991, 1995, 1997. Used by permission of the American College of Rheumatology; (otitis externa: swimmer's ear; cellulitis) Courtesy Lemmi & Lemmi, 2011; (branchial remnant and ear deformity) from Liebert, P. S. (1996). *Color atlas of pediatric surgery* (2nd ed., p. 31, Figure 2-45). Philadelphia: W. B. Saunders.

Art for Table 16-2: (sebaceous cyst) from Liebert, P. S. (1996). *Color atlas of pediatric surgery* (2nd ed., p. 29, Figure 2-40). Philadelphia: W. B. Saunders; (tophi) Reprinted from the Clinical Slide Collection on the Rheumatic Diseases © 1991, 1995, 1997. Used by permission of the American College of Rheumatology; (chondrodermatitis nodularis helicis) from Habif, T. P. (2004). *Clinical dermatology: A color guide to diagnosis and therapy* (4th ed., p. 716, Figure 20-39). St. Louis: Mosby; (keloid) courtesy Lemmi & Lemmi, 2011; (carcinoma) from Callen, J. P., & Greer K. E. (1993). *Color atlas of dermatology.* Philadelphia: W. B. Saunders (p. 111, Figure 3-140A).

Art for Table 16-3: © Pat Thomas, 2010.

Art for Table 16-5: (retracted eardrum) from Adams, G. L., Boies, L. R., & Hilger, P. A. (1989). *Boies fundamentals of otolaryngology: A textbook of ear, nose, and throat diseases* (6th ed., p. 6). Philadelphia: W. B. Saunders; (otitis media with effusion [OME]) from Swartz, M. H. (2009). *Textbook of physical diagnosis: History and examination* (6th ed., p. 320, Figure 11-34A). Philadelphia: W. B. Saunders; (acute purulent otitis media: early stage; acute purulent otitis media: later stage) from Adams, G. L., Boies, L. R., & Hilger, P. A. (1989). *Boies fundamentals of otolaryngology: A textbook of ear, nose, and throat diseases* (6th ed.). Philadelphia: W. B. Saunders; (perforation) from Swartz, M. H. (2009). *Textbook of physical diagnosis: History and examination* (6th ed., p. 318, Figure 11-30A). Philadelphia: W. B. Saunders; (insertion of tympanostomy tubes) from Fireman, P. (1996). *Atlas of allergies* (2nd ed., p. 182, Figure 11-19). London: Mosby; (cholesteatoma; bullous myringitis) from Swartz, M. H. (2009). *Textbook of physical diagnosis: History and examination* (6th ed., pp. 317, 319, Figures 11-27 and 11-31A). Philadelphia: W. B. Saunders; (illustrations of scarred eardrum, blue eardrum, and fungal infection [otomycosis]) © Pat Thomas, 2010.

Chapter 17

Figure 17-1, 17-2, 17-3, 17-6, 17-19: © Pat Thomas, 2006.

Figure 17-4, 17-5: © Pat Thomas, 2010.

Figure 17-7: Martino, R., Silver, F., Teasell, R., Bayley, M., Nicholson G., Streiner, D. L., & Diamant, N. E. (2009). The Toronto Bedside Swallowing Screening Test (TOR-BSST): Development and validation of a dysphagia screening tool for patients with stroke. *Stroke, 40,* 555–561. Retrieved from *http://www.neostrokenetwork.com/newportal/LinkClick.aspx?fileticket=rDVxJ5l9NGo%3D&tabid=299.*

Figure 17-10: Fireman, P. (1996). *Atlas of allergies* (2nd ed., p. 151, Figure 9-27). London: Mosby.

Figure 17-17: Ibsen, O. A. C., & Phelan, J. A. (1996). *Oral pathology for the dental hygienist* (2nd ed., Slide #106). Philadelphia: W. B. Saunders.

Figure 17-18: Courtesy Lemmi & Lemmi, 2011.

Figure 17-24: Zitelli, B. J., McIntire, S.C., & Nowalk, A.J. (2012). *Zitelli & Davis' atlas of pediatric physical diagnosis* (6th ed., p. 780, Figure 20-13). St. Louis: Mosby.

Figures 17-25 and 17-26: Courtesy Lemmi & Lemmi, 2011.

Art for Table 17-1: (foreign body; acute rhinitis; allergic rhinitis; nasal polyps) from Fireman, P. (1996). *Atlas of allergies* (2nd ed.). London: Mosby; (perforated septum) from Hawke, M. (1998). *Diagnostic handbook of otorhinolaryngology.* London: Martin Dunitz (p. 122, Figure 2.60). Reproduced by permission of Taylor & Francis Books UK.

Art for Table 17-2: (cleft lip) from Ibsen, O. A. C., & Phelan, J. A. (1996). *Oral pathology for the dental hygienist* (2nd ed., slide 294). Philadelphia: W. B. Saunders; (herpes simplex 1; angular cheilitis [stomatitis, perlèche]) from Callen, J. P., & Greer K. E. (1993). *Color atlas of dermatology.* Philadelphia: W. B. Saunders; (carcinoma; retention "cyst" [mucocele]) from Hawke, M. (1998). *Diagnostic handbook of otorhinolaryngology.* London: Martin Dunitz (p. 161-62, Figure 3.6 & 3.7). Reproduced by permission of Taylor & Francis Books UK.

Art for Table 17-3: (baby bottle tooth decay) Courtesy F. Ferguson, Department of Children's Dentistry, School of Dental Medicine, State University of New York at Stony Brook, Stony Brook, NY; (dental caries) Courtesy A. McWhorter, Pediatric Dentistry, Baylor College of Dentistry, Texas A&M University System, Dallas, TX; (epulis; gingival hyperplasia) from Ibsen, O. A. C., & Phelan, J. A. (1996). *Oral pathology for the dental hygienist* (2nd ed.). Philadelphia: W. B. Saunders; (gingivitis) from Callen, J. P., & Greer K. E. (1993). *Color atlas of dermatology* (p. 385). Philadelphia: W. B. Saunders; (meth mouth) from Neville, B. W., Damm, D. D., Allen, C. M., & Bouquot, J. E. (2009).

Oral and maxillofacial pathology (3rd ed.). St. Louis: W. B. Saunders.

Art for Table 17-4: (aphthous ulcers) from Sleisinger, M. H., & Fordtran, J. S. (1993). *Gastrointestinal diseases: Pathophysiology, diagnosis, and management* (vol. 1, 5th ed.). Philadelphia: W. B. Saunders; (Koplik's spots) from Feigin, R. D., & Cherry, J. D. (1998). *Textbook of pediatric infectious diseases* (4th ed.). Philadelphia: W. B. Saunders; (leukoplakia) from Sleisinger, M. H., & Fordtran, J. S. (1993). *Gastrointestinal diseases: Pathophysiology, diagnosis, and management* (5th ed., vol. 1). Philadelphia: W. B. Saunders; (candidiasis or monilial infection) from Callen, J. P., & Greer K. E. (1993). *Color atlas of dermatology.* Philadelphia: W. B. Saunders; (herpes simplex 1) courtesy Lemmi & Lemmi, 2011.

Art for Table 17-5: (ankyloglossia) from Ibsen, O. A. C., & Phelan, J. A. (1996). *Oral pathology for the dental hygienist* (2nd ed., slide #28). Philadelphia: W. B. Saunders; (geographic tongue [migratory glossitis]; fissured or scrotal tongue) courtesy Lemmi & Lemmi, 2011; (smooth, glossy tongue [atrophic glossitis]) from Adams, G. L., Boies, L. R., & Hilger, P. A. (1989). *Boies fundamentals of otolaryngology: A textbook of ear, nose, and throat diseases* (6th ed., p. 302). Philadelphia: W. B. Saunders; (black hairy tongue) from Callen, J. P., & Greer K. E. (1993). *Color atlas of dermatology.* Philadelphia: W. B. Saunders (p. 387); (enlarged tongue [macroglossia]) from Zitelli, B. J., & Davis, H. W. (2002). *Atlas of pediatric physical diagnosis* (4th ed.). St. Louis: Mosby. Courtesy Dr. Christine Williams; (carcinoma) from Wenig, B. M., Heffess, C. S., & Adair, C. F. (1997). *Atlas of endocrine pathology.* Philadelphia: W. B. Saunders.

Art for Table 17-6: (cleft palate) from Zitelli, B. J., McIntire, S. C., & Nowalk, A. J. (2012). *Zitelli & Davis' atlas of pediatric physical diagnosis* (6th ed., p. 944, Figure 23-64,BSt. Louis: Mosby. Courtesy Dr. Michael Sherlock, M. D., Lutherville, MD; (bifid uvula) from Hawke, M. (1998). *Diagnostic handbook of otorhinolaryngology.* London: Martin Dunitz (p. 195, Figure 3.67); (oral Kaposi's sarcoma) from Friedman-Kien, A. E. (1989), *Color atlas of AIDS.* Philadelphia: W. B. Saunders (p. 38); (acute tonsillitis and pharyngitis) Courtesy Lemmi & Lemmi, 2011.

Chapter 18

Figure 18-2: © Pat Thomas, 2010.

Figure 18-6: Redrawn from Tanner, J. M. (1962). *Growth at adolescence.* Oxford, UK: Blackwell Scientific.

Figure 18-8: Callen, J. P., & Greer K. E. (1993). *Color atlas of dermatology.* Philadelphia: W. B. Saunders.

Figure 18-19: Courtesy Denise Tarlier.

Figure 18-21: Moore, K. L., Persaud, T.N., & Torchia, M.G. (2013). *Before we are born: Essentials of embryology and birth defects* (8th ed., p. 300, Figure 19-7). Philadelphia: W.B. Saunders. Courtesy Children's Hospital and University of Manitoba, Winnipeg, Manitoba.

Art for Table 18-3: (dimpling) from Evans, A. J., Wilson, A. R. M., Blamey, R. W., Robertson, J. F. R., Ellis, I. O., & Elston, C. W. (1998). *Atlas of breast disease management: 50 illustrative cases.* Philadelphia: W. B. Saunders; (edema [peau d'orange]; fixation; deviation in nipple pointing) from Mansel, R., & Bundred, N.J. (1995). *Colour atlas of breast diseases.* London: Mosby-Wolfe.

Art for Table 18-6: (mammary duct ectasia; intraductal papilloma; Paget's disease [intraductal carcinoma) from Mansel, R., & Bundred, N.J. (1995). *Colour atlas of breast diseases.* London: Mosby-Wolfe; (carcinoma) from Evans, A. J., Wilson, A. R. M., Blamey, R. W., Robertson, J. F. R., Ellis, I. O., & Elston, C. W. (1998). *Atlas of breast disease management: 50 illustrative cases.* Philadelphia: W. B. Saunders.

Art for Table 18-7: (mastitis; breast abscess) from Mansel, R., & Bundred, N.J. (1995). *Colour atlas of breast diseases.* London: Mosby-Wolfe.

Art for Table 18-8: (gynecomastia) from Evans, A. J., Wilson, A. R. M., Blamey, R. W., Robertson, J. F. R., Ellis, I. O., & Elston, C. W.

(1998). *Atlas of breast disease management: 50 illustrative cases.* Philadelphia: W. B. Saunders; (breast carcinoma in men) from Haagensen, C. D. (1986). *Diseases of the breast* (3rd ed., p. 980). Philadelphia: W. B. Saunders.

Chapter 19

Figure 19-1, 19-2, 19-10: © Pat Thomas, 2010.

Figure 19-11: © Pat Thomas, 2006.

Figure 19-12: Nichols, F. H., & Zwelling, E. (1997). *Maternal–newborn nursing: Theory and practice.* Philadelphia: W. B. Saunders.

Chapter 20

Figures 20-2, 20-3, 20-4, 20-8, and 20-9: © Pat Thomas, 2006.

Figure 20-15: Lakatta, E. G. (1985). Cardiovascular function in later life. *Cardiovascular Medicine, 10,* 37–40.

Art for Art for Promoting Health Box (heart truth logo): The Heart Truth: Awareness and Prevention. Retrieved from *http://www.4women.gov/hearttruth.*

Art for Table 20-8: Images © Pat Thomas, 2006.

Art for Table 20-9: Images © Pat Thomas, 2006.

Art for Table 20-10: Stenosis images © Pat Thomas, 2006.

Chapter 21

Figures 21-1, 21-2, 21-3, and 20-5: © Pat Thomas, 2010.

Figures 21-4, 21-6, and 21-23: © Pat Thomas, 2006.

Figure 21-7: Kliegman, R. M., Behrman, R. E., Jenson, H. B., & Stanton, B. (2007). *Nelson textbook of pediatrics* (18th ed.). Philadelphia: W. B. Saunders.

Figure 21-19, B: Bloom, A., Watkins, P. H., & Ireland, J. (1992). *Color atlas of diabetes* (2nd ed.). St. Louis: Mosby.

Figure 21-21, B: Courtesy Lemmi & Lemmi, 2011.

Figure 21-24: © Pat Thomas, 2006.

Art for Table 21-1: (arterial: ischemic ulcer; superficial varicose veins; deep vein thrombophlebitis) from Dockery, G. L. (1997). *Cutaneous disorders of the lower extremity.* Philadelphia: W. B. Saunders. Reprinted with the permission of the author; (venous [stasis] ulcer) from Lookingbill, D. P., & Marks, J. G. (1993). *Principles of dermatology* (2nd ed., p. 267). Philadelphia: W. B. Saunders; (diabetes) courtesy Lemmi & Lemmi, 2011.

Art for Table 21-3: (Raynaud's syndrome; hand cyanosis) courtesy Lemmi & Lemmi, 2011; (lymphedema) Walsh, T. D., Caraceni, A. T., Fainsinger, R., Foley, K. M., Glare, P., Goh, C., …, Rabruch, L. (2009). *Palliative medicine.* Philadelphia: W. B. Saunders (Figure 87-1).

Chapter 22

Figures 22-1, 22-2, 22-3, 22-4, and 22-5: © Pat Thomas, 2006.

Art for Table 22-2: © Pat Thomas, 2006.

Art for Table 22-3: (umbilical hernia) from Zitelli, B. J., & Davis, H. W. (2007). *Atlas of pediatric physical diagnosis* (5th ed.). St. Louis: Mosby. Courtesy Dr. Thomas P. Foley, Jr.; (incisional hernia) courtesy Lemmi & Lemmi, 2011.

Chapter 23

Figure 23-1: © Pat Thomas, 2010.

Chapter 24

Figure 24-2: © Pat Thomas, 2006.

Figures 24-33, C, and 24-34, B: Dieppe, P. A., Cooper, C., & McGill, N. (1991). *Arthritis and rheumatism in practice.* London: Gower Medical Publishing.

Figure 24-38: Courtesy Lemmi & Lemmi, 2011.

Figure 24-51: Zitelli, B. J., McIntire, S.C., & Nowalk, A.J. (2012). *Zitelli & Davis' atlas of pediatric physical diagnosis* (6th ed., pp. 853–854, Figures 21-93B and 21-95). St. Louis: Mosby.

Figures 24-52, B, and Figure 24-55: Courtesy Lemmi & Lemmi, 2011.

Art for Table 24-3: (atrophy; dislocated shoulder; joint effusion) from Bunker, T., & Schranz, P. J. (1998). *Clinical challenges in orthopaedics: The shoulder.* London: Martin Dunitz. Reproduced by permission of Taylor & Francis Books UK. (tear of rotator cuff; frozen shoulder: adhesive capsulitis) from Polley, H. F., & Hunder, G. G. (1978). *Rheumatalogic interviewing and physical examination of the joints* (2nd ed.). Philadelphia: W. B. Saunders.

Art for Table 24-4: (olecranon bursitis) from Dieppe, P. A., Cooper, C., & McGill, N. (1991). *Arthritis and rheumatism in practice.* London: Gower Medical Publishing; (gouty arthritis) from Polley, H. F., & Hunder, G. G. (1978). *Rheumatalogic interviewing and physical examination of the joints* (2nd ed.). Philadelphia: W. B. Saunders; (subcutaneous nodules) from Callen, J. P., & Greer K. E. (1993). *Color atlas of dermatology.* Philadelphia: W. B. Saunders; (epicondylitis—tennis elbow) from Jones, A., & Owen, R. (1995). *Colour atlas of clinical orthopedics* (2nd ed.). London: Mosby-Wolfe.

Art for Table 24-5: (ganglion cyst) from Callen, J. P., & Greer K. E. (1993). *Color atlas of dermatology.* Philadelphia: W. B. Saunders; (carpal tunnel syndrome with atrophy of thenar eminence; Dupuytren's contracture; swan-neck and boutonnière deformity) Reprinted from the Clinical Slide Collection on the Rheumatic Diseases. © 1991, 1995, 1997. Used by permission of the American College of Rheumatology; (ankylosis) from Polley, H. F., & Hunder, G. G. (1978). *Rheumatalogic interviewing and physical examination of the joints* (2nd ed.). Philadelphia: W. B. Saunders; (ulnar deviation or drift; degenerative joint disease or osteoarthritis) Reprinted from the Clinical Slide Collection, 1991, American College of Rheumatology; (syndactyly; polydactyly) from Liebert, P. S. (1996). *Color atlas of pediatric surgery* (2nd ed.). Philadelphia: W. B. Saunders; gout in the thumb: Courtesy Lemmi & Lemmi 2011.

Art for Table 24-6: (mild synovitis; prepatellar bursitis) from Dieppe, P. A., Cooper, C., & McGill, N. (1991). *Arthritis and rheumatism in practice.* London: Gower Medical Publishing; (swelling of menisci) from Jones, A., & Owen, R. (1995). *Colour atlas of clinical orthopedics* (2nd ed.). London: Mosby-Wolfe; (Osgood-Schlatter disease) from Zitelli, B. J., McIntire, S.C., & Nowalk, A.J. (2012). *Zitelli & Davis' atlas of pediatric physical diagnosis* (6th ed., p. 410, Figure 21-97, A) St. Louis: Mosby; (postpolio muscle atrophy) courtesy Lemmi & Lemmi, 2011.

Art for Table 24-7: (Achilles tenosynovitis; acute gout) from Dieppe, P. A., Cooper, C., & McGill, N. (1991). *Arthritis and rheumatism in practice.* London: Gower Medical Publishing; (tophi with chronic gout) from Dockery, G. L. (1997). *Cutaneous disorders of the lower extremity.* Philadelphia: W. B. Saunders. Reprinted with the permission of the author; (hallux valgus with bunion and hammertoes) Reprinted from the Clinical Slide Collection, 1991, American College of Rheumatology; (callus; ingrown toenail; plantar wart) Courtesy Lemmi & Lemmi, 2011.

Art for Table 24-8: (scoliosis *[top]*) Courtesy Lemmi & Lemmi, 2011; (scoliosis *[bottom]*) Zitelli, B. J., McIntire, S.C., & Nowalk, A.J. (2012). *Zitelli & Davis' atlas of pediatric physical diagnosis* (6th ed., p. 840, Figure 21-71, B. St. Louis: Mosby; (herniated nucleus pulposus) from Polley, H. F., & Hunder, G. G. (1978). *Rheumatologic interviewing and physical examination of the joints* (2nd ed.). Philadelphia: W. B. Saunders.

Art for Table 24-9: (congenital dislocated hip) from Zitelli, B. J., McIntire, S.C., & Nowalk, A.J. (2012). *Zitelli & Davis' atlas of pediatric physical diagnosis* (6th ed., p. 850, Figure 21-89, A–B). St. Louis: Mosby; (talipes equinovarus [clubfoot]) Courtesy A. E. Chudley, M.D.; (spina bifida) from Walsh, P. C., Gittes, R. F., Perlmutter, A. D., & Stamey, T. A. (1986). *Campbell's urology* (5th ed.). Philadelphia: W. B. Saunders.

Art for Table 24-10: © Pat Thomas, 2010.

Chapter 25

Figures 25-1, 25-2, 25-3, 25-4, 25-6, and 25-7: © Pat Thomas, 2006.

Figure 25-5: © Pat Thomas, 2010.

Figure 25-54, B: Fenichel, G. M. (1988). *Clinical pediatric neurology.* Philadelphia: W. B. Saunders.

Figure 25-60: Hickey, J. V. (1986). *Neurological and neurosurgical nursing* (2nd ed.). Philadelphia: Lippincott.

Figure 25-61 (Canadian Neurological Scale): Côté, R., Hachinski, V. C., Shurvell, B. L., Norris, J. W., & Wolfson, C. (1986). The Canadian Neurological Scale: A preliminary study in acute stroke. *Stroke, 17*(4), 731–737; Côté, R., Battista, R. N., Wolfson, C., Boucher, J., Adam, J., & Hachinski, V. C. (1989). The Canadian Neurological Scale: Validation and reliability assessment. *Neurology, 39,* 638–643; and Bushnell, C. D., Johnston, D. C. C., & Goldstein, L. B. (2001). Retrospective assessment of initial stroke severity: Comparison of the NIH Stroke Scale and the Canadian Neurological Scale. *Stroke, 32,* 656.

Art for Tables 25-9 and 25-11: © Pat Thomas, 2006.

Chapter 26

Figures 26-1, 26-2 and 26-3: © Pat Thomas, 2006.

Figure 26-4: Redrawn from Marshall, W. A., & Tanner, J. M. (1970). Variations in the pattern of pubertal changes in boys. *Arch Dis Child, 45,* 22.

Figure 26-5: Courtesy Connie Cooper.

Figure 26-13: Sorrentino, S., Wilk, M., & Newmaster, R. (2013). *Mosby's Canadian textbook for the support worker* (3rd ed., p. 702, Figure 31-10, B). Toronto: Elsevier Canada.

Figure 26-10, B: Courtesy Lemmi & Lemmi, 2011.

Art for Table 26-1: Adapted from Tanner, J. M. (1962). *Growth at adolescence.* Oxford, UK: Blackwell Scientific.

Art for Table 26-2: Courtesy Connie Cooper.

Art for Table 26-3: (urethritis [urethral discharge and dysuria]) from Emond, R., Rowland, H.A.K., & Welsby, P. (1995). *Colour atlas of infectious diseases* (3rd ed., p. 161). St. Louis: Mosby-Wolfe.

Art for Table 26-4: (tinea cruris) courtesy Lemmi & Lemmi, 2011; (genital herpes: HSV-2 infection) courtesy Pfizer Laboratories Division, Pfizer Inc., New York. From *A close look at VD: A slide presentation produced as a public service;* (syphilitic chancre) from Emond, R. T., Rowland, H. A. K., & Welsby, P. (1995). *Colour atlas of infectious diseases* (3rd ed., p. 173). London: Mosby-Wolfe; (genital warts) from Habif, T. P., Campbell, J. L., Jr., Chapman, M. S., Dinulos, J. G. H., & Zug, K. A. (2005). *Skin disease: Diagnosis and treatment* (3rd ed.). St. Louis: Mosby; (carcinoma) from Callen, J. P., & Greer K. E. (1993). *Color atlas of dermatology.* Philadelphia: W. B. Saunders.

Art for Table 26-5: (phimosis; hypospadias) from Liebert, P. S. (1996). *Color atlas of pediatric surgery* (2nd ed.). Philadelphia: W. B. Saunders; (epispadias) from Zitelli, B. J., McIntire, S.C., & Nowalk, A.J. (2012). *Zitelli & Davis' atlas of pediatric physical diagnosis* (6th ed., p. 570, Figure 14-14, A). St. Louis: Mosby; (Peyronie's disease) courtesy Dr. Hans Stricker, Department of Urology, Henry Ford Hospital, Detroit, MI.

Art for Tables 26-6 and 26-7: © Pat Thomas, 2006.

Chapter 27

Figure 27-13, A: Courtesy Lemmi & Lemmi, 2011.

Art for Table 27-2: (pediculosis pubis [crab lice]; herpes simplex virus-type 2 [herpes genitalis]) from Callen, J. P., & Greer K. E. (1993). *Color atlas of dermatology.* Philadelphia: W. B. Saunders; (red rash-contact dermatitis) Courtesy Pfizer Laboratories Division, Pfizer Inc., New York. From *A close look at VD: A slide presentation produced as a public service;* (syphilitic chancre;

Credits

abscess of Bartholin's gland) from Emond, R. T., Rowland, H. A. K., & Welsby, P. (1995). *Colour atlas of infectious diseases* (3rd ed.). London: Mosby-Wolfe; (human papillomavirus [HPV] genital warts]) from Habif, T. P., Campbell, J. L., Jr., & Quitadamo, M. J. (2001). *Skin disease: Diagnosis and treatment.* St. Louis: Mosby; (urethral caruncle) from Rimsza, M. E. (1989). An illustrated guide to adolescent gynecology. *Pediatric Clinics of North America, 36*(3), 641.

Art for Table 27-3: (cystocele; uterine prolapse) from Symonds, E. M., & McPherson, M. B. A. (1997). *Diagnosis in colour: Obstetrics and gynecology.* London: Mosby-Wolfe; (rectocele) from Huffman, J. W. (1962). *Gynecology and obstetrics.* Philadelphia: W. B. Saunders.

Art for Table 27-4: (human papillomavirus (HPV, condylomata; polyp; carcinoma) from Symonds, E. M., & McPherson, M. B. A. (1997). *Diagnosis in colour: obstetrics and gynecology.* London: Mosby-Wolfe.

Art for Table 27-5: (candidiasis [moniliasis]) courtesy Lemmi & Lemmi, 2011; (gonorrhea) Courtesy Pfizer Laboratories Division, Pfizer Inc., New York. From *A close look at VD: A slide presentation produced as a public service.*

Art for Table 27-8: (ambiguous genitalia) from Moore, K. L., Persaud, T. N. & Torchia, M. G. (2013). *Before we are born: essentials of embryology and birth defects* (8th ed., p. 184, Fig. 13-25). Philadelphia: W.B. Saunders. Courtesy Dr. Heather Dean, Department of Pediatrics and Child Health, University of Manitoba, Winnipeg, Manitoba.; (vulvovaginitis in child) from Feigin, R. D., & Cherry, J. D. (1998). *Textbook of pediatric infectious diseases* (4th ed.). Philadelphia: W. B. Saunders.

Table 27-1: Adapted from Tanner, J. M. (1962). *Growth at adolescence.* Oxford, UK: Blackwell Scientific.

Chapter 29

Art for unn. figure, centre and bottom of page 809: Sorrentino, S. A. (2011). *Mosby's textbook for long-term care nursing assistants* (6th ed.). St. Louis: Mosby.

Chapter 30

Figures 30-4 and 30-13: Symonds, E. M., & McPherson, M. B. A. (1997). *Diagnosis in colour: Obstetrics and gynecology.* London: Mosby-Wolfe.

Art for Table 30-3: (pre-eclampsia) from Symonds, E. M., & McPherson, M. B. A. (1997). *Diagnosis in colour: Obstetrics and gynecology.* London: Mosby-Wolfe.

Art for Table 30-4: (fetal macrosomia) from Symonds, E. M., & McPherson, M. B. A. (1997). *Diagnosis in colour: Obstetrics and gynecology.* London: Mosby-Wolfe.

Chapter 31

Figure 31-2: Adapted from Katz, S., Downs, T. D., Cash, H. R., & Grotz, R. C. (1970). Progress in the development of the index of ADL. *Gerontologist, 10*(1, Part 1), 20–30.

Figure 31-3: Lawton, M. P., & Brody, E. M. (1969). Assessment of older people: Self-maintaining and instrumental activities of daily living. *Gerontologist, 9*(3, Part 1), 179–186. © The Gerontological Society of America.

Figure 31-4: Thornton, M., & Travis, S. S. (2003). Analysis of the reliability of the Modified Caregiver Strain Index. *The Journal of Gerontology, Series B, Psychological Sciences and Social Sciences, 58*(2), S129. © The Gerontological Society of America.

INDEX

Index

TABLE 1	Serum, Plasma, and Whole Blood Chemistry			
	Normal Values		**Possible Cause of Abnormalities**	
Test	*SI Units*	*Conventional Units*	*Higher Value*	*Lower Value*
Bicarbonate (HCO$_3$)	21-28 mmol/L	21-28 mEq/L	Chronic use of loop diuretics, compensated respiratory acidosis, metabolic alkalosis	Acute renal failure, compensated respiratory alkalosis, diarrhea, metabolic acidosis
Bilirubin • Total • Indirect • Direct	5.1-17 mcmol/L 3.4-12 mcmol/L 1.7-5.1 mcmol/L	0.3-1.0 mg/dL 0.2-0.8 mg/dL 0.1-0.3 mg/dL	Biliary obstruction, hemolytic anemia, impaired liver function, pernicious anemia, prolonged fasting	
Blood gases* • Arterial pH • Arterial partial pressure of carbon dioxide (PaCO$_2$) • Arterial partial pressure of oxygen (PaO$_2$)	7.35-7.45 35-45 mm Hg 80-100 mm Hg	Same as SI unit Same as SI unit Same as SI unit	Alkalosis Compensated metabolic alkalosis, respiratory acidosis Administration of high concentration of oxygen	Acidosis Compensated metabolic acidosis, respiratory alkalosis Chronic lung disease, decreased cardiac output
Carbon dioxide (CO$_2$) content	21-28 mmol/L	21-28 mEq/L	Same as bicarbonate	
Chloride	98-106 mmol/L	98-106 mEq/L	Corticosteroid therapy, dehydration, excessive infusion of normal saline, metabolic acidosis, respiratory alkalosis, uremia	Addison's disease, congestive heart failure, diarrhea, metabolic alkalosis, overhydration, respiratory acidosis, SIADH, vomiting
Cholesterol • High-density lipoprotein (HDL) • Male • Female • Low-density protein (LDL)	<5 mmol/L >0.75 mmol/L >0.91 mmol/L <3.37 mmol/L	<200 mg/dL, age dependent >45 mg/dL >55 mg/dL <60-180 mg/dL	Biliary obstruction, cirrhosis hypothyroidism, hyperlipidemia, idiopathic hypercholesterolemia, renal disease, uncontrolled diabetes	Corticosteroid therapy, extensive liver disease, hyperthyroidism, malnutrition
Glucose, fasting	4-6 mmol/L	72-110 mg/dL	Acute stress, cerebral lesions, Cushing's syndrome, diabetes mellitus, hyperthyroidism, pancreatic insufficiency	Addison's disease, hepatic disease, hypothyroidism, insulin overdosage, pancreatic tumour, pituitary hypofunction, postgastrectomy dumping syndrome
Oxygen saturation, arterial (SaO$_2$)	≥95%	Same as SI unit	Increased inspired oxygen, polycythemia vera	Anemia, cardiac decompensation, decreased inspired oxygen, respiratory disorders
Potassium	3.5-5.0 mmol/L	3.5-5.0 mEq/L	Acute or chronic renal failure, Addison's disease, dehydration, diabetic ketosis, excessive dietary or IV intake, massive tissue destruction, metabolic acidosis	Burns, Cushing's syndrome, deficient dietary or IV intake, diarrhea (severe), diuretic therapy, gastrointestinal fistula, insulin administration, pyloric obstruction, starvation, vomiting
Prostate-specific antigen (PSA)	<4 mcg/L	<4 ng/mL	Benign prostatic hypertrophy, prostate cancer, prostatitis	
Proteins • Total • Albumin • Globulin	64-83 g/L 35-50 g/L 23-34 g/L	6.4-8.3 g/dL 3.5-5 g/dL 2.3-3.4 g/dL	Burns, cirrhosis (globulin fraction), dehydration	Congenital agammaglobulinemia, increased capillary permeability, inflammatory disease, liver disease, malabsorption, malnutrition
Sodium	135-145 mmol/L	135-145 mEq/L	Corticosteroid therapy, dehydration, impaired renal function, increased sodium intake in diet or IV, primary aldosteronism	Addison's disease, decreased sodium intake in diet or IV therapy, diabetic ketoacidosis, diuretic therapy, excessive loss from GI tract, excessive perspiration, water intoxication
T$_4$ (thyroxine), total	64-154 nmol/L	5-12 mcg/dL	Hyperthyroidism, thyroiditis	Cretinism, hypothyroidism, myxedema
T$_4$ (thyroxine), free	10-36 pmol/L	0.8-2.8 ng/dL	Hyperthyroidism, metastatic neoplasms	Hypothyroidism
T$_3$ (triiodothyronine), uptake	24-34 AU	24%-34%		

Continued

Test	Normal Values		Possible Cause of Abnormalities	
	SI Units	*Conventional Units*	*Higher Value*	*Lower Value*
T$_3$ (triiodothyronine), total	1.2-3.4 nmol/L	70-205 ng/dL	Hyperthyroidism	Hypothyroidism
Triglycerides	0.45-1.69 mmol/L	40-150 mg/dL	Diabetes mellitus, hyperlipidemia, hypothyroidism, liver disease	Hyperthyroidism, malabsorption syndrome, malnutrition
Urea nitrogen, blood (BUN)	3.6-7.1 mmol/L	10-20 mg/dL	Burns, dehydration, GI bleeding, increase in protein catabolism (fever, stress), renal disease, shock, urinary tract infection	Fluid overload, malnutrition, severe liver damage, SIADH

*Because arterial blood gases are influenced by altitude, the value for PaO$_2$ decreases as altitude increases. The lower value is normal for an altitude of 1 mile.

GI, gastrointestinal; *IV,* intravenous; *SI,* Système Internationale; *SIADH,* syndrome of inappropriate antidiuretic hormone.

TABLE 2 Hematology

Test	Normal Values		Possible Cause of Abnormalities	
	SI Units	*Conventional Units*	*Higher Values*	*Lower Values*
Bleeding time (Ivy method)	1-9 min	Same as SI unit	Aspirin ingestion, clotting factor deficiency, defective platelet function, thrombocytopenia, vascular disease, von Willebrand's disease	
Activated partial thromboplastin time (aPTT)	30-40 sec*	Same as SI unit	Deficiency of factors I, II, V, VIII, IX and X, XI, XII; hemophilia; heparin therapy; liver disease	
Partial thromboplastin time (PPT)	28-35 sec	Same as SI unit	Deficiency of factors I, II, V, VII, and X; liver disease; vitamin K deficiency; warfarin therapy	
Prothrombin time (protime, PT)	11-12.5 sec*	Same as SI unit	Deficiency of factors I, II, V, VII, and X; liver disease; vitamin K deficiency; warfarin therapy	
International normalized ratio (INR)	0.81-1.2	Same as SI unit	Same causes as for higher PT	
Erythrocyte count[†] (altitude dependent) • Male • Female	4.7-6.1 × 10^{12}/L 4.2-5.4 × 10^{12}/L	4.7-6.1 × 10^6/mcL 4.2-5.4 × 10^6/mcL	Dehydration, high altitudes, polycythemia vera, severe diarrhea	Anemia, leukemia, posthemorrhage status
Hemoglobin (altitude dependent)[†] • Male • Female	140-180 mmol/L 120-160 mmol/L	14-18 g/dL 12-16 g/dL	COPD, high altitudes, polycythemia	Anemia, hemorrhage
Platelet count (thrombocytes)[†]	150-400 × 10^9/L	150,000-400,000/mm^3	Acute infections, chronic granulocytic leukemia, chronic pancreatitis, cirrhosis, collagen disorders, polycythemia, postsplenectomy status	Acute leukemia, cancer chemotherapy, DIC, hemorrhage, infection, SLE, thrombocytopenic purpura
White blood cell (WBC) count[†]	5-10 × 10^9/L	5000-10,000/mm^3	Inflammatory and infectious processes, leukemia	Aplastic anemia, autoimmune diseases, overwhelming infection, side effects of chemotherapy and irradiation

*Values depend on reagent and instrumentation used.

[†]Component of complete blood cell count (CBC).

COPD, chronic obstructive pulmonary disease; *DIC,* disseminated intravascular coagulation; *SI,* Système Internationale; *SLE,* systemic lupus erythematosus.